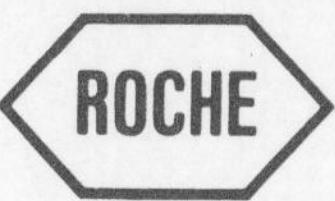

PATHOGENESIS AND TREATMENT OF URINARY TRACT INFECTIONS

PATHOGENESIS AND TREATMENT OF URINARY TRACT INFECTIONS

Thomas A. Stamey, M.D.
Professor of Surgery
Chairman, Division of Urology
Stanford University School of Medicine
Stanford, California

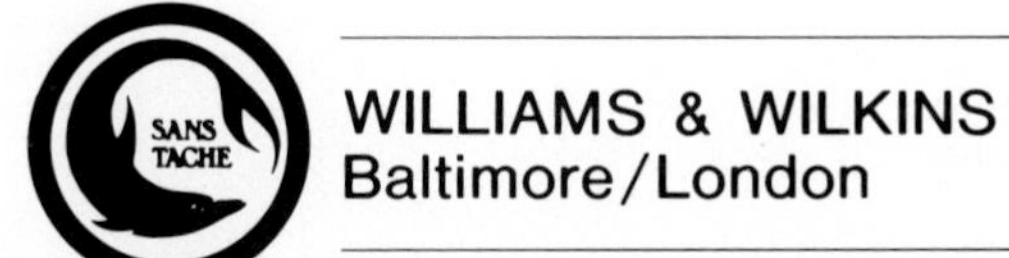

WILLIAMS & WILKINS
Baltimore/London

Made in the United States of America

Library of Congress Cataloging in Publication Data

Reprinted 1981

Stamey, Thomas Alexander.
Pathogenesis and treatment of urinary tract infections.

Includes index.
1. Urinary tract infections. 2. Urinary tract infections—Chemotherapy. I. Title.
[DNLM: 1. Urinary tract infections—Etiology. 2. Urinary tract infections—Therapy. WJ151 S783p]
RC901.8.S73   616.6   79-23178
ISBN 0-683-07909-3

Composed and printed at the
Waverly Press, Inc.
Mt. Royal and Guilford Aves.
Baltimore, Md. 21202, U.S.A.

To my wife, Kathryn

PREFACE

Thomas A. Stamey, M.D.

I wrote in the preface to my first book on urinary tract infections (UTI), published 8 years ago, that I had two reasons for writing a book on this subject[1]. The first was that our experience at Stanford with UTI was not limited to one population group, but included infections in both sexes of all ages. The second was that few, if any, investigators had followed patients with recurrent UTI longitudinally by culturing the colonization sites—the vaginal introitus and urethra in the female, and the prostate and urethra in the male—in between episodes of bacteriuria. To these two reasons, I can add a third, almost a decade later: It is now possible, in 1980, to take any patient with recurrent bacteriuria and successfully solve their problem. It is true that bacterial persistence often requires surgical excision of the infection site (Chapter 9) and that prevention of reinfections will require antimicrobial prophylaxis (Chapter 4), but no patient—adult or child—need suffer from the morbidity and sometimes the mortality of recurrent bacteriuria.

It is also clear in 1980 that the ball game must be played in the physician's office and not in mass screening studies of population groups. While epidemiologic surveys in children and adults have identified bacteriuria in 1–20% of the population under study, and have provided some useful information on such parameters as the incidence of renal scars, the degree of hypertension, and the prevalence of small babies and perinatal mortality, it is amply clear that therapeutic trials applicable to epidemiologic methodology have not altered these morbidity statistics. The heterogeneity of the bacteriuria detected by screening surveys (Chapter 4) is further evidence of the limitation of epidemiologic studies. On the other hand, the morbidity from urinary infections can be virtually eliminated by the interested and informed physician; he needs to recognize the statistical limitation of diagnosing bacteriuria (Chapter 1), that 20% of his symptomatic patients will have less than 100,000 bacteria/ml in their bladder urine (Chapter 4), and that heavy introital colonization can easily lead to a false positive urine culture if the specimen is casually caught without precautions to avoid perineal contamination (Chapters 1, 4, and 5). Once bacteriuria is diagnosed, the urine must be sterilized with appropriate therapy, which means that not one organism of the original infecting strain should be present in the voided urine (Chapter 1 and Chapter 4); otherwise, the infection may have been suppressed rather than sterilized and, if so, it is certain to recur with the same strain. Once the urine is sterile, however, all recurrences can be characterized as either reinfections with new organisms or bacterial persistence of the original strain within the urinary tract (Chapter 1 and Chapter 4).

The diagnosis, natural history, and prevention of reinfections in the adult woman are presented in Chapter 4 and, in the infant and child, in Chapter 6. Because UTI are so common, recognition and proper treatment of the patients at serious risk represent important sections of this book (Chapters 4, 6, and 8). The urethral syndrome is covered extensively in Chapter 4, together with coagulase-negative staphylococcal, anaerobic, and mycoplasmal infections; the recognition and differential diagnosis of sterile pyuria also deserved a subsection, as well as the discussion of when to obtain an intravenous urogram in the adult and child (Chapters 4 and 6). I conclude Chapter 4 with a section indicating the substantial limitation of the 100,000 bacteria/ml concept and a section which shows there is little or no correlation between the site of bacterial infection in the urinary tract and bacterial recurrence with consecutively similar O-serogroups, all of which indicates that the term relapse is very misleading when it is used to imply that the kidney is the cause of the bacterial recurrence.

The physician responsible for individual patients will find within the pages of this book the information required to diagnose and successfully treat recurrent UTI. The causes of bacterial persistence in the presence of a sterile urine while on antimicrobial therapy can be subtle and will often require urologic investigation to identify the specific site of bacterial persistence; 14 examples are presented in detail in Chapter 9, examples which should serve as a check list in searching for the cause of bacterial persistence in any individual patient. There is no doubt that surgical excision of urologic abnormalities which cause bacterial infections to persist in the urinary tract can offer patients a lifetime of freedom from infections. Several case histories in this book, with bacteriologic follow-ups of more than 10 years, attest to this fact. But there is also no doubt that many patients with curable infections are simply labeled as "chronic infections," inappropriately "suppressed" with antimicrobial agents, or simply left as statistical numbers in bacteriuric surveys. There can be no doubt that patients with reinfections far exceed those whose infections are caused by bacterial persistence, but the careful physician should recognize the latter group and seek diligently for the cause of persistence. Reinfections represent a biologic problem and require a medical rather than a surgical solution.

The principles of antimicrobial sensitivity testing and a large section on bacterial resistance are presented in Chapter 2. I am glad to observe that almost all clinicians and most microbiologists in 1980 accept that it is the urinary concentration of antimicrobial agents which determines cure of urinary infections rather than the serum level—an observation that was not easily accepted in 1965[2]. The practical consequences of this concept are presented in Chapter 2.

I have left Chapter 3 from my original book intact because it still stands as the best example in the world's literature of chronic bacterial pyelonephritis uncomplicated by hypertension, diabetes, or glomerulonephritis.

Throughout this book, I have distinguished between those data obtained from patients who present to their physicians with symptoms or signs of urinary tract infections and those data derived from detecting bacteriuric subjects by screening surveys. The latter infections are termed "screening bacteriuria," which I have abbreviated ScBU.

Finally, I hope practicing physicians who treat urinary infections in adults and children will find this book useful so that their patients will suffer less. To this end, I have placed the research aspects which relate to the pathogenesis of UTI into a separate chapter (Chapter 5).

1. Stamey, T. A.: Urinary Infections, Baltimore, Williams & Wilkins Co., 1972.
2. Stamey, T. A., Govan, D. E., and Palmer, J. M.: The localization and treatment of urinary tract infections: The role of bactericidal urine levels as opposed to serum levels. Medicine **44:** 1, 1965.

CONTENTS

CHAPTER 1

The Diagnosis, Localization, and Classification of Urinary Infections

DIAGNOSIS OF BACTERIURIA

Theoretical, Historical, and Observational Basis

Chills, fever, and flank pain, accompanied by dysuria, frequency, and the presence in the urine of many bacilli and leukocytes (with clumps) per high power field of the microscope always indicates a urinary infection. Difficulties in diagnosis arise, however, if the patient forces fluids and voids often or if he is inadequately treated with an antimicrobial agent; although his symptoms may subside, and the leukocytes markedly diminish, the bacteriuria can persist. More importantly, many patients with repeated urinary infections become asymptomatic with their recurrences.

Two observations form the basis for di-

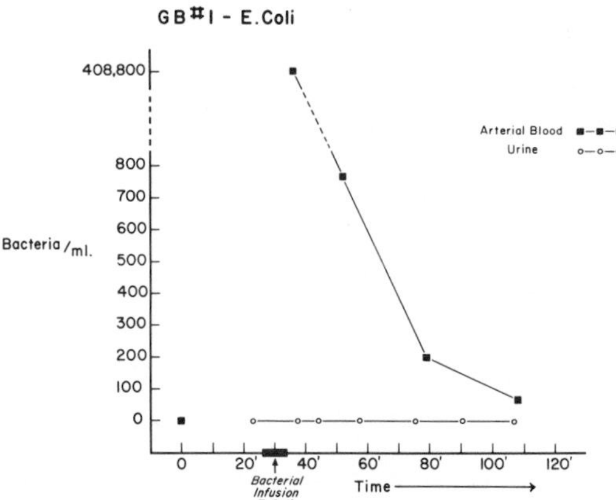

Figure 1.1 Ureteral urine and arterial blood specimens from a dog were cultured after a rapid intravenous infusion of 500 ml of saline solution containing 10^5 *Escherichia coli*/ml. Despite thousands of *E. coli* perfusing the kidney/minute, the ureteral urine specimens remained sterile; a Goldblatt clamp, placed several weeks before this study, partially occluded the left renal artery. (Reproduced by permission from T. A. Stamey and A. Pfau, Calif. Med. **113:** 16, Dec. 1970.)

agnosing urinary infections. First, there is no evidence that bladder urine intermittently contains bacteria. Although transient bacteriemia may be common, the glomeruli do not readily filter these bacteria into the urine. For example, if an anesthetized dog is infused intravenously with millions of bacteria, ureteral urines remain sterile for hours even though thousands of bacteria are perfusing the kidney per minute (Figure 1.1). The bladder urine is normally sterile, and the presence of any bacteria in the bladder urine is an abnormal circumstance. Second, if bacteria are inoculated into normal urines, the organisms double about every 45 minutes,[1] soon approaching 10^8 bacteria/ml of urine. The urine of most patients with urinary infections contains 10^8 bacteria/ml,[2] especially in a nonhydrated or first voided morning urine.

If the physician accepts the data that pyuria (arbitrarily defined as the presence of 5 or more white blood cells per high power field in the centrifuged specimen) occurs in only 50% of asymptomatic female patients with bacteriuria,[3] that pyuria occurs commonly in the absence of bladder bacteriuria,[4] and that the gram stain has an intrinsic error of about 20%,[3] there is no choice other than to count bacteria in the urine. Because of urethral or perineal contamination, the difference between bacteriuria and nonbacteriuria is clearly a statistical consideration in which methodology is of critical importance. Failure to appreciate this point has caused considerable controversy.

Marple at Stanford in 1940,[4] Barr and Rantz of the same university in 1948,[5] and Sanford and his colleagues at Harvard in 1956[6] made the initial observations in quantitating bacterial counts in catheterized urines.

Indeed, Stanford University had an early history of recognizing the importance of quantitating the number of bacteria in the urine. Professor David Rytand showed me a pocket file card from his days as Chief Medical Resident in 1935. As can be seen in Figure 1.2, a 39-year-old woman was admitted with an acute pyelonephritis; observe the notation that "64,000,000 *E. coli* /cc" were found in the urine. It remained for Kass and his co-workers at Boston City Hospital to statistically establish the quantitative basis for diagnosing bacteriuria.[3,7] Initial studies on the frequency distribution of bacterial counts in asymptomatic women from the Boston City Hospital were ob-

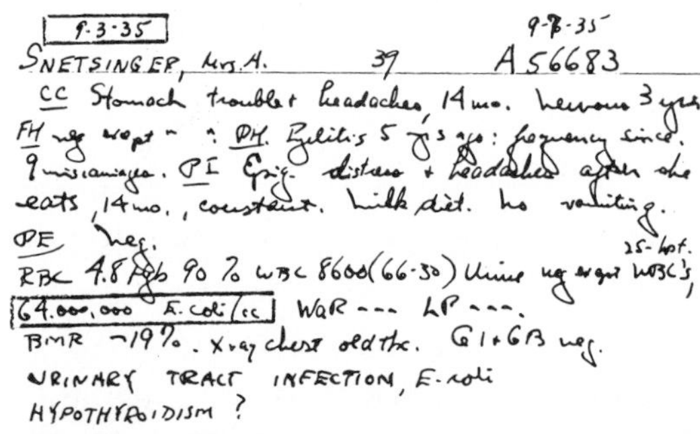
9-3-35 9-[illegible]-35
SNETSINGER, Mrs. A. 39 A 56683
CC Stomach trouble + headaches, 14 mo. Nervous 3 yrs
FH neg [illegible] PH. [illegible] 5 yrs ago: frequency since. 9 miscarriages. PI Epig. distress + headaches after she eats, 14 mo., constant. Milk diet. No vomiting.
PE neg.
RBC 4.8 Hgb 90% WBC 8600 (66-30) Urine [illegible] WBC's, 25-hpf.
64.000,000 E. coli/cc WaR --- LP ---.
BMR −19%. X-ray chest old Tbc. GI + GB neg.
URINARY TRACT INFECTION, E-coli
HYPOTHYROIDISM ?

Figure 1.2 Evidence that the importance of quantitative urine cultures was recognized at least as early as 1935 on the medical service at Stanford University. Professor David Rytand gave me this pocket file-card from his days as chief medical resident.

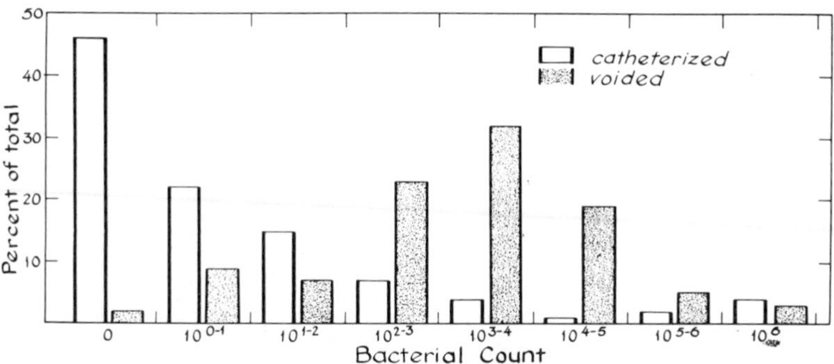

Figure 1.3 The bacterial colony counts in catheterized and whole voided urine specimens obtained from several hundred asymptomatic women, taken at random from an outpatient medical clinic. Modified from Kass.[7] (Reproduced by permission from T. A. Stamey and A. Pfau, Calif. Med. **113:** 16, Dec. 1970.)

tained by catheterization in the clinics under random circumstances (*i.e.*, they were not first morning specimens)[7]; approximately 46% were sterile, 22% contained from 1 to 10 bacteria/ml, 6% had more than 10^5 bacteria/ml, and the remainder of the counts fell into the frequency distribution observed in Figure 1.3. Because the specimens with less than 10^5 bacteria/ml were distributed in frequency toward zero (85% contained less than 100 bacteria/ml), because the bacteria in these low counts were frequently staphylococci, enterococci, diphtheroids, and lactobacilli, and because repeat catheterizations often showed a different flora as well as low numbers inconsistent with the expected growth in urine ($>10^5$/ml), these bacterial counts of less than 10^5/ml were considered to be urethral contaminants. The method of catheterization was not stated in these papers, but the size and type of catheter, the preparation and position of the patient, the attendant doing the catheterization, and, most importantly, the volume of urine that flushes the catheter before collection of the sample for culture all influence contamination of the catheterized urine with urethral bacteria. Undoubtedly, with a more detailed technique of catheterization,[4] one could achieve a higher frequency of sterile urines and smaller numbers of contaminating bacteria. For example, in Marple's study of 100 female patients in the hospital, 69 were sterile, 24 had $>10^5$ bacteria/ml, and only 7 patients had small numbers of bacteria (all <100/ml).[4] In a remarkable study that was well ahead of its time, Philpot obtained catheterized urines from 50 volunteer normal women after washing the introitus with green soap and rinsing with potassium mercuric iodide:66% were sterile, 28% had 1–30 bacteria/ml, and 6% had 30–400 bacteria/ml; none of the contaminating bacteria were Gram-negative bacteria or even enterrococci.[8] Regardless of the technique of catheterization, however, some sterile bladder urines will be contaminated by urethral bacteria; the consideration of a sterile urine, therefore, even with catheterization, must remain on a statistical basis. The catheter cannot offer a categorical delineation between the presence and absence of bacteria.

Only by direct suprapubic needle aspiration of the bladder[9–11] can sterility be defined in terms approaching 99% of confidence limits. The data in Figures 1.4 and 1.5 are from bladder aspirations in two groups of patients with recurrent urinary infections.[11] One group had received no antimicrobial therapy in their recent past history (Figure 1.4), while the second group was on therapy at the time of aspiration (Figure 1.5). In Figure 1.4, only 35 of the 331 aspirations (approximately 10%) contained between 1–10^5 bacteria/ml, but of the 105 patients with bladder bacteriuria, the 35 low counts ($<10^5$/ml) represented 33% of the total infected patients. As expected (Figure 1.5), the error in accepting

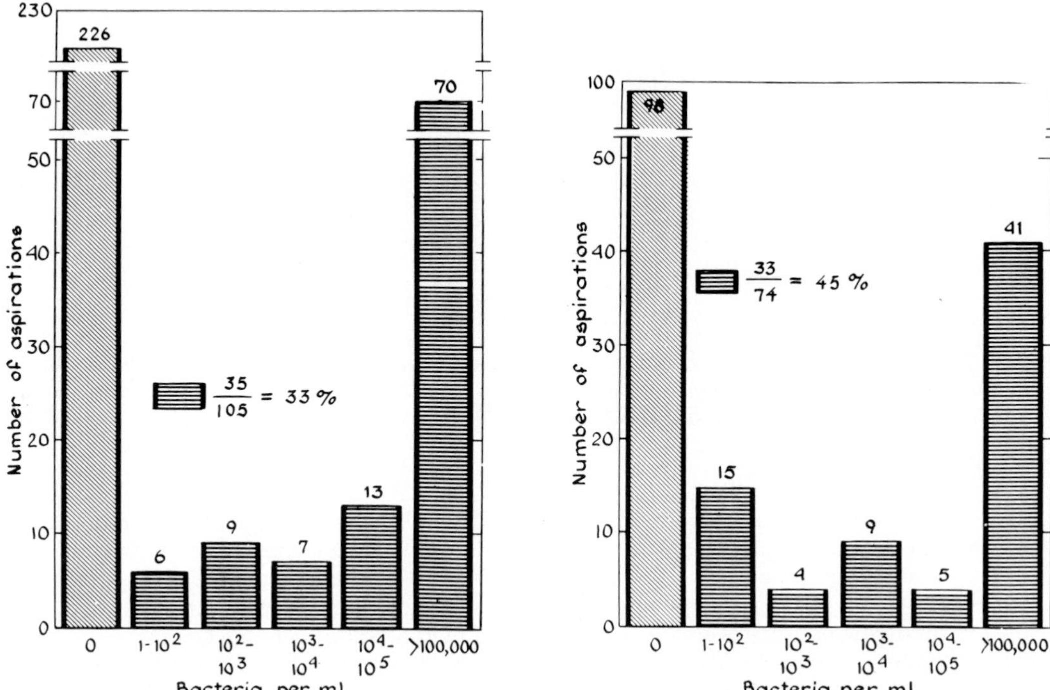

Figure 1.4 (*left*) The bacterial colony counts in urine specimens obtained by direct suprapubic needle aspiration of the bladder. These 331 aspirations were from patients seen in a clinic for urinary infections; none of the patients was receiving antimicrobial therapy. (Reproduced by permission from T. A. Stamey and A. Pfau, Calif. Med. **113:** 16, Dec., 1970.)

Figure 1.5 (*right*) The bacterial colony counts in urine specimens obtained by direct suprapubic needle aspiration of the bladder; these 172 aspirations were from patients receiving antimicrobial therapy at the time of aspiration. (Reproduced by permission from T. A. Stamey and A. Pfau, Calif. Med. **113:** 16, Dec. 1970.)

10^5 bacteria/ml becomes unacceptable in patients receiving antimicrobial therapy; 20% of the total aspirations contained less than 10^5 bacteria/ml, representing 45% of those infected. It is important to point out that these were hydrated patients. Similar data have been obtained by others.[12] While hydration might account for a 10-fold dilution of urine (from 10^5 to 10^4 bacteria/ml), hydration alone cannot explain bacterial counts of 1000 or less/ml. Moreover, Mabeck aspirated 95 women who were not hydrated; 29% of the patients with bacteriuria had $<10^5$ bacteria/ml.[13] Kunz *et al.* found 41.3% of positive aspirations to be $<10^5$ bacteria/ml and 26.7% to be $<10^4$ bacteria/ml.[14]

The real difficulty, and much of the controversy—scientific and emotional—lies not in the interpretation of the catheterized urine in the female, but in interpretation of the voided urine. As seen in Figure 1.3, when asymptomatic women from the same clinic at Boston City Hospital were cultured by collecting voided urines, sterile urines and urines containing less than 1000 bacteria/ml became relatively rare. The average urine thought to be uninfected, cultured 10^3–10^4 bacteria/ml. We obtained a similar distribution curve (Figure 1.6) when midstream voided specimens* were cultured in 54 women who had sterile bladder urine on suprapubic aspiration.[11] The best study of comparing voided urine counts to those obtained by bladder aspiration before voiding is that of Pfau and Sacks[15]; they com-

* The perineums were not cleaned in these studies.

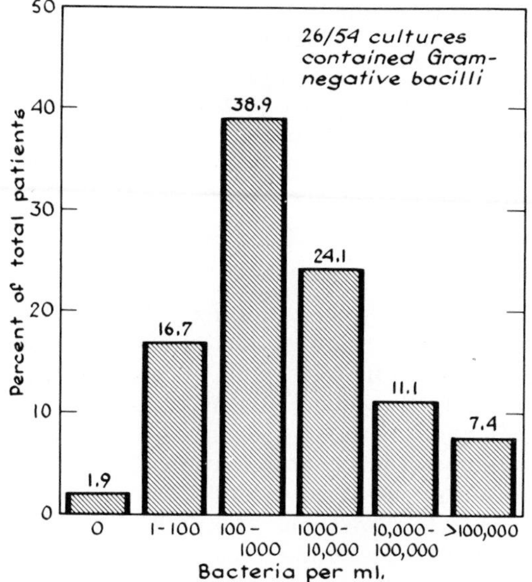

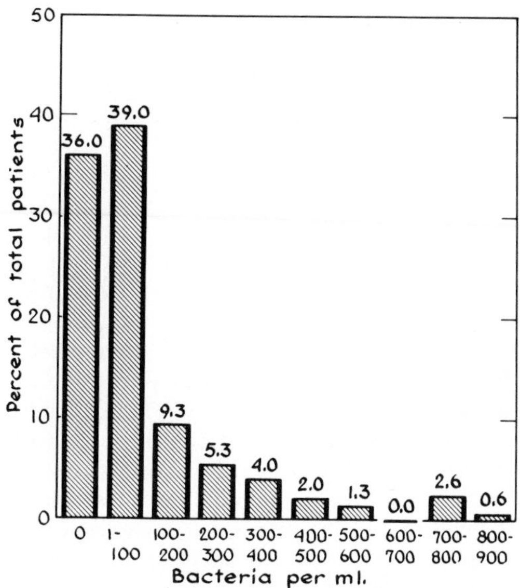

Figure 1.6 (*left*) Bacterial colony counts in 54 midstream, self-caught voided specimens from patients who had sterile bladder urine by direct needle aspiration. (Reproduced by permission from T. A. Stamey, D. E. Govan, and J. M. Palmer, Medicine **44:** 1, 1965.[11])

Figure 1.7 (*right*) Bacterial colony counts in 151 midstream specimens collected by a trained nurse who retracted the labia as the patients voided from a cystoscopy table; all patients had a sterile bladder urine, proven by direct needle aspiration, immediately before voiding. (Reproduced by permission from T. A. Stamey, D. E. Govan, and J. M. Palmer, Medicine **44:** 1, 1965.[11])

pared aspiration to several different techniques of obtaining a voided urine for culture. In the bacteriologic method used by the Boston group,[2] (1) the total voided urine is collected (not midstream specimens), (2) the perineum is washed with four separate 4 × 4-inch sterile gauze sponges soaked with green soap, (3) the soap is not removed before voiding, and (4) the quantitative culture is not performed until the following day after overnight refrigeration of the urine (while awaiting results of a qualitative, screening culture). With this method, Kass and his co-workers have established that a single culture of the whole voided urine, containing 10^5 or more bacteria/ml, has an 80% chance of representing a bladder bacteriuria[7] (in their hands, a single *catheterized* specimen of similar count has a 95% confidence level); two consecutive whole voided specimens containing 10^5 or more bacteria/ml have 91% confidence limits, and three specimens with $>10^5$ bacteria/ml approach the same confidence level as a single catheterized specimen (95%).[2]

By this method, Kass and his group have published a remarkable series of epidemiologic studies on the incidence of bacteriuria in different population groups[7] and on the relationship of bacteriuria to diabetes,[16] pyelonephritis of pregnancy,[2] prematurity,[2] and hypertension.[17]

These same criteria, however, applied to the individual patient in the physician's office or in the hospital, present some serious problems. Neither the practicing physician nor the patient can afford three consecutive whole voided cultures for a 95% reliability. And since one voided culture of 10^5 or greater, using Kass's technique, has *one chance in five* of not representing an infection,[7] the risk and expense of unwarranted antimicrobial therapy based on a single culture becomes a serious consideration. What can be done to avoid three consecutive cultures that still have 1 chance in 20 of not representing an infection even if each culture grows 10^5 bacteria/ml? In order of decreasing complexity, (1) the bladder urine can be directly aspirated, providing the highest degree of reliability[11]; (2) the female patient can be placed on a table in the lithotomy position, the perineum can be cleaned with soap and washed, and the nurse can collect a midstream specimen (Figure 1.7)[11]; and (3) the patient can be catheterized. Bladder aspiration, while neither painful nor dangerous, is not pleasant for the patient. Highly useful in newborn infants,[18] and in patients with paraplegia,[19] bladder puncture should be used freely when the diagnosis remains in doubt in any woman who persists with a questionable culture. Aspiration reveals with a single culture the bacteriologic status of the bladder urine and does not introduce urethral bacteria to initiate a new infection. Despite these advantages, it will probably never be widely used. We have described the second method (Figure 1.7) in detail[11] and continue to use it in both the office and hospital, but most physicians will find this too involved to warrant the effort. But where possible, the nurse should clean the perineum carefully, remove the detergent, retract the labia, and collect the patient's midstream specimen herself. As will be discussed in Chapter 4 on "Urinary Tract Infections in Women," a *single* midstream voided specimen, carefully collected by a trained nurse, probably has the same confidence limits as three consecutive, whole voided specimens.

Finally, it is necessary to emphasize that while the Boston studies established the statistical significance of a whole voided urine containing 10^5 or more bacteria/ml, these important studies did not establish how many patients with less than 10^5 bacteria/ml were also infected. This is an important question for the practicing physician because it is he who sees symptomatic patients who void frequently and are likely to have bacterial counts of $>10^5$/ml. In our own studies on the natural history of symptomatic recurrent bacteriuria in women,[20] we found that 21% of 145 proven urinary infections had colony counts of less than 10^5 bacteria/ml. It is clear, then, that the physician who uses 10^5 bacteria/ml as an absolute diagnostic test for urinary infection will miss one in five urinary infections in his office. Fortunately, most of these patients will have symptoms of urinary infection, most will have pyuria on urinalysis, and the informed physician will treat the patient for infection even if the colony count is 5,000 *Escherichia coli*/ml.

Risk of Urethral Catheterization

From the foregoing, it is easy to understand why catheterization for urine culture will remain an attractive alternative for many practicing physicians. As already emphasized, however, catheterization—regardless of the technique and care—will not prevent urethral contamination of the catheterized urine. With careful technique (using Marple's[4] method), the presence of 10^4 or even 10^3 bacteria/ml should mean, with virtual certainty, the presence of a urinary infection. The objection to the catheter, however, is that it produces a bladder bacteriuria in some patients who have a sterile urine. The incidence of infection varies with the type of patient catheterized. For example, Jackson and Grieble,[21] in an outpatient clinic for hypertensive women, caused bladder bacteriuria in only 2% of single catheterizations; Turck *et al.*[22] catheterized 100 nonhospitalized young women, infecting 1 patient. This low incidence of catheter-induced infections increases in patients who would be expected to carry Enterobacteriaceae (*E. coli*, *Klebsiella*, *Proteus mirabilis*, *Enterobacter*, etc.) on the vaginal introitus and urethra. Brumfitt *et al.*[23] found that the rate of urinary infection in catheterized maternity patients at the time of delivery was twice that of noncatheterized women, while Kaye *et al.*[24] observed that a single catheterization tripled the incidence of infection. When the catheter is used in hospitalized patients, the rate of induced bladder bacteriuria becomes prohibitive. Even Marple,[4] using an aseptic technique unlikely to be duplicated by the best urologists, infected at least 9% of the 69 hospitalized women who had initially sterile urines. In a most convincing study, Thiel and Spühler[25] proved a sterile urine by suprapubic aspiration in 50 hospitalized women, carefully emptied their bladders by catheterization with a glass catheter, and reaspirated the bladder 24 hours after catheterization. Ten of the 50 urines were infected. As summarized in Table 1.1, the incidence of catheter-induced urinary infections is primarily determined by the population at risk, with the lowest incidence occurring in nonhospitalized, healthy women. If an antibacterial solution, such as neomycin and polymyxin, were always left in the bladder after catheterization, the risk might be reduced. Studies on this point would be useful; if catheter-induced infections could be reduced to less than 1% for all population groups, it is at least debatable whether better medicine might be practiced (in a nonhospitalized population) by the correct interpretation of a single catheterized culture than by false interpretation of a single, whole voided culture. J. W. Pearman, in a paper entitled "Prevention of urinary tract infection following spinal cord injury,"[26] presented some remarkable data. Patients were catheterized every 6 hours following acute traumatic spinal cord injury until bladder function returned. At each catheterization the urine was cultured, and 150 mg of kanamycin and 30 mg of colistin sulfate in 25 ml of sterile water were left in the bladder. Of 3036 catheterizations performed in 27 male patients, 16 episodes of bacteriuria occurred (an incidence of 1/190 catheterizations, or 0.5%). Of 1547 catheterizations performed in 9 female patients, 9 instances of bacteriuria occurred (an incidence of 1/172 catheterizations or 0.6%). Almost all the resistant organisms were enterococci and *Staphylococcus epidermidis*.

Table 1.1
Incidence of Catheter-induced Infection in Women[a]

Author	Population	Incidence
		%
Turck *et al.*[22]	Young women without medical illness	1
Jackson and Grieble[21]	Outpatients attending hypertensive clinic	2
Kass[3]	Asymptomatic, untreated outpatients	2.4
	Maternity patients	
Brumfitt *et al.*[23]	Uncomplicated deliveries[b]	4.4
Kaye *et al.*[24]	Nonforceps deliveries[b]	13.5
Marple[4]	Hospitalized on a medical ward[c]	9
Thiel and Spühler[25]	Hospitalized on a medical ward	20

[a] Reproduced by permission from T. A. Stamey and A. Pfau, Calif. Med. **113:** 16, Dec. 1970.

[b] Incidence due to catheter obtained by subtracting the control, uncatheterized incidence from the rate of infection observed following catheterization.

[c] Nine percent is a minimal incidence; 6 of the 69 patients with sterile urine on initial catheterization became acutely symptomatic within 3 days and were found to be infected on repeat catheterization. Determination of the rate of asymptomatic induced infection would have required second catheterizations in all patients 3 to 7 days after the first.

Clinical investigations, on the other hand, are immediately rendered suspect if catheterized specimens are used because the incidence of spontaneous infections (2–6%) is about the same as that from the catheter.

The data in Figure 1.3 are based on random urine samples in patients expected to have a low incidence of infection. The main emphasis has been on the confidence limits that can be placed on the repetition of bacterial counts of 10^5/ml or more. As indicated earlier, except for our study on natural history of recurrent infections in symptomatic women,[20] there are virtually no data on how often urinary infections can be present with $<10^5$ bacteria/ml.[11, 12] Kass clearly stated the major factors that can reduce a bacterial infection in the bladder to numbers less than 10^5/ml.[3, 7] In descending order of importance, (1) frequent voiding, (2) hydration,[12, 27] (3) antimicrobial therapy, (4) fastidious organisms, and (5) the presence of cleansing detergent washed from the perineum into the culture bottle.[27] The presence of contaminating detergent may be particularly important when the urines are refrigerated overnight before quantitative counts are performed.[2] Dr. Kass has reassured me that the green soap used in the Boston studies is not a detergent and did not influence the colony counts.

Laboratory Methods: Office Bacteriology

Sources of Error from Relying Solely upon Microscopic Sediment

Microscopic examination of the urinary sediment adds valuable information to the diagnosis and evaluation of urinary tract disorders, but the microscope can be a trap for the unwary in the diagnosis and follow-up of patients with urinary infections. There are three major sources of error.

The most important error results from the limitation imposed by the microscope on the volume of urine that can be observed. If the volume of urine which can comfortably rest beneath a standard 22-mm cover glass is carefully measured and the number of high dry fields (×570 magnification) present beneath the cover glass is estimated, it is disturbingly apparent that one high dry field represents a volume of approximately 1/30,000 ml. There are excellent studies which show that the bacterial count must be approximately 30,000/ml before bacteria can be found in the sediment, stained or unstained, spun or unspun.[6, 28] For these reasons, a negative urinalysis for bacteria never excludes the presence of bacteria in numbers of 30,000/ml or less. As already pointed out, many circumstances can reduce the bacterial colony count in bladder urine to numbers less than 30,000/ml. Those who adopt the method for office bacteriology presented in this chapter, and who not only look at spun aliquots under the microscope but also culture the urine, will convince themselves in the 1st week that tens of thousands of bacteria/ml can be present on the culture plate that cannot be found in the microscopic sediment.

The second error made by the examiner who relies solely on the microscope is the reverse of the first error: bacteria are seen in the microscopic sediment but the urine culture is reported to be sterile. As will be shown in Chapter 5, the voided urine from the female, even when collected on the cystoscopy table under carefully controlled conditions, can contain many thousands of lactobacilli and corynebacteria. These bacteria are readily seen under the microscope, and, although they are Gram-positive, they often appear Gram-negative (Gram-variable) if stained. They grow poorly under aerobic conditions and are quite properly not reported by bacteriologic laboratories.

The third major error that results from relying solely on the microscope for the diagnosis of urinary infection lies in the interpretation of pyuria. There is probably no more meaningless query in the whole field of medicine than "How many white blood cells (WBC) in the centrifuged urine are significant?" The number of WBC seen under the microscope depends on (1) how the specimen was obtained (especially the degree of vaginal contamination in the female or urethral contamination in the male); (2) the urine flow rate (the degree of hydration) at the time of collecting the specimen; (3) the intensity of the tissue reaction of the uroepithelial surfaces to the disease process; (4) the volume, time, and speed of centrifugation; and (5) the volume in which the physician resuspends the urinary sediment after pouring off the supernatant. Thus, the number of WBC present in the spun sediment can vary so markedly as to be meaningless.

Moreover, many diseases of the urinary tract produce significant pyuria in the absence of bacterial infection. Whereas tuberculosis is the well recognized example of abacterial pyuria, staghorn calculi and stones of smaller size can produce intense pyuria with clumps of WBC in the absence of urinary infection. Almost any injury to the urinary tract, from chlamydial urethritis to glomerulonephritis and nephrosis, can elicit large numbers of fresh polymorphonuclear leukocytes (glitter cells). Depending on the state of hydration, the intensity of the tissue reaction producing the cells, and the method of urine collection, any number of WBC can be seen in the microscopic sediment in the presence of a sterile urinary tract. The presence or absence of pyuria in the centrifuged urine is the worst of all criteria for a urinary infection.

Pyuria, however, can be quantitated in the uncentrifuged urine by measuring either the WBC excretion rate (in a timed urine collection) as WBC/hour or the WBC concentration as WBC/ml in a random, nontimed urine sample. Both methods require that a fresh, unspun sample of urine be placed in a counting chamber of exact volume such as the Neubauer haemocytometer or the Fuchs-Rosenthal chamber that has twice the depth (0.2 mm) and volume of the Neubauer chamber. Mabeck has advocated a timed urine collection where the results are expressed as WBC per hour[29]; he found that women without evidence of urinary tract disease excrete less than 400,000 leukocytes/hour. Gadeholt, however, in a detailed and scientific analysis of the errors involved in counting cells in urine, argues for simply expressing the results as cells/mm^3 of urine in nontimed specimens[30, 31]; he notes that the upper limit of a normal cell count is assumed to be 8 erythrocytes and 13 leucocytes plus nonsquamous epithelial cells/mm^3 of urine. Any clinical investigator who wants to quantitatively count cells in the urine should study Gadeholt's investigations very carefully. Triger and Smith have studied the effect of urinary osmolality, pH, and temperature on the *in vitro* survival of urinary leukocytes[32]; WBC's deteriorated and disappeared the most rapidly in hypotonic alkaline suspensions at 37°C. Interestingly, little change in WBC suspensions occurred in 24 hours if the urine was hypertonic (1200 mOsm/liter) or made very acid (pH 3.0).

We quantitate leukocyte counts in the voided urine of our patients whom we follow closely for research purposes; we use the Fuchs-Rosenthal chamber and report the results as leukocytes/ml of urine. In a careful study of 16 control woman volunteers who had never had urinary infections, the first voided 5–10 ml collected by the nurse on the cystoscopy table (see Figures 1.24 and 1.26) contained 2700 ± 6300 leukocytes/ml (n = 116). In 123 collections in the same 16 volunteers, the midstream urine collected in the same manner (see Figure 1.24) contained 300 ± 700 leukocytes/ml. On the other hand, when volunteer controls collected their own urine samples by voiding from the toilet seat and cleaning their labia twice with a 4 × 4 gauze sponge wet with tap water, the first voided sample from 14 women studied 21 times contained 2300 ± 2600 leukocytes/ml of urine. Midstream samples from the same 14 women, but collected 96 times, contained 900 ± 2400 leukocytes/ml. These latter data, then, indicate that a midstream urine from a normal, premenopausal woman, collected as outlined, should contain less than 7000 leukocytes/ml in 99% of individuals. If the urine specimen is collected from the cystoscopy table as outlined in Figure 1.24, the upper limit of normal should be 2050 leukocytes/ml of urine. This latter figure, where vaginal contamination is minimized, approaches the leukocyte counts reported by Musher *et al.* in 49 of 51 healthy adult men who had 5000 leukocytes/ml or less of urine with a mean WBC count of 1300/ml.[33]

It must be emphasized, however, that as useful as quantitative WBC counts are, the physician must still centrifuge an aliquot and examine it under a good microscope in order to diagnose many diseases of the urinary tract. Indeed, if I were forced to make a choice and could not do both (a quantitative WBC count and a qualitative, centrifuged examination of the urinary sediment), I would choose without hesitation a careful study of the concentrated urinary sediment.

Material and Procedure for Office Bacteriology

In addition to an office incubator, the basic requirements for quantitative office bacteriology include: (1) a sterile disposable culture tube; (2) a calibrated, curved tip, eyedropper type of pipette; and (3) a divided plastic disposable culture plate with blood agar on one side and desoxycholate or eosin-methylene blue (EMB) agar on the other (Figure 1.8). The time required to plate a culture should be less than 1 minute.

The urine specimen is obtained in the plastic culture tube, labeled, and placed in the refrigerator until the end of the day when time is available for culture (the culture must be performed within 24 hours). When possible, the divided agar plates should be removed from the refrigerator a few minutes before culturing to allow the agar time to reach room temperature. The culture tube is gently agitated to assure a uniform distribution of the urine, the cap is removed, and an aliquot of urine is drawn up into the sterile eyedropper pipette. Two drops of urine (0.1 ml) are placed in the corner on each half of the divided culture plate. The curved tip of the eyedropper is used to spread the urine evenly over each half of the plate (Figure 1.9). The culture plate is covered with its plastic top, and the plates are left for at least 15 minutes at room temperature to allow time for the urine to seep into the agar. After 15 minutes, the culture plates are placed in the incubator upside down because moisture accumulates on the dependent half of the culture plate. The following day, after 18–24 hours of incubation, all positive cultures can be observed, recorded, and discarded. If no growth is observed on the culture plates, it is best to incubate for another 24 hours before deciding that the urine culture is sterile, especially if the patient has received an antibacterial drug within 72 hours of the urine culture. Since there are no epidemic bacteria which produce urinary infections, only moderate precautions need be taken in disposing of the used culture plates. It is adequate to place them in a paper bag, seal the top with a stapler or adhesive tape and use the regular trash disposal service.

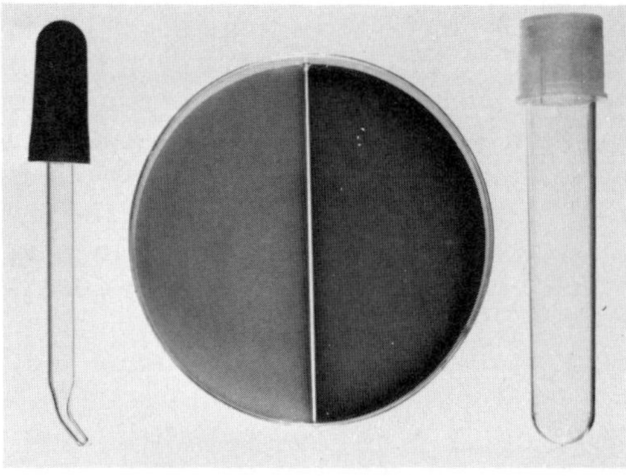

Figure 1.8 Materials required for bacteriologic culture: Calibrated, curved tip pipette, plastic disposable culture plate and sterile disposable culture tube. (Reproduced by permission from T. A. Stamey, J. Urol. **97:** 926, 1967.)

The key to this technique is the curved tip, eyedropper type of pipette which obviates the need for a Bunsen burner and bacteriologic loop for surface streaking the culture plate. This eyedropper pipette can be obtained from Arthur H. Thomas, Philadelphia, PA.

The sterile plastic disposable culture tube, individually wrapped in cellophane, has a cap instead of the routine cotton plug. When the culture tube is removed from the sterile wrapper, the lip beneath the cap remains sterile, making it unnecessary to flame the tube before collecting the culture. The patient's name and source of the culture can be written in crayon directly on the plastic tube. This culture tube can be obtained from Falcon Plastics, a Division

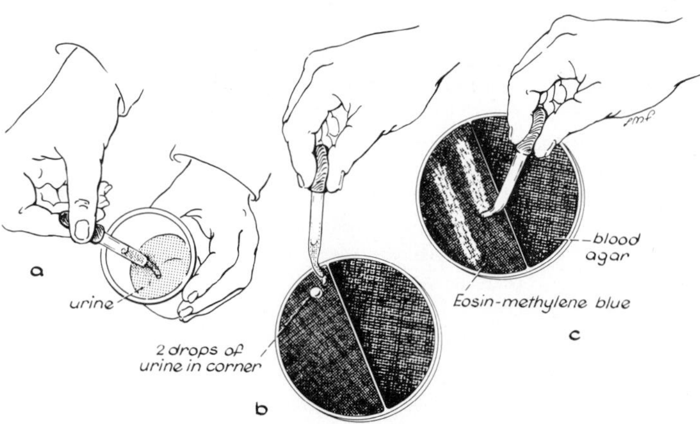

Figure 1.9 Curved tip, eyedropper technique of streaking divided agar plate with 0.1 ml (two drops) of urine. (Reproduced by permission from T. A. Stamey, Prevention of Recurrent Urinary Infections, Science & Medicine Publishing Co., New York 1973.)

of Becton-Dickinson Laboratories, 5500 West 83rd Street, Los Angeles, CA.

The only problem in office bacteriology is the supply of culture plates. The plastic plates, without agar, also can be obtained sterile from Falcon Plastics. The agar which goes into these plates is inexpensive. The final cost, agar and plate, is about 25 cents each (1979), which includes a cost accounting of the technician's time in making the plates. Commercial houses which can supply these plates charge over 90 cents/plate, which is excessive. The best approach is one in which the physician can make arrangements with his own hospital bacteriologic laboratory; 50 cents/plate should be an excellent profit and incentive for the media technician to pour a certain number of extra plates per week. These plates, if stored in the office refrigerator until used for culture, will keep for several weeks. One word of caution if desoxycholate rather than EMB agar is used: whereas the blood agar side of the divided culture plate is standard nutrient agar for any laboratory, several forms of desoxycholate agar are inhibitory for Gram-negative bacilli. The physician should be careful to specify plain desoxycholate agar; for example, Difco's bacto-desoxycholate agar is very satisfactory. On the other hand, certain modifications, *e.g.*, desoxycholate citrate agar, are designed to inhibit coliform bacilli in order to isolate salmonella and shigella. These modifications of the basic bacto-desoxycholate agar (Difco) are not suitable for the culture of bacteria from urinary infections.

Every laboratory catalogue contains examples of suitable incubators, which range in price from $50 to $500, depending on size, degree of temperature control, etc. Since urinary pathogens are not usually fastidious, a costly incubator in which the temperature is controlled to ±0.1°C is unnecessary.

Interpretation of Cultures. The number of bacteria present in the urine is determined by multiplying the number of individual colonies seen on one half of the culture plate (either the blood agar or the desoxycholate) by 10. This number will equal the number of colonies originally present in 1.0 ml of urine (since 0.1 ml was spread over each half of the plate). Quantitative colony counts are based on the theory that each visible colony after incubation began as a single bacterium. As every urologist knows, many bacteria in the urine are joined together in pairs, or occasionally in tight clumps; these bacteria will still appear as one visible colony. Thus, colony counts represent an approximate estimate of the original number of bacteria present. It must be emphasized that, while this method represents excellent bacteriologic practice, the interpretation of the significance of the colony counts is only as meaningful as the method of urine collection is free from contamination. For example, 250 colonies of *Escherichia coli* on the desoxycholate plate (about 3 times the number present in Figure 1.10*A*), representing a colony count of 2500 *E. coli*/ml of the original urine, indicate at least a bladder infection in the male patient, provided the specimen was a good midstream sample from a circumcised patient. However, in the female patient, depending on the method of collecting the midstream voided urine, a bacterial count of 2500/ml could represent introital bacteria in a patient with sterile bladder urine.

In actual office practice where the urologist exercises complete control over the method of collecting urine, the exact colony count assumes less importance. For example, if the culture is performed on an aspirated bladder urine, or from a very careful midstream catheterized specimen in the female patient from whom 200 ml of urine have passed through the catheter before the sample is obtained for culture, it makes no difference whether the colony count is 50, 500, or 50,000 bacteria/ml—the infection is present in the bladder urine. Thus, with a little experience in looking at these plates streaked with 0.1 ml of urine, combined with certain knowledge of the source of the specimen and the method of collection, it is not necessary to do an exacting bacterial count of the number of colonies present on the agar plates. Furthermore, the surface area available on these plates for streaking 0.1 ml of urine is not large. Urine cultures that are heavily infected

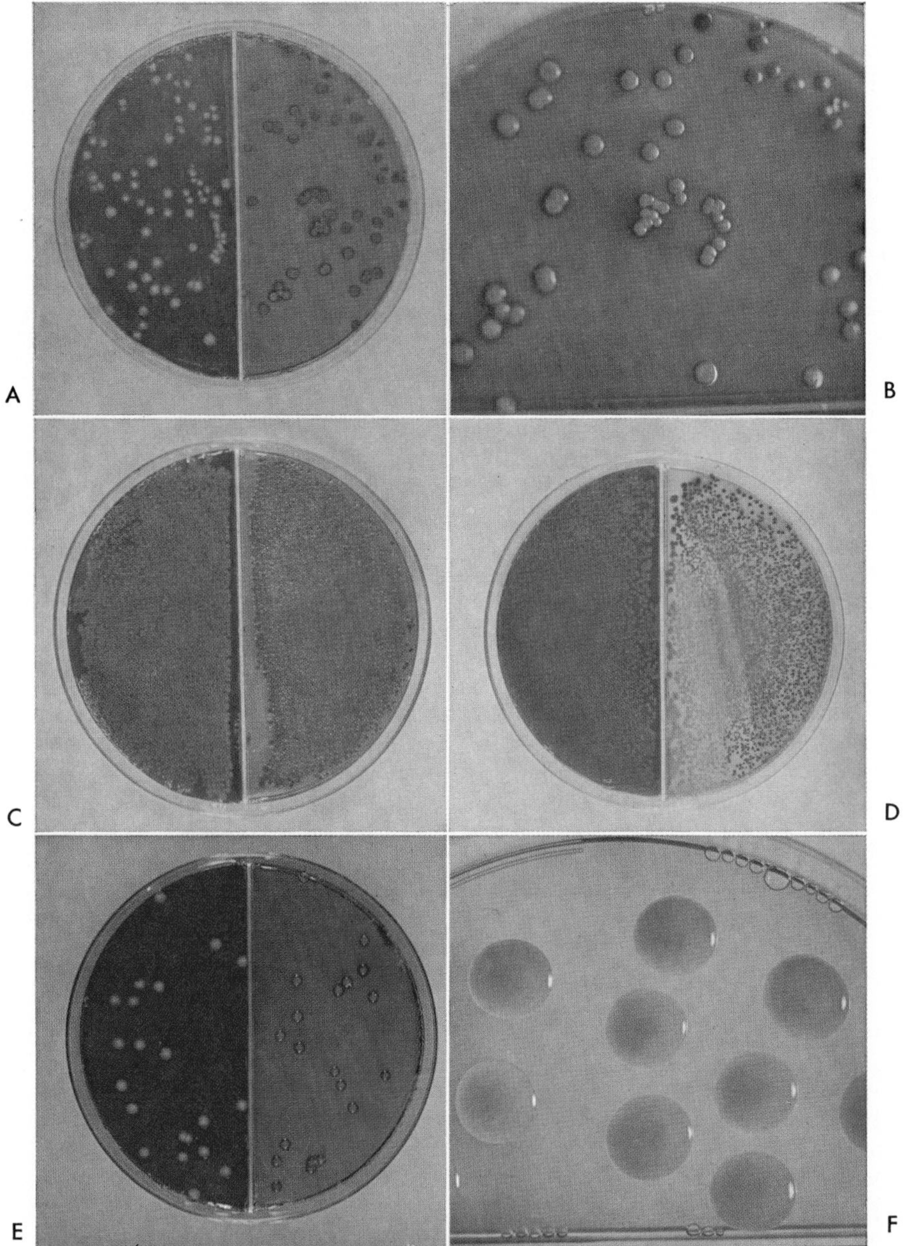

Figure 1.10 *A, Escherichia coli.* Typical example of about 70 colonies of *E. coli* on desoxycholate (700 colonies/ml of original urine). *B, E. coli.* Enlargement of desoxycholate colonies in Figure 1.10*A*. *C, E. coli.* Typical example of heavy growth of *E. coli*; colony count would be greater than 10,000 bacilli/ml of original urine. *D, E. coli.* Characteristic loss of color on desoxycholate when incubation has been prolonged. *E, Klebsiella.* Characteristic mucoid (shiny) appearance to heaped-up colonies of *Klebsiella*. Note, in contrast to *E. coli* in Figure 1.10*A*, that surrounding desoxycholate agar has not changed color. (See text.) *F, Klebsiella.* Enlargement of colonies in Figure 1.10*E*, but plate was 24 hours older. Note mucoid appearance of colonies, less pink than in Figure 1.10*E* but still showing dark center. (Reproduced by permission from T. A. Stamey, J. Urol. **97:** 926, 1967.)

(100,000 bacteria/ml or more) will show a colony growth that covers the entire plate like a blanket without any visible space between the colonies (Fig. 1.10*C*). When this heavy growth of bacteria is observed on the plate the next day, the physician knows that the patient's urine is heavily infected; it is of little importance whether 10,000 or 10 billion bacteria/ml produced the heavy growth. Indeed, when the physician recognizes that bacilli are present in the microscopic sediment—and therefore the colony count will be >30,000 bacterial/ml—he is better off to streak one-tenth or one-hundredth less urine on the plates. Calibrated bacteriologic loops of 0.01 and 0.001 ml are available for this purpose; the number of colonies on the agar is then multiplied by 100 or 1000 for the actual colony count/ml of urine.

The exact colony count also assumes less importance when the urethral aliquot (the first voided 10 ml) of urine is cultured together with the midstream voided specimen; contamination of an otherwise sterile midstream urine by urethral bacteria becomes obvious when the two culture plates are compared side by side.

Identification of Bacteria. Most physicians tend to approach office bacteriology with genuine concern over their ability to identify properly the bacteria producing the infection. However, there are several reassuring aspects in favor of this approach. First, 80% of all urine cultures performed will be either sterile or heavily infected with *E. coli.* Second, 95% of urinary infections are caused by a single infecting organism; thus, the identification of mixed infections is an uncommon problem. Even when mixed infections are present, it is better practice to treat only the predominant pathogen, reculture the urine during therapy, and then therapeutically approach the second pathogen, if it is still present. Third, 99% of urinary infections are caused by less than 10 different major types of bacteria. Thus, the physician soon becomes familiar with the relatively few types of bacteria he needs to recognize on the plates in order to choose antibacterial therapy on an intelligent and statistically successful basis.

Typical examples of six common types of bacteria encountered in urinary infections are presented in Figures 1.10 and 1.11. In general, the Gram-negative bacteria grow on both the desoxycholate agar and the blood agar, while the Gram-positive bacteria encountered in office practice—*Staphylococcus epidermidis, Staphylococcus aureus, Streptococcus faecalis, Streptococcus viridans, diphtheroids,* and *β*-hemolytic streptococci—grow only on the blood agar.

The four common and easily identified Gram-negative bacilli which account for most urinary infections are *E. coli, Klebsiella-Aerobacter,** proteus, and pseudomonas. The advantage of the desoxycholate agar is that *E. coli,* the most common pathogen, and *Klebsiella-Enterobacter* have a characteristic appearance. Since their antibacterial sensitivities are often different, it is important to distinguish between these two bacteria. *E. coli* is a dry, opaque uniformly pink colony; the pink color of the colony diffuses deeply into the desoxycholate medium (Figure 1.10*A–D*). No other colony can be confused with this dry, colorful bacillus. When the growth is heavy from a high bacterial count, or with prolonged incubation, there is a tendency for the indicator in the agar to lose its pink color and become colorless (as in Figure 1.10*D*, near the divider). The identification of *E. coli* colonies on the blood agar side of the plate is nonspecific because many Gram-negative bacilli have the same appearance: the colonies are usually grey and opaque and appear larger than the colonies on the desoxycholate agar.

By contrast, the colonies of *Klebsiella-Enterobacter* are mucoid (shiny), heaped up (grow higher off the agar), and also pink, especially in their centers, but the surrounding desoxycholate agar does not turn

* In the past few years, and since the tube dilution sensitivities represented later in Figures 2.3–2.14, *Klebsiella-Aerobacter* is now divided into two distinct genera: *Klebsiella* (nonmotile) and *Enterobacter* (*Aerobacter aerogenes,* motile). One of the practical reasons for distinguishing between the two species is that *Klebsiella* is usually sensitive to the cephalosporin antibiotics while *Enterobacter* is resistant. The newer cephalosporins, however, show *in vitro* activity against both *Klebsiella* and *Enterobacter.*

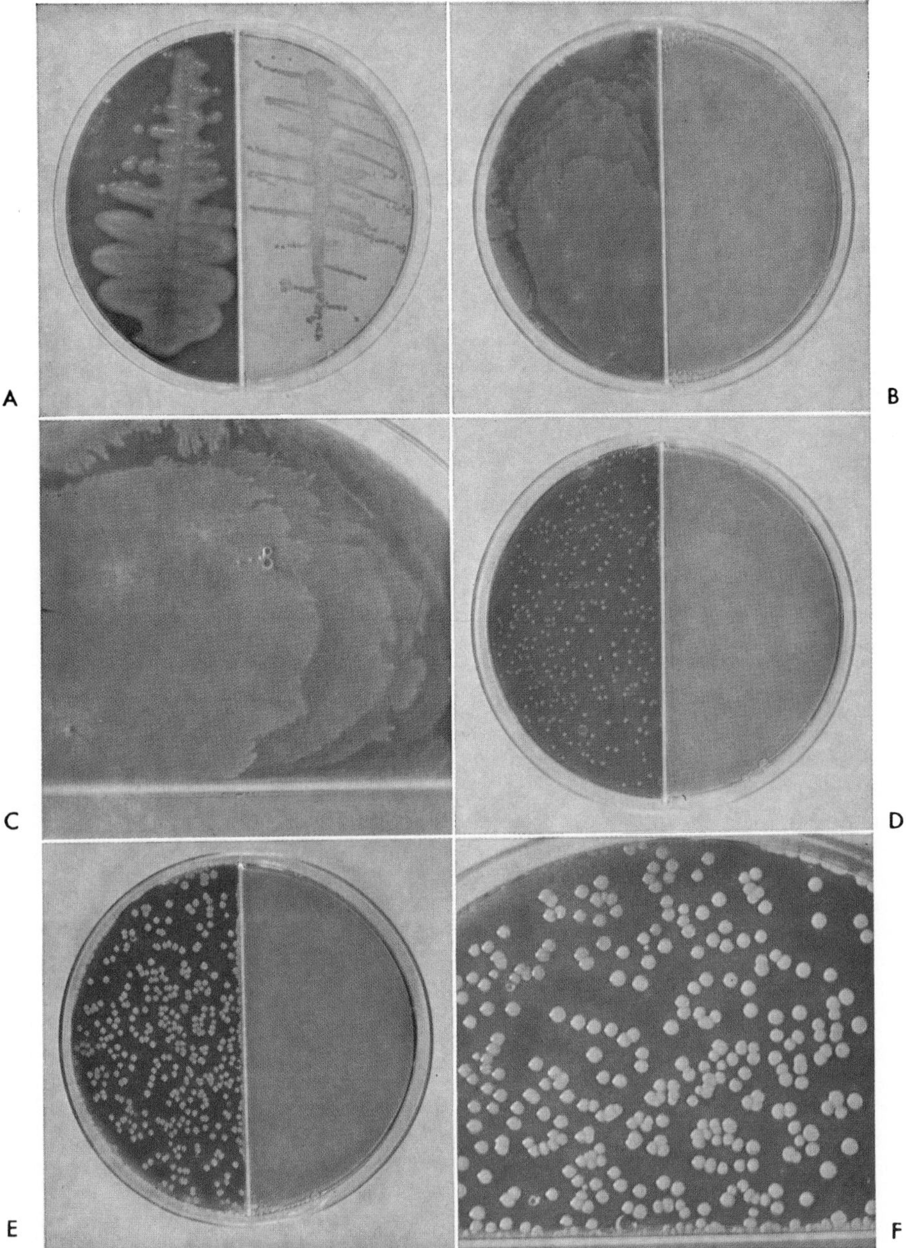

Figure 1.11 *A, Pseudomonas.* Typical metallis sheen is seen on blood agar; note hemolysis. This particular strain of pseudomonas is more mucoid and less green than many strains. Appearance of colonies on desoxycholate can be confused with other nonlactose-fermenting (no pink color) Gram-negative bacilli. *B, Proteus mirabilis.* Characteristic waves of spreading colonies which cover blood agar plate in grey film are emphasized in this photograph. (See text.) *C, P. mirabilis.* Enlargement of spreading proteus on blood agar plate in Figure 1.11*B*. *D, Streptococcus faecalis.* Typical example of small, grey, translucent, dewdrop colonies which do not produce hemolysis on blood agar and do not grow on desoxycholate, except in extremely rare instances. *E, Staphylococcus aureus.* In comparison to Figure 1.11*D*, note that these colonies are larger, much more opaque, and have slight orange color (*aureus*). *Staphylococcus epidermidis* would appear as dead white color as opposed to orange tint in this organism. No growth on desoxycholate. *F, S. aureus.* Enlargement of Figure 1.11*E*. (Reproduced by permission from T. A. Stamey, J. Urol. **97:** 926, 1967.)

pink as is the case with *E. coli* (Figure 1.10*E* and *F*). In some instances, the mucoid appearance of *Klebsiella-Enterobacter* (caused by their capsule characteristics) is so marked that these colonies appear slimy and quite ugly.

Pseudomonas can be identified by its appearance on the blood agar and not on the desoxycholate agar. On the blood agar plate, pseudomonas has a large, greenish grey metallic sheen (Figure 1.11*A*) and has the typical aromatic odor characteristic of pyocyaneus. On the desoxycholate agar, pseudomonas grows as small, translucent, colorless colonies which usually do not have a characteristic appearance and, in fact, are similar to colonies of other Gram-negative bacteria. When incubation is prolonged (48 hours or more), the pseudomonas colonies on desoxycholate can develop a characteristic dark, green-brown center.

Proteus mirabilis appears as colorless colonies on desoxycholate but has a characteristic appearance on blood agar (Figure 1.11*B* and *C*). *Proteus mirabilis* (and *Proteus vulgaris*) spread over the surface of the blood agar as a confluent grey film. Figure 1.11*B* shows the original five colonies from which the *P. mirabilis* started, as well as the five sheets or waves of spreading bacteria derived from the original colonies. It is clear that while identification of *P. mirabilis* can be made from the blood agar appearance and its characteristic putrid odor, the colony counts must be made from desoxycholate agar where proteus is unable to spread. The identification of *P. mirabilis* is important because virtually all urinary infections caused by this organism can be sterilized by 500 mg of oral penicillin-G four times a day.

Streptococcus faecalis is not uncommon in urinary infections (Fig. 1.11*D*). These cocci appear on the blood agar as small, grey, more or less translucent, dewdrop colonies, usually without hemolysis, although sometimes there may be slight α-hemolysis ("green" hemolysis). *S. faecalis*, except in extremely rare instances, does not grow on desoxycholate agar, but will grow in small colonies on EMB.

Staphylococcus aureus and *epidermidis* are larger colonies than *S. faecalis*, are much more opaque, and are either very white (*S. epidermidis*) or orange-appearing (*S. aureus*) depending on the degree of pigment (Figure 1.11*E* and *F*). Some hemolysis may or may not be present around the colonies. Again, for the practical purposes of office bacteriology, it makes no difference whether an infection is *S. aureus* or *epidermidis* because these two staphylococci are equally pathogenic for the urinary tract. In our experience, in fact, *S. epidermidis* is much more common. Penicillin-G is the drug of choice for both staphylococci. Since penicillin-G is also the drug of choice for *S. faecalis*, a good argument can be made for starting oral penicillin-G for any urinary infection that grows on the blood agar side of the plate, but not on the desoxycholate agar.*

Finally, there are urinary pathogens that require biochemical differentiation for more exact identification. These often are the same pathogens that need exact sensitivity determinations in order to choose a proper antibacterial agent for their elimination. Both identification and sensitivity determinations can be obtained readily by taking the culture plate directly to a bacteriologic laboratory. It is also likely that during the first few months of office bacteriology, a sympathetic bacteriologic technician can be of inestimable help to the physician in pointing out further salient characteristics of these common pathogens that have not been covered in this presentation.

For a small effort in time and for a cost of less than 75 cents/culture, office bacteriology offers the physician the following advantages: (1) complete control over the processing of the urine culture, *i.e.*, no opportunity for contaminants to multiply because of inadequate refrigeration, pickup services, etc; (2) an immediate culture report the next day by simply opening the incubator door; (3) a reliable and quantitative method for recognizing the presence or absence of urinary infection without relying

* A fungus growth in the urine will appear as yeast colonies on the blood agar; these colonies can look very similar to staphylococci, but with prolonged incubation the yeast will appear as tiny colorless colonies on the desoxycholate agar.

upon the unavoidable errors associated with the microscope; (4) the identification of the specific pathogen producing the infection, which allows, even without sensitivity determinations, a more intelligent selection of the proper antibacterial agent; (5) the use of disposable culture materials; and (6) a meaningful culture available to the patient and physician at a fraction of the usual cost.

Other Methods of Bacteriologic Cultures

Techniques other than the surface streaking method just described can be used for counting bacteria in urine, but, because they do not offer a qualitative identification of the bacteria, they are greatly inferior to the surface streaking method in Figures 1.10 and 1.11.

Pour Plates. A known quantity of urine, usually a diluted aliquot, is mixed with a measured volume of molten agar and allowed to harden. After incubation, the colonies appear within the depths of the agar and can be counted. This method, with proper dilutions, can be highly accurate, but it must always be combined with surface streaking for qualitative identification of the bacteria; most all bacteria appear similar when growing as deep colonies in agar. Because of this disadvantage, it is simpler to streak a known quantity (or dilution) of urine onto surface plates of diagnostic agar, as in Figures 1.10 and 1.11.

Miniature Agar Plates. Filter paper dip sticks are used to absorb a constant quantity of urine, very small agar trays are touched with the filter paper, and the colonies are counted after incubation. Available from Ayerst Laboratories under the commercial name of Testuria, this method is probably useful for detecting bacteriuria when the colony count is 10^5 bacteria/ml or more,[34] but it has not been tested adequately in clinical practice. Because such a small quantity of urine is absorbed on the filter paper strip and transferred to the agar surface, urines with 10^4 bacteria/ml or less will appear to be sterile. Moreover, the use of a single, all-purpose growth medium prevents preliminary identification of the organism and contributes to false-positive cultures by elevating the bacterial count from contaminating normal flora (micrococci, yeasts, and diphtheroids).

Dip Inoculum Methods. Mackey and Sandys[35] developed a spoon with an oval bowl (Figure 1.12) containing a constant surface area of agar. The spoon is dipped into urine, the excess urine is allowed to drain off, and the spoon is suspended in the center of a transport bottle. Although this method also will not detect smaller numbers of bacteria because of the limited agar surface area, it has the advantage of not requiring immediate incubation; the spoon can be mailed to a laboratory and incubated 2 or 3 days later.[35]

The most appealing dip inoculum method is the agar-coated microscopic slide described by Guttmann and Naylor (Fig. 1.12)[36] and studied in detail by Cohen and Kass.[37] An ordinary glass microscope slide is coated for a length of 2 inches with nutrient agar on one side and EMB or MacConkey's agar on the other. The coated four-fifths of the slide is dipped into fresh urine, the excess is allowed to drain off for a few seconds, and the slide is returned to the close-fitting plastic container that prevents the agar from touching the side of the bottle (Figure 1.13). There is a direct relationship between the number of colonies that appear on the dip-slide after incubation and the number of bacteria in the urine. Because the surface area (13 cm^2) is greater than that of Mackey and Sandys' spoon, the dip-slide can detect smaller colony counts (the volume of urine absorbed

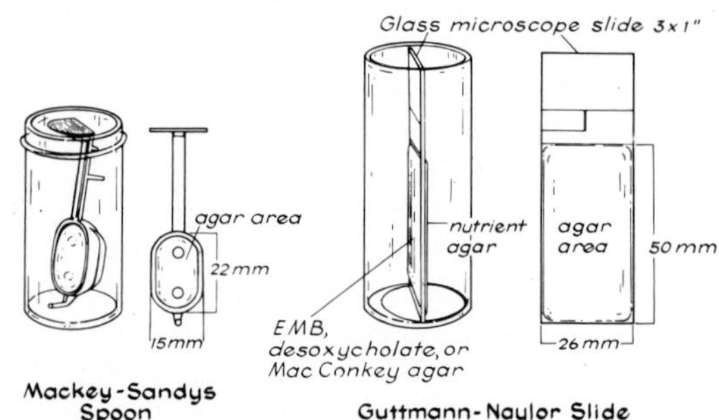

Figure 1.12 Dip inoculum methods: The Mackey-Sandys spoon and the Guttmann-Naylor slide.

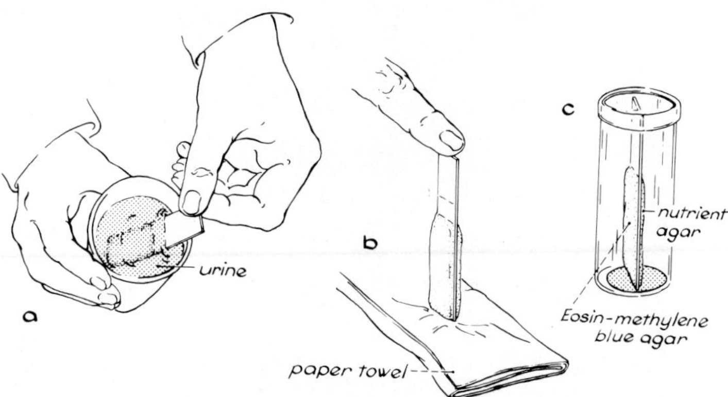

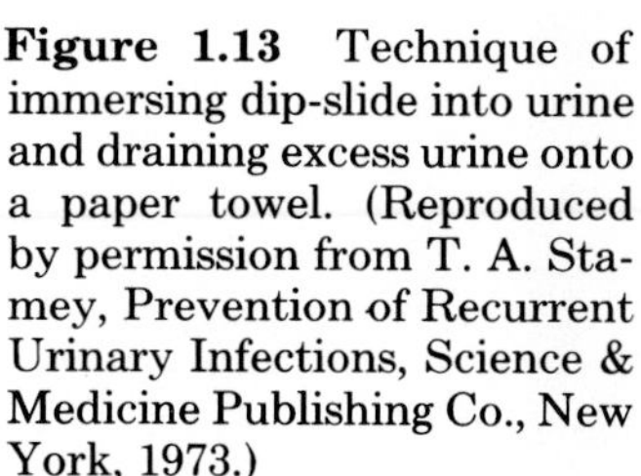
Figure 1.13 Technique of immersing dip-slide into urine and draining excess urine onto a paper towel. (Reproduced by permission from T. A. Stamey, Prevention of Recurrent Urinary Infections, Science & Medicine Publishing Co., New York, 1973.)

on the slide is estimated by Cohen and Kass[37] to be 0.01–0.02 ml). Thus, one colony would represent 100–200 bacteria/ml, which also represents the lower limit of sensitivity.

There is only a 10-fold difference in the volume of urine cultured on the dip-slide and the quantity (0.1 ml) used to culture the urines in Figures 1.10 and 1.11. The two methods are shown side-by-side in Figure 1.14; a broth culture of *Klebsiella* was diluted in saline to 10^3, 10^4, and 10^5 bacteria/ml. We have used the Uricult dip-slide for several years with EMB agar on one side and CLED (cystine-lactose-electrolyte deficient) agar on the other. They can be obtained from Medical Technology Corp., 497 Hacksensack Avenue, Hackensack, NJ 07606, and have been very satisfactory. In terms of accuracy of quantitative counts, the dip-slide is comparable to the surface plate technique using the eyedropper or a pipette to spread the 0.1 ml of urine, as observed also by others.[38–40] McAllister is particularly enthusiastic, entitling his paper "The Day of the Dipslide."[40] Some investigators have observed little difference between incubation of the dip-slide at room temperature compared to incubation at 37°C,[41] while others have shown a substantial rate of false negative cultures at room temperature.[38] It makes more sense to incubate, but one of the advantages with the dip-slide is that patients can culture their first voided urine and bring the cultures into the clinic or even mail it if great distances are involved. The disadvantage to the dip-slide, in comparison to routine agar surface streaking (Figures 1.10 and 1.11), is that the bacteria are more difficult to identify for species differentiation (*E. coli*, pseudomonas, etc.). Indeed, Vejlsgaard and Justesen could demonstrate by dip-slide only 56% of the species found by spreading 0.5 ml of diluted urine on blood agar.[38] Except for these reservations in easily identifying the bacterial species on the dip-slide agar, Uricult is an excellent way to practice office bacteriology in an efficient and inexpensive way (one box of 10 Uricult dip-slides cost $5.80, or 58 cents/culture).

Chemical Indices of Bacteriuria. Chemical tests, such as nitrate reduction to nitrites (the Greiss test)[42, 43] and the triphenyltetrazolium chloride reduction (T.T.C. test),[44] have been shown to have a high percentage of false-negative results, although Finnerty and Johnson[45] reported better results by combining the Greiss nitrate test with a measurement of sufficient nitrate. Most promising of all, theoretically, is the reduction of normal urinary glucose in the presence of bacteriuria.[46, 47] Unfortunately, as with the other chemical indices, an unacceptable rate of false-negative results—about 50%—has been reported by different authors.[38, 48] Moreover, all of these chemical indices of bacteriuria require retention of urine in the bladder for about 6 hours before micturition. Kunin has reported that a plastic strip containing both dehydrated culture media and a chemical to detect nitrite in the urine ("Microstix," Ames Company) detected 90% of urines

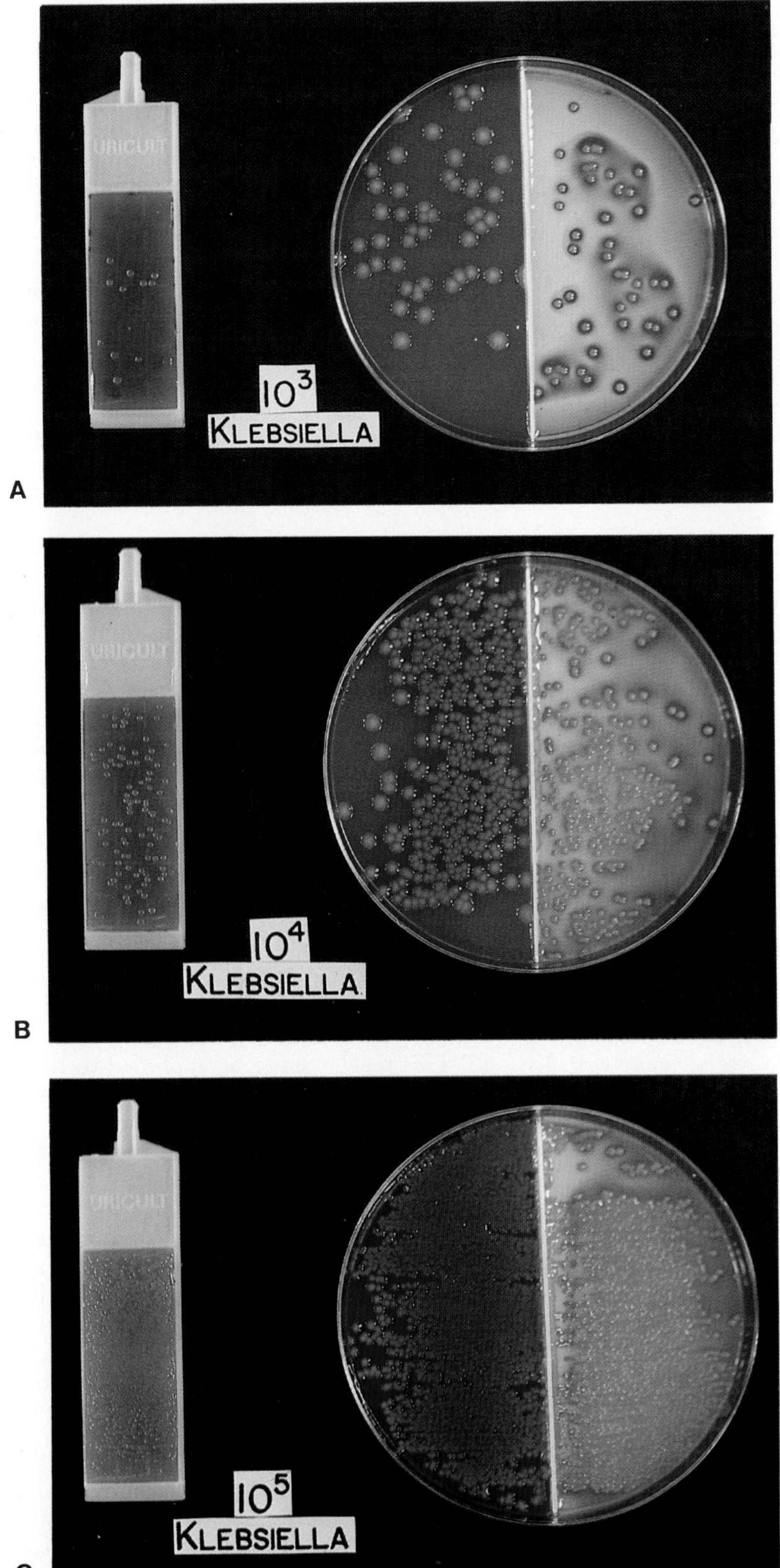

Figure 1.14 A comparison of the dip-slide agar technique to the surface streak method (0.1 ml) presented in Figures 1.9–1.11.

with greater than 10^5 bacteria/ml.[49] While a dip-stix has some storage advantages, it still requires 6 hours of urine retention and does not qualitatively identify the infecting organism or allow for sensitivity testing. It is not likely to prove very useful.

It should be emphasized, however, that none of these chemical methods will be able to quantitate smaller numbers of bacteria, so necessary in localizing urinary infections. As initial screening studies for population surveys and for use in the busy general practitioner's office, the dip-slide inoculum methods are adequate. But the urologist, who is responsible for more exacting bacteriologic studies when he attempts to localize the source of the bacteriuria, must not use these methods for localization studies. The surface streaking technique in Figures 1.10 and 1.11 quantitates the bacteria in 0.1 ml of urine; to culture a smaller volume means a greater percentage of false-negative cultures. In terms of the individual patient, a false-negative culture means to miss the source of his infection.

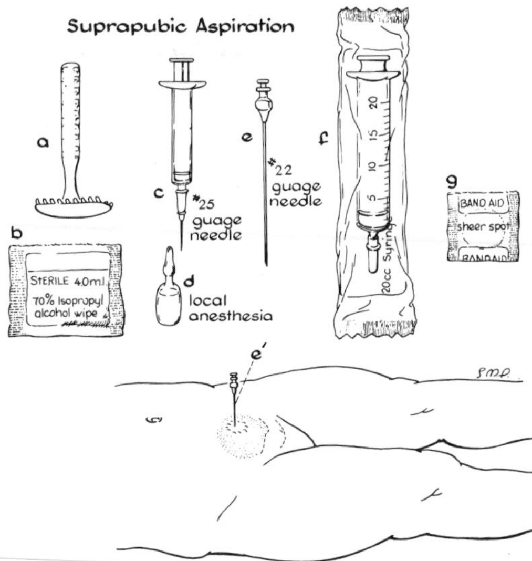

Figure 1.15 Technique of suprapubic aspiration of the bladder (SPA). (Reproduced by permission from T. A. Stamey, Prevention of Recurrent Urinary Infections, Science & Medicine Publishing Co., New York, 1973.)

LOCALIZATION OF INFECTION SITE

The following sections, especially the bacteriologic localization studies, establish the techniques and methodology upon which most of the data presented in this book are based. These methods are important.

Bacteriologic Localization Studies: Bladder or Kidney?

Suprapubic Needle Aspiration of the Bladder (SPA)

Before a suprapubic needle aspiration is performed, the patient should force fluids until the bladder is full. The site of the needle puncture is in the midline, between the symphysis pubis and the umbilicus, and directly over the palpable bladder. The full bladder in the male is usually palpable because of its greater muscle tone; unfortunately, the full bladder in the female is frequently not palpable. In such patients, the physician performing the aspiration must rely on the observation that suprapubic pressure directly over the bladder produces an unmistakable desire to urinate. After determining the approximate site for needle puncture, the local area is shaved and the skin is cleansed with an alcohol sponge; a cutaneous wheal is raised with a 25-gauge needle and any local anesthetic (Figure 1.15). A 3½-inch, 22-gauge needle is introduced through the anesthetized skin; the progress of the needle is arrested just below the skin within the anesthetized area and, with a quick plunging action, similar to any intramuscular injection, the needle is advanced into the bladder. Most patients experience more discomfort from the initial anesthetization of the skin than they feel with the second stage when the needle is advanced into the bladder. After the needle has been introduced, a 20-ml syringe is used to aspirate 5 ml of urine for culture and 15 ml of urine for centrifugation and urinalysis. The obturator is reintroduced into the needle, and both needle and obturator are withdrawn. A small strip-dressing is placed over the needle site in the skin. If urine is not obtained with complete introduction of the needle, the patient's bladder is not full and is usually deep within the retropubic area. When no urine is obtained with the first try, it is probably wiser to desist until the bladder is full. Nevertheless, we have often made several attempts without complications, but it is uncomfortable to the patient.

As I have already emphasized, SPA is critically important in infants,[18] in patients with spinal cord injury,[19] and it has even been strongly recommended as a safe, reliable, and well tolerated method for obtaining specimens from women in a general practice.[50] Interestingly, Dove and his collaborators cultured the SPA urine with a dip-slide[50]; this combination of SPA and a dip-slide is clearly ideal because it avoids the problem of interpreting bacteria on the dip-slide which represents contaminants from the female perineum. Because our technique of collecting a voided urine from patients on the cystoscopy table avoids substantial perineal contamination, we perform SPA only on those patients in whom we cannot interpret the midstream culture. SPA is also useful in any patient (male or female) who has pyuria without positive aerobic cultures. In this situation, SPA can confirm the pyuria does not arise from the lower urinary tract below the internal vesical neck. Lastly, as I will show later in Chapter 4, SPA is the only technique that can prove urinary infection with *Ureaplasma urealyticum.*

Differentiation between Bladder Bacteriuria and Renal Bacteriuria by Ureteral Catheterization Studies

Although three consecutive whole voided urine cultures in the female of 10^5 or $>10^5$ bacteria/ml of urine, a single culture of a carefully catheterized urine of 10^3 bacteria or more/ml, and probably any number of bacteria in a suprapubic aspiration of the bladder all serve to confirm the presence of a bladder infection, the kidneys may or may not be infected. Thus, bacteriuria only confirms the presence of bacteria in bladder urine; the renal urines may be sterile. Both Rantz[5] and Sanford[6] recognized the importance of establishing the bacteriologic status of renal pelvic urine in patients with bacteriuria; they observed that ureteral urines collected at cystoscopy often contained much smaller numbers of bacteria than the bladder urine. The ureteral catheters, however, had to pass through an infected bladder, making it difficult to interpret the significance of single ureteral cultures, especially with low counts. About 1960, we developed a technique of cystoscopy (based on extensive washing of the bladder, a control culture of the ureteral catheters before entering the ureteral orifices, and multiple serial cultures from each kidney) that distinguished between bladder and renal pelvic bacteriuria.[51]

The technical problem is to pass ureteral catheters through infected bladder urine and be sure that the subsequent ureteral cultures represent uncontaminated samples of renal urine. To accomplish this, the patient is well hydrated prior to cystoscopy, given a saddle or caudal anesthesia, and prepared for cystoscopy with the usual sterile precautions. The cystoscope (obturator in place) is passed into the bladder; a representative sample of bladder urine is obtained from the open stopcock. This sample is labeled CB, the symbol for "catheterized bladder." The bladder is washed with 2–3 liters of sterile irrigating solution and then emptied. Size 5 French (Fr) polyethylene ureteral catheters (Stamey Ureteral Catheters, ACMI) are introduced with the catheterizing element into the cystoscope, but passed only to the bladder. About 50–100 ml of irrigating fluid are run into the bladder; the inflow stopcock is then closed. The irrigating fluid passing from the bladder through the ureteral catheters is collected for culture by holding the ends of both catheters over the open end of a sterile culture tube. This culture (labeled WB, the symbol for "washed bladder") indicates the number of bacteria/ml carried within the lumina of the catheter as they are advanced to the midureter. These bacteria represent the maximal contamination possible in the first serial kidney culture if the total volume of urine collected from the kidney is equal to the volume of irrigating fluid displaced from the ureteral catheter (approximately

1.0 ml for a No. 5 Fr polyethylene catheter). Since, in actual practice, the first 5–10 ml from each catheter are never cultured, and since cultural aliquots are always several times (5–10 ml) the volume of the ureteral catheter lumen, the bacterial count in this WB culture represents a theoretical maximum. Nonetheless, if the bladder wash leaves many bacteria in the irrigating water within the ureteral catheter, and if the patient has an antidiuresis (0.2 ml/minute/kidney) rather than a brisk water diuresis, large numbers of bacteria may be recovered from the ureteral catheter when the kidney urine is sterile.

The ureteral catheters are then quickly passed to each midureter or renal pelvis without introducing additional irrigating fluid. Both stopcocks of the cystoscope are then opened to ensure an empty bladder; this prevents reflux of urine from the bladder around the ureteral catheters to the renal pelvis during the kidney collections. The first 5–10 ml of urine from each ureteral catheter are discarded. Four consecutive paired cultures (5–10 ml in volume) are collected from the ureteral catheters directly into sterile culture tubes; these ureteral specimens are labeled LK_1, RK_1, LK_2, RK_2, etc. If the urine flow rate is too slow, mannitol can be given intravenously to produce a diuresis. Renal urines are collected for microscopic study before removing the ureteral catheters. If the diuresis is brisk, I centrifuge 5–10 ml of urine from each kidney; microscopic examination of the sediment often localizes pyuria to one side or the other and usually agrees with the bacteriologic cultures. *It is mandatory that the patient be started on the appropriate antibacterial agent before leaving the cystoscopy room.*

The specific gravity, urine creatinine concentration, and sometimes urine osmolality were occasionally determined on several pairs of renal samples since the major functional defect in pyelonephritis is a failure to reabsorb water in the medulla of the kidney.[52, 53] Because a water diuresis, when compared with an antidiuresis, tends to mask this functional defect in concentrating ability,[53] some patients had one or two urine samples collected before their water diuresis. These concentrated aliquots were never used for culture, although they were useful for sediment studies.

Representative localization patterns from patients whose bacteriuria was limited to the bladder are presented in Table 1.2, to the bladder and one kidney in Table 1.3, and to the bladder and both kidneys in Table 1.4. Specific gravity was measured by a Refractometer (American Optical Company), creatinine by Auto-Analyzer, and osmolality by the Fiske osmometer. An accurate specific gravity—rapidly performed on a single drop of urine with the Refractometer—is just as useful as urinary creatinine or osmolality in comparing urinary concentration between the two kidneys, or in following serial changes in urinary concentration during bacteriologic collections. In Figure 1.16 urine creatinine is compared to specific gravity in 33 different samples.

The localization patterns in patients with lower urinary infections (Table 1.2) present few diagnostic difficulties. The data indicate the remarkable facility with which bacteria in the bladder are washed down to low counts, an observation that formed the basis for Fairley's method of distinguishing between bladder and renal infections.[54] This potential of washing virtually all of the bacteria from the bladder enhances the validity of localization studies by reducing the magnitude of ureteral contamination. In addition, it indicates that most of the bacteria in the bladder are in the urine and not in bladder tissues. These patterns (Table 1.2) show that the first ureteral collection may contain a few contaminating bacteria carried by the catheter into the ureter. Actually, about half of the first ureteral specimens will contain some bacteria as contaminants, depending on the urine flow rate from the kidney, the number of bacteria carried up the ureter within the catheter, and the time interval between ureteral catheterization and the collection of urine. In occasional instances, where a gross abnormality of the bladder is present, the final wash culture (WB) of the bladder may contain several thousand bacteria/ml. In such patients, even the second ureteral specimen

Table 1.2
Localization Patterns in Patients with Sterile Renal Urines[a]

Source[b]	Bacteria/ml	Organism	Specific Gravity	Urine Creatinine	Urine Osmolality
				mg/100 ml	*mOsm/liter*
Patient P.G.					
CB	69,000,000	*Proteus mirabilis*	1.014	91	—
WB	94	*P. mirabilis*	1.000	1.5	—
LK_1	0	0	1.002	9	—
RK_1	0	0	1.002	9	—
LK_2	0	0	1.002	10	—
RK_2	0	0	1.002	9	—
LK_3	0	0	1.002	10	—
RK_3	0	0	1.002	11	—
Patient J.A.					
CB	3,900	*Escherichia coli*	—	—	—
WB	59	*E. coli*	—	—	—
LK_1	0	0	1.006	24	272
RK_1	1	*E. coli*	1.005	25	279
LK_2	0	0	1.005	18	228
RK_2	0	0	1.005	20	232
LK_3	0	0	1.004	16	190
RK_3	0	0	1.005	21	225
Patient L.D.					
CB	>10,000	*E. coli*	1.001	7	45
WB	900	*E. coli*	1.000	1	—
LK_1	0	0	1.001	8	55
RK_1	10	*E. coli*	1.001	7	54
LK_2	0	0	1.001	9	56
RK_2	0	0	1.001	9	56
Patient J.M.					
CB	292,000,000	*E. coli*	1.015	53	—
WB[c]	0	0	1.000	0	—
LK_1	0	0	1.009	29	246
RK_1	0	0	1.007	21	164
LK_2	0	0	1.005	6	143
RK_2	0	0	1.004	7	113
LK_3	0	0	1.004	5	111
RK_3	0	0	1.004	5	97
Patient S.B.					
CB	>100,000	*E. coli*	1.004	15	—
WB	155	*E. coli*	1.000	<1	—
LK_1	0	0	1.011	42	—
RK_1	1	0	1.013	52	—
LK_2	0	0	1.007	28	—
RK_2	0	0	1.008	32	—
LK_3	0	0	1.003	10	—
RK_3	0	0	1.003	11	—

[a] Reproduced by permission from T. A. Stamey, D. E. Govan, and J. M. Palmer, Medicine **44:** 1, 1965.[11]

[b] CB = catheterized bladder urine; WB = washed bladder (after 2–3 liters of sterile water irrigation); LK_1 to LK_3 = serial left renal urines; RK_1 to RK_3 = serial right renal urines.

[c] Bladder washed with 5 liters of irrigating water; patient was an 8-year-old girl carrying 400 ml of residual urine in her bladder.

Table 1.3
Localization Patterns in Patients with Unilateral Renal Bacteriuria[a]

Source	Bacteria/ml	Organism	Specific Gravity	Urine Creatinine	Urine Osmolaity
				mg/100 ml	*mOsm/liter*
Patient S.I.					
CB	1,260,000	*Escherichia coli*	—	—	—
WB	3,720	*E. coli*	—	—	—
RK_1	394,000	*E. coli*	1.008	37	354
LK_1	91	*E. coli*	1.009	62	613
RK_2	228,000	*E. coli*	1.003	12	127
LK_2	2	*E. coli*	1.005	22	263
RK_3	33,400	*E. coli*	1.002	9	88
LK_3	0	0	1.002	11	123
Patient L.C.					
CB	3,300	*Proteus mirabilis*	—	—	—
WB	258	*P. mirabilis*	—	—	—
LK_1	1,980	*P. mirabilis*	1.001	9	78
RK_1	0	0	1.001	9	79
LK_2	2,400	*P. mirabilis*	1.001	9	84
RK_2	0	0	1.002	9	84
LK_3	2,880	*P. mirabilis*	1.002	11	99
RK_3	0	0	1.002	11	98
Patient J.G.					
CB	>100,000	*E. coli*	—	—	—
WB	600	*E. coli*	—	—	—
RK_1	Not cultured	—	1.008	32	395
LK_1	Not cultured	—	1.009	35	425
RK_2	>100,000	*E. coli*	1.007	—	—
LK_2	15	*E. coli*	1.007	—	—
RK_3	>100,000	*E. coli*	1.006	—	—
LK_3	12	*E. coli*	1.006	—	—
RK_4	>100,000	*E. coli*	1.004	—	—
LK_4	1	*E. coli*	1.005	—	—
Patient C.C.					
CB	>100,000	*E. coli*	—	—	—
WB	1,000	*E. coli*	—	—	—
RK_1	Not cultured	—	1.009	80	376
LK_1	Not cultured	—	1.019	176	738
RK_2	178	*E. coli*	1.006	53	—
LK_2	0	0	1.017	128	—
RK_3	170	*E. coli*	1.008	52	—
LK_3	0	0	1.016	111	—
RK_4	166	*E. coli*	1.009	62	—
LK_4	0	0	1.016	117	—
Patient L.S.					
CB	3,180	*E. coli*	—	—	—
WB	0	0	—	—	—
RK_1	Not cultured	—	1.021	179	666
LK_1	Not cultured	—	1.020	180	667
RK_2[b]	125	*E. coli*	1.025	33	565
LK_2	0	0	1.025	31	537
RK_3	130	*E. coli*	1.026	—	526
LK_3	0	0	1.027	—	528
RK_4	177	*E. coli*	1.029	—	590
LK_4	0	0	1.030	—	600

[a] Abbreviations and source as in Table 1.2.
[b] Collections made with mannitol as a diuretic.

Table 1.4
Localization Patterns in Patients with Bilateral Renal Bacteriuria[a]

Source	Bacteria/ml	Organism	Specific Gravity	Urine Creatinine	Urine Osmolaity
				mg/100 ml	*mOsm/liter*
Patient O.S.					
CB	>100,000	*Escherichia coli*	—	—	—
WB	2,760	*E. coli*	—	—	—
RK_1	Not cultured	—	1.0048	17	245
LK_1	Not cultured	—	1.0053	25	342
RK_2	Not cultured	—	1.0053	20	334
LK_2	Not cultured	—	1.0068	32	371
RK_3	162,000	*E. coli*	1.0043	—	—
LK_3	55,000	*E. coli*	1.0043	—	—
RK_4	144,000	*E. coli*	1.0035	—	—
LK_4	48,000	*E. coli*	1.0038	—	—
RK_5	90,000	*E. coli*	1.0035	—	—
LK_5	30,000	*E. coli*	1.0038	—	—
Patient D.M.					
CB	>100,000	*Proteus mirabilis*	—	—	—
WB	3,420	*P. mirabilis*	—	—	—
RK_1	Not cultured	—	1.018	151	672
LK_1	Not cultured	—	1.018	154	704
RK_2	23,760	*P. mirabilis*	1.024	42	—
LK_2	7,440	*P. mirabilis*	1.025	44	—
RK_3	65,000	*P. mirabilis*	1.024	58	—
LK_3	21,600	*P. mirabilis*	1.025	57	—
RK_4	>100,000	*P. mirabilis*	1.022	59	—
LK_4	>100,000	*P. mirabilis*	1.023	62	—
Patient B.L.					
CB	>100,000	*E. coli*	—	—	—
WB	2,400	*E. coli*	—	—	—
RK_1	>10,000	*E. coli*	1.015	77	644
LK_1	1,800	*E. coli*	1.015	80	664
RK_2	>10,000	*E. coli*	1.014	—	—
LK_2	1,300	*E. coli*	1.014	—	—
RK_3	>10,000	*E. coli*	1.014	—	—
LK_3	780	*E. coli*	1.014	—	—
Patient J.C.[b]					
CB	>100,000	*E. coli*	—	—	—
WB	2,160	*E. coli*	—	—	—
RK_1	Not cultured	—	1.009	41	332
LK_1	Not cultured	—	1.010	42	340
RK_2	Not cultured	—	1.009	39	313
LK_2	Not cultured	—	1.009	41	335

[a] Abbreviations and source as in Table 1.2.

[b] A 72-year-old white woman with diabetes of 4 years duration; her BUN was 43 and creatinine clearance 17 ml/minute. An intravenous urogram showed no stones or obstruction and no postvoiding residual urine. The urinary infection was sterilized with nitrofurantoin.

[c] A 61-year-old white man with a 1-year history of resistant urinary infection; his serum creatinine was 2.2 mg/100 ml. An intravenous urogram showed no stones, obstruction, or bladder residual; a cystogram showed no reflux. At the time of open wedge biopsy of the right kidney 2.5 g of renal cortex were ground in sterile soy broth; all cortical tissue cultures were sterile. Microscopic sections showed marked arteriosclerotic narrowing of the small arteries, focal tubular atrophy, but no pyelonephritis. His urinary infection was sterilized with colistin methane sulfonate.

[d] Repeat studies performed immediately prior to open wedge biopsy of the right kidney.

Table 1.4, *Continued*

RK_3	>100,000	*E. coli*	1.006	20	—
LK_3	>100,000	*E. coli*	1.006	21	—
RK_4	>100,000	*E. coli*	1.006	17	—
LK_4	>100,000	*E. coli*	1.006	18	—
RK_5	>100,000	*E. coli*	1.006	17	246
LK_5	>100,000	*E. coli*	1.006	19	267
Patient L.P.[c]					
3/13/63					
CB	>100,000	*E. coli*	—	—	—
WB	>50,000	*E. coli*	—	—	—
RK_1	>100,000	*E. coli*	1.013	65	—
LK_1	>100,000	*E. coli*	1.013	64	—
RK_2	>100,000	*E. coli*	1.011	52	—
LK_2	>100,000	*E. coli*	1.012	52	—
RK_3	>100,000	*E. coli*	1.010	49	—
LK_3	>100,000	*E. coli*	1.010	51	—
4/24/63[d]					
CB	>100,000	*E. coli*	1.005	—	186
WB	6,000	*E. coli*	—	—	—
RK_1	>100,000	*E. coli*	1.003	13	100
LK_1	>100,000	*E. coli*	1.002	14	95
RK_2	>100,000	*E. coli*	1.004	20	161
LK_2	>100,000	*E. coli*	1.004	21	161
RK_3	>100,000	*E. coli*	1.004	18	159
LK_3	>100,000	*E. coli*	1.004	18	153

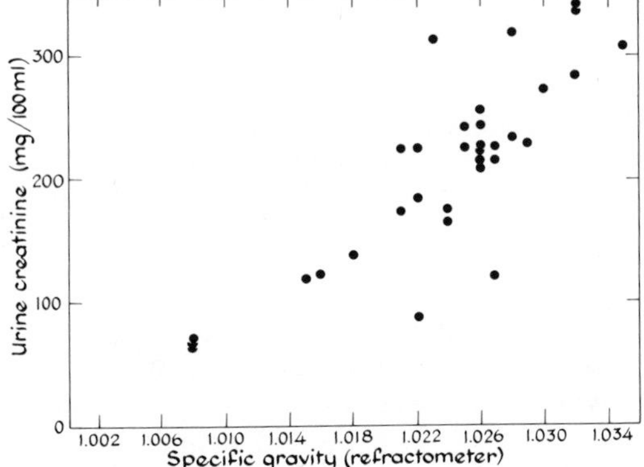

Figure 1.16 A comparison of refractometric specific gravity with urinary creatinine in 33 urines.

may contain a few bacteria before the third culture demonstrates sterility of the renal urine.

Representative examples of patients with unilateral renal bacteriuria are presented in Table 1.3. The diagnosis of unilateral renal bacteriuria is important; 50% of the upper urinary tract infections in our patients are limited to one kidney (see Table 1.6). Furthermore, when unilateral pyelonephritis is accompanied by abnormalities which render permanent cure of the infection impossible, despite adequate and repeated antibacterial treatment, unilateral localization of the infection offers a chance for permanent cure if a nephroureterectomy is performed.[51] This course of action, however, must be taken with caution and with indisputable bacteriologic data.

Bacteriologic data from five representative patients with bilateral renal bacteriuria illustrate some distinctive differences (Table 1.4). Although unilateral renal bacteriuria may occur with high bacterial counts in the hydrated renal urine, bilateral renal bacteriuria is nearly always associated with higher bacterial counts. In 22 consecutive patients reported in 1965[11] with documented bacteriologic patterns of bilateral renal bacteriuria, the average bacterial counts in three consecutive ureteral specimens from each kidney showed greater than 100,000 bacteria/ml in 10 patients and greater than 10,000 bacteria/ml in 9 additional patients; the remaining 3 had average counts of 7830, 8000, and 9300, respectively. By contrast, 18 of 25 patients with unilateral renal bacteriuria had less than 10,000 bacteria/ml in their ureteral urines. These high bacterial counts in renal urines explain the higher WB counts in patients with upper tract infections.

The presence of high colony counts in urine specimens obtained directly from the kidneys should not "be taken as almost certain evidence that there is some degree of hydronephrosis and pooling of urine above the site from which the specimen was obtained."[55] None of the patients in Table 1.4 had upper urinary tract obstruction. Of the 22 consecutive patients referred to above with bilateral renal bacteriuria, only 3 had obstructions. Of the remaining 19 patients, 4 had renal stones without obstruction, and 1 had bilateral reflux with excellent drainage from the ureters on intravenous urography; 14 patients had anatomically normal intravenous urograms. Thus, it is clear that urines with high bacterial counts from the renal pelvis do not suggest hydronephrosis. As further evidence, Table 1.5 and Figure 1.17 represent studies from a 32-year-old Negro female who had had an asymptomatic childhood.

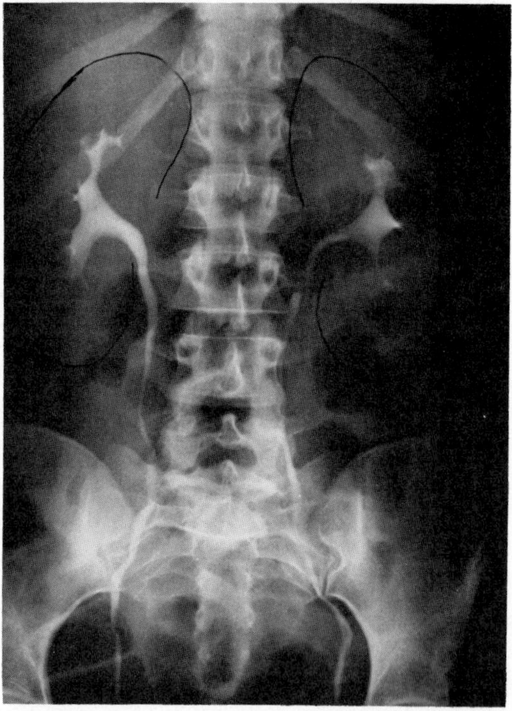

Figure 1.17 A retrograde urogram on a 32-year-old female performed at the end of the bacteriological localization studies presented in Table 1.5. In spite of severe bilateral renal bacteriuria, the calyces were delicate. Although the bacterial counts in both kidneys were greater than 10,000,000 *Escherichia coli*/ml of urine, there was no evidence of obstruction or pooling of urine.

Table 1.5
Typical Bacteriologic Pattern in Bilateral Nonobstructive Pyelonephritis in a 32-year-old Female without Reflux or Residual Urine[a]

Source	Bacteria/ml	Organism	Specific Gravity	Urine Creatinine
				mg/100 ml
CB	91,800,000	*Escherichia coli*	1.011	133
WB	64	*E. coli*	—	—
LK_1	>10,000,000	*E. coli*	1.006	54
RK_1	>20,000,000	*E. coli*	1.011	90
LK_2	>10,000,000	*E. coli*	1.007	57
RK_2	>20,000,000	*E. coli*	1.011	90
LK_3	>10,000,000	*E. coli*	1.007	62
RK_3	>20,000,000	*E. coli*	1.011	95
LK_4	>10,000,000	*E. coli*	1.008	73
RK_4	>20,000,000	*E. coli*	1.012	—

[a] Abbreviations and source as in Table 1.2.

Her first urinary infection was in 1957, 4 months after the birth of her third child; she was hospitalized and treated for a left pyelonephritis. The second attack was in June 1958. One week before the studies in this table (January 14, 1964), she developed back pain, malaise, chills, and fever; there was no dysuria or frequency. Her residual urine was 1 ml. There was no reflux on a voiding cystourethrogram, and the retrograde urogram (Figure 1.17), performed at the end of the studies in Table 1.5, was normal. Nitrofurantoin, 100 mg every 6 hours, was started after these localization studies; 72 hours later, the urine was sterile on suprapubic needle aspiration of the bladder. Thus, it is clear that high bacterial counts in renal urines are not indicative of hydronephrosis.

The bacterial count in consecutive renal samples bears a direct relationship to urine flow rate. This relationship is striking in the infected renal urines with smaller bacterial numbers, but it is present also in renal infections with high bacterial counts. It suggests either that an infected kidney elaborates bacteria at a constant rate, which seems unlikely, or that most of the bacteria in renal tissue are in surface contact with the urine. Since the bacteria are in the medulla of the kidney and not in the cortex,[51] an increasing urine flow rate, originating as sterile glomerular filtrate, could readily dilute the number of bacteria in surface contact with the infected medulla. The usual pattern is a progressively falling bacterial count with an increasing urine flow rate. In Table 1.4, the data on patient D.M. illustrate an *increase* in bacterial counts with a falling urine flow rate (a rising creatinine concentration), confirming the inverse relationship between urine flow rate and renal bacterial counts.

Whitworth *et al.*, after localizing bacteria to the renal pelvis by ureteral catheterization, lavaged the pelvis with gentamicin followed by a Frusemide diuresis[56]; in only 2 of 25 patients were they able to obtain sterile urines. They concluded, correctly I think, that pyelitis must be rare.

Tables 1.4 and 1.5 show that the degree of renal bacteriuria cannot be recognized by a functional disparity between the two kidneys in their concentrating mechanism. Patients B.L. and D.M. in Table 1.4 had gross bacteriologic differences with no significant difference in urine creatinine concentration. The data in Table 1.4 on L.P., a patient with severe bilateral pyelonephritis, show no differences in urine creatinine concentration at creatinine levels of 60 mg/100 ml or in a second study, when the urine was more dilute (creatinine 13 mg/100 ml). It is true that in unilateral renal bacteriuria there are usually significant differences between the infected and uninfected kidney. We are unable to explain Brod *et al.'s* report that his patients with chronic pyelonephritis showed an average difference of 78% in urine creatinine concentration between the two kidneys.[52] It is, perhaps, a matter of definition, stage of the disease, and the degree of dehydration.

History and physical examination are rarely of value in predicting the bacteriologic involvement of the kidneys. Many patients with urinary infections and low back pain have no kidney infection. Patients who complain of tenderness in one renal area frequently have equal bacteriologic involvement of the contralateral kidney. Many patients with renal bacteriuria have only lower urinary tract symptomatology.

In 1965, using these cystoscopic and bacteriologic localization techniques, we reported the sites of infection in 95 women and 26 men who had bacteriuria.[11] Table 1.6 shows that 40% of the women had a bladder infection only, 28% had unilateral renal bacteriuria, and 32% had bilateral renal bacteriuria. Only 10 of the men had upper tract infection, and in 6 of these it was unilateral. Most of these 95 patients had intravenous urograms that were nonsurgical; that is, only rarely was there obstruction, stones, or gross loss of renal cortex. Reflux was rare in those patients who had cystograms. Since 1965, many more patients have had localization studies. The data remain about the same: any adult woman with recurrent bladder bacteriuria, studied at one point in time, has about a 50% chance of the bacteria being present in either one or both renal pelvic urines. These studies have been confirmed by other investigators.[57, 58] We called these upper tract localizations "pyelonephritis" in 1965,[11] but renal bacteriuria would have been a better term. If destruction of renal tissue by bacteria is an acceptable definition of pyelonephritis, then most of the patients in Table

Table 1.6
Localization of Urinary Tract Infections in 95 Females and 26 Males with Bacteriuria[a]

Number and Sex	Bladder Only	Unilateral Renal Bacteriuria	Bilateral Renal Bacteriuria
95 females	38 (40%)	27 (28%)	30 (32%)
26 males	16 (62%)	6 (26%)	4 (15%)

[a] Source as in Table 1.2.

1.6 who had renal bacteriuria did not have pyelonephritis.

The usefulness of this bacteriologic localization technique has been amply confirmed by other investigators, including Fairley *et al.*,[57] Brumfitt and co-worker,[58] Turck and colleagues,[59] and Eykyn and her colleagues at St. Thomas's Hospital, London.[60] The last group has recently published their experience from a series of 212 patients and presented a convincing argument for the value of accurate bacteriologic localization studies "in determining treatment, both medical and surgical, and in assessing prognosis." The correlation in their studies between the intravenous urogram and the site of infection is shown in Table 1.7.

While it would clearly be useful to have an easier clinical measurement of the presence or absence of renal bacteriuria, accurate localization by cystoscopy and ureteral catheterization is the cornerstone for evaluation of other techniques indicative of renal involvement. In a careful assessment of homologous serum antibody (both 19S and 7S), urinary concentrating ability, urinary β-glucuronidase excretion, and the intravenous urogram, Turck and co-workers[61, 62] reluctantly concluded that none of these measurements provided a separation between upper and lower tract bacteriuria as clinically useful as that determined by ureteral catheterization. Pfau *et al.* also found β-glucuronidase activity to be useless.[63]

Table 1.7
Intravenous Urogram and Site of Infection in 212 Patients[a]

The site of infection, proven by bilateral ureteral catheterization in 212 patients with bacteriuria, is compared to the findings on intravenous urography.

Intravenous Urogram	No.	Site of Infection	
		Bladder	Upper Tract
Normal	69	51	18
Abnormal	140	24	116
Stone(s)	75	5	70
Chronic pyelonephritis[b]	29	4	25
Congenital abnormality	17	11	6
Hydronephrosis and/or pelvi-ureteric obstruction	16	4	12
Renal calcification	3	0	3
No urogram	3	0	3

[a] Reproduced by permission from S. Eykyn, R. W. Lloyd-Davies, and K. E. D. Shuttleworth, Invest. Urol. **9:** 271, © 1972.[60]

[b] Radiological diagnosis based on small scarred kidney, narrowing of renal cortex, and clubbing of calyces.

Fairley Bladder Washout Test

As I pointed out, when Ken Fairley observed the ease with which infections localized to the bladder (Table 1.2) were washed free of bacteria by the irrigating fluid, he astutely realized this might be accomplished with a Foley catheter followed by serial cultures that would essentially represent ureteral urine. He modified his original 1967 procedure[54] in 1971 to the following protocol[64]:

"After collecting the initial specimen, the bladder is emptied through a urethral catheter and 40 ml of 0.2% neomycin, together with one ampoule of "Elase," is introduced into the bladder. After 10 minutes, the bladder is distended with 0.2% neomycin to reduce the folds in the mucosa and the catheter is clipped off for 20 minutes. The bladder is then emptied and washed out with 2 liters of sterile saline solution. Some of the saline of the final washout is collected for culture and, after emptying the bladder, a further three, timed, specimens are collected at 10-minute intervals. Bacterial counts are done on all specimens."[64]

"Elase," a combination of two lytic enzymes—fibrinolysin and desoxyribonuclease—was apparently added to produce a cleaner bladder surface in terms of potential exudative mucosal lesions. The truth is that, except for acute hemorrhagic cystitis, almost all bacteriuric patients have a surprisingly clean and normal-appearing bladder mucosa; it is unlikely that the addition of these enzymes plays any role in changing the bladder mucosa, and I know of no studies that have demonstrated a beneficial effect of these enzymes in reducing bacteria that may be stuck to the mucosa. The neomycin, on the other hand, is probably important. In his 1971 paper, Fairley gave specific criteria for separating bladder from renal infection: "Renal infection was assumed to be present when the timed specimen collected 20–30 minutes after bladder washout contained more than 3000 bacteria/ml, and in addition this 20–30 minute specimen contained more than 5 times as many bacteria as were present in the final bladder washout specimen. Bladder infection was assumed to be present when the final timed specimen (20–30 minutes after the bladder washout) was sterile."[64] Using these criteria, 21 of 48 patients in this general practice study showed evidence of renal infection, 22 showed the infection was limited to the bladder, and only 5 studies were equivocal.[64] The published patterns of these five doubtful studies all would have represented renal infections based on the patterns seen by ureteral catheterization studies (Tables 1.2 to 1.5). The fact that these five patients were considered doubtful, however, is a credit to the rigid separation of upper from lower tract infections, and there can be little, if any, doubt as to the validity of this procedure and these criteria.

The Fairley washout test has been used widely throughout the world, undoubtedly with some modifications and not always spelled out as they should be. Allan Ronald's group at Winnipeg, Canada has used the Fairley test in a number of excellent publications, and it is worthwhile quoting from their most recent publication[65]:

"Under aseptic conditions, a three-way No. 18 Foley catheter is inserted into the bladder, and a specimen collected (Specimen Number 1). The bladder is then emptied. One hundred mls of normal saline solution containing 10 mg of gentamicin sulfate and 125,000 International Units of streptokinase-streptodornase are instilled and left in the bladder for 45 minutes. The bladder is then emptied. Three liters of normal saline is continuously flushed through the bladder to wash out any residual gentamicin sulfate. The final 5 ml is collected (Specimen Number 2). Then five specimens are collected at 10-minute intervals, and labeled three through seven. All seven specimens are serially diluted and absolute quantitative bacterial counts are determined with calibrated platinum loops aliquoting 0.001 ml and 0.01 ml of urine onto blood agar and MacConkey broth. The infecting pathogens are identified by standard microbiological methods. The patient is said to have a lower-tract infection if the catheterized specimen grew at least 10^4 organisms/ml and the bladder washout specimen plus all subsequent specimens were sterile. The patient is said to have an upper-tract infection if there is a one log increase in urine bacterial count between the bladder washout specimen (Specimen 2) and four of the five specimens (specimens three through seven)."[65]

I like the addition of two extra serial specimens, but I again doubt that the streptokinase-streptodornase is really needed. It also should be noted for those who use this simple test that substantial hydration should be avoided because the data in Tables 1.3 and 1.4 make it amply clear that renal bacterial concentrations are proportional to urine flow rate. Dr. Fairley recognized this and had to discontinue the use of a frusemide diuresis which was a part of his original protocol.[54] On the other hand, an adequate urine flow rate, probably moderate hydration, is necessary to collect the serial urines. It is somewhat surprising that a refractometric index of specific gravity (urine creatinine concentration would be better but more expensive) is not done on the serial urine collections because the third urine collection in Fairley's technique[64] (the 20–30 minute specimen) and the four of five urines in Ronald's modification[65] all could become falsely low from a rising water diuresis. In the end, there is probably no ideal way to control urine flow rate, but the physician should be aware that a rapidly changing urine flow rate is to be avoided.

Antibody-Coated Bacteria in Urinary Infections

In 1974, Thomas, Shelokov, and Forland reported what I believe to be the most significant advance in the diagnosis of urinary tract infections in the past 10 years.[66] They observed that if the bacteria in the urine of a patient with urinary infection

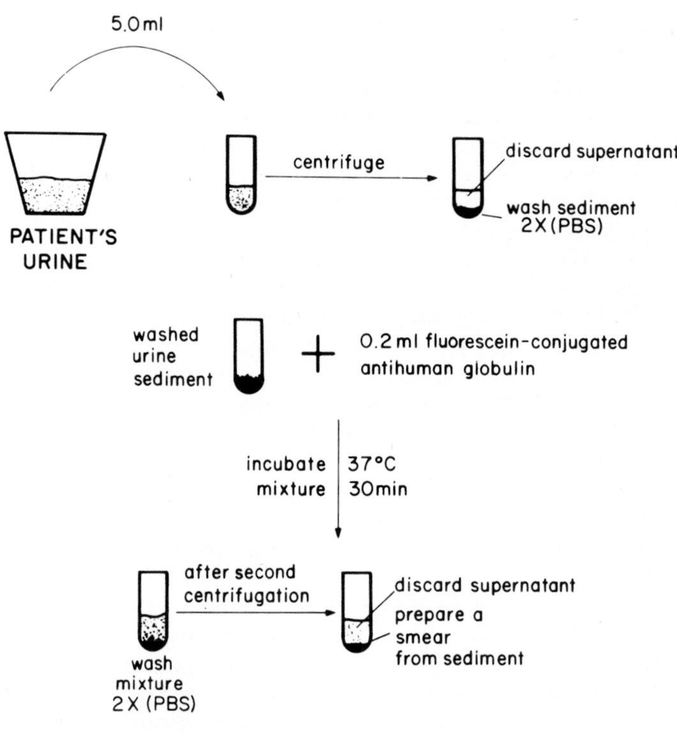

Figure 1.18 Procedure for detecting antibody-coated bacteria by direct immunofluorescence. (Reproduced by permission from V. L. Thomas, M. Forland, and A. Shelokov, Kidney Int. **8:** S20, 1975.[77])

were centrifuged, washed and mixed with fluorescein-conjugated antihuman globulin (Figure 1.18), antibody-coating of the bacteria could be observed under a fluorescence microscope; the typical apple-green fluorescence of a *Klebsiella* coated with antibody is seen in Figure 1.19. More importantly, Thomas and her colleagues reported that 34 of 35 patients with pyelonephritis had antibody-coated bacteria that were fluorescent antibody positive (FA+), while 19 of 20 patients with cystitis were not antibody-coated (FA−). Except for 12 patients in the pyelonephritis group who had either a renal biopsy (3 patients) or direct bacterial localization studies (ureteral catheters or the Fairley washout test), the diagnosis of pyelonephritis was made on sound clinical criteria using conventional radiologic and renal function studies.[66] Jones, Smith, and Sanford, in the same issue of the same journal, and using Thomas' technique, used the Fairley washout method to localize the site of bacterial infection in 23 of 26 patients; the antibody-coating technique correctly predicted the site of infection (18 renal, 8 bladder) in 25 of 26 patients.[67]

Since these studies were reported in 1974, the validity of this immunofluorescent technique in separating renal from bladder infection has been confirmed in adults by several studies.[65, 68] In children, however, the reported results have shown less of a correlation[69]; 8 of 12 upper tract localizations showed that 20% or more of the bacteria in the urinary sediment were FA+, while 13 of 35 lower tract localizations had FA+ bacteria. Forsum *et al.*[70] also found a poor correlation in children. Perhaps the bladder of children is more likely to produce immunoglobulins to infection than occurs in adults. Scherf *et al.* reported 61% of 75 lower tract localizations by the Fairley test in children were FA+.[117]

The careful study by Allan Ronald's group from Winnipeg, Canada is probably the best[65] because they were meticulous with both the Fairley washout technique as well as Thomas' immunofluorescent

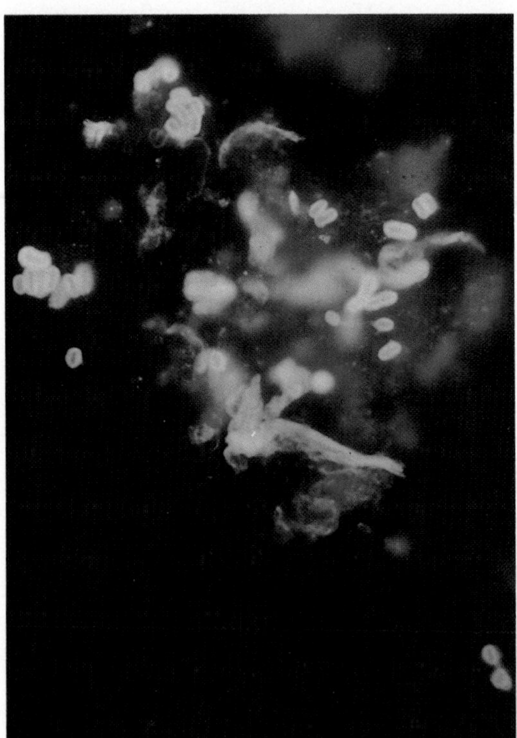

Figure 1.19 Antibody-coated bacteria, prepared by the method outlined in Figure 1.18, and viewed with the fluorescence microscope. Observe the typical, apple-green fluorescence which represents specific antibody-coating of the infecting Klebsiella strain.

method of antibody-coated bacteria. These investigators studied 51 adult females. All 31 patients who had FA+ bacteria localized to the kidney, but 6 of the 20 women who were FA− also localized to the kidney. Of these six women with renal infections and FA− bacteria, three had upper tract symptoms for 2–7 days, one had lower tract symptoms for 8 days, and two were asymptomatic. One of the asymptomatic patients was infected with a *Streptococcus faecalis.* Since antibody-coating of bacteria depends on local production of immunoglobulin, it is feasible that the symptomatic patients had not yet raised local renal antibody to the invading bacteria. For example, Thomas, *et al.* observed that 3 of 15 obstetrical patients with acute pyelonephritis were FA−[71]; since these 3 patients were not immunodeficient, it is likely that some patients require a longer time to produce local antibodies. Despite these few exceptions to FA− bacteriuric women, it seems well documented that FA+ bacteriuric patients indicate renal infection. Does the bladder ever produce immunoglobulins that could coat bacteria in the absence of renal involvement? We do know in the experimental animal that the bladder can produce immunoglobulin (IgG),[72] and I have often observed (and biopsied) lymphoid follicles on the mucosa of human bladders that have been infected for many months; in fact, we called these brownish, raised 1–2 mm nodules "bacteriuric bumps" for years before we proved they were lymphoid follicles. In the rare patient, I have documented the appearance of lymphoid follicles in the bladder within a few weeks of becoming bacteriuric; for example, in a 50-year-old woman followed cystoscopically at 3-month intervals for recurrent stage A bladder tumors, she acquired an asymptomatic *E. coli* bacteriuria in between her 3-month examinations and her bladder mucosa became florid with lymphoid follicles. Her *E. coli* were FA+, but unfortunately she was not bacteriologically localized. I mention this only because there is bound to be an occasional FA+ bacteriuric patient whose infection will be limited to the bladder, but this does not detract from the overall significance of detecting antibody-coated bacteria in the urine. Indeed, Hawthorne *et al.*[73] reported 5 of 15 patients with lower tract infection had FA+ urines.

The determination of antibody-coated bacteria in patients will allow the physician to decide without an invasive technique whether the kidneys are involved or not, and ultimately whether it makes any real therapeutic difference or not. As I said in the first edition of this book in 1972, I do not believe it makes a lot of difference whether the kidneys are involved or not in the adult woman with a nonproteus urinary infection and a nonobstructed urinary tract who is neither diabetic nor an analgesic abuser. But this is certainly the technique to answer these therapeutic questions in the adult patient. In two fascinating studies by the San Antonio group, one on antibody-coating in urinary infections in diabetic patients[74] and the other in pregnant patients with asymptomatic bacteriuria,[75] it is clear that reinfection with a different organism is just as likely in diabetic patients whose previous infection was renal (FA+) as it is in those whose previous infection was limited to the bladder (FA−). In asymptomatic bacteriuria of pregnancy, urinary infection recurred in 10 of the 35 patients who were FA+ at their original infection and in 8 of the 35 patients who were FA−; interestingly, all 10 recurrences from the originally FA+ patients were FA− recurrences and were actual reinfections with different bacteria. Indeed, of the 8 patients who originally had lower tract infection, half of their recurrences were FA+. I interpret these data to mean that in terms of bacteriologic recurrences, it makes little difference whether the kidneys are involved or not, a view also supported by the ureteric localization data of Cattel *et al.*[76] In terms of other morbidity factors, however, such as intrauterine growth retardation, FA+ bacteriuria may make a significant difference.[75] The important point, however, is that Dr. Virginia Thomas[66] has given us a method to get the answers.

Before leaving the subject, it is important to point out that the physician who uses this technique of antibody-coated bacteria will have to face the question of how many fluorescent bacteria on the slide constitute a FA+ test. Neither Thomas *et al.*[66] nor Jones *et al.*[67] were explicit about this in their original publication, undoubtedly because in most bacteriuric specimens the bacteria are either all fluorescent or all nonfluorescent (a negative control, where a subculture of the bacteria which cannot have antibody on their surface is also treated with the fluorescein conjugate, is mandatory). But there are some urines which are not all or none in fluorescence and how are they to be read? Thomas *et al.* clarified this issue in a later publication by requiring 25% or more of the bacterial cells to fluoresce in order to be FA+,[77] but Jones in a Letter to the Editor argued that only 2 uniformly fluorescent (apple-green) bacteria/200 oil immersion fields (×100 objective, and ×15 ocular) was sufficient to indicate antibody coating and therefore FA+.[78] Thomas decided that an FA test should be read as negative if less than 25% of the bacteria in each field were fluorescing because small numbers of fluorescent bacteria often were observed in voided specimens from women who had never had urinary infections.[79] Jones, on the other hand, observed upper tract localizations that had only a few fluorescent bacteria in the bladder urine, and he felt they should be called positive.[78] From our own studies on local vaginal antibody, there is no doubt that women have vaginal antibody directed against their fecal Enterobacteriaceae and that antibody-coated bacteria can be present on the vaginal vestibule and therefore easily contaminate the voided urine.[80] For this reason, I am afraid that 2 fluorescent bacteria/200 oil immersion fields will open up false positives from vaginal contamination of the voided urine, and accordingly we have adopted Thomas' criteria. One can also argue that if upper tract localizations occur with only two fluorescent bacteria, the local renal antibody response must be so negligible that such a specimen had just as well be considered negative in terms of serious renal infection. After all, it is already clear that even with Thomas' criteria only 25% of asymptomatic patients with FA+ bacteriuria have serum antibody titers above normal control sera[75]; to reduce the amount of locally produced urinary antibody to such a small amount required to coat a fraction of the bacteria will surely remove antibody-coating as an indicator of renal infection to even less systemic significance.

It is interesting that in the excellent study by Harding *et al.*[65] an FA+ urine was one that had only five or more uniformly fluorescing bacteria after examining multiple fields for 5 minutes. Since catheterized bladder urines were used for the FA studies, they probably avoided FA+ vaginal and urethral contamination. Nevertheless, it would be important to know how many FA+ specimens had few fluorescent bacteria compared to the 25% requirement by Thomas. In a letter from Dr. Ronald, 2

April 1979, he informed me that only 2 of their 31 patients with FA+ bacteria contained less than 25% fluorescing bacteria.

Lastly, there are a few minor exceptions to the significance of FA^+ bacteria. Jones has raised the question of whether FA+ urines in patients with chronic bacterial prostatitis might not be from prostatic immunoglobulins coating the bladder bacteria rather than upper tract local immunoglobulin[81]; to date the question remains unanswered as to its statistical significance. Proteinuria may also give a false positive FA test in about 30% of specimens with urinary protein.[79] And yeasts (*Candida species* and *Torulopsis species*) are apparently always antibody-coated regardless of the site where they are found, although no urinary localization studies were done[82]; it is possible, for example, that all the cases of funguria actually involved the kidney as the source of urinary immunoglobulin. A highly mucoid layer of *P. aeruginosa* can interfere with antibody-coating.[83] With these latter few exceptions, which for the most part are rare and not really proven to be of significance, it is clear that the detection of antibody-coated bacteria in the urine is a powerful new research tool that may prove clinically useful.

Other Techniques Indicative of Renal Infection

Histologic Evidence for Pyelonephritis from Renal Biopsies

Needle biopsy of the kidney carries a small, but definite risk to the patient. The major reason, however, that needle biopsy is contraindicated as a means of obtaining evidence of renal involvement in the presence of bacteriuria is the patchy nature of renal cortical involvement in pyelonephritis (Chapter 3). Thus, a negative biopsy does not exclude pyelonephritis, and a positive one may grossly misrepresent the extent of the disease. I recall once asking Dr. Robert Heptinstall whether he would prefer a needle or open wedge biopsy of a kidney in order to make the diagnosis of pyelonephritis. He replied, on a national panel, that he "would prefer the whole kidney and a bloody good history!" The Ciba Foundation Symposium on *Renal Biopsy*, held in 1961, and published by Little, Brown and Company, Boston, MA., contains three papers with excellent discussions on the difficulties of renal biopsy in pyelonephritis.

Effect of Bacteriuria on Renal Concentrating Mechanism

A defect in concentrating ability has long been recognized in pyelonephritis.[84, 85] Since upper tract bacteriuria in women is as often unilateral as it is bilateral, effects on the renal concentrating mechanism are best studied at the time of bacteriologic localization with ureteral catheters. In an excellent study, Ronald, Cutler, and Turck[59] showed that patients with renal bacteriuria concentrated less well than those whose infection was limited to the bladder, and that the noninfected side in patients with unilateral bacteriuria concentrated better than the contralateral, infected kidney. Seven of 12 patients with renal infection improved their overall concentrating ability by at least 100 mOsm/kg after eradication of bacteriuria. All patients had serum creatinines of less than 1.5 mg/100 ml. Thus, the presence of renal pelvic bacteriuria is accompanied by a functional defect in renal concentrating ability. But does this mean pyelonephritis? Minimal edema at the papillary tip, well within the renal pelvis, could influence greatly the counter-current concentrating mechanism. There is a tendency in the current literature, especially in pregnancy studies, to equate a decreased concentrating ability with "pyelonephritis" in patients with bacteriuria; nevertheless, impaired concentration may mean nothing more than the presence of pelvic bacteriuria.

In a valiant effort to distinguish between bladder and renal bacteriuria, Clark *et al.*[61] measured the maximal urinary concentration (U_{max}) of the voided urine in 66 patients during a 36-hour period of fluid deprivation. Bilateral ureteral catheterization studies to localize the site of the bacteriuria were performed after the maximal concentrating test. The results are reproduced in Figure

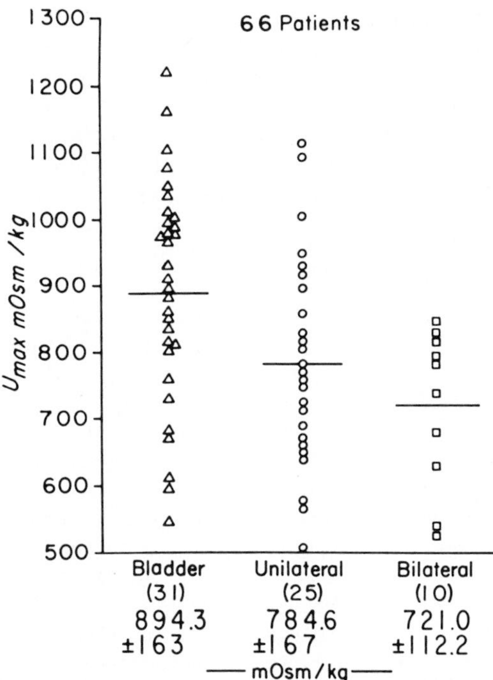

Figure 1.20 Maximal concentrating ability in 66 patients with recurrent bacteriuria correlated with the site of infection. (Reproduced by permission from H. Clark, A. R. Ronald, R. E. Cutler, and M. Turck, J. Infect. Dis. **120:** 47, 1969.[61])

1.20. Normal individuals achieve a U_{max} of 900 mOsm/kg or greater while values less than 800 mOsm/kg are abnormal.[86] In Figure 1.20, 7 of the 31 patients whose infections were limited to the bladder (at least at the time of that localization) could not concentrate to 800 mOsm/kg while 11 of 25 patients with unilateral renal bacteriuria concentrated above 800 mOsm/kg. Thus, the overlap is so significant that the use of this test to distinguish upper from lower tract bacteriuria is probably not warranted, at least not for the individual patient.

Serologic Antibody Titers as an Indicator of Renal Disease

Siede and Luz[87] were the first to use immune responses to differentiate patients with pyelonephritis from those with cystitis. Following Neter's[88, 89] introduction of the hemagglutination technique for measuring serum antibody, Needell *et al.*[90] used this technique to study the serum antibody response of patients with infections of the urinary tract. Ten years later, Williamson *et al.*[91] and Percival, Brumfitt, and de Louvois[92] published their studies in adults, while Winberg and associates[93] measured antibodies in children. In general, patients with acute urinary infections associated with chills, fever, and flank pain have high serologic titers; patients with classic cystitis have low titers. The major difficulty is that the grey zone is enormous, as emphasized by Sanford and Barnett.[94] For example, Ehrenkranz and Carter[95] found a 4-fold rise in antibody titers in 13 of 18 patients with acute lower urinary tract infections. More importantly, if the patients are not selectively divided into those with obvious upper tract disease on the basis of overt history or radiologic findings, but are studied nonselectively on the basis of bacteriologic localization studies, serum antibody titers are not very helpful.[62, 96] For example, Clark, Ronald, and Turck[62] localized the site of infection by ureteral catheterization in 77 patients, measuring both hemagglutinating activity of whole (19S antibody) and 2-mercaptoethanol-treated (7S antibody) serum collected at the time of ureteral catheterization. Figure 1.21 is reproduced from their studies; as can be seen, the overlap in antibody titers between patients with renal bacteriuria and bladder bacteriuria is substantial.

It should be noted, however, that these serum antibody titers were either hemagglutination or bacterial agglutination, techniques that we know now measure mainly IgM and not IgG or IgA. Whether newer techniques for measuring serum antibodies, such as solid phase radioimmunoassay as used in Chapter 7, Figure 7.9, will make a difference in detecting renal bacteriuria remains to be seen. The indirect immunofluorescence technique for measuring serum antibodies, which does measure IgG and IgA as well as IgM, suggests that renal bacteriuria as measured by antibody-coated bacteria is not usually accompanied by elevated serum titers[75]; only 8 out of 32 FA+ bacteriuric obstetrical patients had serum antibody titers higher than those found in normal control sera.

Radiologic Evidence of Pyelonephritis

If histology, bacterial localization, urinary concentration, and serologic titers all fail as adequate criteria for chronic pyelonephritis, what measures should the clinician use as evidence for chronic, progressive disease? We believe the intravenous urogram. In the absence of stones, obstruction, and tuberculosis, and with the single exception of analgesic nephritis with papillary necrosis—readily excluded by history—pyelonephritis is virtually the only disease that will produce a localized scar over a deformed calyx; in advanced pyelonephritis, calyceal distortion and irregularity, together with cortical scars, complete the picture (Figure 1.22). C. J. Hodson,[97] in a review of some 12,000 pyelographic examinations, clearly defined gross cortical scars as well as the case for the rarity of such scars developing in adults. As Hodson pointed out, renal infarction (an extremely rare condition) may closely resemble pyelonephritic scars, but the renal pyramid remains in renal infarction, in contradistinction to pyelonephritis.

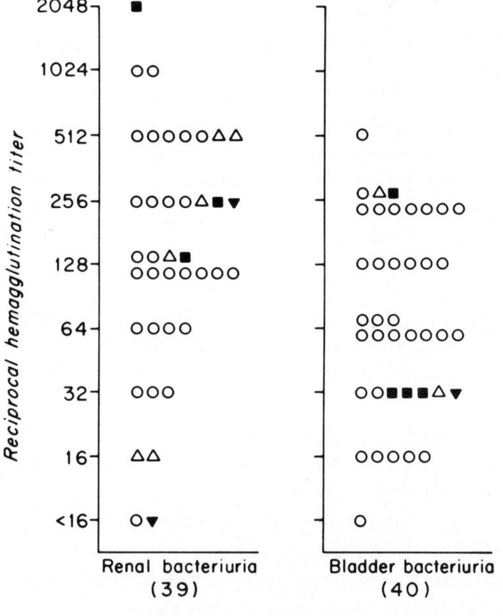

Figure 1.21 Reciprocal hemagglutination titer in whole serum from 77 patients at the time of bilateral ureteral catheterization (79 localizations). A similar overlap in the two groups of patients occurred when the serum was treated with 2-mercaptoethanol (to measure 7S antibody). (Reproduced by permission from H. Clark, A. R. Ronald, and M. Turck, J. Infect. Dis. **123:** 539, 1971.[62])

Unfortunately, most intravenous urograms are grossly inadequate for showing the relationship of calyces to the cortical outline; for this reason, the clinician should insist upon either an early nephrogram phase (60 seconds after the start of intravenous injection) or tomographic films with every intravenous urogram in patients investigated for urinary infections. Tomographic films are almost unique in defining cortical outlines, but the primary reason for poor urograms is inadequate preparation. The routine in the Department of Radiology at Stanford, based on the principle of using a cathartic on the small and large intestine (magnesium citrate)—thereby filling the colon with fluid—and followed by colonic mucosal stimulation (bisacodyl), is as follows. At lunch and supper the day before the intravenous urogram, food is limited to bouillon soup, plain Jello, plain chicken or turkey sandwich at lunch, and apple or grape juice. Water must be encouraged during the day and evening, and 11 oz of magnesium citrate (in adults) are taken at 8 PM and three Ducolax tablets (bisacodyl) at 10 PM. Nothing is taken by mouth after midnight. At 7 AM on the day of examination, a Ducolax rectal suppository is inserted (for direct stimulation of the rectosigmoid) and retained for 20 minutes–1 hour. This regimen for preparing the patient produces nearly perfect films.

C-Reactive Protein

The Göteborg group studied 25 girls, age 5–17 years, who presented to the emergency room with an acute urinary infection[98]; 14 patients were thought clinically to have acute pyelonephritis with fever >39°C together with loin or high abdominal pain. Ten patients had acute cystitis (tempera-

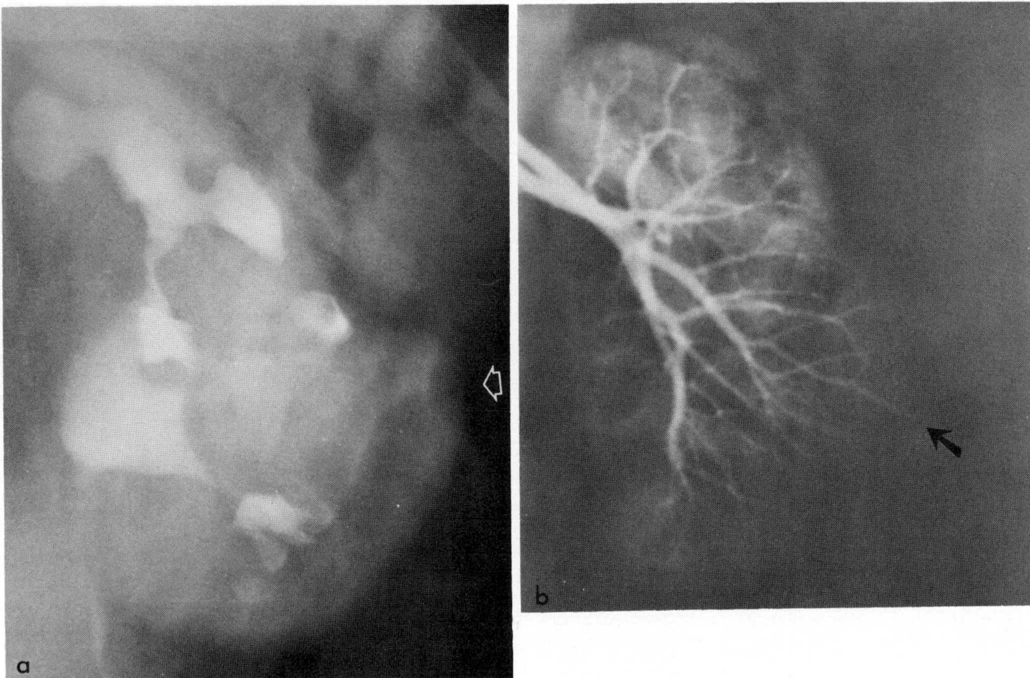

Figure 1.22 An intravenous urogram (*a*) and arteriogram (*b*) of the left kidney in a 41-year-old female with a 14-year documented history of continuous *Enterobacter* urinary infection. The dilated, irregular calyces with loss of cortex (*a*) are the classic radiologic findings of pyelonephritis. The intervening hypertrophied tissue in the middle of the kidney was so striking it suggested a tumor; the arteriogram, however, showed normal cortical tissue. This patient was cured of her urinary infection and has maintained a sterile urine for the past 5 years; the details of her course and therapy are presented in Chapter 10.

ture <38°C) with dysuria and frequency and one patient's symptoms were indeterminate. A Fairley washout test was done at the time of presentation. Each patient had the following determinations: C-reactive protein, sedimentation rate, maximum urine concentrating capacity, and indirect hemagglutination serum antibody titers. Only the C-reactive protein was elevated in all 14 patients with acute pyelonephritis and normal or undetectable in those patients with cystitis. In a further publication, Jodal and Hanson followed the time course of the elevated C-reactive protein in 19 patients with acute pyelonephritis[99]; in those patients who were adequately treated with effective antimicrobial therapy, the C-reactive protein returned to normal within 1 week, even before the sedimentation rate which required 2–4 weeks to reach normal values.

Although C-reactive protein is nonspecific for acute pyelonephritis and will reflect any parenchymal infection, its rapid return to normal within 7 days could be useful as a measure of adequate antimicrobial therapy. It is doubtful if C-reactive protein will be helpful in asymptomatic renal bacteriuria; for one thing, two of the afebrile patients with symptoms of cystitis clearly had positive Fairley washout studies and undetectable levels of C-reactive protein.[98]

In a recent report in children,[100] C-reactive protein was superior to the antibody-coated bacteria test as an indication of clinically apparent pyelonephritis.

Lower Urinary Tract Localization Studies

We published in 1963 the bacteriologic technique for distinguishing between bladder and renal bacteriuria by cystoscopy and ureteric catheterization,[51] and in 1965 we reported localization data on 121 patients[11] (Table 1.6), but between 1964 and 1970, we became less interested in this distinction and more concerned with how the bacteria gain access to the bladder. There were several reasons for this. First, there seemed to be equal difficulty in preventing recurrent infections, in the absence of stones and obstruction, whether renal bacteriuria was present or not. Second, the ability to serotype *E. coli* had led several different investigators, studying little girls and adult women, to conclude that the major problem in recurrences was reinfection, not relapse from persistence of the same bacteria.[101–103] And third, several general practice studies began to appear in 1965, beginning with Gallagher, Montgomerie, and North,[104] that showed about half of the women presenting with dysuria, frequency, and suprapubic cramps actually had a sterile bladder urine, at least at that point in time.

For these reasons, we began to develop techniques, based on segmenting the voided urine into sequential aliquots, that allowed bacteriologic assessment of the urethra and prostate in the male, and the urethra and vaginal vestibule in the female, without the artifacts and morbidity introduced by instrumentation. These techniques require multiple cultures, and the bladder urine must be sterile at the time of sampling.

Male: Urethra and Prostate

Technique for Obtaining Routine Cultures When the Bladder Urine is Sterile. For bacteriologic localization, the voided urine and expressed prostatic secretions are labeled as follows: the first voided 5–10 ml (VB_1, the symbol for "voided bladder 1"); the midstream aliquot (VB_2, for "voided bladder 2"); the pure prostatic secretion expressed by prostatic massage (EPS, for "expressed prostatic secretions"); and the first voided 5–10 ml immediately after prostatic massage (VB_3, for "voided bladder 3"). These aliquots are illustrated in Figure 1.23.

The patient must be well hydrated with a full bladder to ensure proper collections.

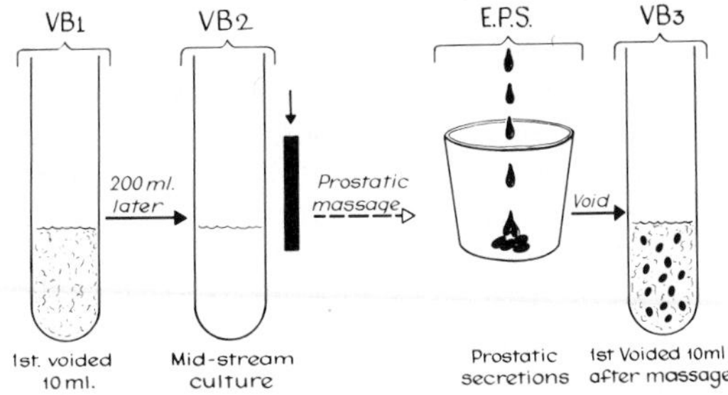

Figure 1.23 Segmented cultures of the lower urinary tract in the male. (Reproduced by permission from E. M. Meares and T. A. Stamey, Invest. Urol. **5:** 492, 1968.)

The foreskin is fully retracted; it should be maintained in this position throughout all collections if contamination is to be prevented. So important is this maneuver that the foreskin should be taped back in the retracted position by a circular strip of adhesive around the midshaft of the penis. The glans is cleaned with a detergent soap, all of the soap is removed with a wet sponge, and the glans is then dried carefully with a sterile sponge. The VB_1 is collected by holding the sterile culture tube directly in front of the urethral meatus. As the patient continues to void, the physician quickly removes the VB_1 culture tube from the stream of urine. When the patient has voided approximately 200 ml (about one half of the bladder urine), the second culture tube (VB_2) is inserted into the stream of urine for a 5- to 10-ml sample. The patient is immediately instructed to stop voiding. After shaking any residual urethral urine from the shaft of the penis, he bends over with his elbows on the examining table and his legs separated but straight. The physician removes any residual drops of urine from the meatus with tissue paper and I usually press the bulbar urethra posteriorly with blunt but gentle pressure in case more residual urine is retained along the bulbar urethra. By sitting on a chair in a sideways position to the patient, the examiner can massage the prostate with his right hand and hold the sterile container to collect the EPS in his left hand; in this way, drops of prostatic secretion can be observed directly to appear at the meatus and to fall uncontaminated into the sterile container. The first drop to appear should be pure opalescent prostatic fluid without any yellow tint of urine. Occasionally when there has been little or no prostatic fluid, pressure with the right thumb on the bulbar urethra will produce a few drops that have accumulated in the wide part of the urethra. Sometimes a steady, increasingly firm digital pressure on one lateral lobe will empty the prostatic glands better than massage from base to apex. Immediately after massage, the patient voids again and the VB_3 is collected in similar manner to the VB_1. Throughout the collections, contamination of the specimens must be prevented in the uncircumcised male; if the foreskin slips over the meatus during the collections, the results can be meaningless. Thousands of Gram-negative bacteria can reside under the uncircumcised foreskin even though it is easily retractable and seemingly clean; the presence of these foreskin bacteria can be a major source of confusion in localizing the site of infection in the lower urinary tract. Equally important, all of the detergent must be removed before collecting any of these cultures, especially the VB_1; if the 5–10 ml of urine for culture are contaminated by even a small amount of detergent, the quantitative colony counts will not be valid.[27] If the patient is circumcised, it is not necessary to cleanse the glans before collecting the cultures.

Where possible, 0.1 ml or even more of EPS should be surface streaked onto the appropriate agar plates; when the volume is too small, a bacteriologic loop, quantitated to deliver 0.01 ml, can be used. The loop should be avoided if possible because the volume cultured is too small to detect less than 100 bacteria/ml.

Importance of Culturing the First Voided 5 to 10 ml of Urine (VB_1). Although even a casual study of our bacteriologic data shows that the bacterial count in the VB_1 aliquot is greatly reduced a few milliliters later in the midstream sample, the point is worth emphasizing for three reasons. First, if the clinician wishes to study urethral bacteria, it is almost pointless to culture the midstream urine. In Table 1.8, I have selected a few representative examples to re-emphasize the washing effect of sterile bladder urine on urethral bacteria. Second, even though the wash-down count is very low in a midstream urine, when the patient stops voiding in preparation for a prostatic massage, and then reinitiates voiding a minute or two later, large numbers of urethral bacteria will reappear in the first voided aliquot (Chapter 7, Table 7.3). Third, failure to collect the first 3 or 4 ml, which is easy to do if the stream splays at the meatus, probably accounts for some of the false, Gram-positive bacterial localizations to the prostate. The density of the normal urethral flora—*Staphylococcus epidermidis*, streptococci, and diphtheroids—at the fossa navicularis surely is concentrated in the first few drops of urine to come from the urethral meatus. If these drops are missed by splaying of the initial stream but not missed in the VB_3, and of

Table 1.8
Washing Effect of Sterile Bladder Urine on Urethral Bacteria in Male Patients

Patient	First Voided 10 ml	Midstream Sample	Organism
	bacterial/ml		
P.E.	44,000	0	*Streptococcus faecalis*
M.P.	14,850	5	*Staphylococcus epidermidis; α-streptococcus*
R.P.	10,230	60	*β-Hemolytic streptococcus*
B.M.	10,092	6	*Streptococcus faecalis*
H.Z.	1,380	0	*Staphylococcus aureus*
A.W.	1,188	3	Pseudomonas
J.K.	1,904	12	*Klebsiella*
B.B.	1,920	13	*Enterobacter*
L.W.	2,660	10	Pseudomonas; *Proteus mirabilis*
R.S.	6,090	18	*Klebsiella*

course they are never missed in the EPS, then the localization counts will suggest the prostate rather than the urethra as the source of these Gram-positive bacteria. The importance of collecting all of the first few milliliters of urine of the VB_1 is so important that a good argument can be made for collecting the VB_1 in a wide-mouth culture cup rather than the test tube shown in Figure 1.23.

Value of the EPS Culture Compared with the VB_3. When a sterile bladder urine assures a low bacterial count in the VB_2, localization of the infection to the urethra or prostate depends upon a comparison of the quantitative colony counts in the VB_1 with the counts in the VB_3. When the VB_1 count far exceeds that of the VB_3, and this is reproducible, the bacteria originate in the anterior urethra (Chapter 7, Table 7.27). When the colony count of the VB_3 greatly exceeds the VB_1, as in acute bacterial prostatitis before the bladder becomes infected, the bacteriologic pattern leaves no doubt as to the source of the infection (Chapter 7, Table 7.2).

Unfortunately, patients who have chronic bacterial prostatitis as the cause of their recurrent bladder infections do not have large numbers of bacteria in their prostatic fluid, as will be seen in Chapter 7. For this reason, the diagnosis is more subtle and the bacteriologic demonstration more difficult. It is here that a direct culture of the EPS, when it can be obtained, is extremely helpful, as shown by the data in Table 1.9. Patient S.T. repeatedly produced enough prostatic fluid for culture. His cultures showed that the EPS colony count always exceeded the VB_3 count; indeed, the VB_3 was actually sterile in the first set of cultures when bacteria were cultured from the EPS. In fact, the bacterial counts in the EPS in Table 1.9 are about 10–100 times greater than the counts in the VB_3. If the volume of prostatic fluid remaining along the urethra after prostatic massage is about 0.1 ml., and if the VB_3 volume of collection is 10 ml, a 100-fold dilution of the prostatic fluid occurs, accounting for the difference in bacterial counts between EPS and VB_3 observed in Table 1.9. Indeed, these differences in counts allow calculation of the residual prostatic fluid along the urethra after massage. For example, the last two patients in Table 1.9, T.L. and J.T., show that if the VB_3 volume was 10 ml, the volume of EPS washed into the VB_3 collection had to be exactly 0.1 ml to produce final counts of 50 and 1000 bacteria/ml in the VB_3 aliquots. If the volume of VB_3 was 5 ml, the amount of EPS left along the

Table 1.9
Value of the EPS Culture Over the VB_3 Culture[a,b]

Patient	Drug	VB_1	VB_2	EPS	VB_3	Organism
				colonies/ml		
S.T.	No	0	0	120	0	*Escherichia coli*
S.T.	No	0	0	4,000	120	*E. coli*
S.T.	No	0	0	10,000	600	*E. coli*
S.T.	Yes	0	0	2,000	120	*E. coli*
S.T.	Yes	0	0	700	10	*E. coli*
S.T.	Yes	0	0	900	220	*E. coli*
I.A.	Yes	250	0	100,000	8,000	*Klebsiella-Enterobacter*
I.A.	Yes	120	0	100,000	200	*Klebsiella-Enterobacter*
I.A.	Yes	0	0	10,000	1,000	*Klebsiella-Enterobacter*
P.P.	No	60	0	1,000	20	*Enterobacter*
P.P.	No	640	40	10,000	220	*Enterobacter*
E.McC.	Yes	0	0	10,000	250	*Klebsiella-Enterobacter*
T.L.	Yes	20	0	5,000	50	*Klebsiella-Enterobacter*
J.T.	Yes	50	0	100,000	1,000	*Klebsiella-Enterobacter*

[a] VB_1 = first voided 10 ml of urine (urethral); VB_2 = midstream urine aliquot (bladder); EPS = expressed prostatic secretion (prostatic); VB_3 = first voided 10 ml of urine after prostatic massage (prostatic).

[b] Reproduced by permission from E. M. Meares and T. A. Stamey, Invest. Urol. **5:** 492, © 1968.

urethra after massage would be 0.05 ml. In some of our patients, the volume of residual EPS in the urethra has been only 0.01 ml, in which case the difference in EPS and VB_3 counts is 1000-fold. These volumetric and bacteriologic calculations readily explain how the VB_3 culture can be sterile when the EPS contains small numbers (<200) of bacteria/ml. They also emphasize not only the importance of obtaining EPS when possible but the equal necessity of culturing a substantial volume of EPS on the agar culture plates; at least 0.1 ml should be cultured and the calibrated bacteriologic wire loops of 0.01 and 0.001 ml should never be used. As useful as the EPS culture is, however, I have pointed out in Chapter 7 the theoretical and sometimes practical advantage of comparing the VB_1 directly to the VB_3 culture; the interested reader should consider the discussion in Chapter 7.

Technique for Detection of Bacterial Prostatitis at the Time of Cystoscopy and Ureteral Catheterization in the Presence of an Infected Bladder Urine. Once the bladder urine is infected, it is impossible to detect the few bacteria originating from the prostate; thus, in the presence of bladder bacteriuria, the diagnostic technique of partitioning the voided urine into urethral and prostatic segments cannot be used.

There is one additional maneuver at the completion of the cystoscopic localization for renal pelvic bacteriuria that can be suggestive of prostatic infection. After collecting the urines from each kidney, the ureteral catheters are advanced well into each renal pelvis. The stopcocks of the cystoscope are closed, and 30–60 ml of irrigating fluid are run into the bladder. The outflow stopcock is then opened and a bladder sample is quickly obtained directly into a sterile culture tube; most of the 30–60 ml are left in the bladder. This sample is labeled WB_2, the symbol for "washed bladder 2." With both stopcocks closed and a finger in the rectum, the cystoscope (with ureteral catheters attached) is withdrawn to a point just distal to the verumontanum of the prostate. The prostate is massaged vigorously. The inflow stopcock is then opened briefly to allow not more than 20–30 ml of irrigating fluid to wash the accumulated prostatic secretions back into the bladder. The cystoscope is then readvanced into the bladder with the ureteral catheters still in position, and a bladder sample is again obtained through the outflow stopcock directly into a culture tube. This sample is labeled WB_3, the symbol for "washed bladder 3." If the WB_3 bacterial count significantly exceeds the WB_2 count, the prostate is probably the source of the extra bacteria.

Under the best of circumstances, this technique is fraught with potential errors. First, the renal urines must be sterile lest ureteral leakage at the time of prostatic massage add bacteria to the WB_2 reservoir; in opposite error, gross leakage of sterile urine around the ureteral catheters could mask an increase in bacteria in the WB_3 produced by prostatic massage. Second, the initial washout of infected bladder urine must be carefully (and successfully) accomplished so that the bacterial counts in WB_1 and WB_2 are less than 500 bacteria/ml. Third, the amount of irrigating fluid used to establish the WB_2 reservoir, as well as the irrigation used to wash the prostatic secretion back into the bladder, must be carefully controlled. Even with perfect success in these procedural details, this method will not detect those patients with chronic bacterial prostatitis who have the lowest bacterial counts in their prostatic secretion; thus, it should not be used to exclude bacterial prostatitis when the WB_3 count is similar to the WB_2.

As always after ureteral catheterization in the presence of bacteriuria, the appropriate antibacterial therapy must be started before the patient leaves the cystoscopy room.

Female: Vaginal Vestibule and Urethra

Data will be presented in Chapter 4 to show that recurrent urinary infections in the female are preceded by colonization of the vaginal introitus and urethra with enterobacteria from the rectal flora. For this reason, the technique of collecting these specimens as well as the bacteriologic, serologic, and bacterial banking methodology will be presented in detail to prevent repetition in later chapters.

Technique for Obtaining Specimens. Bacteriologic cultures of the vagina, urethra, and midstream urine (Figure 1.24) are obtained by a carefully trained nurse in the following manner.

Vaginal Vestibule Cultures. The woman is placed on the cystoscopy table in a semisitting position with her legs in stirrups. The nurse, wearing sterile rubber gloves, spreads the labia and swabs the vaginal vestibule with two sterile cotton applicator sticks held together (Figure 1.25); this maneuver is performed in a circular motion covering all four quadrants at the level of the hymenal ring. The cotton tip of the applicator sticks always remains in view. The cotton applicator sticks are then placed in a test tube containing 5 ml of transport broth (Earle's balanced salt solution, 10-528, Microbiological Associates, Bethesda, MD) or sterile saline (Figure 1.24) and immediately refrigerated. This culture of the vaginal vestibule at the level of the hymenal membrane is labeled "E. vag." for "external vagina" in most of the illustrations throughout this book. The bacteria are reported as bacteria/ml of transport broth or saline.

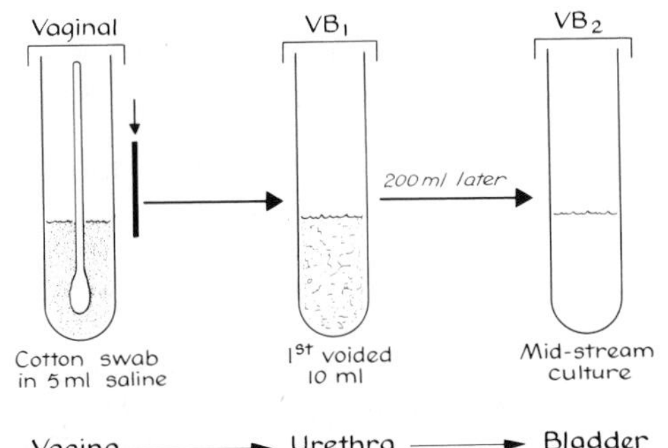

Figure 1.24 Segmented cultures of the lower urinary tract in the female.

Urethral and Midstream Urine Cultures. After the vaginal specimen is obtained, the nurse spreads the labia with one hand and collects the first voided 5–10 ml by holding a culture tube 1 cm from the urethral meatus (Figure 1.26); this culture, representative of the urethral flora, is labeled VB_1, the symbol for voided bladder 1. As the woman continues to void, the midstream aliquot (VB_2, voided bladder 2) is collected in a similar fashion. The perineum is not cleaned before or after collecting these cultures. The urine is refrigerated within 3 minutes and cultured within 4 hours.

About 10% of our women are unable to void on the cystoscopy table with a nurse in attendance. These women are carefully instructed in the collection technique and permitted to obtain their own specimens by

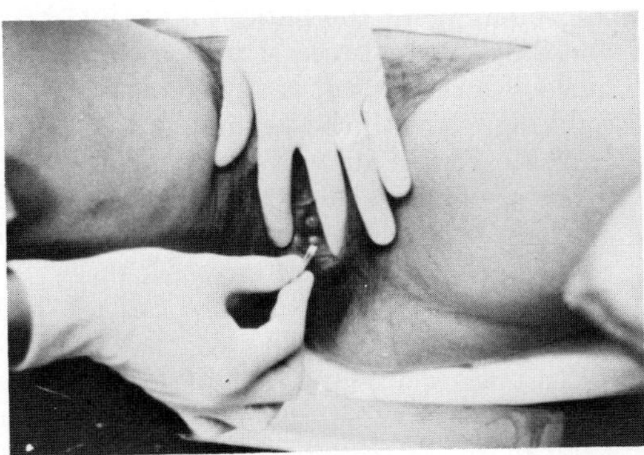

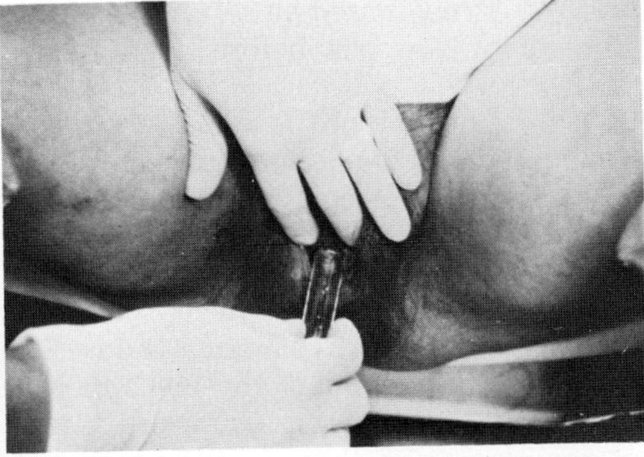

Figure 1.25 (*left*) A photograph of the technique used to collect vaginal vestibule cultures.
Figure 1.26 (*right*) A photograph of the technique used to collect the first voided urine from the urethra (VB_1).

sitting on the back edge of the toilet seat, holding the labia apart with one hand, and collecting the specimens as described above.

Anal Swab Cultures. To sample the fecal bacteria of the rectum, a cotton swab stick moistened with transport broth is inserted into the anal canal until coated with yellow, fecal material. The swab stick is then placed in 5 ml transport broth and immediately refrigerated.

Bacteriologic Methods. The culture fluid from the vaginal vestibule is vigorously agitated on a laboratory mixer, and the cotton applicator sticks are discarded. Cultures of the 5 ml of transport broth or saline (vaginal vestibule), VB_1 (urethral), and VB_2 (midstream) urines are performed as follows.

Aerobic Cultures. First, 0.1 ml of the vaginal vestibule transport broth and VB_1 and VB_2 specimens are cultured on whole plates of sheep blood and EMB agars. All cultures are incubated in 5% CO_2 at 35°C for 24 hours and rechecked at 48 hours after standing at room temperature for 24 hours. If no growth is present at 24 hours, they are reincubated for an additional day.

Anaerobic Cultures. Sheep blood agar plates are innoculated for anaerobic incubation in sealed GasPak jars placed at 35°C for 3 days. Plates are read immediately after removal from the GasPak jars.

Mycoplasma Cultures. A 0.2-ml sample from the vaginal vestibule and VB_1 and VB_2 specimens are inoculated into Shepard's U-9 broth,[105, 106] incubated at 35°C in 5% CO_2, and held for 2 weeks before counting as negative.

A 0.01-ml portion of the three specimens is inoculated as a single drop on a confined area of Shepard's A-5c agar[105, 107] and incubated in 5% CO_2 (in a humid atmosphere to prevent drying of plates) at 35°C for 72 hours. The agar area is removed as a block and stained with methylene blue, and a 22-mm cover slip is applied; the mycoplasma units are counted under ×100 magnification and reported as colony forming units of *Ureaplasma urealyticum*/ml.

Banking of Gram-negative Bacteria. As will be seen in Chapter 4, the VB_1 culture usually reflects the vaginal vestibule flora. In 10 patients without bladder infections, but with *E. coli* on the vaginal vestibule and in the VB_1 culture, five individual colonies were picked and serotyped from each site; about 90% of the individual colonies proved to be of the same serotype. Thus, any strains of Gram-negative bacilli found in the vaginal culture are banked for serotyping and other studies. Each different organism is banked by touching 5–10 similar appearing colonies, chosen at random, which are then streaked in duplicate on nutrient agar slants. The slants are incubated for 24 hours at 35°C, sealed with a cork dipped in melted paraffin, and stored in a box free from direct light. When Gram-negative bacteria are occasionally found in the urine but are not present on the vaginal vestibule, the urine bacteria are banked. In the presence of a bladder bacteriuria, organisms are banked in duplicate from both the VB_2 and the vaginal vestibule. When Gram-negative bacteria of the same species seem to vary in colonial morphology, sensitivity, or biochemical pattern, they are banked as separate organisms.

After mixing the anal swab culture and discarding the cotton applicator stick, the fecal bacteria are plated on blood agar, EMB, MacConkey, phenylethyl alcohol and Mueller-Hinton agar plates. The latter contain either 50 μg/ml of nitrofurantoin, 50 μg/ml of nalidixic acid, 20 μg/ml of trimethoprim-sulfamethoxazole, or 1.0 μg/ml of trimethoprim, depending on which antimicrobial agent the patient is taking. From these plates, resistant strains of Gram-negative bacteria are easily recognized for banking. As with the vaginal and urine cultures described above, 5–10 colonies of each different species of Gram-negative bacilli present are touched and banked on duplicate nutrient agar slants.

Serologic Classification of E. Coli. Rabbit antisera, prepared by immunization with standard O-antigens of *E. coli*, were obtained from the Communicable Disease Center, U. S. Public Health Center, Atlanta, GA. Sera for 143 O-groups are available.

The technique for O-grouping is that reported by Edwards and Ewing[108] and is identical to the procedure used by Vosti and his colleagues.[109] Strains which could not be grouped due to self-agglutination were classified as "self-agglutinating" (SA), while those strains which failed to be agglutinated by any antisera were classified as "nontypable" (NT).

The banked bacteria to be serotyped are innoculated directly from the nutrient agar slants into tryptose broth. During the serotyping, bacterial strains will occasionally agglutinate in two different antisera. While this is usually due to O-antigen cross reactivity, it occasionally is caused by banking together two different O-serogroups that could not be distinguished by their colonial morphology; this is confirmed by subculturing the banking slant and serogrouping individual colonies. By our technique of touching 5–10 colonies of each strain during the initial banking procedure, the possibility of completely missing a serotype present in significant numbers in proportion to the total Gram-negative population is minimized.

Antigenic identity or difference for strains of *Proteus mirabilis* was determined by the swarming technique of Dienes[110] and confirmed by serogrouping through the courtesy of Dr. Norman Hinton, Professor and Chairman, Department of Bacteriology, Banting Institute, University of Toronto, Toronto, Canada.

Tissue and Stone Cultures

Using sterile technique at the operating table, the surgeon places the stone or fragment of tissue into a sterile culture tube containing 5 ml of saline; the culture tube is packed in ice and sent to the bacteriologic laboratory where, after agitation of the stone or tissue in the 5 ml of saline, 0.1 ml of the saline is surface streaked on both blood agar and EMB agar. The saline is then poured off the specimen; with sterile pickups, the stone or tissue is transferred to a second 5 ml of sterile saline. After agitation to ensure a reasonable washing action, the saline is again decanted and the specimen is transferred to a third 5 ml of saline and finally to a fourth 5 ml of saline. This last saline wash is cultured quantitatively in the same manner as the first. The remainder of this fourth 5 ml of saline is poured with the stone or tissue into a sterile mortar and pestle. After crushing the stone or grinding the tissue in the fourth saline wash, 0.1 ml is again cultured on both blood agar and EMB. The difference in colony counts between the first and fourth saline wash represents the washing effect of the saline transfers on the surface bacteria of the stone or tissue. The difference between the fourth saline wash before and after crushing (or grinding) represents the difference between surface bacteria and bacteria within the specimen.

CLASSIFICATION OF URINARY INFECTIONS

In 1975 I presented a classification of urinary tract infections that is mainly based on therapeutic and, to some extent, etiologic alternatives.[111] It avoids meaningless terms such as "chronic" and imprecise terms such as "relapse." It has been very helpful to us at Stanford and will be used throughout this book.

All urinary infections can be divided into four categories:

1. First infections
2. Unresolved bacteriuria
3. Bacterial persistence } Recurrent
4. Reinfections } infections

First Infections

Since there is no way to determine a first asymptomatic infection, unless cultures are routinely performed at regular intervals throughout an individual's lifetime, first infections are of necessity symptomatic infections. For obvious reasons, nothing is known about the causes of domiciliary first infections, but presumably the etiology is similar to recurrent infections in the same population group. A first infection has an 80% chance of being an *E. coli*, will be highly sensitive to almost any antimicrobial agent (provided the patient has not taken oral antimicrobial agents in the preceding 3 months), and only about one-fourth of adult women with their first infection will have a recurrence in the next 18 months.[112] Five days of sulfonamide therapy, or any other inexpensive antimicrobial agent, represents adequate therapy.

Unresolved Bacteriuria

The term "unresolved", at first consideration, seems clumsy but a word is needed to include any bacteriuria that continues unabated despite therapeutic attempts, medical or surgical, to sterilize the urine. "Persistent" bacteriuria might serve equally well but the word persistence is a better microbiological term when used to indicate bacterial persistence in the presence of a sterile urine.

"Unresolved" bacteriuria is an excellent action word because not only does it indicate failure to sterilize the urine and continued bacteriuria despite therapeutic efforts, but unresolved carries the clear connotation that the bacteriuria must be *resolved* before a cure of the urinary infection can occur. Moreover, until the physician sterilizes the urine and resolves the bacteriuria at least during therapy, the type of recurrent bacteriuria—bacterial persistence or reinfection—which the patient may experience cannot be ascertained; the type of recurrence is very important, because bacterial persistence often requires surgery to cure the recurrent infections while reinfections require antimicrobial prophylaxis. It is clear, then, that bacteriuria must be resolved as the first step in the treatment of urinary infections.

The causes of unresolved bacteriuria during antimicrobial therapy are important. The physician often fails to sterilize the urine during therapy and does not recognize it because he either does not culture the urine during therapy or he misinterprets numbers of bacteria <100,000/ml in the voided urine as representing contaminants. It is clear that if a single colony of the original infecting strain is present in the midstream voided specimen during treatment—and regardless of how low the number—the physician cannot be certain that he has actually sterilized the urine (*i.e.*, resolved the bacteriuria) without a suprapubic needle aspiration of the bladder. The causes of unresolved bacteriuria during antimicrobial therapy are presented in Table 1.10. They are briefly considered here, but excellent clinical examples of each cause are found in the chapters that follow.

Table 1.10
Causes of Unresolved Bacteriuria in Descending Order of Importance

1. Bacterial resistance to the drug selected for treatment
2. Development of resistance from initially sensitive bacteria
3. Bacteriuria caused by two different bacterial species with mutually exclusive sensitivities
4. Rapid reinfection with a new, resistant species during initial therapy for the original sensitive organism
5. Azotemia
6. Papillary necrosis from analgesic abuse
7. Giant staghorn calculi in which the "critical mass" of sensitive bacteria is too great for antimicrobial inhibition

The most common cause of unresolved bacteriuria during treatment is the presence of organisms resistant to the antimicrobial agent selected to treat the infection. The clinical setting is almost invariably one in which the patient has a recent history of antimicrobial therapy, a treatment that has produced resistant organisms among the fecal flora which have reinfected the urinary tract. Tetracyclines and sulfonamides are notorious for producing resistance in the fecal bacteria. Moreover, through resistance transfer factors (R factors), a single course of treatment with one of these drugs may produce bacteria which are simultaneously resistant to several other agents such as ampicillin, cephalosporins, streptomycin, and chloramphenicol. Thus, a recent history (3 months or less) of antimicrobial therapy increases the likelihood that resistant fecal flora have colonized the vaginal introitus and produced a urinary tract infection which will require sensitivity testing to select a drug capable of sterilizing the urine.

The second but a less common cause of unresolved bacteriuria is the development of resistance in a previously sensitive population of organisms infecting the urinary tract. This form of resistance is easy to recognize clinically because within 48–72 hours of starting therapy a previously sensitive population of 10^5 or more bacteria/ml of urine is replaced by an equal population of completely resistant bacteria of the same species through selection of a resistant clone undetected in the original sensitivity testing. Selection of resistant clones from dense bacterial populations (10^8 bacteria or more) occurs in about 8% of patients treated with 1 g/day of tetracycline[113] and about 7% of patients treated with 4 g/day of nalidixic acid.[114] These percentages are not insignificant. The subject of bacterial resistance, both R-factor mediated through fecal resistance and selection of chromosomal resistant clones within the urinary tract, is treated in considerable detail in Chapter 2.

The third cause of unresolved bacteriuria is the presence of a second unsuspected species which is resistant to the antimicrobial agent chosen to treat the predominant infecting organism. In these mixed infections, one of the two organisms acquires dominance over the other and often appears on culture plates as a pure culture of the dominant species. Treatment of the dominant organism unmasks the presence of the second strain. Before the advent of nalidixic acid and the cephalosporins, it was not uncommon to treat a *Klebsiella* urinary infection with colistin (Colymycin) only to find on the 2nd or 3rd day of therapy a *Proteus mirabilis*. With the broader spectrum antimicrobial agents, this is much less of a problem than it was 10 years ago.

The fourth cause is rapid reinfection with a new, resistant species before the completion of 5–10 days of therapy for the original infecting organism. Fortunately, most reinfections, even in highly susceptible females, do not recur this quickly. Nevertheless, the physician will have the urine sterile within 48 hours of starting therapy and a new, resistant strain can infect the bladder from introital carriage by the 5th–10th day of therapy, appearing as if the original bacteriuria was unresolved. This subject of reinfection is covered extensively in later chapters of this book.

The fifth cause of unresolved bacteriuria is azotemia where the bacteriuria continues with sensitive bacteria; the urine cannot be sterilized because the antimicrobial agent cannot be delivered into the urine by the diseased kidney. Bioassay of urinary antimicrobial concentration in these cases usually shows the level of the drug is below the minimal inhibitory concentration of the infecting organism.

The sixth cause is related to azotemia and papillary necrosis ("analgesic" nephritis) but these patients have serum creatinine concentrations less than 2 mg percent accompanied by severe defects in medullary concentrating capacity; they can be bacteriuric while taking an antimicrobial agent to which the organism is sensitive. Sometimes the antimicrobial agent can be switched to one with even higher urinary concentrations, the patient encouraged *not* to force fluids, and the bacteriuria can be resolved.

The last cause of unresolved bacteriuria relates to those rare patients with giant staghorn calculi who have such an inordinate mass of bacteria near the surface of the stone that even urinary levels of bactericidal drugs in nonazotemic patients are inadequate to sterilize the urine. The phenomenon of a "critical density" is well known in sensitivity testing where it is recognized that even sensitive bacteria cannot be inhibited once they reach a certain critical density on the agar plate.[115] Although these giant staghorn calculi are rare, and smaller calculi do not interfere with sterilization of the urine, this is the only circumstance (other than renal failure and the occasional patient with analgesic nephritis) in which sensitive bacteria can continue to cause an unresolved bacteriuria in the presence of proper antimicrobial therapy.

Bacterial Persistence

Once the bacteriuria has been resolved for several days and the antimicrobial agent stopped, recurrence with the same organism from a site within the urinary tract can be identified in only a few circumstances. These circumstances, however, are important because they represent the only surgically curable causes of recurrent urinary tract infections.

The causes of bacterial persistence are listed in Table 1.11. They will not be discussed here because they are well documented throughout this book; indeed, entire chapters are devoted to the two most common causes of bacterial persistence: infected renal calculi and chronic bacterial prostatitis.

Reinfections

Considering the relative rarity of patients with bacterial persistence (Table 1.11), and the enormous number of women and children with recurrent urinary infections, it is probably not an exaggeration to conclude that at least 99% of all infections in females are reinfections of the urinary tract. It is for this reason that the biologic cause of recurrent urinary infections in women is so important. Chapter 4 is devoted exclusively to the pathogenesis and natural history of recurrent urinary infections in women, and Chapter 6 to urinary infections in infancy and childhood.

To complete this classification, vesicointestinal and vesicovaginal fistulae fall under reinfections of the urinary tract because the changing bacterial flora within the urinary tract can reflect the variable intestinal and vaginal flora.

Table 1.11
Causes of Bacterial Persistence in Urinary Infections

1. Infected renal calculi
2. Chronic bacterial prostatitis
3. Unilateral, infected atrophic pyelonephritis
4. Infected pericalyceal diverticulae
5. Infected, nonrefluxing ureteral stumps following nephrectomy for pyonephrosis
6. Medullary sponge kidneys
7. Infected urachal cysts
8. Infected necrotic papillae from papillary necrosis

Other Terms Requiring Clarification

Prophylaxis is the prevention of recurrent bacteriuria by continuous antimicrobial therapy after the preceding bacteriuria has been *cured*.

The word "suppressive" must not be confused with prophylaxis. Suppressive antimicrobial therapy is to give antimicrobials in the presence of bacterial persistence within the urinary tract. For example, for an "infection" staghorn calculus where the patient cannot be operated upon and yet the urine needs to be sterilized even though the bacteria persist in the staghorn calculus. Another example of suppressive therapy would be chronic bacterial prostatitis where the bacteria persist in the prostate while the antimicrobial therapy prevents the organism from infecting the bladder. In this example I admit that continuous therapy might be considered "prophylactic" for the bladder, but with the advent of drugs that diffuse into the prostate it is more reasonable that such therapy is suppressive, but not curative, to the prostatic bacteria. Lastly, the term "suppressive" might have some meaning in the clinical situation in which the physician is unable to sterilize the urine with an oral antimicrobial agent (for example, a *Pseudomonas* urinary tract infection associated with a stone), but he uses some agent anyway in the hope of suppressing (not sterilizing) bacterial growth and preventing clinical symptoms. In this situation, it is an admission of defeat in failing to sterilize the urine; in my experience, clinical applicability is limited almost exclusively to a few *Pseudomonas* infections.

Thus, the term suppressive has very limited use and since it is an admission of failure to cure a urinary infection, the less it is used the more successful is our practice of medicine. It must not be confused with prophylaxis where the urinary infection, including bacterial persistence, has been cured and the antimicrobial agent is used exclusively to prevent a reinfection of the urinary tract with a new organism.

The term "relapse" should be avoided; it is imprecise and misleading. The advent of serogrouping *E. coli* two decades ago allowed investigators to determine whether two successive *E. coli* infections were of the same serotype ("relapse") or of different serotypes ("reinfection"),[116] and it was a useful distinction at that time. The difficulty with the term relapse is that in the United States it came to imply persistence of the infection within the kidney during the interval between two successive infections of the same serotype. This forced those who found the term useful to use a qualifying period of time, usually defined as the recurrence of the same organism within 2 weeks of stopping antimicrobial therapy. The weakness of this definition is apparent because detection of the recurrence with the same serotype on the 16th day after therapy makes it a reinfection whereas detection 2 days earlier makes the infection a relapse. As will be seen in Chapter 4, recurrences with a different serotype within the first 2 weeks of therapy are just as common as recurrences with an identical serotype. Moreover, the major cause of bacterial recurrence with the same serotype (or a different one) is persistence of that serotype on the vaginal introitus during and after antimicrobial therapy. If the term relapse were used to indicate two successive infections of the same serotype, regardless of elapsed time and without implication of renal persistence, it would be a biologically useful term. This is the way most Europeans use the term but this is not true in this country. Accordingly, I believe communication in the field of urinary infections is served better if the term relapse is dropped. In the classification I have proposed, if one means bacterial persistence as a cause of two consecutive recurrences of the same serotype, then it is called exactly that: bacterial persistence. On the other hand, if the successive recurrences of the same serotype are reinfections, then reinfection is the correct term. It makes life much simpler to say exactly what you mean.

REFERENCES

1. Asscher, A. W., Sussman, M., Waters, W. E., Davis, R. H., and Chick, S.: Urine as a medium for bacterial growth. Lancet **2:** 1037, 1966.
2. Savage, W. E., Hajj, S. N., and Kass, E. H.: Demographic and prognostic characteristics of bacteriuria in pregnancy. Medicine **46:** 385, 1967.
3. Kass, E. H.: Asymptomatic infections of the urinary tract. Trans. Am. Phys. **69:** 56, 1956.
4. Marple, C. D.: The frequency and character of urinary tract infections in an unselected group of women. Ann. Intern. Med. **14:** 2220, 1941.
5. Barr, R. H., and Rantz, L. A.: The incidence of unsuspected urinary tract infection in a selected group of ambulatory women. Calif. Med. **68:** 437, 1948.
6. Sanford, J. P., Favour, C. B., Mao, F. H., and Harrison, J. H.: Evaluation of the "positive" urine culture. Am. J. Med. **20:** 88, 1956.
7. Kass, E. H.: The role of asymptomatic bacteriuria in the pathogenesis of pyelonephritis. In E. L. Quinn and E. H. Kass (Eds.), Biology of Pyelonephritis. Boston, Little Brown & Co., 1960, p. 399.
8. Philpot, V. B., Jr.: The bacterial flora of urine specimens from normal adults. J. Urol. **75:** 562, 1956.
9. Guze, L. B., and Beeson, P. B.: Observations on the reliability and safety of bladder catheterization for bacteriologic study of the urine. N. Engl. J. Med. **255:** 474, 1956.
10. Monzon, O. T., Ory, E. M., Dobson, H. L., Carter, E., and Yow, E. M.: A comparison of bacterial counts of the urine obtained by needle aspiration of the bladder, catheterization and midstream voided methods. N. Engl. J. Med. **259:** 764, 1958.
11. Stamey, T. A., Govan, D. E., and Palmer, J. M.: The localization and treatment of urinary tract infections: The role of bactericidal urine levels as opposed to serum levels. Medicine **44:** 1, 1965.
12. Goldberg, L. M., Vosti, K. L., and Rantz, L. A.: Microflora of the urinary tract examined by voided and aspirated urine culture. In E. H. Kass (Ed.), Progress in Pyelonephritis. Philadelphia, F. A. Davis & Co., 1965, p. 545.
13. Mabeck, C. E.: Studies in urinary tract infections: I. The diagnosis of bacteriuria in women. Acta Med. Scand. **186:** 35, 1969.
14. Kunz, H. H., Sieberth, H. G., Freiberg, J., Pulverer, G. and Schneider, F. J.: Zur bedeutung der blasenpunktion für den sicheren nachweis einer bakteriurie. Dtsch. Med. Wochenschr. **100:** 2252, 1975.
15. Pfau, A., and Sacks, T. G.: An evaluation of midstream urine cultures in the diagnosis of urinary tract infections in females. Urol. Int. **25:** 326, 1970.
16. Pometta, D., Rees, S. B., Younger, D., and Kass, E. H.: Asymptomatic bacteriuria in diabetes mellitus. N. Engl. J. Med. **276:** 1118, 1967.
17. Miall, W. E., Kass, E. H., Ling, J., and Stuart, K.

L.: Factors influencing arterial pressure in the general population in Jamaica. Br. Med. J. **2:** 497, 1962.
18. Newman, C. G. H., O'Neill, P., and Parker, A.: Pyuria in infancy, and the role of suprapubic aspiration of urine in diagnosis of infection of urinary tract. Br. Med. J. **2:** 277, 1967.
19. Govan, D. E., Butler, E. D., and Engelsgjerd, G. L.: Pathogenesis of urinary tract infections in patients with neurogenic bladder dysfunction. Urol. Digest **7:** 16 (July), 1968.
20. Kraft, J. K., and Stamey, T. A.: The natural history of symptomatic recurrent bacteriuria in women. Medicine **56:** 55, 1977.
21. Jackson, G. G., and Grieble, H. G.: Pathogenesis of renal infection. Arch. Intern. Med. **100:** 692, 1957.
22. Turck, M., Goffe, B., and Petersdorf, R. G.: The urethral catheter and urinary tract infection. J. Urol. **88:** 834, 1962.
23. Brumfitt, W., Davies, B. I., and Rosser, E. I.: Urethral catheter as a cause of urinary tract infection in pregnancy and puerperium. Lancet **2:** 1059, 1961.
24. Kaye, M., de Vries, J., and MacFarlane, K. T.: The initiation of urinary tract infection following a single bladder catheterization. Can. Med. Assoc. J. **86:** 9, 1962.
25. Thiel, G., and Spühler, O.: Urinary tract infection by catheter and the so-called infectious (episomal) resistance. Schweiz. Med. Wochenschr. **95:** 1155, 1965.
26. Pearman, J. W.: Prevention of urinary tract infection following spinal cord injury. Paraplegia **9:** 95, 1971.
27. Roberts, A. P., Robinson, R. E., and Beard, R. W.: Some factors affecting bacterial colony counts in urinary infection. Br. Med. J. **1:** 400, 1967.
28. Kunin, C. M.: The quantitative significance of bacteria visualized in the unstained urinary sediment. N. Engl. J. Med. **265:** 589, 1961.
29. Mabeck, C. E.: Studies in urinary tract infections: IV. Urinary leukocyte excretion in bacteriuria. Acta Med. Scand. **186:** 193, 1969.
30. Gadeholt, H.: Quantitative estimation of urinary sediment, with special regard to sources of error. Br. Med. J. **1:** 1547, 1964.
31. Gadeholt, H.: The cellular content in non-timed specimens of urine. Acta Med. Scand. **184:** 323, 1968.
32. Triger, D. R., and Smith, J. W. G.: Survival of urinary leucocytes. J. Clin. Pathol. **19:** 443, 1966.
33. Musher, D. M., Thorsteinsson, S. B., and Airola, V. M. II: Quantitative urinalysis. Diagnosing urinary tract infection in men. J. Am. Med. Assoc. **236:** 2069, 1976.
34. Hobday, J. D.: A simplified culture method for detecting asymptomatic bacteriuria in children. Pediatrics, **38:** 903, 1966.
35. Mackey, J. P., and Sandys, G. H.: Laboratory diagnosis of infections of the urinary tract in general practice by means of a dip-inoculum transport medium. Br. Med. J. **2:** 1286, 1965.
36. Guttmann, D., Naylor, G. R. E.: Dip-slide: An aid to quantitative urine culture in general practice. Br. Med. J. **3:** 343, 1967.
37. Cohen, S. N., and Kass, E. H.: A simple method for quantitative urine culture. N. Engl. J. Med. **277:** 176, 1967.
38. Vejlsgaard, R., and Justesen, T.: Quantitative bacterial culture of urine. II. Evaluation of 10 different screening methods for the diagnosis of bacteriuria compared with results obtained by the dilution technique. Acta Med. Scand. **193:** 147, 1973.
39. Edwards, P. D., Burke, E. A., and Wear, J. B., Jr.: A new method for outpatient culture and sensitivity of urine. J. Urol. **109:** 689, 1973.
40. McAllister, T. A.: The day of the dipslide. Nephron **11:** 123, 1973.
41. Arneil, G. C., McAllister, T. A., and Kay, P.: Detection of bacteriuria at room temperature. Lancet **1:** 119, 1970.
42. Kincaid-Smith, P., Bullen, M., Mills, M., Fussell, U., Huston, N., and Goon, F.: Reliability of screening tests for bacteriuria in pregnancy. Lancet **2:** 61, 1964.
43. Guignard, J. P., and Torrado, A.: Nitrite indicator strip test for bacteriuria. Lancet **1:** 47, 1978.
44. Neter, E.: Evaluation of the tetrazolium test for the diagnosis of significant bacteriuria. J. Am. Med. Assoc. **192:** 769, 1965.
45. Finnerty, F. A., Jr., and Johnson, A. C.: A simplified accurate method for detecting bacteriuria. Am. J. Obstet. Gynecol. **101:** 238, 1968.
46. Schersten, B., and Fritz, H.: Subnormal levels of glucose in urine. A sign of urinary tract infection. J. Am. Med. Assoc. **201:** 949, 1967.
47. Scherstén, B., Dahlqvist, A., Fritz, H., Köhler, L., and Westlund, L.: Screening for bacteriuria with a test paper for glucose. J. Am. Med. Assoc. **204:** 205, 1968.
48. Alwall, N., and Lohi, A.: Factors affecting the reliability of screening tests for bacteriuria. I. Nitrite test (Urnitest®), Uriglox® and dip-slide (Inculator®). Acta Med. Scand. **193:** 499, 1973.
49. Kunin, C. M.: New methods in detecting urinary tract infections. Urol. Clin. N. Am. **2:** 423, 1975.
50. Dove, G. A., Bailey, A. J., Gower, P. E., Roberts, A. P. and de Wardener, H. E.: Diagnosis of urinary-tract infection in general practice. Lancet **2:** 1281, 1972.
51. Stamey, T. A., and Pfau, A.: Some functional, pathologic, bacteriologic, and chemotherapeutic characteristics of unilateral pyelonephritis in

man. II. Bacteriologic and chemotherapeutic characteristics. Invest. Urol. **1:** 162, 1963.
52. Brod, J., Prat, V., and Dejdar, R.: Early functional diagnosis of chronic pyelonephritis with some remarks on the pathogenesis of the pyelonephritic contracted kidney. In E. L. Quinn and E. H. Kass (Eds.), Biology of Pyelonephritis. Boston, Little Brown & Co., 1960, p. 311.
53. Stamey, T. A., and Pfau, A.: Some functional, pathologic, bacteriologic and chemotherapeutic characteristics of unilateral pyelonephritis in man. I. Functional and pathologic characteristics. Invest. Urol. **1:** 134, 1963.
54. Fairley, K. F., Bond, A. G., Brown, R. B., and Habersberger, P.: Simple test to determine the site of urinary tract infection. Lancet **2:** 427, 1967.
55. Kass, E. H.: Letters to the Journal. J. Am. Med. Assoc. **184:** 142, 1963.
56. Whitworth, J. A., Fairley, K. F., O'Keefe, C. M., and Johnson, W.: The site of renal infection: pyelitis or pyelonephritis? Clin. Neophrol. **2:** 9, 1974.
57. Fairley, K. F., Bond, A. G., and Adey, F. D. The site of infection in pregnancy bacteriuria. Lancet **1:** 939, 1966.
58. Reeves, D. S., and Brumfitt, W.: Localization of urinary tract infection. A comparative study of methods. In F. W. O'Grady and W. Brumfitt (Eds.), Urinary Tract Infection. London, Oxford University Press, 1968, p. 53.
59. Ronald, A. R., Cutler, R. E., and Turck, M.: Effect of bacteriuria on renal concentrating mechanisms. Ann. Intern. Med. **70:** 723, 1969.
60. Eykyn, S., Lloyd-Davies, R. W., and Shuttleworth, K. E. D.: The localisation of urinary tract infection by ureteric catheterisation. Invest. Urol. **9:** 271, 1972.
61. Clark, H., Ronald, A. R., Cutler, R. E. and Turck, M.: The correlation between site of infection and maximal concentrating ability in bacteriuria. J. Infect. Dis. **120:** 47, 1969.
62. Clark, H., Ronald, A. R., and Turck, M.: Serum antibody response in renal versus bladder bacteriuria. J. Infect. Dis. **123:** 539, 1971.
63. Pfau, A., Ashkenazi, A., and Sacks, T. G.: The value of urinary β-Glucuronidase activity in the assessment of urinary tract infections. Isr. J. Med. Sci. **4:** 1249, 1968.
64. Fairley, K. F., Grounds, A. D., Carson, N. E., Laird, E. C., Gutch, R. C., McCallum, P. H. G., Leighton, P., Sleeman, R. L., and O'Keefe, C. M.: Site of infection in acute urinary-tract infection in general practice. Lancet **2:** 615, 1971.
65. Harding, G. K. M., Marrie, T. J., Ronald, A. R., Hoban, S., and Muir, P.: Urinary tract localization in women. J. Am. Med. Assoc. **240:** 1147, 1978.
66. Thomas, V., Shelokov, A., and Forland, M.: Antibody-coated bacteria in the urine and the site of urinary tract infection. N. Engl. J. Med. **290:** 588, 1974.
67. Jones, S. R., Smith, J. W., and Sanford, J. P.: Localization of urinary tract infections by detection of antibody-coated bacteria in urine sediment. N. Engl. J. Med. **290:** 591, 1974.
68. Kohnle, W., Vanek, E., Federlin, K., and Franz, H. E.: Lokalisation eines Harnwegsinfektes durch Nachweis von antikörperbesetzten Bakterien im Urin. Dtsch. Med. Wochenschr. **100:** 2598, 1975.
69. Hellerstein, S., Kennedy, E., Nussbaum, L., and Rice, K.: Localization of the site of urinary tract infections by means of antibody-coated bacteria in the urinary sediments. J. Pediatr. **92:** 188, 1978.
70. Forsum, U., Hjelm, E., and Jonsell, G.: Antibody-coated bacteria in the urine of children with urinary tract infections. Acta Paediatr. Scand. **65:** 639, 1976.
71. Thomas, V. L., Harris, R. E., Gilstrap, L. C., III, and Shelokov, A.: Antibody-coated bacteria in the urine of obstetrical patients with acute pyelonephritis. J. Infect. Dis. **131:** S57, 1975.
72. Hand, W. L., Smith, J. W., Miller, T. E., Barnett, J. A., and Sanford, J. P.: Immunoglobulin synthesis in lower tract infection. J. Lab. Clin. Med. **75:** 19, 1970.
73. Hawthorne, N. J., Kurtz, S. B., Anhalt, J. P., Segura, J. W.: Accuracy of antibody-coated-bacteria test in recurrent urinary tract infections. Mayo Clin. Proc. **53:** 651, 1978.
74. Forland, M., Thomas, V., and Shelokov, A.: Urinary tract infections in patients with diabetes mellitus. Studies on antibody coating of bacteria. J. Am. Med. Assoc. **238:** 1924, 1977.
75. Harris, R. E., Thomas, V. L., and Shelokov, A.: Asymptomatic bacteriuria in pregnancy: Antibody-coated bacteria, renal function, and intrauterine growth retardation. Am. J. Obstet. Gynecol. **126:** 20, 1976.
76. Cattell W. R., Charlton, C. A. C., McSherry, A., Fry, I. K., O'Grady, F. W.: The localization of urinary tract infection and its relationship to relapse, reinfection and treatment, In W. Brumfitt and A. W. Asscher (Eds.), Urinary Tract Infection, London, Oxford University Press, 1973, p. 206.
77. Thomas, V. L., Forland, M., and Shelokov, A.: Antibody-coated bacteria in urinary tract infection. Kidney Int. **8:** S-20, 1975.
78. Jones, S. R.: Antibody-coated bacteria in urine (letter). N. Engl. J. Med. **295:** 1380, 1976.
79. Thomas, V. L., Forland, M., LeStourgeon, D., and Shelokov, A.: Antibody-coated bacteria in persistent and recurrent urinary tract infections. Kidney Int. **14:** 607, 1978.
80. Stamey, T. A., Wehner, N., Mihara, G., and

Condy, M.: The immunologic basis of recurrent bacteriuria: Role of cervicovaginal antibody in enterobacterial colonization of the introital mucosa. Medicine **57:** 47, 1978.
81. Jones, S. R.: Prostatitis as cause of antibody-coated bacteria in urine. N. Engl. J. Med. **291:** 365, 1974.
82. Harding, S. A., and Merz, W. G.: Evaluation of antibody coating of yeasts in urine as an indicator of the site of urinary tract infection. J. Clin. Microbiol. **2:** 222, 1975.
83. Marrie, T. J., Harding, G. K. M., Ronald, A. R., Dikkema, J., Lam, J., Hoban, S., and Costerton, J. W.: Influence of mucoidy on antibody coating of *Pseudomonas aeruginosa.* J. Infect. Dis. **139:** 357, 1979.
84. Longcope, W. T., and Winkenwerder, W. L.: Clinical features of the contracted kidney due to pyelonephritis. Bull. Johns Hopkins Hosp. **53:** 255, 1933.
85. Brod, J.: Chronic pyelonephritis. Lancet **1:** 973, 1956.
86. DePalma, J. R., and Cutler, R. E.: Maximum urinary concentration (U_{max}) and free water reabsorption (T_mc H_2O) reproducibility in hydropenic subjects. Clin. Res. **14:** 152, 1966.
87. Siede, W., and Luz, K.: Agglutinabilität und Pathogenität des Bacterium coli bei Erkrankungen der Harnwege. Klin. Wochenschr. **20:** 241, 1941.
88. Neter, E., Bertram, L. F., Zak, D. A., Mumdock, M. R., and Arbesman, C. E.: Studies on hemagglutination and hemolysis by *Escherichia coli* antisera. J. Exp. Med. **96:** 1, 1952.
89. Neter, E., Westphal, O., Lüderitz, O., Gino, R. M., and Gorzynski, E. A.: Demonstration of antibodies against enteropathogenic *Escherichia coli* in sera of children of various ages. Pediatrics **16:** 801, 1955.
90. Needell, M. H., Neter, E., Staubitz, W. J., and Bingham, W. A.: The antibody (hemagglutinin) response of patients with infections of the urinary tract. J. Urol. **74:** 674, 1955.
91. Williamson, J., Brainerd, H., Scaparone, M., and Chueh, S. P.: Antibacterial antibodies in coliform urinary tract infections. Arch. Intern. Med. **114:** 222, 1964.
92. Percival, A., Brumfitt, W., and de Louvois, J.: Serum-antibody levels as an indication of clinically inapparent pyelonephritis. Lancet **2:** 1027, 1964.
93. Winberg, J., Andersen, H. J., Hanson, L. A., and Lincoln, K.: Studies of urinary tract infections in infancy and childhood. I. Antibody response in different types of urinary tract infections caused by coliform bacteria. Br. Med. J. **2:** 524, 1963.
94. Sanford, J. P., and Barnett, J. A.: Immunologic responses in urinary tract infections: Prognostic and diagnostic evaluation. J. Am. Med. Assoc. **192:** 587, 1965.
95. Ehrenkranz, N. J., and Carter, M. J.: Immunologic studies in urinary tract infections: I. The hemagglutinin response to *Escherichia* O antigens in infections of varying severity. J. Immunol. **92:** 798, 1964.
96. Bremner, D. A., Fairley, K. F., Kincaid-Smith, P., and O'Keefe, C.: The serum antibody response in renal and bladder infections. Med. J. Aust. **1:** 1069, 1969.
97. Hodson, C. J.: Coarse pyelonephritic scarring or "atrophic pyelonephritis." Proc. R. Soc. Med. **58:** 785, 1965.
98. Jodal, U., Lindberg, U., and Lincoln, K.: Level diagnosis of symptomatic urinary tract infections in childhood. Acta Paediatr. Scand. **64:** 201, 1975.
99. Jodal, U., and Hanson, L. A.: Sequential determination of C-reactive protein in acute childhood pyelonephritis. Acta Paediatr. Scand. **65:** 319, 1976.
100. Wientzen, R. L., McCracken, G. H. Jr., Petruska, M. L., Swenson, S. G., Kaijser, B., and Hanson, L. A.: Localization and therapy of urinary tract infections of childhood. Pediatrics **63:** 467, 1979.
101. McGeachie, J.: Recurrent infection of the urinary tract: Reinfection or recrudescence? Br. Med. J. **1:** 952, 1966.
102. Kunin, C. M., and Halmagyi, N. E.: Urinary tract infections in school children. II. Characterization of invading organisms. N. Engl. J. Med. **266:** 1297, 1962.
103. Bergström, T., Lincoln, K., Ørskov, F., Ørskov, I., and Winberg, J.: Studies of urinary tract infections in infancy and childhood. VIII. Reinfection vs. relapse in recurrent urinary tract infections. Evalution by means of identification of infecting organisms. J. Pediatr. **71:** 13, 1967.
104. Gallagher, D. J. A., Montgomerie, J. Z., and North, J. D. K.: Acute infections of the urinary tract and the urethral syndrome in general practice. Br. Med. J. **1:** 622, 1965.
105. Shepard, M. C.: Cultivation and properties of T-strains of mycoplasma associated with nongonococcal urethritis. Ann. N. Y. Acad. Sci. **143:** 505, 1967.
106. Shepard, M. C.: U9 urease color test medium for detection of T-strains of mycoplasma in clinical material. U. S. Naval Med. Field Res. Lab., Camp Lejeune, N. C., November 7, 1967.
107. Shepard, M. C.: Medium A-5C for the primary isolation of T-strains of mycoplasma from clinical sources. U. S. Naval Med. Field Res. Lab., Camp Lejeune, N. C., January 21, 1969.
108. Edwards, P. R., and Ewing, W. H.: Identification of Enterobacteriaceae. Minneapolis, Burgess, 1955.

109. Vosti, K. L., Goldberg, L. M., Monto, A. S., and Rantz, L. A.: Host-parasite interaction in patients with infections due to *Escherichia coli.* I. The serogrouping of *E. coli* from intestinal and extraintestinal sources. J. Clin. Invest. **43:** 2377, 1964.
110. Dienes, L.: Reproductive processes in proteus cultures. Proc. Soc. Exp. Biol. Med. **63:** 265, 1946.
111. Stamey, T. A.: A clinical classification of urinary tract infections based upon origin (editorial). South. Med. J. **68:** 934, 1975.
112. Harrison, W. O., Holmes, K. K., and Belding, M. E.: A prospective evaluation of recurrent urinary tract infection in women. Clin. Res. **22:** 125A, 1974.
113. Stamey, T. A., Fair, W. R., Timothy, M. M., Millar, M. A., Mihara, G., and Lowery, Y. C.: Serum versus urinary antimicrobial concentrations in cure of urinary-tract infections. N. Engl. J. Med. **291:** 1159, 1974.
114. Stamey, T. A., and Bragonje, J.: Resistance to nalidixic acid. A misconception due to underdosage. J. Am. Med. Assoc. **236:** 1857, 1976.
115. Cooper, K. E., Linton, A. H., and Sehgal, S. N.: The effect of inoculum size on inhibition zones in agar media using staphylococci and streptomycin. J. Gen. Microbiol. **18:** 670, 1958.
116. Turck, M., Anderson, K. N., and Petersdorf, R. G.: Relapse and reinfection in chronic bacteriuria. N. Engl. J. Med. **275:** 70, 1966.
117. Scherf, H., Kollermann, M. W., and Busch, R.: Nachweis antikorperbeladener bakterien im ursediment bei kindlichen harnwegsinfektionen. Monatssch. Kinderheilk. D. **126:** 23, 1978.

CHAPTER 2

Antimicrobial Sensitivity Testing and Bacterial Resistance

ANTIMICROBIAL SENSITIVITY TESTING

General Principles

SENSITIVITY testing is based on the principle that bacterial resistance or sensitiveness can be determined *in vitro* under conditions that simulate closely the environment of the bacteria in the host. Infections of the urinary tract are ideally suited to test this principle because urine, in contrast to blood, has few, if any, effective bacterial inhibitors. For example, we tested the question of whether normal urine is inhibitory to small numbers of bacteria by collecting midstream urines from females who voided from the cystoscopy table as described in the first chapter. These urines were obtained from patients and normal volunteers who were known to have uninfected urinary tracts and who were on no antimicrobial therapy. This technique of collecting the voided urine meant that small numbers of perineal bacteria from the urethra and vaginal introitus would be self-inoculated into a sterile bladder urine. By culturing the voided urine before and after incubation for 24 hours at 37°C, it was possible to answer the question of whether a normal urine is inhibitory or not when small numbers of bacteria reach the bladder.[1] In Table 2.1, only three of 113 patients (2.6%) showed inhibitory activity during incubation; all the rest of the urines supported bacterial growth as expected (*Escherichia coli* better than the Gram-positive flora). One-tenth milliliter of urine was the largest volume cultured; thus, those patients who showed <10 bacteria/ml (9 who grew *E. coli*, 18 enterococci, 10 *Staphylococcus epidermidis*, and 7 other Gram-positive species) actually had no bacteria detectable in the 0.1 ml of urine cultured. The inoculum had to be extremely low, perhaps even as low as one single bacterium in these cases, and yet there was no inhibition to growth. For practical purposes, and despite a single *in vitro* report on a few first voided AM urines to the contrary,[2] there seem to be no effective antibacterial inhibitors in the urine, chemical or immunological.

Of first importance in understanding sensitivity testing, however, is to recognize that the terms "sensitive" and "resistant" have no meaning without reference to a specific concentration of the antimicrobial agent under consideration. All bacteria can probably be killed by some agent at some concentration (table salt is bactericidal in high enough concentrations); on the other hand, highly potent antibiotics that readily kill bacteria can be used in such low concentrations that they have no effect on the bacteria. Thus, the terms sensitive and resistant must be used only in reference to a specific concentration. Unfortunately, in clinical practice, this is seldom done, misleading students and practitioners of medicine to believe that bacteria are inherently sensitive or resistant to specific drugs. Perhaps because penicillin-G was the first antibiotic and was used almost exclusively for tissue infections, bacterial "sensitivity" is defined in terms of the concentration that can be expected in the blood serum. Furthermore, since protein binding prevents antimicrobial activity of the bound fraction in the serum,[3] I agree with Ericsson that sensitivity should mean that the "concentration of antibiotic in the blood should many times exceed the level corresponding to the sensitivity of the causal organism."[4] For example, a β-hemolytic group A streptococcal pharyngitis is usually inhibited by 0.01 μg of penicillin-G/ml. If 250 mg of oral penicillin-G, given by mouth every 6 hours, is expected to produce a concentration in the serum of 0.25 μg of unbound penicillin-G/ml, then the group A streptococcus in question would be considered "sensitive" to penicillin-G; *i.e.*, the serum concentration (0.25 μg/ml) well exceeds the minimal concentration (0.01 μg/ml) *in vitro* required to inhibit the bacteria. Observe, however, that this definition of sensitivity not only requires reference to a specific concentration of penicillin-G, but also implies considerable information on the pharmacology of the drug, including the dosage route and schedule of administration, not to mention individual variations in the clinical status of the patient that might sharply alter the usual pharmacodynamics of the drug. Moreover, is it the peak level of the administered drug, usually occurring 1–2 hours after oral dosage, that is important, or is it the average level maintained between dosages? The average level will be much less than the peak concentration for most drugs taken every 6 hours. Answers to this basic question simply are not available. Nevertheless, if the general serum level of free drug exceeds by several fold the minimal amount required *in vitro* to inhibit bacterial growth, the bacteria can be considered sensitive. Unfortunately, however, this *modus operandi* finds little consistency when we consider the broad spectrum antimicrobial agents used for Gram-negative bacterial infections. As will be seen when the Kirby-Bauer method of sensitivity testing is dis-

Table 2.1
Bacterial Counts in Urine Before and After 24 Hours of Incubation

No. of Patients	Organism	Before Incubation	After Incubation
		(*bacteria/ml*)	(*bacteria/ml*)
9	*Escherichia coli*	<10	≥10^5
21	*E. coli*	10–100	≥10^5
18	Enterococci	<10	≥10^4
4	Enterococci	10–100	≥10^4
10	*Staphylococcus epidermidis*	<10	≥10^4
7	*S. epidermidis*	10–100	≥10^4
7	Other Gram positive	<10	≥10^4
16	Other Gram-positive	10–10^4	≥10^4
18	None	Sterile	Sterile
1	*S. epidermidis*	500	Sterile
1	*E. coli*	40	Sterile
1	*Proteus morganii*	30	Sterile
113			

Other Gram-positive organisms include α, β, γ-streptococci, corynebacteria and yeast.

cussed, 5 μg of tetracycline/ml is considered the serum level to which bacterial sensitivity should be related.[5] But 250 mg of oral tetracycline hydrochloride every 6 hours achieve a peak concentration of only 2–4 μg/ml, averaging 1–2 μg/ml,[6–9] and 56% of this is inactive because of binding to serum albumin.[10] Even with 500 mg orally every 6 hours, the average serum level of active drug will not exceed 2 or 3 μg/ml.[6, 9] Under no circumstances, short of intravenous dosage, can the physician achieve 5 μg/ml of free tetracycline in the serum.

One of the best infectious disease laboratories in the country 18 years ago used the "test" concentrations indicated in Table 2.2 as the end point for determining sensitivity or resistance; agar plates were poured with the antimicrobial concentrations indicated under the column "Test Concentration." I have indicated in the adjacent column to the right what the average concentration will be in plasma, including free and bound drug, when adult patients receive the usual standard dosage. Why did these levels of *in vitro* sensitivity testing ("Test Concentration") so exceed what could be obtained in the serum with conventional dosage? One wonders if the reason why sensitivity levels usually represent unrealistic concentrations is that the broad spectrum antibiotics were commonly used for urinary tract infections, unlike penicillin-G and erythromycin where the discrepancy between test concentrations and *in vivo* level is minimal. But the best indication of *in vitro* validity is whether the patient is cured of his infection by the drug under consideration. If the bacteriologist reported sensitivities actually based on the true serum level, as in the case of penicillin-G, few Gram-negative urinary pathogens would ever be reported as sensitive. Yet, clinicians were often observing cure of the infection with the very drug reported to be ineffective on *in vitro* testing, and so the level of the drug used to indicate sensitivity was gradually increased until more of the bacteria were reported as sensitive and the sensitivity listings correlated better with results in patients.

Serum versus Urinary Levels

The definition of bacterial resistance, based on sensitivity to the serum concentration of the drug, is often artificial; for example, the treatment of urinary tract in-

Table 2.2
Discrepancy Between Test and Actual Concentration Achieved in Plasma

Drug	Dosage	Test Concentration	Average Concentration Achieved in Plasma
		μg/ml	*μg/ml*
Penicillin-G	250 mg q.i.d.	0.6	0.3
Erythromycin	250 mg q.i.d.	2.0	1.0
Oxytetracycline	250 mg q.i.d.	10.0	1.0–2.0
Coly-Mycin	75 mg q 12 hr i.m.	5.0	1.0–2.0
Chloramphenicol	500 mg q.i.d.	10.0	3.0–4.0
Ampicillin	250 mg q.i.d.	10.0	2.0
Streptomycin	500 mg q 12 hr i.m.	10.0	6.0–8.0
Furadantin	100 mg q.i.d.	100.0	1.0

Antibacterial concentrations in agar dilutions used by a major university infectious disease laboratory (test concentration) compared to the actual, average concentrations achieved in plasma.

Table 2.3
Antimicrobial Concentrations in the Serum and Urine of Adults with Normal Renal Function

Drug	Dosage	Average Serum Concentration	Average Urine Concentration[a]
	q 6 hr p.o.		
Penicillin-G	500 mg	<1.0	300
Nitrofurantoin	100 mg	<2.0	150
Tetracycline	250 mg	1.0–2.0	500
Colistin methane sulfonate	75 mg (i.m. q 12 hr)	0.5–1.0	34
Ampicillin	250 mg	1–2	350
Nalidixic Acid	1000 mg	20–50[b]	75
Gentamicin	1.0 mg/kg/8 hr (i.m. q 8 hr)	2–3	125
Cephalexin	250 mg	4–6	800

[a] These values for the average antibiotic concentration in the urine are derived from the best available excretion data and are based on a 24-hour urine output of 1200 ml.
[b] Eighty-five percent bound to serum albumin.

fections has the advantage that low serum levels become high concentrations in the renal tubule and urine. Table 2.3 shows the difference between the average serum and average urine concentration achieved in normal subjects on standard dosage. The argument over the importance of serum versus urinary concentrations of antimicrobial agents in determining cure of urinary infections still occurs. Despite numerous emotional statements, there are only three groups, to our knowledge, that have tried to investigate the problem. McCabe and Jackson treated 252 patients with "pyelonephritis"[11]; they concluded that antimicrobial activity in the serum did not separate the cures from the failures, but that inhibitory activity in the urine did relate to cure of bacteriuria. Our group at Stanford first localized urinary infections to the kidneys and then used either oral penicillin-G or nitrofurantoin for treatment[12]; since neither agent is active in serum against Gram-negative bacteria, the resulting cures were attributed to urinary levels. Klastersky *et al.* serially diluted serum and urine from patients with urinary infections, inoculated their infecting organism, and determined the bacteriostatic titers.[13] Despite using three antibiotics (gentamicin, doxycycline, and cephalexin) that have high serum concentrations, they concluded that the "response to therapy of patients with urinary tract infections correlated best with the inhibitory level found in the urine."[13]

In a major clinical effort to resolve this issue, we designed a study with a broad spectrum antibiotic, oxytetracycline, that is widely used in the treatment of urinary tract infections. Bacteriuria was diagnosed in 33 consecutive women by microscopic study of the urinary sediment; none was receiving antimicrobial therapy. The clinical characteristics of these 33 women are presented in Table 2.4. A control blood serum was drawn, a urine culture was obtained, and the infecting organism was banked; all patients were started on 250 mg of oxytetracycline four times a day for 10 days (Figure 2.1). Between the 5th and 10th days of therapy, the patients returned to the out-patient unit; they were given an additional 250 mg of oxytetracycline regardless of the time of their last medication, and a blood serum and urine were obtained 1 hour later. This urine sample, in addition to being cultured, was Millipore-filtered and inoculated with the original, pretreatment infecting organism at a final concentration of 500–2000 bacteria/ml. At the same time, the pretreatment and on-treatment blood serums were heated to 56°C for 60 minutes, a maneuver that destroyed the natural serum-cidal effect of serum, but did not change the antimicrobial activity of oxytetracycline (Table 2.5); these experiments were conducted by dipping 10-mm filter-paper discs into both heated and unheated aliquots of normal serum to which oxytetracycline was added in concentrations of 5.0, 7.5, and 10 μg/ml (Table 2.5). The excess serum was shaken off the discs which were placed on the surface of Mueller-Hinton agar plates previously inoculated with a *S. epidermidis* assay organism (minimal inhibitory concentration of 0.5 μg/ml of oxytetracycline). The surface inoculum was dense but not confluent, as recommended by Ericsson.[14] After 20 minutes of prediffusion at room temperature, the plates were incubated at 37°C. As seen in Table 2.5, the zone sizes after 24 hours incubation (15.5–24.5 mm) showed no difference between the heated (56°C for 1 hour) and the unheated serums. These preliminary studies were important and clearly showed that heating serum containing oxytetracycline to 56°C for 1 hour did not change the antimicrobial activity of the oxytetracycline; moreover, the tetracyclines are known to be heat stable.[15]

Table 2.4
Clinical Characterization

(Age: 14–78 years (mean = 37))

Number of Infections	
First	7
<6	11
>6	15
	33
Symptoms	
None	15
Dysuria, frequency	15
Flank pain	1
Hematuria	1
Malodorous urine	33
Intravenous urogram	
Normal	12
Obstruction	2
Renal scars	4
Renal calculi	2
Renal transplant	1
Neurogenic bladder	1
Unknown	11
	33

Table 2.5
The Effect on Oxytetracycline Activity of Heating Serum to 56°C for 60 Minutes

Serum	Concentration of Oxytetracycline	Zone Size
	μg/ml	*mm*
Heated	10	23.5
Unheated	10	24.5
Heated	7.5	21.0
Unheated	7.5	21.0
Heated	5.0	15.5
Unheated	5.0	15.5

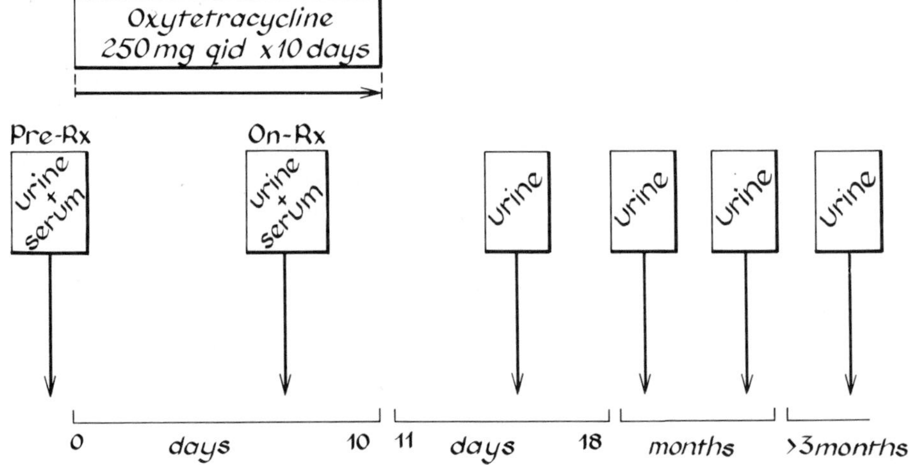

Figure 2.1 Clinical protocol; 33 female patients with bacteriuria.

Table 2.6
Bacterial Species Responsible for Urinary Infection

Genus and Species	Number
Escherichia coli	26
Proteus mirabilis	3
Klebsiella	2
Staphylococcus aureus	1
Escherichia intermedia	1
Total	33

The pretreatment blood serum, the on-treatment serum containing maximal levels of oxytetracycline, and the Millipore-filtered urine obtained at the same time as the on-treatment serum were inoculated with the original infecting organism at concentrations of 500–2000 bacteria/ml of serum or urine. Large inocula (10^5) were avoided, not only because renal tissue infections occur with much smaller numbers of bacteria than grow in the urine, but also because we did not want to handicap the possibility of antibacterial activity in the serum. Subcultures were performed at 0, 6, 24, and 48 hours after inoculation and incubation at 37°C.

All patients were followed with repeat cultures for at least 3 months. Recurrent infections with *E. coli* were serogrouped to distinguish reinfections with the same or different bacteria. The results of these studies were published in late 1974,[16] but are reproduced here in detail. The bacterial species responsible for the 33 urinary infections are listed in Table 2.6.

The original bacterial species causing the bacteriuria was eradicated in 20 of the 33 patients by the oxytetracycline therapy. Not a single serum was inhibitory to the infecting organism, whereas the urine obtained during therapy was bactericidal in 18 of the 20 cures (Table 2.7). Indeed, bacterial growth in the treatment serum was virtually identical in every subculture to growth in the pretreatment serum.

There were 13 patients whose bacteriuria was not eradicated by oxytetracycline therapy. In 8 of the 13 cases the bacteriuria was unresolved because the original infecting organism was resistant to oxytetracycline (minimal inhibitory concentration (MIC)

Table 2.7
Antibacterial Activity of Serum and Urine in 18/20 Cures

Source	Bacteria/ml on Subculture		
	0 Hr	*6 Hr*	*24/48 Hr*
Pretreatment serum	1000	10^4	$>10^5$
On-treatment serum	1200	$>10^4$	$>10^5$
On-treatment urine	1200	320	40/0

Table 2.8
Antibacterial Activity of Serum and Urine in Failures

Source	Bacteria/ml on Subculture		
	0 Hr	*6 Hr*	*24/48 Hr*
Pretreatment serum	1500	10^4	$>10^6$
On-treatment serum	1500	$>10^4$	$>10^6$
On-treatment urine	1200	10^5	$>10^6$

>150 μg/ml), and in all 8 instances the Millipore-filtered urine obtained during therapy supported bacterial growth (Table 2.8). The serums of all 13 failures, as in the 20 cures (Table 2.7), were noninhibitory to the infecting strains. In 5 of the 13 failures, the urine was inhibitory to the original infecting strain and the causes of failure in these 5 cases are very instructive: two patients had renal calculi, one infected with *Klebsiella* (MIC = 2.6 μg/ml) and the other with *Staphylococcus aureus* (MIC = 4.5 μg/ml), and both organisms recurred on the first culture after completion of therapy; a third patient, whose urine became sterile during therapy, was a heavy introital carrier of a nontypable *E. coli* and her bacteriuria recurred by the 5th day after therapy; the remaining two patients in whom the on-treatment urine was inhibitory are examples of unresolved bacteriuria due to chromosomal selection of resistant mutants. In these two examples, an *E. coli* 07 (MIC = 2.2 μg/ml) and a nontypable *E. coli* (MIC = 10 μg/ml) continued in the urine during therapy but their MIC increased to >150 μg/ml; the on-treatment urine was inhibitory (bactericidal) to the pretreatment sensitive strain but was noninhibitory to the on-treatment resistant mutant.

As summarized in Table 2.9, not a single serum was inhibitory to the infecting strain whether the patient was cured or not, while

Table 2.9
Antibacterial Activity of Serum and Urine

Results	Serum Inhibitory	Urine Inhibitory
20 Cures	0/21	18/20
13 Failures	0/13	5/13

18 of 20 urines in the cured cases were inhibitory. As just discussed in detail, the 5 inhibitory urines in the 13 failures are exactly what would be expected and hardly represent exceptions to the general premise that the cure of urinary infections is directly dependent upon urinary concentrations and independent of serum levels. To be sure, if oral antimicrobial agents were available that achieved inhibitory concentrations in the serum as well as in the urine then, theoretically, we would choose such agents, all else being equal. But the facts are that the cure of urinary infections clearly requires inhibitory urinary levels, is actually independent of the serum levels, and recognition of this dependence on urinary concentrations gives the physician access to some very useful antimicrobial agents that would otherwise be excluded from his armamentarium.

I believe there is a now general acceptance of this thesis among practicing members of the medical profession. Unfortunately, some bacteriologists still cling to the historical concept of tissue concentrations in urinary infections. For example, P. Naumann, without presenting any data of his own,[17] strongly criticizes our original 1965 work[12] on the basis that we did not consider spontaneous cure of upper tract infections, and the 1974 oxytetracycline data[16] I have just presented on the basis that fresh human serum enhances the action of tetracycline, an enhancement we could not have detected because we inactivated our sera by heating to 56°C. Not only do these comments seem moot almost to the point of being contrived, but Naumann seems unaware that tetracyclines actually *interfere* with the bactericidal effect of serum *in vivo*,[18] making his criticism even more pointless.

The question of serum versus urinary levels, unfortunately, is a practical one because the policy of sensitivity testing antibacterial agents at concentrations obtainable in serum prevents the physician from using drugs which are effective only at the urinary levels, for example, oral penicillin-G (as a broad spectrum antibiotic) for *Escherichia coli* and *Proteus mirabilis*, or tetracycline for *Pseudomonas*. Until the U.S. Food and Drug Administration allows the manufacture of antimicrobial discs for urinary sensitivity testing, the practicing physician is denied an intelligent selection of these useful drugs for his patients.

Before leaving the subject of serum versus urinary concentrations, the interested reader may find the data in Table 2.10 useful. I have compiled the best data I could find, based on the references cited, on the serum and urine concentrations of 12 antimicrobial agents useful in the treatment of urinary infections. Observe that with a specific dosage regimen, I have listed the peak serum concentration, the percent bound to plasma proteins, and the time required for the serum level to fall to one-half its peak concentration. Because of large variations in urine flow rate during urinary infections (some physicians force fluids, others do not), diurnal variations in urine flow, and often diminished concentrating ability in upper tract infections, it is impractical (if not impossible) to plot standard concentration curves in urine against dosage regimens. The best way to solve this problem is to take the total amount of biologically active drug excreted in the urine during the specific dosage regimens. In order to use these data in terms of urinary concentrations, it is necessary to assume normal renal function and an average urine flow rate of 1200 ml/24 hours. In Table 2.10, the column "Mean (Active) Urine Levels" indicates the average urinary concentration based on the biologically active drug excreted in the presence of normal renal function and a urine flow rate of 1200 ml/24 hours. These data are derived by multiplying the total daily dose by the percent of the dose excreted in the urine in biologically active form and dividing the product in micrograms by 1200 ml.

The available data for urinary concentra-

Table 2.10
Serum and Urinary Antimicrobial Levels in Adults

Antibiotic	Dose	Peak Serum	% Bound to Protein	T ½ Serum Peak	Mean (Active) Urine Levels	Percentage of Dose Excreted in Urine	Percentage of Dose Active in Urine (if Different)
	mg	*μg/ml*		*hr*	*μg/ml*		
Ampicillin[19, 20]	250 p.o. q 6 hr	3 at 2 hr	15	1	350	42	
Carbenicillin[21–23]	764 p.o. q 6 hr	11–17 at 1.5 hr	60	1.2	1000	40	
Cephalexin[24, 25]	250 p.o. q 6 hr	9 at 2 hr	12	0.9	800	98	
Colistin[26, 27]	75 i.m. q 12 hr	1.8 at 4 hr	≃10	2	34	75	50
Gentamicin[28]	1 mg/kg i.m. q 8 hr (200 mg/day)	4 at 1 hr	Negligible	2	125	80	
Kanamycin[29]	500 i.m. q 12 hr	18 at 1 hr	Negligible	2	750	94	
Nalidixic acid[30]	1000 p.o. q 6 hr	34 at 2–3 hr	85	1.5	75	79	5
Nitrofurantoin[31]	100 p.o. q 6 hr	<2		0.3	150	42	
Penicillin-G[32–34]	500 p.o. q 6 hr	1 at 1 hr	60	0.5	300	20	
Sulfamethizole[35, 36]	250 p.o. q 6 hr		98	10	700	95	85
Tetracycline HCl[37, 38]	250 p.o. q 6 hr	2–3 at 4 hr	31	6	500	60	
Trimethoprim/Sulfa-methoxazole[39–41]	160/800 p.o. q 12 hr	1.7/32 at 2 hr	45/66	10/9	150/400	55/50	—/37
Trimethoprim[42]	100 μg p.o. q 12 hr	1.0 at 2–4 hr	45	10	92	55	

tions of trimethoprim (TMP) show considerable variation in the literature.[39, 40, 42] Some of this variation may be explained by the pH dependancy observations of Craig and Kunin[41] who found that acid loading increased the recovery of TMP, probably by ion trapping, while alkali loading decreased the urinary recovery of TMP and increased the amount of nonacetylated sulfamethoxazole (SMX). Thus, in acid urines the ratio of SMX/TMP was about 1.0, but in alkaline urines the ratio was 3.8 to 16.8.

The Reliability of Sensitivity Testing in Determining The Clinical Outcome of Urinary Infections

The basic concept behind *in vitro* sensitivity testing is that determination of the MIC of the infecting organism will be useful in choosing the correct antimicrobial agent and in predicting the outcome of therapy. Because all 33 patients in the oxytetracycline study (Figure 2.1, Tables 2.4–2.9) were prospectively treated on the basis of bacteriuria and without knowledge of the minimal inhibitory concentration (MIC) to oxytetracycline, the clinical course of these patients allows an evaluation of the predictive value of the MIC determination.

First, the clinical characteristics of the 20 patients who were cured and the 13 who failed therapy are documented in Tables 2.11 and 2.12. Except for the observation that the failure group contained no patients with first infections and apparently had less abnormalities on intravenous urography, the differences are not impressive. The MIC data for oxytetracycline to the original infecting strains are presented in Table 2.13. Only 1 of the 20 cures had an MIC of >150 μg/ml and 15 were 3.5 μg/ml or less. As can be seen in Table 2.10, the urinary concentrations of tetracycline (oxytetracycline is about 20% higher) can average 500 μg/ml of urine. The reinfection pattern of these 20 cured patients is shown in Table 2.14.

More can be learned about the MIC data and subsequent bacteriologic course of the 13 failures. Of the 10 who had unresolved bacteriuria during therapy, 8 had bacteria resistant to >150 μg/ml and the other 2 selected resistant mutants within the urinary tract. It is important that 9 of these 10

Table 2.11
The 20 Cures and 13 Failures Compared to Number of Infections in Each Group

Infections	Cures	Failures
1st	7	0
<6	5	6
>6	8	7
Total	20	13

Table 2.12
The 20 Cures and 13 Failures Compared to Abnormalities on Intravenous Urography

Abnormalities	Cures	Failures
None	9	3
Not done	7	4
Renal scars	2	2
Ureteral obstruction	0	2
Renal transplant	1	0
Neurogenic bladder	1	0
Renal calculi	0	2
Total	20	13

Table 2.13
Minimal Inhibitory Concentration (MIC) of Oxytetracycline to Original Infecting Organism

20 Cures
- 15 = 3.5 μg/ml
- 1 = 7 μg/ml
- 1 = 14 μg/ml
- 1 = 90 μg/ml
- 1 = 108 μg/ml
- 1 = >150 μg/ml

13 Failures
- 10 unresolved bacteriuria
  - 8/10 MIC > 150 μg/ml (Before treatment)
  - 2/10 MIC → > 150 μg/ml (On treatment[a])
- 3 sterile on treatment
  - 1/3 MIC >150 μg/ml[b]
  - 1/3 MIC = 2.2 μg/ml[c]
  - 1/3 MIC = 4.5 μg/ml[c]

[a] Patients who selected resistant mutants in the urine during therapy.
[b] The heavy introital carrier who recurred by the 5th day of therapy.
[c] Patients with renal calculi.

patients were cured by further treatment for 10 days with a different antimicrobial agent to which the bacteria were sensitive and which produced a sterile urine on therapy. The single exception was one of the two patients with ureteral obstruction secondary to metastatic carcinoma of the breast whose clinical status required a left nephrostomy and who died 7 months after receiving the oxytetracycline therapy. Of the 3 patients whose urine became sterile during treatment, the two with infected (MIC = 2.2/4.5 μg/ml) renal calculi required surgical removal for cure of their infection; the third patient, the heavy introital carrier who recurred by the 5th day of therapy (MIC >150 μg/ml), was subsequently cured with 10 days of nalidixic acid therapy (follow-up period of 19 months).

It is clear from these studies that sensitivity testing, in the absence of renal calculi and ureteral obstruction, was highly predictive of the clinical outcome. It is also apparent, as emphasized in Chapter 1, that the major cause of unresolved bacteriuria (10/33 patients) is the presence of resistant bacteria to the antimicrobial agent chosen to treat the infection (8/10 patients) and the second most common cause (2/10 patients) is the selection of resistant mutants from among the millions of sensitive bacteria infecting the urinary tract. The therapeutic rate at which resistant mutants are selected during tetracycline treatment of sensitive urinary infections is 2/25 patients, or 8%.

Table 2.14
Bacteriuria Eradicated ("Cured") in 20 Patients

Number	Condition
10	Remained sterile (>3 months)
7	Reinfected with different organism (10–210 days)
2	Reinfected with same organism (92, and 120 days)
1	Changed organism during treatment (*Escherichia coli* → *Proteus mirabilis*)

Methods of Sensitivity Testing

Tube Dilution

Of the three major methods of sensitivity testing—tube dilution, agar dilution, and discs—tube dilution is theoretically the most applicable to *in vivo* conditions. For one thing, the antimicrobial agent is suspended in liquid media, permitting a more uniform concentration of the agent. The effect of serum binding can be controlled by adding serum (though this is rarely done since it is easier to correct for known binding), and, perhaps more importantly, bacteriostatic effects can be differentiated from bactericidal activity in tube dilutions. For the first 7 years at Stanford (1961–1968), we used exclusively the following tube dilution method: a representative series of tubes were prepared containing 0.8 ml of trypticase soy broth and 0.1 ml of an appropriate saline dilution of an antibiotic. After the antibiotic powder was weighed and corrected for base activity, antibiotic dilutions were made so that the final concentrations were 0.2, 1, 5, 10, 20, 50, 100, 250, and 500 μg/ml. These tubes were prepared in large numbers and stored in a freezer. The following antibacterial agents were used in the tube dilutions: penicillin-G (potassium crystalline), streptomycin sulfate, chloramphenicol (Chloromycetin), colistin sodium methane sulfonate (Coly-Mycin), nitrofurantoin sodium (Furadantin), polymyxin-B sodium methane sulfonate (Thiosporin, a derivative of polymyxin-B that was never marketed), oxytetracycline hydrochloride (Terramycin), tetracycline hydrochloride, and neomycin sulfate (Mycifradin).

After isolation and identification of the infecting bacterium, the organism was inoculated into soy broth and grown at 37°C. The tube dilution results were the same whether the soy broth culture was incubated for 6 or 18 hours. A 1:1000 dilution of this incubated culture was made in soy broth if a 6-hour culture was used, and a 1:10,000 dilution if the soy broth culture was 18 hours old; 0.1 ml of this dilution, representing between 10^5 and 10^8 bacteria, was added to each of the 0.9-ml soy broth tubes containing the various antibacterial concentrations. Because either dilution of the inoculum produced a clear solution, all of the final tubes were clear after the addition of the bacteria. The tubes were then incubated for 24 hours at 37°C; turbidity in any tube after 24 hours of incubation indicated bacterial growth and showed that the concentration of antibiotic in that tube was ineffective. The clear tubes, however, presented a problem because the initial inoculum of 10^5 to 10^8 bacteria/ml might be only inhibited rather than killed. For this reason, all clear tubes were subcultured at 24 hours by withdrawing a standard loop containing approximately 0.004 ml of the soy broth and surface streaking it on blood agar. The tubes were further read at 48 hours to see if any clear tube had become cloudy with 24 hours of additional incubation; in such instances, the subculture from the clear tube at 24 hours showed a confluent growth (too numerous to count as individual colonies). Figure 2.2 is representative of a typical tube dilution study of *E. coli* in the presence of penicillin-G. Note that the tube containing 5 μg of penicillin-G/ml inoculated with 10^5 *E. coli*/ml was almost as cloudy as the control soy broth tube containing no penicillin-G. Thus, at 5 μg/ml concentration of penicillin-G, this representative *E. coli* was resistant to penicillin-G. The remainder of the tubes were

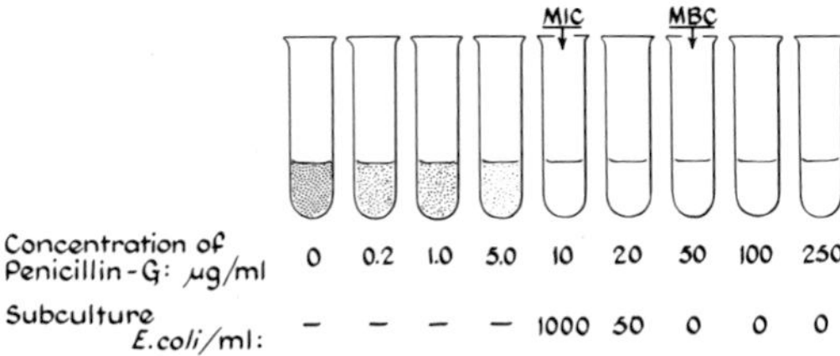

Figure 2.2 A representative tube dilution sensitivity. The minimal inhibitory concentration (*MIC*) and minimal bactericidal concentration (*MBC*) of penicillin-G for an average strain of *Escherichia coli* are illustrated in the figure. Penicillin-G is virtually never inhibitory for *E. coli* at 5 μg/ml but is bactericidal at 100 μg/ml for 80% of strains of *E. coli* (Figures 2.3 and 2.8). In fact, the *MIC* and *MBC* usually occur in the same tube, within the step dilutions illustrated in this figure, for most *E. coli* with penicillin-G (Figures 2.3 and 2.8).

clear, as were all of the tubes, including the control, immediately following inoculation of 10^5 *E. coli*/ml; for this reason, it was necessary to subculture the clear tubes. As seen in Figure 2.2, the 10 and 20 μg/ml tubes contained some viable *E. coli* 18–24 hours after incubation at 37°C. The 10 μg/ml tube—the first tube to remain clear after incubation—is referred to as the minimal inhibitory concentration (MIC) of penicillin-G for the strain of *E. coli* tested. Because the 10 and 20 μg/ml tubes allowed some residual bacteria to survive, these tubes were bacteriostatic only; *i.e.*, these concentrations did not kill all the inoculum. The first tube to show no bacteria on subculture was the one containing 50 μg of penicillin-G/ml; this is called the minimal bactericidal concentration (MBC).

What is the clinical significance of the difference between the MIC and MBC? Most tube dilution data are reported in terms of the MIC, not the MBC; and the other methods of sensitivity testing, both agar dilution and discs, indicate only the MIC. There are no data, to my knowledge, that show a clinical difference in success or failure in treating infections based on the *in vitro* MIC as opposed to the MBC; we had the impression, and I emphasize the word impression, that when the expected urinary levels of a therapeutic regimen were based on MIC concentrations, sterilization of the urine was difficult or even impossible with that particular drug if there was a wide discrepancy between the MIC and MBC concentrations. This is worth further investigation; drugs like chloramphenicol have substantial differences between the first MIC tube and the MBC tube and would be ideal to test this hypothesis. For most drugs, however, and especially for Gram-negative bacilli treated on the basis of urinary concentrations, the MIC end point and the MBC are usually the same tube.

The disadvantages of the tube dilution technique are the expense and the time-consuming manipulations; of some help are recent innovations in tube dilution automation.[43] Although the reproducibility observed in Table 2.15, where tube dilutions are performed on the same bacterium at weekly intervals, is reasonably impressive,

Table 2.15
Reproducibility of the Tube Dilution Technique at Weekly Intervals on the Same *Escherichia coli* Using a 1:1000 Dilution of a 6-hour Broth Culture[a]

April 22, 1963

Drug	Time of Reading	Control	Drug Concentration (μg/ml)								
			0.2	1	5	10	20	50	100	250	500
	hr										
Penicillin	24/48	+	+/+	+/+	+/+	+/+	+/+	+/+	$0/0^{0}_{0}$	$0/0^{0}_{0}$	$0/0^{0}_{0}$
Streptomycin	24/48	+	+/+	+/+	+/+	+/+	+/+	+/+	+/+	+/+	+/+
Chloramphenicol	24/48	+	+/+	+/+	+/+	+/+	+/+	+/+	$0/0^{34}_{34}$	$0/0^{1}_{1}$	$0/0^{0}_{0}$
Coly-Mycin	24/48	+	+/+	$0/+^{C}_{C}$	$0/0^{0}_{0}$	$0/0^{C}_{C}$	$0/0^{0}_{0}$	$0/0^{0}_{0}$	$0/0^{0}_{0}$	$0/0^{0}_{0}$	$0/0^{0}_{0}$
Furadantin	24/48	+	+/+	+/+	+/+	+/+	+/+	+/+	+/+	+/+	$0/0^{0}_{0}$
Polymyxin-B	24/48	+	+/+	+/+	$0/0^{0}_{0}$	$0/0^{0}_{0}$	$0/0^{0}_{0}$	$0/0^{0}_{0}$	$0/0^{0}_{0}$	$0/0^{0}_{0}$	$0/0^{0}_{0}$
Terramycin	24/48	+	+/+	+/+	+/+	+/+	+/+	+/+	+/+	+/+	$0/+^{C}_{C}$
Neomycin	24/48	+	+/+	+/+	+/+	+/+	+/+	$0/0^{0}_{0}$	$0/0^{0}_{0}$	$0/0^{0}_{0}$	$0/0^{0}_{0}$
Tetracycline	24/48	+	+/+	+/+	+/+	+/+	+/+	+/+	+/+	+/+	$0/+^{10}_{10}$

April 29, 1963

	Time of Reading	Control	Drug Concentration (μg/ml)								
			0.2	1	5	10	20	50	100	250	500
	hr										
Penicillin	24/48	+	+/+	+/+	+/+	+/+	+/+	$0/+^{C}_{C}$	$0/0^{0}_{0}$	$0/0^{0}_{0}$	$0/0^{0}_{0}$
Streptomycin	24/48	+	+/+	+/+	+/+	+/+	+/+	+/+	+/+	+/+	+/+
Chloramphenicol	24/48	+	+/+	+/+	+/+	$0/+^{C}_{C}$	$0/0^{20}_{20}$	$0/0^{4}_{4}$	$0/0^{1}_{1}$	$0/0^{0}_{0}$	$0/0^{0}_{0}$
Coly-Mycin	24/48	+	+/+	$0/+^{C}_{C}$	$0/0^{0}_{0}$	$0/0^{0}_{0}$	$0/0^{0}_{0}$	$0/0^{0}_{0}$	$0/0^{0}_{0}$	$0/0^{0}_{0}$	$0/0^{0}_{0}$
Furadantin	24/48	+	+/+	+/+	+/+	+/+	+/+	+/+	+/+	$0/+^{C}_{C}$	$0/0^{0}_{0}$
Polymyxin-B	24/48	+	+/+	+/+	$0/0^{0}_{0}$	$0/0^{0}_{0}$	$0/0^{0}_{0}$	$0/0^{0}_{0}$	$0/0^{0}_{0}$	$0/0^{0}_{0}$	$0/0^{0}_{0}$
Terramycin	24/48	+	+/+	+/+	+/+	+/+	+/+	+/+	+/+	+/+	+/+
Neomycin	24/48	+	+/+	+/+	+/+	+/+	$0/0^{0}_{0}$	$0/0^{0}_{0}$	$0/0^{0}_{0}$	$0/0^{0}_{0}$	$0/0^{0}_{0}$
Tetracycline	24/48	+	+/+	+/+	+/+	+/+	+/+	+/+	+/+	$0/0^{15}_{15}$	$0/0^{0}_{0}$

May 6, 1963

	Time of Reading	Control	Drug Concentration (μg/ml)								
			0.2	1	5	10	20	50	100	250	500
	hr										
Penicillin	24/48	+	+/+	+/+	+/+	+/+	+/+	+/+	$0/0^{6}_{6}$	$0/0^{0}_{0}$	$0/0^{0}_{0}$
Streptomycin	24/48	+	+/+	+/+	+/+	+/+	+/+	+/+	+/+	+/+	+/+
Chloramphenicol	24/48	+	+/+	+/+	+/+	+/+	$0/0^{0}_{0}$	$0/0^{0}_{0}$	$0/0^{0}_{0}$	$0/0^{0}_{0}$	$0/0^{0}_{0}$
Coly-Mycin	24/48	+	+/+	$0/0^{20}_{20}$	$0/0^{0}_{0}$	$0/0^{0}_{0}$	$0/0^{0}_{0}$	$0/0^{0}_{0}$	$0/0^{0}_{0}$	$0/0^{0}_{0}$	$0/0^{0}_{0}$
Furadantin	24/48	+	+/+	+/+	+/+	+/+	+/+	+/+	+/+	+/+	$0/0^{0}_{0}$
Polymyxin-B	24/48	+	+/+	+/+	$0/0^{0}_{0}$	$0/0^{0}_{0}$	$0/0^{0}_{0}$	$0/0^{0}_{0}$	$0/0^{0}_{0}$	$0/0^{0}_{0}$	$0/0^{0}_{0}$
Terramycin	24/48	+	+/+	+/+	+/+	+/+	+/+	+/+	+/+	+/+	+/+
Neomycin	24/48	+	+/+	+/+	+/+	$0/0^{0}_{0}$	$0/0^{0}_{0}$	$0/0^{0}_{0}$	$0/0^{0}_{0}$	$0/0^{0}_{0}$	$0/0^{0}_{0}$
Tetracycline	24/48	+	+/+	+/+	+/+	+/+	+/+	+/+	+/+	$0/+^{C}_{C}$	$0/0^{0}_{0}$

[a] All tubes were clear following the inoculation of 10^{5-8} bacteria/ml before incubation. + = cloudy tube (gross evidence of bacterial growth); 0 = clear tube after incubation. 0/0 indicates the tubes are clear at both 24 and 48 hours of incubation. If tubes are clear at 24 hr (0), a loop subculture is transferred to the appropriate agar to determine presence or absence of bacterial growth. The superscript in the right upper corner indicates the number of bacteria present in the subculture at 24 hr; the number in the right lower corner is a 48-hour reading of the 24-hour subculture. C = confluent growth.

Ericsson's comment that the error of tube dilution ranges between −50 and 150% (±1 tube at two-fold dilutions) is surely correct. The apparent reproducibility in Table 2.15 is somewhat artifactual because the dilution steps are much greater than two-fold (1–5 μg/ml is a five-fold step); indeed, for neomycin and chloramphenicol, reproducibility is clearly poor. Differences in the size of the inoculum influence greatly the MIC and MBC. In Table 2.16, the same *E. coli* used in the weekly studies presented in Table 2.15 was inoculated undiluted into the tube dilutions; there was no bacterial inhibition at any concentration of antimicrobial agent. In Table 2.17 the same *E. coli* were diluted one to a million before inoculation; compared with the 1:1000 dilution in Table 2.15, an additional 1000-fold dilution shifted the MIC and MBC end points to much lower concentrations. A further, but minor, disadvantage to tube dilutions is that broth cultures are more amenable to contamination than agar dilution or disc methods and, unless the cloudy tubes are subcultured, there is no assurance that the growth is produced by the pathogen thought to be inoculated. And, as Er-

Table 2.16
Effect of Using an Undiluted 6-hour Broth Culture on the Tube Dilution Pattern of the Same *Escherichia coli* as in Table 2.15[a]

Drug	Time of Reading	Control	Drug Concentration (μg/ml)								
			0.2	1	5	10	20	50	100	250	500
	hr										
Penicillin	24/48	+	+	+	+	+	+	+	+	+	$\pm/+^{60}_{63}$
Streptomycin	24/48	+	+	+	+	+	+	+	+	+	+
Chloramphenicol	24/48	+	+	+	+	+	+	+	+	+	+
Coly-Mycin	24/48	+	+	+	+	+	+	+	+	+	+
Furadantin	24/48	+	+	+	+	+	+	+	+	+	+
Polymyxin-B	24/48	+	+	+	+	+	+	+	+	+	+
Neomycin	24/48	+	+	+	+	+	+	+	+	+	+
Tetracycline	24/48	+	+	+	+	+	+	+	+	+	+
Terramycin	24/48	+	+	+	+	+	+	+	+	+	+

[a] See footnote to Table 2.15 for explanation of symbols.

Table 2.17
Effect of 1:1,000,000 Dilution[a] of the 6-hour Broth Culture on the Tube Dilution Pattern of the Same *Escherichia* coli as in Table 2.15[b]

Drug	Time of Reading	Control	Drug Concentration (μg/ml)								
			0.2	1	5	10	20	50	100	250	500
	hr										
Penicillin	24/48	+	+/+	+/+	+/+	+/+	+/+	$0/0^{0}_{0}$	$0/0^{0}_{0}$	$0/0^{0}_{0}$	$0/0^{0}_{0}$
Streptomycin	24/48	+	+/+	+/+	+/+	+/+	+/+	+/+	+/+	$0/0^{0}_{0}$	$0/0^{23}_{24}$
Chloramphenicol	24/48	+	+/+	+/+	+/+	$0/0^{0}_{0}$	$0/0^{0}_{0}$	$0/0^{0}_{0}$	$0/0^{0}_{0}$	$0/0^{0}_{0}$	$0/0^{0}_{0}$
Coly-Mycin	24/48	+	+/+	$0/0^{0}_{0}$	$0/0^{0}_{0}$	$0/0^{0}_{0}$	$0/0^{0}_{0}$	$0/0^{0}_{0}$	$0/0^{0}_{0}$	$0/0^{0}_{0}$	$0/0^{0}_{0}$
Furadantin	24/48	+	+/+	+/+	+/+	+/+	+/+	+/+	+/+	$0/+^{C}_{C}$	$0/0^{80}_{C}$
Polymyxin-B	24/48	+	+/+	$0/0^{0}_{0}$	$0/0^{0}_{0}$	$0/0^{0}_{0}$	$0/0^{0}_{0}$	$0/0^{0}_{0}$	$0/0^{0}_{0}$	$0/0^{0}_{0}$	$0/0^{0}_{0}$
Neomycin	24/48	+	+/+	+/+	+/+	$0/0^{0}_{0}$	$0/0^{0}_{0}$	$0/0^{0}_{0}$	$0/0^{0}_{0}$	$0/0^{0}_{0}$	$0/0^{0}_{0}$
Tetracycline	24/48	+	+/+	+/+	+/+	+/+	+/+	+/+	+/+	$0/0^{1}_{1}$	$0/0^{0}_{0}$
Terramycin	24/48	+	+/+	+/+	+/+	+/+	+/+	+/+	+/+	+/+	$0/0^{0}_{0}$

[a] Final inoculum represented 150 *E. coli*/tube.
[b] See footnote to Table 2.15 for explanation of symbols.

icsson pointed out,[4] tube dilution measures the maximal resistance within the bacterial population in the inoculum, but this may be as much of an advantage as a disadvantage.

Figures 2.3–2.7 are representative of our results from the years 1961 to 1964.[12] Interestingly, as we became more involved with the penicillin analogues (sodium ampicillin, penicillin-V, and methicillin), the data in Figures 2.8–2.11 were obtained in the years 1965 to 1967.[34] Eighty percent of *E. coli* causing urinary tract infections on our service were sensitive to penicillin-G at 100 μg/ml in the 1961–1964 period (Figure 2.3); despite a wide spread use of oral penicillin-G on our service, 80% of new strains causing urinary infections were sensitive at the 100-μg level in the years 1965–1967 (Figure 2.8). Not only does this negate resistance as an increasing problem in urinary tract infections treated with penicillin-G, but it shows the reproducibility of the tube dilution method in testing *in vitro* sensitivity 2 years later on a similar population of patients.

The data from tube dilution studies using

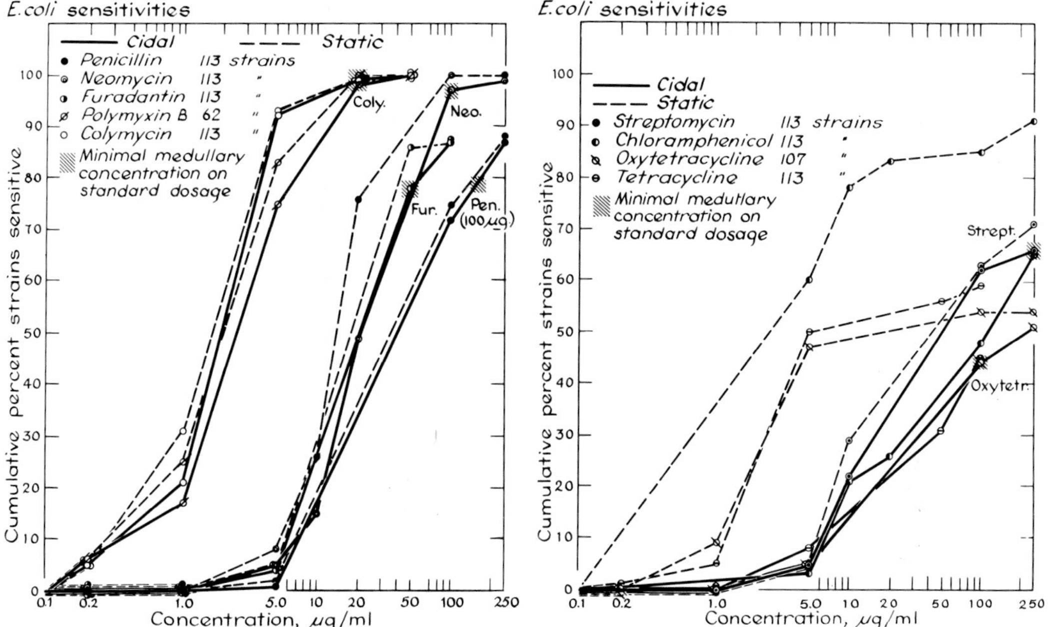

Figure 2.3 Tube dilution sensitivities (minimal inhibitory concentration (MIC) and minimal bactericidal concentration (MBC)) of penicillin-G, neomycin sulfate, nitrofurantoin (Furadantin), polymyxin-B, colistin methane sulfonate (Coly-Mycin), streptomycin sulfate, chloramphenicol, oxytetracycline, and tetracycline for *Escherichia coli.* The percentage of strains sensitive to the various antibiotics is indicated along the vertical axis as a cumulative number. The bacteria were tested at serum and medullary (urinary) concentrations for each antibiotic; these concentrations are indicated on the horizontal axis and are plotted on a semilogarithmic scale to expand the serum concentrations. All concentrations are in micrograms/ml except for penicillin-G, which is in units/ml. Bactericidal activity is indicated by the *solid lines*, bacteriostatic by the *interrupted lines.* The minimal urinary concentration of each antibiotic for adult patients on standard dosage regimens is shown by the *shaded square.* The effectiveness of the various antibacterial agents in the cure of urinary tract infections caused by these specific organisms can be assessed by comparing the *shaded squares.* (Reproduced by permission from T. A. Stamey, D. E. Govan, and J. M. Palmer, Medicine **44:** 1, 1965.[12])

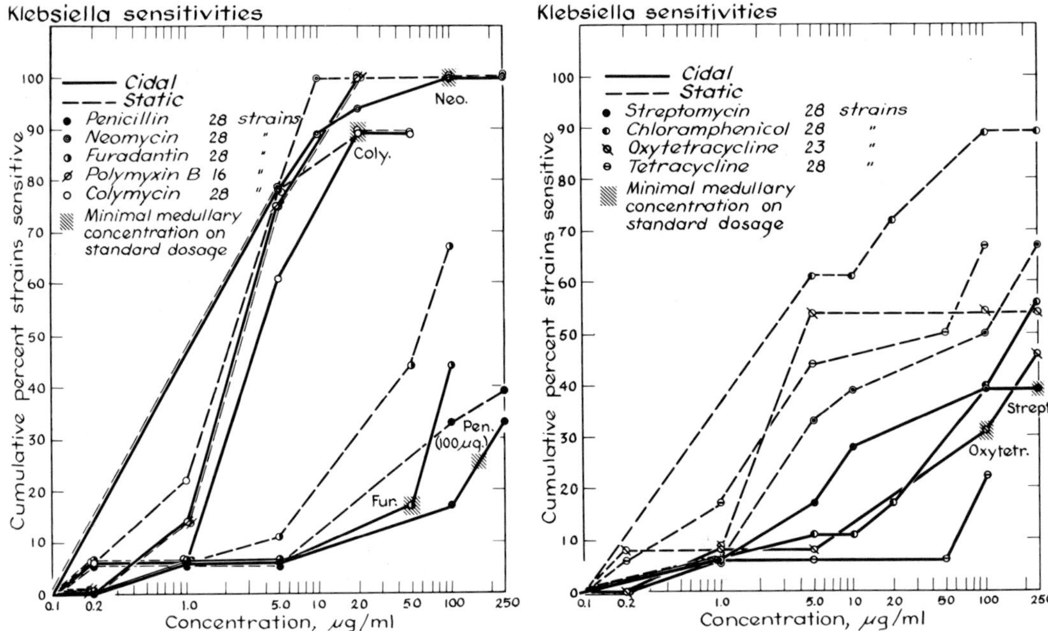

Figure 2.4 Same as Figure 2.3 except that organism is *Klebsiella-Enterobacter* rather than *Escherichia coli.* (Reproduced by permission from T. A. Stamey, D. E. Govan, and J. M. Palmer, Medicine **44:** 1, 1965.[12])

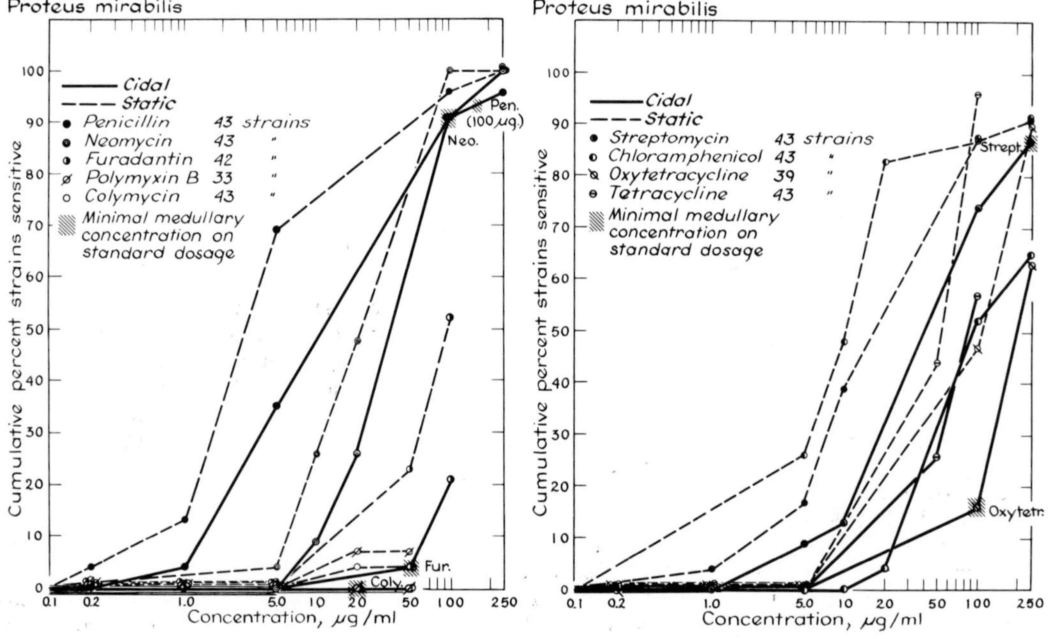

Figure 2.5 Same as Figure 2.3 except that organism is *Proteus mirabilis.* (Reproduced by permission from T. A. Stamey, D. E. Govan, and J. M. Palmer, Medicine **44:** 1, 1965.[12])

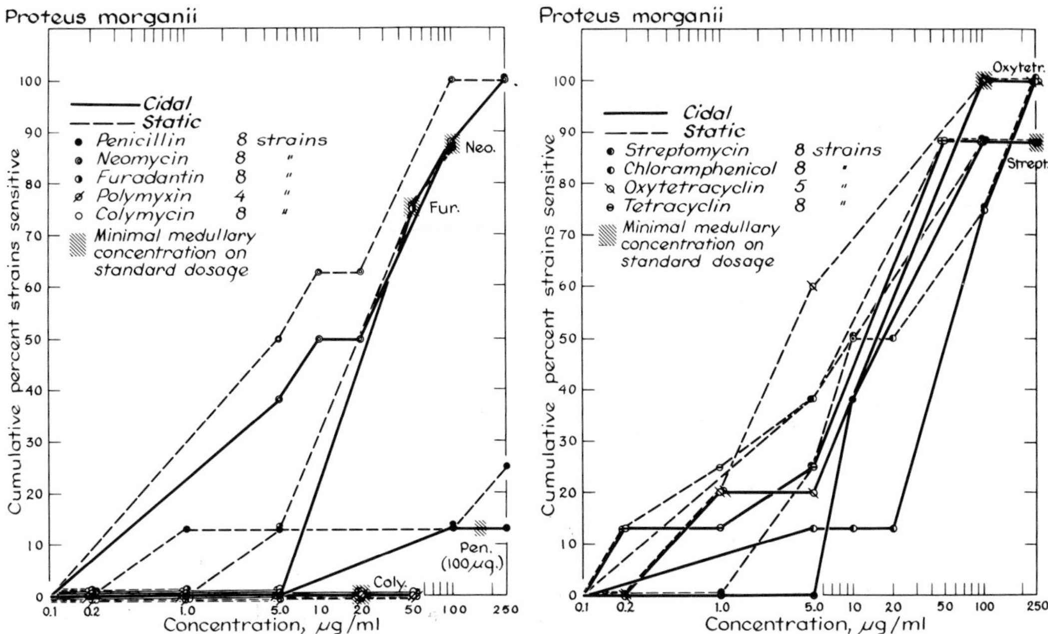

Figure 2.6 Same as Figure 2.3 except that organism is *Proteus morganii.* (Reproduced by permission from T. A. Stamey, D. E. Govan, and J. M. Palmer, Medicine **44:** 1, 1965.[12])

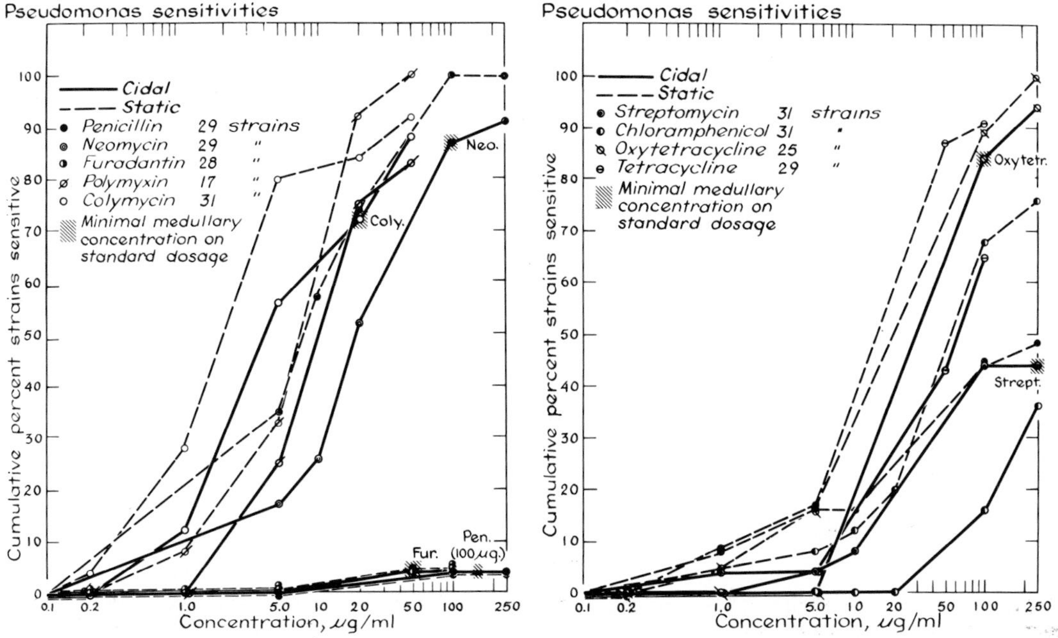

Figure 2.7 Same as Figure 2.3 except that organism is *Pseudomonas.* (Reproduced by permission from T. A. Stamey, D. E. Govan, and J. M. Palmer, Medicine **44:** 1, 1965.[12])

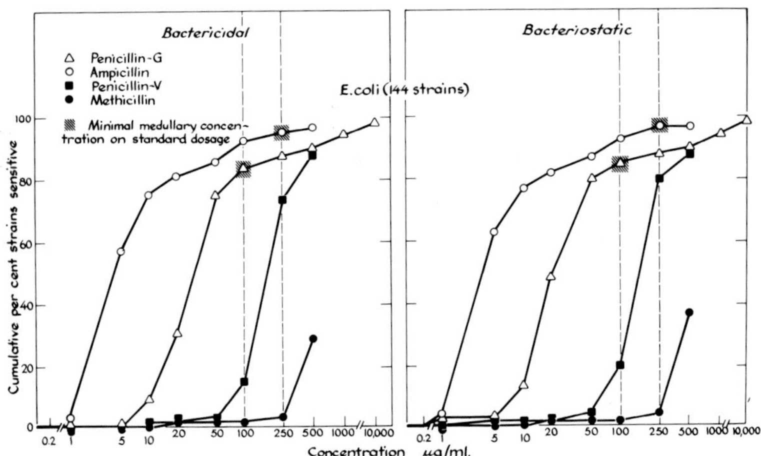

Figure 2.8 Tube dilution sensitivities (minimal inhibitory concentration (MIC) and minimal bactericidal concentration (MBC)) of penicillin-G, ampicillin, penicillin-V, and methicillin for *Escherichia coli*. The cumulative percentage of strains sensitive to the four antibiotics is shown on the vertical scale with the corresponding concentration of antibiotic in$the tube tested on the horizontal. The *left-hand vertical dotted line*, intersecting the *shaded square*, represents the minimal urinary concentration of penicillin-G expected to be present in renal urine; the *right-hand vertical dotted line* represents the minimal urinary concentration for ampicillin. (Reproduced by permission from J. M. Palmer, J. F. Neal, and T. A. Stamey, In Proceedings of 6th International Congress of Chemotherapy, 1969. Vol. 1, Baltimore, University Park Press, 1970, p. 902.[34])

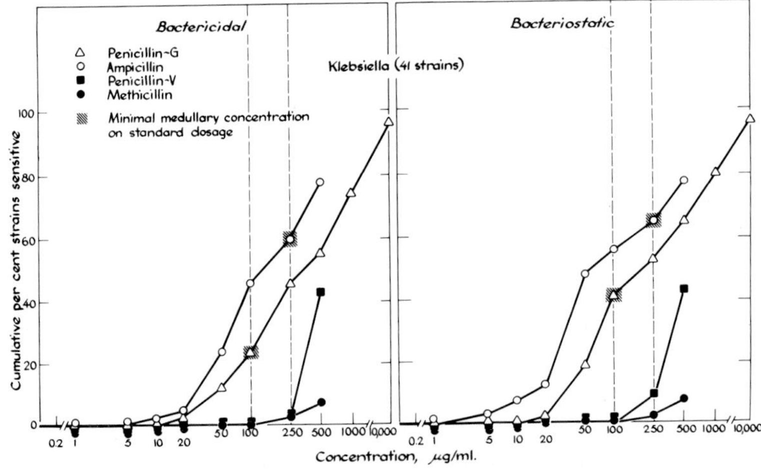

Figure 2.9 Same as Figure 2.8 except that organism is *Klebsiella-Enterobacter*. (Reproduced by permission from J. M. Palmer, J. F. Neal, and T. A. Stamey, In Proceedings of 6th International Congress of Chemotherapy, 1969. Vol. 1, Baltimore, University Park Press, 1970, p. 902.[34])

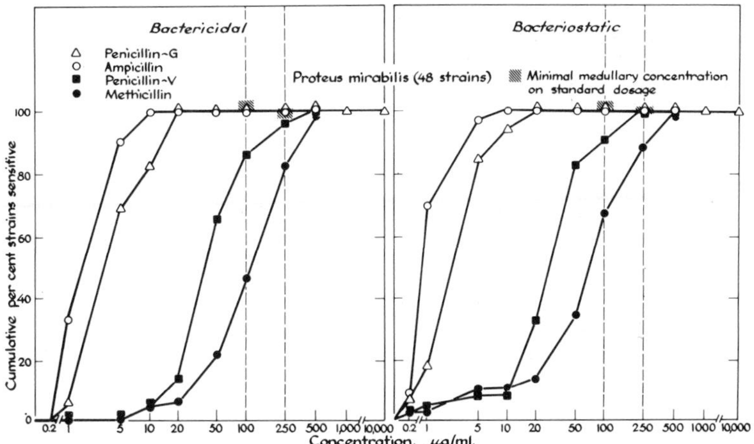

Figure 2.10 Same as Figure 2.8 except that organism is *Proteus mirabilis*. (Reproduced by permission from J. M. Palmer, J. F. Neal, and T. A. Stamey, In Proceedings of 6th International Congress of Chemotherapy, 1969. Vol. 1, Baltimore, University Park Press, 1970, p. 902.[34])

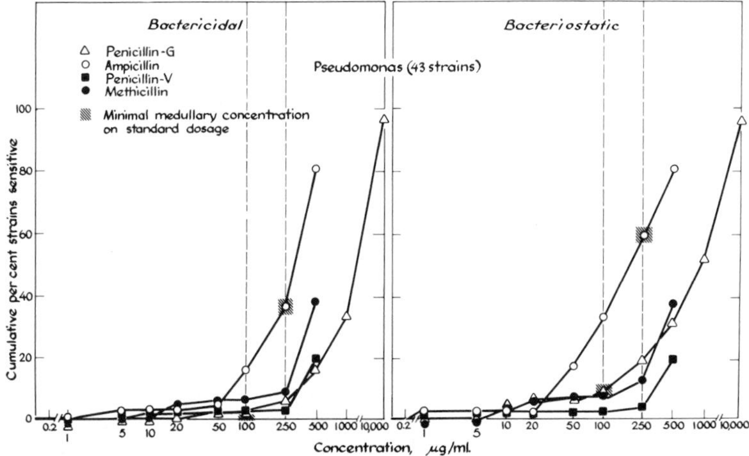

Figure 2.11 Same as Figure 2.8 except that organism is *Pseudomonas*. (Reproduced by permission from J. M. Palmer, J. F. Neal, and T. A. Stamey, In Proceedings of 6th International Congress of Chemotherapy, 1969. Vol. 1, Baltimore, University Park Press, 1970, p. 902.[34])

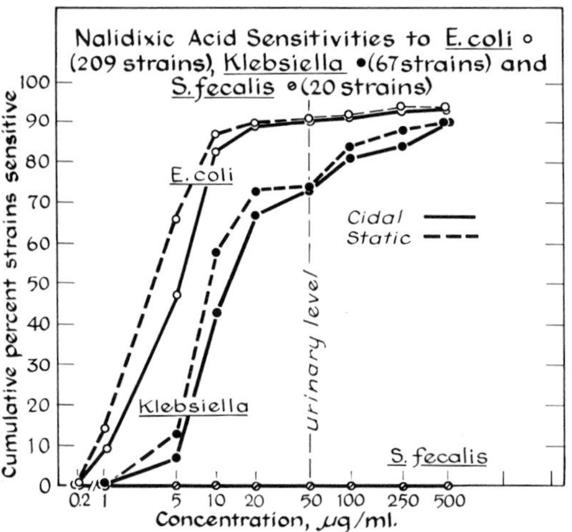

Figure 2.12 Tube dilution sensitivities of 209 strains of *Escherichia coli*, 67 *Klebsiella-Enterobacter* and 20 *Streptococcus faecalis*. (Reproduced by permission from T. A. Stamey, N. J. Nemoy, and M. Higgins, Invest. Urol. **6:** 582, 1969.[44])

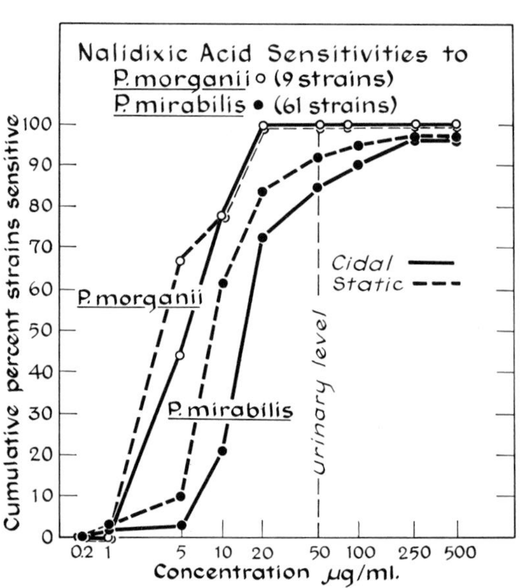

Figure 2.13 Tube dilution sensitivities of 61 strains of *Proteus mirabilis* (indole-negative) and 9 strains of *Proteus morganii* (indole-positive). (Reproduced by permission from T. A. Stamey, N. J. Nemoy, and M. Higgins, Invest. Urol. **6:** 582, 1969.[44])

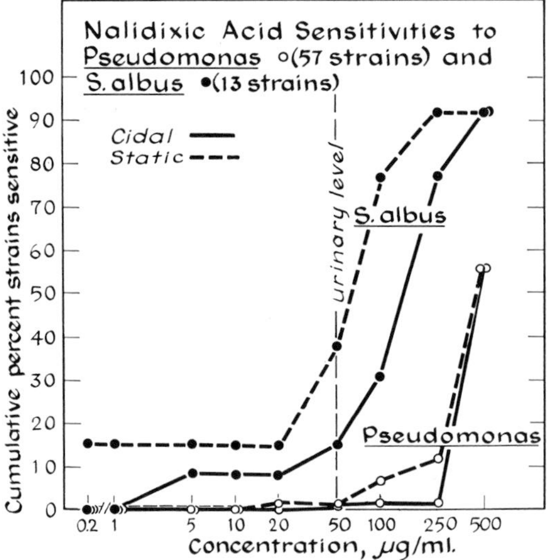

Figure 2.14 Tube dilution, sensitivities of 57 strains of pseudomonas and 13 strains of *Staphylococcus epidermidis*. (Reproduced by permission from T. A. Stamey, N. J. Nemoy, and M. Higgins, Invest. Urol. **6:** 582, 1969.[44])

nalidixic acid are presented in Figures 2.12 to 2.14.[44]

The Micro-Media System of Tube Dilution. Because of the time-consuming expense in standard tube dilution studies, an inexpensive and efficient technique based on prefilled plastic microdilution trays and an 80-pronged inoculator lid is now marketed and carries FDA approval (Micro-Media Systems, Inc., 1435 Kall Circle, San Jose, California 95112). Each set contains a seed trough (an empty lid) into which the diluted bacteria are poured in a specific volume, an 80-pronged "replicating" transfer lid, and the prefilled microdilution tray that contains the antimicrobial agent in frozen nutrient medium. The microdilution trays are thawed at room temperature and the bacterial inoculum diluted and poured into the seed trough. As seen in Figure 2.15, the 80-pronged transfer lid is dipped into the seed trough, lifted free, and the 80 prongs—containing about 10^5 bacteria/prong—are lowered into the 80 wells for inoculation. After overnight incubation, the microdilution trays are read through a

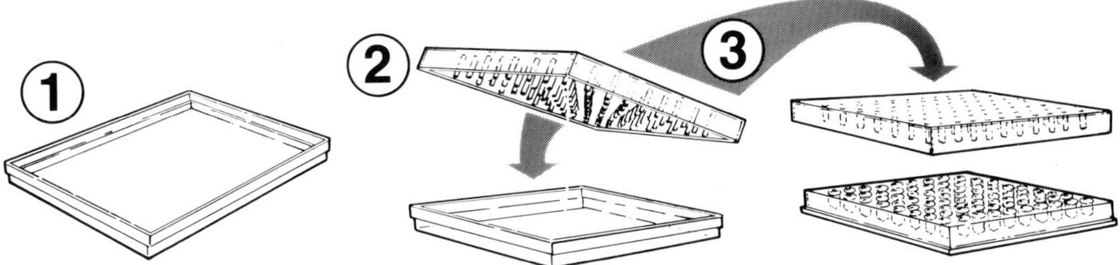

Figure 2.15 The seed trough is filled with the diluted bacteria to be tested for sensitivities. The 80-pronged transfer lid is dipped into the seed trough, lifted free, and transferred into the 80 wells of the test panel, thereby inoculating all antimicrobial agents and biochemicals simultaneously.

mask in a back-lighted viewer that indicates the antibacterial agent and concentration in each row. Various combinations of antimicrobial agents at both serum and urine levels as well as biochemical wells for species identification (biotyping) are available for both Gram-positive and Gram-negative bacteria. The one for Enterobacteriaceae at both serum and urine concentrations is most useful for urinary infections (Figure 2.16). The system has been studied well by experts in the field[45] and, surprisingly, hospital bacteriologic technicians find the technique simpler and faster than the standard Kirby-Bauer method which reports bacteria only as sensitive, intermediate, or resistant.

The Choice of Specific *In Vitro* Concentrations of Antimicrobial Agents for Urinary Sensitivity Testing. When cost, convenience, and other factors dictate that the number of tube dilutions be limited—rather than continuous dilutions from low to high concentrations as in Figures 2.3–2.14—what specific concentrations should be used for *in vitro* sensitivity testing at urinary levels? For example, let's take penicillin-G which has a mean urinary concentration of 300 μg/ml if the patient is on a regimen of 500 mg every 6 hours. I propose that the three tube dilutions be 128 μg/ml (about ½ the mean level, allowing for convenient dilutions), 32 μg/ml (1/10th the mean), and 16 μg/ml (1/20th the mean). If the MIC is 128 μg/ml (the 16 and 32 μg/ml tubes are turbid from bacterial growth), the MIC of the infecting strain will be exceeded at least two-fold by the mean urinary level and probably 2–5 times by the peak urine level if the patient is not forcing fluids. At this MIC of 128 μg/ml, there is a reasonable chance of sterilizing the urine. But, as will be discussed in the last section on Bacterial Resistance in this chapter, the MIC of the infecting strain should ideally be exceeded by at least 10-fold, and concentrations of penicillin-G 20 to 100 times the MIC would be even better in reducing the chances of selecting resistant clones.

For these reasons, the second highest concentration in urinary tube dilutions should be 10 times less than the average urinary level. Continuing the same example of penicillin-G, if 300 μg/ml is the mean urinary level, 32 μg/ml would be the second highest tube (32 μg/ml is the most convenient dilution close to 1/10th of the 300 μg/ml). If the infecting strain now has an MIC of 32 μg/ml (both the 128 and the 32 μg/ml tubes were clear on incubation with the infecting strain), then therapy with oral penicillin-G has an even better chance of sterilizing the urine without selecting resistant clones.

Now, what about a third tube that would be 20 times less than the mean urinary concentration of penicillin-G? One-twentieth of 300 μg/ml is 15 μg/ml, which is

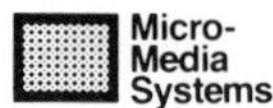

MIC TEST PANEL

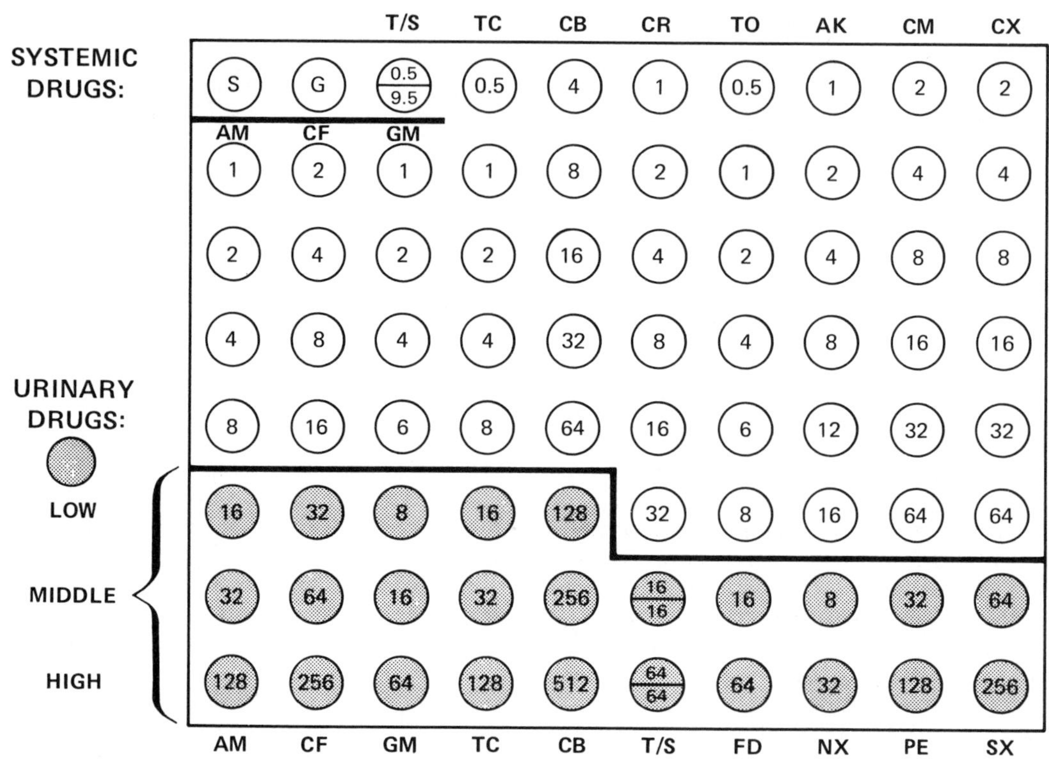

Figure 2.16 Layout of antimicrobial concentrations to encompass both serum and urinary concentrations. The urinary concentrations are the same as in Table 2.18; the reader should consult the text for the reasons for selecting these concentrations. *T/S* = trimethoprim-sulfamethoxizole, *TC* = tetracycline, *CB* = carbenicillin, *CR* = chloramphenicol, *TO* = tobramycin, *AK* = amikacin, CM = cefamandole, *CX* = cefoxitin, *AM* = ampicillin, *CF* = cephalothin, GM = gentamicin, *FD* = nitrofurantoin, *NX* = nalidixic acid, *PE* = penicillin-G, and *SX* = sulfisoxazole.

technically an inconvenient dilution, but a 16 μg/ml tube is about 19 times less than the mean urinary concentration. From Figure 2.3 and 2.8, however, observe that 16 μg/ml of penicillin-G is bacteriostatic (MIC) to only about 25–30% of all strains of *E. coli* (5 μg/ml is ineffective against all strains). Thus, when the general sensitivity pattern of infecting strains is considered, one can sometimes make an argument for omitting the lowest tube (1/20th the average urinary level) of the proposed three-tier urinary tube dilution system. In the case of penicillin-G, however, I believe the 16 μg/ml tube is worthwhile; the physician would recognize that the MIC of 25–30% of all *E. coli* would be exceeded 19 times by penicillin-G and virtually exclude the selection of resistant mutants. One can, moreover, see the immediate advantage of combining a serum level tube dilution with these selected urinary concentrations in the same dilution tray as illustrated in Figure 2.16. This combination will often allow recognition of a MIC within the serum dilution tubes, especially the highest serum tube; in such instances, the average urinary concentration may exceed the MIC of the infecting strain by 100 or more times, as in the case of gentamicin. As the reader will recognize, however, the inclusion of penicillin-G serum level tubes offers no advantage for Enterobacteriaceae.

In Table 2.18, I have taken the antimicrobial agent, dosage, and mean urinary concentration values from Table 2.10 and suggested a convenient high tube dilution equal to one-half the mean urinary antimi-

Table 2.18
Urinary Sensitivity Testing

Antimicrobial Agent and Dosage	Mean Urinary Concentration[a]	Suggested Tube Dilution Concentrations			80% Sensitivity[b]		
		High	Middle (1/10)	Low (1/20)	*Escherichia coli*	*Proteus mirabilis*	*Klebsiella*
mg	*μg/ml/24 hr*		*μg/ml*		*Minimal inhibitory concentration (μg/ml)*		
Ampicillin 250 mg q 6 hr	350	128	32	16	64	8	500
Carbenicillin 2 tabs (764 mg) q 6 hr	1000	512	128	64	64	4	>256
Cephalexin 250 mg q 6 hr	800	256	64	32	32	16	16
Colistin 75 mg q 12 hr	35	16	4	2	2	>256	4
Gentamicin 1 mg/kilo/8 hr 200 mg/day	125	64	16	8	4	8	2
Kanamycin 500 mg q 12 hr	750	256	64	32	32	32	8
Nalidixic Acid 1.0 gm q 6 hr	75	32	8	4(?)[c]	10	32	32
Nitrofurantoin 100 mg q 6 hr	150	64	16	8(?)[c]	64	>128	>128
Penicillin-G 500 mg q 6 hr	300	128	32	16(?)[c]	64	8	1000
Sulfamethizole 250 mg q 6 hr	700	256	64	32[d]	64	128	128
Tetracycline: HCl 250 mg q 6 hr	500	128	32	16	64	64	8
Trimethoprim sulfamethoxazole 160/180 mg q 12 hr	150/150	64/64	16/16	8/8	0.5/0.5	0.5/0.5	0.5/0.5[e]
Trimethoprim 100 mg q 12 hr	90	32	8	4	2	4	6

[a] Based on dosage given, normal renal function in a 70-kg adult, and 1200 ml/day of urine output. Mean urinary concentrations are rounded off to nearest 10, 25, or 50 μg at levels of <100, <1000, or >1000 μg/ml.

[b] Approximate minimal inhibitory concentration (MIC) at which 80% of strains are inhibited. Will vary with domicilliary or hospital infections. Data obtained primarily from Cleveland Clinic Microdilution Antimicrobial Data (1971–1974) and our Stanford Tube Dilution data (Figures 2.3–2.14). Small variations should not be taken seriously; these are approximations.

[c] For nalidixic acid, nitrofurantoin, and penicillin-G, (?) indicates that these lowest concentrations for tube dilutions (1/20 of the mean urinary concentration) may or may not be useful, depending on whether it is helpful to detect the 50% of *E. coli* (nalidixic acid, Figure 2.12), 40% of *E. coli* (nitrofurantoin, Figure 2.3) or 27% of *E. coli* (penicillin-G, Figure 2.3) inhibited by these lower concentrations.

[d] Data taken from tube dilutions of sulfamethizole performed in urine (Reproduced by permission from T. A. Stamey, Urinary Infections, Baltimore, Williams & Wilkins, 1972, p. 281[35]).

[e] *In vitro*, inhibits 98% of all three species (Reproduced by permission from S. R. M. Bushby, J. Infec. Dis., **128:** S442, 1973).

crobial concentration, followed by tube dilutions that will allow MIC readings whereby the mean urinary concentration exceeds the MIC by 10 times (middle tube) and by 20 times (lowest tube). In the right hand columns, I have tried to estimate the antimicrobial concentrations that will be inhibitory for 80% of *E. coli*, *P. mirabilis*, and *Klebsiella*. With these MIC sensitivity data, the physician can make an intelligent decision as to whether or not the lowest of the three tube dilutions is worthwhile. When the 80% sensitivity level is less than the lowest suggested urinary tube dilution ($^1/_{20}$ the mean urinary concentration), the low level tube should certainly be included because the physician will know that when the MIC falls within this tube, he has the best of all chances for successful therapy and avoidance of resistant mutants. When, however, the 80% sensitivity level exceeds the low level tube, he should carefully consult the tube dilution pattern (the cumulative percent sensitivity at increasing concentrations as in Figures 2.3–2.14) in order to decide whether the percentage of bacterial strains likely to have a MIC at the lower tube level warrants inclusion of this tube for urinary sensitivity testing. The urinary tube dilution concentrations selected by Micro-Media in Figure 2.16 were taken from Table 2.18. Hence, this system exactly reflects the considerations presented here. Note that carbenicillin appears different but is not because the 64 μg/ml level is included as the high serum concentration, thereby allowing selection of MICs at the 64, 128, and 512 concentrations. Also observe in Figure 2.16 that if TMP/SMX is to be combined in MIC studies (and a good argument can be made for separating them and using the concentrations in Table 2.18), the urinary concentration ratios of TMP/SMX are 1:1 in the urine but 1:19 in the serum. As already discussed, a 1:1 ratio for normally acid urine is approximately correct.[41]

Agar Dilutions

Agar dilutions are similar to tube dilutions except that the antimicrobial agent is poured directly into the liquid agar before solidification. The bacteria are then inoculated onto the surface of the plate. Visible colonies after 18–24 hours of incubation mean that the specific concentration of drug in the agar was not inhibitory; failure of colony growth indicates an inhibitory concentration. By convention, if only one or two colonies are visible on the surface streak, when hundreds were inoculated, that particular agar dilution is considered the MIC end point. Agar dilution plates are reported only as MICs. Theoretically, the MBC could be determined by subculturing the area of the bacterial streak to see if the inoculum was killed after incubation, rather than inhibited, but in practice this is not done.

In general, if agar dilution MICs are compared to broth dilution MICs, either they are the same or the broth dilution MIC is higher by one dilution step.[46] With tetracycline, however, greater chelation of the antibiotic occurs in agar than in broth, and therefore broth MICs are usually lower than those in agar.

Disc Methods

Ericsson Quantitative Disc Technique. The factors determining the size of antibiotic inhibition zones in agar media were established and described by Cooper, Linton, and Sehgal[47] in a series of papers between 1946 and 1958. In 1951, Lund *et al.*[48] made a valiant attempt to correlate the size of the inhibition zone surrounding antibiotic discs of known content with the MIC by a broth dilution method. But it remained for Ericsson in 1954 and 1960 to show that under certain conditions to be discussed, the inhibition zone surrounding an antibiotic disc is proportional to the MIC of the antimicrobial agent as determined by agar dilution.[49–51]

The reason antibiotic discs can be quantitated is that most drugs, when placed on an absorbent filter paper in good contact with the agar surface, establish a linear concentration gradient as they diffuse from the center of the discs to some peripheral point in the agar. Thus, the concentration in the agar will be highest near the disc and dissipate in the periphery. Bacteria, on the

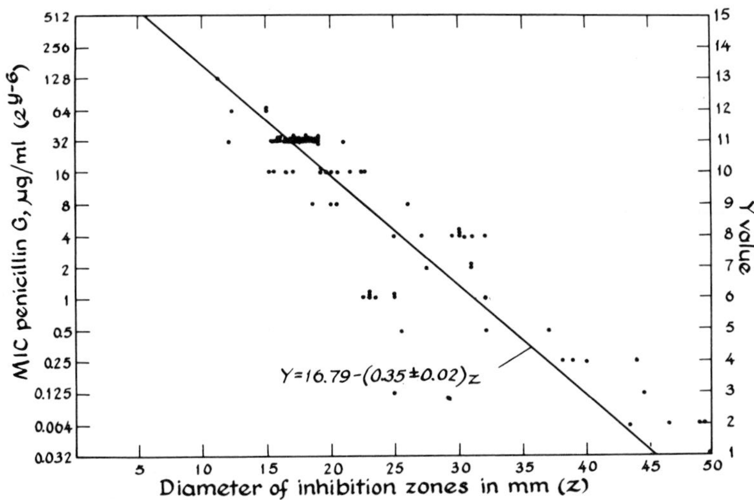

Figure 2.17 The minimal inhibitory concentration (MIC) of penicillin-G (vertical axis), as determined by agar dilution for 93 strains of bacteria, is compared to the inhibition zone diameters of a 100 µg disc of penicillin-G (horizontal axis). The computer-derived regression line (described in the text) fits the experimental points.

surface or in the agar, will be presented with a continuous gradient of increasing concentration, similar to minutely spaced antibiotic agar dilutions; the outer edge of the zone of inhibition represents that concentration at which the bacteria would be inhibited if that same antibiotic concentration were distributed uniformly in an agar dilution pour plate. But since the actual concentration at the point (outer zone edge) of gradient inhibition (the MIC) is unknown and is difficult to determine mathematically because of diffusion complexities (although Schlesinger,[52] using Lund's method[48] and Cooper's derivations,[47] came close), Ericsson[49-51] determined the concentration (the MIC) indirectly by simultaneously performing antibiotic agar dilution pour plates. If this is done for large numbers of bacteria of varying sensitivity, a reasonably straight line can be obtained and a regression slope calculated (Figure 2.17 (penicillin-G) and Figure 2.18 (oxytetracycline)).

Some antibiotics are more suitable for quantitating the inhibitory zone around the disc than others. For example, the polymyxins (Figure 2.19) diffuse so poorly that the concentration gradient from the center of the disc to the periphery decreases very little, yielding too small a gradient to differentiate bacteria of varying sensitivities (at least within the ± 1-mm error of measuring inhibitory zones). The concentration of antibiotic surrounding each disc varies with the amount of drug in the disc, the solubility and other physicochemical properties of the antibiotic, as well as the depth, concentration, chemical composition, and permeability of the agar.* Because of the different diffusion characteristics of each antibiotic, widely different zone sizes surrounding two different antibiotic discs of similar content may not indicate a difference in sensitivity. Each antimicrobial agent has its own characteristic regression curve (Figs. 2.19 and 2.20).

But the physical chemistry of difusion concentration gradients of each antibiotic is only one determinant of zone size.

* An important concept, as emphasized by Ericsson, is that one should never refer to the amount of antibiotic in a disc as "the concentration/disc." To do so is to misunderstand the principle of gradient diffusion. The concentration of drug in the agar adjacent to the disc may be greater/ml than the total content of the disc. Indeed, it is for this reason that a 30-µg antibiotic disc can be used to determine that a bacterial strain is sensitive to 100 µg of the antibiotic/ml.

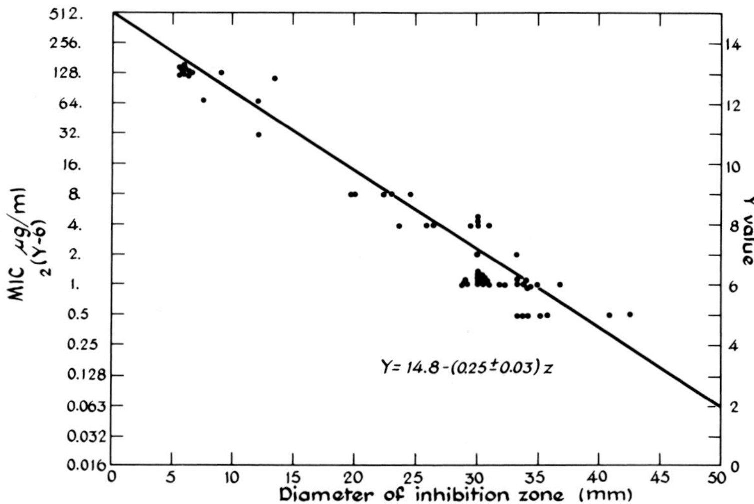

Figure 2.18 The minimal inhibitory concentration (MIC) of oxytetracycline (vertical axis), as determined by agar dilution for 58 strains of bacteria, is compared to the inhibition zone diameters of a 100 µg disc of oxytetracycline (horizontal axis). The computer-derived regression line (described in the text) fits the experimental points.

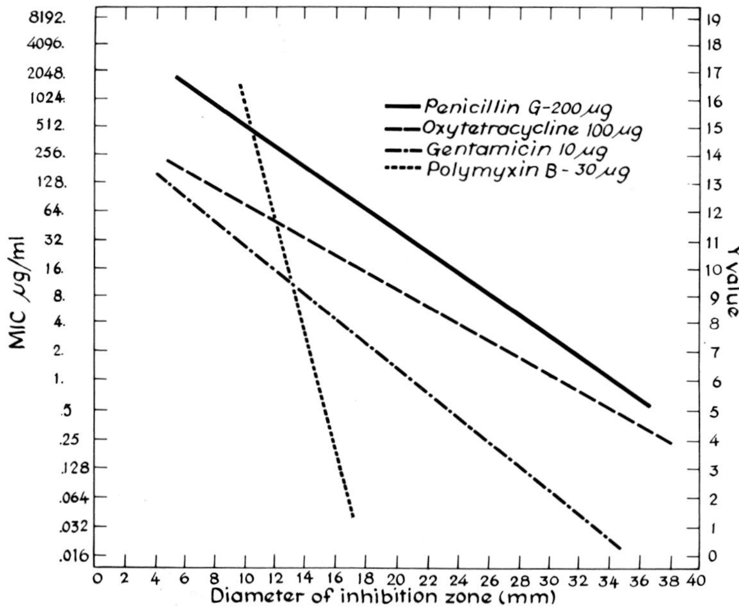

Figure 2.19 Regression lines for minimal inhibitory concentration and inhibitory zone diameter for *penicillin-G* (200 µg), *oxytetracycline* (100 µg), *gentamicin* (10 µg), and *polymyxin B* sulfate (30 µg).

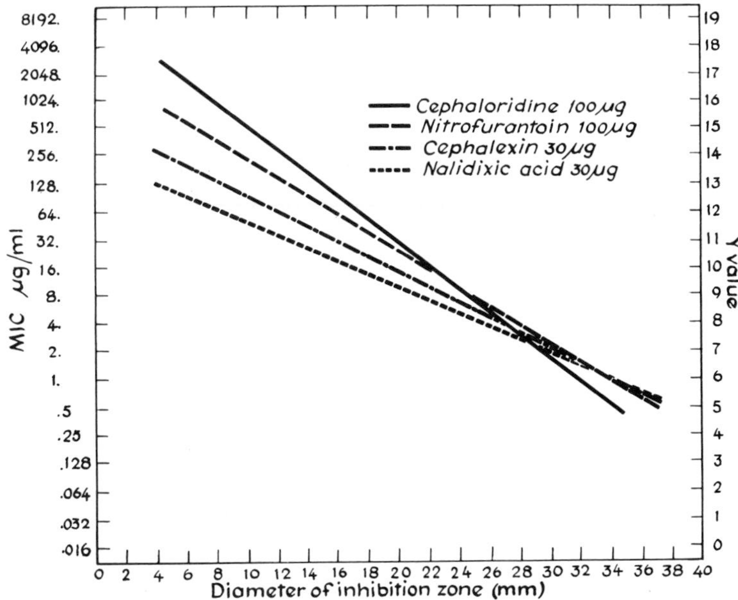

Figure 2.20 Regression lines for minimal inhibitory concentration and inhibitory zone diameter for *cephaloridine* (100 µg), *nitrofurantoin* (100 µg), *cephalexin* (30 µg), and *nalidixic acid* (30 µg).

Cooper[47] showed that the effect of an antibiotic on bacteria is a function of not only the concentration of the antibiotic but also the density and metabolic activity of the organisms. For example, he found that a substantial increase in antibiotic concentration did not inhibit the bacteria once the population had reached a certain critical density; the time required by bacteria to reach this critical density, called the critical time, was found to be approximately equal to the lag phase plus three or four generation cycles. Since the lag phase for most bacteria is about 60 minutes, and the generation time between 20 and 40 minutes, the antibiotic concentration must be established in the agar within 3 or 4 hours of the start of the bacterial growth. Because bacteria differ in their lag phase, Ericsson relied on 3 hours of prediffusion whereby the discs were allowed to remain on the agar at room temperature before placing the plates in the incubator for maximal bacterial growth. The workshop group of the World Health Organization (WHO), of which Ericsson was chairman, decided on 30 minutes of prediffusion, for practical rather than theoretical reasons. They also decided to use Mueller-Hinton agar for sensitivity testing, a decision that offers a chance to standardize disc testing.[46]

From the many variables studied by Ericsson that influence the zone size, such as glucose content, agar depth, pH, etc., all can be standardized by using Mueller-Hinton agar poured to a reasonably constant depth of about 4 mm. Since most antimicrobial agents will establish their gradients in agar well before the critical time of 3 or 4 hours after incubation, preincubation is not terribly important, but it should be controlled. Because a large inoculum reaches the critical density sooner than a small inoculum, the most important variable in determining zone diameters is the size of the inoculum; it must be constantly watched. We use Ericsson's method of plate flooding for inoculation because it allows us to pick 10 colonies from our initial culture plates and begin the sensitivity at once, without growing the bacteria in broth. His technique gives a reproducible inoculum of

Table 2.19
Disc Content and Regression Equations for Determining the MIC of Eight Antimicrobial Agents

For each antimicrobial agent and disc content, the regression equation relating minimal inhibitory concentration and zone diameter is given. In this equation, Y is a function of the minimal inhibitory concentration (MIC), related by the formula MIC = $2(Y - 6)$; z is the zone diameter in millimeters. The MIC and zone diameter relationships for relatively resistant bacteria ($z = 10$ mm) and highly sensitive bacteria (MIC = 1 μg/ml) are given for comparison with the urinary and serum levels of each antibacterial agent when administered as a specific regimen. The number of bacteria used to establish each regression line is shown. For those who do not wish to use the regression equation to calculate the MIC or draw the regression line, the same line can be drawn as follows. Select 5 cycle X 70 division semilogarithmic paper and use the vertical logarithmic axis for MIC values and the horizontal linear axis for zone diameter. The practical range for these scales covers the region from 0.01 μg/ml to 1000 μg/ml on the vertical and 0 to 35 mm zone diameter on the horizontal axis. Plot the MIC value at 10 mm and the zone diameter at 1 μg/ml MIC; join the two points by a straight line from one end of the paper to the other. Thus, for a given zone diameter selected on the horizontal axis, the MIC can be found on the vertical axis of the logarithmic scale. Difco Mueller-Hinton agar was used for all studies.

Antimicrobial Agent	Disc Content	Number of Bacteria Tested	Regression Equation	MIC at Zone Diameter of 10 mm	Zone Diameter at MIC of 1 μg/ml	Suggested Guidelines for Serum and Urine Concentration in Adults with Normal Renal Function and Standard Dosage Regimens		
						Dosage	Peak serum concentration	Urine concentration
	μg			*μ/ml*	*mm*		*μg/ml*	
Gentamicin	10[a, b]	63	$Y = 15.3 - (0.43 \pm 0.02)z$	32	21.5	1.0 mg/kg i.m. q 8 hr	4	125
	20	68	$Y = 15.3 - (0.41 \pm 0.02)z$	36.5	22.5			
	40	68	$Y = 17.25 - (0.47 \pm 0.02)z$	93.5	24			
	200	68	$Y = 23.3 - (0.59 \pm 0.032)z$	>100	29.5			
Nalidixic acid	15	85	$Y = 13 - (0.23 \pm 0.049)z$	26	30.5	1000 mg p.o. q 6 hr	20–50 (85% bound to serum albumin)	75
	30[a, b]	87	$Y = 14.2 - (0.24 \pm 0.03)z$	55.5	34			
	60	87	$Y = 15 - (0.27 \pm 0.02)z$	79	33.5			
Oxytetracycline	50	58	$Y = 13.25 - (0.26 \pm 0.04)z$	25	28	250 mg p.o. q 6 hr	2–3	500
	100†	58	$Y = 14.8 - (0.25 \pm 0.03)z$	79	35			
Nitrofurantoin	30	64	$Y = 16.24 - (0.30 \pm 0.05)z$	151	34	100 mg p.o. q 6 hr	<2	150
	100[a, b]	64	$Y = 17 - (0.32 \pm 0.02)z$	223	34			
	200	64	$Y = 18.15 - (0.32 \pm 0.03)z$	494.5	38			
Penicillin-G	12[a]	93	$Y = 13.91 - (0.37 \pm 0.058)z$	18.5	21	250 mg p.o. q 6 hr	0.5	150
	50	93	$Y = 14.82 - (0.31 \pm 0.02)z$	53	28.5			
	100	93	$Y = 16.79 - (0.35 \pm 0.02)z$	156.5	31	500 mg p.o. q 6 hr	1.0	300
	200[b]	93	$Y = 18.68 - (0.37 \pm 0.02)z$	505	34			

Colistin sulfate	10	66	$Y = 30.4 - (2 \pm 0.001)z$	21	12	Colymycin	1–2	34
	30[a–c]	66	$Y = 36.8 - (2.09 \pm 0.02)z$	955	15	75 mg		
	100	66	$Y = 34.95 - (1.78 \pm 0.001)z$	>1000	16	i.m. q 12 hr		
	250	66	$Y = 42.05 - (1.91 \pm 0.25)z$	>1000	19			
Cephaloridine	30[a]	92	$Y = 15.25 - (0.34 \pm 0.019)z$	57.5	27	1000 mg	20–30	1600
	100[b]	92	$Y = 19.1 - (0.41 \pm 0.05)z$	512	32	i.m. q 8 hr		
	200	92	$Y = 18.8 - (0.37 \pm 0.03)z$	548	34.5			
	400	92	$Y = 19.78 - (0.38 \pm 0.029)z$	1009	36			
Cephalexin	30[b]	57	$Y = 15.5 - (0.28 \pm 0.03)z$	104	34	250 mg	9	800
	100	57	$Y = 17 - (0.28 \pm 0.046)z$	294	39	p.o. q 6 hr		

[a] Available commercially.

[b] Disc contents used in our laboratory for determining MIC.

[c] Colisitin sulfate, polymyxin-B sulfate, and colistin methane sulfonate discs of 30 μg content all showed identical zones of inhibition against Gram-negative organisms. Only polymyxin-B sulfate is available commercially as the 30 μg disc. For the regression curve, colistin sulfate was used in the agar dilutions.

"dense, but not confluent" colonies, and the correctness of this inoculum is easy to judge after incubation. For Gram-negative urinary pathogens, 10 colonies are collected with a platinum loop from the culture plates and emulsified in 1 ml of lactated Ringer's solution. One drop of this suspension is added to 5 ml of lactated Ringer's solution, and 1 drop of the 5-ml suspension is placed in a second 5 ml of lactated Ringer's solution. This latter 5-ml suspension is poured over the surface of a 15-cm Petri plate containing Mueller-Hinton agar poured to a depth of about 4 mm. The plate is then tipped in various directions until the inoculum covers the entire surface; the excess fluid is suctioned off by sharply slanting the Petri plate to one side, rotating the plate during suctioning. After the inoculated plate is dried for 30 minutes at room temperature, the discs are firmly applied to the surface of the agar with sterile forceps. The plates are allowed to stand at room temperature for another 30 minutes (prediffusion) before incubation at 37°C for 18–24 hours. The zone diameters are measured after incubation to the nearest 1 mm by using sliding calipers applied to the bottom surface of the Petri plate.

Using 30 minutes prediffusion, Mueller-Hinton agar, and dense but not confluent inocula, we have established regression curves for several clinically useful antimicrobial agents, as illustrated in Figures 2.17–2.20. Each regression curve is based on the simultaneous determination of zone size to a specific antibiotic disc content and the MIC of the same antibiotic in two-fold agar dilution plates; 57–93 different species of bacteria, providing a wide range of varying sensitivity, were used to establish each regression curve. If the same disc, agar, prediffusion time, and inoculum density are followed, these regression curves can be used by any laboratory desiring to report sensitivities in terms of the actual concentration of antimicrobial agent required to inhibit the bacteria. For this reason, the antibiotic disc contents and the regression equations are presented in Table 2.19. Regression curves for each antibiotic were determined at different disc contents, in-

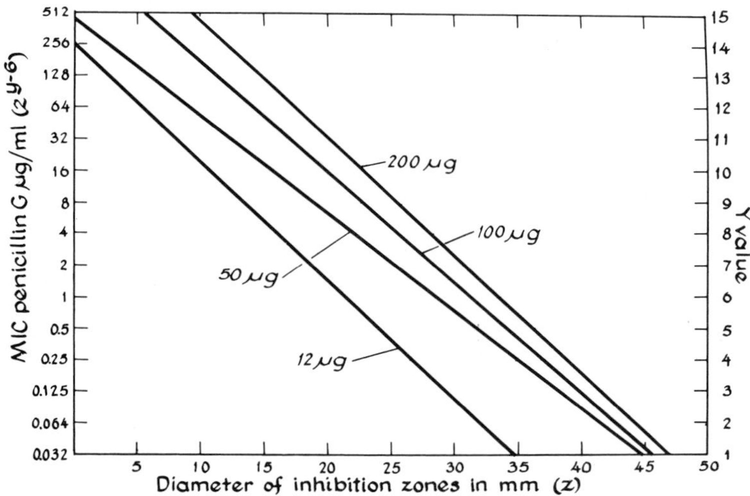

Figure 2.21 Regression lines for penicillin-G disc contents of *12, 50, 100,* and *200 µg* (see Table 2.5).

cluding the commercial disc with the highest content. For example, the regression curves for penicillin-G were determined for disc contents of 12, 50, 100, and 200 µg (Figure 2.21). Note that each increase in disc content results in a reasonably parallel regression line. For each antibiotic, we use the commercially available disc, provided the regression curve intercepts the 10-mm zone at MIC concentrations representative of antimicrobial concentrations readily obtainable in the urine. In Figure 2.21, since the urinary concentration of penicillin-G averages about 300 µg/ml and will rarely fall below 100 µg/ml on standard oral dosage,[33, 34] it is clear that penicillin disc contents of less than 100 µg are not useful in predicting bacterial sensitivity for urinary infections. Since the highest content available in commercial penicillin discs is 10 µg, the commercial discs are useless. We are thus forced, until the FDA allows manufacture of "urinary discs," to make our own penicillin-G disc of 100 or 200 µg content. Where possible, however, we have used the commercial disc. Thus, the 30 µg nalidixic acid (NA) commercial disc produces an MIC intercept at the 10-mm zone of approximately 50 µg/ml, which is close to the 75 µg/ml concentration achieved in urine when adults take 1000 mg by mouth every 6 hours (see Table 2.10). Even when the commercial disc did not allow MIC determinations at urinary levels, if the regression curve intersected the 10-mm zone diameter at a MIC concentration that would be expected to kill 90% of the organisms found in urinary infections, we settled for the commercial disc rather than make our own in order to detect the 10% of more resistant organisms. For example, although the regression curve for the 10 µg gentamicin sulfate commercial disc intercepts the 10-mm zone at only 32 µg/ml, and although the urinary concentration for a normal adult receiving 1.0 mg/kg/8 hours will average 125 µg/ml, [53, 54] 32 µg/ml exceeds the gentamicin MIC for over 90% of urinary pathogens.[54, 55]

Although the discs are 6 mm in diameter, we chose the 10-mm zone for these intercept decisions because the ±1 mm error in measuring zone diameters constitutes a larger percentage error in the smaller zones (the more resistant bacteria).

We believe that the Ericsson quantitative disc is almost as useful as the more time-consuming tube or agar plate dilutions. As will be discussed, if the major work of establishing the regression curves is done by someone else,* any laboratory can determine the MIC of a given bacterial strain with no more laboratory effort than is involved in the Kirby-Bauer sensitivity method.

Kirby-Bauer Single Disc Technique. Using Mueller-Hinton agar, commercial discs of the highest available antimicrobial content, and a heavy inoculum (compared to the dense but not confluent inoculm of the Ericsson method) of staphylococci, Bauer, Perry, and Kirby[56] showed that tube dilution definitions of sensitivity and resistance could be correlated with the zone size around the disc. A plot of the resulting zone sizes of a large number of staphylococci showed two different populations—a "resistant" and a "sensitive" group—with very few strains falling in between; less than 3–5% of all strains fell into the "intermediate" range with chloramphenicol, tetracycline, and erythromycin. This bimodal distribution defined the standards for zone sizes of the resistant and sensitive bacteria. These standard zones, because of the differences in diffusion for each antibiotic, varied with each drug. These authors also showed that, when single disc results were compared with tube dilution results, there was a good correlation "regarding the quality sensitive or resistant."[56] But, as they noted, there was little correlation as to the degree of sensitivity or resistance in the two methods; that is, zones of widely varying diameters were associated with the same MIC within the sensitive or resistant range.

Turck, Lindemeyer, and Petersdorf[5] applied the same criteria to a study of Gram-negative bacteria. They performed tube dilutions and simultaneously measured the agar zone size for single discs of the highest available antibiotic content. Five antibiotics were studied. Bacteria were considered sensitive on tube dilution studies if they were inhibited by 5 μg of tetracycline/ml, 10 μg of chloramphenicol/ml, 25 μg of streptomycin/ml, 25 μg of kanamycin/ml, and 5 μg of polymyxin-B/ml. Figure 2.22 is reproduced from their paper to show the tube dilution MICs of tetracycline with *E. coli*, and Figure 2.23 for *Pseudomonas*, together with the corresponding zones of inhibition surrounding the 30-μg tetracycline disc.

Several points are worth considering. First, with the Gram-negative bacteria, the bimodal distribution into a sensitive and resistant population was rarely as clear cut as with the staphylococci. Second, although Turck, Lindemeyer, and Petersdorf[5] argue that a good correlation exists between tube dilution and disc definition of sensitivity, I have already discussed the difficulties inherent in choosing 5 μg of tetracycline/ml as a definition of sensitivity. If 2–3 μg/ml, a much more reasonable[6–10] serum level of free tetracycline, were chosen in Figure 2.22, half of the sensitive (large zones) *E. coli* would then be considered resistant and no correlation would exist between the 30-μg disc of tetracycline and tube dilution results. Moreover, from Figure 2.23, no strains of *Pseudomonas* are considered by these authors to be sensitive. This is true for concentrations of tetracycline at 5 μg/ml, but 250 mg orally every 6 hours produces an average urinary level of at least 500 μg/ml (*see* Table 2.10); 100 μg of tetracycline/ml is bacteriostatic for 90% of pseudomonas strains (as we pointed out in our early studies[12] seen in Figure 2.7, and as can be observed in the MIC data of Turck *et al.*[5] in Figure 2.23). In the absence of stones, obstruction, and azotemia, tetracycline is one of the most useful of all drugs for pseudomonas urinary infections. The Kirby-Bauer method will indicate resistance (Figure 2.23) for virtually all strains of *Pseudomonas.*

The Kirby-Bauer method is an important advance in the art and science of *in vitro* sensitivity testing. The Seattle group, by showing the gross inferiority of the multi-disc method, by standardizing the agar

* An excellent monograph, "The Paper Disc Method in Quantitative Determination of Bacterial Sensitivity to Antibiotics," can be obtained from AB Biodisk, Grevgatan 50, S-114 58, Stockholm, Sweden. This monograph presents in an abbreviated and practical form principles, recommended methods, and the regression curves for quantitative disc sensitivity testing. It is based on the conclusions of the World Health Organization published as supplement 217 to Acta Pathologica et Microbiologica Scandinavica, Section B: Microbiology and Immunologi.[46]

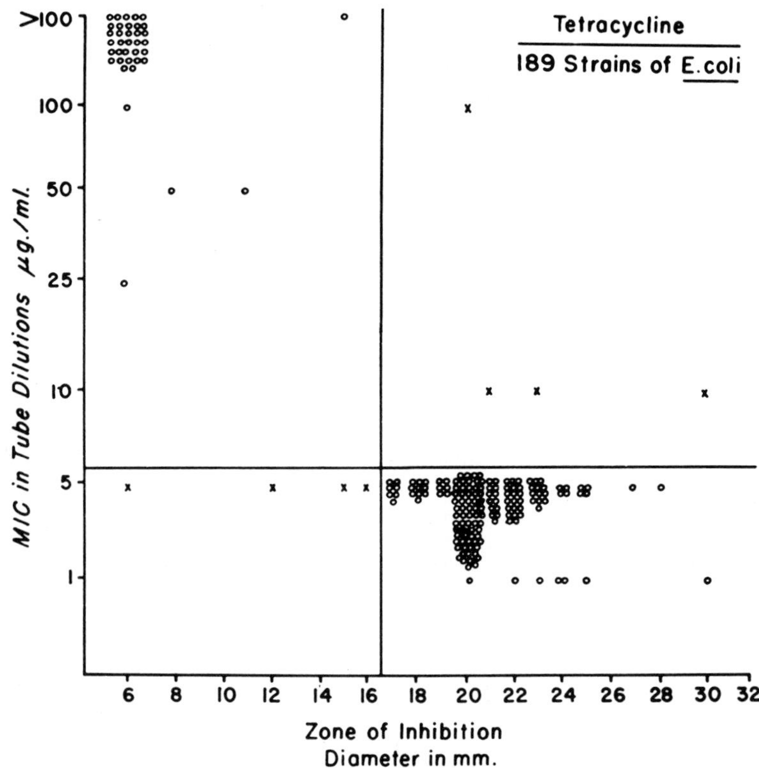

Figure 2.22 Correlation of results of single disc (30 μg) and tube dilution sensitivities of 189 strains of *Escherichia coli* tested with tetracycline. (Reproduced by permission from M. Turck, R. I. Lindemeyer, and R. G. Petersdorf, Ann. Intern. Med. **58:** 56, 1963.[5])

(Mueller-Hinton) and the inoculum size, by establishing standards of different zone sizes for each antimicrobial agent, and by emphasizing that the majority of bacteria are either sensitive (large zones) or resistant (small zones), have made a great contribution.

But the disadvantages are equally clear. While the vast majority (95%) of staphylococci fall into the bimodal distribution of two distinct populations, the Gram-negative urinary pathogens show a much higher percentage of strains with intermediate sensitivity, and, for some genera, there is no bimodal distribution at all for certain antimicrobial agents (*Proteus mirabilis* and *Pseudomonas aeruginosa* against tetracycline[5]). Since sensitivity and resistance are defined in terms of concentrations obtainable in the serum, these definitions may be artificial (as I have argued for tetracycline) and, in any event, exclude the choice of useful urinary level drugs for bacteria which are resistant at serum concentrations.

Once the regression curves have been determined in a standardized method, the Ericsson quantitative disc is no more trouble to perform than the Kirby-Bauer, since inoculum size must be controlled in both methods. By reporting disc sensitivity directly in terms of the concentration of antimicrobial agent required to inhibit the organism (MIC), the three disadvantages to the Kirby-Bauer method are avoided. First, there is no artifactual division into categories where 2- or 3-mm differences in zone size force a categorical definition of sensitive, intermediate, or resistant. Second, no pharmacologic decisions in terms of drug concentrations in body fluids are implied by the bacteriologic laboratory. Third, bacteria resistant at serum levels are not cate-

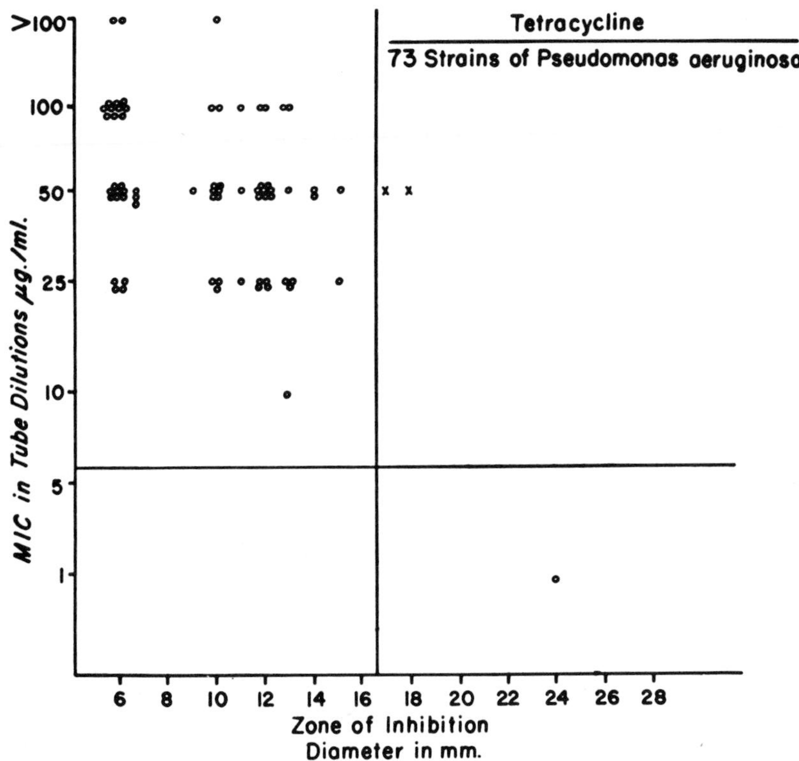

Figure 2.23 Correlation of results of single disc (30 µg) and tube dilution methods with 73 strains of *Pseudomonas aeruginosa* tested with tetracycline. Seventy-one of 73 strains resistant by serial tube dilution assays had zone diameters of less than 16 mm. (Reproduced by permission from M. Turck, R. I. Lindemeyer, and R. G. Petersdorf, Ann. Intern. Med. **58:** 56, 1963.[5])

gorized as resistant but are interpreted in terms of the exact MIC needed to inhibit the organism, thereby allowing the intelligent use of antibacterial drugs that achieve inhibitory concentrations in the urine. For example, the urinary level often exceeds by severalfold the MIC of bacteria termed "resistant" by the Kirby-Bauer method, but some bacteria truly are resistant to even urinary concentrations. The term "resistant" allows no distinction between these varying degrees of resistance. By reporting the true MIC of bacteria, using the quantitative Ericsson disc, inconsistencies are avoided. True, the clinician must know whether or not he is likely to achieve a concentration of drug that will exceed the MIC in the body fluid harboring the infection, but if rational therapy is ever to be practiced in clinical medicine, is there a better way to educate practicing physicians than to report bacterial sensitivities in terms of the MIC?

There is a further advantage to the Ericsson quantitative disc. I emphasized earlier that, since most antibiotics establish their diffusion gradients from disc to agar before the time (about 3½ hours) the inoculum reaches the critical concentration, prediffusion is not critical. But inoculum size is critical and remains the biggest variable in determining the size of the inhibition zone. The inoculum size for the Kirby-Bauer method, while representing a semicontrolled dilution, is a confluent growth and is considerably heavier than the "dense, but not confluent" inoculum used in the Ericsson method. Obviously, it is much harder, if not impossible, to tell the difference between degrees of confluent growth, whereas variations in a dense but not confluent inoculum are immediately recognizable, whether they be too light or too dense. For these reasons, the proper density of the Ericsson inoculum is more recognizable (and therefore more correctly interpretable as to standards of reference). Indeed, the rather heavy inoculum of the Kirby-Bauer plates may be in part responsible for the insensitivity of the zone size to increasingly high disc contents reported by Bauer[57]; however, as shown in Figure 2.21, when the Ericsson inoculum was tested with discs of increasingly high penicillin-G content, the size of the inhibition zones responded logarithmically, as expected. Our experience has been the same with all antibiotics in Table 2.19, even including the polymyxins; when zone sizes are arithmetically plotted against the logarithm of increasingly higher disc contents, a straight line results, indicating a proportional response of inhibition zones to these high disc contents.

Table 2.20
Tabulation of MICs for Penicillin-G from 200 μg Disc Regression Curve ($Y = 18.68 - [0.37 \pm 0.02]z$) at 0.5-mm Zone Size Intervals

MIC (*μg/ml*)	Zone Size (*mm*)	MIC (*μg/ml*)	Zone Size (*mm*)
1408.55	6.0	15.83	23.5
1239.02	6.5	13.93	24.0
1089.90	7.0	12.25	24.5
958.74	7.5	10.78	25.0
843.35	8.0	9.48	25.5
741.86	8.5	8.34	26.0
652.57	9.0	7.34	26.5
574.04	9.5	6.45	27.0
504.95	10.0	5.68	27.5
444.18	10.5	4.99	28.0
390.72	11.0	4.39	28.5
343.70	11.5	3.86	29.0
302.33	12.0	3.40	29.5
265.95	12.5	2.99	30.0
233.94	13.0	2.63	30.5
205.78	13.5	2.31	31.0
181.02	14.0	2.03	31.5
159.23	14.5	1.79	32.0
140.07	15.0	1.57	32.5
123.21	15.5	1.39	33.0
108.38	16.0	1.22	33.5
95.34	16.5	1.07	34.0
83.86	17.0	0.94	34.5
73.77	17.5	0.83	35.0
64.89	18.0	0.73	35.5
57.08	18.5	0.64	36.0
50.21	19.0	0.56	36.5
44.71	19.5	0.50	37.0
38.85	20.0	0.44	37.5
34.18	20.5	0.38	38.0
30.06	21.0	0.34	38.5
26.45	21.5	0.30	39.0
23.26	22.0	0.26	39.5
20.46	22.5	0.23	40.0
18.00	23.0		

Lastly, it is more practical in the laboratory to construct tables of increasing zone sizes at 0.5-mm intervals from each regression curve so that MICs can be read directly from a table rather than the regression line. For example, in Table 2.20, the MICs to penicillin-G have been tabulated for zone sizes around a 200 μg penicillin-G disc at 0.5-mm intervals, thereby facilitating direct conversion of zone sizes to MICs.

BACTERIAL RESISTANCE

In the classification of urinary infections presented in Chapter 1, I emphasized that bacterial resistance accounts for the two most common causes of unresolved bacteriuria. Since the clinician must first sterilize the urine if the infection is to be cured or if the type of recurrent infection is to be therapeutically solved as either bacterial persistence or reinfection, he must understand the mechanisms and implications of bacterial resistance.

From the therapeutic view of the physician who treats urinary infections, bacterial resistance can be divided into three categories:*

1. "Natural" resistance
2. Selection of resistant mutants within the urinary tract during therapy
3. Transferable ("infectious"), extrachromosomal resistance (R-factor)

"Natural" Resistance

Of the three categories, natural resistance is the easiest to recognize and simply

* Parts of this presentation have been previously published in T. A. Stamey: Urinary tract infections in women. In Campbell's Urology, Ed. 4, Chap. 11, Philadelphia, W. B. Saunders Co., 1978.[58]

refers to the lack of drug-sensitive substrate (i.e., substrate sensitive to certain classes of antimicrobial agents) in some species of bacteria. For example, all species of *Proteus* are resistant to the polymyxin antibiotics. The same is true of *Streptococcus faecalis* resistance to nalidixic acid. It is also true of most strains of *P. mirabilis* to nitrofurantoin and of *Pseudomonas* species to nitrofurantoin and penicillin-G, but here the distinction is not as categorical as for *Proteus* species to polymyxin or *S. faecalis* to nalidixic acid. Nevertheless, for all practical purposes of even maximum urinary concentrations, no rational use of antimicrobial therapy should ever include these agents for these organisms. If *in vitro* sensitivities are obtained before resolution of a case of bacteriuria, then gross mistakes relating to natural resistance can be avoided. On the other hand, if office bacteriologic testing identifies the species, then clearly, nitrofurantoin should not be used for a *Psuedomonas* or *P. mirabilis* infection, even if *in vitro* sensitivities are not obtained.

Selection of Resistant Mutants Within the Urinary Tract During Therapy

Selection of resistant mutants during therapy is more complicated but has important therapeutic implications. The clinical setting is simple. *In vitro* sensitivities show that the bacteriuric population is highly sensitive to a specific antimicrobial drug, but within 3 days of a 10-day course of therapy the urine is infected with 10^5 or more bacteria/ml of the same strain, but now the entire population is highly resistant to the antimicrobial agent (*in vitro* studies would now require several hundred times as much drug to inhibit the organism!). It can be shown that the resistant organism was present *before* contact with the drug, but only in numbers of one resistant bacterium/10^5–10^{10} organisms, making it impossible to detect its presence clinically before therapy. The actual frequency rate of spontaneous mutation to resistance varies both with the bacterial species and the antimicrobial agent. For example, with streptomycin and *Mycobacterium tuberculosis*, the rate of mutation is about 10^{-10} but for isoniazid and *M. tuberculosis* the rate is much higher, 10^{-6}. This pattern of early replacement, within 5 days and often within 2, corresponds to laboratory studies with what is called the one-step, or streptomycin, pattern of selection of mutants[59]; this type of resistance is easily illustrated *in vitro* (Figure 2.24 and Table 2.21). This basically means that although the entire population of sensitive organisms in the urinary tract is eliminated within a few hours, upon exposure to the drug the resistant mutant or its early progeny has the chromosomal capability of resisting several hundred times the original antimicrobial concentration that selected the mutant in the first place.

The penicillin, or multiple-step, pattern of mutation selection also occurs in urinary infections, is more subtle than the one-step pattern, and fortunately is much less fre-

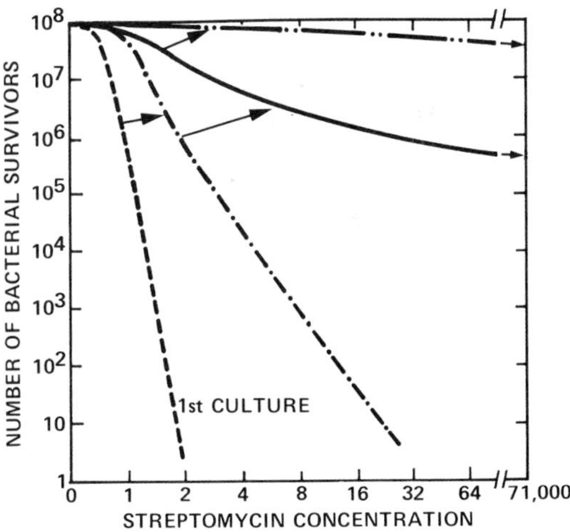

Figure 2.24 Streptomycin one-step pattern of resistance. Stepwise increase in bacterial resistance to streptomycin. *First culture curve* represents the survival of the original stock culture. Strains were selected from the sublethal concentrations indicated by the *arrows*. It should be noted, however, that highly resistant strains can be isolated from the first culture as well as the fourth (· · — · ·) even though the percentage of highly resistant colonies is very small in the first culture (see Table 2.21). (Modified from M. Demerec, J. Bacteriol. **56:** 53, 1948.[59])

Table 2.21
Proportions of Fully Resistant Colonies Obtained when Sensitive Populations of *Escherichia coli* Are Plated with Increasing Concentrations of Streptomycin[a]

Concentration of Streptomycin	No. of Colonies Tested	No. of Colonies Resistant to 1000 μg/ml	Percentage of Resistant Colonies
(*μg/ml*)			
8	14	1	7
16	13	5	38
32	5	5	100
64	41	41	100

[a] Modified from H. B. Newcombe and R. Hawirko, J. Bacteriol. **57:** 565, 1949.[60]

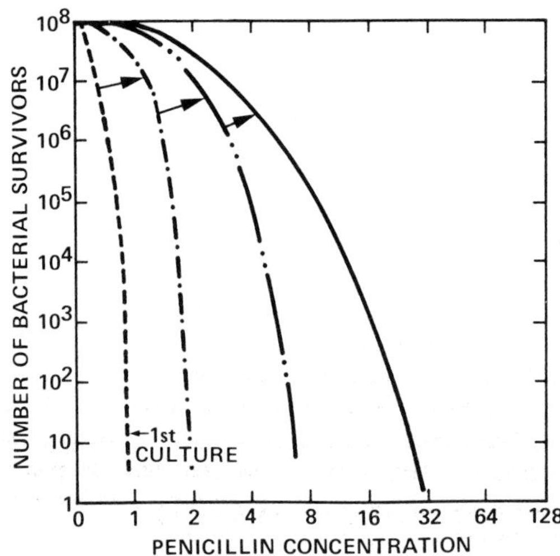

Figure 2.25 Penicillin, multiple-step, pattern of resistance. Stepwise increase in bacterial resistance to penicillin-G. Strains were selected from the sublethal concentrations indicated by the *arrows*. Observe the constant, geometric increase in resistance to penicillin-G without the early appearance of highly resistant strains. (Modified from M. Demerec, J. Bacteriol. **56:** 53, 1948.[59])

quent (Figure 2.25). A clinical example will illustrate the difference. A 39-year old mother of three children was seen at Stanford in 1966 for treatment of bacteriuria due to *Klebsiella* that was highly sensitive to polymyxin-B sulfate (1.25 μg/ml was bactericidal). Cystoscopic studies localized the infection to the right kidney and also showed a few inflammatory "polyps" in the proximal urethra at the vesical neck. An intravenous urogram was normal and demonstrated no postvoiding residual urine. The patient received 75 mg of polymyxin-E sulfate ever 12 hours for 9 days. Daily cultures showed a sterile urine by the 3rd day, but 80 *Klebsiella*/ml on the 8th day, 1000/ml on the 9th day, and more than 10,000 *Klebsiella*/ml 2 days after stopping therapy—all resistant to greater than 20 μg/ml of polymyxin-B. She was then treated with kanamycin, which was bactericidal to *Klebsiella* at 5 μg/ml, for 10 days at 0.5 gm every 12 hours. The urine was sterile on the first culture obtained on the 5th day of therapy and remained so for the 3 1/2 years she was followed.

The difference between the one-step pattern of streptomycin resistance and the multiple-step pattern of penicillin resistance is contrasted in Table 2.22. The latter type, as shown in the polymyxin example, is due to chromosomal changes in degrees of resistance in small, multiple steps of gradually increasing resistance, thereby preventing overgrowth in the early days of therapy but nevertheless inexorably selecting with time the eventual emergence of strains resistant to even the urinary concentrations. In contrast to the penicillin pattern where resistance occurs in geometric, stepwise movements and where mutants only appear when sensitive bacteria face low concentrations of antimicrobials, the streptomycin pattern is strikingly different: one-step mutants resistant to the highest attainable urinary concentrations occur, usually from large populations of bacteria (10^{10}), but mutants also appear at lower concentrations of antimicrobials and, at least *in vitro*, arise at different rates of mutation.[59–61]

Table 2.22
Two Clinical Patterns of Mutational Resistance in Bacteriuric Patients[a, b]

Days on Therapy	One-step, Streptomycin Pattern (*Escherichia coli*/ml bladder urine)	MIC to NA	Multiple-step, Penicillin Pattern (*Klebsiella*/ml bladder urine)	MIC to PmB
	(Rx = NA)	*(μg/ml)*	*(Rx = PmE)*	*(μg/ml)*
0	$>10^5$	5.0	$>10^5$	1.25
3	$>10^5$	>1000	0	
8	$>10^5$	>1000	80	>22
9	$>10^5$	>1000	1000	>22
−2	$>10^5$	>1000	$>10^5$	>22

[a] RX = treatment; NA = nalidixic acid; PmE = polymyxin-E; PmB = polymyxin-B. MIC = minimal inhibitory concentration in tube dilutions.

[b] Reproduced by permission from Campbell's Urology, Ed. 4, Philadelphia, W. B. Saunders, 1978.[58]

How often will the urologist experience the selection of resistant strains in the course of therapy for a previously sensitive bacteriuric population? Somewhere between 5–10% of the time, which is clearly not insignificant, and a factor that must be considered in resolving bacteriuria. In personally studied series, we selected resistant mutants in 8% of 25 consecutive patients treated with 250 mg of oxytetracycline four times a day,[16] and 7.4% of 27 consecutive patients treated with 1 gm of nalidixic acid four times a day,[62] figures which are probably comparable to other antimicrobial agents. In all instances, resistance was of the one-step, streptomycin, pattern.

What can the urologist do to prevent the selection of resistant mutants among the apparently sensitive bacteriuric population? He must avoid underdosage with antimicrobial therapy. Stated in microbiologic terms, he must exceed the minimal inhibitory concentration (MIC) of the antimicrobial agent for the infecting strain by as wide a margin as possible (10 times is good, but 100 times is even better). Nowhere is this principle of therapy better illustrated than in the case of nalidixic acid. An early, but influential, clinical report indicated that in 25% of bacteriuric patients, treated with nalidixic acid, selection of resistant mutants occurred.[63] However, the dosage used was 2 gm/day, not the usual 4 gm/day. Several recent investigators, all using 4 gm/day, have reported selection of resistant mutants at an average rate of only 5.3%.[62] Perhaps this can be appreciated better in the test tube. If 100 sensitive strains are placed in broth containing nalidixic acid at concentrations close to their MIC, 10 times the MIC, and 100 times the MIC, it is clear that the selection of resistant mutants is dependant upon how much the MIC is exceeded (Table 2.23). Although more mutants will be selected at 10^8 than 10^5 bacteria/ml (1000 times more bacteria), the percentage reduction in successful mutations by increasing the concentration of nalidixic acid by 10-fold (from 1 to 10 times the MIC) is the same in both concentrations of bacteria. The data in Table 2.23 can perhaps be appreciated better in Figure 2.26; the preincubation MIC to nalidixic acid for the 100 strains is shown in Figure 2.27.

Table 2.23
Development of Resistance to Nalidixic Acid in Broth in 75 Strains of *Escherichia coli*, 12 *Klebsiella* and 13 *Proteus mirabilis*

Inoculum Bacteria/ml	Percent Resistant Strains at:[a]		
	1 MIC	10 MIC	100 MIC
	(5 μg/ml)	*(50 μg/ml)*	*(500 μg/ml)*
10^5	7	2	0
10^8	50	14	3

[a] See Figure 2.27 for pre-incubation minimal inhibitory concentration (MIC) to nalidixic acid.

The clinical message is clear. Since the mean urinary concentration of nalidixic acid in the normal adult on 4 gm/day is only 75 μg/ml, the urologist cannot afford underdosage. This is especially true in the azotemic patient, in the very young, and in the very old, in whom the pharmacody-

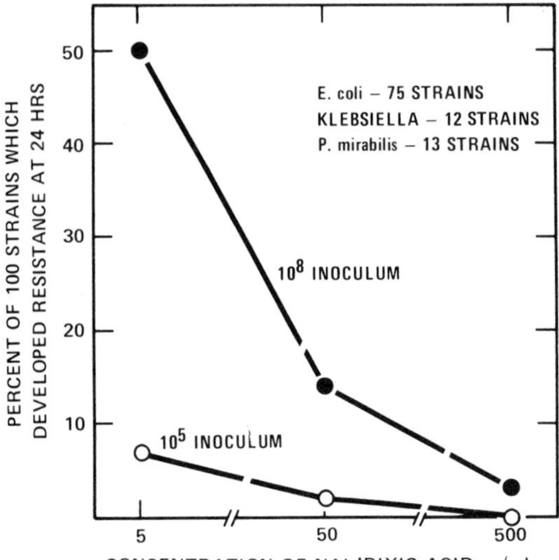

Figure 2.26 Development of resistance in 100 sensitive strains of Enterobacteriaceae exposed to one minimal inhibitory concentration (MIC) of nalidixic acid (5 μg/ml), 10 MICs (50 μg/ml), and 100 MICs (500 μg/ml). Note equivalent effect of decreasing resistance regardless of inoculum size (10^5 or 10^8 bacteria/milliliter). (Reproduced by permission from T. A. Stamey and J. Bragonje, J. Am. Med. Assoc., **236:** 1857, © 1976.[62])

SPECIES	NUMBER	MEAN MIC μg/ml TO NALIDIXIC ACID (RANGE)
E. coli	75	4.4 (1.7 – 11.0)
Klebsiella	12	6.6 (4.0 – 11.0)
P. mirabilis	13	6.2 (1.7 – 9.0)

Figure 2.27 Preincubation minimal inhibitory concentration (MIC) of 100 strains to nalidixic acid.

namics of renal excretion can deviate quite widely from the norm. The same principle, however, applies to all antimicrobial agents: the MIC of the infecting strain should be exceeded by as much as 10-fold if possible, and 100 times is even better. We have performed similar *in vitro* studies with 50 strains of *E. coli* and ampicillin (mean MIC = 1.3 μg/ml). Observe in Table 2.24, in comparison to nalidixic acid, how important it is to exceed the ampicillin MIC by 100 times. Fortunately with ampicillin's very high urinary concentrations, unlike those of nalidixic acid, it is not difficult to exceed the MIC by 100-fold.

It is theoretically true that therapy with antimicrobial agents that produce the multiple-step, penicillin type of resistance may offer some advantage, since the likelihood of overcoming small, multiple increases in resistance is greater with high urinary concentrations. In truth, however, the difference between the two types of chromosomal resistance is quantitative and one of degree rather than a qualitative distinction. For example, although nalidixic acid can certainly produce one-step increases in resistance by several hundred-fold, it is clear that there are intermediate and small-step increases in Table 2.23 at 1 time the MIC which are sharply reduced at 10 times MIC and largely prevented at 100 times the MIC. Indeed, from the clinical standpoint, as seen in Table 2.22, there are some advantages to the one-step pattern (if resistance has to occur), in that recognition can occur early in therapy, rather than later, and appropriate changes be made in treatment.

The classic way to prevent either form of resistance is to treat a sensitive infection with two, or even three, antimicrobial agents, thereby reducing the chance of selection of a resistant mutant from 1×10^{-10}

Table 2.24
Development of Resistance to Ampicillin and Nalidixic Acid in *Escherichia coli* in Broth

Drug and Inoculum	Percentage of Resistant Strains at:		
	1 MIC	10 MIC	100 MIC
Ampicillin			
10^5	26	0	0
10^8	26	4	0
Nalidixic acid			
10^5	1	2	0
10^8	52	12	4

[a] 50 Strains *E. coli*, ampicillin, mean minimal inhibitory concentration (MIC) = 1.3 μg/ml; 75 strains *E. coli*, nalidixic acid, mean MIC = 4.4 μg/ml.

to 1×10^{-20} or even 1×10^{-30} with three agents. While this is necessary in the therapy of tuberculosis in which a chronic tissue infection imposes great difficulties in exceeding the MIC of the infecting strain, it is almost never required in urinary infections, in which the opportunity to exceed the MIC by 10–100 times occurs with many antimicrobial agents.

Lastly, it is true that many patients with bacteriuria can be cured with minimal amounts of an antimicrobial drug. However, the favorable variables here are usually small bacterial populations, often less than 5000 bacteria/ml from urinary frequency and forced hydration, and an infection reservoir in which the residual bacterial population reduces dramatically with each voiding. These occasional successes should not lull the urologist into trying to resolve a fully developed case of bacteriuria with suboptimal dosage. The effectiveness of single-tablet nightly prophylaxis with nitrofurantoin is almost certainly related to the small size of the bacterial inoculum which enters the bladder, an inoculum that has virtually no chance of including a resistant mutant for selection.

In theory, ideal therapy for bacteriuria in reinfections of the urinary tract would include acute hydration and diuresis to reduce the total bacterial population before commencing drug therapy (to reduce the chance of resistant mutants), double or triple dosage therapy in the first 48 hours (also to reduce the chance of resistant mutants), and probably only 3 or 4 days of regular dosage therapy. Indeed, although we have conventionally treated bacteriuric episodes with 10 days of therapy, it is likely that 5 days of therapy is fully adequate.

Transferable, Extrachromosomal Drug Resistance

This third and last form of resistance is important in the urologist's understanding of how resistant strains, and especially strains with multiple resistance, are acquired in the course of recurrent bacteriuria. Transferable drug resistance, first postulated by the Japanese in 1957 to explain the large increase in multiple drug resistance in *Shigella* isolates from patients with bacillary dysentery, relates to sexual conjugation among Enterobacteriaceae (and *Pseudomonas*) in which the "male" transfers extrachromosomal DNA along conjugation bridges to the female. These single strands of DNA carry the genetic determinanants (R factors) for enzymes that inactivate antimicrobial agents. These R factors self-replicate independently of the bacterial chromosome and can be transferred even from one species to another, for example, from *Klebsiella* or *P. mirabilis* to *E. coli*.

The importance of R factors relates to the fecal flora, in which it explains the occurrence of multiple drug resistance in single species. Since fecal bacteria represent the ultimate reservoir for urinary infections in females, it is not surprising that multiple-resistant bacteria sometimes appear in patients with bacteriuria. R factor resistance also explains the occurrence of resistant strains in patients who have not personally received antimicrobial agents ("natural" resistance, of course, must first be excluded in any such analysis). For example, Moorhouse isolated resistant strains from 81 of 100 healthy infants less than 2 years of age living in an urban community.[64] While 32% of these infants had received antimicrobial therapy earlier in life (4 to 44 weeks before collection of the stool specimen), and 10% had contacts with individuals who had received therapy, 57% had neither treatment nor contacts. The antimicrobial agents to which these strains (71 *E. coli*, 6 *Klebsiella*, and 4 *P. mirabilis*) were resistant are interesting (see Table 2.25), as well as the number of different agents to which each strain was resistant (Table 2.26). As can be seen in Table 2.26, strains resistant to two and three, or more, antimicrobials all transferred their resistance, and over 50% of the strains resistant to a single agent were also resistant because of R factor.

While at first glance this specter looks like a terrible problem for urologists treating urinary infections, it is clearly not of this magnitude. I have reviewed the sensitivities to 65 consecutive outpatient bacter-

Table 2.25
Enterobacterial Resistance in 81/100 Fecal Specimens from Healthy Infants (<2 Years)[a]

Antimicrobial Agent	Percentage Resistant
Tetracycline	67
Streptomycin	63
Ampicillin	62
Neomycin	17
Chloramphenical	16
Furazolidone	1
Nalidixic acid	0

[a] From E. C. Moorhouse, Br. Med. J. **2:** 405, 1969.[64]

Table 2.26
Resistant Patterns in 81 Strains: 71 *Escherichia coli*, 6 *Klebsiella*, and 4 *Proteus mirabilis*[a]

Number of Strains	Number of antibiotics	R Factors
29	1	17
25	2	24
27	3 or more	27[b]
81		68

[a] From E. C. Moorhouse, Br. Med J. **2:** 405, 1969.[64]
[b] 13 Transferred total pattern.

Table 2.27
Resistance Patterns of 100 Consecutive Outpatient Bacteriurias at Stanford, 1974

Organism	No. of Strains
Escherichia coli	65
Proteus mirabilis	9
Klebsiella	11
Pseudomonas	11
Proteus morganii	1
Staphylococcus epidermidis	1
Staphylococcus aureus	1
Streptococcus faecalis	1
Resistance Patterns	
Pan-sensitive:	42 strains
(40 *E. coli*, 1 *Klebsiella*, 1 *S. epidermidis*)	
Resistant to 1 agent:	9 strains
(5 *E. coli*, 3 *Klebsiella*, 1 *S. aureus*)	
Resistant to 2 or more:	49 strains

iurias due to *E. coli*, 9 due to *P. mirabilis*, 11 caused by *P. aeruginosa* and 11 due to *Klebsiella* at Stanford University Hospital in 1974 (Table 2.27). The antimicrobial agents used in quantitative disc determinations of MICs (the Ericsson method as presented in this chapter) were ampicillin, cephalexin, cephaloridine, polymyxin-B, gentamicin, kanamycin, nalidixic acid, nitrofurantoin, oxytetracycline, penicillin-G, and sulfamethizole. As seen in Table 2.28, even though many of these patients had received antimicrobial agents in the recent past, 40 of the 65 *E. coli* were pansensitive (*i.e.*, sensitive to all agents), 8 were resistant to one drug only, and only 17 of the 65 resistant to two or more drugs. All nine strains of *P. mirabilis* were sensitive to all drugs if one excludes the "natural" resistance of this organism to nitrofurantoin and oxytetracycline. The 11 infections due to *P. aeruginosa* were all resistant to ampicillin, penicillin-G, cephalexin, nitrofurantoin, and cephaloridine, but here again this resistance is "natural" and does not infer R factors. However, 9 of the 11 were sensitive to sulfonamide, 10 of 11 sensitive to oxytetracycline (MIC, 0.72–37 μg/ml), 7 of 11 partially sensitive to nalidixic acid (MIC, 0.46–34 μg/ml), and all 11 of 11 exquisitely sensitive to gentamicin and polymyxin-B sulfate. The klebsiella pattern is always the most variable in natural chromosomal resistance, making it difficult to judge without actual R factor transfer studies to a recipient female whether R factor resistance played a role. Even so, one strain was pansensitive, four strains were resistant to one antimicrobial only, five strains resistant to two, and only one strain was resistant to 3 of the 11 antimicrobials.

It seems fair to say that although trans-

Table 2.28
Resistance Patterns of 65 Consecutive Outpatient Bacteriurias Due to *Escherichia coli*, (Stanford, 1974)

Number of Strains	Number of Antimicrobials to Which Strains are Resistant
40	0
8	1
6	2
9	3
1	4
1	5
17/65	2 or more

ferable drug resistance in the bowel is a critically important mechanism in explaining the occurrence of multiple-resistant strains in the urinary tract, *in vitro* antimicrobial sensitivities will *always* indicate one or several drugs with which the urologist can resolve the bacteriuria. Moreover, it is worth pointing out that transfer of R factor resistance to nitrofurantoin almost never occurs and has never been demonstrated with nalidixic acid. Indeed, of the 65 strains of *E. coli* in Table 2.28, regardless of multiple resistance, all were inhibited by 5.6 μg/ml, or less, of nalidixic acid.

Thus, for the clinician who is faced with the problem of resolving bacteriuria and who uses *in vitro* sensitivity testing, the 5–10% selection of resistant mutants based on chromosomal resistance imposes a greater handicap in achieving sterile urine in the patient than do the difficulties imposed by transferable drug resistance.

REFERENCES

1. Stamey, T. A., and Mihara, G.: Observations on the growth of urethral and vaginal bacteria in sterile urine. J. Urol., 1980 (in press).
2. Kaye, D.: Antibacterial activity of human urine. J. Clin. Invest. **47:** 2374, 1968.
3. Kunin, C. M.: Clinical significance of protein binding of the penicillins. Ann. N. Y. Acad. Sci. **145:** 282, 1967.
4. Ericsson, H.: Rational use of antibiotics in hospitals. Scand. J. Clin. Lab. Invest. **12**(Suppl. 50): 1, 1960.
5. Turck, M., Lindemeyer, R. I., and Petersdorf, R. G.: Comparison of single disc and tube dilution techniques in determining antibiotic sensitivity of gram negative pathogens. Ann. Intern. Med. **58:** 56, 1963.
6. Pulaski, E. J., and Isokane, R. K.: Tetracycline concentrations in blood serum, bile, and prostatic and spinal fluids following oral administration of tetracycline phosphate complex and tetracycline hydrochloride. Antibiot. Med. Clin. Ther. **4:** 408, 1957.
7. Kaplan, M. A., Dickison, H. L., Hubel, K. A., and Buckwalter, F. H.: A new, rapidly absorbed, complex salt of tetracycline. Antibiot. Med. Clin. Ther. **4:** 99, 1957.
8. Milberg, M. B., Kamhi, B., and Banowitch, M. M.: Pharmacology and therapeutic efficacy of tetracycline. Antibiot. Chemother. **4:** 1086, 1954.
9. Dowling, H. F.: Tetracycline. New York, Medical Encyclopedia, Inc., 1955, p. 23.
10. Schach von Wittenau, M., and Yeary, R.: The excretion and distribution of body fluids of tetracyclines after intravenous administration in dogs. J. Pharmacol. Exp. Ther. **140:** 258, 1963.
11. McCabe, W. R., and Jackson, G. G.: Treatment of pyelonephritis: Bacterial, drug and host factors in success or failure among 252 patients. N. Engl. J. Med. **272:** 1037, 1965.
12. Stamey, T. A., Govan, D. E., and Palmer, J. M.: The localization and treatment of urinary tract infections: The role of bactericidal urine levels as opposed to serum levels. Medicine *44:* 1, 1965.
13. Klastersky, J., Daneau, D., Swings, G., and Weerts, D.: Antibacterial activity in serum and urine as a therapeutic guide in bacterial infections. J. Infect. Dis. **129:** 187, 1974.
14. Ericsson, H.: Assay of antibiotics in small amounts of fluid. Scand. J. Clin. Lab. Invest. **12,** 423, 1960.
15. Regna, P. P., and Solomons, I. A.: The chemical and physical properties of terramycin. Ann. N. Y. Acad. Sci. **53:** 229, 1950.
16. Stamey, T. A., Fair, W. R., Timothy, M. M., Millar, M. A., Mihara, G., and Lowery, Y. C.: Serum versus urinary antimicrobial concentrations in cure of urinary-tract infections. N. Engl. J. Med. **291:** 1159, 1974.
17. Naumann, P.: The value of antibiotic levels in tissue and in urine in the treatment of urinary tract infections. J. Antimicrob. Chemother. **4:** 9, 1978.
18. Forsgren, A., and Gnarpe, H.: Tetracycline interference with the bactericidal effect of serum. Nature **244:** 82, 1973.
19. Kunin, C. M., and Finkelberg, Z.: Oral cephalexin and ampicillin: Antimicrobial activity, recovery in urine, and persistence in blood of uremic patients. Ann. Intern. Med. **72:** 349, 1970.
20. Howell, A., Sutherland, R., and Rolinson, G. N.: Effect of protein binding on levels of ampicillin and cloxacillin in synovial fluid. Clin. Pharmacol. Ther. **13:** 724, 1972.
21. Fabre, J., Burgy, C., Rudhardt, M., and Herrera, A.: The behaviour in man of C. P. 15,464, a carbenicillin absorbed following oral administration. Chemotherapy **17:** 334, 1972.
22. Knirsch, A. K., Hobbs, D. C., and Korst, J. J.: Pharmacokinetics, toleration, and safety of indanyl carbenicillin in man. J. Infect. Dis. **127:** S105, 1973.
23. Hansen, I., Jacobsen, E., and Weis, J.: Pharmacokinetics of sulbenicillin, a new broad-spectrum semisynthetic penicillin. Clin. Pharmacol. Ther. **17:** 339, 1975.
24. Meyers, B. R., Kaplan, K., and Weinstein, L.: Cephalexin: Microbiological effects and pharmacologic parameters in man. Clin. Pharmacol. Ther. **10:** 810, 1969.

25. Gower, P. E., and Dash, C. H.: Cephalexin: Human studies of absorption and excretion of a new cephalosporin antibiotic. Br. J. Pharmacol. **37:** 738, 1969.
26. Sande, M. A., and Kaye, D.: Evaluation of methods for determining antibacterial activity of serum and urine after colistimethate injection. Clin. Pharmacol. Ther. **11:** 873, 1970.
27. Schwartz, B. S., Warren, M. R., Barkley, F. A., and Landis, L.: Microbiological and pharmacological studies of colistin sulfate and sodium colistinmethanesulfonate. *In* Antibiotics Annual. New York, Antibiotica, Inc., 1960, p. 41.
28. Regamey, C., Gordon, R. C., and Kirby, W. M. M.: Comparative pharmacokinetics of tobramycin and gentamicin. Clin. Pharmacol. Ther. **14:** 396, 1973.
29. Clarke, J. T., Libke, R. D., Regamey, C., and Kirby, W. M. M.: Comparative pharmacokinetics of amikacin and kanamycin. Clin. Pharmacol. Ther. **15:** 610, 1974.
30. Männistö, P. T.: Pharmacokinetics of nalidixinic acid and oxolinic acid in healthy women. Clin. Pharmacol. Ther. **19:** 37, 1976.
31. Conklin, J. D., and Hailey, F. J.: Urinary drug excretion in man during oral dosage of different nitrofurantoin formulations. Clin. Pharmacol. Ther. **10:** 534, 1969.
32. Kunin, C. M.: Clinical pharmacology of new penicillins. I. The importance of serum protein binding in determining antimicrobial activity and concentration in serum. Clin. Pharmacol. Ther. **7:** 166, 1966.
33. Hulbert, J.: Urinary tract infection and oral penicillin G. J. Clin. Pathol. **25:** 73, 1972.
34. Palmer, J. M., Neal, J. F., and Stamey, T. A.: The use of oral sodium benzylpenicillin in the urinary tract: A study of urinary levels and in vitro activity. In Progress in Antimicrobial and Anticancer Chemotherapy. Proceedings of the 6th International Congress of Chemotherapy Vol. 1, Baltimore, University Park Press, 1970, p. 902.
35. Stamey, T. A.: Urinary infections. Baltimore, Williams & Wilkins Co., 1972, p. 280.
36. Agren, E.: Sulfa-protein binding. Scand. J. Urol. Nephrol. Suppl. **18:** 19, 1973.
37. Steigbigel, N. H., Reed, C. W., and Finland, M.: Absorption and excretion of five tetracycline analogues in normal young men. Am. J. Med. Sci. **255:** 296, 1968.
38. Kunin, C. M.: The tetracyclines. Pediatr. Clin. N. Am. **8:** 1001, 1961.
39. Schwartz, D. E., and Rieder, J.: Pharmacokinetics of sulfamethoxazole + trimethoprim in man and their distribution in the rat. Chemotherapy **15:** 337, 1970.
40. Bach, M. C., Gold, O., and Finland, M.: Absorption and urinary excretion of trimethoprim, sulfamethoxazole, and trimethoprim-sulfamethoxazole: Results with single doses in normal young adults and preliminary observations during therapy with trimethoprim-sulfamethoxazole. J. Infect. Dis. **128:** S584, 1973.
41. Craig, W. A., and Kunin, C. M.: Trimethoprim-Sulfamethoxazole: pharmacodynamic effects of urinary pH and impaired renal function. Studies in humans. Ann. Intern. Med. **78:** 491, 1973.
42. Kasanen, A., Anttila, M., Elfving, R., Kahela, P., Saarimaa, H., Sundquist, H., Tikkanen, R., and Toivanen, P.: Trimethoprim. Pharmacology, antimicrobial activity and clinical use in urinary tract infections. Ann. Clin. Res. **10**(Suppl. 22)**:** 1, 1978.
43. MacLowry, J. D., and Marsh, H. H.: Semiautomatic microtechnique for serial dilution-antibiotic sensitivity testing in the clinical laboratory. J. Lab. Clin. Med. **72:** 685, 1968.
44. Stamey, T. A., Nemoy, N. J., and Higgins, M.: The clinical use of nalidixic acid: A review and some observations. Invest. Urol. **6:** 582, 1969.
45. Barry, A. L., Jones, R. N., and Gavan, T. L.: Evaluation of the Micro-Media system for quantitative antimicrobial drug susceptibility testing: a collaborative study. Antimicrob. Agents Chemother. **13:** 61, 1978.
46. Ericsson, H., and Sherris, J. C.: Antibiotic sensitivity testing—Report of an international collaborative study. Acta Pathol. Microbiol. Scand. Suppl. 217, Sect. B, 1971.
47. Cooper, K. E., Linton, A. H., and Sehgal, S. N.: The effect of inoculum size on inhibition zones in agar media using staphylococci and streptomycin. J. Gen. Microbiol. **18:** 670, 1958.
48. Lund, E., Funder-Schmidt, B., Christensen, H., and Dupont, A.: Sensitivity test with the tablet method. Acta. Pathol. Microbiol. Scand. **29:** 221, 1951.
49. Ericsson, H., Högman, C., and Wickman, K.: A paper disk method for determination of bacterial sensitivity to chemotherapeutic and antibiotic agents. Scand. J. Clin. Lab. Invest. **6:** 21, 1954.
50. Ericsson, H.: The paper disc method for determination of bacterial sensitivity to antibiotics. Studies on the accuracy of the technique. Scand. J. Clin. Lab. Invest. **12:** 408, 1960.
51. Ercisson, H., Tunevall, G., and Wickman, K.: The paper disc method for determination of bacterial sensitivity to antibiotics. Relationship between the diameter of the zone of inhibition and the minimum inhibitory concentration. Scand. J. Clin. Lab. Invest. **12:** 414, 1960.
52. Schlesinger, F. G.: Sensitivity tests by means of diffusion methods and their clinical interpretation. Acta Med. Scand. **148:** 357, 1954.
53. Black, J., Calesnick, B., Williams, D., and Weinstein, M. J.: Pharmacology of gentamicin, a new broad-spectrum antibiotic. Proceedings of the 3rd Interscience conference on Antimicrobial Agents

& Chemotherapy Pubs. by American Society for Microbiology, 1963, p. 138.

54. Jao, R. L., and Jackson, G. G.: Gentamicin sulfate, a new antibiotic against gram-negative bacilli. Laboratory, pharmacological, and clinical evaluation. J. Am. Med. Assoc. **189:** 817, 1964.
55. Bulger, R. J., Sidell, S., and Kirby, W. M. M.: Laboratory and clinical studies of gentamicin. A new broad-spectrum antibiotic. Ann. Intern. Med. **59:** 593, 1963.
56. Bauer, A. W., Perry, D. M., and Kirby, W. M. M.: Single-disk antibiotic-sensitivity testing of staphylococci. An analysis of technique and results. Arch. Intern. Med. **104:** 208, 1959.
57. Bauer, A. W.: The significance of bacterial inhibition zone diameters. A study of the factors influencing antibiotic disc sensitivity tests. In proceedings of the 3rd International Congress of Chemotherapy. Stuttgart, Germany, New York, Hafner Publishing Co., 1964, p. 466.
58. Stamey, T. A.: Urinary tract infections in women. In Campbell's Urology, Ed. 4, Chap. 11, Philadelphia, W. B. Saunders Co., 1978, p. 451.
59. Demerec, M.: Origin of bacterial resistance to antibiotics. J. Bacteriol. **56:** 63, 1948.
60. Newcombe, H. B., and Hawirko, R.: Spontaneous mutation to streptomycin resistance and dependence in *Escherichia coli.* J. Bacteriol. **57:** 565, 1949.
61. Bryson, V., and Demerec, M.: Bacterial resistance. Am. J. Med. **18:** 723, 1955.
62. Stamey, T. A., and Bragonje, J.: Resistance to nalidixic acid. A misconception due to underdosage. J. Am. Med. Assoc. **236:** 1857, 1976.
63. Ronald, A. R., Turck, M., and Petersdorf, R. G.: A critical evaluation of nalidixic acid in urinary tract infections. N. Engl. J. Med. **275:** 1081, 1966.
64. Moorhouse, E. C.: Transferable drug resistance in enterobacteria isolated from urban infants. Br. Med. J. **2:** 405, 1969.

CHAPTER 3

Pyelonephritis—A Case Study in Depth

PYELONEPHRITIS is relatively uncommon unless the infection occurs in the presence of urinary tract obstruction, analgesic abuse or diabetes, severe ureteral reflux in girls under two years of age, or sometimes with overt mismanagement of urinary infections. Moreover, "pyelonephritis" means different things to different people. The best description of the clinical and pathological difficulties associated with the terms acute and chronic pyelonephritis is that of Dr. Paul Beeson, when he was Professor of Medicine at Oxford University.[1] The interested clinician or pathologist should read his thoughtful, careful, and sensible analysis.

Because most descriptions of pyelonephritis were based on necropsy findings where superimposed hypertension, nephrosclerosis, and a variety of terminal events made it difficult to see the true consequences of bacterial disease in the kidney, we published in 1963 a unique case.[2] In July of 1962, a 28-year-old, white mother of two children was admitted to Stanford University Hospital because of recurrent, symptomatic pyelonephritis. Because a nephrectomy was ultimately required to stop her infections, and because her disease represents an example of pure pyelonephritis in a young, symptomatic woman uncomplicated by superimposed hypertension, nephrosclerosis, or glomerulonephritis, her case is presented in detail in this chapter. She has been followed by us at Stanford from 1962 to 1979. This chapter seems as timely in 1980 as it did in 1972 when my first book on urinary infections appeared.[3] For this reason, Chapter 3 is the only chapter from the original book that is not substantially altered and updated.

CLINICAL, BACTERIOLOGIC, AND THERAPEUTIC INVESTIGATIONS

The first attack of cystitis in C.B. occurred 4 days after her marriage in 1952; she was asymptomatic for the next 5 years. In 1954, she delivered a healthy full term baby; there were no urinary tract symptoms during the pregnancy. In 1957, she experienced the first of many acute illnesses that always followed the same pattern: chills, fever (usually to 105°F), backache, urinary urgency and frequency, and urinary tenesmus. The backache frequently localized in the area of the right kidney. These episodes were remarkably similar and generally responded within 3–7 days to a variety of different antimicrobial agents including penicillin, streptomycin, nitrofurantoin, chloramphenicol, and several sulfa preparations. There were two to three attacks a year between 1957 and 1960. A second, full term, pregnancy terminated with a healthy baby in November, 1961; however, one urinary tract infection required hospitalization in the first trimester, and, despite her remaining in bed for the remainder of the pregnancy, three additional episodes required vigorous antibiotic therapy. In the first 6 months of 1962, there were three symptomatic infections. The patient passed no stones during these years, and gross hematuria never occurred. Her blood pressure was always normal. The patient's mother, father, four brothers, and one sister were alive and well; there was no history of renal disease.

Physical examination when the patient was first seen by us on July 8, 1962 revealed a healthy appearing afebrile, 48-kg woman. Her blood pressure was 115/80 mm Hg; the fundi were normal. Except for minimal tenderness in the right kidney on deep palpation, there were no positive physical findings.

Laboratory examinations upon admission in 1962 revealed the following: serum creatinine (S_{Cr}) 0.9 and 0.8 mg/100 ml, blood urea nitrogen (BUN) 15 mg/100 ml, serum sodium (S_{Na}) 139 and 140 mEq/liter, serum potassium (S_K) 4.2 mEq/liter, serum calcium (S_{Ca}) 9.9 and 9.3 mg/100 ml, serum phosphorus (S_P) 3.9 mg/100 ml, total protein 6.8 mg/100 ml, uric acid 5.8 mg/100 ml, fasting blood glucose 83 mg/100 ml, and alkaline phosphatase 1.7 and 2.0 Bessy Lowry units (normal range, 0.2–2.3). The white blood cell count (WBC) was 6300 with 1 banded, 44 segmented, 6 eosinophils, 5 monocytes, and 44 lymphocytes. The hematocrit (Hct) was 42% and the hemoglobin(Hb) 14.2 g. The 15-minute phenolsulfonphthalein (PSP) excretion was 29% in a volume of 160 ml. The urine pH was 5.5, protein 0; microscopic analysis of the fresh centrifuged sediment showed 5–25 fresh neutrophils ("glitter" cells)/high power field (hpf). Bacilli were visible. There were no casts on repeated examinations.

An intravenous urogram (IVU) was performed at another hospital in August of 1960. The 15-minute film (Figure 3.1) showed a dilated pelvic ureter on the right, clubbing of the calyces in the right kidney, and a delicate left renal architecture and ureter. Cystoscopy also was performed in August, 1960; contrast medium was injected into the right kidney, the ureteral catheter was removed, and an x-ray was taken after 10 minutes in the upright position. This film (Figure 3.2) demonstrated retention of the contrast medium in the pelvic ureter. Multiple, small calcifications were present in the renal medulla (indicated by the *arrows* in Figure 3.4). A 5-minute IVU (Figure 3.3) in April, 1962, indicated the atonicity of the right renal calyces; the small medullary calcifications were visible. The right kidney measured 10.5 cm and the left 11.4 cm. A cystogram in July, 1962, showed no

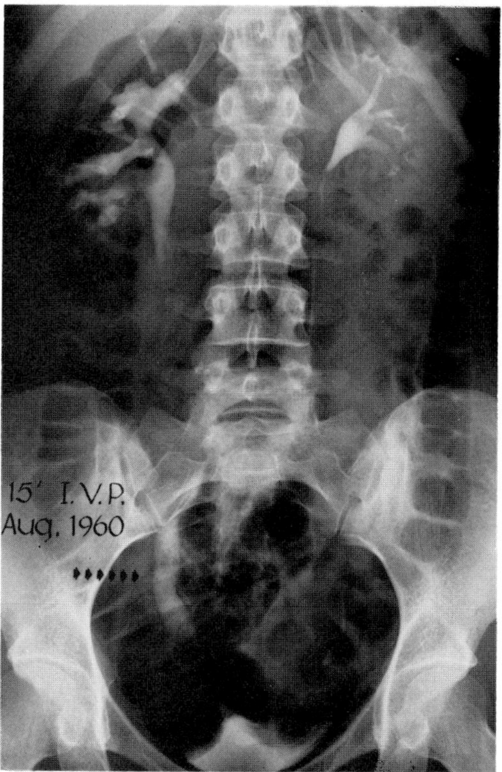

Figure 3.1 Intravenous urogram (15 minute) performed in August, 1960. The *arrows* indicate the dilated pelvic ureter. (Reproduced by permission from T. A. Stamey and A. Pfau, Invest. Urol. **1:** 134, 1963.)[2]

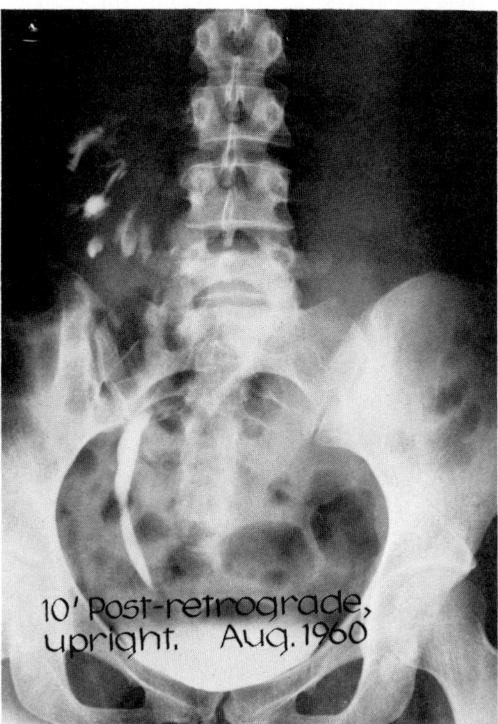

Figure 3.2 A retrograde urogram made 10 minutes after injecting contrast medium and removing the ureteral catheter. The patient was in the upright position during the 10-minute interval following removal of the catheter. (Reproduced by permission from T. A. Stamey and A. Pfau, Invest. Urol. **1:** 134, 1963.)[2]

reflux (Figure 3.4) to either kidney; the postvoiding x-ray demonstrated complete emptying of the bladder without reflux. Two direct catheterizations for postvoiding residual urine in the bladder yielded less than 5 ml each.

Bacteriologic localization studies (Table 3.1) and differential renal function studies were performed at 9:00 AM on July 13, 1962, using a Nupercaine saddle anesthesia. Both ureteral orifices were normal. A No. 8 French (Fr) polyethylene catheter passed easily up the right ureter, and a No. 6 catheter was passed up the left ureter. Pure cultures of *Pseudomonas aeruginosa* were present in the bladder and the right kidney. Tube dilution sensitivities of the *Pseudomonas* isolated from the right kidney are presented in Table 3.2. The left kidney was not infected. The ureteral catheterization studies were completed by 12:15 PM; the patient's urine output was in excess of 1000 ml the night of July 13, and on July 14 the urine output was 2650 ml. She remained afebrile for 24 hours; her temperature at 4:00 PM on July 14 (28 hours after the study) was 100.4°F and 4 hours later was 104.6°F (Figure 3.5). She complained of chills and discomfort in the right kidney. These symptoms were exactly similar to those of her previous episodes. Blood cultures, taken three times, were sterile. At 12:30 AM on July 15, 1962 she was started on 60–80 mg of sodium colistin methane sulfonate (Coly-Mycin) every 8 hours (3.8–5 mg/kg/day). On July 16, 1962, her WBC was 20,400 with 9 banded, 84 segmented, 3 monocytes, and 4 lymphocytes. Her S_{Cr} was 1.4 mg/100 ml, and her urine output 3000 ml per day. Because the febrile course and tenderness in the right flank continued, a No. 5 Fr polyethylene catheter was passed up the right ureter (without difficulty). Clear urine was obtained under a constant flow. Both bladder and right kidney cultures were sterile (32 hours after the first injection of Coly-Mycin). The supernatant of the right renal urine contained 10 mg of protein/100 ml; the spun sediment contained many "glitter" cells. The right ureteral catheter was removed on July 18; the patient's WBC was 8800 (13 banded, 62 segmented, 2 basophils, 15 monocytes, and 8 lymphocytes), S_{Cr} 0.9 mg/100 ml, S_{Na} 141 mEq/liter, S_K 3.6 mEq/liter, Hct 35% and Hb 11.8 g.

On July 23, 1962, after 8 days of Coly-Mycin therapy the S_{Cr} was 0.8 mg/100 ml, the BUN 11 mg/100 ml, and the WBC 6200 with a normal differential. A radiomercury (Hg^{203}) scan of the kidney was performed (Figure 3.6); the left kidney measured 13 × 8 cm and the right kidney 10.5 × 6.5 cm. The patient was discharged the following day and placed on Coly-Mycin, 50 mg every 8 hours.

On August 1, 1962, she weighed 46.5 kg and her blood pressure was 110/70 mm Hg. She complained of slight dizziness on arising and of some numbness of the lips. Her S_{Cr} was 0.8 mg/100 ml, BUN 9 mg/100 ml, WBC 7400, Hb 12.4 g, and a culture of the

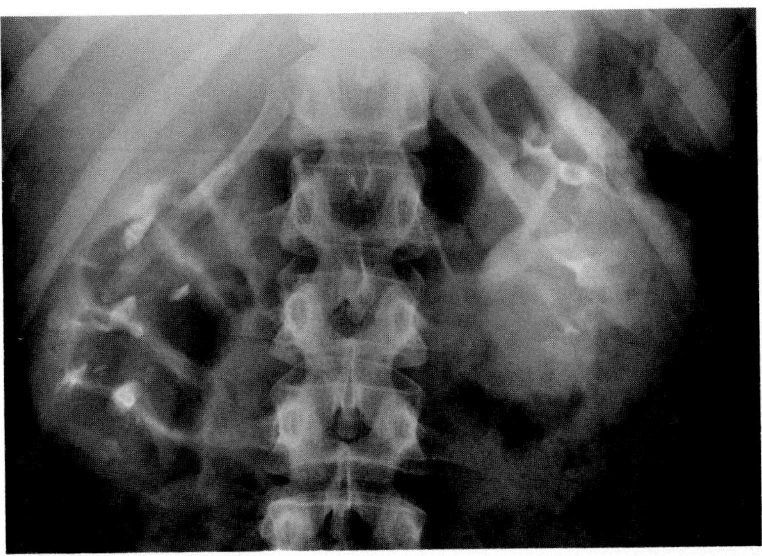

Figure 3.3 Intravenous urogram (5-minute) performed in April, 1962. The left kidney measures 11.4 cm; the right kidney 10.5 cm. The atonicity of the right renal calyces is apparent. Several small perimedullary calcifications can be seen. (Reproduced by permission from T. A. Stamey and A. Pfau, Invest. Urol. **1:** 134, 1963.)[2]

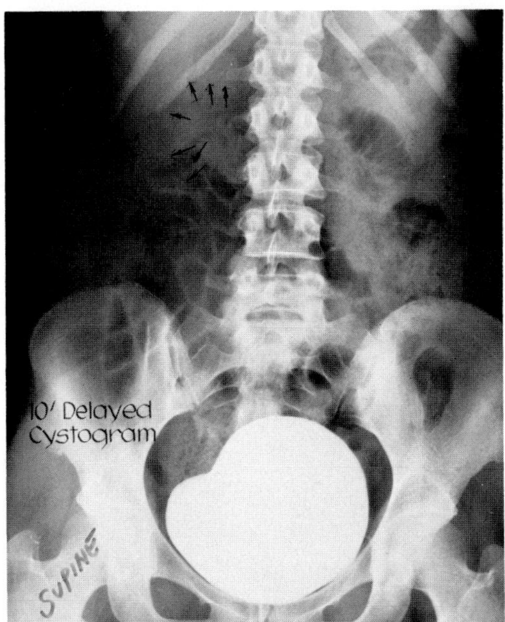

Figure 3.4 Delayed cystogram (10-minute) showing no reflux. The postvoiding film showed complete emptying of the bladder without reflux. The *arrows* in the hilum of the right kidney indicate small calcifications. (Reproduced by permission from T. A. Stamey and A. Pfau, Invest. Urol. **1:** 134, 1963.)[2]

midstream voided urine grew 250 enterococci/ml. Coly-Mycin, 50 mg every 8 hours, was continued.

On August 8, 1962, the patient's blood pressure was 100/70 mm Hg, S_{Cr} 0.9 mg/100 ml, and the BUN 13 mg/100 ml. She was asymptomatic on Coly-Mycin, 50 mg every 8 hours. Culture of her voided urine showed 80,000 enterococci/ml. She was started on *dl*-methionine, 2 g, four times a day.

On August 15, 1962, her blood pressure wa 102/80 mm Hg; she weighed 45 kg. Urine pH was 5.0. A culture of the midstream urine grew 400 *Staphylococcus epidermidis*/ml. She has experienced some right flank aching on August 13, 1962. Coly-Mycin was stopped on August 15, 4 weeks after the initial therapy. One gram of methenamine mandelate (Mandelamine) four times a day was added to the methionine therapy. She developed urinary urgency and frequency, nocturia, and cloudy urine within 3 days of stopping the Coly-Mycin. A midstream culture on August 27 grew 25,000 *Pseudomonas*/ml. The Mandelamine and methionine therapy were continued; the pH of the urine remained less than 6.0. She did

Table 3.1
Bacteriologic Studies Performed July 13, 1962[a]
C.B., 28-year-old, white, female patient.

Source	Urine Flow		Bacterial Count	Specific Gravity[b]	Urine Creatinine		Urine Inulin	
	ml/min		*bacilli/ml*		*mg/100 ml*		*mg/100 ml*	
Cystoscopic bladder urine			220,000					
Bladder count after washing			1					
RK_1[c]	3.92	> 0.81	1,334	1.002	5.15	> 0.75	155	> 0.84
LK_1	4.85		2	1.002	6.86		185	
RK_2	3.94	> 0.76	1,160	1.002	4.93	> 0.79	146	> 0.81
LK_2	5.20		1	1.002	6.22		180	
RK_3	4.01	> 0.81	1,392	1.002	5.23	> 0.72	137	> 0.79
LK_3	4.93		0	1.003	7.29		173	
RK_4	1.01	> 1.02	1,276	1.011	Lab. accident		495	> 0.45
LK_4	0.99		0	1.014			1,105	
RK_5	3.14	> 0.85	1,102	1.008	4.93	> 0.76	162	> 0.74
LK_5	3.68		0	1.010	6.61		220	

[a] Reproduced by permission from T. A. Stamey and A. Pfau, Invest. Urol. **1:** 162, 1963.[2]
[b] Refractometer, American Optical Company.
[c] RK and LK = right and left kidney; subscript denotes the serial order of separate collection periods.

Table 3.2
Tube Dilution Data for *Pseudomonas* before Therapy July 13, 1962[a]
All tubes were clear following the inoculation of 10^{6-8} bacteria/ml before incubation. + = cloudy tube (gross evidence of bacterial growth). 0 = clear tube after incubation. If tubes are clear at 24 hours (0), a loop subculture is transferred to the appropriate agar to determine presence or absence of bacterial growth. The superscript indicates the number of bacteria present in the subculture. C indicates confluent growth on subculture (too numerous to count).

	Time of Reading	Control	Drug Concentration (μg/ml)								
			0.2	1	5	10	20	50	100	250	500
	hr										
Primary pseudomonas											
Penicillin	24/48	+	+/+	+/+	+/+	+/+	+/+	+/+	+/+	+/+	+/+
Streptomycin	24/48	+	+/+	+/+	+/+	+/+	+/+	+/+	+/+	+/+	$0/+^{C}$
Chloramphenicol	24/48	+	+/+	+/+	+/+	+/+	+/+	+/+	+/+	+/+	+/+
Coly-Mycin	24/48	+	+/+	+/+	+/+	$0/0^{0}$	$0/0^{0}$	$0/0^{0}$	$0/0^{0}$	$0/0^{0}$	$0/0^{0}$
Furadantin	24/48	+	+/+	+/+	+/+	+/+	+/+	+/+	+/+	+/+	+/+
Thiosulfil	24/48	+	+/+	+/+	+/+	+/+	+/+	+/+	+/+	+/+	+/+
Neomycin	24/48	+	+/+	+/+	$0/+^{C}$	$0/+^{C}$	$0/+^{C}$	$0/+^{12}$	$0/0^{0}$	$0/0^{0}$	$0/0^{0}$
Tetracycline	24/48	+	+/+	+/+	+/+	+/+	+/+	+/+	$0/+^{C}$	$0/0^{41}$	$0/0^{15}$
Oxacillin	24/48	+	+/+	+/+	+/+	+/+	+/+	+/+	+/+	+/+	+/+
Mucoid pseudomonas variant											
Streptomycin	24/48	+	+/+	+/+	$0/+^{C}$	$0/+^{C}$	$0/0^{0}$	$0/0^{0}$	$0/0^{0}$	$0/0^{0}$	$0/0^{0}$
Chloramphenicol	24/48	+	+/+	+/+	+/+	+/+	+/+	+/+	+/+	+/+	+/+
Coly-Mycin	24/48	+	+/+	+/+	+/+	$0/0^{0}$	$0/0^{0}$	$0/0^{0}$	$0/0^{0}$	$0/0^{0}$	$0/0^{0}$

[a] Reproduced by permission from T. A. Stamey and A. Pfau, Invest. Urol. **1:** 162, 1963.[2]

not develop chills or fever. On September 12, 1962, a suprapubic needle aspiration of the bladder urine grew 18,000 *Pseudomonas*/ml. The spun sediment was loaded with "glitter" cells; the supernatant contained no protein.

Tube dilution sensitivities (Table 3.3) indicated that the Coly-Mycin was still bactericidal for the *Pseudomonas* at a concentration of 5 μg/ml and that increased resistance had not developed.

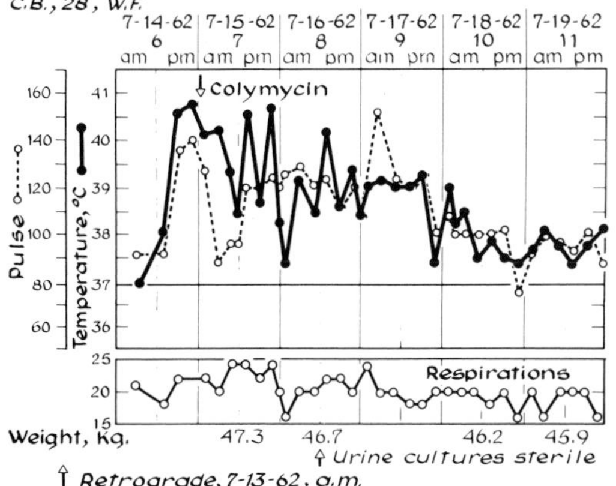

Figure 3.5 Temperature record indicating the time of ureteral catheterization, the onset of fever, the start of Coly-Mycin therapy, the sterilization of the urine, and the persistence of the fever in the presence of a sterile urine. (Reproduced by permission from T. A. Stamey and A. Pfau, Invest. Urol. **1:** 134, 1963.)[2]

The patient was readmitted to the hospital on September 16, 1962. Her S_{Cr} was 0.9 mg/100 ml, WBC 5000 (62 segmented, 4 eosinophils, 2 monocytes, and 32 lymphocytes), Hct 41.5%, and Hb 13.7 g. Bacteriologic studies on the bladder and ureteral urine were performed on September 17, 1962 (Table 3.4). These collections were made with No. 5 Fr polyethylene catheters in the midureter; a water diuresis was obtained by oral hydration. Ureteral peristalsis was measured simultaneously in each ureter with venous pressure strain gauges (Statham) and a Honeywell Visicorder (Figures 3.7–3.8).

One hour after completion of the cystoscopic studies (2:00 PM) on September 17, the patient received 75 mg of Coly-Mycin.

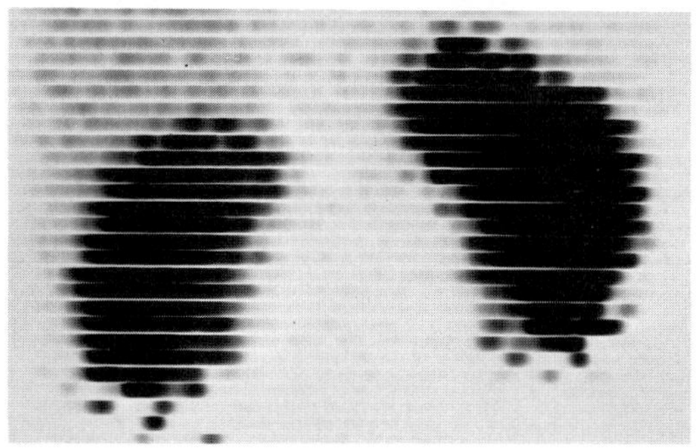

Figure 3.6 Radiomercury (Hg^{203}) scan of the kidneys. (Reproduced by permission from T. A. Stamey and A. Pfau, Invest. Urol. **1:** 134, 1963.)[2]

Table 3.3
Tube Dilution Data for *Pseudomonas* after Coly-Mycin Therapy September 9, 1962[a]

	Time of Reading	Control	Drug Concentration (μg/ml) 0.2	1	5	10	20	50	100	250	500
		hr									
Penicillin	24/48	+	+/+	+/+	+/+	+/+	+/+	+/+	+/+	+/+	+/+
Streptomycin	24/48	+	+/+	+/+	+/+	+/+	+/+	+/+	+/+	+/+	+/+
Chloramphenicol	24/48	+	+/+	+/+	+/+	+/+	+/+	+/+	+/+	$0/+^{C}$	$0/+^{C}$
Coly-Mycin	24/48	+	+/+	+/+	$0/0^{0}$	$0/0^{0}$	$0/0^{0}$	$0/0^{0}$	$0/0^{0}$	$0/0^{0}$	$0/0^{0}$
Furadantin	24/48	+	+/+	+/+	+/+	+/+	+/+	+/+	+/+	+/+	+/+
Thiosulfil	24/48	+	+/+	+/+	+/+	+/+	+/+	+/+	+/+	+/+	+/+
Neomycin	24/48	+	+/+	+/+	$0/+^{C}$	$0/+^{C}$	$0/+^{C}$	$0/+^{12}$	$0/0^{0}$	$0/0^{0}$	$0/0^{0}$
Tetracycline	24/48	+	+/+	+/+	+/+	+/+	+/+	+/+	$0/+^{C}$	$0/0^{41}$	$0/0^{15}$
Oxacillin	24/48	+	+/+	+/+	+/+	+/+	+/+	+/+	+/+	+/+	+/+

[a] Reproduced by permission from T. A. Stamey and A. Pfau, Invest. Urol. **1:** 162, 1963.[2]
[b] See legend to Table 3.2 for explanation of symbols.

A second 75 mg were given at 10:00 PM on September 17; on September 18, she received 75 mg of Coly-Mycin at 6:00 AM and 10:00 PM. She remained afebrile and comfortable.

Table 3.4
Bacteriologic Studies Performed September 17, 1962

Source	Bacterial Count	Specific Gravity[a]	Urine Creatinine	
	bacilli/ml		*mg/100 ml*	
Cystoscopic bladder urine	2,500	1.005	30	
Bladder count after washing	1	1.000	<1	
RK_1[b]	3,016	1.005	22	>0.27
LK_1	1	1.013	82	
RK_2	1,160	1.003	13	>0.48
LK_2	0	1.006	27	
RK_3	754	1.002	9	>0.53
LK_3	0	1.003	17	

[a] Refractometer, American Optical Company.
[b] RK and LK = right and left kidney; subscript denotes the serial order of separate collection periods.

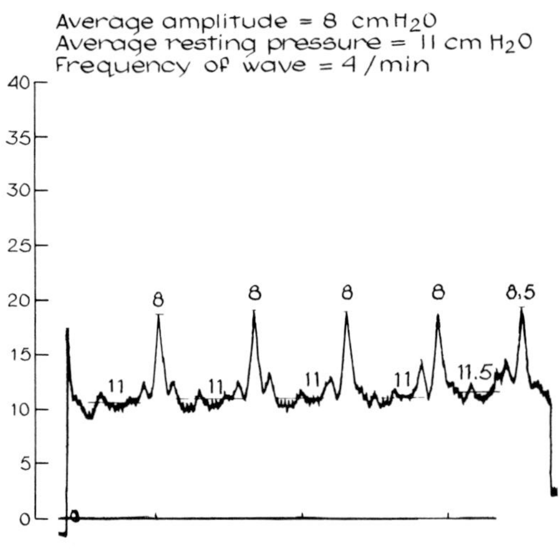

Figure 3.7 Honeywell Visicorder pressure tracing of ureteral peristalsis, right upper ureter. The "resting pressure" reflects baseline intra-abdominal pressure plus the unknown distance between the recording end of the catheter and the "zero" setting of the strain gauge. The average amplitude of ureteral peristalsis in 8 cm of water, 4 waves/minute of frequency. (Reproduced by permission from T. A. Stamey and A. Pfau, Invest. Urol. **1:** 134, 1963.)[2]

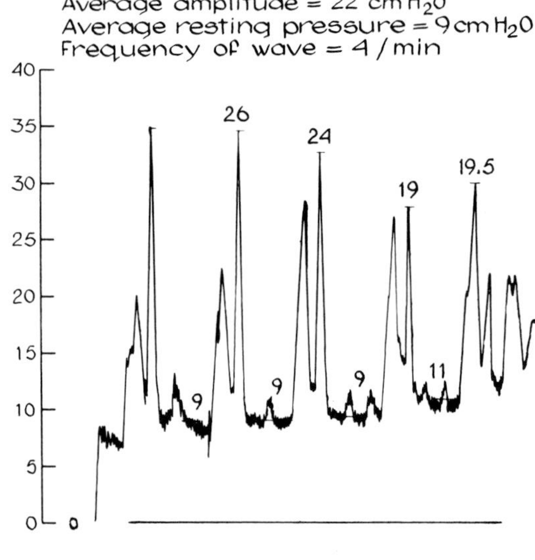

Figure 3.8 Ureteral pressure tracing, left upper ureter. The average amplitude of ureteral peristalsis is 22 cm of water, 4 waves/minute frequency. (Reproduced by permission from T. A. Stamey and A. Pfau, Invest. Urol. **1:** 134, 1963.)[2]

The abdomen was explored at 7:30 AM on September 19, 1962. A midline, transperitoneal incision allowed full exploration of the abdominal contents. The bladder was aspirated for culture from within the abdomen; 1218 *Pseudomonas*/ml were recovered despite the previous 48 hours of Coly-Mycin at 150 mg/day. The right kidney moved easily beneath the posterior peritoneum; the capsule was smooth, and there were no perirenal adhesions. The kidney appeared entirely normal, although somewhat small. The kidney, all of the ureter, and a cuff of the bladder containing the ureteral orifice were excised and placed in a sterile basin. The capsule was washed with saline. Several grams of cortex were removed and placed in sterile saline; the kidney was opened in the longitudinal axis, and several grams of medullary tissue were excised. Both cortex and medulla were pulverized in a sterile tissue blending apparatus. The cortex, per gram of tissue, was sterile; the medulla contained 2784 *Pseudomonas*/g of tissue. Coly-Mycin tube dilution sensitivities on the *Pseudomonas* isolated from the medulla of the kidney showed a bacteriostatic effect at a concentration of 5 μg/ml and a bactericidal effect at 10 μg/ml.

The patient had an uneventful postoperative course. An indwelling Foley catheter was left in the bladder for 48 hours. She received Coly-Mycin, 75 mg every 12 hours, until September 26. A midstream voided urine culture on September 24 grew 82 million *Proteus morganii*/ml. The tube dilution sensitivities showed an unexpected sensitivity to tetracycline (Table 3.5), and so she was started on 250 mg of tetracycline every 6 hours on September 26. A midstream voided urine on September 28, 1962 was sterile. She was discharged on September 28 and told to continue the tetracycline for 7 days. Her S_{Cr} at the time of discharge was 1.0 mg/100 ml.

The patient returned for an outpatient visit 2 weeks after discharge (October 9, 1962); she had received no medication for 1 week. A midstream voided urine obtained on the cystoscopy table was sterile.

On November 6, 1962, a voided urine culture grew 165 colonies of *Staphylococcus epidermidis*/ml.

She remained asymptomatic and felt extremely well. On December 4, 1962, a catheterized urine specimen was sterile. Inulin and *p*-aminohippuric acid (PAH) clearances were performed under an oral water diuresis to study the glomerular filtration rate (GFR), renal plama flow (RPF), and free water clearances ("C_{H_2O}") of the remaining left kidney.

On March 5, 1963, a midstream voided urine was sterile; the patient's blood pressure was 110/80 mg Hg, and she was asymptomatic.

She was seen again on May 9, 1963 for a study of inulin and PAH clearances from her remaining kidney. The bladder was catheterized with a Foley catheter for these clearances; the catheterized urine was sterile.

One year later, in 1964, she had her first postnephrectomy episode of urinary frequency and tenesmus, but no dysuria. A urine culture showed 10^5 *Escherichia coli*/ml, and she was treated with oral penicillin-G for 10 days. Although her bladder urine became sterile and remained so, her vaginal vestibule and urethal cultures grew thousands of *E. coli*; because of this, she was started on a regimen of taking 250 mg of penicillin-G after sexual intercourse. Urine cultures in September, 1966 and August, 1967 were sterile even though pathogenic flora persisted on the perineum. In November 1967, she was found to have an asymptomatic *E. coli* bacteriuria that was treated with nalidixic acid, after which she was changed to nalidixic acid as a postintercourse regimen.

Between 1967 and December 1970, she had two to three episodes each year characterized by urinary frequency and tenesmus, always responding to a few days of continuous nalidixic acid. Her next infec-

Table 3.5
Tube Dilution Data for *Proteus morganii* after Surgery September 24, 1962[a]

	Time of Reading	Control	Drug Concentration (μg/ml)								
			0.2	1	5	10	20	50	100	250	500
		hr									
Penicillin	24/48	+	+/+	+/+	+/+	+/+	+/+	+/+	+/+	+/+	+/+
Streptomycin	24/48	+	+/+	+/+	+/+	$0/0^0$	$0/0^0$	$0/0^0$	$0/0^0$	$0/0^0$	$0/0^0$
Chloramphenicol	24/48	+	+/+	+/+	$0/0^C$	$0/0^4$	$0/0^4$	$0/0^3$	$0/0^0$	$0/0^0$	$0/0^0$
Coly-Mycin	24/48	+	+/+	+/+	+/+	+/+	+/+	+/+	+/+	+/+	+/+
Furadantin	24/48	+	+/+	+/+	+/+	+/+	+/+	$0/0^0$	$0/0^0$	$0/0^0$	$0/0^0$
Thiosulfil	24/48	+	+/+	+/+	+/+	+/+	+/+	+/+	+/+	+/+	+/+
Neomycin	24/48	+	+/+	+/+	+/+	+/+	+/+	$0/0^7$	$0/0^0$	$0/0^0$	$0/0^0$
Tetracycline	24/48	+	+/+	+/+	$0/0^{10}$	$0/0^4$	$0/0^2$	$0/0^0$	$0/0^0$	$0/0^0$	$0/0^0$
Oxacillin	24/48	+	+/+	+/+	+/+	+/+	+/+	+/+	+/+	+/+	+/+

[a] See legend to Table 3.2 for explanation of symbols

tion occurred on December 19, 1970. She was seen at Stanford University for reevaluation on December 22. Over 7 days had elapsed since the last capsule of postintercourse nalidixic acid; she had forced fluids for relief of her symptoms between December 19 and 22. Upon examination, there was no abdominal or pelvic tenderness. Examination of a hydrated urine indicated no protein or bacilli, but two "glitter" cells (fresh polymorphonuclear leukocytes) per high power field were found in the centrifuged sediment. The vaginal vestibule culture showed no Gram-negative bacteria for the first time, the urethral aliquot 500 *Proteus mirabilis*/ml, and the midstream urine 500 *P. mirabilis*/ml, all collected with the patient voiding from the cystoscopy table. The *P. mirabilis* was highly sensitive to nalidixic acid. She voided 350 ml; a catheterized urine 5 minutes later was 20 ml, and again it grew 500 *P. mirabilis*/ml, confirming the low count bacteriuria. A serum creatinine was 0.9 mg/100 ml. An intravenous urogram obtained on December 23 was unremarkable and compared in every way to the examination in 1962. The left kidney measured 12.8 cm, the cortical border was well outlined and smooth (Figure 3.9), and the calyces were delicate (Figure 3.10).

Her infections seemed to cease after 1970. Cultures were sterile at Stanford in 1973 and 1975. There was a single episode of left flank, groin, and inner thigh pain with nausea but no fever or dysuria in July 1975. A routine intravenous urogram in October 1975, was exactly comparable to her previous examinations; no stones were visible in the left kidney. Between 1975 and January 1979 she received no antimicrobial agents and urine cultures every 6 months have shown no infection.

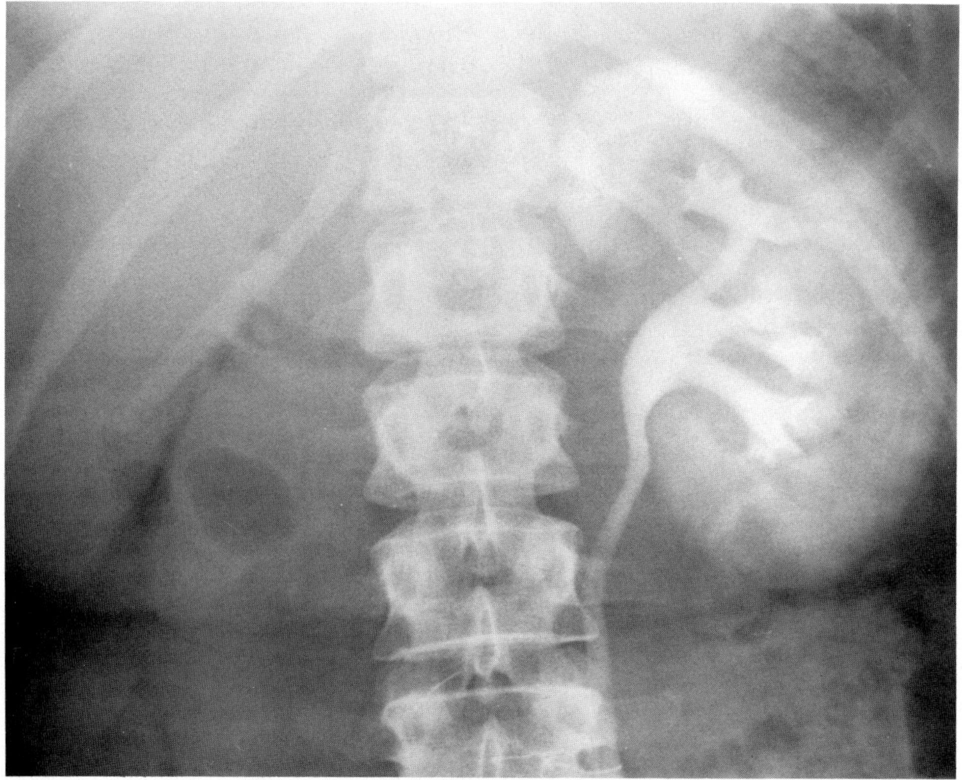

Figure 3.9 A 10-minute compression film from an intravenous urogram on C.B. in October, 1975. The calyces are delicate, the cortical margins are well seen; there are no scars.

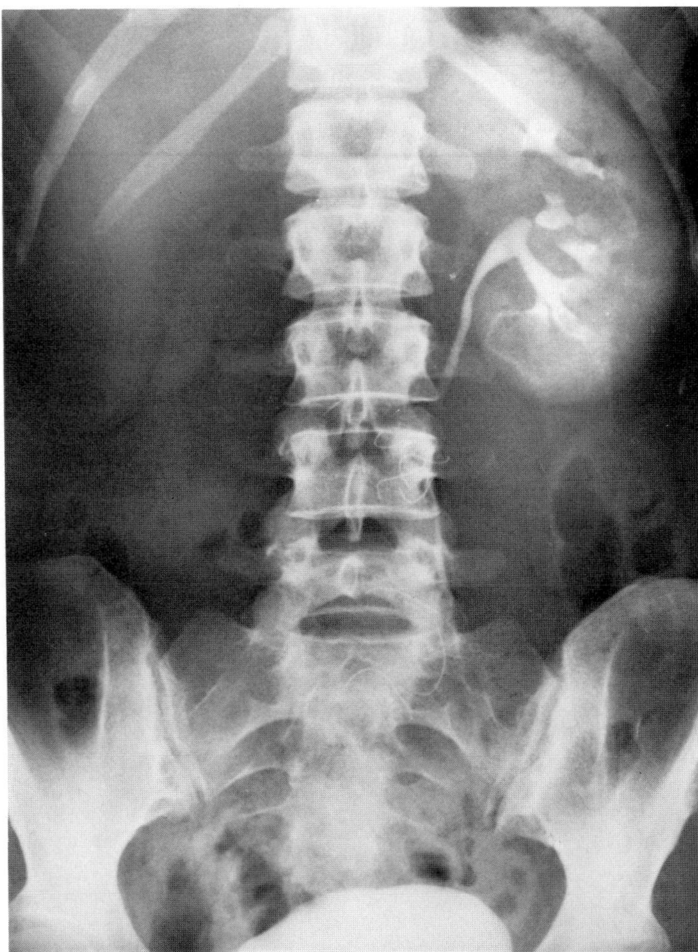

Figure 3.10 Film from intravenous urogram on C.B. after release of compression in Figure 3.9.

Some Observations On the Pathogenesis and Clinical Course of Her Disease

The right kidney was removed in 1962 because Coly-Mycin, 50 mg every 8 hours for 4 weeks, sterilized the urine but did not prevent recurrence of the *Pseudomonas* 3 days after stopping therapy. At that time, Coly-Mycin was the only drug really useful for pseudomonas infections. Between 1957 and 1962, numerous infections were documented by her history and urinalysis, but the only culture obtained during her hospitalizations was in September 1960, which showed *Pseudomonas* in pure culture. Since *Pseudomonas* is usually a hospital-acquired organism, it is possible that her early infections were *E. coli* and that the *Pseudomonas* occurred following one of her instrumentations.

The pericalyceal calcifications may have been the reason for her bacteriologic persistence. As will be seen in Chapter 8, infection stones harbor the bacteria deep inside the interstices of the stone and cannot be killed with antimicrobial therapy. Thus, bacterial persistence in recurrent bacteriuria usually occurs because of renal calculi rather than renal tissue.

Her subsequent course after nephrectomy indicates that the basic problem was the establishment of a pathogenic Gram-negative flora on the vaginal vestibule and urethral mucosa, followed by introduction of these bacteria into the bladder. It was very likely her original problem. The establishment of pathogenic Gram-negative bacteria on the vaginal vestibule and their subsequent entry into the bladder are discussed in the following chapter.

PATHOLOGIC CHARACTERISTICS

The excised right kidney weighed 100 g. Representative microscopic sections of the cortex (Figures 3.11–3.16), medulla (Figures 3.17–3.20), and ureter (Figure. 3.21) were

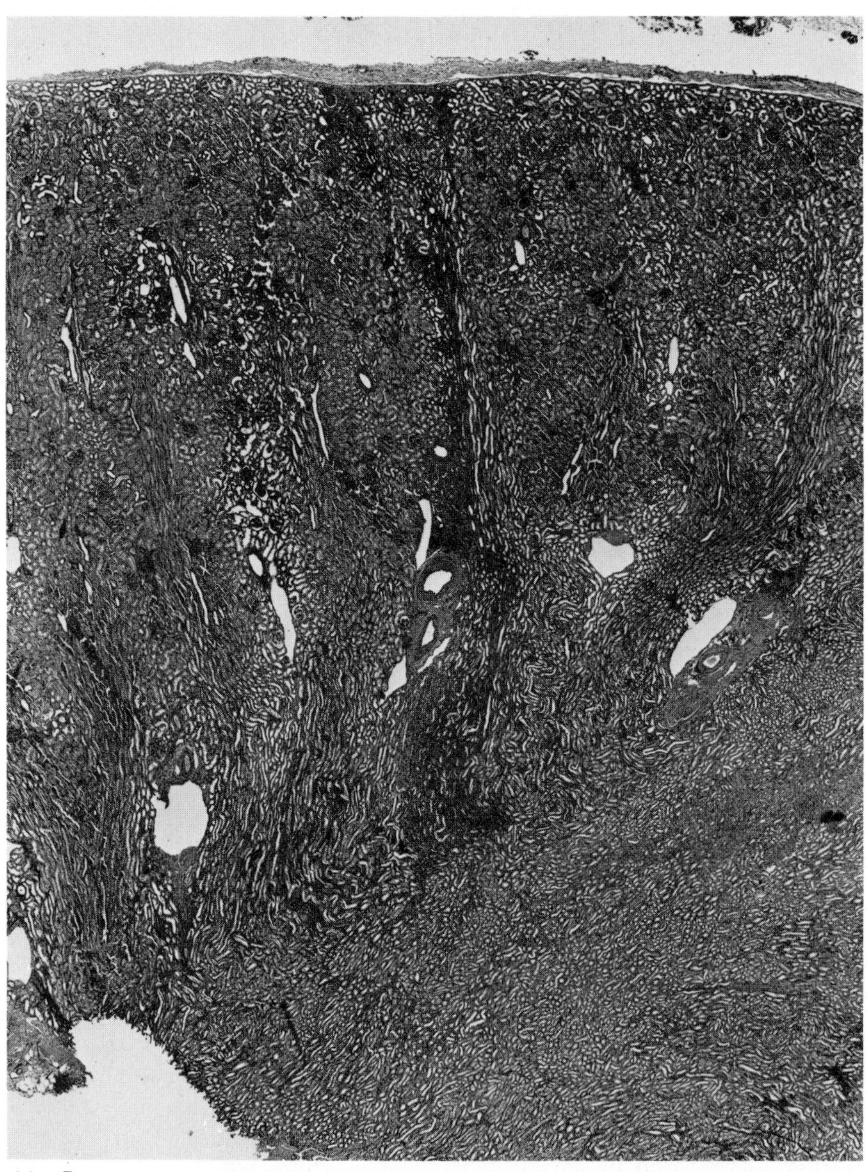

Figure 3.11 Low power section (×10) of the renal cortex and medulla showing a linear band of chronic inflammation extending from the medulla to the capsule. Most of the renal cortex was less involved than this figure. The two large arteries at the junction of the middle and lower one-third of the linear band are shown in Figure 3.16. Despite being in contact with the inflammatory area, there is no arteritis of these large vessels. (Reproduced by permission from T. A. Stamey and A. Pfau, Invest. Urol. **1:** 134, 1963.)[2]

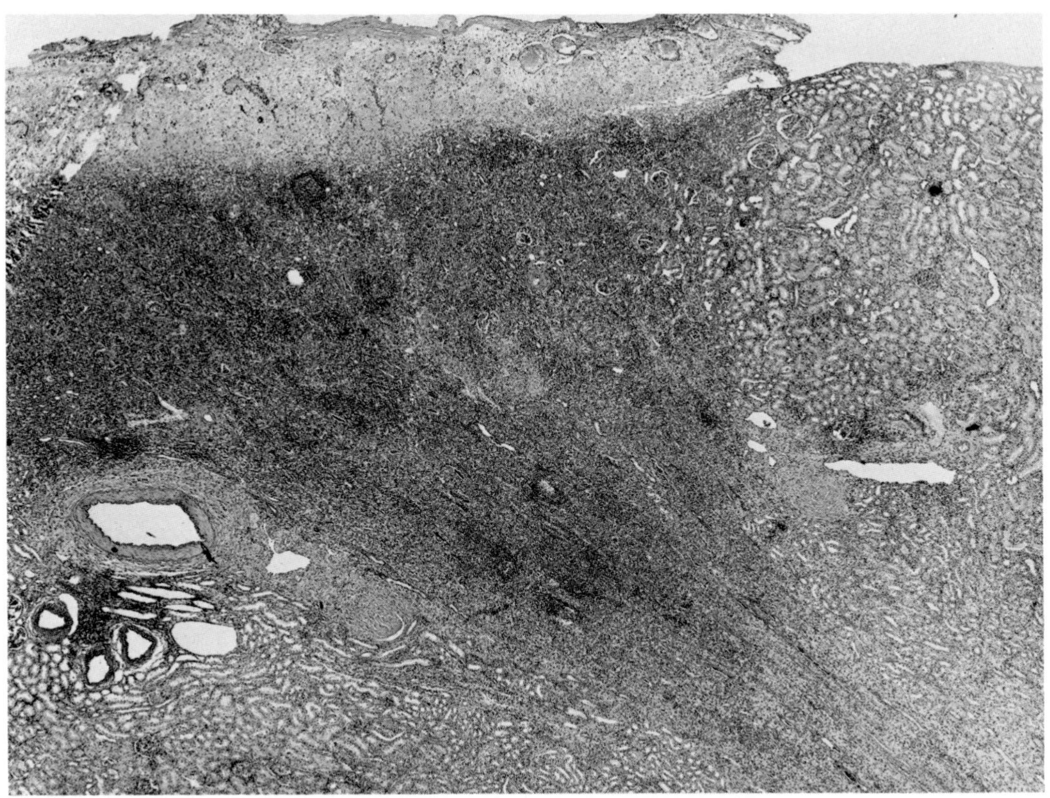

Figure 3.12 Section (×18) of the renal cortex showing a large wedge-shaped area of the acute and chronic inflammation extending from the medulla to the cortex. The large vessels are not involved with inflammatory reaction. (Reproduced by permission from T. A. Stamey and A. Pfau, Invest. Urol. **1:** 134, 1963.)[2]

studied in 10 random blocks of kidney tissue.

Figure 3.11 is a low power (×10) section of the renal cortex showing the linear bands of inflammation extending from the medullary area to the renal capsule. Most of the renal cortex was less involved than the portion shown in Figure 3.11, and 75% of the renal cortex showed no inflammatory disease. An occasional area of the cortex (Figure 3.12) was more severely involved in a classical wedge of inflammatory tissue. Figure 3.13 shows the demarcation between the wedge of inflammatory tissue of Figure 3.12 and the adjacent normal cortex. Figures 3.14 and 3.15 are sections (×200) from the cortical wedge of inflammation (Figure 3.12) which show the presence of polymorphonuclear leukocyte casts (Figure 3.14) and typical proliferative changes in the interlobular arteries and arterioles (Figure 3.15). Figure 3.16 shows the large normal arcuate arteries immediately adjacent to the linear band of inflammation in the center of Figure 3.11.

The medulla of the kidney was uniformly involved. The calyceal epithelium was thickened and infiltrated with leukocytes; fibroblastic proliferation was prominent (Figure 3.17). Figure 3.18 shows the involvement of a calyceal fornix adjacent to a pyramid seen on the right. Figure 3.19 is a higher magnification (×200) of the tissue reaction in the medulla, and Figures 3.17 and 3.19 show polymorphonuclear leukocyte casts. Local foci of calcification were present in both the cortex (*right upper corner* of Figure 3.12) and corticomedullary

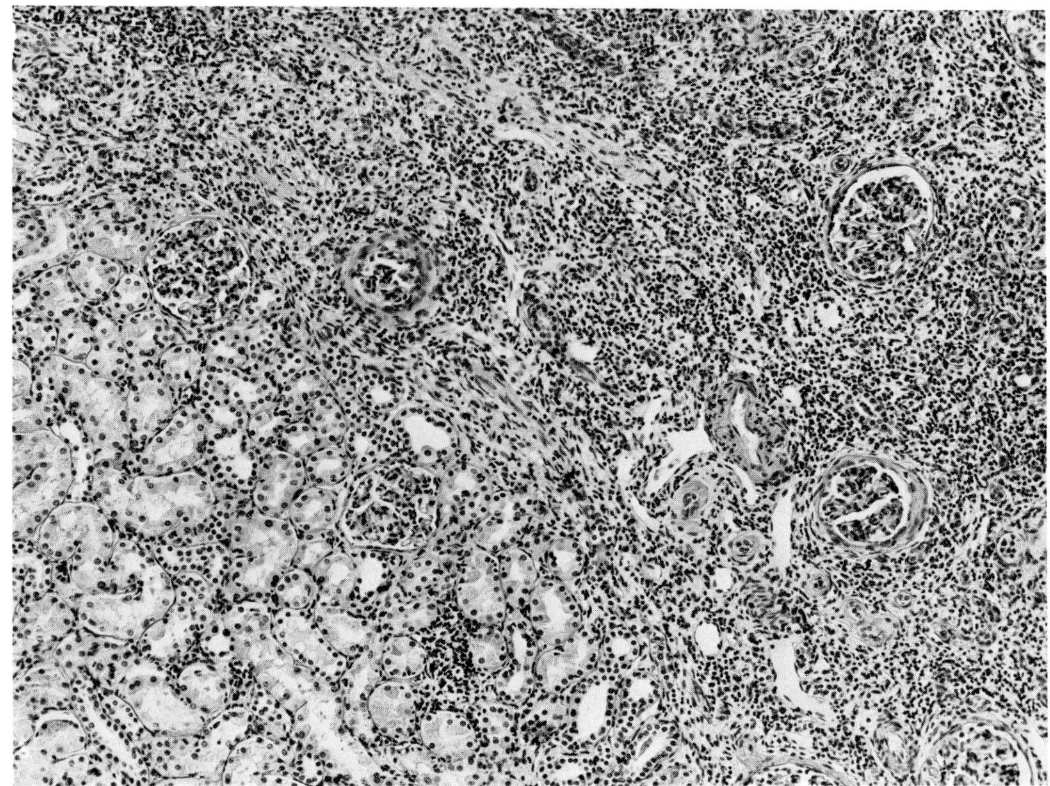

Figure 3.13 Higher magnification (×90) of the right edge of the wedge-shaped lesion in Figure 3.12. Some glomeruli show true periglomerular fibrosis, while others show collagen laid down internally to Bowman's capsule with pronounced cellular components resembling crescents. The interstitial tissue is densely infiltrated with lymphocytes, some eosinophils, and occasional polymorphonuclear leukocytes. (Reproduced by permission from T. A. Stamey and A. Pfau, Invest. Urol. **1:** 134, 1963.)[2]

junction (Figure 3.20). These calcifications were not associated with the areas of inflammation.

The ureter was moderately involved, and subepithelial cysts (ureteritis cystica) were present (Figure 3.21).

Dr. Robert H. Heptinstall, Professor and Chairman of the Department of Pathology, The Johns Hopkins Hospital, kindly reviewed these sections for me in 1963 and had this to say:

The kidney shows evidence of a patchy pyelonephritic lesion which is mainly chronic but with some evidence of active inflammation. There are numerous chronic inflammatory foci mainly confined to the cortex but in places involving the medulla. In between these areas there is normal renal tissue. The uninvolved areas as judged by these sections account for approximately three-quarters of the kidney substance. The changes in the inflammatory zones are as follows.

Glomeruli. These show a variety of changes. Some are normal, others show thickening of Bowman's capsule, and others show mild degrees of true periglomerular fibrosis. A number show collagen being laid down internal to Bowman's capsule, and some of these have a very pronounced cellular component resembling crescents. These changes probably represent a response both to local inflammation and to ischemia. The glomerular tufts usually merely show

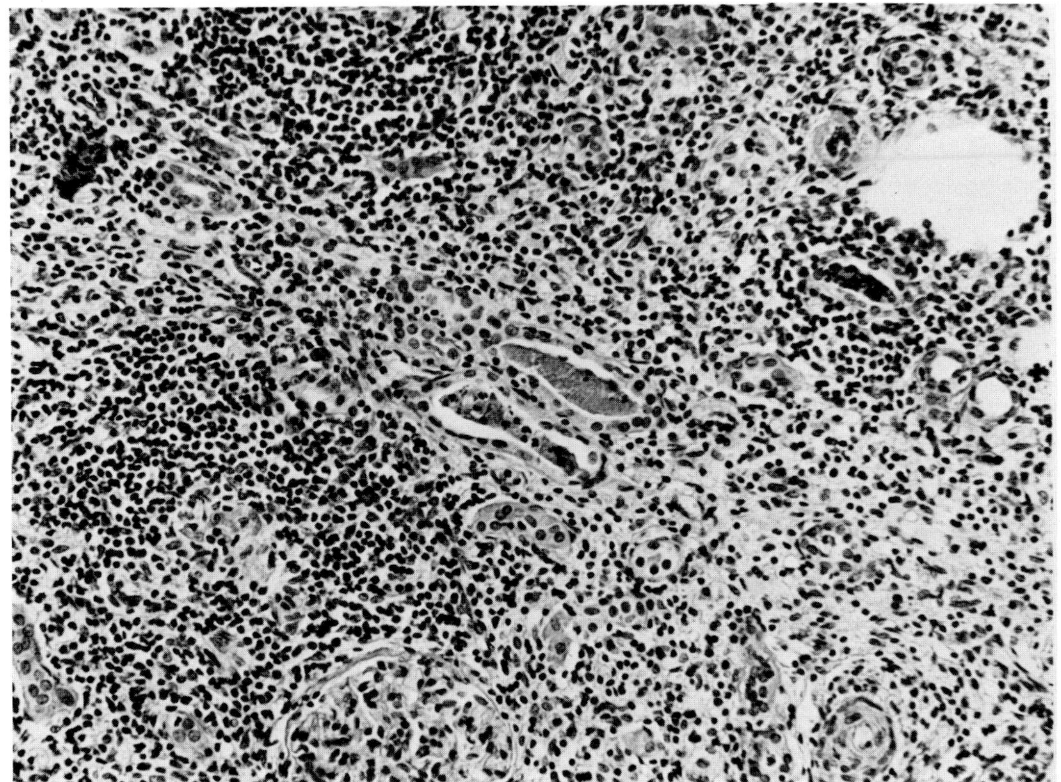

Figure 3.14 Polymorphonuclear leukocyte cast (×180) present in the cortical inflammation of Figure 3.12. Only a few atrophic tubules remain. (Reproduced by permission from T. A. Stamey and A. Pfau, Invest. Urol. **1:** 134, 1963.)[2]

shrinkage in those glomeruli with changes in relation to Bowman's capsule.

Tubules. Proximal tubules and limbs have largely disappeared, and some are undergoing atrophy with much basement membrane thickening. Some collecting tubules show polymorphs in their lumen and probably indicate some active inflammation. In places there are atrophic tubules containing hyaline casts, but this is not pronounced.

Vessels. There is an early but definite intimal thickening in small arteries and larger arterioles.

Interstitial Tissue. There is dense infiltration by lymphocytes and to lesser degree by eosinophiles. Occasional polymorphs are seen, and fibrosis is not pronounced.

Intervening areas, apart from changes consequent on surgical ligation of pedicle, show no remarkable change.

There are some calcific foci in tubules, usually in the medulla.

The calyces are widened and lined by rather thickened epithelium. There is a pronounced cellular reaction under the epithelium. Some of the pelvic epithelium is much thickened, and polymorphs are present between the cells. Tissue under the pelvis shows lymphocytes, lymphoid follicles, plasma cells, eosinophiles, and some polymorphs.

The feature which impresses me in this case is that so much of the parenchyma has been spared by the inflammatory process. Apart from this it is a patchy chronic pyelonephritis with some evidence of acute reaction.

The classical pathologic description of pyelonephritis is that of Weiss and Parker.[4] Their autopsy studies, however, included late stages of the disease which are often complicated by hypertension and vascular changes. Because the patient reported here

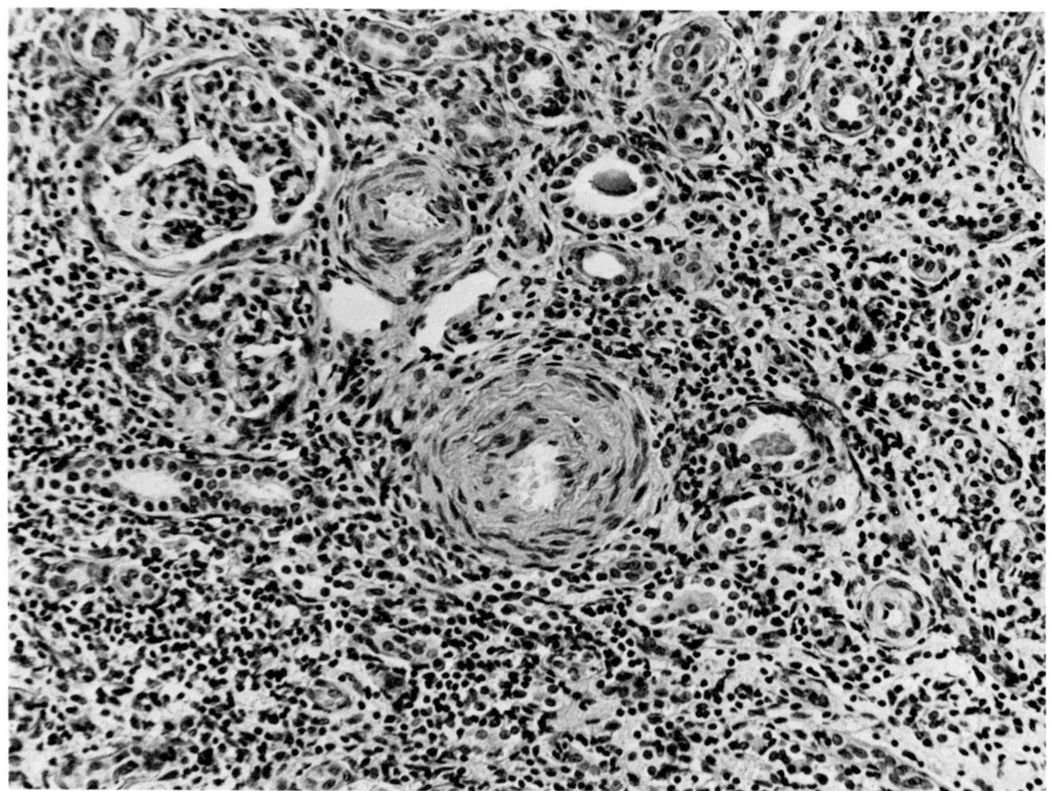

Figure 3.15 Section (×180), also from the cortical wedge of inflammation in Figure 3.12, showing the intense proliferative arteritis and arteriolitis described by Weiss and Parker.[4] These vascular changes are seen only in the inflammatory areas. The tubules are virtually destroyed. (Reproduced by permission from T. A. Stamey and A. Pfau, Invest. Urol. **1:** 134, 1963.)[2]

is an example of pure symptomatic pyelonephritis, incurable with drug therapy and uncomplicated by vascular hypertension, the microscopic sections (Figures 3.11–3.21) together with Dr. Heptinstall's comments represent an unusual opportunity to study the pathologic characteristics of this disease in its purest form. The important pathologic findings are indicated in the legends of each figure.

FUNCTIONAL CHARACTERISTICS

Over the past years, Bricker and his associates,[5, 6] using an experimental model which allows the study of a diseased kidney in comparison to the contralateral normal kidney in the dog, have supported the theory of the "intact nephron" in the diseased kidney. This theory implies that "the pathologic processes do not destroy specific functional sites in the tubule"[6] and that the surviving nephrons in the diseased kidney, regardless of the type of renal disease, remain essentially intact. Bricker *et al.*,[5] from serial studies on unilateral pyelonephritis in the dog, concluded that, "per unit of glomerular filtrate, concentrating capacity and diluting capacity remain comparable to the intact kidney. These observations fail to demonstrate a functional pattern distinguishing pyelonephritis from other forms of progressive renal disease and suggest that the persisting nephrons in pyelonephritic kidneys retain normal functional characteristics."[5]

Our own studies on unilateral pyelonephritis in man, of which the patient presented in this paper is representative, do not support the "intact nephron" theory. The data in this paper not only show a specific functional defect in the surviving nephrons, but also indicate that the site of this functional lesion is clearly in the medulla of the kidney, while proximal tubular function remains normal. This medullary functional defect is important because it (1) explains the clinical observations relating to sodium, water, and extracellular fluid balance presented by the pyelonephritic pa-

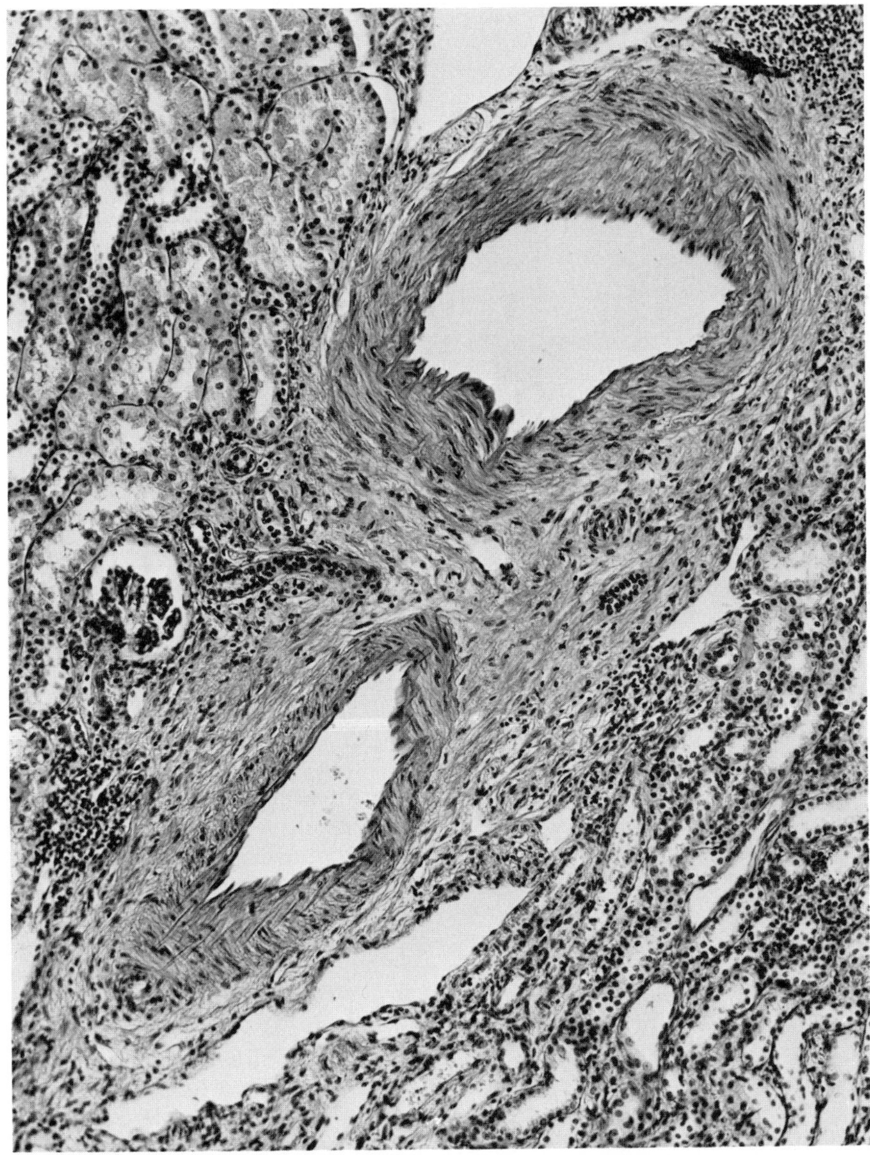

Figure 3.16 The two vessels (×100) referred to in Figure 3.11. There is no vascular reaction even though the arteries are in immediate juxtaposition to the inflammatory area. (Reproduced by permission from T. A. Stamey and A. Pfau, Invest. Urol. **1:** 134, 1963.)[2]

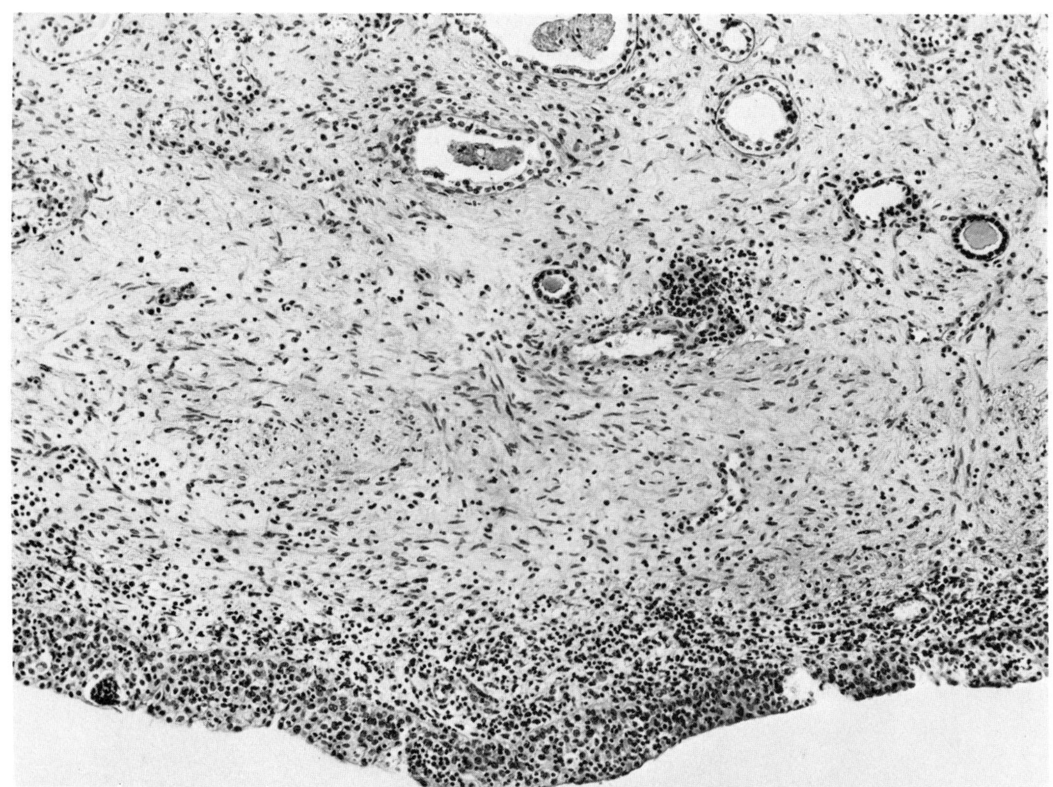

Figure 3.17 Typical section (×90) of the calyceal epithelium showing a pronounced cellular reaction with lymphocytes, plasma cells, polymorphonuclear leukocytes, eosinophils, and fibroblastic thickening. Casts are visible in the distal collecting ducts. (Reproduced by permission from T. A. Stamey and A. Pfau, Invest. Urol. **1:** 134, 1963.)[2]

tient and (2) confirms the functional defect in concentrating ability long recognized as characteristic of pyelonephritis.[7, 8]

The technique used in this patient for performing reproducible differential renal function studies is published in detail elsewhere.[9, 10] Three consecutive collection periods with oral water hydration are presented and averaged in Table 3.6 (20–55 minutes). These initial collections with a water diuresis were followed by an infusion of 8% urea in saline at 10 ml/minute. Antidiuretic hormone (ADH, Pitressin) was added to the infusion to deliver 5 mU/kg/hour, and a single loading dose of 5 mU of ADH/kg was injected intravenously. After 250 ml of this infusion, three consecutive collection periods were obtained (Table 3.6, 90–125 minutes); the patient received 0.58 g of urea/kg by the start of the collections with urea, and 1.17 g/kg by the end of the last collection period.

The following comparisons can be made between the pyelonephritic, infected right kidney and the normal, uninfected left kidney:

1. The infusion of urea-ADH-saline, superimposed on a water diuresis, decreases the differences between the two kidneys in urine flow rates (column 1, Table 3.6). These changes are the reverse of renal ischemia; when a kidney with functionally significant arterial occlusion is compared with a contralateral nonoccluded kidney, an infusion of urea-ADH-saline always produces a greater disparity in urine flow rate

differences.[9, 10] The data in column 15 indicate that the pyelonephritic kidney excretes a greater fraction of the filtered water, in comparison with the contralateral kidney, during the infusion of urea-ADH-saline. In effect, this greater increase in the fraction of filtered water excreted by the right kidney decreases the difference between the two kidneys in urine flow rates. The comparative 10% increase in excretion of the filtered water during the urea-ADH-saline diuresis (1.33–1.23 in column 15) explains the 11% change in urine flow rate ratios from 0.79 during the water diuresis to 0.90 during the urea infusion (column 1).

2. The concentration of inulin (A comparative index of total water reabsorption) is less in the urine from the infected kidney (column 2). The differences between the two kidneys in U_{In} (column 2) are the same as the differences in U_{PAH} (column 4). For this reason, in normotensive patients with pyelonephritis, inulin and PAH *equally* reflect the degree of renal damage; furthermore, the comparison of PAH concentration ratios is a valid measure for comparing total water reabsorption in normotensive patients with unilateral renal disease, as well as in hypertensive patients with renal artery occlusion.[9]

The infusion of urea-ADH-saline produces greater differences between the two kidneys in U_{In} and U_{PAH} than are present during a water diuresis (columns 2 and 4); the infected kidney, excreting 10% *more* of the filtered water (in *comparison* with the contralateral normal kidney) during the infusion of urea-ADH-saline (1.33–1.23 in col-

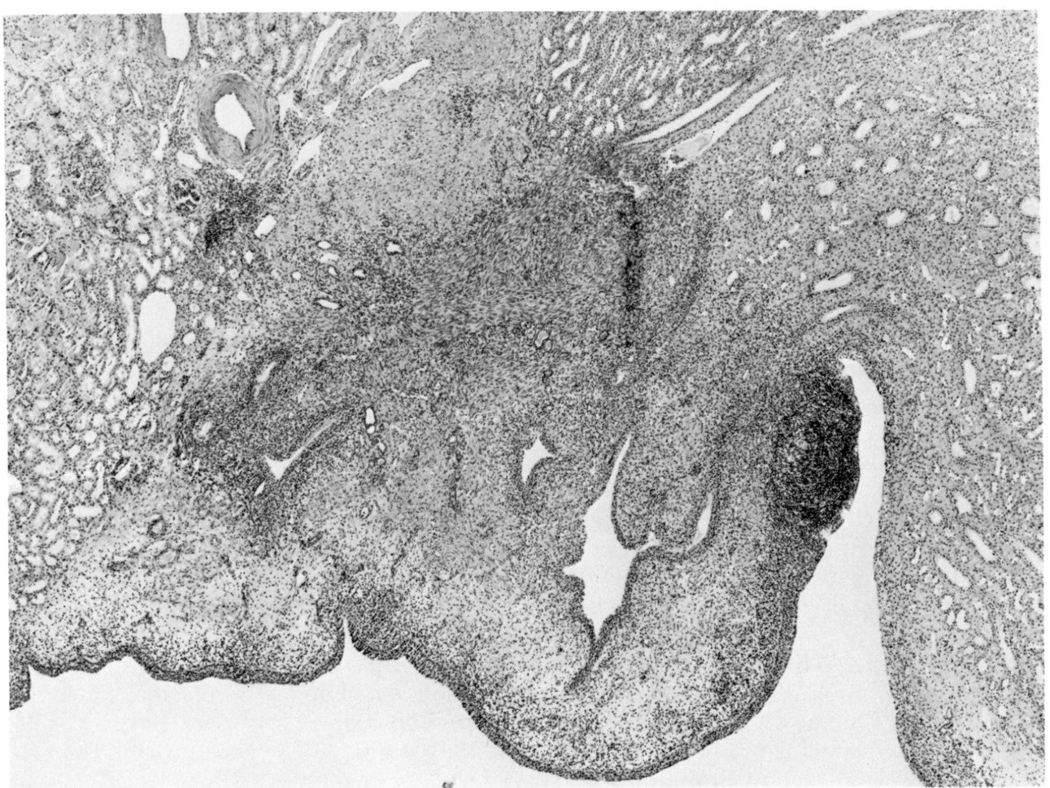

Figure 3.18 A particularly severe inflammatory area in a calyceal fornix immediately adjacent to a pyramid (×27). (Reproduced by permission from T. A. Stamey and A. Pfau, Invest. Urol. **1:** 134, 1963.)[2]

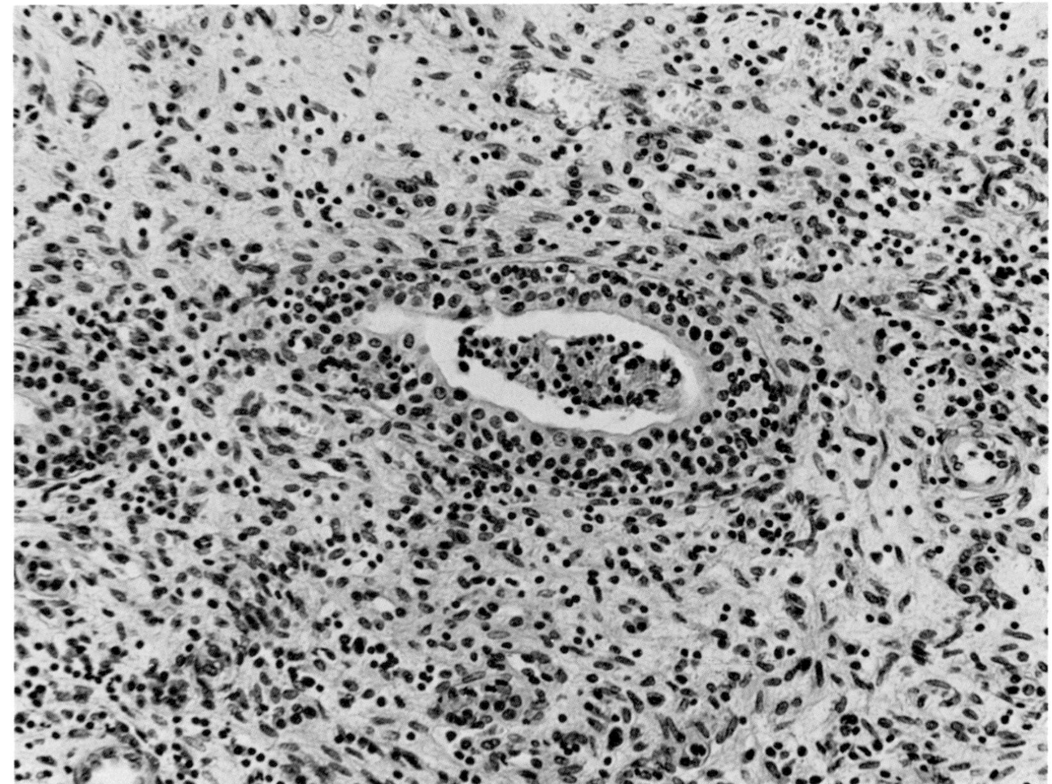

Figure 3.19 A ×180 magnification of the thickened and inflamed tissue surrounding the collecting ducts in the medulla. A polymorphonuclear leukocyte cast is clearly visible. (Reproduced by permission from T. A. Stamey and A. Pfau, Invest. Urol. **1:** 134, 1963.)[2]

umn 15), shows a greater failure to concentrate the nonreabsorbable inulin and PAH during the latter infusion. In the left kidney, U_{In} increases from 179 mg/100 ml during the water diuresis to 291 mg/100 ml during the urea diuresis (an increase of 62%). The pyelonephritic right kidney, however, reabsorbs 10% less water (column 15) and increases the concentration of inulin by only 51% (from a U_{In} of 146 to 221 mg/100 ml, column 2).

3. Columns 3 and 5 seem to indicate that the infusion or urea-ADH-saline produces a small fall in C_{In} and C_{PAH}. This apparent decrease, however is a mathematical artifact. The infusion rate of inulin and PAH was slightly greater than the rate of excretion by the kidneys. The PAH concentrations in plasma samples, 2, 3, and 4 (Table 3.6) were 2.31, 3.09, and 3.12 mg/100 ml; the inulin concentrations were 22.0, 26.0, and 26.2 mg/100 ml. Although P_2 and P_3 were averaged to calculate the plasma concentration during the time period 20–55 minutes, the true concentration may have been closer to P_3, thereby lowering the calculated plasma clearances during the water diuresis.

Columns 3 and 5 suggest a slightly greater fall in GFR and RPF in the left kidney; this difference could not be explained by changes in plasma concentration. The disproportionate fall in the left kidney is only 4%, which is within the error of the chemical method.

4. The filtration fractions (C_{In}/C_{PAH}, column 6) are equally elevated in both kidneys (0.27 as compared with a normal value of

0.194 ± 0.039 [9]) and do not change when an infusion of urea-ADH-saline is superimposed on a water diuresis.

5. The excretion rate of Na (column 8) is less from the pyelonephritic kidney because there is less tissue (C_{In} and C_{PAH} are reduced, columns 3 and 5). However, when the initial differences in GFR (C_{In}) are compensated for by calculating the percentage of the filtered sodium excreted ((C_{Na}/C_{In}) $\times$ 100) by each kidney (column 10), it is clear that the pyelonephritic kidney excretes 34% more of the filtered sodium during a water diuresis.

This difference in (C_{Na}/C_{In}) $\times$ 100 between the two kidneys decreases to 19% during the urea-ADH-saline infusion. The right kidney increased the (C_{Na}/C_{In}) $\times$ 100 from 2.38% with a water diuresis to 8.18% with urea (an increase of 344%). The left kidney increased from 1.77 to 6.87 (an increase of 388%). The left kidney increased by (388/344) $\times$ 100, or 13% more than the right kidney. Because the right kidney was originally excreting 34% more of the filtered sodium than the left kidney, this 13% disproportionate increase from the left kidney exactly accounts for the change in ratio from 1.34 in column 10 under water diuresis to 1.19 with the urea-ADH-saline infusion.

The sodium concentration differences (column 7) do not reflect the magnitude of this saluresis from the infected kidney; there is a 10% increase in the concentration of sodium from the infected kidney during a water diuresis, and an 11% *decrease* in concentration during the urea-ADH-saline infusion.

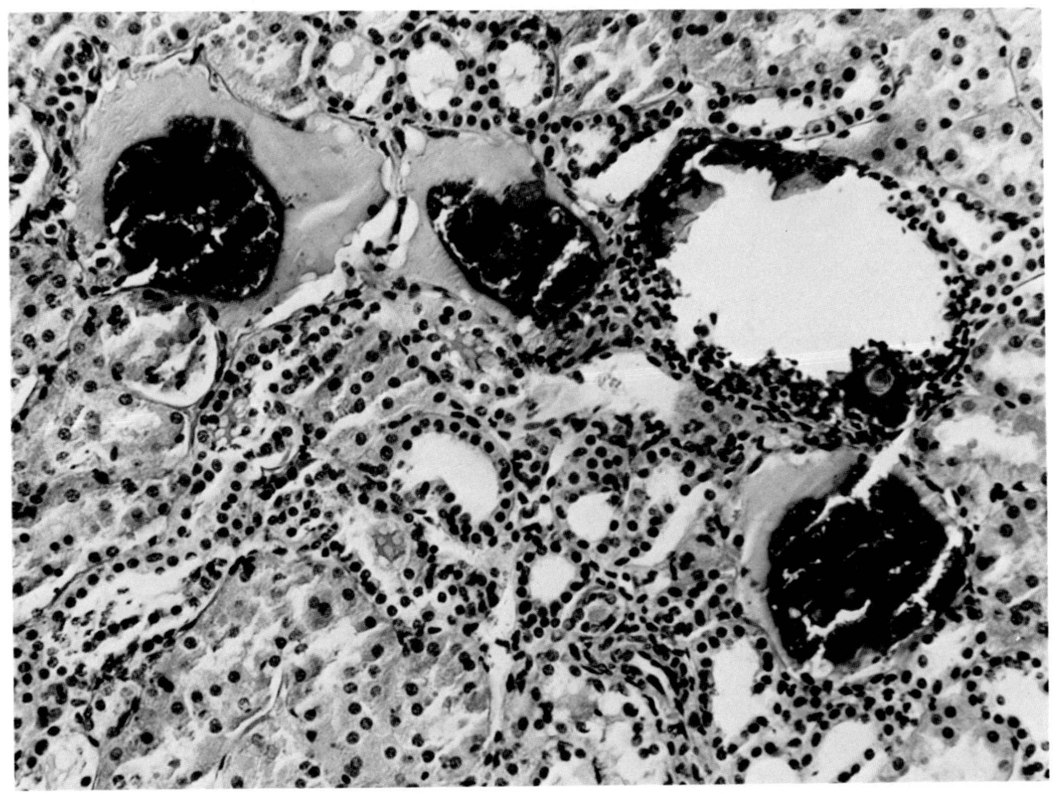

Figure 3.20 Area of calcification (×180) near the corticomedullary junction. These calcific foci occurred in relatively normal areas of the kidney. (Reproduced by permission from T. A. Stamey and A. Pfau, Invest. Urol. **1:** 134, 1963.)[2]

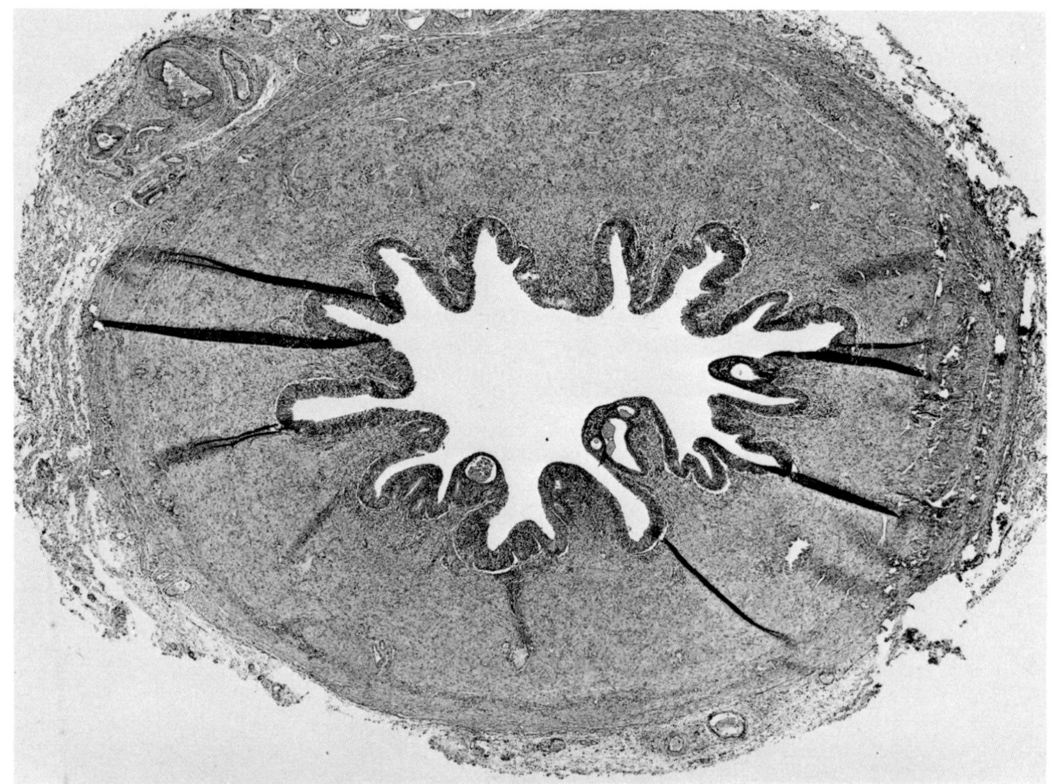

Figure 3.21 Section of the upper ureter (×18) showing considerable chronic inflammation with formation of subepithelial cysts ("ureteritis cystica"). (Reproduced by permission from T. A. Stamey and A. Pfau, Invest. Urol. **1:** 134, 1963.)[2]

6. The pyelonephritic kidney and the normal kidney clear the plasma of osmotically active substances (column 12) in the same proportion whether the plasma is influenced by a water load or by urea-ADH-saline infusion (that is, the urea-ADH-saline infusion does not impair either kidney in its ability to clear the plasma of osmolals).

The infected kidney, under a water diuresis, excretes 14% more of the filtered osmolals (column 13) than the normal kidney, and 5% more during the urea-ADH-saline infusion. The same mathematics apply to column 13 as applied to column 10; the $(C_{Osm}/C_{In}) \times 100$ increases 8% more in the left kidney than the right. This increase explains the change in ratio from 1.14 during the water diuresis to 1.05 during the urea infusion (column 13).

The differences in urine osmolality between the infected and normal kidney are greater during the infusion of urea-ADH-saline than during the oral water diuresis (column 11).

7. During a water diuresis, the pyelonephritic kidney excretes per 100 ml GFR (or per unit nephron) 25% more solute-free water than the normal kidney (column 14).

During a urea-ADH-saline diuresis, the pyelonephritic kidney reabsorbs 43% *less* solute-free water than the contralateral, normal kidney; this represents the greatest single difference between the pyelonephritic nephron and the contralateral, normal nephron (column 14).

Functional changes in the remaining left kidney were measured at 10 weeks after the right nephrectomy (Table 3.7) and on May 9, 1963, 8 months after surgery. In Table

3.8, the preoperative studies with water diuresis are compared to the postoperative studies at 10 weeks and at 8 months. Three consecutive 45-minute clearance periods were obtained during the study at 8 months, similar to the studies in Table 3.7.

The postoperative studies at 8 months (Table 3.8), when compared to the preoperative data during the water diuresis, show that (1) GFR increased by 60% and RPF by 44%; (2) the filtration fraction increased from 0.26 to 0.29; (3) the hypertrophied kidney excreted 51% more of the filtered sodium ($C_{Na}/C_{In} \times 100$) which, together with the 60% increase in GFR, approximated the 141% enhanced ability of the kidney to clear the plasma of Na (C_{Na}); and (4) the osmolal excretion fractions ($C_{Osm}/C_{In} \times 100$) increased by 44% and C_{Osm} by 131%. These studies suggest that the hypertrophied solitary kidney maintains Na and water homeostasis not only by an increase in GFR, but also by an equivalent increase in solute excretion fractions.

It is possible that the higher filtration fraction increases the flow rate of the glomerular filtrate down the nephron; an increase in flow rate would allow less time for reabsorption and could increase the solute excretion fractions.

Some Observations on Renal Function Studies

The technique of bilateral ureteral catheterization used in this patient has several quantitative advantages in studying tubular transport, especially the transport of sodium and water. These advantages, based on the qualitative similarity of the glomerular filtrate in both the diseased and contralateral normal kidney, were discussed in a previous publication.[10] In this patient, it is important to emphasize that 75% of the renal cortex of the pyelonephritic kidney was free of inflammatory disease. All the nephrons, however, must pass through the diseased medulla.

The data in Table 3.6 indicate that the functional lesion in the pyelonephritic kidney is a specific defect in the tubular handling of sodium and water.

Water

The 23% increase in the excretion of filtered water (column 15) during the water diuresis can be accounted for completely by the 25% increase in solute-free water (column 14); this identity localizes the site of this functional defect to the medulla of the kidney. Water which is not osmotically obligated is called solute-free water. The volume of urine per minute that is osmotically obligated is equal to the milliliters of plasma cleared of osmotically active substances in the urine excreted during 1 minute of time (column 12). Thus, to the extent that urine flow rate exceeds C_{Osm} (column 12), solute-free water is generated, $V - C_{Osm}$ (the + sign in column 14). During the water diuresis, the pyelonephritic kidney generates 25% more solute-free water than the contralateral kidney. When, however, the infusion of urea-ADH-saline is superimposed on the water diuresis, the urine becomes concentrated above the plasma osmolality, indicating that solute-free water has been *reabsorbed* against the osmotic gradient in the distal tubule (the − sign in column 14). Dividing $V - C_{Osm}$ by the C_{In} (column 14) corrects for differences in GFR; this correction allows a comparison of the free water generated as if both the pyelonephritic and normal kidney contained equal numbers of nephrons (actually per 100 ml GFR per kidney).

When an infusion of urea-ADH-saline is superimposed on the water diuresis, the ability of the pyelonephritic nephron to reabsorb solute-free water (column 14) is 43% less than the contralateral, normal nephron. This striking inability of the pyelonephritic nephron to reabsorb solute-free water under a maximal ADH stimulus (1) again points to the medulla as the site of the specific functional lesion and (2) constitutes the best diagnostic index for pyelonephritis. The magnitude of the medullary failure to reabsorb solute-free water (column 14) explains the relatively greater increase in the excretion of filtered water by the pyelonephritic kidney (column 15) during the urea-ADH-saline infusion; this relative increase in excretion of filtered wa-

Table 3.6
Renal Function Data of Patient with Unilateral Pyelonephritis, July 13, 1962[a]
C.B., 28-year-old white female.

Time	Column 1 Urine Flow			Column 2 Concentration of Inulin (U_{In})			Column 3 Clearance of Inulin, (C_{In})			Column 4 Concentration of PAH (U_{PAH})			Column 5 Clearance of PAH (C_{PAH})			Column 6 Filtration Fraction (C_{In}/C_{PAH})			Column 7 Concentration of Sodium (U_{Na})		
	R	L	R/L	R	L	R/L	R	L	R/L	R	L	R/L	R	L	R/L	R	L	R/L	R	L	R/L
min	*ml/min*			*mg/100 ml*			*ml/min*			*mg/100 ml*			*ml/min*						*µEq/ml*		
−80	Blood pressure 110/82 mm Hg. 600 ml of H_2O, p.o., followed by 400 ml H_2O/hr prior to the urea infusion																				
−60	Plasma #1 drawn.																		Plasma #1 = 136.9		
−55	15 ml of 10% inulin and 1.7 ml of 20% PAH injected i.v.; infusion started of 5% D/W at 1.1 ml/min, to deliver 13.6 mg/ml inulin and 7.27 mg/ml PAH.																				
−45	Blood pressure 112/84 mm Hg; 1 ml of 0.25% heavy Nupercaine injected into the fourth lumbar space for saddle anesthesia.																				
0	No. 8 or 7 Fr polyethylene catheters would not enter the left ureteral orifice. No. 6 Fr polyethylene catheter passed easily to left midureter; no. 8 Fr polyethylene catheter passed easily to right midureter.																				
18	Plasma #2 drawn. Blood pressure 120/86 mm Hg.																		Plasma #2 = 132		
20–30	3.92	4.85	0.808	154.7	184.5	0.838	25.27	37.28	0.678	52.4	79.9	0.656	76.07	143.52	0.530	0.33	0.26	1.27	20.00	17.91	1.117
30–40	3.94	5.20	0.758	146.4	180.0	0.813	24.03	39.00	0.616	63.1	78.6	0.803	92.07	151.37	0.608	0.26	0.26	1.00	18.86	17.52	1.076
45–55	4.01	4.93	0.813	136.9	172.6	0.793	22.88	35.45	0.645	74.9	77.4	0.968	111.22	141.33	0.786	0.21	0.25	0.84	18.63	16.80	1.109
(Avg 20–55)	3.96	4.99	0.794	146.0	179.0	0.816	24.06	37.24	0.646	63.5	78.6	0.808	93.12	145.41	0.640	0.27	0.26	1.04	19.16	17.41	1.101
55	Infusion changed to 8% urea in saline at 10 ml/min to deliver 1.50 mg/ml inulin, 0.80 mg/ml PAH, and 5 mU/kg/hr of ADH. 5 mU/kg of ADH injected i.v.																				
70	Blood pressure 116/90 mm Hg.																				
78	Plasma #3 drawn.																		Plasma #3 = 132		
90–100	2.41	2.49	0.968	291.6	367.7	0.793	26.93	35.08	0.768	118.6	157.2	0.754	92.19	126.26	0.730	0.29	0.28	1.04	85.72	95.43	0.898
100–110	2.74	3.00	0.913	210.6	285.6	0.773	22.11	32.83	0.673	96.1	127.3	0.755	84.94	123.19	0.690	0.26	0.27	0.96	86.75	97.03	0.894
110–125	3.14	3.68	0.853	161.8	220.2	0.735	19.47	31.05	0.627	73.6	101.1	0.728	74.55	120.00	0.621	0.26	0.26	1.00	86.75	97.72	0.888
(Avg 90–125)	2.76	3.06	0.902	221.3	291.2	0.760	22.84	32.99	0.692	96.1	128.5	0.748	83.89	123.15	0.681	0.27	0.27	1.00	86.41	96.73	0.893
126	Plasma #4 drawn. Blood pressure 116/80 mm Hg.																		Plasma #4 = 131.6		
127	600 ml of 8% urea in saline absorbed.																				

Time	Column 8 Excretion Rate of Sodium ($U_{Na}V$)			Column 9 Clearance of Sodium (C_{Na})			Column 10 Filtered Sodium Excreted [$(C_{Na}/C_{In}) \times 100$]			Column 11 Urine Osmolality (U_{Osm})			Column 12 Clearance of Osmolals (C_{Osm})			Column 13 Filtered Osmolals Excreted [$(C_{Osm}/C_{In}) \times 100$]			Column 14 Free Water Generated per 100 ml GFR [$(\text{“}C_{H2O}\text{”}^{c}/C_{In}) \times 100$]			Column 15 Filtered Water Excreted [$(1/U_{In}/P_{Im}) \times 100$]		
	R	L	R/L	R	L	R/L	R	L	R/L	R	L	R/L	R	L	R/L	R	L	R/L	R	L	R/L	R	L	R/L
min	*μEq/min*			*ml/min*			%	%		*μOsm/g H₂O*			*ml/min*			%	%		*ml:min:100 ml GFR*			%	%	
−80																								
−60										Plasma #1 = 280														
−55																								
−45																								
0																								
18										Plasma # 2 = 277														
21–30	78.40	86.86	0.90	0.59	0.66	0.89	2.33	1.77	1.32	62	64	0.97	0.86	1.10	0.78	3.40	2.95	1.15	+12.11	+10.06	1.20	15.50	13.00	1.19
30–40	74.31	91.10	0.82	0.56	0.69	0.81	2.33	1.77	1.32	58	61	0.95	0.81	1.12	0.72	3.37	2.87	1.17	+13.03	+10.46	1.25	16.39	13.33	1.23
45–55	74.71	82.82	0.90	0.57	0.63	0.90	2.50	1.78	1.40	53	61	0.87	0.75	1.06	0.72	3.28	2.99	1.10	+14.25	+10.92	1.30	17.54	13.91	1.26
(Avg 20–55)	75.80	86.93	0.87	0.57	0.66	0.86	2.38	1.77	1.34	58	62	0.94	0.81	1.09	0.74	3.35	2.94	1.14	+13.13	+10.48	1.25	16.48	13.41	1.23
55																								
70																								
78										Plasma #3 = 289														
90–100	206.59	237.62	0.87	1.57	1.80	0.87	5.83	5.13	1.14	400	512	0.78	3.22	4.26	0.76	11.96	12.14	0.99	−3.01	−5.05	0.65	8.95	7.10	1.26
100–110	237.70	291.09	0.82	1.80	2.21	0.81	8.14	6.73	1.21	365	480	0.76	3.34	4.73	0.71	15.11	14.41	1.05	−2.71	−5.27	0.51	12.39	9.14	1.36
110–125	272.40	359.61	0.76	2.06	2.72	0.76	10.58	8.76	1.21	366	450	0.81	3.84	5.54	0.69	19.72	17.84	1.11	−3.60	−5.99	0.60	16.13	11.85	1.36
(Avg 90–125)	238.90	296.11	0.81	1.81	2.24	0.81	8.18	6.87	1.19	377	481	0.78	3.47	4.84	0.72	15.60	14.80	1.05	−3.11	−5.44	0.57	12.49	9.36	1.33
126										Plasma #4 = 309														
127																								

[a] Reproduced by permission from T. A. Stamey and A. Pfau, Invest. Urol. **1:** 134, 1963.[2]

[b] R = right kidney; L = left kidney.

[c] “C_{H_2O}” is enclosed with quotation marks because C_{H_2O} is an unfortunate symbol in renal literature. There is no solute-free water in the plasma, and hence there can be no plasma clearance (C) of solute-free water. Solute-free water must be “generated” by the kidney, in the same sense that NH_4 is produced by the distal tubules; thus, the symbol C for C_{H_2O} in column 14 is clearly different from the remainder of the C symbols.

Table 3.7
Renal Function Studies 10 Weeks After Right Nephrectomy
All values represent function of the remaining left kidney.

Time	Column 1 Urine Flow	Column 2 Concentration of Inulin (U_{In})	Column 3 Clearance of Inulin (C_{In})	Column 4 Concentration of PAH (U_{PAH})	Column 5 Clearance of PAH (C_{PAH})	Column 6 Filtration Fraction (C_{In}/C_{PAH})	Column 7 Concentration of Sodium (U_{Na})	Column 8 Excretion Rate of Sodium (U_{Na} V)
min	*ml/min*	*mg/100 ml*	*ml/min*	*mg/100 ml*	*ml/min*		*μEq/ml*	*μEq/min*
−59	Blood pressure 110/75 mm Hg.							
−55	Plasma #1 drawn.						Plasma #1 = 131.4	
−52	15 ml of 10% inulin and 1.7 ml of 20% PAH injected i.v.							
−49	Infusion started of normal saline at 1.1 ml/min to deliver 9.43 mg/ml inulin and 5.28 mg/ml PaH.							
−48	No. 18 Fr red rubber catheter inserted into bladder per urethra.							
−3	Plasma #2 drawn.						Plasma #2 = 131.4	
0–45	9.00	125.0	54.6	59.5	273.2	0.20	15.5	139.50
50–95	8.51	131.3	54.2	65.1	282.7	0.19	17.8	151.48
97–142	8.64	133.8	56.1	64.1	282.6	0.20	21.8	188.35
(Avg 0–142)	8.72	130.0	55.0	62.9	279.5	0.20	18.4	159.78
143	Plasma #3 drawn.						Plasma #3 = 132.8	
145	265 ml of normal saline absorbed.							

Time	Column 9 Clearance of Sodium (C_{Na})	Column 10 Filtered Sodium Excreted $\left(\frac{C_{Na}}{C_{In}} \times 100\right)$	Column 11 Urine Osmolality (U_{Osm})	Column 12 Clearance of Osmolals (C_{Osm})	Column 13 Filtered Osmolals Excreted $\left(\frac{C_{Osm}}{C_{In}} \times 100\right)$	Column 14 Free Water Generated per 100 ml GFR $\left(\frac{\text{"}C_{H_2O}\text{"}}{C_{In}} \times 100\right)$	Column 15 Filtered Water Excreted $\left(\frac{1}{U_{In}/P_{In}} \times 100\right)$
min	*ml/min*	%	*μOsm/g H_2O*	*ml/min*	%	*ml/min:100 ml GFR*	%
−59							
−55			Plasma #1 = 279				
−52							
−49							
−48							
−3			Plasma #2 = 274				
0–45	1.06	1.94	63	2.06	3.77	+12.71	16.47
50–95	1.15	2.12	55	1.70	3.14	+12.47	15.70
97–142	1.43	2.55	59	1.85	3.30	+12.10	15.38
(Avg 0–142)	1.21	2.20	59	1.87	3.40	+12.43	15.85
143			Plasma #3 = 275				
145							

ter explains the increasing differences in U_{In}, U_{PAH}, U_{Na}, U_{Osm} (columns 2, 4, 7, and 11) and the decreasing differences in urine flow rates (column 1).*

* In renal ischemia, where the functional lesion is *excessive* water reabsorption, the urea-ADH-saline infusion produces exactly the opposite effect, as occurs in columns 1, 2, 4, 11, and 15. In effect, pyelonephritis produces a specific functional lesion at the distal end of the nephron, while vascular occlusion produces an equally specific functional change beginning at the proximal end of the nephron.

The concentrating mechanism, which determines solute-free water reabsorption, depends in part on the interstitial medullary tissue concentrations of sodium and urea.[11] Several investigators[12, 13] have shown that the osmolality of the water in the medullary tissue near the papillae is identical to the osmolality of the final elaborated urine. Sodium, together with its attendant univalent anion, and urea account for 75% of the medullary osmolality.[12] The concentration of urea was not determined in these studies, but if the sodium content is doubled to account for the matching anions and subtracted from the osmolal concentration, the difference approximates the urea content. Columns 7 and 11 show that the concentrations of Na, osmolals, and, by difference, urea, are all reduced in the urine from the pyelonephritic kidney during the urea-ADH-saline infusion; this reduced concentration in the urine presumably reflects decreased concentration gradients in the water of the diseased medullary tissue (Figures 3.17–3.19). In addition to the diminished concentration of Na and urea in the medullary interstitial water, the fibrosis and inflammation (Figure 3.19) probably impair the action of ADH in facilitating water reabsorption in the collecting ducts.

Column 11 shows that, although the diagnostic differences between the two kidneys in U_{Osm} are enhanced by the urea-ADH-saline infusion, these differences do not compare with the differences in reabsorption of solute-free water (column 14, urea-ADH-saline infusion).

Sodium

The 34% increase in the excretion of filtered sodium is the most striking characteristic of the pyelonephritic kidney during the water diuresis. Because increased osmotic loads were not present during the water diuresis, this observation of increased sodium excretion emphasizes, as Kleeman realized from quite different evidence,[14] that an increased osmotic load in the remaining nephrons of azotemic patients with pyelonephritis is not the basic explanation for the defect in sodium conservation. Kleeman, Hewitt, and Guze[14] in a magnificent comparison of two azotemic groups of patients with pyelonephritis and glomerulonephritis, showed that sodium wasting occurred in only 4 of 33 patients with glomerulonephritis; all 4 patients had serum creatinines above 7 mg/100 ml. On the other hand, 19 of 55 patients with azotemia secondary to pyelonephritis could not conserve sodium. In the occasional patient, a marked failure to conserve sodium may constitute a salt-wasting clinical syndrome.[15–18]

The increased excretion of the filtered sodium in the pyelonephritic nephron explains why patients with pyelonephritis, except those in terminal failure, rarely present problems in sodium and water retention. By contrast, patients with comparable degrees of renal damage from nephrosclerosis and glomerulonephritis frequently present problems in sodium and water retention; their functional lesion is one of *excessive* sodium and water reabsorption in the nephron,[9] a condition exactly opposite to that occurring with the functional defect in pyelonephritis. Kleeman *et al.*[14] reported that they had never observed a patient with the nephrotic syndrome caused by pyelonephritis; neither have we observed such a patient.

The magnitude of the saluresis from the pyelonephritic kidney is not proportional to

Table 3.8
Renal Function Studies, Left Kidney: Water Diuresis

	Preoperative	Postoperative	
		10 weeks	8 months
V (ml/min)	4.99	8.72	9.53
$[1/(U_{In}/P_{In})] \times 100$ (%)	13.41	15.84	15.95
C_{In} (ml/min)	37.24	55.00	59.50
C_{PAH} (ml/min)	145.41	279.50	209.00
Filtration fraction	0.26	0.20	0.29
C_{Na} (ml/min)	0.66	1.21	1.59
$C_{Na}/C_{In} \times 100$ (%)	1.77	2.20	2.67
C_{Osm} (ml/min)	1.09	1.87	2.52
$C_{Osm}/C_{In} \times 100$ (%)	2.94	3.40	4.23
"C_{H_2O}"$/C_{In} \times 100$ (%)	+10.48	+12.43	+11.75

the Na concentration differences (Table 3.6). In fact, during the urea-ADH-saline diuresis, Na concentration from the pyelonephritic kidney was 11% *less* than that from the contralateral kidney (column 7), whereas the percentage of filtered sodium excreted was greater than that from the contralateral kidney by 19% (column 10).

Although 34% more of the filtered sodium (column 10) is excreted from the pyelonephritic kidney compared with the normal kidney, only 14% more of the filtered osmolals are excreted (column 13). This discrepancy suggests that some filtered solute other than sodium is being disporportionately reabsorbed in the pyelonephritic kidney. This solute is probably urea, but, unfortunately, urea was not determined in these studies.

Column 12 indicates that the pyelonephritic and the contralateral, normal kidney both clear the plasma of osmotically active substances in the same proportion during the urea-ADH-saline diuresis as during the water diuresis (0.74 difference during the water diuresis and 0.72 during the urea infusion). This similarity is equally true for the plasma clearance of sodium (column 9). Despite these similarities in the plasma clearances of sodium and osmolals, the differences between the two kidneys in the percentage of *filtered* sodium (column 10) and osmolals (column 13) *excreted* decrease during the infusion of urea-ADH-saline. This diminishing difference is caused by a greater proportional increase in filtered solute excreted by the normal left kidney. It is reasonable that the extra solute excreted by the normal kidney is produced by an osmotic washout of the high solute concentration in the medulla of the kidney. The medullary interstitial disease in the right kidney could retard a proportional washout of medullary solute, which, as has already been pointed out, is probably lower than that of the contralateral, normal kidney prior to the osmotic diuresis. Malvin and Wilde[19] have shown that a mannitol diuresis in the dog dissipates the sodium concentration gradient between the base and apex of the renal pyramid. The data in Table 3.6 on solute excretion fractions (columns 10 and 13) suggest that these fractions, at least for sodium, urea, and osmolals, are not valid calculations during osmotic loading; that is, the excreted solute is not derived exclusively from the filtered solute.

"Intact" Proximal Tubule

Columns 2 and 4 and columns 3 and 5 show that inulin and PAH, and GFR and RPF are completely proportional in both the diseased kidney and the contralateral kidney. Thus, there is no doubt that pyelonephritis destroys complete nephrons on a functional basis; *i.e.*, the remaining tubules within the diseased kidney exhibit no imbalance between glomerular and proximal tubular function when compared with the proximal tubules of the contralateral kidney. GFR and RPF are measurements of proximal tubular function only; they cannot detect even massive changes in the transport of salt and water after the glomerular filtrate is formed. Michie and Michie,[20] studying renal function in unilateral pyelonephritis in man, concluded that the remaining nephrons functioned normally; their measurements, however, consisted of GFR, RPF, and maximal tubular excretory capacity for PAH (TmPAH), all indices of proximal tubular function.

The data in Table 3.6 show that the proximal tubule is indeed "intact"; the functional defect is in the distal tubule within the medulla of the kidney (columns 7, 10, 11, 13, 14, and 15).

Since these studies were published in 1963, Bank and Aynedjian,[21] using both renal clearance and micropuncture techniques in rats with pyelonephritis, also concluded that the concentrating defect cannot be accounted for by a simple reduction in the number of functioning nephrons.

SUMMARY

The functional lesion in pyelonephritis is a specific medullary defect characterized by a marked loss of filtered water and sodium. This defect (1) explains several clinical characteristics of these patients, and (2) argues against the "intact nephron theory" of chronic renal disease.

The proximal tubules of the pyelonephritic kidney show no imbalance between glomerular (GFR) and proximal tubular (RPF) function and are "intact."

The failure of the pyelonephritic kidney to reabsorb solute-free water in the presence of maximal antidiuretic hormone activity and a urea diuresis constitutes the greatest diagnostic difference when a pyelonephritic kidney is compared to a contralateral, normal kidney.

The pathologic material, presented in detail, represents an example of pure, symptomatic pyelonephritis, incurable with bactericidal drug therapy, and uncomplicated by generalized vascular disease, hypertension, or glomerulonephritis.

REFERENCES

1. Beeson, P. B.: Urinary tract infection and pyelonephritis. In D. A. K. Black (Ed.), Renal Disease, Ed. 2, Chap. 15. Philadelphia, F. A. Davis & Co., 1967, p. 382.
2. Stamey, T. A., and Pfau, A.: Some functional, pathologic, bacteriologic, and chemotherapeutic characteristics of unilateral pyelonephritis in man. Invest. Urol. **1:** 134, 1963.
3. Stamey, T. A.: Urinary Infections. Baltimore, The Williams & Wilkins Co., 1972.
4. Weiss, S., and Parker, F., Jr.: Pyelonephritis: Its relation to vascular lesions and to arterial hypertension. Medicine **18:** 221, 1939.
5. Bricker, N. S., Dewey, R. R., and Lubowitz, H.: Studies in experimental pyelonephritis. Simultaneous and serial investigation of a pyelonephritic and intact kidney in the same animal. Clin. Res. **6:** 292, 1958.
6. Bricker, N. S., Dewey, R. R., Lubowitz, H., Stokes, J., and Kirkensgaard, T.: Observations on the concentrating and diluting mechanisms of the diseased kidney. J. Clin. Invest. **38:** 516, 1959.
7. Longcope, W. T., and Winkenwerder, W. L.: Clinical features of the contracted kidney due to pyelonephritis. Bull. Johns Hopkins Hosp. **53:** 255, 1933.
8. Brod, J., and Prague, M. D.: Chronic pyelonephritis. Lancet **1:** 973, 1956.
9. Stamey, T. A., Nudelman, I. J., Good, P. H., Schwentker, F. N., and Hendricks, F.: Functional characteristics of renovascular hypertension. Medicine **40:** 347, 1961.
10. Stamey, T. A.: Renovascular Hypertension. Baltimore, The Williams & Wilkins Co., 1963.
11. Levinsky, N. G., and Berliner, R. W.: The role of urea in the urine concentrating mechanism. J. Clin. Invest. **38:** 741, 1959.
12. Ullrich, K. J., and Jarausch, K. H.: Untersuchungen zum Problem der Harnkonzentrierung und Harnverdünnung. Pflueger. Arch. Ges. Physiol. **262:** 537, 1956.
13. Ullrich, K. J., Kramer, K., and Boylan, J. W.: Mechanism of urinary concentration. In D. A. K. Black (Ed.), Renal Disease. Philadelphia, F. A. Davis Co., 1962, p. 49.
14. Kleeman, C. R., Hewitt, W. L., and Guze, L. B.: Pyelonephritis. Medicine **39:** 3, 1960.
15. Enticknap, J. B.: The condition of the kidneys in salt-losing nephritis. Lancet **2:** 458, 1952.
16. Knowles, H. C., Levitin, H., and Bridges, A.: Salt-losing nephritis with fixed urinary composition. Am. J. Med. **22:** 158, 1957.
17. Peterson, V. P.: Renal function and electrolyte metabolism in salt-losing nephritis. Acta Med. Scand. **154:** 187, 1956.
18. Thorn, G. W., Koepf, G. F., and Clinton, M., Jr.: Renal failure simulating adrenocortical insufficiency. N. Engl. J. Med. **231:** 76, 1944.
19. Malvin, R. L., and Wilde, W. S.: Washout of renal countercurrent Na gradient by osmotic diuresis. Am. J. Physiol. **197:** 177, 1959.
20. Michie, A. J., and Michie, C. R.: Kidney function in unilateral pyelonephritis. I. Clinical data. Am. J. Med. **22:** 179, 1957.
21. Bank, N., and Aynedjian, H. S.: Individual nephron function in experimental bilateral pyelonephritis. II. Distal tubular sodium and water reabsorption and the concentrating defect. J. Lab. Clin. Med. **68:** 728, 1966.

CHAPTER 4

Urinary Tract Infections in Women

PREVALENCE OF BACTERIURIA

URINARY infections in women are common, varying with both the age of the patient and the population under study. In house to house population surveys in Wales and Jamaica, about 2% of adult women were found to be bacteriuric in the 15- to 24-year-old age group, increasing 1 or 2%/decade to a prevalence rate of 10% in the 55- to 64-year decade.[1] Freedman *et al.*[2] found young and middle-aged Japanese women to have about the same frequency of bacteriuria: 1–3%. Thus, about 4–6% of women of childbearing age will be bacteriuric at any one survey. Because the turnover is substantial, with cure of bacteriuria in some and new infections in others, it is estimated that about 10–20% of women experience a urinary infection in their lifetime.[1]

Kunin and McCormack,[3] however, reported that the frequency of bacteriuria in nuns is stikingly less (0.4–1.6% in the four decades from 15 to 54 years), clearly suggesting that sexual intercourse plays a significant role in urinary infections. These surprising differences between the two populations are reproduced in Figure 4.1. In the 15- to 34-year age group, bacteriuria was 12.8 times higher in white control women than in nuns ($P < 0.001$). This difference in frequency became less marked in the age group of 55 years or over, but even in the 35- to 54-year age group the prevalence of bacteriuria in nuns was as low as in schoolgirls of age 6 (about 1%). This study is important also because Kunin and McCormack analyzed the effect of marriage, pregnancy, oral contraceptives, and menstrual protection on the frequency of bacteriuria in the control women; except for the suggestion that bacteriuria was half as frequent in single women 15–24 years of age (2.7%) as in married women of the same age (5.9%), prevalence was not affected by these factors. The accentuated frequency of bacteriuria in Negro women in the control population, 8.5% in Figure 4.1, was interpreted by Kunin and McCormack to be mostly related to availability of medical care rather than to personal hygiene.

Hospitalized women on general medical

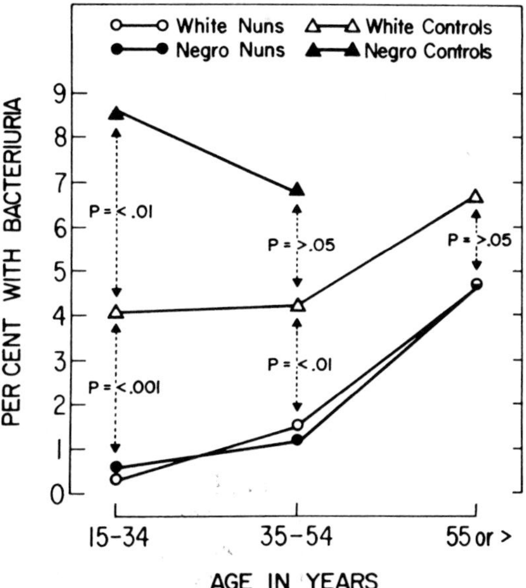

Figure 4.1 Prevalence of bacteriuria in white and Negro nuns and control women according to 20-year age groups. (Reproduced by permission from C. M. Kunin and R. C. McCormack, N. Engl. J. Med. **278:** 635, 1968.[3])

units, as originally shown by Marple,[4] have a much higher rate of infection (24%); Kass[5] reported that 30% of 76 female patients on the medical wards at Boston City Hospital had bacteriuria.

Screening Bacteriuria (ScBU)

These prevalence studies are based on screening populations for the presence or absence of bacteriuria; indeed, the bacteriuria detected in such surveys has been conventionally called "asymptomatic bacteriuria," but this is not a very satisfactory term. Some of these patients are not totally asymptomatic at the time of the screening culture; more importantly, few remain completely asymptomatic over long periods of time. In addition, many patients who present with symptomatic bacteriuria, especially those who are untreated or inadequately treated, may become asymptomatic, and the term asymptomatic bacteriuria is needed for this aspect of their otherwise symptomatic history. Thus, "screening bacteriuria" is clearly a more accurate term for bacteriuria detected during population surveys; I will use it throughout this book even though it sounds somewhat clumsy and less sophisticated than "asymptomatic bacteriuria"; ScBU, the abbreviation I will use for bacteriuria detected during the screening surveys, may avoid some of the verbal harshness.

The really important point is not one of semantics. The student and clinician should try to distinguish in the literature those studies which relate to patients who come to the physician with symptomatic infections in contrast to those patients whose infections are detected by screening populations for the presence of bacteriuria; I will try to keep this distinction clear throughout the chapters of this book. In the final analysis, however, I expect most readers will conclude, as I have, that both symptomatic and ScBU are integral parts of the same disease process, *i.e.*, urinary tract infections. Indeed, it is likely that there will be little practical merit, in the long run, to separating symptomatic bacteriuria from ScBU.

Screening Bacteriuria and Symptomatic Urinary Infections

The only prospective study of which I am aware that assesses the prevalence of both ScBU and symptomatic urinary infections, and their interrelationship, in a closed population is that by Gaymans, *et al.*[6] In this admirable general practice study, the authors screened 1758 women over the age of 14 (which represented 94.4% of their total practice population) for ScBU. The prevalence of ScBU ranged from 2.7% in the age group 15–24 years to 9.3% in women 65 years and older; the overall prevalence of ScBU was 4.7%. Ninety percent of the infections were caused by *Escherichia coli.* The critical part of this study was that all patients with ScBU were followed for 1 year while the physicians simultaneously observed the presentation of women with symptomatic urinary tract infections (UTI) from the population study group. During these 12 months, 105 women presented with a symptomatic infection, for an annual incidence rate of 59/1000 population; 29% of these symptomatic infections came from the women with pre-existing ScBU. Thus, the probability of acquiring a symptomatic infection was about 7 times greater in women with known ScBU compared to persons without bacteriuria ($P < 0.0001$). The acquisition rate of both symptomatic and ScBU patients for 1 year in this closed, general practice, setting was 12% of the total population.

NATURAL HISTORY OF SYMPTOMATIC, RECURRENT BACTERIURIA

First Infections

Little is known about women who present with their first known symptomatic urinary infection. In a prospective study of women over age 15 who came to an outpatient clinic with symptoms of urinary infection, 60 women presented with their first symptomatic infection.[7] After treatment for 7–10 days with sulfisoxazole, only 28% of these 60 women experienced a recurrence in the following 18 months. Of 106 women seen in the same clinic with UTI who had previously experienced documented UTI, 83% had a recurrent infection in the following 18 months. In my own experience with first infections in women, they are almost always pansensitive to all antimicrobial agents with the single exception of tetracycline. A short course of sulfonamides clearly represents excellent therapy.

Recurrent Symptomatic Infections

In a remarkable study of 219 women with symptoms of UTI referred by general practitioners to a medical outpatient clinic, Mabeck[8] observed that 60% of those placebo-treated obtained a sterile urine spontaneously within 4 weeks and 80% were sterile within 5 months; one-half, however, had recurrent infections within 12 months. Of those treated successfully with short term therapy (2–4 weeks), only 45% maintained sterile urine for 2 years; the recurrence rate was highest during the first 2 months after treatment and thereafter was fairly constant for the next 2 years.

About one-sixth of Mabeck's patients (37 of 219), presenting with symptoms of UTI and proven bacteriuria, had four or more infections in the 16–41 months (average, 30.5 months) of follow-up. These 37 women accounted for 244 recurrences, which represented a frequency 8 times that of the other 182 patients; in addition, placebo treatment of 13 of these 37 patients resulted in spontaneous cures in only 38% compared to 80% in the overall group.

Surely it is from this highly susceptible 16% (one-sixth) of all patients with symptomatic UTI that cause the greatest medical morbidity and public health cost to society, and it is these patients on whom I would like to present our natural history data from Stanford.

Stanford Data on Natural History

We analyzed our experience with 23 patients who were followed very closely by our research unit, who took antimicrobial agents *only* under our direction, and who reported to us all symptoms even suggestive of UTI.[9]

Patients

Adult females with a history of at least two symptomatic episodes of urinary tract infection in the previous 12 months and at least two prior infections documented by a clean catch culture showing $\geq 10^5$ bacteria/ml of a single species were accepted for study (specimens were collected from the cystoscopy table as described in Chapter 1).

All patients agreed to monthly cultures while asymptomatic and immediate cultures whenever symptoms occurred. Patients with underlying conditions which might increase susceptibility to infection such as diabetes mellitus or immunosuppressive medication were excluded. Any patient followed less than 1 year or who had no infections during follow-up (one patient) was excluded from the analysis.

The 23 patients included in this study had a mean age of 35.7 years and were followed an average of 36.3 months. Eighteen patients had normal intravenous urograms (IVU). Six of 23 had some additional urologic disease; 3 had scars of previous pyelonephritis on IVU; 1 had had a urethral diverticulectomy; and 1 had passed a calcium oxalate stone a year prior to the study, but had a normal IVU at the time of entering the study.

Symptoms

The most common symptoms were frequency, dysuria, and suprapubic pain. Tenesmus and nocturia were often present. Flank pain and fever were rare. Any symptomatology which caused the patient to come to the Stanford Urology Clinic for evaluation of infection was considered a symptomatic episode.

Infections

Infections were judged to be present whenever a clean catch midstream specimen contained $\geq 10^5$ bacteria of a single species or whenever nurse-collected lithotomy table specimens showed no decrease in colony count between the first voided and midstream cultures and both contained $\geq 10^3$ organisms of a single species. Three infections included for analysis did not meet the colony count criteria above but were judged to represent bacteriuria because of single species cultures and the presence of significant pyuria on urine microscopy. Occasionally a suprapubic urine aspirate was used to confirm or deny low count bacteriuria. A negative culture off antimicrobial treatment was obtained between each infection.

Treatment

The Urology Clinic was available without charge at any time during the study. Each infection was treated with a 10-day course of an oral antimicrobial to which the organism was sensitive, as determined by a quantitative disc technique as described in Chapter 2.

Results

During this study, 23 patients were followed for 836 months and 1317 cultures were performed. All patients had at least one infection. The mean number of infections per patient was 6.3 (Table 4.1). All patients had two or more symptomatic episodes and these averaged 8.2/patient.

Twenty-two of 23 patients had one or more infection-free periods lasting 26 weeks or longer. These remissions from infection averaged 55 weeks. The mean number of remissions per patient was 2.1 (Table 4.1).

There were 145 infections, 138 of which had associated symptoms (94%) (Table 4.2). A plot of each patient's infections against time is seen in Figure 4.2; the frequency distribution of the 122 recurrences shows the number of infections per 30-day period (Figure 4.3). The cumulative frequency of recurrences and cumulative percent of patients with recurrences per 30-day period of observation is presented in Table 4.3. By subtracting the date of last therapy from

Table 4.3
Frequency Distribution of 122 Recurrent Infections[a]

Days Between Recurrences	Frequency	Cumulative Frequency	Cumulative Percent
360 and above	12	122	100
330–359	5	110	90
300–329	3	105	86
270–299	1	102	84
240–269	8	101	83
210–239	5	93	76
180–209	6	88	72
150–179	2	82	67
120–149	10	80	66
90–119	12	70	57
60–89	11	58	48
30–59	23	47	39
0–29	24	24	20
	122		

[a] From Kraft and Stamey.[9]

Table 4.1
Summary of Patient Data[a]

Variable/Patient	Mean	Std. Error of Mean	Range
Age	35.7yr	2.8	19–63 yr
Months on Study	36.3	5.0	15–110 mo
No. of Cultures	57.3	6.2	24–125
No. of Symptomatic Episodes Prompting Culture	8.2	0.9	2–19
No. of Infections	6.3	0.7	1–14
No. of Infection Remissions[b] ≥6 months	2.1	0.3	0–7

[a] From Kraft and Stamey.[9]
[b] Remissions averaged 55.4 wks. in length (range 26–289 weeks).

Table 4.2
Infections[a]

	Total	With Symptoms	Without Symptoms	Followed by ≥6-Mo Remission	Followed by ≥12-Mo Remission
Number of Infections	145	138	7	49	14

[a] From Kraft and Stamey.[9]

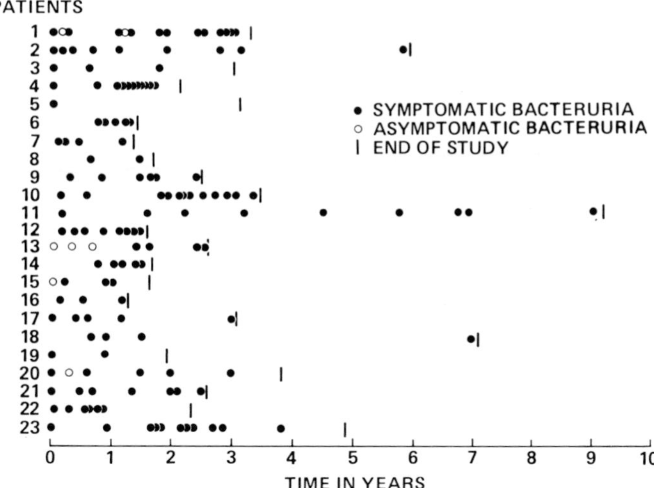

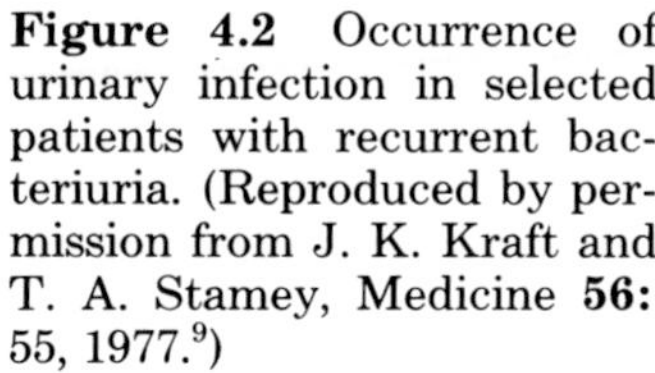
Figure 4.2 Occurrence of urinary infection in selected patients with recurrent bacteriuria. (Reproduced by permission from J. K. Kraft and T. A. Stamey, Medicine **56:** 55, 1977.[9])

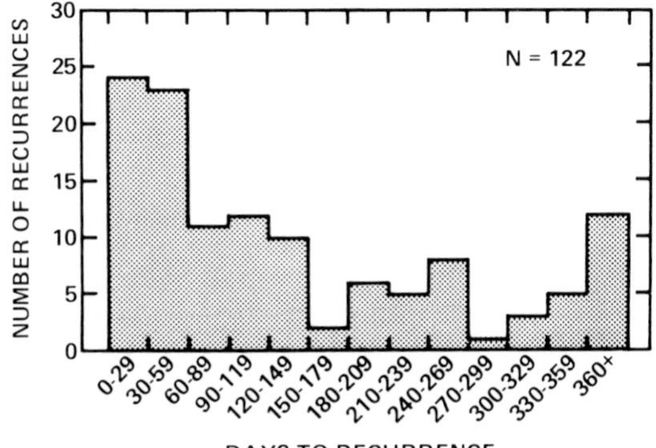

Figure 4.3 Time between urinary infections grouped by 30-day intervals. (Reproduced by permission from J. K. Kraft and T. A. Stamey, Medicine **56:** 55, 1977.[9])

the date of next infection, the time between infections was found to average 23 weeks; however, the median time between infections was only 13 weeks. Intervals lasting 26 weeks or longer occurred 49 times. Fourteen of these were longer than 1 year.

The patients reported 213 symptomatic episodes (Table 4.4) but 24 of these were so minor that they resolved quickly at home and did not prompt a clinic visit or treatment. The 189 cultures taken during symptomatic episodes showed significant bacteriuria was present in 138 instances and no infection in 51 instances.

The causative organism and antimicrobial treatment used during 145 infections are summarized in Tables 4.5 and 4.6. *Escherichia coli* accounted for 82% of all infections. Thirty of 145 infections had cultures with colony counts less than 10^5/ml from the midstream specimen. Nitrofurantoin, nalidixic acid, and sulfonamides were the most commonly used antimicrobials.

Discussion

The attack rate of urinary infections in this selected group of women is 0.17 infections/month. This rate correlates well with figures reported by Guttmann[11] of 0.13 infections/month and by Vosti[12] of 0.13 infections/month in selected groups with recurrent urinary tract infections. Guttmann showed also that the attack rate of infections in women is independent of the patient's urologic status as determined by intravenous urography. In 119 women, the attack rate was not significantly different for patients with normal intravenous urograms when compared with the attack rates in four groups of patients with progressively more abnormal urograms.

In the present study, 94% of all infections had associated symptoms. Only 6% of the infections were asymptomatic bacteriurias identified by monthly screening cultures. Further, 73% of symptomatic episodes had associated bacteriuria. That most infections were symptomatic and that most symptomatic episodes were accompanied by infection are important findings in this study. The screening of women susceptible to

Table 4.4
Symptomatic Episodes[a]

	Total	Prompting Visit and Culture	Infection Present	Infection Absent
Number of Symptomatic Episodes	213	189	138	51

[a] From Kraft and Stamey.[9]

Table 4.5
Organisms Causing 145 Infections[a]

Organism	Total Incidence	Percent of 145	No. with $<10^5$ Organisms	Percent of Incidence
Escherichia coli	119	82	24	20
Proteus mirabilis	15	10	3	20
Klebsiella	7	5	1	14
Enterococcus	3	2	1	33
Staphylococcus aureus	1	1	1	100
Total	145	100	30	21

[a] From Kraft and Stamey.[9]

symptomatic recurrent urinary tract infections is unlikely to identify infection unless the patient is symptomatic. Less than 1% of cultures performed while the patients were asymptomatic showed an infection.

To perform cultures while the patient is symptomatic will identify > 90% of all infections but about one-fourth of these cultures will be negative. The patients analyzed in this study all had confirmed infections at some time; yet 27% of the symptomatic episodes occurred without infection and represent what can be called the "urethral syndrome." Gallagher, Montgomerie, and North[13] catheterized women who presented to their family practitioner with symptoms of a urinary tract infection; 41% had sterile urine. They used the term "urethral syndrome" for these episodes. Twenty-eight percent of the women presenting with urethral syndrome subsequently had a documented infection during a short follow-up period (3 months). They concluded that the urethral syndrome is definitely common and is likely to be related to infection of the urethra or surrounding glands.[13] The present study shows that even in patients selected for recurrent urinary infections, the urethral syndrome is common and accounts for 27% of symptomatic episodes. This syndrome is discussed in detail in a later section in this chapter.

Asymptomatic bacteriuria represented 6% of the infections in this series. These asymptomatic infections occurred in 4 of 23 patients (17%). In Gallagher's study cited above, 17% of the patients had asymptomatic bacteriuria at some time during the 3-month follow-up period. These asymptomatic infections occurred in a similar proportion of patients who initially presented with symptoms and bacteriuria as in those who had only the urethral syndrome. O'Grady *et al.*,[14] in analyzing cultures from 330 women referred for "cystitis," found that 17% had either occasional or persistent asymptomatic bacteriuria. In the present study, asymptomatic bacteriuria accounts for only a small portion (6%) of the total infections but it does occur in a substantial percentage of the patients (17%).

Remission from infection for periods of 6 months or longer was not uncommon for our patients. When the data were analyzed for remissions lasting ≥ 26 weeks and ≥ 52 weeks, 49 of 145 infections (34%) were followed by an infection-free interval of at least 26 weeks. Fourteen remissions lasted more than 52 weeks. The median duration of remissions was 43 weeks. Of the 836 months of total study time, 631 months were spent in remission from infection. However, even lengthy remissions were followed by more infections and this study does not identify a cure rate or drop out rate for women having recurrent urinary infections.

The 34% 6-month or longer remission

rate from infection found in this study is useful for designing future studies. For studies having a short follow-up period, *i.e.*, under 2 years, change in the attack rate could be explained simply by the predicted remission rate for patients. This factor must also be considered in studies designed to determine the efficacy of one form of urinary tract infection therapy against another.

When the infections occurring during this study are plotted longitudinally against time, areas of lengthy remission are seen (Figure 4.2). Between these remissions, infections often occur in close proximity. Frequently, these infections were caused by serotypically identical organisms, but since each infection was separated by negative urine cultures while the patient was off antimicrobial therapy, each occurrence is singular for treatment purposes.

As will be seen in the following section, vaginal carriage of pathogenic organisms precedes infection of the bladder urine.[10, 15, 16] During periods of persistent vaginal carriage of bacteria, urinary tract infections are more likely to occur. Therefore, the clustering of recurrent infections as often seen during this study is not a surprising finding.

The clustering of infection means that since patients spent 75% of the time in remission, the remaining time was a period of high morbidity caused by multiple recurrences. The attack rate of infections while the patients were not in a 6-month or longer remission was 0.47 infections/month. This

Table 4.6
Treatment of 145 Infections[a]

Agent	Times Used
Nitrofurantoin	47
Nalidixic Acid	23
Sulfonamide	20
Tetracycline	18
Penicillin-G	15
Cephalosporin	10
Ampicillin	5
Oxytetracycline-sulfamethizole	2
Penicillin-G—sulfamethizole	1
Trimethoprim-sulfamethoxazole	1
Unknown	3
Total	145

[a] From Kraft and Stamey.[9]

is almost three times the overall attack rate observed in this study. These periods of frequent infections were not adequately controlled by a successful 10-day antimicrobial treatment. Analysis could not predict when a cluster of infections would begin, how long it would last, or when it would end.[17–21] Because of these findings some other treatment regimen, for example, antimicrobial prophylaxis, may be indicated for better control during periods of frequent infections.

The present analysis adds some information in determining when to begin a prophylactic antimicrobial regimen. The attack rate pattern for all patients was examined to determine the nature and number of sets of infection preceded and followed by a remission lasting 6 months or longer. Once 6 months pass without infection, the next infection initiates a new set. This set lasts until another 6 months pass without an infection. Thirty-two sets of infection were observed during this study. Twenty-two of these contained only a single infection. The remaining sets contained two to eight infections each. Figure 4.4 is a plot of the risk of additional infections without an intervening remission based on the set sizes found in this analysis. Sixty-nine percent of the sets contained a single infection. The remaining sets show a consistent drop out rate approximating a 33% decay curve. If a patient has two or more infections without 6 months passing between any two of them, then there is a two-thirds probability of having another infection during the next 6 months. Applying this observation to prophylactic antimicrobial regimens, it is clear that if prophylaxis is begun after the second or any succeeding infection within a set, about one-third of the patients will be treated unnecessarily since they will be in remission. The remaining two-thirds of the patients would still be at risk of more infections.

Since effective antimicrobial prophylaxis is available in the form of nightly doses of either 100 mg of nitrofurantoin or one-half tablet of trimethoprim-sulfamethoxazole, it is possible to compare the cost of treating individual infections versus the cost of prophylaxis.[22–24] The assumptions in this analysis include the following:

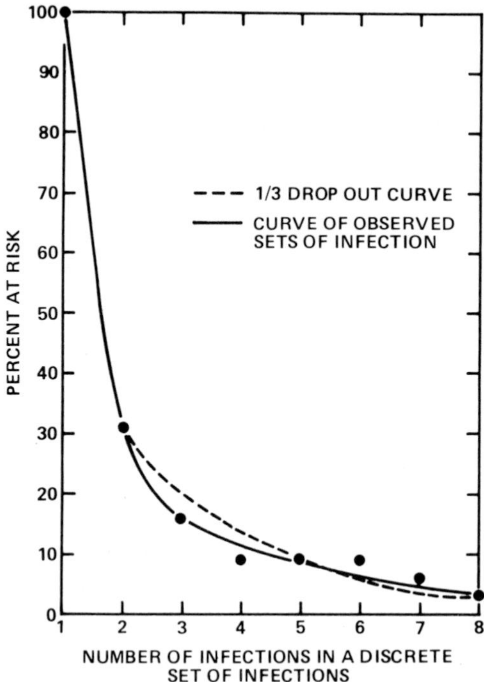

Figure 4.4 Sets of urinary infections plotted as a declining fraction of the total number of sets. A set is defined as any infection or group of infections preceded and followed by 6 months of remission. (Reproduced by permission from J. K. Kraft and T. A. Stamey, Medicine **56:** 55, 1977.[9])

1. Complete control of infection by prophylactic therapy
2. Cost of an infection (estimated minimum)
   - A. Initial culture and urinalysis. $12.00
   - B. Trimethoprim-sulfamethoxazole or nitrofurantoin, 40 tablets 11.00
   - C. Physician's visit fee 10.00
   - D. Culture after completion of treatment 10.00
   - TOTAL $43.00
3. Cost of prophylaxis (based on three pharmacies in our area).
   - A. Trimethoprim-sulfamethoxazole, ½ tablet nightly × 6 months $26.50
   - B. Nitrofurantoin, 100 mg generic 18.00
   - C. Macrodantin, 100 mg 41.00
   - AVERAGE $28.50
4. All patients have two infections treated prior to prophylaxis

These cost figures show that prophylaxis costs about two-thirds as much as treating an infection. Since two-thirds of the patients having two infections will have a third infection, the cost of treating a group with prophylaxis is about the same as delaying and treating the next infection. Because those having more than two infections are still at 66% risk of more infections and because a six-month prophylactic regimen may protect against more than one subsequent infection, the costs of treating the entire population increases whenever prophylaxis is delayed. The least expensive time to begin prophylaxis is after the second infection within 6 months.

Lastly, these data on natural history in a selected group of women referred because of at least two symptomatic infections in the preceding 12 months, and therefore representing a substantial problem to them, may explain why many physicians avidly believe that invasive procedures such as urethral dilations, internal urethrotomies and urethroplasties, etc., alter susceptibility to recurrent infection. Since 10 days of effective antimicrobial therapy alone results in a 6-month or longer remission in 34% of all infections and a mean remission of 55 weeks, it is understandable why these invasive procedures are often considered therapeutic. After all, a 34% "cure" rate, which occurs by natural history alone when accompanied by antimicrobial therapy, is a fairly impressive therapeutic effect. It is clear that any regimen which claims to alter susceptibility to recurrent infections must be controlled by similar patients simply treated with 10 days of effective antimicrobial therapy.

Summary

In 23 adult women having uncomplicated recurrent urinary tract infections treated with 10 days of appropriate antibiotic for each infection, the following findings were noted.

1. The attack rate was 0.17 infections/month.
2. 94% of infections had associated symptoms.
3. 73% of symptomatic episodes had an associated infection.
4. 21% of infections had less than 10^5 bacteria/ml.
5. 34% of all infections were followed by an infection-free interval of at least 6 months, and averaged 12.8 months. All but one patient had at least one infection-free interval.
6. Long infection-free intervals were followed by further infections; a remission is not a cure.
7. Between infection-free intervals the infections tended to occur in clusters with an attack rate of 0.47 infections/month.
8. Prophylaxis is less costly if begun at the second infection within a 6-month period.

BIOLOGIC BASIS OF RECURRENT BACTERIURIA

If longitudinal studies are performed with frequent cultures of the vaginal vestibule and urethra in women with recurrent bacteriuria, colonization of the vaginal vestibule and distal urethral mucosa with enterobacteria can be shown to precede the occurrence of bacteriuria.[10, 15, 16] Since the fecal reservoir is apparently the same in women with and without urinary infections,[25] these observations suggest that characterization of susceptibility lies in colonization of the vaginal vestibule with Enterobacteriaceae from the rectal flora.

Urethral colonization is determined by the introital bacteria of the vagina. Not only are these two moist, mucosal surfaces confined anatomically by the distal labia minora, but both are derived embryologically from the urogenital sinus. They are under the same hormonal control (Papanicolaou smears of the urethra show estrogen variation identical to that of vaginal epithelial cells),[26] and several thousand of our introital and urethral cultures have shown bacteriologic similarity. Thus, the physician needs to culture only the introital mucosa to determine the urethral bacteriology. Our technique, as reviewed in Chapter 1, is simple. Two cotton applicator sticks are held together, and the vaginal vestibule in the area of the hymenal ring, including the posterior vaginal wall as well as the anterior vaginal wall immediately below the urethral orifice, is swabbed in a circular motion (Chapter 1, Figure 1.25). The two cotton sticks are placed in 5 ml of transport broth (or saline) and agitated on a laboratory vibrator, the sticks discarded, and the transport medium cultured; bacteria on the introital mucosa are reported as organisms per milliliter of transport medium. The vaginal introitus and vaginal vestibule are interchangeable terms, both referring to the area inside the labia minora at the entrance to the vaginal canal.

I would like to present several clinical examples representative of over 100 patients we have closely followed.

First Clinical Example

K.S., a 26-year-old white woman, is representative of the general results. Without any childhood history of urinary infections, she experienced frequency, dysuria, bilateral flank pain, and fever to 104°F 2 months after her marriage. Although she responded well to antibiotics, 4 similar episodes occurred in the next 14 months, causing her to withdraw from a training school of nursing. We saw her in December 1968 shortly after the fifth episode of acute urinary infection. An excretory urogram showed only a dilated calyx in the middle of the right kidney. She was bacteriuric with *E. coli.* The urine was easily sterilized with 10 days of nitrofurantoin and she was placed on a postintercourse regimen of a single 500 mg. capsule of nalidixic acid. No further infections occurred on this regimen, even though the introital cultures remained positive for *E. coli* which maintained their sensitivity to nalidixic acid. In August 1969, a rash developed owing to the nalidixic acid and the medication was changed to 250 mg oral penicillin-G after intercourse. For the next year all bladder cultures remained sterile, although *E. coli* persisted on the introitus. On August 27, 1970 she was found to have an asymptomatic *E. coli* bacteriuria resistant to penicillin-G. Minimal inhibitory concentration (MIC) was greater than 1,200 μg/ml.

With this culture, she agreed to stop all drugs and to enter our protocol of close follow-up with frequent cultures. The *E. coli* bacteriuria proved to be serologically nontypable (NT) (Figure 4.5). Seven days of oxytetracycline (MIC greater than 150 μg/ml) failed to clear the infection but 10 days of nitrofurantoin (MIC equaled 13 μg/ml) was successful. The first culture after stopping nitrofurantoin showed a sterile bladder urine but the NT *E. coli* persisted on the vaginal vestibule and urethra together with some colonies of an *E. coli* 039 (Figure 4.5). However, the following cultures showed the appearance of an *E. coli* 04 on the vaginal vestibule. The *E. coli* 04 persisted and apparently grew to substantial numbers before the occurrence of the *E. coli* 04 bladder infection. This *E. coli* 04 bacteriuria occurred about 50 days after the start of the 10-day course of nitrofurantoin therapy and 32 days after the establishment of the *E. coli* 04 on the introitus. She was symptomatic with frequency and nocturia at the time of the *E. coli* 04 bladder infection. Immediate treatment with sulfamethizole probably prevented the development of chills and fever from upper tract infection. The small numbers of *E. coli* 04 in the midstream urine urine prior to the *E. coli* 04 bladder infection (Figure 4.5) represent contaminants of a sterile bladder urine caused by heavy introital and urethral colonization.

On the last day of sulfamethizole therapy, the bladder urine was sterile; a few NT *E. coli* were found on the introitus at this as well as the subsequent culture. Thereafter, the introital cultures reverted to normal and remained so for 6 months; during this time, she received no antibiotics and remained asymptomatic as well as free from recurrent bladder infections. However, an *E. coli* 04 eventually reappeared on the vaginal vestibule (Figure 4.6) and was present in the bladder 27 days later (June 1, 1971). Four days prior to this culture, suprapubic cramps, urinary frequency during the day and a constant pressure in the urethra developed. Some flank aching was

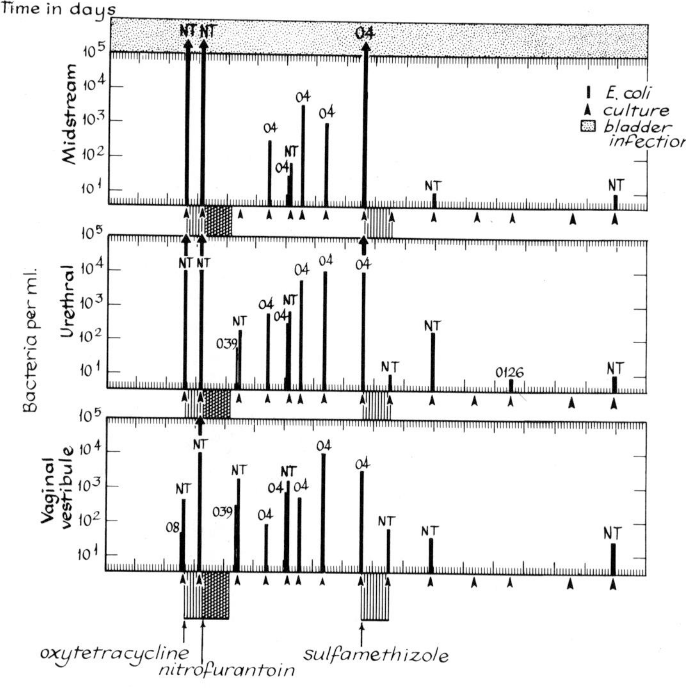

Figure 4.5 Enterobacterial relationship of vaginal vestibule, urethral and midstream cultures in K.S. a 26-year-old white married woman. Gram-negative enterobacteria cultured were *Escherichia coli.* Culture symbol (▲) without overlying vertical bars indicates complete absence of Gram-negative enterobacteria. Serogroup of *E. coli* appears at top of each solid bar. NT is nontypable *E. coli.* Patient had 3-year history of recurrent chills, fever, and flank pain. Data show that two, *E. coli* 04 bacteriuric episodes were preceded by establishment of large numbers of introital *E. coli* 04 before occurrence of each bacteriuria. Six months remission was associated with return of introital bacteriologic flora to normal.

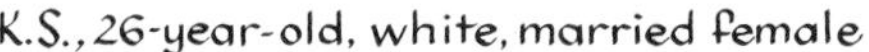

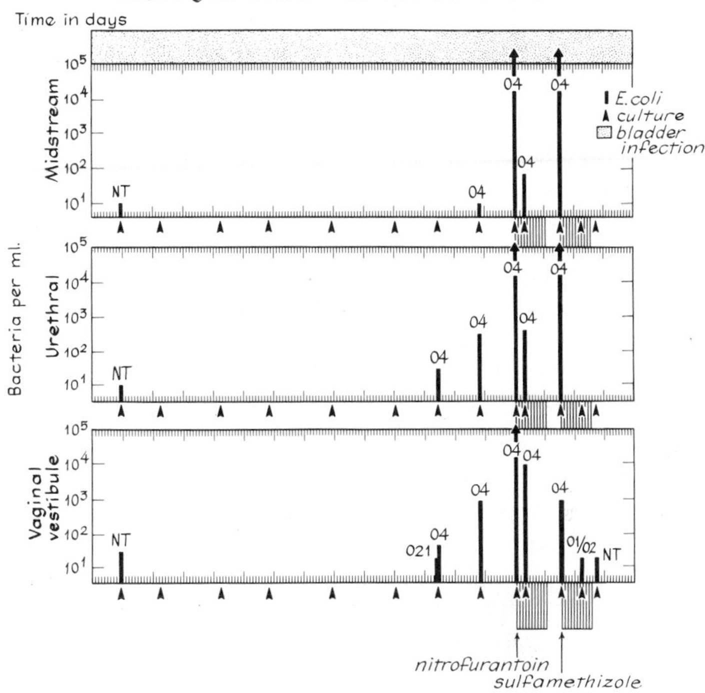

Figure 4.6 Enterobacterial relationship of vaginal vestibule, urethral and midstream cultures in K.S. a 26-year-old white, married woman which is continuous with Figure 4.5. Gram-negative enterobacteria cultured were *Escherichia coli*. Culture symbol (▲) without overlying vertical bars indicates complete absence of Gram-negative enterobacteria. Serogroup of *E. coli* appears at top of each solid bar. NT is non-typable *E. coli*. Patient had 3-year history of recurrent chills, fever and flank pain. Data show that two, *E. coli* 04 bacteriuric episodes were preceded by establishment of large numbers of introital *E. coli* 04 before occurrence of each bacteriuria.

present in both sides, especially when she was in the sitting position. A strong odor to the urine was observed 1 day prior to the June 1 culture. Urinalysis on that day showed in the spun urine only 2–4 white blood cells/high power field but many bacilli. Treatment with nitrofurantoin (MIC equaled 11 μg/ml) was followed by reinfection 15 days later; introital carriage of the same *E. coli* 04 was extremely heavy on the one culture obtained during the 4th day of nitrofurantoin therapy. With the recurrence of the *E. coli* 04 bacteriuria 5 days after therapy, she was again treated with 10 days of sulfamethizole. Both on, and 3 days off, sulfonamide therapy, the bladder urine was sterile and the *E. coli* 04 disappeared from the introitus (Figure 4.6). Because she moved 60 miles distant to Stanford, she was dropped from our study but placed on 500 mg methenamine twice a day. She was seen 9 months later (February 1972) with a sterile bladder urine but 300 colonies of an *E. coli* 018/ml were present on the vaginal vestibule. A rectal culture at the same visit (10 colonies randomly selected) showed 50% 018, 30% 025, and 10%/% NT *E. coli.* She remained uninfected for the next 5½ years, but maintained the methenamine, 500 mg twice a day except during her 9 months of pregnancy in 1976. One year after the birth of her son she had one episode of urinary frequency, flank pain, and high fever for which she was seen in a hospital emergency room. After the infection was cleared with an antibiotic, she was restarted on methenamine 500 mg once a day until April 1979, and had no further infections. She was last contacted in June 1979, some 11 years after we first saw her. She is now off the methenamine and asymptomatic. She is very likely to have further infections at some time in the future.

The data in Figures 4.5 and 4.6 show that her infections were preceded by colonization of the introital mucosa with the infecting strain of *E. coli*.

Second Clinical Example

The bacteriologic course of C.S., a 29-year-old white married female, followed through eight urinary infections over a period of 27 months is especially informative.

Her first urinary infection occurred in 1963 when she was 20 years old. The next 5 years were free from infection, years that included marriage and two full-term pregnancies. The following 4 years, however, were characterized by four to five urinary infections each year. An intravenous urogram and voiding cystourethrogram were normal. Because of the unremitting pattern of her recurrences and the failure of a variety of therapeutic regimens, including urethral dilatation, she was referred to us in September, 1972. Her bacteriologic course is presented in Figures 4.7 and 4.8; cultures of the vaginal vestibule are shown, together with the specific episodes of bacteriuria.

An intrauterine device was in place throughout the first nine months of our observations (until June 26, 1973); a vasectomy was performed on her husband on June 8, 1973. Vaginal douches were not done either before or after removal of the intrauterine device.

She experienced symptoms, including urgency, frequency, and suprapubic cramping ("bladder spasm") at every infection, although on one occasion we detected bacteriuria 24 hours before the onset of her symptoms. Dysuria never occurred. Although her symptoms (especially urgency) often persisted for several days after the start of antimicrobial therapy and even in the presence of a sterile urine, she was always asymptomatic in between episodes of bacteriuria. Pyuria was usually but not invariable present, and it always cleared a few days later. She was never catheterized,

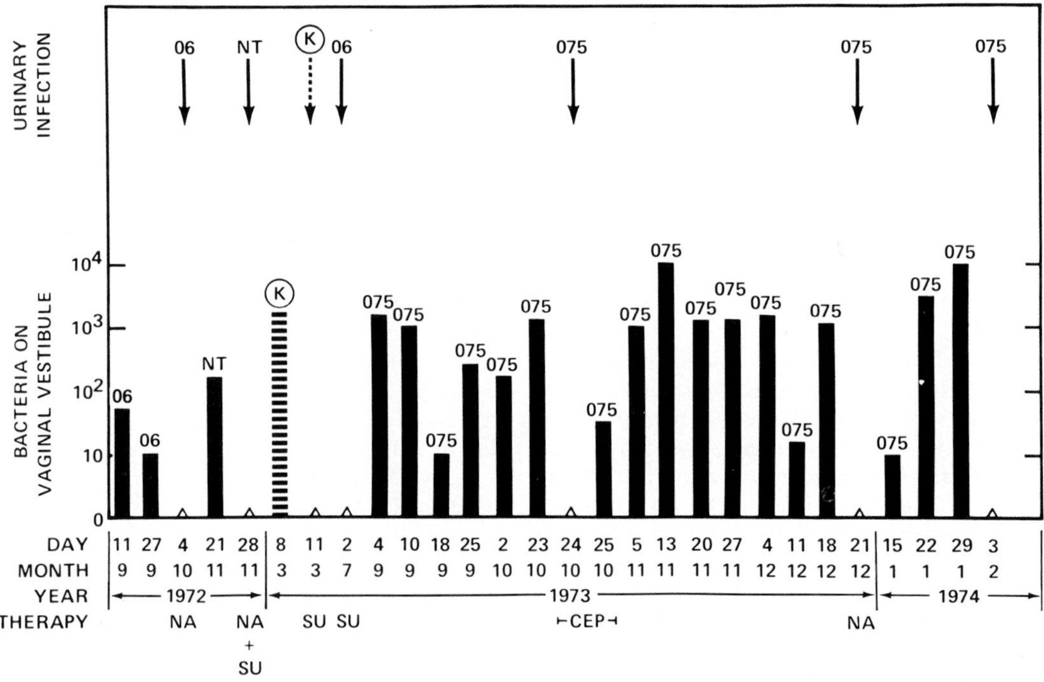

Figure 4.7 Clinical course of a 29-year-old married Caucasian woman followed through eight urinary infections in 27 months. Bacteriuric episodes are shown, together with every consecutive culture preceding the bacteriuria in which the same strain producing the infection was found on the vaginal vestibule. △ without overlying bars, indicates vaginal vestibule cultures without any detectable Enterobacteriaceae; *NA* stands for nalidixic acid; *SU*, sulfonamide; and *CEP*, cephalexin. *K* refers to *Klebsiella*; *NT*, to nontypable *Escherchia coli*; and numbers at top of bars, to specific serogroups of *E. coli*. (Reproduced by permission from J. H. Harrison, R. F. Gittes, A. D. Perlmutter, T. A. Stamey, and P. C. Walsh, Campbells Urology, Ed. 4, Chap. 11, Philadelphia, W. B. Saunders, 1978.)

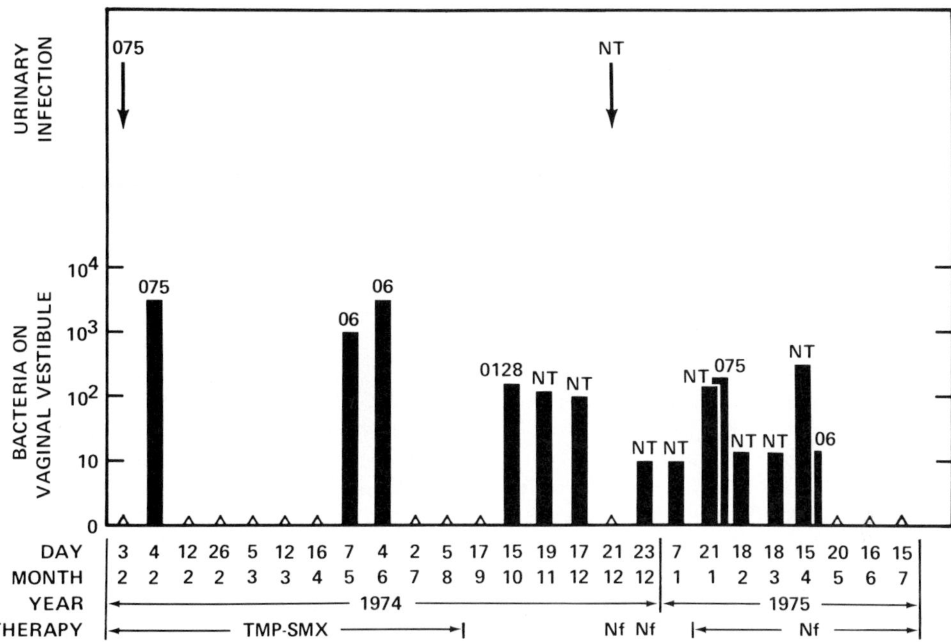

Figure 4.8 Same patient as shown in Figure 4.7, but illustrating the next 13 months, when continuous prophylaxis with trimethoprim-sulfamethoxazole (*TMP-SMX*, 6 months) and nitrofurantoin (*Nf*, 6 months) was used to prevent reinfections. All vaginal cultures are shown, as well as the episodes of bacteriuria.

nor was instrumentation employed. Each infection was treated for 10 days.

As seen in Figure 4.7, with the exception of the second *E. coli* 06 bacteriuria on July 2, 1973, every infection was preceded by colonization of the vaginal vestibule with the responsible pathogen. The culture immediately preceding this infection was obtained on June 26, 1973, a few hours after her gynecologist had removed an intrauterine device for prevention of pregnancy; this culture contained *Klebsiella* but no *E. coli.*

Although her first four infections showed a different organism at each succeeding bacteriuria, note that three consecutive infections were caused by *E. coli* 075 (Figure 4.7). More importantly, observe that the vaginal carriage of *E. coli* 075 persisted at every culture between the first and second 075 bacteriuria (a period of 8 weeks) and between the second and third 075 infection (a period of 6 weeks). Anal cultures in between each 075 infection showed the same *E. coli* 075 to be the predominant strain in the feces.

The reason for pointing out these consecutive infections at close intervals with the same serogroup of *E. coli* is that not only do they clearly show the vaginal route of pathogenesis through persistence of the pathogenic strain on the vaginal mucosa, but they equally show why the term "relapse" should not be used in defining the nature of recurrent bacteriuria (see Chapter 1). Those who use the term in this country imply persistence within the urinary tract (kidney), while these data show persistence outside the urinary bladder. It is clear that most consecutive infections with the identical organism, except in the patient with infection stones (Chapter 8) or bacterial prostatitis (Chapter 7) are actually reinfections from vaginal persistence.

During the 18 months of observation shown in Figure 4.7 before continuous prophylactic therapy was started on, February 3, 1974, there were 66 cultures obtained when she was not bacteriuric. It is important to note that 22 of the 66 did not contain a single detectable colony of Enterobacteriaceae. I have shown in Figure 4.7, for simplicity, every *consecutive* culture preceding each bacteriuric episode in which the identical strain causing the bacteriuria was found on the vaginal vestibule. We have pointed out repeatedly that colonization with Enterobacteriaceae is often intermittent in these susceptible patients.[16, 27, 28] The longest period of time this patient's vaginal mucosa was cultured without finding colonization with Enterobacteriaceae was from December 1, 1972 to January 17, 1973 (six cultures). On the other hand, her longest period of consecutive carriage of Enterobacteriaceae was from March 12, 1973 to June 8, 1973 (13 cultures).

As can be observed in Figure 4.8, following the last *E. coli* 075 infection, the patient was treated for 10 days with trimethoprim-sulfamethoxazole (TMP-SMX) at full dosage of two tablets every 12 hours, but followed on the 11th day with one-half tablet each evening at bedtime for the next 6 months. Bacteriuria did not recur while she was on prophylaxis or during the first 4 months after she stopped taking nightly doses of TMP-SMX (Figure 4.8). Moreover, while she was on prophylaxis (February 14, 1974 to August 5, 1974), only two of nine cultures showed transient vaginal colonization with enterobacteria (*E. coli* 06). Following the bacteriuria due to nontypable (NT) *E. coli* on December 21, 1974 (which incidentally was again preceded by vaginal colonization with the same NT *E. coli*), she was treated with nitrofurantoin for 10 days (until December 31, 1974); nitrofurantoin prophylaxis, 100 mg each night, was begun after the culture on January 21, 1975. During the 6 months of nitrofurantoin prophylaxis (Figure 4.8) there were no episodes of bacteriuria, but three of six vaginal cultures showed carriage of Enterobacteriaceae, all sensitive to nitrofurantoin. The prophylactic prevention of bacteriuria is presented in some detail in the following section in this chapter.

After completing 6 months of nitrofurantoin prophylaxis in July 1975, she was asymptomatic and free from infection until February 1976 when she became infected with a self-agglutinating *E. coli*. She responded to a short course of TMP-SMX and was well until October 1976; a nontypable *E. coli* caused the October infection. She was then well for over 1 year until December 1977 when the onset of acute lower tract symptoms caused her to self-treat herself with 5 days of TMP-SMX. In 1978, and until July 1979, she has remained off all medication and has been asymptomatic.

Third Clinical Example

S.W., a 27-year old, married, white female consulted me in April of 1970 for recurrent episodes of frequency, urgency, and dysuria of three year's duration. She had documented infections with *Proteus mirabilis* in 1968, *Klebsiella* in February, 1969 and *E. coli* in November, 1969; an intravenous urogram was normal.

Her bacteriologic course through the first three of her five infections in our studies are shown in Figure 4.9. When first cultured, her vaginal introitus and urethra were colonized with *P. mirabilis* 048; 14 days later she was symptomatic and bacteriuric with the same organism. Observe that at the time of this bacteriuria, about 150 colonies/ml of an *E. coli* 08 were also detected on the introital culture and that this *E. coli* was sensitive to tetracycline, penicillin-G, and sulfonamides (Figure 4.9). When the *P. mirabilis* bacteriuria was treated with 10 days of oxytetracycline, cultures on the 5th day of treatment showed clearance of all the *P. mirabilis* both from the bladder and the introitus, but the *E. coli* 08 was firmly established on the introitus although it was now resistant to all three antimicrobial agents. The presence of this multiple resistance strongly suggests that these 290 colonies of *E. coli* 08 present on the introitus during oxytetracycline therapy represent rapid colonization from the fecal flora rather than a resistant change in the previously sensitive *E. coli* 08 originally present on the vagina (see Chapter 2). By the 10th day of oxytetracycline therapy, she was severely symptomatic and infected with the resistant *E. coli* 08. These data indicate the rapidity with which an *E.*

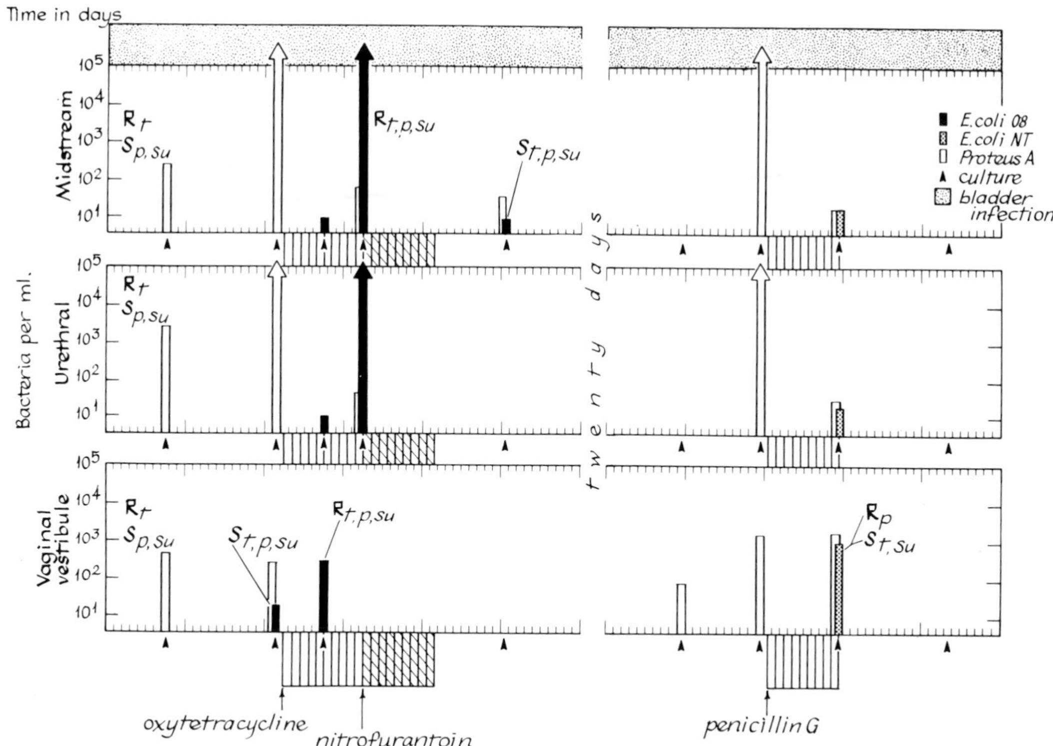

Figure 4.9 Enterobacterial and antimicrobial relationship of the vaginal vestibule, urethral, and midstream cultures in a 27-year-old, white, married female (S.W.) with recurrent bladder infections. All Gram-negative enterobacteria cultured are shown, except for *Klebsiella pneumoniae* which appeared transiently in the introitus on four occasions: <20/ml three times and 4000/ml once; the culture symbol (▲), without overlying vertical bars, indicates the complete absence of Gram-negative enterobacteria. *Escherichia coli* 08 is indicated by the solid bars. See text for the antimicrobial relationship of the *E. coli* 08 on the introitus before and during oxytetracycline therapy. The open bars represent identical strains of *Proteus mirabilis* as shown by Dienes swarming; all strains were found to be of the same O-antigen serogroup (048). R = resistant, S = sensitive, t = oxytetracycline, p = penicillin-G, and su = sulfonomide.

coli from the fecal flora can colonize the introitus and infect the bladder; 10 days at the most in this instance and possible within 5 days. The *E. coli* 08 bacteriuria was cured with nitrofurantoin, and approximately 2 months later she was again bacteriuric with *P. mirabilis* 048; as with the first proteus infection, the *P. mirabilis* 048 was detected on the vaginal vestibule several days before reaching the bladder. Note also in Figure 4.9 the transient appearance of a penicillin-G resistant (> 100 μg/ml) nontypable *E. coli* on the introitus at the end of 10 days of therapy with penicillin-G for the *P. mirabilis* infection.

These data in Figure 4.9 further show the fallacy of defining a relapse as a recurrent infection with the same serotype within 14 days of completing therapy. To be sure, this recurrence in Figure 4.9 with the *E. coli* 08 was a different organism from the *P. mirabilis* and clearly a reinfection, but the rapidity with which an organism from the fecal flora can colonize the introitus and infect the bladder must offer little comfort to those who believe a recurrence within 14 days indicates the kidney as the source of bacterial persistence. Since most symptomatic UTIs in women can be shown to have the same *E. coli* as the predominant orga-

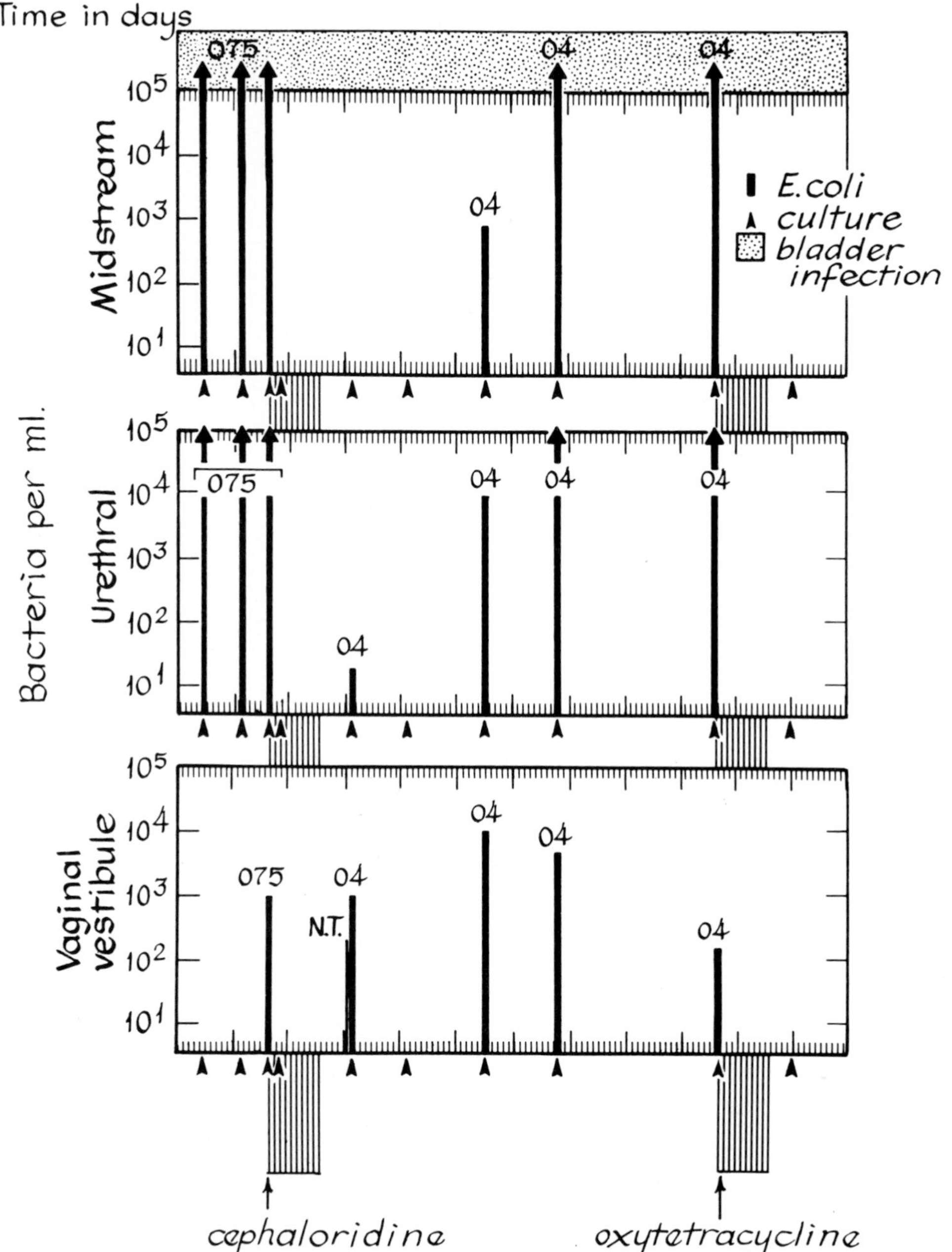

Figure 4.10 Enterobacterial relationship of the vaginal vestibule, urethral, and midstream cultures in a 32-year-old white married female (G.W.). The only Gram-negative enterobacteria cultured were *Escherichia coli*; the culture symbol (▲), without overlying vertical bars, indicates the complete absence of Gram-negative enterobacteria. The serogroup of *E. coli* appears at the top of each solid bar; *NT* is nontypable *E. coli*. Except for one hospitalization with her first pregnancy at the age of 17, she was free from urinary infections until age 31 when a series of recurrences resulted in her referral to Stanford. She was found to have a congenital left ureteral stump (Figure 4.11) and a urethral diverticulum. Despite these two anatomical abnormalities, her recurrences were

nism in the fecal flora,[25] and since these bacteria can infect the bladder in a very few days as shown in Figure 4.9, I believe many, if not most, infections thought to be relapses from the kidney after 5–10 days of adequate therapy are actually reinfections from the introitus and rectum with the same O-serogroup.

Patient S.W., after the three infections in Figure 4.9, had one further infection 4 months later with the *P. mirabilis* 048 and 1 month after that a single infection with an *E. coli* 075, in December 1970. She was then free from infection for 13 months when, in January 1972, she had a second infection with an 075 *E. coli*. In the past 7 years she has had no further infections or symptoms. From 1972 to 1976, she was cultured on 9 occasions; her introital cultures did not contain a single colony of Enterobacteriaceae during this period. When last cultured on December 20, 1978, there were 30 colonies of a nontypable *E. coli* on the introitus, her midstream urine was sterile, and nontypable *E. coli* were also found in the rectum.

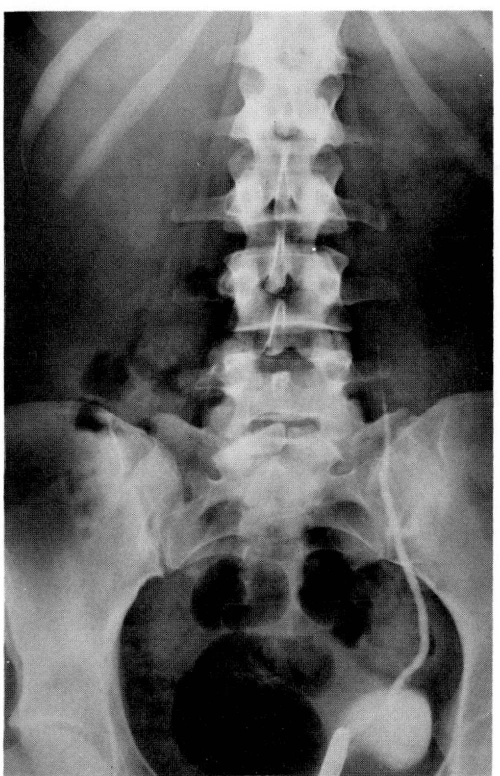

Figure 4.11 Left retrograde ureterogram in G.W. (Figure 4.10) showing a blind ending and irregular left ureter.

Fourth Clinical Example

G.W. (Figure 4.10), was a 32-year-old married female referred in February of 1970 because of recurrent bacteriuria of 1–2 years' duration, bilateral low back and suprapubic pain, and some subcostal discomfort in the left anterior upper quadrant. The presence of bacteriuria usually correlated with her low back and suprapubic discomfort. Her referring urologist was concerned whether the blind-ending left ureter at the fourth lumbar vertebra (Figure 4.11) was the cause of her recurrent infections. Cystoscopy and bacteriologic localization studies at the time of her 075 infection (Figure 4.10), using the technique outlined in Chapter 1, showed that the right kidney was sterile, but the bladder wash counts were too high (3000/ml) to decide if the bacteria recovered from the left ureter (180–1000/ml), obtained by irrigation with sterile saline, were real or contaminants from the bladder urine in the ureteral catheter. Cystoscopy also revealed a 3–4 cm urethral diverticulum in the middle one-third of the urethra. An arteriogram showed no evidence of a left renal artery (Figure 4.12) and no evidence of a nephrogram on the left side (Figure 4.13).

---

reinfections. The *E. coli* 04 responsible for her second bacteriuric episode appeared on the introitus first, similar to other infections in women without congenital abnormalities. Following the single post-treatment culture for her 04 bladder infection in Figure 4.10, she was seen 91 days later, without interval introital cultures, and had an *E. coli* 016 bladder infection. Treatment with cephaloglycin cleared the 016 bacteriuria, her introital cultures reverted to normal, and she had no further infections in the 6 months after the 016 bacteriuria. Not only were her introital cultures devoid of any Gram-negative enterobacteria, but copious fluid from the urethral diverticulum—obtained by urethral massage—was sterile.

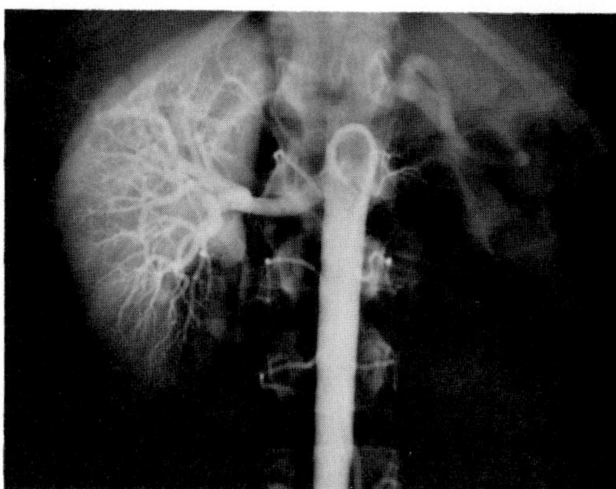

Figure 4.12 Arteriogram in G.W. showing no evidence for a left renal artery.

Following cephaloridine therapy for the *E. coli* 075, an *E. coli* 04 appeared on the introitus and was responsible for the next urinary infection on May 7, 1970 (Figure 4.10). After treatment of the *E. coli* 04, the next bacteriuria was caused by *E. coli* 016, but the time lapse between the last culture in Figure 4.10 and the 016 bacteriuria was 13 weeks. Thus, the left ureter was clearly not the cause of her recurrent infections because the serogroup was different with each infection and, for the one infection where serial introital cultures were obtained (Figure 4.10), the *E. coli* 04 was established on the vaginal vestibule before it appeared in the bladder. The possibility that the urethral diverticulum was the cause of her recurrent infections was equally unlikely in view of the changing serogroups. In the 6 months after the *E. coli* 016 bladder infection, she received no antimicrobial therapy and remained asymptomatic. Cultures in January and March of 1971 contained no enterobacteria in any of the introital or urinary cultures. In fact, urethral massage of the diverticulum produced 2.0 ml of cloudy, yellow thick fluid, containing many large leukocytes per high power field, but no bacteria on culture.

In July 1971, she was again bacteriuric with an *E. coli* 075. On September 30, 1971 and October 14, 1971, catheterized urine cultures were sterile, but discharge from the urethral diverticulum showed a heavy growth of *Haemophilus influenzae* and many white blood cells (WBC). A urethral diverticulectomy was done on November 1, 1971 without complications; gentamicin sterilized the diverticulum before surgical excision. Since the diverticulectomy, she has had about one infection per year, including *E. coli* 016, 04, and a self-agglutinating *E. coli* in August 1976, treated with nitrofurantoin macrocrystals. She remained sterile between August 1976 and September 1978 when she was once again infected with an *E. coli*.

These data should serve as a clear warning to all urologists who find an anatomical defect in the urinary tract in the presence of recurrent urinary infections; neither the left ureter nor the urethral diverticulum was related to the bacteriuric episodes in this patient.

Conclusions and Comments

These four longitudinal studies on young women with UTI illustrate the biologic basis of recurrent bacteriuria, *i.e., that colonization of the introital mucosa with enterobacteria precedes the bacteriuric episode.* It is reasonable that, if we knew the factors responsible for this colonization, we might prevent UTI and all its consequences. Our past 10 years of research into the causes of introital colonization are pre-

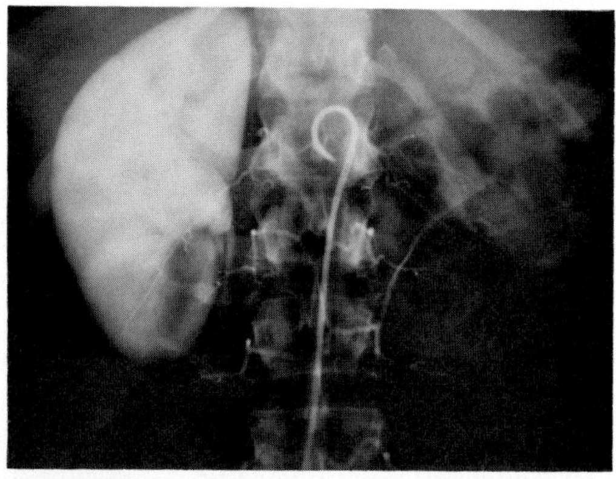

Figure 4.13 Nephrogram phase of the arteriogram in G.W. There is no nephrogram on the left side to indicate the presence of renal tissue. The right renal cortex shows no evidence of renal scars from her history of recurrent bacteriuria.

Table 4.7
Periurethral Aerobic Gram-Negative Rods in 13 Girls, 4-12 Years[a]

Condition	No. of Girls	Time in Days	No. of Cultures	Percent with 10^3 Gram-negative rods or >/cm^2 of periurethral mucosa
Infection	7	3–30	59	75
No Infection	6	9–123	235	10

[a] Modified from I. Bollgren & J. Winberg.[29]

sented in Chapter 5; the interested reader may find these investigations informative. The basic observation, however, for both the clinician and the investigator, is that enterobacteria from the rectal reservoir must first colonize the introital mucosa of the vagina before bacteriuria can occur. The implication of the corollary of this observation is clinically important: in the absence of introital colonization, bacteriuria should not occur. The critical student will notice, I hope, that these observations do not mean that introital colonization with enterobacteria invariably leads to bacteriuria, a concept we have been credited with in some uncritical publications. Our observation that introital colonization precedes bacteriuria has been confirmed by Bollgren and Winberg[29] who sampled the periurethral and midstream bladder urine almost daily in 13 girls who stopped nitrofurantoin prophylaxis. Seven girls developed a UTI in 3–30 days of stopping nitrofurantoin prophylaxis; all were heavily colonized periurethrally with Gram-negative rods which ultimately caused their UTI (Table 4.7). On the other hand, 6 girls remained uninfected; they had normal periurethral flora with only rare colonization with Gram-negative bacteria.

Summary

1. Introital colonization with Enterobacteriaceae precedes bacteriuria (clinical examples 1 (K.S.), 2 (C.S.), 3 (S.W.) and 4 (G.W.).
2. Even in highly susceptible patients, introital colonization is clearly intermittent. Thus, whatever the real cause of introital colonization turns out to be, it does not appear to be a constant defect (K.S., S.W., and G.W.).
3. *E. coli* from the rectal reservoir can colonize the introitus and gain entry into the bladder very quickly; in the case of S.W., clinical example 3, we have demonstrated the time interval to be as short as 5 days, which must indicate that even shorter intervals can occur in some patients.
4. In the American literature, recurrent infections with the same organism within 2 weeks are termed "relapse" and imply renal persistence. The almost constant introital colonization of C.S. with an *E. coli* 075, the second clinical example, and the astonishingly short 5 days between colonization of the introitus with a resistant *E. coli* 08 and the *E. coli* 08 bacteriuria in S.W., the third clinical example, argues strongly against the concept and implications of "relapse."
5. Congenital anomalies, though frequently blamed for recurrent UTI, are often unrelated; infections in most patients with congenital anomalies are caused by the same biologic defect that allows introital colonization and thereby causes most urinary infections in females without congenital anomalies (G.W., fourth clinical example).

PROPHYLACTIC PREVENTION OF RECURRENT BACTERIURIA

Since the basic cause of recurrent UTI appears to be a biological problem related to colonization of the introital mucosa, it is not surprising that surgical approaches to the urinary tract such as urethral dilatations, antireflux operations on the ureters, and operations designed to open the internal vesical neck of the bladder have had little or no bacteriologic evidence to support their efficacy (see Chapters 6 and 9); fortunately for the patient, there appears to be an increasing awareness among urologists of the lack of efficacy from these procedures.

As noted in Figure 4.4 and discussed earlier in this chapter, the best time to begin antimicrobial prophylaxis is immediately after the second infection of any series provided it occurs within a 6-month period.

Antimicrobial Effect on Bowel and Vaginal Flora

Effective prophylaxis depends in large part on whether the antimicrobial drug has an adverse or favorable effect on the introital and fecal reservoirs of pathogenic bacteria. Winberg and his colleagues,[30, 31] to my knowledge, were the first to emphasize the relationship between resistant strains in the fecal flora, caused by oral antimicrobial therapy, and the occurrence of resistant urinary infections. They had shown earlier that 60 days of sulfonamide therapy was no better than 10 days in preventing recurrent infections but, more importantly, that the infections which occurred during the 60 days of therapy were usually resistant to sulfonamides[32]; these latter observations undoubtedly suggested the adverse effect of sulfonamides on the fecal reservoir.

I have summarized the data from three different studies in Table 4.8 on the effect of sulfonamide therapy in promoting resistant *E. coli* in the fecal flora.[31, 33, 34]

In short term therapy, 10 days or less, a resistant fecal flora is not as great a disadvantage because rapid reinfections (as in Figure 4.9) are relatively uncommon. Nevertheless, the increase in resistant strains of *E. coli* as well as the proliferation of *Klebsiella* and *Candida albicans* in the fecal and vaginal flora that accompanies even short term, oral administration of tetracyclines, ampicillin, sulfonamides, and amoxicillin are well documented[30–39]; these ecologic changes are potentially serious and should be considered in the administration of these antimicrobial agents. Before considering the effect of continuous, low dosage prophylaxis, however, it is worth reviewing some instructive studies on short term therapy of ampicillin, TMP-SMX, and nalidixic acid; the biologic pressure of these antimicrobial agents on the fecal and vaginal flora has been studied in detail at full dosage therapy.

Effect of Full Dosage, Short Term Therapy

Effect of Ampicillin on Vaginal and Fecal *E. coli*. In a small, but carefully done, unpublished study, we treated four volunteers who were healthy, young premenopausal women, ages 20–40, with 250 mg of ampicillin four times a day. They had vaginal and anal canal swab cultures placed in 5 ml of Earle's transport medium (see Chapter 1) at weekly intervals for 5–7 weeks before beginning therapy, and at least once

Table 4.8
Sulfonamide Effect on Fecal *Escherichia coli*

Drug	Percent Resistant					
	Before	During	After Week			
			1	*2*	*3*	*4*
Sulphamethoxydiazine-Sulphamethoxazole (350 mg/day)[a 34]	1.0	77	27	11	1	0
Sulphisoxazole Hospital[b] (50–200 mg/kg/day[31]	10	95				
Outpatient[b] (50–200 mg/kg/day[31]	10	66				
Sulphadimidine (1/4–1.0 gm/day)[33]		'66	Continuous Prophylaxis			

[a] 3 weeks of therapy.
[b] 10 days of therapy.

Trimethoprim-sulfamethoxazole (Septra). In the first half of 1973, before TMP-SMX was approved by the FDA for use in this country, we performed experiments on the diffusion and concentration of TMP from plasma into prostatic fluid of the dog[44] (see Chapter 7). We observed that TMP achieved concentrations in prostatic fluid which exceeded the plasma by 8–10 times (canine prostatic fluid in the anesthetized dog was acid to plasma by 1.0–1.5 pH units, or 10–50 times more hydrogen ions). While discussing these experiments one day in our laboratories, as well as considering some of our female patients with heavy introital colonization, we suddenly realized that human vaginal secretion was 3 full pH units more acid than plasma (1000 times more hydrogen ions). Since TMP, a lipid-soluble base with a favorable pKa (see Chapter 7), will move by nonionic diffusion across noninflamed epithelial membranes almost in proportion to the pH gradient, we knew the human vagina was the perfect secretory surface for ion trapping of TMP.

Accordingly, we took two of our most difficult women in terms of uncontrollable recurrent urinary infections and, after sterilizing their urine, placed them on one-half a tablet of TMP-SMX (40 mg of TMP and 200 mg of SMX) nightly, which represented one-eighth of the regular, full dosage. Because the result was not only gratifying, but astonishing in terms of vaginal clearance of Enterobacteriaceae,[45] their clinical and bacteriologic course is of some interest.

The first patient was a 39-year old diabetic Caucasian mother of two children who had experienced multiple recurrences of bacteriuria, often with chills and fever, following a hysterectomy in 1971. She was referred to Stanford in April 1973, where, despite antimicrobial therapy based on quantitative disc sensitivity testing, we too were unable to prevent her recurrent bacteriuria between April and July 1973. An intravenous urogram showed papillary necrosis without cortical scars or calcifications. The longest interval without medication between infections was 11 days. Attempts to follow successful eradication of her bacteriuria with nitrofurantoin prophylaxis were thwarted by nitrofurantoin-resistant *E. coli*. As seen in Figure 4.14, 9 of 13 cultures of the vaginal vestibule were colonized with the same *E. coli* causing her infections; similar *E. coli* were found in the rectal flora. In July, she began a 10-day course of TMP-SMX (2 tablets every 12 hours) for her self-agglutinating *E. coli* bacteriuria, followed by one-half tablet each evening at bedtime. Not a single aerobic Gram-negative bacteria was cultured from the mucosa of the introitus after starting TMP-SMX, and, of course, the bacteriuric episodes ceased (Figure 4.14). Measurements of TMP and SMX in her vaginal fluid during full dosage therapy showed 5–8.5 μg of TMP/ml; SMX was not detectable in her vaginal fluid. The mean concentrations of TMP and SMX in the serum and vaginal fluid of seven patients on both full dosage and prophylactic therapy is shown in Table 4.13. Note that the SMX was virtually undetectable in vaginal fluid.[45]

Three months after stopping TMP-SMX prophylaxis on April 8, 1974 (9 months of prophylaxis), she became reinfected with a self-agglutinating (SA) *E. coli*, for which she received 10 days of TMP-SMX at full dosage. Ten days after completing TMP-SMX therapy, she was infected with *Streptococcus faecalis* and received 10 days of nitrofurantoin, 400 mg/day. On the 11th day, she began nitrofurantoin prophylaxis, 100 mg each night. After 107 days of nitrofurantoin prophylaxis, *E. coli* bacteriuria again occurred, for which she received a short, effective course of sulfasoxazole and then resumed nitrofurantoin prophylaxis. Seventeen days later a nontypable *E. coli*, resistant to nitrofurantoin, caused an infection that was treated with oxytetracycline for 10 days, and prophylaxis with nitrofurantoin was continued. Five weeks later, having completed 6 months of nitrofurantoin prophylaxis, all therapy was stopped. However, within 2 months she was again infected with another SA *E. coli*, for which she was treated with TMP-SMX and restarted on TMP-SMX prophylaxis, one-half tablet each night. For the past 4 years, she has done well on TMP-SMX prophylaxis. About every 6 months to 1 year she

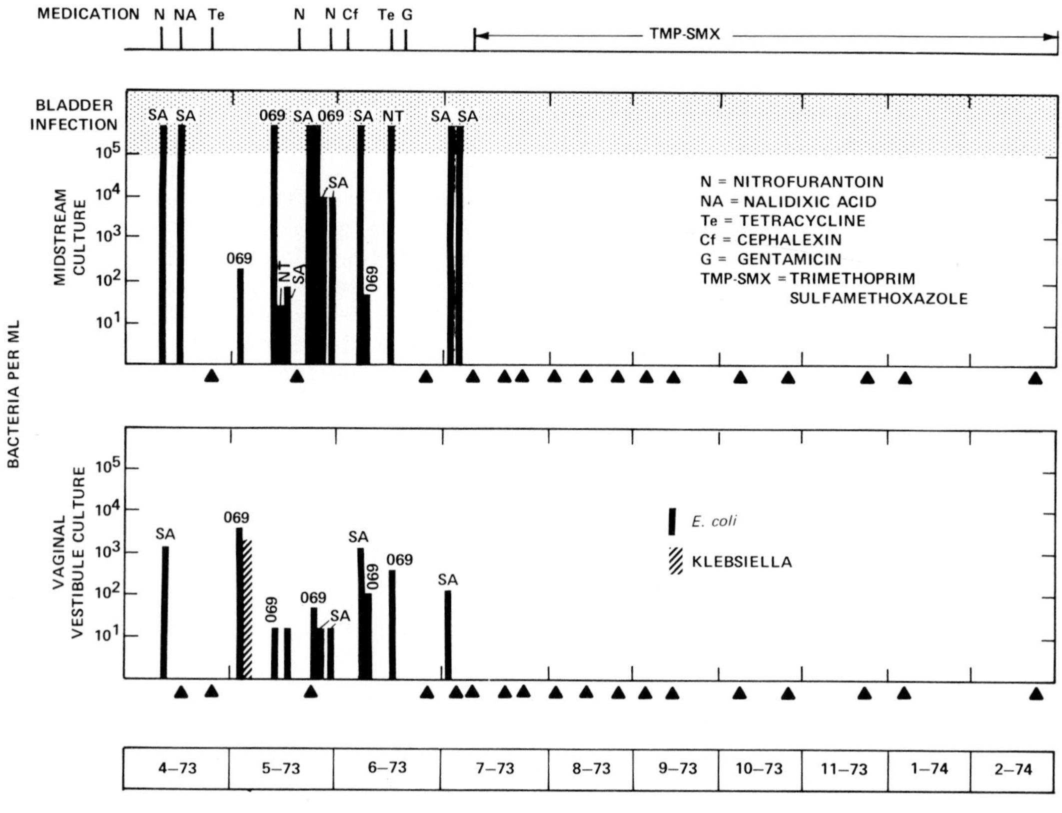

Figure 4.14 Clinical course of recurrent infections of the urinary tract in a 39-year-old diabetic woman. Quantitative cultures of the vaginal vestibule and midstream voided urine are shown with the serotypes of *Escherichia coli*. ▲ indicates a culture in which no Gram-negative bacteria were detectable in 0.1 ml of vaginal transport fluid or urine. Small colony counts of Gram-positive organisms are not shown. *SA* refers to self-agglutinating *E. coli*, and *NT*, to nontypable *E. coli*. (Reproduced by permission from T. A. Stamey, and M. Condy, J. Infect. Dis., **131:** 261, 1975, The University of Chicago Press, 1975 by The Journal of Infectious Diseases.[45])

stops TMP-SMX prophylaxis, but becomes symptomatic everytime within 3 weeks with a UTI, almost always *E. coli*. Her last serum creatinine in April 1978, was 1.0 mg%. This patient clearly indicates how these reinfections simply will not cease in some patients and that nightly prophylaxis, especially with TMP-SMX, can be extraordinarily effective.

A 48-year-old Caucasian mother had her first urinary infection in 1957 and a second in 1966. Hysterectomy and bilateral oophorectomy were performed in 1967 and followed by 0.6 mg of conjugated estrogen daily. Between 1968 and 1973, symptomatic bacteriuria recurred at 4-month intervals, always with dysuria and frequency, but occasionally with fever. An intravenous urogram showed only dilatation of the right upper calix and infundibulum, without evidence of a cortical scar. After we saw her in August 1973, she had four urinary infections in 3 months, three caused by *E. coli* 06 and one in September caused by *P. mirabilis* (Figure 4.15). The vaginal vestibule was heavily colonized at every culture with *E. coli* of several types (including the *E. coli* 06 that caused her bacteriuria), as well as *P. mirabilis* and later a species of *Klebsiella*. Three rectal cultures showed the same *E. coli* 06 and *P. mirabilis* in large numbers. TMP-SMX prophylaxis was started in November 1973, 10 days after starting treatment with tetracycline for the low-count *E. coli* 06 bacteriuria that had persisted with the initial cephalexin therapy. Although her prophylactic dosage was one tablet every other night (one-half tablet each night is a better regimen), the immediate and remarkable clearance of all Enterobacteriaceae from the vaginal vestibule and the prevention of further infections is readily seen in Figure 4.15. She continued the TMP-SMX prophylaxis for 9 months, until August 1974; not a single colony of Enterobacteriaceae was ever detected on the vaginal vestibule during prophylaxis. Two collections of vaginal fluid during prophylaxis showed concentrations of 0.42 μg and 0.25 μg of TMP/ml, respectively. SMX was not detectable.

In the first 4 weeks after stopping TMP-SMX prophylaxis, two cultures showed small numbers of nontypable *E. coli* on the vaginal vestibule. However, the next seven monthly cultures showed no colonization, and she remained free of bacteriuria. Eight months after stopping TMP-SMX prophylaxis, she became bacteriuric with *E. coli* 013. Although the problem was not as severe as that in the preceding patient during the period immediately after stopping TMP-SMX prophylaxis, it is clear that 9 months without Enterobacteriaceae on the vaginal vestibule during prophylaxis did not suffice to prevent further reinfections.

Six months after the *E. coli* 013 UTI in 1975, she was reinfected with NT *E. coli* that caused both symptoms and pyuria. Eighteen months later, in March 1977, she was infected again with an *E. coli* that was not serotyped. Since March 1977 she has been completely asymptomatic, has received no antimicrobial agents, and has had no UTI. Her last culture at Stanford on August 2, 1979 showed no Enterobacteriaceae or enterococci on the introital culture and her midstream urine was sterile.

These two difficult patients show the extraordinary effectiveness of TMP-SMX in clearing the vaginal introitus of Enterobacteriaceae. Since the SMX is barely detectable in vaginal fluid and occurs at insignificant concentrations, the introital clearance of Enterobacteriaceae is surely related to the TMP. The interested reader will find a full discussion of the principles governing the nonionic diffusion and ion trapping of TMP on the acid side of epithelial membranes in Chapter 7. It is worth noting that the concentration of TMP measured in the vaginal secretions (Table 4.13) are bactericidal for most urinary pathogens.

Paul Madsen and his colleagues[46, 47] at Wisconsin presented some ingenious experiments demonstrating the diffusion of trimethoprim, erythromycin, rosamicin, and ampicillin from the plasma into the female urethra and vagina of the dog. Only the first three basic, highly lipid soluble, antimicrobial agents were iontrapped on the urethral and vaginal mucosa in concentrations that exceeded the plasma level by severalfold.

It is also worth noting that all these months of keeping the introital mucosa totally free of all Enterobacteriaceae was insufficient for the normal introital flora to prevent recolonization with Enterobacteriaceae once the TMP-SMX was stopped.

Table 4.13
Concentration of TMP[a] and SMX in Serum and Vaginal Fluid in Seven Patients

Dosage	TMP			SMX		
	Serum	Vaginal	Ratio V/S	Serum	Vaginal	Ratio V/S
		μg/ml			*μg/ml*	
Full Dosage (4 tabs/day)	2.72	4.84	1.8	83	0.41	0.005
Prophylactic Dosage (1/2 tab/day)	0.39	0.64	1.6	13	0.05	0.004

[a] TMP = Trimethoprim; SMX = sulfamethoxazole; V/S = ratio of the vaginal concentration to the serum concentration.

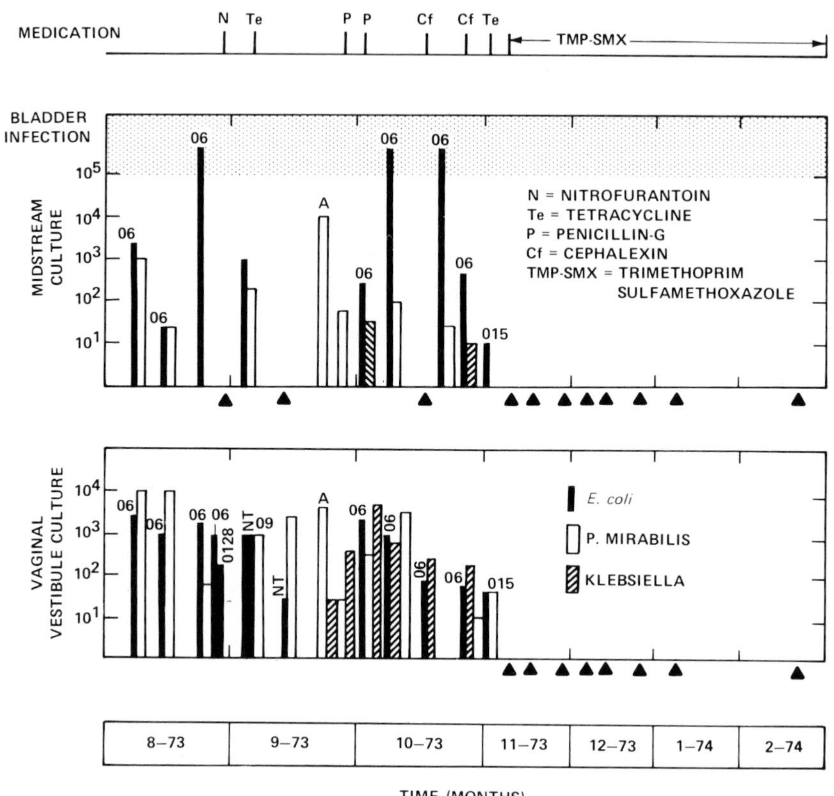

Figure 4.15 Clinical course of recurrent bacteriuria in a 48-year-old woman. Quantitative cultures of the vaginal vestibule and midstream voided urine are shown with the serotypes of *Escherichia coli*. ▲ indicates a culture in which no Gram-negative bacteria were detectable in 0.1 ml of vaginal transport fluid or urine. Small colony counts of Gram-positive organisms are not shown. *NT* refers to nontypable *E. coli*, and *A*, to *Proteus mirabilis* bacteriuria, even though the colony count in the midstream urine was 10^4/ml. The patient had been symptomatic for only a few hours, and marked pyuria accompanied infection with *P. mirabilis*. (Reproduced by permission from T. A. Stamey and M. Condy, J. Infect Dis., **131:** 261, 1975, The University of Chicago Press, 1975 by The Journal of Infectious Diseases.[45])

This observation means that microbial interference or protection by the normal vaginal flora is not biologically active enough to prevent subsequent recolonization and UTI. The biologic defect that allows colonization, therefore, appears to be a substantial one in terms of overcoming the normal introital flora.

I would now like to report a patient who did equally well on nitrofurantoin prophylaxis; she is also most instructive in terms of (1) resistance of the adult kidney to renal scarring in the face of horrendous clinical episodes of acute pyelonephritis, (2) the role of childhood infections in accounting for adult renal scarring, and (3) the role of ureteral reflux and its disappearance with the passage of time in the presence of a sterile urine. All three of these points are important principles in the management of UTI and are considered in some detail in other sections of this book (the "pyelonephritis" section later in this chapter, and Chapter 6). Nowhere, however, are these three principles better illustrated than in patient D.B. whose description follows in the next section.

Nitrofurantoin (Furadantin or Macrodantin). Nitrofurantoin, either because of its complete absorption in the upper intestinal tract or its degradation and inactivation in the intestinal tract, does not produce fecal resistance. Thus, although vaginal colonization may persist during long term prophylaxis[24, 50] the bacteria remain susceptible to the urinary concentrations and are undoubtedly killed by the evening dosage if they gain entrance into the bladder.

A good example of nitrofurantoin prophylaxis, with ultimate disappearance of susceptibility to recurrent infections is illustrated by the following patient: D.B., a 23-year-old California girl, was first seen by me in September 1970. She had just experienced a horrendous 4 months of recurrent urinary infections, characterized by chills, fever, and flank pain; these infections had required multiple hospitalizations in Europe. All of her symptoms began within a few weeks of her marriage and were definitely related to the onset of sexual intercourse. An intravenous urogram showed good cortex bilaterally, but a calyceal deformity in the upper pole was present extending toward the capsule of the left kidney, diminutive calyces could be seen in the left kidney below the deformed calyx, and

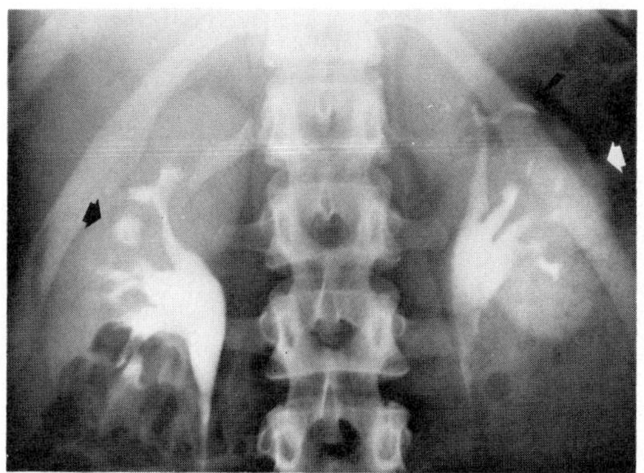

Figure 4.16 An intravenous urogram from D.B., a 22-year-old, white female with documented bilateral ureteral reflux present since infancy. This film was taken after 5 minutes of abdominal compression. The *arrows* indicate the dilated calyx in the right kidney, a peculiar calyx in the left kidney that almost extends to the capsule (*upper arrow*), and a diminutive calyx (*lower arrow*) just below the capsular calyx.

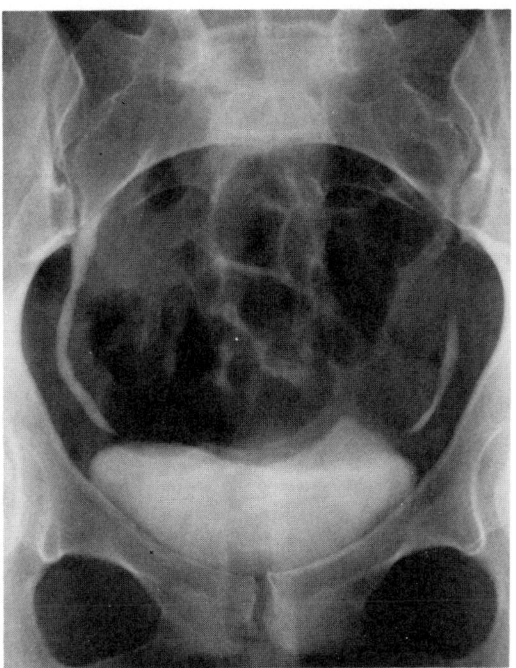

Figure 4.17 The lower ureters, 10 minutes after the release of the abdominal compression in Figure 4.16.

a dilated calyx was visible in the middle of the right kidney (Figure 4.16). The right kidney measured 12.5 cm and the left kidney 12.1 cm, but the mass of the right kidney was considerably larger than the left. The lower ureters were not remarkable (Figure 4.17). Her serum creatinine was 1.2 mg/100 ml. Although asymptomatic when I first saw her, she was bacteriuric with an *E. coli* 050; ureteral catheterization studies showed bilateral renal bacteriuria (Table 4.14). The bladder was normal except that both ureteral orifices were somewhat "U" shaped or "stadium" in appearance, rather than slit-like; they were normally placed on the trigone. Before passing the cystoscope, the urethra was carefully calibrated with No. 22, 24, and 26 Fr. bougie á boules; no resistance was felt at the internal vesical neck, the distal urethra, or at the urethral meatus. Agglutination antibodies in her serum could not be detected against the *E. coli* in her urine. The strain of *E. coli* was highly sensitive to all drugs except oxytetracycline and penicillin-G, with which she

Table 4.14
Bacterial Localization Studies in D.B., 22-year-old, White Woman

Source[a]	Cultures	Specific Gravity[b]	Creatinine
	Escherichia coli/ml		*(mg/100 ml)*
CB	> 100,000		
WB	20		
LK_1	10,000	1.018	128
RK_1	>10,000	1.019	126
LK_2	1,000	1.019	116
RK_2	10,000	1.018	111
LK_3	540	1.019	118
RK_3	10,000	1.018	106
LK_4	610	1.019	
RK_4	8,000	1.017	99

[a] CB = catheterized bladder urine; WB = washed bladder (after 2–3 liters of sterile water irrigation); LK_1 to LK_4 = serial left renal urines; RK_1 to RK_4 = serial right renal urines.

[b] Measured by refractometry.

had been treated in the recent past. Her urine was readily sterilized with nalidixic acid.

The patient recalled a letter, given to her by her mother, from a urologist written 20 years ago. This letter was obtained, and it documented recurrent chills and fever beginning at the age of 6 weeks. When she was 2½ years old, a complete urological evaluation had been performed; the bladder appeared normal at cystoscopy, but reflux into the left ureter and kidney was demonstrated on a cystogram. The intravenous urogram, which was obtained for review, showed *the same three abnormal calyces* that were present 20 years later (Figure 4.16) and which I had originally interpreted as being secondary to her recent episodes of pyelonephritis following her marriage.

A voiding cystourethrogram obtained at

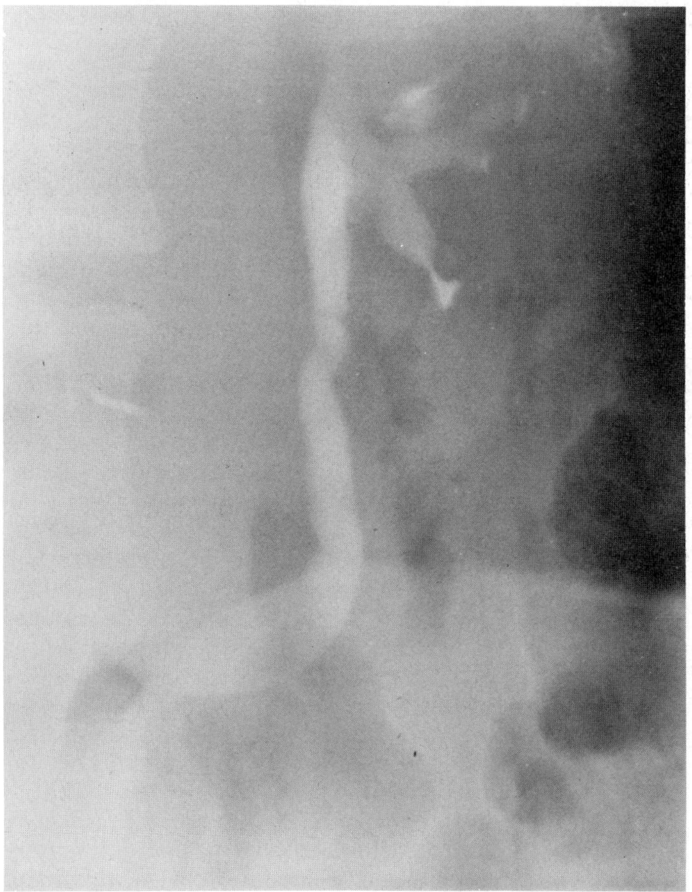

Figure 4.18 A fluoroscopic spot film, showing gross reflux to the left kidney, during a voiding cystourethrogram in patient D.B. There was also reflux to the middle of the right ureter, but not into the kidney.

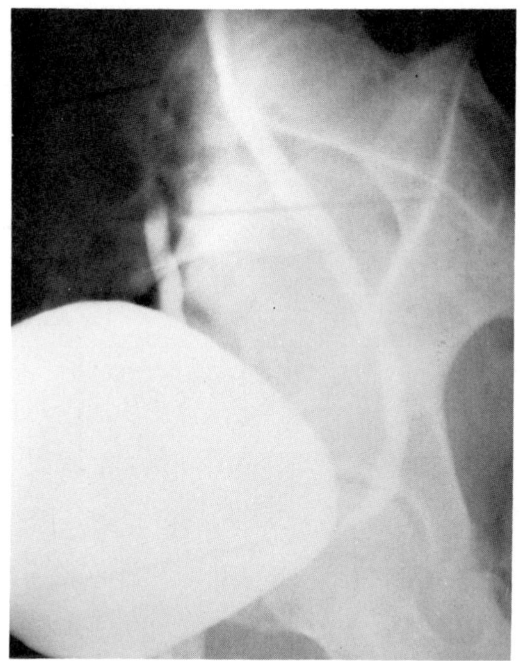

Figure 4.19 A cystogram from D.B., made 3 weeks after clearing the bacteriuria, showing bilateral reflux. Fluoroscopy and spot films showed reflux extending to the left kidney without dilatation of the calyces; the reflux up the right ureter stopped at the middle lumbar segments.

Stanford, after the urine was sterile for 3 weeks, showed reflux extending to the calyces of the left kidney (Figure 4.18) and to the middle segment of the right ureter (Figure 4.19). Thus, the renal damage found on intravenous urogram in 1970 had occurred in 1950 before the age of 30 months. Furthermore, despite the presence of rather marked reflux for 22 years, there has been no appreciable change in her kidneys.

After 6 weeks, the nalidixic acid was stopped and she promptly became reinfected with *E. coli* 078. From that time on, as seen in Figure 4.20, each reinfection was treated with nitrofurantoin for a few days at full dosage, followed by nightly prophylaxis. The *S. faecalis* infections toward the end of her susceptibility were treated with very short courses.

The introital and urethral cultures in relation to the bacteriuric and midstream cultures are shown in Figures 4.21 and 4.22. The The *E. coli* 011 infection was clearly preceded by introital colonization, but the several days of elapsed time without cultures before the *E. coli* 06 and 078 bacteriurias were apparently too long to detect introital colonization. A repeat intravenous urogram in late 1972 was identical to that in Figure 4.16. A voiding cystourethrogram, performed exactly as the one in 1970 was, showed no reflux to the right ureter and only 4 cm of reflux in the terminal left ureter during voiding.

This patient illustrates (1) the effectiveness of nitrofurantoin in long term prophylaxis in preventing bacteriuria, (2) the gradual loss of susceptibility to recurrent urinary infections with prophylactic prevention of recurrences. Indeed, she has been seen twice a year since 1973. A single symptomatic *E. coli* infection occurred in August 1973, for which she received a few days of nitrofurantoin therapy. Between August 1973 and our last culture in July 1979, she has remained totally asymptomatic and has received no antimicrobial therapy. A full term pregnancy occurred in 1977 without any complications; bacteriuria was not present before, during, or after this pregnancy. Her last culture on July 12, 1979, showed no infection but the introital culture had 20 colonies each of *Klebsiella* and *E. coli*/ml of transport broth.

With the presentation of these two patients on TMP-SMX prophylaxis (Figures 4.14–4.15) and the one on nitrofurantoin prophylaxis (Figure 4.20–4.22), it is time to compare these two antimicrobial agents as to their effects on the vaginal and rectal flora.

A Comparison of Nitrofurantoin Macrocrystals and TMP-SMX in Their Effects On Vaginal and Fecal Flora. Twenty-eight patients at Stanford who had experienced 92 episodes of symptomatic UTI in the preceding 12 months were placed on either half a tablet of TMP-SMX (40 mg of TMP, 200 mg of SMX)* or 100 mg of nitrofurantoin macrocrystals**

*Septra
**Macrodantin

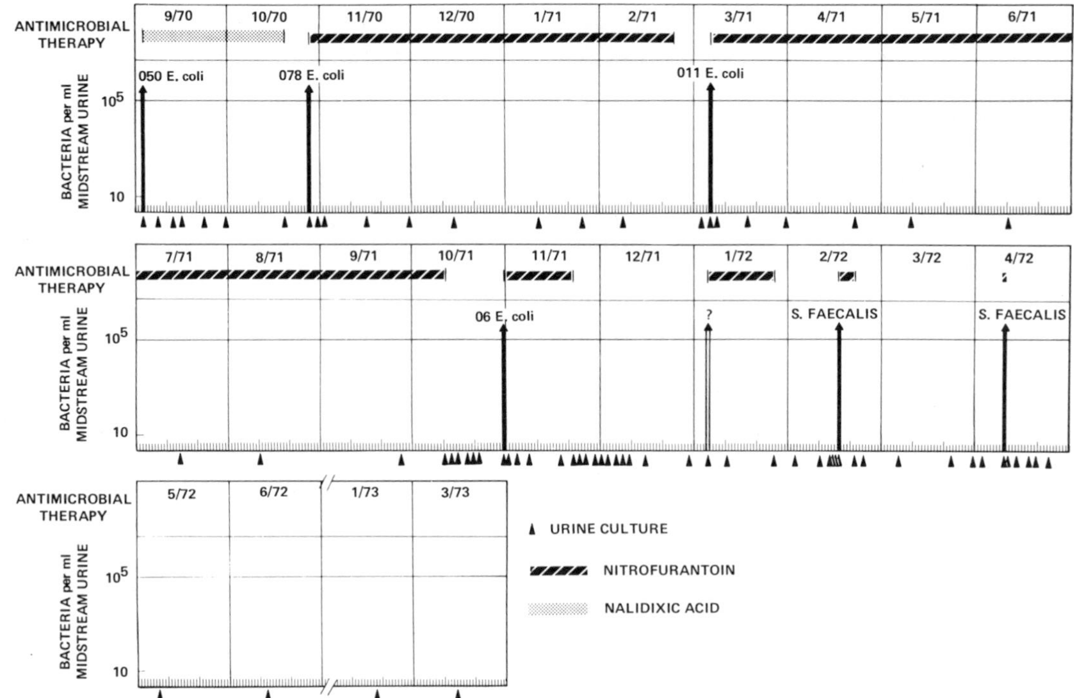

Figure 4.20 Bacteriologic course of the patient shown in Figures 4.16 to 4.19. At each reinfection, after therapy was discontinued, nitrofurantoin was given for a few days at full dosage and then immediately followed by nightly prophylaxis of 100 mg. Cultures twice a year since 1973 have shown neither bacteriuria nor enterobacterial carriage on the vaginal vestibule.

nightly for 6 months.[24] At the end of 6 months of prophylaxis, recurrences in 10 patients were followed by an additional 6 months of prophylaxis with the opposite agent. Thus, these 28 patients had 38 episodes of prophylaxis (Table 4.15). The patients on nitrofurantoin averaged 6.4 months of prophylaxis/patient, while the patients on TMP-SMX averaged 6.7 months of prophylaxis/patient.

Introital, anal, and midstream cultures before starting prophylaxis and at monthly intervals during prophylaxis were obtained by the techniques discussed in Chapter 1. One-tenth milliliter of both the fecal and introital cultures were spread on blood and eosin-methylene-blue agar plates as well as Mueller-Hinton agar plates which contained either nitrofurantoin at 50 μg/ml of agar or TMP-SMX at 1 μg/ml of agar of TMP combined with 20 μg/ml of agar of SMX. Any bacteria growing on the Mueller-Hinton agar plate containing nitrofurantoin or TMP-SMX were considered resistant; resistance was confirmed by isolation and quantitative disc sensitivity testing as described in Chapter 2.

There were 95 vaginal and rectal cultures for analysis during prophylaxis with nitrofurantoin and 188 vaginal and 182 rectal cultures during TMP-SMX prophylaxis (Table 4.16).

As can be seen in Table 4.17, of 182 fecal cultures during TMP-SMX therapy, only 27% showed *E. coli* compared to 96% of fecal cultures during nitrofurantoin prophylaxis. Thus, virtually all fecal cultures during nitrofurantoin prophylaxis contained *E. coli* and the density of these *E. coli* was similar to the preprophylactic cultures. For example, 85% of cultures during nitrofurantoin prophylaxis contained greater than 1000 *E. coli*/ml, whereas only 15% of the 182 cultures during TMP-SMX prophylaxis contained *E. coli* of this magnitude. Of the nitrofurantoin cultures, 2.1% showed resistant *E. coli* compared to 8.8% of the TMP-SMX cultures, but over half of the latter cultures occurred in a single patient.

The vaginal carriage of *E. coli* is shown in Table 4.18. Only 8.5% of the 188 cultures during TMP-SMX therapy showed *E. coli* while 36% showed *E. coli* during nitrofurantoin prophylaxis; resistance was negligible in both groups.

In Tables 4.19 and 4.20, colonization with *Klebsiella* and *Proteus* species is shown in both the fecal and vaginal cultures. There was virtually no carriage of these organisms on the introitus during TMP-SMX prophylaxis, but 14% of all nitrofurantoin cultures showed colonization with *Klebsiella* or *Proteus* species. The fecal carriage in Table 4.19 probably represents the natural recovery rate of *Klebsiella* and *Proteus* species from the feces with or without nitrofurantoin therapy; TMP-SMX prophylaxis shows a marked reduction in carriage rate of these organisms.

Tables 4.21 and 4.22 show no difference in the carriage rate of enterococci in the vagina or feces during nitrofurantoin or TMP-SMX prophylaxis, nor is there a difference in the carriage of *Pseudomonas* in the feces during either form of prophylaxis (Table 4.23). Five of 188 introital cultures during TMP-SMX therapy were positive for pseudomonas; 2 of 95 introital swabs were positive during nitrofurantoin prophylaxis.

These studies show that TMP-SMX prophylaxis is accompanied by a low order of bacterial resistance in the feces, as reported also by Grünenberg *et al.*[48] in children. These authors also observed that fecal *E. coli* were eliminated in 71% of their rectal swabs, as compared with 73% in our studies (Table 4.17); their children, however, were treated with one-third the full pediatric dosage of TMP-SMX whereas our regimen represented one-eighth of the adult dosage.

Harding and Ronald[49] found only 1 of 105

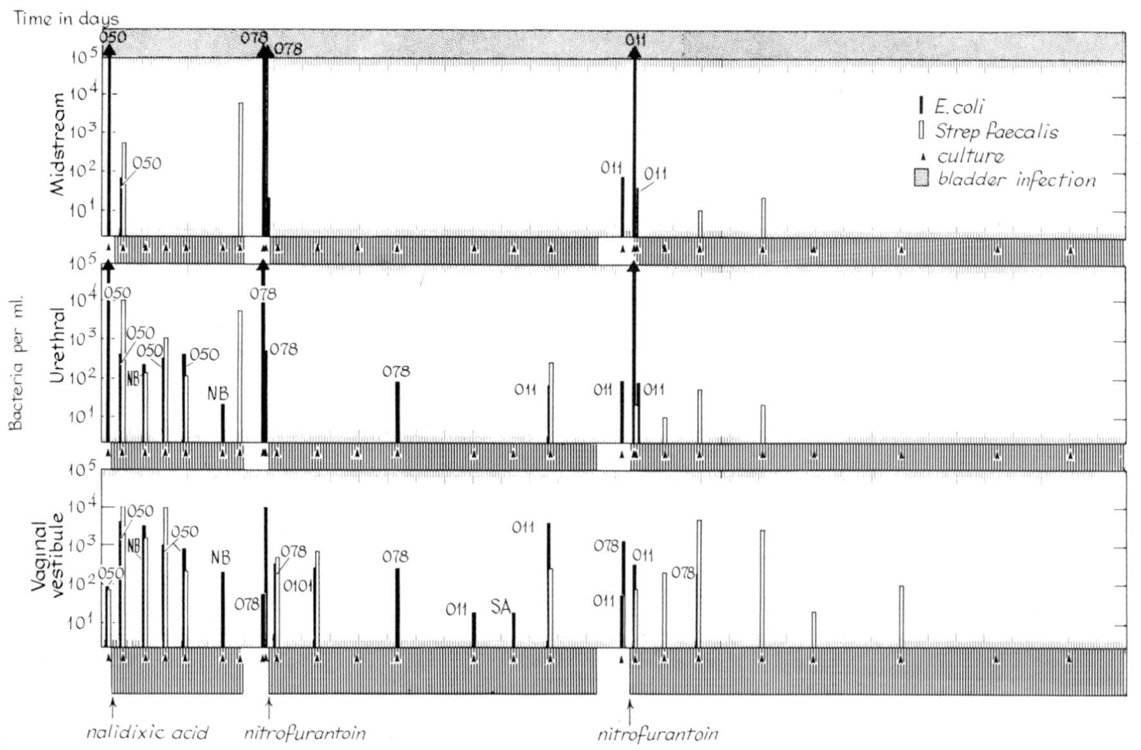

Figure 4.21 D.B., 23-year-old, white, married female.

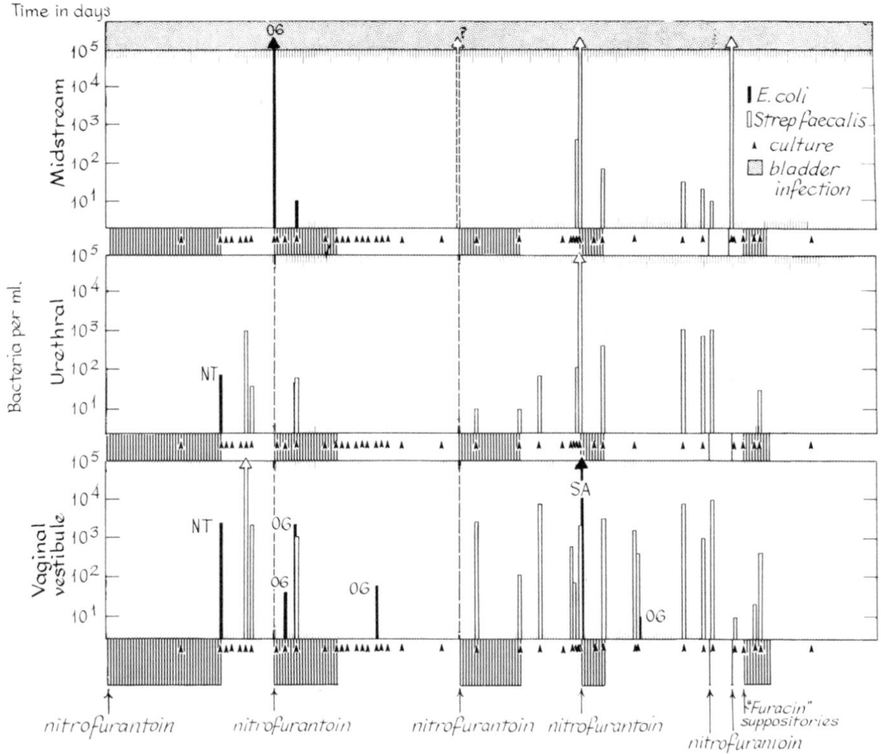

Figure 4.22 D.B., 23-year-old, white, married female (continued)

Table 4.15
Prophylactic Efficacy of Nitrofurantoin and TMP-SMX
28 Women (mean age, 36 years); 38 prophylactic periods[a] (253 months).

Treatment	Months/Patient
Nitrofurantoin (100 mg/day)	6.4
TMP-SMX (1/2 Tab/Day)	6.7

[a] 10 "Cross-Over" Periods

Table 4.16
38 Prophylactic Periods (253 Months)

No. of Periods	Treatment and Culture	
23	TMP-SMX (156 Months)	
	Vaginal Cultures	188
	Fecal Cultures	182
15	Nitrofurantoin (97 Months)	
	Vaginal Cultures	95
	Fecal Cultures	95

Table 4.17
Fecal *Escherichia coli* During Prophylaxis

Treatment	No. of Cultures	Percent *E. coli*	Percent Resistant *E. coli*
Nitrofurantoin	95	96	2.1
TMP-SMX	182	27[a]	8.8[b]

[a] 24/50 Strains = 3 Patients
[b] 9/16 Strains = 1 Patient

Table 4.18
Vaginal *Escherichia coli* During Prophylaxis

Treatment	No. of Cultures	Percent *E. coli*	Percent Resistant *E. coli*
Nitrofurantoin	95	36	0
TMP-SMX	188	8.5	1.1

periurethral swabs positive for *E. coli* (as compared to 30% positive swabs in the control group) during daily prophylaxis with ½ tablet of TMP-SMX.

The 36% carriage rate of vaginal *E. coli* during nitrofurantoin prophylaxis is not too different from the 26% rate reported by Bailey *et al.*,[50] especially since our patients were selected with greater susceptibility to UTI. The virtual absence of resistant fecal *E. coli* during nitrofurantoin prophylaxis is in agreement with the data of Grünenberg, *et al.*[33] in 18 children examined during nitrofurantoin prophylaxis.

Because these 28 patients were so carefully followed during their 253 months of prophylaxis, I have reproduced the quantitative results of their fecal and introital cultures in Tables 4.24–4.27.

Effect of Trimethoprim (Proloprim) Alone on Fecal and Vaginal Flora. Although our data are preliminary, and trimethoprim (TMP) alone has just become available for clinical use, the effect of TMP on fecal and vaginal flora is important and will ultimately determine its usefulness in the prophylactic treatment of UTI.

Table 4.19
Fecal *Klebsiella* and *Proteus* Species During Prophylaxis

Treatment	No. of Cultures	Percent Strains	Percent Resistant Strains
Nitrofurantoin	95	34	21
TMP-SMX	182	12	2.7

Table 4.20
Vaginal *Klebsiella* and *Proteus* Species During Prophylaxis

Treatment	No. Cultures	Percent Strains	Percent Resistant Strains
Nitrofurantoin	95	14	9.5
TMP-SMX	188	1.6	0

Table 4.21
Fecal Enterococci During Prophylaxis

Treatment	No. of Cultures	Percent Enterococci	Percent Resistant Enterococci
Nitrofurantoin	95	41	0
TMP-SMX	182	51	6

Table 4.22
Vaginal Enterococci During Prophylaxis

Treatment	No. of Cultures	Percent Enterococci	Percent Resistant Enterococci
Nitrofurantoin	95	42[a]	1.1
TMP-SMX	188	36[b]	1.1

[a] Randomly distributed
[b] 27/67 = 2 patients

Table 4.23
Fecal *Pseudomonas* During Prophylaxis

Treatment	No. Cultures	Percent *Pseudomonas*	Percent Resistant *Pseudomonas*
Nitrofurantoin	95	22	22
TMP-SMX	182	21	20

Kasanen *et al.*[51] from Finland reported on the effects of TMP on the fecal flora in 10 volunteers who took 100 mg/day for 3 weeks and on 20 patients treated for 6–36 months on the same dosage. In both studies, they determined TMP resistance to 10 lactose-fermenting colonies selected from fecal samples taken "at appropriate intervals." Six hundred thirty-three strains from the 3-week study showed only one resistant "coliform" organism; resistance was defined as no zone of inhibition to a 1.2 μg of TMP disc. In the long term study, 11 of the 20 patients had coliform organisms in their feces, but 4 of these 11 contained resistant coliforms to 8 μg/ml of TMP or greater in agar dilution plates; 91 strains were isolated from these 11 patients, 39% of which were resistant to TMP. Six of 11 strains of *Enterobacter* and all 10 strains of *Citrobacter* isolated were highly resistant to TMP (≥16 μg/ml). Thus, in the long term study, as opposed to the short term one, resistance appeared to be substantial even though 9 of 20 patients lost their coliform organisms.

Our studies are presented in Table 4.28. Fifty-eight cultures of the introitus and anal canal were obtained at monthly intervals during 63 months of TMP prophylaxis in 10 patients who received 50 mg of TMP once daily. TMP resistance was determined by

Table 4.24
Bacteria in Fecal Culture During 156 Months (182 Cultures) of TMP-SMX Prophylaxis

Organism	Bacteria/milliliter				Total Positive Cultures	Percent Positive Cultures (of 182)	No. of Resistant Strains	Distribution of Positive Cultures	Distribution of Resistant Strains
	0	10–99	100–999	>1000					
								Per patient	
Enterobacteriaceae									
Escherichia coli	132	13	10	27	50	27.4	16	10 8 6	9
Proteus mirabilis	166	4	5	7	16	8.8	4	8 7	4
Klebsiella	177	1	3	1	5	2.7	1	Random	
Other	175	4	2	1	7	3.7	0	Random	
Pseudomonas	144	15	8	15	38	20.8	37	9 15	9 15
Enterococci	90	8	19	65	92	50.5	11	14 11 8	Random
Acinetobacter	178	3	1	0	4	2.1	0		

Table 4.25
Bacteria in Fecal Culture During 97 Months (95 Cultures) of Nitrofurantoin Prophylaxis

Organism	Bacteria/milliliter				Total Positive Cultures	Percent Positive Cultures (of 95)	No. Resistant Strains	Distribution of Positive Cultures	Distribution of Resistant Strains
	0	10–99	100–999	>1000					
								Per patient	
Enterobacteriaceae									
Escherichia coli	4	1	9	81	91	95.7	2	Random	
Proteus mirabilis	79	10	2	4	16	16.8	14	7	6 5
Proteus vulgaris	92	1	1	1	3	3.1	3		
Proteus morganii	94	0	0	1	1	1.1	0		
Klebsiella	83	3	4	5	12	12.6	3	Random	
Other	85	4	1	5	10	10.5	0	Random	
Pseudomonas	74	6	6	9	21	22.1	21	9	9
Enterococci	56	6	9	24	39	41.0	0	Random	
Acinetobacter	89	2	4	0	6	6.3	2	5	

culturing the anal and introital cultures on Mueller-Hinton agar containing 1 μg of TMP/ml of agar; organisms that grew on the TMP agar were then checked against a 5-μg disc of TMP. Those with zone sizes of 8 mm or less were considered resistant to TMP. Although this study is still in progress and the numbers are clearly too small, it is of some interest to compare Table 4.28 with Tables 4.24 and 4.26. *E. coli* carriage in the anal canal appears to be increased from 27% on TMP-SMX prophylaxis to 40% with TMP alone; there is minimal *E. coli* resistance, only one resistant strain was isolated in the TMP study. The major difference with TMP prophylaxis seems to lie with an increase in *Klebsiella*; a 24% carriage rate appears substantially higher than the 2.7% incidence found with TMP-SMX (Table 4.24). Eight of the 14 *Klebsiella* strains were present in numbers >1000 bacteria/ml of transport broth. The number of resistant Enterobacteriaceae during TMP prophylaxis does not appear to be statistically different from that with TMP-SMX prophylaxis, but larger numbers are needed for adequate assessment.

Prophylactic Efficacy

In the 28 patients described above, who experienced 92 episodes of recurrent UTI in the 12 months before prophylaxis, only 6 infections occurred during the 253 months of prophylactic therapy (Table 4.29).[24] These six infections occurred in three patients; thus, 25 of the 28 patients had no infections during prophylactic therapy. All six infections occurred during nitrofurantoin prophylaxis (none occurred during TMP-SMX therapy); four infections were due to *E. coli* sensitive to nitrofurantoin, one infection was due to a sensitive enterococcus, and one was due to a resistant *Acinetobacter*. All three of these patients in whom the six infections occurred partic-

Table 4.26
Bacteria on the Vaginal Introitus During 156 Months (188 Cultures) of TMP-SMX Prophylaxis

Organism	Bacteria/milliliter				Total Positive Cultures	Percent Positive Cultures (of 188)	No. of Resistant Strains	Distribution of Positive Cultures	Distribution of Resistant Strains
	0	10–99	100–999	>1000					
								Per patient	
Enterobacteriaceae									
Escherichia coli	172	9	2	5	16	8.5	2	Random	
Proteus mirabilis	186	2	0	0	2	1.1	0		
Klebsiella	187	0	1	0	1	0.5	0		
Pseudomonas	183	4	1	0	5	2.7	3	Random	Random
Enterococci	121	16	29	22	67	36.0	2	13 14	
Acinetobacter	187	1	0	0	1	0.5	0		

Table 4.27
Bacteria on the Vaginal Introitus During 97 Months (95 Cultures) of Nitrofurantoin Prophylaxis

Organism	Bacteria/milliliter				Total Positive Cultures	Percent Positive Cultures (of 95)	No. of Resistant Strains	Distribution of Positive Cultures	Distribution of Resistant Strains
	0	10–99	100–999	>1000					
								Per patient	
Enterobacteriaceae									
Escherichia coli	61	13	8	13	34	35.7	0	Random	
Proteus mirabilis	84	6	1	4	11	11.5	8	5	4
Klebsiella	93	1	1	0	2	2.1	1		
Other	93	1	1	0	2	2.1	0		
Pseudomonas	93	1	1	0	2	2.1	2		
Enterococci	55	15	13	12	40	42.1	1	Random	
Acinetobacter	92	2	1	0	3	3.1	1		

Table 4.28
Bacteria in Fecal and Introital Cultures During 63 Months (58 Cultures) of Trimethoprim Prophylaxis (10 Patients)

Organism	Bacteria/milliliters				Total Positive Cultures	Percent Positive Cultures (of 58)	No. of Resistant Strains	Distribution of Positive Cultures	Distribution of Resistant Strains
	0	10–99	100–999	>1000					
								Per patient	
BACTERIA IN FECAL CULTURES									
Enterobacteriaceae									
Escherichia coli	35	7	6	10	23	40	1	5 4	
Proteus mirabilis	57	0	0	1	1	2	1		
Klebsiella	44	3	3	8	14	24	4	5 4	Random
Other	53	2	1	2	5	9	1	Random	
Pseudomonas	52	4	1	1	6	10	4	3	3
Enterococci	38	3	2	15	20	34	0	Random	
BACTERIA ON THE VAGINAL INTROITUS									
Enterobacteriaceae									
E. coli	54	1	1	2	4	7	1	Random	
P. mirabilis	57	0	0	1	1	2	1		
Klebsiella	55	2	1	0	3	5	2	1	1
Other	58	0	0	0	0	0	0		
Pseudomonas	58	0	0	0	0	0	0		
Enterococci	49	4	1	4	9	16	0	Random	

Table 4.29
Bacteriuric Episodes in 28 Women

	No. of Patients[a]	No. of Infections
12 Months Before Prophyl	28	92(3.3/Patient)
During Prophylaxis	3	6

[a] 25/28 Patients had no infections during prophylaxis

Table 4.30
Reinfections in 32 of 38 Periods Followed for 6 Months After Prophylaxis

No. Periods	Treatment	Months
9/14	Nitrofurantoin = 64%	
	Mean time to recurrence	2.0
10/18	TMP-SMX = 56%	
	Mean time to recurrence	3.2

ipated in the cross over study in which each was on TMP-SMX and nitrofurantoin for 6 months.

In 32 of the 38 periods of prophylaxis, each patient was followed for at least 6 months after discontinuing antimicrobial therapy (Table 4.30). Nine of the 14 periods of nitrofurantoin prophylaxis were followed by a recurrent UTI with a mean time to recurrence of 2.0 months. Ten of the 18 TMP-SMX prophylactic periods were followed by recurrent urinary infections with a mean time to recurrence of 3.2 months.

The effectiveness of nitrofurantoin in the prevention of recurrent UTI has been reported by several investigators,[12, 22, 52] and the prophylactic efficacy of low dose TMP-SMX therapy is well established.[24, 34, 49, 52, 53] It is clear from these investigations, as well as the data presented above, that prophylaxis with either agent is extraordinarily effective in preventing UTI recurrences.

Our data here at Stanford, however, indicate that the prophylactic efficacy of nitrofurantoin and TMP-SMX is through two entirely separate mechanisms. Nitrofurantoin has no effect on either the bowel flora or the introital carriage rate of Enterobacteriaceae and therefore must exert its effectiveness *after* the pathogenic organism has entered the bladder urine. TMP-SMX prophylaxis, on the other hand, exerts a profound effect, firstly in vaginal secretions by ion trapping of trimethoprim at bactericidal concentrations to Enterobacteriaceae and secondly, by clearing all Enterobacteriaceae from the fecal flora in about 70% of cultures without exerting an inordinate degree of bacterial resistance.

ASYMPTOMATIC URINARY TRACT INFECTION DETECTED DURING SCREENING SURVEYS

The prevalence rates for screening bacteriuria (ScBU) were reviewed in the opening paragraphs of this Chapter. There are at least two important questions relevant to patients who have ScBU. Is there evidence of substantial renal disease associated with their bacteriuria? Can ScBU be successfully treated within a public health approach to disease containment?

Asscher *et al.*[54] have pointed out that the two basic requirements for a useful screening procedure are that it "detects disease before irreversible damage has occurred and that the disease so detected may be effectively treated."

What about autopsy data on the incidence of pyelonephritis as supporting evidence that ScBU is damaging to the kidney?

Histologic Evidence for Pyelonephritis

Attempts to correlate bacteriuric prevalance with general autopsy data[55] have not been accepted by most workers in this field,[56–59] largely because so many different diseases of the kidney produce similar morphologic pathology. The interested reader should consult Chapter 14 (Robert Heptinstall[56]) and Chapter 15 (Paul Beeson[57]) in the 1967 edition of D. A. K. Black's book, *Renal Disease*, and the 1961 and 1964 papers of Paul Kimmelstiel.[58, 59] Beeson,[57] in his careful and searching analysis of the histologic and clinical data, had this to say: "The suggestion being offered here is that true chronic pyelonephritis may be far less common than most autopsy data suggest, and that the figures based on autopsy findings are misleading because they result from inclusion of a heterogeneous group of disorders with similar morphologic features under the single heading of chronic pyelonephritis. Freedman,"[60] in a review of autopsies at 2-year intervals between 1957 and 1964 at Yale University, showed a progressive decline in the frequency of the pathologic diagnosis of chronic pyelonephritis. He attributed this decline to a growing appreciation of the nonspecificity of the histologic features.

Even the pathologic diagnosis of "active" chronic pyelonephritis, characterized by fresh polymorphonuclear leukocytes as well as plasma cells and lymphocytes, was seriously questioned as a histologic hallmark of bacterial pyelonephritis by Angell, Relman, and Robbins.[61]

Cardiff Studies

I have reviewed in Chapter 1 the evidence that renal biopsy, ureteral catheterization studies, urinary concentration, and serologic bacterial agglutination titers are all inadequate to diagnose chronic pyelonephritis. With these limitations, how does the clinical investigator or physician decide if adult women with ScBU are at serious risk? One of the real limitations has been that most epidemiologic studies on the 4–6% of adult women with bacteriuria have included such demographic parameters as age, blood pressure, concentrating ability, serologic titers, proteinuria, etc., but have never answered two critical questions: What do the kidneys look like? What is the history of these patients in relation to their bacteriuria?

Fortunately, Asscher, Sussman, and their colleagues[62, 63] at Cardiff, Wales, have answered these questions on a group of nonpregnant women with ScBU between ages

20 and 65. They screened 3578 asymptomatic hospital visitors for significant bacteriuria defined as two consecutive *midstream* specimens of $>10^5$ bacteria/ml of the *same serotype*. The perineum was cleaned three times with green soap. One hundred and seven subjects were found to have bacteriuria (3%); they were matched with 100 nonbacteriuric women of the same age, parity, and marital status who served as controls. All 107 of the bacteriuric subjects and 88 of the nonbacteriuric controls consented to a detailed history by a medical epidemiologist who was unaware of the culture results. Sixty-nine percent of the bacteriuric subjects gave a history of urinary symptoms within the years preceding the detection of bacteriuria, but only 18% of the controls gave a similar story. Asymptomatic bacteriuria, then, in epidemiologic surveys is not very asymptomatic.

Ninety-three of the 107 bacteriuric subjects (87%) and 50 of the 88 controls (57%) consented to an excretory urogram (surely a tribute to the persistence of the Welsh!). The excretory urograms were read independently by two radiologists. I had the unique opportunity to review all of these urograms in the spring of 1968. *Every patient had more than an adequate amount of renal cortex.* Abnormalities were found in 34% of bacteriuric subjects and in 12% of controls.[62] There were occasional scars, but most were minor and rarely involved more than a single calyx. Eight patients had small stones, four of them in the same kidneys that had scars. The hydroureter and hydronephrosis reported[62] in 9 patients were, to me, definitely nonsurgical; the problem seemed to be more calyceal and pelvic atonicity than actual obstructive disease. The remainder of the abnormalities were congenital, such as kidney rotation, cysts, etc. In short, I did not see one excretory urogram of a patient who seemed in serious trouble from loss of renal cortex, even though half the bacteriuric women were over 45 years old. Of equal importance was the comparative delicacy and lack of collecting system abnormalities observed in the 50 urograms from nonbacteriuric women. In summary, the collecting systems in the bacteriuric women were more atonic and contained more stones and scars; it was easy to believe that half of these women had pelvic bacteriuria to accompany their bladder infection. It was not easy to believe that they had chronic, progressive pyelonephritis.

From these considerations, it is difficult to believe that the nonpregnant woman with recurrent bacteriuria in the absence of stones and in the presence of a nonobstructive intravenous urogram is at serious risk from her bacteriuria.

If she is not at serious risk from renal failure, what about the secondary consequences of renal involvement such as hypertension or anemia? The hematocrits of bacteriuric and nonbacteriuric women are essentially the same.[62] Differences in blood pressure, while statistically higher in bacteriuric women,[2, 64] are simply not impressive enough to believe that urinary infections constitute a major, preventable cause of hypertension. In the Cardiff studies, no significant difference was found between the bacteriuric and control subjects in systolic blood pressure, although the diastolic pressure was significantly higher in the bacteriuric population (86 ± 10.7 mm of Hg compared to 83.1 ± 9.0 mm of Hg).[54]

The Cardiff studies included measurements of the serum urea as an estimate of renal function. In the bacteriuric group, serum urea was 25.7 ± 7.8 mg/100 ml and 23.2 ± 7.7 mg/100 ml in the control group,[62] a difference that was barely significant ($0.05 > P > 0.02$). Serum creatinine, especially if determined by autoanalysis, would have been preferable to the serum urea because creatinine is uninfluenced by dietary protein or urine flow rate. Nevertheless, these studies suggest that screening populations for ScBU does detect enough renal disease in some patients to be reflected by an elevated serum urea; this reduction in renal function, however, could clearly be from pyelonephritis of childhood detected in the screening survey.

In an interesting follow-up, 90% of the 107 bacteriuric subjects and 65% of the 88 nonbacteriuric controls were restudied 3–5 years later (mean, 47 and 52 months, respectively).[65] There was no evidence that bacteriuria had led in the intervening years to a rise in blood pressure, an increase in serum urea concentration, or renal scarring on intravenous urography.

Effect of Treatment on Natural History of ScBU

In the Cardiff studies, 94 of the 107 bacteriuric subjects were treated with either nitrofurantoin for 7 days (49 subjects) or placebo (45 subjects).[54] The bacteriuria was cured in 39 of the 49 subjects treated with nitrofurantoin (80%); neither resistance to nitrofurantoin nor radiological abnormalities accounted for the 20% failures. It is interesting that in contrast to Mabeck's placebo treatment of symptomatic UTI where 80% achieved a sterile urine within 5 months,[8] only 5 of 45 subjects (11%) with ScBU in the Cardiff series spontaneously cleared their infection.

At the completion of 1 years follow-up, only 27 of the 49 treated bacteriurics (55%) were still free of infection, while 16 of the 45 placebo subjects had undergone spontaneous remission (35.5%). This difference was not significant ($0.1 > P > 0.05$) and Asscher concluded that successful therapy in ScBU was little different in the long run from the natural history of spontaneous remissions.[54]

In addition, 37% of the treated subjects developed UTI symptoms, mainly dysuria and frequency, within 12 months of nitrofurantoin therapy as compared to 36% of the placebo treated group. The 36% development of symptomatic UTI from an untreated ScBU group of subjects compares favorably with the 29% found by Gaymans *et al.*[6] in their 1976 general practice study.

Heterogeneity of Women with ScBU

Gaymans and his colleagues[6] have made an important contribution in dividing their women with ScBU into three groups: those with transient bacteriuria, those who developed symptomatic bacteriuria (29% of the total group with ScBU), and the third and largest group, those who remained bacteriuric and asymptomatic at follow-up cultures obtained at frequent intervals (termed "persistent" ScBU). They make the important point that at least 6 months of follow-up are required to separate any screening survey into these three different groups.

Nothing could make more sense than this proposal because the first group are surely unimportant in terms of serious disease, the second group who developed symptomatic ScBU will probably seek and receive medical treatment anyway, and it is only the third and last group who represent the reservoir of silent, persistent bacteriuria. Although the numbers are small, Gaymans' paper[6] indicates that the symptomatic group with ScBU had a higher percentage of abnormalities on intravenous urograms, more upper tract symptoms, and higher bacterial agglutination titers in their serum than the group with persistent ScBU; in addition, the symptomatic patients were younger (41 versus 51.2 years). Indeed, they close what is clearly a major contribution to ScBU by noting that the results of treatment in the group with persistent ScBU may not justify the therapeutic attempts to cure the bacteriuria, a view surely shared by Asscher *et al.*[54] Except for bacteriuria of pregnancy, they conclude from their data that screening programs to detect asymptomatic bacteriuria are not advocated in the adult female population for the following reasons: "(1) Screening would have to be repeated too frequently in order to detect all cases with significant asymptomatic bacteriuria; (2) a simple detection of asymptomatic bacteriuria without follow-up of at least 6 months yields only limited information as to the type of asymptomatic bacteriuria present; (3) persistent asymptomatic bacteriuria in our study predominantly showed lower tract involvement as opposed to symptomatic asymptomatic bacteriuria."[6]

Comment

I cannot conclude this section on ScBU without making a few historial comments.

Once the diagnosis of asymptomatic bacteriuria was placed on a firm statistical basis (however unsatisfactory that basis is for dealing with symptomatic infections) in 1956,[66] a powerful tool was placed in the hands of epidemiologic investigators for door to door population surveys. Spurred on by the high, but false, incidence of histologic changes in kidneys suggestive of pyelonephritis,[55] there were great hopes in the late 1950s and early 1960s that the serious consequences of diseases related directly or indirectly to pyelonephritis,[67] such as renal failure, hypertension,[68] pyelonephritis of pregnancy,[69] and diabetes[70] might be averted by early detection and treatment.

It is fair to comment in 1980 that these high hopes have not materialized; indeed, it is probably true that the work by Asscher's group[54, 62, 63, 65] and the general practice investigation by Gaymans and his colleagues[6] have done more than any other studies to place asymptomatic bacteriuria detected during screening surveys in proper perspective. To that perspective, however, one must add that: (1) the adult kidney is astonishingly resistant to renal destruction by bacteria in the absence of stones, obstruction, and analgesic abuse (see section on Pyelonephritis); (2) that hypertension, if effected at all in patients with ScBU, is a very minimal effect indeed and the physician will do better to treat the hypertension than to treat the bacteriuria[13, 65, 71]; (3) that if prematurity or intrauterine growth retardation is increased in pregnant patients with ScBU (see next section), prevention of bacteriuria does not reverse birthweight; and (4) that even in progressive renal failure, the presence of bacteriuria cannot be shown to be responsible for the progression.[72]

Many of us who spent much of our time seeing patients with UTI could not believe even in the 1960s that there was this great reservoir of silent, asymptomatic renal disease in the population at large. My own concerns were converted to certainty when Bill Asscher of Cardiff in 1968 allowed me the opportunity to review each one of the 143 intravenous urograms he obtained in his patients and control subjects; serious renal disease, caused by bacteriuria, simply was not present in these patients.

Lastly, in long term follow-up, the failure of short term, curative therapy to be much better than spontaneous cures argues against detection of ScBU by epidemiologic surveys.[54] While some might argue that long term therapy in patients with ScBU might show more benefit, patient compliance would be impossible in an asymptomatic population. Moreover, it is unlikely to be successful. As I have reviewed earlier in this chapter, trimethoprim-sulfamethoxazole is the ideal drug for returning the introital flora to normal for many months and completely preventing recurrent bacteriuria; discontinuance of therapy, however, is associated with a high order of introital recolonization and reinfection (56% in Table 4.30). Although these studies are in symptomatic patients, it is unlikely to be any different in asymptomatic ones.

All of these issues surely lead to the conclusion that public health money is better spent in educating the physician on how to diagnose, treat, and assess the renal risk to the symptomatic patient in his office, rather than screening and treating asymptomatic populations.

As will be seen in Chapter 6 on Urinary Infections in Infancy and Childhood, the same conclusion also applies to children, despite their great susceptibility to renal scarring from bacteriuria in the presence of ureteral reflux.

BACTERIURIA OF PREGNANCY

Introduction, Prevalence, and Acute Symptoms

Interest increased in bacteriuria of pregnancy (1) when Kass and colleagues[73] showed that symptomatic episodes of acute pyelonephritis in later stages of pregnancy could be prevented by detecting and treating asymptomatic bacteriuria in the early stages of gestation, (2) when Kass suggested that the incidence of prematurity and perinatal deaths in bacteriurics could be reduced by early treatment,[74] and (3) when

Kincaid-Smith[75] and Whalley[71] reported a strikingly high incidence of radiologic abnormalities in bacteriuric women evaluated after delivery. Several investigators have studied the prevalence of bacteriuria in pregnant women, the incidence of acute pyelonephritis, the incidence of prematurity, and the radiologic abnormalities found on intravenous urography after delivery. These statistics have been abstracted from each publication and are presented in Table 4.31, together with the methods used by each group in collecting the urine specimens for culture.

Only the prevention of acute episodes of pyelonephritis by early treatment has been amply confirmed (Table 4.31). Some of the statistical differences in Table 4.31 may depend on population selection, on relative differences in rigidly defining the bacteriuric population at risk, and on interpretation of radiologic abnormalities. As pointed out in Chapter 1, confidence limits in interpreting voided cultures vary considerably with the method of collecting the specimen; these limits, of course, determine the number of cultures required to admit a pregnant woman as a true bacteriuric. Since the actual number of bacteriurics with 10^5 or greater bacteria/ml in any pregnant population is only about 4% (Table 4.31), a relatively few nonbacteriurics mistakenly admitted as true infections could readily lead to false conclusions. Some investigators used midstream specimens collected by trained nurses,[71, 77, 78] and others used the whole voided specimen collected by the patients themselves.[73, 78] In some studies,[77, 79, 80] sterile water was used to rinse off the detergent after cleaning the introitus, but in others this was not done.[73, 79] Of interest is the 4% prevalence of bacteriuria (three consecutive whole voided specimens collected by the patient) in Savage's studies,[73] which is similar to that found by Brumfitt[81] using one midstream specimen collected by the nurse; this suggests that one careful midstream specimen collected by a nurse has the same confidence limits as three whole voided urines collected by the patient (see Chapter 1). In Eykyn's[82] study of 1000 consecutive pregnancies, urine obtained by suprapubic bladder puncture indicated a greater prevalence of 5.9%. Her figures may serve as further evidence that confidence limits based on $>10^5$ bacteria/ml do not allow detection of the total bacteriuric population (*i.e.*, those with less than 10^5 bacteria/ml).

As shown in Table 4.31, the prevalence of bacteriuria in these different investigations varied from 4 to 6.9%, and the incidence of acute pyelonephritis in pregnant women can be reduced from about 25 to 35% in untreated bacteriuric women to less than 10% in treated women. In a much later study, however, Kass's group[83] reported only 18% pyelonephritis in 148 placebo-treated, pregnant women who were bacteriuric. Bacteriuria increases with gravidity from about 5% at the first pregnancy to 7% in women with 5 or more pregnancies,[73] but because bacteriuria increases with age in nonpregnant women, it is difficult to separate the effects of age from multigravida. Socioeconomic factors may also influence the distribution of bacteriuria in the population. For example, Turck, Goffe, and Petersdorf[84] catheterized 1727 women at the time of delivery. Women from a low financial, educational, and social status were 3 times as bacteriuric (6.5%) as women from a middle income, well educated group (2.0%); these differences, however, may simply reflect better medical care during early pregnancy in the middle income group rather than some basic factor in pathogenesis.

Kass[74] reported a small increase (1%) in the incidence of bacteriuria in relation to the duration of pregnancy, but McFadyen *et al.*,[85] using suprapubic needle aspiration of the bladder, found only one infection to develop in 186 women who had sterile urine in early pregnancy.

Bacteriuric pregnant women are reported to be more anemic than nonbacteriuric pregnant women at their first antenatal visit; there was also some evidence of increasing anemia as pregnancy progressed.[86]

Although the prevalence of screening bacteriuria in pregnant women is apparently no different than the prevalence in nonpregnant women of the same age, Gay-

Table 4.31
Prevalence of Bacteriuria, Acute Pyelonephritis, Prematurity, and Radiologic Abnormalities in Pregnancy[a]

Reported by	Methods	No. of Pregnant Patients Screened	Bacteriurics	Incidence of Acute Clinical Pyelonephritis			Prematurity			Radiologic Abnormalities on IVP after Delivery	Treatment
				Bacteriurics		Nonbacteriurics[b]	Nonbacteriurics	Bacteriurics			
				Treated	Untreated			Treated	Untreated		
			%	%	%	%	%	%	%	%	
Savage, Hajj, and Kass[73]	3 whole voided specimens $>10^5$ bacteria after preparation and collection by patient. No rinse of soap with water. Pregnancy less than 32 weeks	6202	4.0	0	26.4	1.4	11.5	7.5	15.3		Long term (single or multiple) up to delivery
Condi, Williams, Reeves, and Brumfitt[80]	2 "clean-catch" (probably midstream) specimens $>10^5$ bacteria after preparation and probably collected by nurse. Rinse of soap with water.	4590	4.6	10.3	23.3	2	5	12.8			Short term
Eykyn and McFadyen[82]	2 specimens obtained by suprapubic aspiration of bladder.	1000	5.9								Short term
Kincaid-Smith and Bullen[75]	1 midstream specimen $>10^5$ bacteria without preparation plus 1 midstream $>10^5$ after preparation and collection by nurse. No rinse of soap with water. Pregnancy less than 26 weeks.	4000	4.0	2.8–3.3	28.7–36.6		5	12.5–14.8	17.8–21.5	51.4	Long term up to delivery

Little[77]	2 midstream specimens $>10^5$ after preparation and collection by nurse. Rinse of detergent with water. Pregnancy less than 14 weeks.	5000	5.3	3.2	24.8	0.4	7.6	8.1	9.2	18			Long term up to delivery
Whalley[71, 76, 78]	2 "clean whole voided" specimens $>10^5$ after preparation and collection by patient. No rinse of soap with water. Pregnancy less than 28 weeks.	4357	6.9		25.7	0	11.9	14.8		47			No treatment except in symptomatic infections
Brumfitt, Grüneberg, and Leigh[81]	1 midstream specimen $>10^5$ bacteria after preparation and collection by nurse.	8907	4.4	2.8			5.5	7.2		37			Short term
										Responded to one course of therapy	Responded to repeated therapy	Did not respond to repeated therapy	
										23	35	65	
Wilson, Hewitt, and Monzon[79]	2 midstream specimens $>10^5$ bacteria after preparation and collection, probably by patient. Rinse of soap with water. Pregnancy less than 32 weeks.	6048	6.5										Short term only when symptomatic

[a] Reproduced by permission from T. A. Stamey and A. Pfau, Calif. Med. **113:** 16, 1970.

[b] These patients who developed acute pyelonephritis after being screened initially as nonbacteriuric either were missed because of infections with less than 10^5 bacteria/ml or became infected after the initial cultures.

mans *et al.*[6] in their general practice study have shown that symptomatic infections in women during pregnancy (15%) occurred at 3 times the rate of nonpregnant women followed over the same time interval (5.3%). I believe these data confirm the impressions of many physicians who treat pregnant women with recurrent UTI.

In a careful and instructive study, Mortimer *et al.*[87] studied the bacterial content of the female urethra in 100 pregnant women by obtaining swabs at the external urethral meatus, and at points ½ and 1 inch up the urethra from the meatus; the latter cultures were obtained through glass tubes that prevented contact of the swab tips with the surrounding urethral tissue. Twenty-four to 26% of these pregnant women had *E. coli* at the external meatus during the first 30 weeks of gestation, but only 6% had *E. coli* during the last trimester of pregnancy. A total of 18 out of 100 women had *E. coli* at the external meatus; four had *E. coli* ½ inch from the external meatus, and two had *E. coli* 1 inch from the urethral meatus.

These data do not suggest an increasing susceptibility to bacteriuria as pregnancy advances.

Prematurity

Whereas the incidence of prematurity in Table 4.31 seems to be increased in bacteriurics compared with nonbacteriuric pregnant women (which does not mean the bacteriuria causes the prematurity), most investigators failed to show a reduction in the rate of prematurity by treating the bacteriurics.[75,77] Even the rigidly defined studies of Kass and his associates[73] showed a reduction in prematurity that was only suggestive ($P > 0.1$). Wilson *et al.*[79] concluded that prematurity was more often associated with obstetrical abnormalities than with bacteriuria in either symptomatic or asymptomatic pregnant women.

Radiologic Abnormalities

That substantial dilatation and tortuosity of the ureters with pyelocaliectasis, especially on the right side, occur in the course of most normal pregnancies is well recognized. Hundley and his colleagues[88] performed intravenous urograms on 27 normal pregnant women who had no evidence of urinary infection. Between the 15th week of pregnancy and term, 24 of the 27 had dilatation of the renal pelvis and calyces, often accompanied by severe tortuosity of the ureters. Ureteral dilatation always began at the brim of the pelvis, was always worse on the right side than the left, and never involved the pelvic ureters. In only 8 patients did the dilatation return to normal by the 7th day postpartum, and 8 of the 26 were still abnormal on the 28th day, 1 requiring 56 days for complete resolution. This study, and other similar ones reviewed by Hundley *et al.*[88] establish that severe dilatation of the urinary tract in the last trimester of pregnancy is normal. It is surely no surprise that untreated bacteriuria in the first trimester is accompanied by a substantial incidence of acute pyelonephritis, especially in view of Fairley's[89] documentation that half of these women have upper tract bacteriuria. Untreated bacteriuria involving these dilated upper tracts would be expected to produce a significant number of abnormalities that should be radiologically apparent. Kincaid-Smith and Bullen[75] cultured 4000 women at their first antenatal visit. Of 240 bacteriuric women, 148 returned for intravenous urography 6 weeks after delivery. The radiological abnormalities are reproduced in Table 4.32. Except for the four cases of "duplex kidney" without evidence of localized chronic pyelonephritis, and perhaps the seven cases of simple disparity in renal length of more than 2 cm, thereby excluding 11 of the 76 abnormal urograms, I believe most observers would accept these radiologic abnormalities as evidence of bacterial disease or analgesic nephritis. Whalley's[71] report, on the other hand, contains far too many instances of simple congenital variations, such as eight cases of ureteral duplication and two cases of bifid renal pelvis, to believe that the abnormalities were significant. Their ureteral catheterization data are questionable because serial cultures of ureteral urines were not obtained; more-

Table 4.32
Radiologic Abnormalities in 148 of 240 Patients with Bacteriuria[a]

Radiologic Finding	No. of Patients
Normal intravenous pyelogram	72 (48.6%)
Abnormal intravenous pyelogram	76 (51.4%)
Calyceal abnormality including papillary necrosis	15
Chronic pyelonephritis	14
Circumscribed loss of renal substance (probable chronic pyelonephritis, 6 with difference in renal length of more than 2 cm in addition)	14
Calculi	10
Duplex kidney (3 with localized chronic pyelonephritis)	7
Disparity in renal length of more than 2 cm	7
Gross hydronephrosis	4
Miscellaneous	5

[a] Reproduced by permission from P. Kincaid-Smith and M. Bullen, Lancet 1: 395, 1965.[75]

over, their report that the bladder fluid was sterile in all 23 bacteriuric patients after washing with 1000 ml of sterile irrigating fluid[71] is simply impossible (see Chapter I). Gower *et al.*[90] found that 82% of their bacteriuric women had no renal abnormality on intravenous urography, but their study is complicated because the radiologic examination was often performed years after the pregnancy.

Brumfitt's[81] observations may be relevant; he showed that the incidence of radiologic abnormalities in bacteriuria of pregnancy is proportional to the difficulty in curing the infection. Those patients easily cured of their bacteriuria by a single course of therapy had a 23% incidence of radiologic abnormalities, but those who remained bacteriuric despite repeated therapeutic efforts had a 65% incidence of radiologic changes (Table 4.31).

Renal Function

Kincaid-Smith and Bullen[75] observed an elevation in the blood urea levels of bacteriuric pregnant women compared to nonbacteriuric women; as pointed out, however, an elevation of blood urea has been reported for bacteriuric nonpregnant women as well.[62] Kaitz[91] could not show a difference in serum creatinines between 20 bacteriuric pregnant women and 21 nonbacteriuric women, but his series is obviously small when compared to that of Kincaid-Smith and Bullen.[75]

St. Thomas' Hospital Studies

In a unique study of bacteriuria in pregnancy, McFadyen, Eykyn, Gardener, and their colleagues[85] at St. Thomas' Hospital in London obtained urines from 2000 pregnant women by suprapubic needle aspiration of the bladder. The prevalence rate for bacteriuria was 6.6%. I have reproduced in Table 4.33 the organisms they found in the 132 patients who were not sterile on suprapubic aspiration. Only three aspirated urines contained two organisms, all the rest had a single species. *E. coli* accounted for 77% of the patients with bacteriuria; coagulase-negative staphylococci, enterococci, β-hemolytic streptococci (group B) and *P. mirabilis* accounted for all the remainder with the exception of three organisms. The reader should note that the staphylococci, β-hemolytic streptococci, and enterococci found on suprapubic aspiration could easily be interpreted as contaminants had the urine been obtained by voided techniques, especially the whole voided urine. Their technique of suprapubic bladder aspiration undoubtedly accounts for the lower inci-

Table 4.33
Bacterial Species in Bladder-Aspirated Urine From 132 Pregnant Patients with Bacteriuria At First Antenatal Visit[a]

Organism	No. of Patients
Escherichia coli	101
Coagulase-negative staphylococci	11
Enterococci	8
Proteus mirabilis	6
β-haemolytic streptococci, group B	6
Enterobacter	1
Klebsiella	2
Total	135[b]

[a] Adapted from I. R. McFadyen *et al.*[85]

[b] Three of the 132 aspirates contained two species of bacteria.

dence (77%) of *E. coli* found in this study. Moreover, 27% of all bacterial counts in these infected urines were less than 10^5 bacteria/ml of urine.

Thirty percent of these 132 patients with proven bacteriuria had symptoms suggestive of UTI, but so also did 25% of the age and parity matched, uninfected controls. The authors concluded that neither bacteriuria nor recurrence of infection after therapy could be diagnosed by symptoms.

One hundred eighty-six patients who had sterile urine on their first visit before the 20th week of gestation were reaspirated between the 24th and 28th week of gestation and again between the 32nd and 36th week of gestation. Only two patients, one with 10^4 *E. coli*/ml of urine which disappeared spontaneously 2 weeks later and the other with 10^5 β-hemolytic group B streptococci/ml developed a urinary infection later during their pregnancy. These findings surely confirm that screening for bacteriuria at the first antenatal visit will detect bacteriuria of pregnancy in all but about 1% of patients.

Ninety-five of the infected patients were treated with 10-day courses of antimicrobial agents to which the infecting organisms were sensitive. Sixty-two percent required only one course of treatment to eliminate the bacteriuria, 21% required two courses and 17% required three or more courses. The amount of treatment required was unrelated to the patient's age, parity, or social class. Indeed, unlike the studies by Savage *et al.*,[73] the St. Thomas' study did not show a progressive rise in bacteriuria with increasing age and parity.

Suprapubic bladder aspiration was performed after delivery in 104 patients who had proven bacteriuria in pregnancy, 95 of whom had been treated and 9 untreated. Eighteen of 67 patients aspirated 3–5 days after delivery were infected while 17 of 61 patients aspirated 6 weeks after delivery were infected. The recurrence rate of bacteriuria after delivery was directly related to the amount of treatment required during pregnancy; it was unrelated to either catheterization at the time of delivery or to complicated delivery.

Fifty intravenous urograms were done at 10–14 weeks following delivery; four showed dilatation of the right ureter and three showed "changes suggestive of pyelonephritis." Two of these latter three patients had required three courses of antimicrobial therapy during pregnancy, and one had required two courses, to achieve a bacteriuric-free status. Finally, it is of interest that nine patients had ureteral catheterization studies to locate the site of infection after delivery. In only one instance was bacteria found in the ureteral urine, the ureters could not be catheterized in one patient, and in the remaining 7, the infection was confined to the bladder; four of these seven were patients who had required three or more courses of antimicrobial agents during pregnancy.

I believe any practicing obstetrician will find these data from St. Thomas' Hospital extremely useful because each bacteriuria was proven and followed by suprapubic needle aspiration. The urinary tract abnormalities found on intravenous urography were minor indeed.

Antibody-Coated Bacteria in Pregnant Patients with ScBU

Harris, Thomas, and Shelokov[92] in San Antonio, Texas have made a substantial contribution to the risk of bacteriuria of pregnancy by detecting those patients with screening bacteriuria (ScBU) who have antibody-coated bacteria in their urine. They screened 1400 pregnant women, 70 of whom were found to have bacteriuria (5%); 35 of the 70 had fluorescent antibody-coated bacteria (FA+), and 35 did not (FA−). The FA+ patients had an increased serum creatinine and a decreased creatinine clearance compared to the FA− bacteriuric patients, as well as when compared to 55 matched obstetric patients who served as nonbacteriuric controls ($P < 0.05$). Although the median weights of the infants at birth did not differ among these three groups, intrauterine growth retardation (IUGR) (an infant weight below the 10th percentile of the hospital's "normal-weight" infant for the corresponding gestational age) was present in four of the mothers with FA+ bacteriuria and none of the mothers with FA− bacteriuria. This 15% incidence of IUGR in FA+ patients was 9 times the incidence in 1330 nonbacteriuric patients (1.6%).

Since the Fa− bacteriuric patients did not differ from the nonbacteriuric matched controls in either renal function or the incidence of IUGR, these authors make a case for detecting FA+ bacteriuria during pregnancy. Since all Fa+ bacteriuric episodes, however, were treated successfully when initially detected, including 14 recurrences in 10 patients that all proved to be reinfection with different bacteria, it appears that successful therapy in the treatment and prevention of bacteriuria of pregnancy does not prevent IUGR.

Long Term Follow-Up on Bacteriuria of Pregnancy

In a 10–14 year follow-up of bacteriuria of pregnancy reported in 1971, Zinner and Kass[93] determined maximal urinary osmolality of 51 patients who had been bacteriuric in 1955 and were still bacteriuric in 1970; they compared the osmolality in the 51 patients to 50 subjects who were neither bacteriuric in 1955 nor 1970. The mean osmolality of the bacteriuric group was 793 ± 156 and of the nonbacteriuric subjects 846 ± 163, which was statistically different ($P \lessapprox 0.05$).[93] Interestingly, however, the maximal osmolality of 81 patients who were bacteriuric in 1955 but uninfected in 1970 was 889 ± 186 which represents a better osmolality than even those pregnant women who presumably were never bacteriuric. Zinner and Kass found no difference in the blood pressures between those who were bacteriuric initially and at follow-up 10–14 years later in comparison to those who had never shown bacteriuria during these years. These authors reported a 28% incidence of "pyelonephritis" on intravenous urography in those patients who were presumably bacteriuric throughout the years of follow-up; two of the nine patients with pyelonephritis had renal papillary necrosis. We are not told whether the radiologic evidence of "pyelonephritis" involved as little as a single calyx or multiple calyces in both kidneys. Since creatinine clearances were similar in all three groups of women, and since the osmolality differences are small even though significant, it is likely that changes on the intravenous urograms in this important follow-up study were not very significant.

Reflux and Residual Urine

There are two remarkable papers that not only add to our knowledge of radiologic physiology in normal and bacteriuric pregnancies, but must also be counted as significant contributions toward the understanding of urinary tract infections in adult women. Heidrick, Mattingly, and Amberg[94] obtained single film cystograms during voiding in 200 patients randomly chosen in the last trimester of pregnancy. Catheterized urines were carefully obtained for culture at the time of the cystogram. A group of 121 additional patients had a cineradiographic study of the entire act of voiding within the first 30 hours postpartum. Of the 321 patients, 9 (2.8%) showed vesicoureteral reflux while 20 (6.2%) were bacteriuric. Of the nine patients showing vesicoureteral reflux only one was infected, but three had a previously documented episode of acute pyelonephritis. There was, however, "conspicuous absence of radiographic changes consistent with chronic pyelonephritis in all cases of reflux."

Williams, Davies, Evans, and Williams,[95] in a most thorough study, investigated, 4–6 months after delivery, 100 of 115 women who had proven coliform bacteriuria during pregnancy. When the bacteriuria was detected at the first antenatal visit, each patient was treated in succession with sulphadimidine, nitrofurantoin, and ampicillin until the urine became sterile. In six patients the bacteriuria persisted despite repeated courses of ampicillin. No patient was treated after delivery. Four to six months following delivery, residual urine, urine culture, intravenous urogram and voiding cystourethrography were performed on all 100 patients. Thirty-two patients were infected and 68 were sterile; there was no difference in residual urine between the two groups, and the "majority had residual volumes of less than 10 ml." Vesicoureteral reflux was found in 21 patients (21%), and coliform bacteriuria was present in 13 of these 21 (62%). Ten of the 21 patients with reflux had renal scarring, but again 7 of these were bacteriuric. Eleven of the 21 patients with reflux were normal radiologically even though 6 were bacteriuric. A substantial increase in all radiologic abnormalities was present in those patients who required multiple courses of antimicrobial therapy in order to maintain sterile urine during the antenatal period. Moreover, vesicoureteral reflux or renal scarring or both were present in 19 of the 32 bacteriuric patients (59%) at the time of the postpartum study, whereas these radiologic abnormalities were present in only 9 of the 68 patients (13%) whose urine was sterile. I believe that these data mean that prolonged bacteriuria of pregnancy represents the primary danger unless there are scars of childhood pyelonephritis.

Therapy

Since the prevalence of bacteriuria is already established at the first prenatal visit of the pregnant woman,[73] and since the incidence of 4–6% is about the same as in the nonpregnant female population of the same age, it is reasonable to believe that most women carry their infections into pregnancy. From the point of view of simply preventing clinical episodes of pyelonephritis in late pregnancy, it seems justifiable to detect these bacteriuric women and treat them. Even so, however, not all episodes can be prevented.[95] Data are insufficient to judge the advantage of long term therapy up to term[73, 75, 77] or short term therapy,[80, 85] but with long term therapy the incidence of acute pyelonephritis in treated bacteriuric pregnant women varied from 0–3.3%, whereas the rate rose to 10.3% for a similar group receiving short term therapy. Brumfitt's early report of 2.8% incidence of acute pyelonephritis in one group of short term treated bacteriuric patients[81] compared to a later publication of 10.3%[80] is confusing to us. Whalley *et al.*[71] thought that more patients were bacteriuric after delivery if untreated during the pregnancy, which seems reasonable, but Gower *et al.*[90] could detect no difference in postpartum bacteriuria between treated and untreated bacteriurics.

I would prefer short term therapy with close follow-up and reserve a complete urologic investigation 3 months after delivery for those patients who prove resistant to therapy. Antimicrobial drugs that are safe to use, even in early pregnancy, include oral penicillin-G, the short acting sulfonamides (sulfamethizole or sulfisoxazole), and nitrofurantoin.

Elder *et al.*,[83] in an interesting report on the effect of tetracycline on the clinical course and outcome of bacteriuria of pregnancy, treated 148 bacteriuric patients with placebo. Ninety-eight remained bacteriuric and asymptomatic throughout their pregnancy, 20 spontaneously cleared their bacteriuria (14%) and 27 patients developed symptomatic pyelonephritis (18%). The 11% rate of spontaneous disappearance of ScBU during pregnancy compares well with the 11% spontaneous clearance in the Cardiff series of nonpregnant patients with ScBU.[54] In the tetracycline study of Elder *et al.*,[83] it is of substantial interest, especially in designing treatment trials, that the administration of tetracycline to nonbacteriuric, pregnant patients decreased the rate of prematurity and increased the duration of gestation!

ROLE OF SEXUAL INTERCOURSE IN RECURRENT BACTERIURIA

Many women with recurrent cystitis believe their infections are related to sexual intercourse, and some are very clear that their first infection coincided with or shortly after the onset of sexual activity. This latter relationship was absolutely certain in patient D.B., Figures 4.16 to 4.22, even though she had experienced severe enough infections in infancy to produce renal scarring; her infections ceased at age 2½ years until the onset of sexual activity.

Despite this apparent relationship between sexual activity and urinary infection, there are no conclusive data to document the relationship or its frequency of occurrence. It is clear that most women who have frequent sexual intercourse never have urinary infections; for this reason, it is difficult to believe that sexual intercourse is the primary cause of urinary tract infections. It is easier to believe that sexual activity may be the precipitating cause in some women who have other susceptibility factors in operation, *i.e.*, such as introital colonization with Enterobacteriaceae. Moreover, it is absolutely certain that many women get UTIs without sexual activity and that sexual intercourse is surely not the cause of recurrent infections in infants and children. I suspect that the basic cause of recurrent bacteriuria in females will be the same in both children and adults.

With these reservations, what is the evidence that sexual intercourse plays a role in women with recurrent bacteriuria? Suggestive, but certainly not conclusive, evidence must include the following:

1. Almost every epidemiologic survey has shown a greater prevalence of bacteriuria in married women than among single females of the same age group.
2. Kunin and McCormack[3] showed that the frequency of bacteriuria was 13 times greater in white control women than among nuns in the 15–34 age group; see Figure 4.1.
3. In 1965, we advocated a postintercourse regimen of a single tablet of antimicrobial agent, usually penicillin-G,[96] which was remarkably effective in our practice. Vosti[97] documented this nicely in 1975; fourteen patients on postintercourse prophylaxis experienced 19 infections in 761 months of follow-up compared to 90 infections during 705 months while they were off therapy ($P < 0.001$). Moreover, 394 of 571 cultures (69%) contained small numbers of Gram-negative bacteria from the voided urine during the period they were off therapy; this compared to 181 of 384 cultures (47%) which contained Gram-negative bacteria in small numbers while on prophylaxis ($P < 0.001$). Thus, not only did postintercourse prophylaxis substantially reduce their episodes of recurrent infection, but it also reduced the number of Gram-negative bacteria contaminating the voided urine from the perineum.
4. Using suprapubic bladder aspiration before and after urethral massage in women under anesthesia, Bran *et al.*[98] found urethral bacteria in the bladder following massage in 9 of 24 women.
5. Buckley *et al.*[99] examined clean catch urines before sexual intercourse, 1 hour afterwards, 6–10 hours later, and 30–48 hours later in 20 women, 17 of whom had a history of UTI. Seventy-six intercourse episodes were studied; 23 of the 76 showed a rise in bacterial counts greater than one log in the postintercourse urines. Midstream urine counts of greater than 10^5 bacteria/ml occurred in 7 episodes, but *E. coli* as a single species occurred only once. Because the bladder was not aspirated, the authors point out it is uncertain whether bacteriuria actually occurred or not. None of the 23 episodes of intercourse-induced rises in bacterial counts in the urine were symptomatic. The one log rise or greater in colony counts was always transient; it occurred with pathogens and nonpathogens alike.

   Whether or not bacteriuria actually occurred after these 76 episodes of sexual intercourse is unknown; nevertheless, this study does establish that intercourse at least causes an increase in bacteria in the voided urine which could presumably be due to an increased density of bacteria in the introital or external urethral area.
6. Perhaps the most suggestive study is some recent work by Allan Ronald's group in Winnipeg, Canada.[100] Somewhat reminiscent of Bollgren and Winberg's study[29] shown in Table 4.7, the Winnipeg group obtained daily voided urine cultures (by dip-slides) in nine

women highly susceptible to UTI who discontinued prophylaxis. Three women had a mean frequency of sexual intercourse once every 3.8 days, acquired no infections during follow-up (mean, 4 weeks), had no evidence of introital colonization with Enterobacteriaceae, and remained asymptomatic.

Six women had nine episodes of bacteriuria (10^5 bacteria/ml) during a mean surveillance of 5 weeks; *E. coli* was responsible for five of the nine infections. The mean frequency of sexual intercourse was once every 3.7 days, the same frequency as in those who remained abacteriuric. Seven of the nine infections were acquired during 61 postsexual intercourse days (within 24 hours of sexual intercourse); two infections occurred during the 169 days that sexual intercourse did not occur. The perineum was colonized with the infecting organism in all six patients.

PYELONEPHRITIS

In earlier sections in this chapter, Asymptomatic Bacteriuria Detected During Screening Surveys and Bacteriuria of Pregnancy, I reviewed the evidence for the lack of serious renal involvement in patients with nonobstructive UTI. I want to make a few comments here, however, about pyelonephritis in general.

Schechter, Leonard, and Scribner analyzed the cause of renal failure in 173 patients referred to them for dialysis. Chronic pyelonephritis was the primary cause of end-stage renal failure in 13% and was "almost always associated with an underlying structural defect. Unequivocal nonobstructive chronic pyelonephritis was not found."[101] They also observed that symptomatic infections tended to occur prior to the onset of azotemia in those patients with chronic pyelonephritis.

Murray and Goldberg[102] looked at 101 patients with chronic renal disease who were azotemic (serum creatinine >1.3 mg%) and who did not have evidence of primary glomerular disease. Thirty-one patients had anatomical, obstructive disease of the urinary tract, 20 had analgesic nephropathy, 11 had hyperuricemia, 10 had nephrosclerosis, and 9 had obstructive renal calculi. The cause of renal disease was indeterminate in 11 and 7 had multiple causes; they felt that UTI—although documented in 27 patients—was never the primary cause of the azotemia. For example, in the 11 men and 16 women with UTI, all 27 had other primary causes of renal disease prior to the first documentation of bacteriuria; these causes were obstructive abnormalities in 14, stones in 7, gout in 2, nephrosclerosis in 1, and analgesic abuse nephropathy in 3. Murray and Goldberg[102] not only concluded that UTI is seldom the cause of chronic renal disease in the adult, but they observed that 89% of their azotemic patients had a readily identifiable primary cause of their disease, a point of view to which I heartily subscribe. Gower[103] drew similar conclusions from a prospective study of 26 patients with radiological unilateral chronic pyelonephritis, 36 with bilateral chronic pyelonephritis, 14 patients with papillary necrosis, and 9 with obstructive atrophy who were followed for a total of 374 patient years. Bacteriuria was not associated with deteriorating renal function. Analgesic abuse was the most common cause of either a decline in renal function or a change in serial radiographs of the kidney. Hypertension was clearly associated with higher levels of plasma creatinine. Gower[103] concluded that control of blood pressure and analgesic intake is the best way to preserve renal function, a view we have emphasized with our patients for the past decade. In the azotemic patient who is hypertensive and bacteriuric, it is far more important to control the blood pressure than it is to control the bacteriuria.

Johnson and Smythe[72] measured renal function annually in 47 patients who had chronic bacteriuria, 41 of whom had additional evidence of "pyelonephritis." About half the patients lost renal function during a 5-year follow-up. In 26 patients, however, the bacteriuria disappeared early in the study either spontaneously or in response to therapy. When the 21 patients whose bacteriuria persisted were compared with the 26 whose bacteriuria disappeared, no differences in the degree of loss of renal function could be detected. The authors concluded that factors other than bacteriuria determined the rate of nephron destruction in chronic pyelonephritis.

All of the above studies, therefore, point to the absolute rarity with which nonobstructive UTI causes serious renal damage in adults. A. W. Asscher[104] has tabulated 8 long-term follow-up studies from the literature on kidneys of adults with UTI (Table 4.34). These reports include follow-ups on 901 patients with UTI; as seen in Table 4.34, the renal changes are either nonexistent or extremely minimal.

The resistance of the adult kidney to renal scarring—even in the presence of acute flank pain with chills and fever accompanying the UTI—is remarkable. I have pointed this out in patient D.B. who had renal scarring from infections in infancy, Figures 4.16–4.22, but I would like to briefly review an even more common problem seen in practice. A 51-year-old Caucasian woman was seen at Stanford University Hospital for the first time in February 1979. She had no infections as a child or as an adolescent until after her marriage when she experienced one or two episodes per year of suprapubic discomfort, urinary urgency, and frequency for which she learned to self-treat herself with antimicrobial agents. In 1971 she had a total abdominal hysterectomy followed in 1973 by a cholecystectomy; from 1973 to 1979, she was hospitalized twice each year for fever, severe shaking chills, right flank discomfort, urgency, frequency, and dysuria; her bladder symptoms usually preceded the flank pain and fever by 18–24 hours. Pyuria and

Table 4.34
Long-Term Follow-Up Studies of Urinary Tract Infections in Adults[a]

Author	Number of Cases	Study Group	Follow-Up Years	Findings
Freedman (1960)[105]	111	Symptomatic infections in adult women	0.5–3	No progression of kidney damage
Pratt (1963)[106]	84	Symptomatic infections in adults	1–6	12% showed a fall in glomerular filtration rate (GFR)
Little *et al.* (1965)[107]	16	Symptomatic infections in adult women	0.25–2	No scarring. Decrease in kidney size after acute infection in 75%
Freedman (1972)[108]	250	Symptomatic infections in adult women	12	No reduction of kidney function or rise of blood pressure
Asscher *et al.* (1973)[109]	107	Symptomless infection in women aged 21–65	4	No progression in kidney damage
Bullen (1975)[110]	106	Adult women with infections detected in pregnancy	10	No progression of kidney damage
Freeman *et al.* (1975)[111]	137	Elderly men with bacteriuria	2–4	No kidney damage except in presence of obstruction
Gower (1976)[103]	52	Symptomatic adult women with unilateral or bilateral chronic pyelonephritis and UTI	0.4–11	No progression of kidney damage

[a] Reproduced by permission from A. W. Asscher, The Challenge of Urinary Tract Infection, New York, Academic Press, 1980.[104]

a positive urine culture, usually *E. coli*, was always present; she was usually admitted to the hospital for intravenous antibiotic therapy. Her last episode before being seen at Stanford in February 1979 was in November 1978 when she was hospitalized with an *E. coli* UTI and symptoms of pyelonephritis. On discharge she was maintained on nitrofurantoin 50 mg three times a day. On this therapy, she had remained asymptomatic, her blood pressure was 140/80 mm Hg, her urine contained neither protein nor sediment, and a midstream urine culture was sterile. Her intravenous urogram from 1973 was completely normal, but I thought with so many hospitalizations for documented *E. coli* pyelonephritis that the urogram should be repeated. The 10-minute film, shown in Figure 4.23, obtained a few minutes after release of the ureteral compression bag, is entirely normal without any evidence of renal scarring or even calyceal disease. A voiding cystourethrogram showed neither ureteral reflux nor residual urine. In 38 patients who presented with documented UTI and clinical symptoms of acute pyelonephritis, Mabeck[112] reported that the intravenous urogram showed "signs of chronic pyelonephritis" in only 7 of the 38; 26 out of these 38 patients

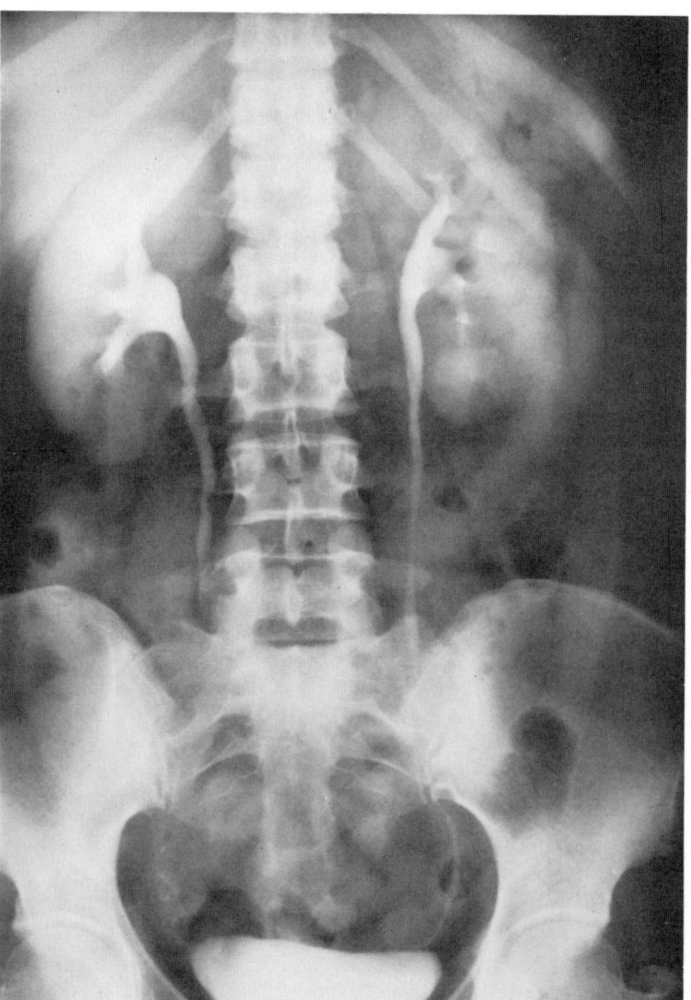

Figure 4.23 A 10-minute, intravenous urogram after release of ureteral compression in a 51-year-old Caucasian woman with multiple admissions to the hospital for recurrent, acute *Escherichia coli* pyelonephritis.

received antidiuretic hormone and had a reduction in maximal urinary concentrating ability.

I would like to present two adults with childhood pyelonephritis who are representative of the clinical spectrum in this disease. B.T., a 49-year-old, Caucasian female had frequent urinary infections as a child until age 11; she was asymptomatic from age 11 until age 20 when, after her marriage, she was again troubled by frequent *E. coli* UTI. Although her symptoms were usually dysuria and frequency, chills and fever with back pain were occasionally present. An intravenous urogram at age 33 was reported to show "clubbing of calyces with parenchymal thinning of the right upper pole kidney." In 1966, a voiding cystourethrogram showed moderate bilateral vesico-ureteral reflux; her ureters were reimplanted that same year when she was 43 years old. Repeat cystograms after reimplantation showed no further reflux but she continued to have recurrent episodes of urinary infections with frequency and dysuria; at least three episodes were accompanied by chills, fever, and flank pain between the reimplantation in 1966 and when I first saw her in 1972. Indeed, she was personally certain that the ureteral reimplantations had not changed the morbidity or her susceptibility to recurrent urinary infections. A creatinine clearance in 1970 was 91 ml/minute; her blood pressure was noted to be 150/100 mm Hg in 1971. When I saw B.T. in June of 1972, her blood pressure was 160/100 mm Hg without medication, the serum creatinine was 1.1 mg%, and her urinalysis showed neither protein nor urinary sediment; urine culture was sterile. She had completed a short course of nitrofurantoin 2 weeks before my consultation. I obtained an intravenous urogram on June 9, 1972, which was comparable in every way to the one I had for review from 1968. The right kidney measured 11 cm and the left 11.6 cm; Figures 4.24, *A* and *B* and 4.25, *A* and *B* show the classic changes of childhood pyelonephritis. I placed her on 50 mg of nitrofurantoin each night, a regimen that completely stopped all of her infections between 1972 and 1976. She ceased taking the nitrofurantoin prophylaxis in 1976; my last follow-up in September 1977 indicated that she had been well without any further urinary infections. A telephone call in July 1979 confirmed that she remained free of UTI.

Both D.B. (Figures 4.16–4.22) and B.T. (Figures 4.24 and 4.25) clearly had pyelonephritis of childhood, both show the radiologic hallmarks of that disease, and both became symptomatic as adults when sexual activity began. It is interesting that each showed moderate degrees of renal reflux at the height of their infections as adults; successful reimplantation of the ureters in B.T. did not change the course of her infections, not even her episodes of clinical pyelonephritis. D.B., on the other hand, spontaneously lost her reflux with time (or 95% of it), has had no infections since 1973, and went through a full term pregnancy in 1977 without any complications or urinary infections. She was last cultured on July 12, 1979; the midstream urine was sterile but the introital culture showed 20 *Klebsiella* and 20 *E. coli*/ml of transport broth.

These two patients did not sustain enough damage from pyelonephritis of childhood to change their life expectancy although B.T. has some mild, labile hypertension which has been present since 1971. Unfortunately, not all adults with childhood pyelonephritis have such a benign course. E.B. was 33 years old when I first saw her in October 1975; her blood pressure was 184/110 mm Hg, her serum creatinine was 3.3 mg % and the creatinine clearance was 22 ml/minute. She arrived with an intravenous urogram from November 1971, which showed an atrophic, pyelonephritic right kidney and a severely damaged left kidney classic of childhood pyelonephritis (Figure 4.26). A cystogram, performed in August 1975, showed no reflux on multiple films taken during filling, but voiding produced reflux to the pelvic brim (Figure 4.27). Her bladder capacity was 500 ml, there was no residual urine, and her bladder pressure during voiding rose only 15 cm of H_2O. Her urine was sterile, 30 mg% protein

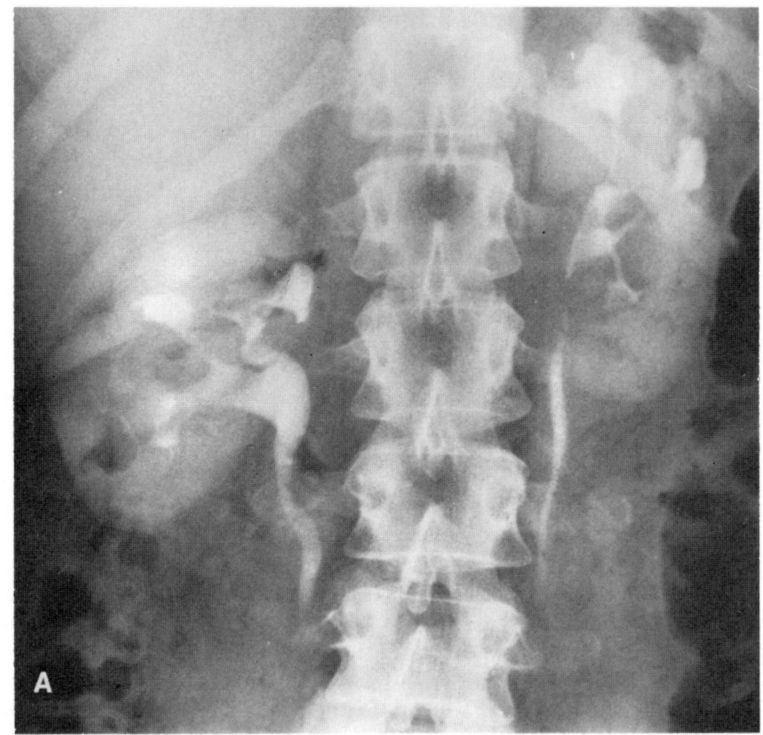

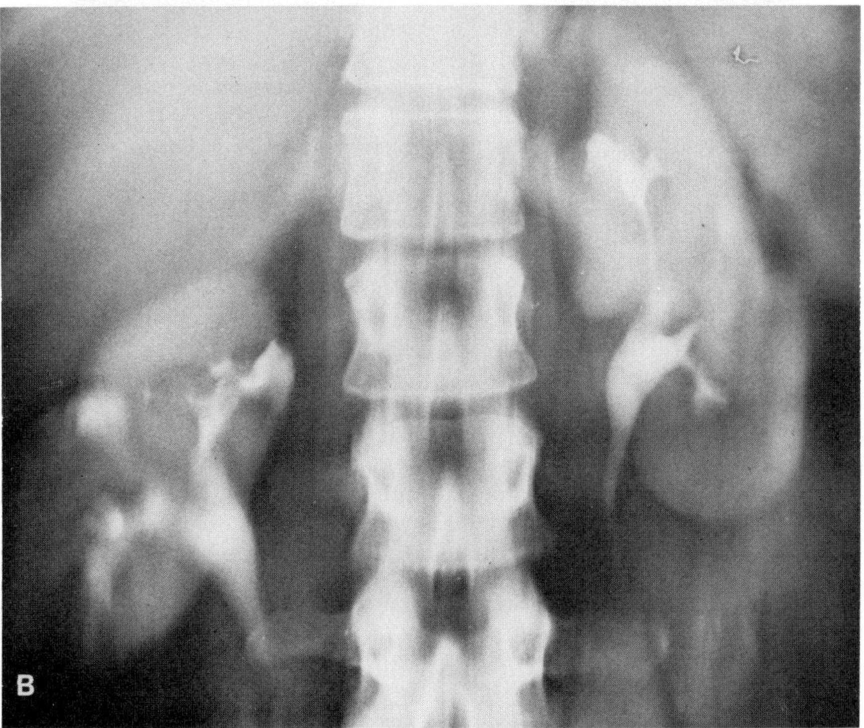

Figure 4.24 *A*, A 15-minute intravenous urogram from June 1972 on B.T., a 49-year-old white female who had many urinary infections as a child. The right kidney measures 11.0 cm and the left 11.6 cm. *B*, A 7-cm tomographic film from the same study. Her serum creatinine at age 49 was 1.1 mg%. She weighed 53 kg, her blood pressure was 160/100 mm Hg, her urine contained no protein, and the urinalysis was normal.

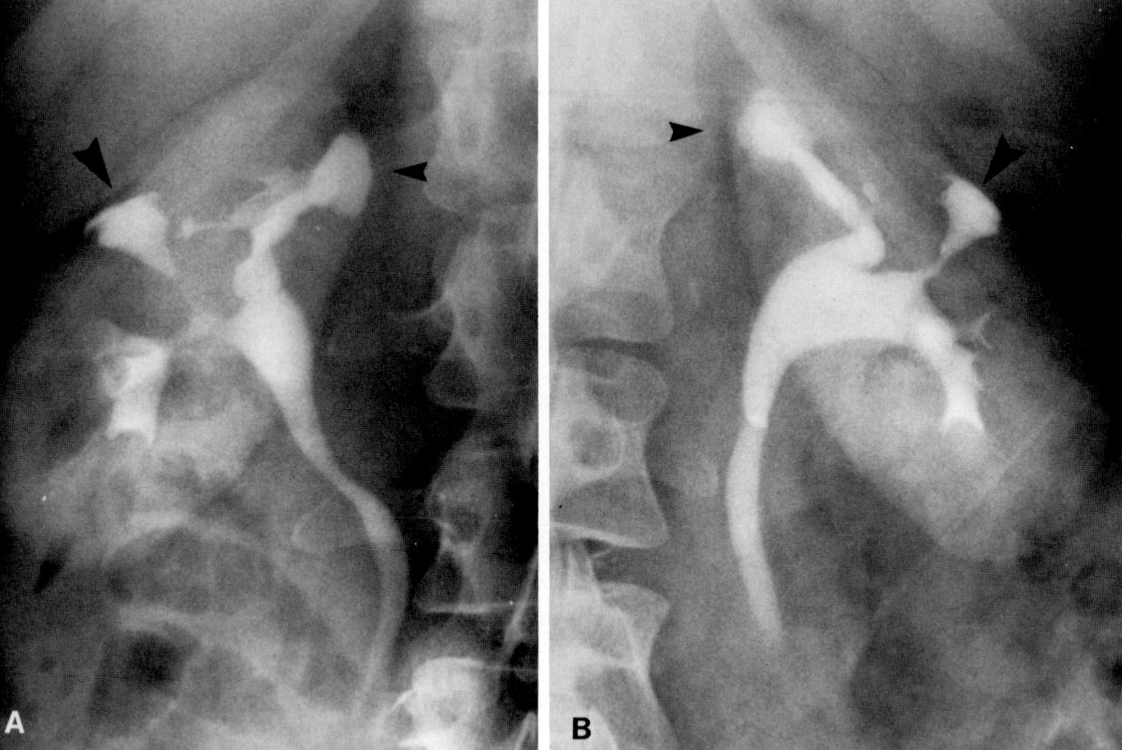

Figure 4.25 Oblique intravenous urograms from same study as Figure 4.24. *A*. Right kidney. The upper medial calyx (*small arrow*) and middle calyx (*large arrow*) show complete obliteration of the renal cortex; the calyx extends to the capsule. *B*. Left kidney. The upper medial calyx (*small arrow*) and middle calyx (*large arrow*) show total loss of overlying renal cortex with extension of the calyx to the capsule. It is interesting that the areas of renal atrophy involved the same calyces in each kidney, suggesting the genetic determinants of intra-renal reflux and atrophy (see Chapter 6).

was present, and her urinary sediment was insignificant; subsequent urines contained no protein. A repeat intravenous urogram on October 14, 1975 was similar in every respect to the urogram in 1971; contrast excretion was poor to be sure, but a 7-cm tomographic cut with ureteral compression shows the architecture essentially unchanged from earlier films (Figure 4.28). Her childhood history was one of recurrent chills and fever to 104°F., often lasting 3–5 days; she especially recalled the episodes of right flank pain. After puberty, these infections diminished and by the time I saw her in 1975 she was having about one episode of acute pyelonephritis per year. I started her on propranolol 40 mg and hydrochlorothiazide 100 mg each day. I also placed her on one-half tablet of TMP-SMX each night for prophylaxis. After her blood pressure was controlled, she was seen every 6 months; in October of 1977 her blood pressure was 120/70 mm Hg, and her serum creatinine 4.3 mg%. Thereafter, partly because of personal problems, she was reluctant to take her antihypertensive medications. By March 1978, her creatinine was 5.9 mg%, in April it was 6.9 mg%, and by October 1978, it was 12.1 mg%. She was begun on dialysis in October 1978, and transplanted in early 1979, after a bilateral nephrectomy. At the present time her renal function is normal.

In a follow-up on 74 women admitted to hospitals in Madison, WI, 10–20 years previously for acute pyelonephritis, Parker and

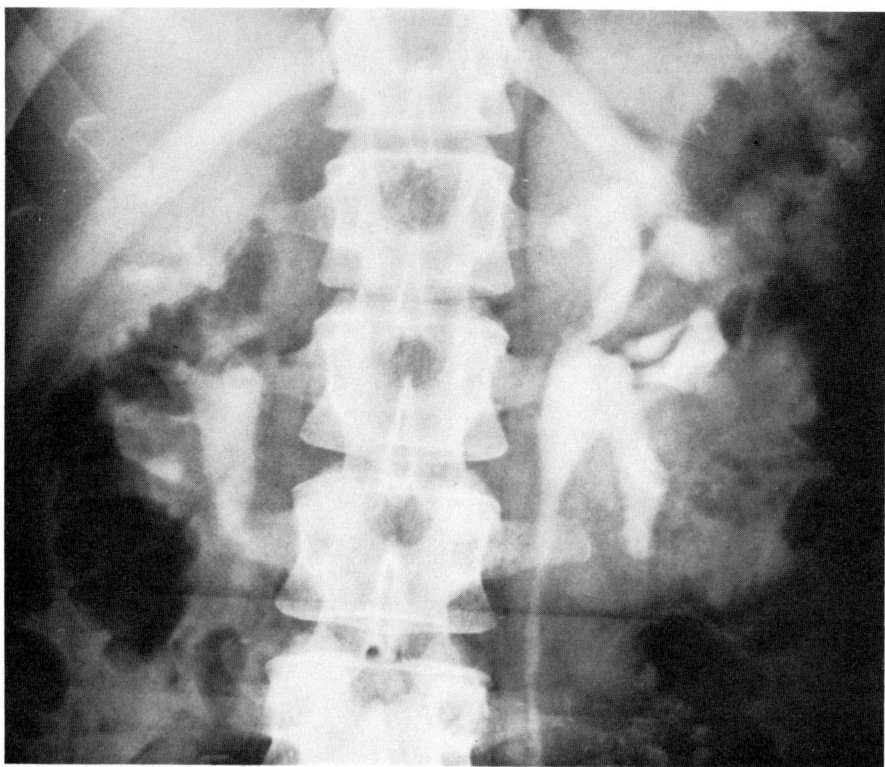

Figure 4.26 15-minute intravenous urogram from November 1971 on E.B., a 33-year-old white female with a severe history of childhood pyelonephritis. The right renal atrophy and distortion of all calyces is seen in both kidneys. The renal outlines are not well seen. Her serum creatinine at age 33 was 3.3 mg%. She weighed 51 kg, her blood pressure was 184/110 mm Hg, her urine contained 30 mg% protein, and her urinalysis was unremarkable.

Kunin[113] found that clinical illness for most of these patients had begun in association with marriage, pregnancy, or the postpartum period. Only 17% were bacteriuric at the time of follow-up, and only 10% had elevated blood pressure. Only four patients had suffered severely from their disease; two had mild azotemia, one had a renal transplant because of azotemia and nephrolithiasis, and one had died from complications of uremia with multiple abscesses. The authors pointed out that the relative benignity of this disease, with the important exception of a few patients, was in agreement with the pregnancy studies by Crabtree and his associates in the late 1930s.[114–116]

There is, however, a rare adult patient with nonobstructive pyelonephritis who develops substantial renal atrophy in the absence of analgesic abuse or renal artery stenosis. Bailey *et al.*[117] and Davies *et al.*[118] have each reported a single case. Whether these represent unusual sensitivities of the renal parenchyma to specific bacterial antigens is unknown.

The Ask-Upmark kidney is now thought to be a form of pyelonephritic atrophy from childhood UTI. It is considered in some detail in Chapter 6 on Urinary Infections in Infancy and Childhood. Most of these patients have hypertension. Pfau and Rosenmann[119] believe that unilateral chronic pyelonephritis is a rare cause of hypertension, a view with which I am in agreement, but it does occur and we have all overlooked the fact that the Ask-Upmark kidney is probably secondary to early infection and ureteral reflux in infancy without evidence of infection later in life.

RECOGNITION OF ADULT PATIENTS AT SERIOUS RISK FROM RECURRENT BACTERIURIA

Although the morbidity, medical cost, and time lost by patients with recurrent UTI is a major public health problem, it is equally clear from the preceding sections that the number of adult patients at serious risk of loss of renal cortex is relatively small. Nevertheless, to these few the risk is great and the major burden of solving their problem falls to the urologist.

The conditions in which we recognize increased risk to the patient in terms of loss of renal cortex are listed in Table 4.35. To these eight categories might be added the immunosuppressed patient and patients with recurrent bacteriuria who have valvular cardiac disease or prosthetic implants; I have not added these potentially catastrophic conditions because loss of renal cortex is not the major morbidity. Before reviewing these categories in Table 4.35, it will be worthwhile for the reader to briefly review the classification of UTI presented in Chapter 1; all infections are divided into first infections, unresolved bacteriuria, bacterial persistence, and reinfections of the urinary tract. While the first three categories in Table 4.35—struvite infection stones, infected congenital anomalies, and infected obstructions—are examples of bacterial persistence in terms of their bacterial recurrence, the next four

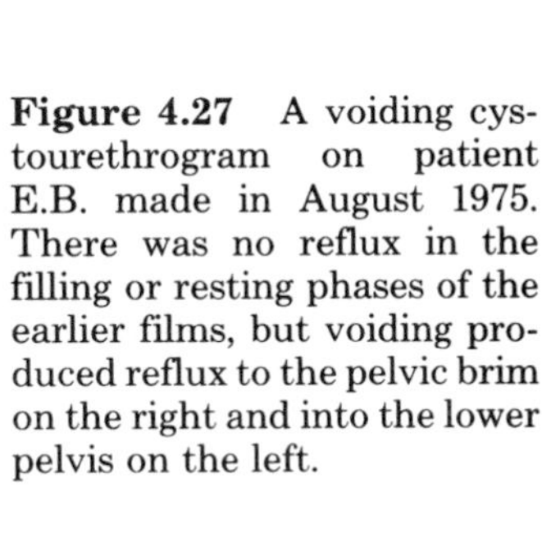

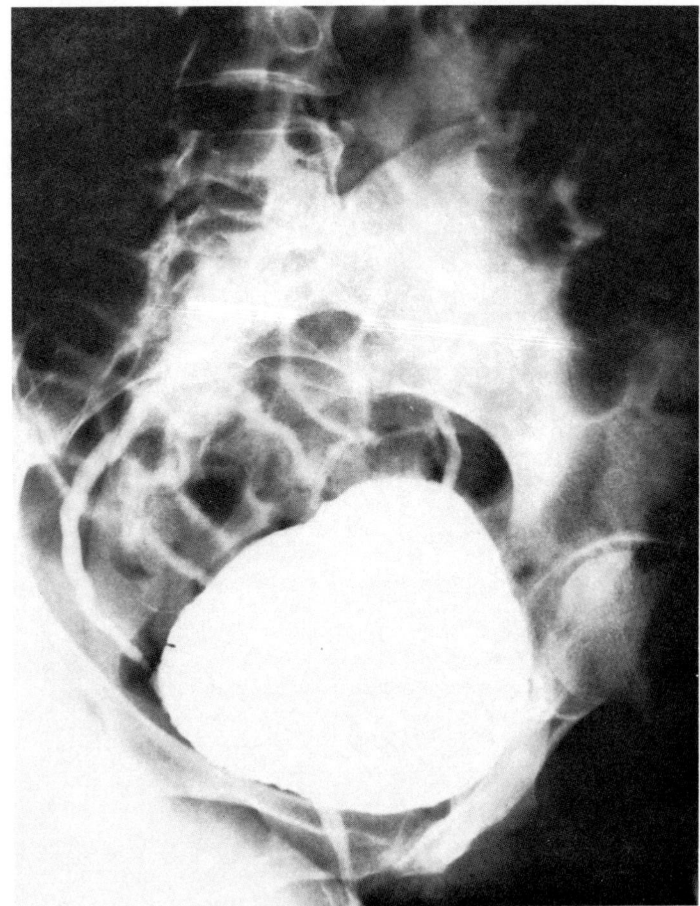

Figure 4.27 A voiding cystourethrogram on patient E.B. made in August 1975. There was no reflux in the filling or resting phases of the earlier films, but voiding produced reflux to the pelvic brim on the right and into the lower pelvis on the left.

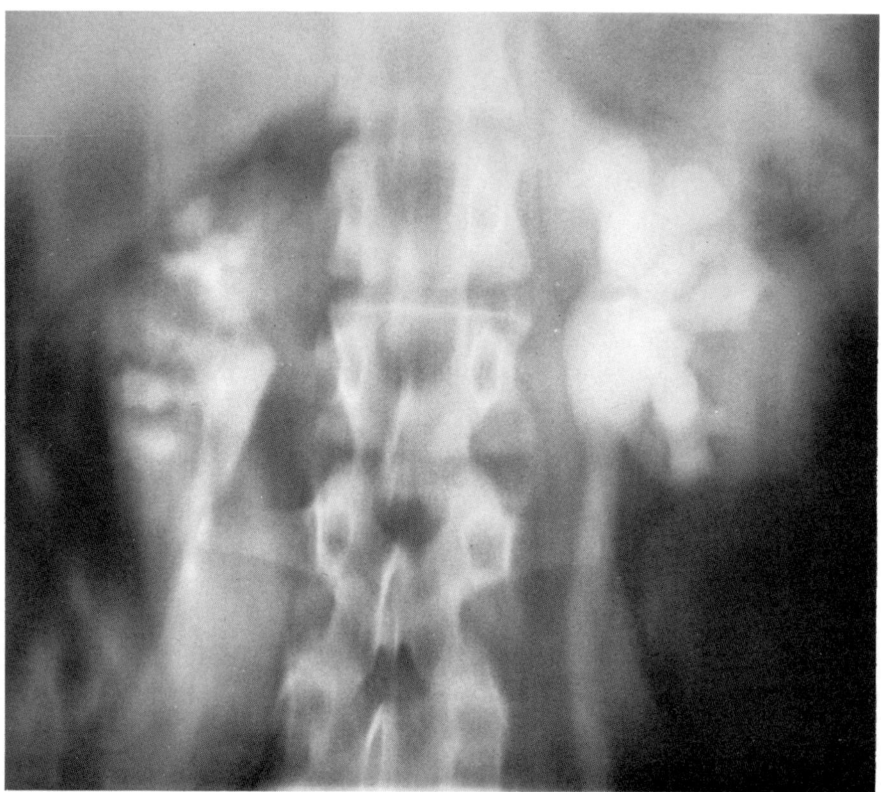

Figure 4.28 A 7-cm tomographic cut from a compression film during an infusion nephrotomogram on patient E.B. made in October 1975. The renal architecture and renal scarring are unchanged from the 1971 study (Figure 4.26). Observe the severe atrophy with all calyces extending to the capsule of the right kidney. The spared area of renal hypertrophy in the left lower pole appears as a pseudotumor.

Table 4.35
Major Categories of Increased Risk in Women With Recurrent Bacteriuria

1. Urea-splitting bacteria that cause struvite renal stones
2. Congenital anomalies that become secondarily infected
3. Bacteriuria in the presence of urinary tract obstruction, acute or chronic
4. Analgesic abuse
5. Diabetes
6. Neurogenic bladder, especially spinal cord injury
7. Pregnancy
8. Perinephric abscess

categories—analgesic abuse, diabetes, neurogenic bladder, and pregnancy—derive their bacteriuric morbidity from reinfections. Recurrent bacteriuria with a perinephric abscess is, of course, an example of bacterial persistence.

Urea-Splitting Bacteria That Cause Struvite Renal Stones

As long as recurrent infections in the adult women are caused by *E. coli*, the consequences other than symptomatic morbidity are not usually serious. Urea-splitting bacteria, however, especially the common *Proteus mirabilis*, cause intense alkalinization of the urine with precipitation of calcium, magnesium, ammonium, and phosphate salts and the subsequent formation of branched, struvite renal stones. The bacteriologic consequences are substantial because the bacteria presist inside these soft stones, even though the urine is readily sterilized. Indeed, struvite infection stones, together with the occasional oxalate or apatite stone—which can also become secondarily infected—constitute the major cause of bacterial persistence in women in the absence of azotemia. The bacteriuria in most of these patients with struvite stones recurs almost immediately upon stopping antimicrobial therapy, and certainly recurs within 5–7 days. These patients with struvite stones are so important to diagnose and treat properly that Chapter 8 is devoted exclusively to this problem.

All of the residual particles of struvite stones must be removed at the time of surgery if recurrent bacteriuria from bacterial persistence in the calculus is to be prevented. Rocha and Santos[120] have shown that even soaking these stones in iodine and alcohol for 6 hours will not kill the bacteria in the interior of the stone. The importance of recognizing this fact is two-fold: (1) the bacteria cannot be killed by antimicrobial therapy, even though the urine may be kept sterile for months and (2) any fragments left behind at the time of surgical removal leave residual bacteria and assure recurrence of the stone together with the morbidity which occurs from further bacteriuria.

The physician should beware of the patient with recurrent bacteriuria due to *P. mirabilis*. To be sure, *P. mirabilis* is not an uncommon cause of bacteriuria (about 25% of us carry *P. mirabilis* in our fecal flora), and most *P. mirabilis* infections are not associated with formation of struvite stones. Most of these latter instances, however, are of short duration, while struvite formation is associated with a protracted infection with *P. mirabilis*.

While the bacteriologic, biochemical, and surgical management of these patients is presented in Chapter 8, I would emphasize two further points. One, these struvite stones, usually 80% struvite, 20% apatite, often contain little calcium and are easily obscured on plain films of the abdomen unless the kidneys are absolutely free of overlying gas and feces. Therefore, any patient with recurrent *P. mirabilis* infection deserves plain film tomography of the kidneys. Second, once all fragments are removed or dissolved and the patient has sterile urine while off antimicrobial therapy (the final test of successful surgery), she must be followed bacteriologically at close intervals to detect reinfection with a new strain of urea-splitting bacteria. With early detection and treatment, or continuous prophylaxis, recurrent stones and more renal surgery can be prevented.

Congenital Anomalies That Become Secondarily Infected

As noted in the classification of UTI presented in Chapter 1, the other major cause of bacterial persistence occurs when any woman with a biologic susceptibility to recurrent bacteriuria also has a congenital anomaly that becomes secondarily infected. At that point in her history, recurrences will be characterized by the same organism until the anomalous infected structure is surgically removed. But almost invariably after resection, if she is followed long enough, simple reinfections with enterobacteria will appear again. Such anomalies include nonfunctioning duplications of the renal collecting system, such as the one we reported in which bacteriuria due to *Pseudomonas aeruginosa* had been constantly present for several years[121]; complete resection of the ureteral duplication cured the *P. aeruginosa* urinary infection, but this patient has had several simple *E. coli* infections in the 5 years since this case report.

Other anomalies include pericalyceal diverticula that lose their free communication with pelvic urine, urachal cysts of the dome of the bladder, medullary sponge kidney, and an occasional congenital obstruction that has produced a nonfunctioning kidney into which effective urinary concentrations of antimicrobial agents cannot be delivered. Several interesting patients with unusual causes of bacterial persistence are presented in Chapter 10.

Bacteriuria in Presence of Acute or Chronic Urinary Tract Obstruction

This group of patients at serious risk are mainly iatrogenic and largely preventable. I include here those sterile calcium oxalate stones causing acute obstruction that become secondarily infected in the course of unsuccessful efforts to remove the calculus. The most tragic examples of chronic obstruction and bacteriuria causing serious loss of renal cortex is the child with minimal reflux who develops ureteral obstruction following an unsuccessful ureteral reimplantation. The tragedy is even greater when one observes the normal kidneys present preoperatively, usually in the presence of minimal to moderate reflux, and compares these normal kidneys to the scarred, shrunken kidneys of the postoperatively obstructed and infected urinary tracts. I have seen the same tragedy in the male adult with megaloureters who had adequate to good renal function and sterile urine before he was operated upon to "improve" renal drainage; postoperatively he becomes obstructed, infected, and eventually requires dialysis and transplantation. It should not be forgotten that 15 of the 22 patients who presented to Scribner's[101] dialysis unit with end stage renal failure, in whom the primary cause was chronic pyelonephritis, were due to "significant obstructive or calculus disease which preceded the initial episode of urinary tract infection in each."

Analgesic Abuse with Papillary Necrosis and Subsequent Obstruction

In the preceding section on Pyelonephritis, I have already reviewed the evidence that control of an elevated blood pressure and avoidance of analgesic drugs represent the two most useful therapeutic tools in preventing further deterioration of renal function in the presence of renal disease. Indeed, although renal disease is commonly thought to predispose the patient to urinary infections, there are almost no data to support this impression. In fact, Leonard *et al.*[122] followed 82 patients with parenchymal renal disease for 26 months, obtaining an average of 17 cultures/patient, and only two patients (2.4%) acquired bacteriuria.

Acute urinary obstruction caused by necrotic papillae, superimposed on an unresolved bacteriuria, and occurring in the presence of kidneys already damaged from analgesic abuse, clearly constitutes a urologic emergency if further nephron loss is to be prevented. Since many of these patients are already azotemic, early intervention by ureteral catheterization to bypass the soft, obstructing papillus, or by percutaneous nephrostomy, is all the more critical. Obviously, careful and effective antimicrobial sterilization of the urine in the face of azotemia should go hand in hand with immediate relief of the obstruction.

Whether UTI in patients with analgesic abuse nephropathy causes renal parenchymal damage in the absence of obstruction from a free papillus is unclear to me. Since papillary necrosis *per se* probably causes intratubular obstruction, common sense would dictate the necessity of getting the urine sterile and keeping it sterile. Most patients with analgesic abuse nephropathy do not have bacteriuria,[102] but those that do need careful bacteriologic control to reduce this additional morbidity. Arger and Goldberg[123] have an excellent review and further update in their 1976 paper. One of the most detailed analyses on 288 patients from Essen, Germany, has just been presented by K. D. Bock and T. Nitzsche: Analgesic nephrology—symptomatology and clinical course, 4th International Symposium on Pyelonephritis at Münster, Germany, October 1979, published by Thieme, Stuttgart, 1980.

Although any bacteriuric patient with chronic renal disease deserves to have their urine sterilized if drug toxicity can be avoided, the physician should be cautious in assuming that all such patients have renal infection. In our own experience, we have observed a number of patients with bacteriuria and severe renal disease, such as polycystic kidneys in the presence of azotemia, whose infections were limited to the bladder when ureteral catheterization studies were performed to localize their bacteriuria. Thus, bacteriuria in the presence of noninfectious parenchymal disease cannot be assumed to always involve the kidneys.

Diabetes

The increased prevalence of asymptomatic UTI among diabetic women, with no substantial increase among diabetic men, has been shown by several investigators.[124-126] Forland *et al.*[124] surveyed 333 patients attending a diabetes mellitus outpatient clinic over a 1-year period; they found that 19% of the women and 2% of the men had urinary tract infections. Vejlsgaard[125] reported a prevalence rate of 18.2% in 132 diabetic women who were followed throughout pregnancy.

The determination of antibody coating of bacteria in the study of Forland and his colleagues[124] has added significant information; antibody-coated bacteria were initially present in 43% of the patients but rose to 79% within a mean pretreatment period of 7 weeks. This evidence of an increasing immunologic response in diabetic patients who acquire bacteriuria suggest renal parenchymal involvement and a potential increase in morbidity. Papillary necrosis as well as perinephric abscess are well recognized hazards in the diabetic patient.

Emphysematous Pyelonephritis

Emphysematous pyelonephritis occurs only in diabetics. It is characterized by parenchymal and perirenal infection with gas-forming bacteria in the presence of necrotic renal cortex and medulla. It is usually lethal if treated medically; emphysematous pyelonephritis is a surgical emergency. Our group at Stanford has presented recently a diabetic patient with nonobstructive, emphysematous pyelonephritis that is carefully documented with surgical, radiologic, and histologic photographs.[127] Freiha, Messing, and Gross[127] emphasize in this report that the tissue gas is distributed in the parenchyma and perinephric tissues in association with the necrotic tissue; this distribution of gas should not be confused with cases of pyelonephritis where the air is in the collecting system of the kidney, a condition which also occurs in nondiabetics and is usually nonlethal. In Figure 4.29, *A* and *B*, one can see the characteristic pattern of retroperitoneal air with both perinephric and parenchymal gas; it should be carefully noted because recognition of this gas pattern in a diabetic with clinically acute pyelonephritis can be life-saving. The interested clinician should also consult the excellent papers by Schainuck *et al.*,[128] Turman and Rutherford,[129] and Dunn *et al.*[130]

Neurogenic Bladder, Especially Spinal Cord Injury

Of all patients with bacteriuria, no group compares in severity and morbidity to those with spinal cord injury. Nearly all require catheterization early after their injury because of bladder spasticity or flaccidity, and significant numbers develop ureterectasis, hydronephrosis, reflux, or renal calculi. Although pelvic floor spasticity with the obstructed bladder under high pressure is easier to manage in the female than in the male, these women are nevertheless at increased risk precisely because of high intravesical and intrarenal pressures in the presence of bacteriuria. Bacteriologic management of these patients with spinal cord injury is discussed in Chapter 9 on obstructive urologic abnormalities.

Pregnancy

The major renal complication we see in our pregnant patients with bacteriuria is secondary to *Proteus* infections with struvite stone formation. Nevertheless, as reviewed in the preceding section on Bacteriuria of Pregnancy, the fact that acute pyelonephritis can be prevented in the last trimester by early treatment in a substantial percentage of patients, justifies inclusion of bacteriuria in pregnant women. Although clinical pyelonephritis in the last trimester probably causes little permanent renal damage, this morbidity to pregnant mothers is surely needless and should be prevented.

Perinephric Abscess

In 1974, Thorley, Jones, and Sanford[131] made a substantial contribution by review-

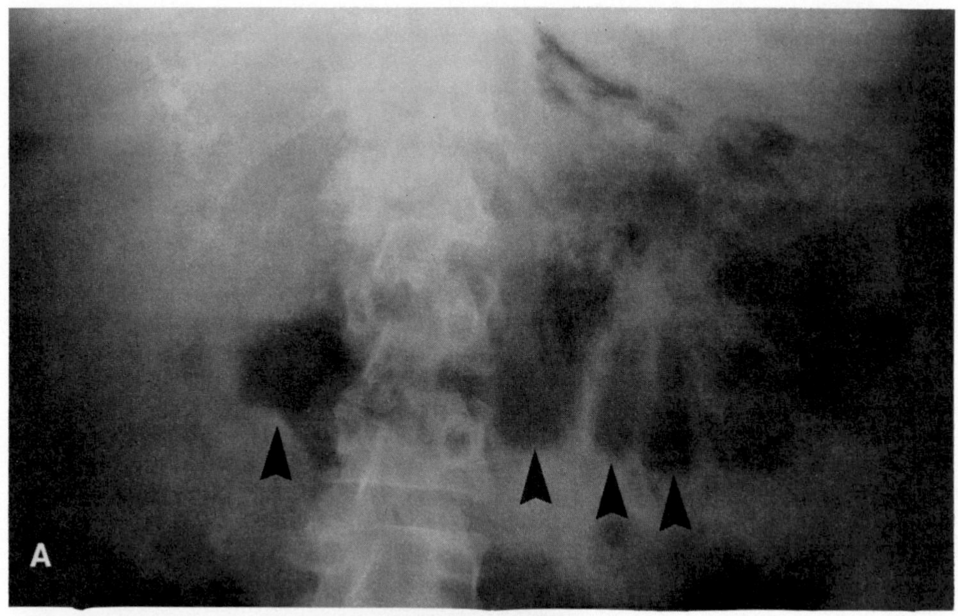

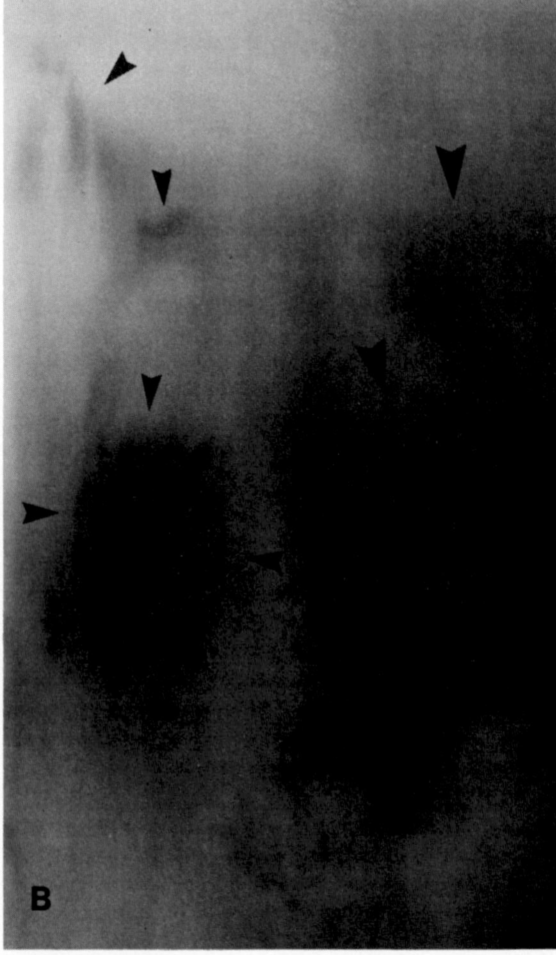

Figure 4.29 *A*, A plain-film radiograph 3 days after the first onset of symptoms of acute pyelonephritis in a 37-year-old black, diabetic woman with emphysematous pyelonephritis. Her white blood cell count was 10,000/cu mm, her blood glucose 425 mg%, and her serum creatinine 2.5 mg%. Note the retroperitoneal air which conforms to the boundaries of Gerota's fascia. Except for the air in the transverse colon (marked by the *4 arrows*), the remainder of the gas is retroperitoneal. *B*, A tomographic cut at 8 cm, through the plane of the kidney, shows that the gas is both perinephric (*small arrows*) and intraparenchymal (*large arrows*). This tomogram was made immediately after the plain-film in *A*.

ing 52 cases of perinephric abscess seen at the Parkland Memorial Hospital in Dallas, TX. The mortality rate was 50%; moreover, one-third of the cases were undiagnosed before necropsy. The clinical features and radiographic findings in these 52 cases are presented in Tables 4.36 and 4.37.

The most difficult clinical decision is often the distinction between perinephric abscess and acute pyelonephritis. In a discerning analysis of the distinctive features which would allow differentiation between these two diagnoses, Thorley *et al.*[131] observed that 33 of 37 patients with acute uncomplicated urinary tract infections were symptomatic for fewer than 5 days; 7 of 9 patients with perinephric abscess, initially admitted with the diagnosis of acute pyelonephritis, were symptomatic for longer than 5 days. Moreover, no patient with acute pyelonephritis was febrile for more than 4 days; all patients with perinephric abscess were febrile for a minimum of 5 days with a median febrile period of 7 days (median febrile period for pyelonephritis was 2 days).

The treatment of perinephric abscess is surgical drainage. Medical procrastination usually results in death of the patient. Ultrasonography should represent a genuine advance in the early diagnosis of perineph-

Table 4.36
Clinical Features of Perinephric Abscess[a]

Symptoms and Signs	No. of Patients	Percent
Symptoms		
Fever	47	90
Unilateral flank pain	38	73
Abdominal pain	31	60
Chill	28	54
Dysuria	21	41
Signs		
Unilateral flank tenderness	38	73
Abdominal tenderness	33	63
Temperature 100°F	28	54
102°F	3	6
Abdominal mass	18	35
Flank mass	14	27

[a] Reproduced by permission from J. D. Thorley, S. R. Jones, and J. P. Sanford, Medicine, **53:** 441, Baltimore, Williams & Wilkins 1974.[131]

Table 4.37
Radiographic Features of Perinephric Abscess[a]

	No. of Patients	Percent
Abdominal supine film	48/52	92
Normal	19	40
Abnormal unilaterally (abscess side)	20	46
Absent psoas shadow	10	50
Upper quadrant "mass"	9	45
Absent renal shadow	6	30
Genitourinary stone	5	25
Retroperitoneal gas	2	10
Multiple unilateral abnormalities	12	60
Abnormal bilaterally	9	19
Absent renal shadows	4	44
Absent renal and psoas shadows	2	22
Absent psoas shadows	1	11
Peritonitis	1	11
Paralytic ileus	1	11
Chest radiogram	48/52	92
Normal	26	54
Abnormal unilaterally (abscess side)	20	42
Pleural effusion	8	40
Lower lobe infiltrate	6	30
Elevated diaphragm	4	20
Lower lobe atelectasis	3	15
Upper lobe infiltrate	1	5
Multiple unilateral abnormalities	2	10
Abnormal bilaterally	2	4
Elevated diaphragms	1	50
Apical scarring	1	50
Intravenous pyelogram (IVP)	37/52	71
Normal	7	19
Abnormal unilaterally (abscess side)	28	76
No function	11	39
Diminished function	7	25
Calyectasis	6	21
Calyceal stretching	5	18
Genitourinary stone	4	14
Renal displacement	1	4
Multiple unilateral abnormalities	6	21
Abnormal bilaterally	2	5
Diminished function	1	50
Calyceal stretching	1	50

[a] Reproduced by permission from J. D. Thorley, S. R. Jones, and J. P. Sanford, Medicine, **53:** 441, Baltimore, Willliams & Wilkins, 1974.[131]

ric abscess. Any patient with acute pyelonephritis who fails to resolve as expected should have an ultrasound; on rare occasions, a computerized tomographic scan may be required for diagnosis.

URETHRAL SYNDROME

Syndrome in Patients Susceptible to Recurrent Bacteriuria

Gallagher and his associates[13] first showed that 41% of women in general practice presenting with symptoms suggestive of UTI—suprapubic aching and cramping, urinary frequency, or a variety of related bladder complaints, such as dysuria, urinary urgency or tenesmus, low backache, and even unilateral flank discomfort—actually had sterile urine. They suggested the term "urethral syndrome." Their belief that urethral infection caused this syndrome was based on the similarity of symptoms in patients with and without bacteriuria as well as the observation that bladder infection developed within a short period of follow-up (3 months) in 13 of 46 patients with the urethral syndrome. O'Grady *et al.*[132] observed that 58 percent of 122 abacteriuric patients who presented initially with frequency and/or dysuria subsequently developed bacteriuria within 9 months of follow-up. In our own studies of women with recurrent symptomatic bacteriuria, about 30% of all symptomatic episodes were accompanied by sterile urine.[9]

Definition of Urethral Syndrome and Difficulty Imposed in Ascertaining a Sterile Urine

If we define the urethral syndrome as any symptom or combination of symptoms suggestive of UTI but occurring in the presence of a sterile urine, we are immediately faced with serious problems in interpreting some otherwise excellent studies in the literature. A sterile urine means *no* bacteria in the bladder urine which therefore must be obtained either by catheterization or suprapubic aspiration of the bladder. Moreover, sterility should ideally include cultures for organisms such as anaerobes and *Ureaplasma urealyticum*, as well as the routine aerobic bacteria. Additionally, there is no place for culturing minute quantities of urine with calibrated bacteriologic loops; even a calibrated loop as large as 0.01 ml could not detect the presence of 99 bacteria/ml of urine. These limitations suggest that investigations into the etiology of the urethral syndrome cannot include midstream voided urines as the sole method of examination; there is no way, using the voided urine, to exclude, with certainty, bladder infections due to low counts of pathogenic bacteria. For example, even in the classic study by Gallagher *et al*,[13] 23% of the patients they included as urethral syndrome had catheterized urine counts of less than 10,000 bacteria/ml; thus, one out of four patients may actually have been bacteriuric (the remaining 77% were truly sterile). So we can conclude early in this discussion that, depending upon the investigator's certainty that the bladder urine really is sterile, some patients with bladder infections who have low counts of bacteria will be mistakenly included as the urethral syndrome. In addition, since 80% of women with acute UTIs spontaneously achieve a sterile urine within a few weeks of the infection, there must be some who do so rapidly. Thus a woman who has been acutally symptomatic for a few days may have spontaneously achieved a sterile urine before she was examined by the physician. We have documented several such patients who also manifest pyuria for a few days after the infection has spontaneously cleared, and thus may falsely appear also as examples of "sterile pyuria."

Fortunately, these patients with either low count bacteriuric episodes or those who have just spontaneously cleared their bacteriuria, recognizably fall into the group of women who have documented recurrent bacteriuria. In our own studies where 30% of all symptomatic episodes in women with recurrent bacteriuria were accompanied by sterile urine, antimicrobial prophylaxis—as outlined in an earlier section of this chapter—not only prevented their episodes of bacteriuria but also seemed to alleviate their symptoms of the urethral syndrome.

Etiology of Urethral Syndrome in Patients with Recurrent Bacteriuria

Do we know the cause of this syndrome in women with recurrent bacteriuria? Is it due to bacterial colonization of the urethra with Enterobacteriaceae prior to the bacteria reaching the bladder? In our longitudinal studies on patients with recurrent bacteriuria, we have not been able to identify any relationship between colonization of the introitus with Enterobacteriaceae and the occurrence of the urethral syndrome. We have observed the urethral syndrome without colonization of the introitus and, even more often, our patients have been asymptomatic with extensive colonization of the introitus by Enterobacteriaceae. Bruce *et al.*[133] observed that introital cultures for Enterobacteriaceae did not correlate with the urethral syndrome in their patients. Colleen *et al.*[134] aspirated the bladder in 25 consecutive women who had documented UTI in the past, 19 of whom were symptomatic. *E. coli* was grown from the bladder aspirates of three patients (one in very low counts), two had heavy growth of *Bacteroides* (both of which were reproducible after methanamine hippurate therapy), and one had *U. urealyticum* before and after therapy; thus, three of 22 aspirates which otherwise would have been judged as sterile by conventional aerobic cultures, were infected with unusual pathogens.

Maskell *et al.*[135] have suggested recently that slow growing, CO_2-dependent, Gram-positive organisms—mainly *Lactobacillus* species and a few corynebacteria species—may be the cause of the urethral syndrome. By incubating routine urine specimens in 7% CO_2 for 24–48 hours, they isolated these anaerobes in counts of 10^7 or greater/ml in "pure culture" from 73 women, 93% of whom were symptomatic; 61–64% of these women had pyuria (5 or more WBC/hpf). One hundred ninety-seven out of 200 urines "sent to the lab for a variety of reasons" failed to grow lactobacilli species in pure culture. Since this was a laboratory bench study of isolating fastidious bacteria, apparently little is known about the method of collecting the midstream urine. It is quite possible that the technique allowed extensive vaginal contamination. Moreover, even less is known about the 200 control urines sent to the lab for a "variety of reasons" (were most control urines from males?). Despite these reservations, if these results can be confirmed by suprapubic aspiration of the bladder (which is the *only* way to prove this proposal), then *Lactobacillus* species could be a major cause of the urethral syndrome in women with recurrent bacteriuria. I am concerned, however, that despite the apparent differences from the control urines, these large numbers of fastidious lactobacilli may simply be introital contaminants of an otherwise sterile bladder urine. We have proven *Lactobacillus* species in a few patients by suprapubic needle aspiration of the bladder, but they have been asymptomatic and pyuria was not a prominent feature.

The report by Maskell and her associates[135] is somewhat reminiscent of the study by Geckler *et al.*[136] who found pure anaerobic cultures in 20% of 153 midstream voided urines that contained $>10^5$ bacteria/ml. Although males rather than females were investigated, localization studies by segmenting the voided urine showed that the urethra rather than the bladder was the source of these large numbers of anaerobic bacteria. Indeed, bladder aspiration demonstrated anaerobes in only 2 of 10 patients who had large numbers of anaerobes in the voided samples.[136] It is possible that these high bacterial counts of anaerobes in voided urines in the report by Maskell are related to the colonization density of anaerobes in the urethra and introitus of the female either in health or disease. Just as the density of anaerobes is 1000 times greater than *E. coli* in the bowel, the same relationship may occur on the urethral mucosa of the male and introitus of the female. In fact, Bartlett *et al.*[137] have shown that vaginal anaerobes far outnumber the aerobes. If such is the case, midstream counts of anaerobes might be expected to occur in the 10^5 bacteria/ml range which almost never happens when *E. coli* is the colonizing organism on the urethra or the introitus.

It is possible, of course, that the anaerobic bacteria found by Maskell really are on the urethra in enormous numbers rather than the bladder and might still be the cause of the urethral syndrome. If so, the fact that 61–64% of the urines contained pyuria would indicate that her symptomatic patients fall into the category of the urethral syndrome in women with recurrent bacteriuria (see below). Since all of her lactobacilli were resistant to TMP-SMX, I cannot explain our excellent results with TMP-SMX prophylaxis in preventing the urethral syndrome in women with UTI.

Gynecological Abnormalities as a Cause of Urethral Syndrome

Brooks and Maudar[138] divided all females in their general practice who consulted them with symptoms of UTI into those with 10^5 bacteria/ml of urine or greater and those with 10^4 bacteria/ml or less. Sixty-seven of 138 patients (49%) had 10^5 bacteria/ml or more ("infected") while 50 patients had 10^4 bacteria/ml or less ("uninfected"). Eighty-four women who had never experienced urinary symptoms or infection served as controls, and 91% had no growth of bacteria on the dip-spoon culture. Cervical erosion or cervicitis was demonstrated in 28% of the infected females, 34% of the noninfected women, and 37% of the control subjects. Uterine prolapse was demonstrated equally among the three groups. Vaginal discharge occurred in 21% of infected females and 26% of the controls.

Gordon *et al.*[139] has shown that a normal bacterial flora accompanies erosions of the cervix.

From these two excellent studies, we can conclude that gynecological abnormalities play no role in the urethral syndrome.

In 84 women presenting with the dysuria syndrome, Dans and Klaus[140] found UTI in 33, nothing bacteriologically in 29, but *Neisseria gonorrhoeae* in 5, *Trichomonas vaginalis* in 4, *Candida albicans* causing vaginitis in 6, and *Herpes simplex* type 2 vulvitis in one. Thus, in these latter 16 patients—representing almost one of five who presented with dysuria—routine bacterial cultures would have failed to diagnose the cause of the dysuria.

Urethral Syndrome in Patients Resistant to Recurrent Bacteriuria

Just as it is important to distinguish bacteriuria detected on screening surveys from bacteriuria in symptomatic women presenting to the physician, it is no less vital to separate out those patients with the urethral syndrome who are not susceptible to recurrent UTI. Some women may have had UTI in the remote past, but it is usually clear that they are now symptomatic in the presence of a sterile urine which has not been infected for many, many months. These patients with the urethral syndrome are the most difficult to treat and undoubtedly represent more than one etiology. Zufall[141] reviewed his results in treating 150 women with 498 episodes of the urethral syndrome. His paper "Ineffectiveness of Treatment of Urethral Syndrome in Women," reviews the many different procedures used to treat this syndrome; he shows the results of nine different modalities of therapy in his own practice, with no clear cut advantage of one over the other. With almost any form of therapy, 60% of his patients were able to go for over 3 months without sufficient symptoms to warrant a repeat office visit; he concludes "it would appear that treatment should be supportive and harmless."[141] Richardson[142] claimed 90% cures, 6% good results, and only 4% unsatisfactory results in 300 women undergoing an external urethroplasty.

I believe that most, but certainly not all, patients with the urethral syndrome who do not have recurrent bacteriuria have interstitial cystitis. This disease is considered in greater detail in the section below on clinical management of the urethral syndrome.

The Question of Inflammatory Cells in Urine of Patients With Urethral Syndrome

The difficulty with the published literature on the presence of inflammatory cells is the failure to clearly separate those patients with the urethral syndrome who have recurrent bacteriuria from those patients who do not. Inflammatory cells are understandable in the former group, either as a consequence of bladder infection with low numbers of bacteria or even perhaps from urethral inflammation caused by pathogenic colonization of the urethra. I have trouble with the latter possibility, as advocated by Moore *et al.*,[143] because we have obtained first voided urine specimens before and after urethral massage in dozens of patients with recurrent bacteriuria due to Enterobacteriaceae; we have never once proved infection of the periurethral glands. To be sure, our massages were not done to study the urethral syndrome and we looked only at Enterobacteriaceae and not anaerobes, *Chlamydia*, *Ureaplasma urealyticum*, or other fastidious bacteria. It is likely that the symptomatic patients in whom Moore *et al.* reported their "differential urethro-vesical cell-counts" (a voided bladder (VB_1 and VB_2) urine collected to 50-ml volumes after cleaning the external genitalia) were actually patients with recent or even actual UTI; the findings of edema and "polypoid formation at the bladder neck" is also a characteristic of bladders with recurrent bacteriuria.

In the general practice study of Brooks and Maudar,[138] 80% of their 67 subjects with $\geqslant 10^5$ bacteria/ml had pyuria compared to only 18% of the 50 patients $\leqslant 10^4$ bacteria/ml. The latter group, however, surely contains some patients who were highly susceptible to bacteriuria; indeed, 26% of them developed bacteriuria within 3 months.

O'Grady *et al.*[14] made a valiant effort to study the inflammatory response in women presenting to a cystitis clinic. When they separated out their patients with the "abacteriuric urethral syndrome," whether symptomatic or asymptomatic when seen on multiple occasions, pyuria was not a distinguishing feature; in contrast, those patients who were intermittently bacteriuric with the urethral syndrome had substantial pyuria in comparison to women with the abacteriuric urethral syndrome (*i.e.*, those who had never had bacteriuria or who at least had not done so for many months or years).

The question of pyuria is obviously important in sorting out patients with bladder symptoms, and I deal with the broader question of "sterile pyuria" in a later section of this chapter. I would like to briefly relate the history of an instructive patient who was referred to me with the urethral syndrome, and in whom the presence of pyuria proved to be crucial. She is all the more instructive because I, too, was confident she had the urethral syndrome; I placed her into a special protocol for urethral syndrome patients whereby we would quantitate the leukocytes in the first voided 10 ml of urine as well as a midstream aliquot of the same volume. Unlike the report of Moore *et al.*[143] where the patient collected her own specimens, in our study the nurse kept the labia retracted and obtained the specimens under direct vision with the patient in a semisitting position on the cystoscopy table (see Figure 1.26, Chapter 1). We first determined with this technique the normal leukocyte counts in volunteer women who were asymptomatic and who had never had urinary infections. We obtained 121 paired specimens from 16 volunteers; 1–10 collections were made on each volunteer, with 10 of the 16 women studied at least eight times. The leukocytes were counted in a Fuchs-Rosenthal counting chamber using uncentrifuged urine. All counts were performed on undiluted urines except where the cells were too numerous to count. The mean ± one standard deviation for leukocytes in the first voided 5–10 ml of urine was 2700 ± 6300 cells/ml while the midstream aliquot of approximately the same volume contained 300 ± 700 cells/ml. The variation is clearly great and for obvious reasons, but it is apparent that normal women have a substantially greater number of WBCs in their first voided aliquot than in their midstream sample even when the labia are retracted during voiding.

With these normal counts reasonably established, our first patient with the urethral syndrome was a 37-year-old, married, Caucasian secretary whom I first saw in October 1971 with severe, episodic dysuria and urinary frequency with urgency. She had experienced about one documented UTI per year since her marriage 13 years before. She had been seen at least twice a month in 1971 for episodes of hourly frequency during the day, nocturia one time, urgency, and severe dysuria which was often unrelieved by voiding but helped by sitz baths. Although 6–10 cultures had been sterile off antimicrobial therapy, she had been helped for short periods of time by a variety of antimicrobial agents, especially erythromycin. An intravenous urogram was normal. Her cultures when I first saw her showed 10,000 *E. coli* on the introitus, 640 *E. coli* in the urethral aliquot, and none in the midstream urine. Her urethral and midstream leukocyte counts, however, were 100,000 leukocytes/ml of urine without any difference in the two aliquots. She was obviously pyuric, which I confirmed by suprapubic aspiration of the bladder; about half of the leukocytes in the aspirated urine were mononuclear and half were polymorphonuclear. To be brief, she was shown to be tuberculin positive. At cystoscopy, there was edema of the right ureteral orifice and ureter; ureteral catheterization specimens showed all the pyuria was coming from the right kidney. The bladder and right renal urines grew *Mycobacterium tuberculosis*; the left kidney was sterile. Except for minimal ureteriectasis of the lower right ureter, bilateral retrogrades were normal. She was started on triple drug therapy after several voided specimens were obtained to measure her WBC excretion/hour (Figure 4.30). She became asymptomatic almost immediately on therapy, treatment was stopped after 2 years, and she has remained asymptomatic without pyuria since early in 1972 (last follow-up, 1979). In Figure 4.30, 20 days into triple drug therapy, an aspirated urine showed 5–10 large glitter cells/hpf in the centrifuged sediment; 50 days into therapy, I could find only 1–2 WBC/hpf in the spun aspirate; 100 days into therapy—the last entries in Figure 4.30—I could not find a single WBC in 15 ml of aspirated, centrifuged urine. 10^4 and 10^5 WBC per hour represents her baseline excretion rate because she has remained at this level for the past 7 years; leukocyte excretions of this magnitude clearly represent WBC from the urethra and introitus, because they are not from the normal bladder or kidney.

Repeat cystoscopy 22 months into therapy showed a normal bladder, right ureteral orifice, and right ureter on retrograde ureterogram.

I realize that any patient with persistent sterile pyuria, confirmed either by bladder puncture or urethral catheterization, should have first voided morning cultures for *M. tuberculosis*. This had not been done before I saw her, probably because of the normal intravenous urograms, her urethral syndrome symptoms, and the fact that she temporarily seemed to improve on antibiotics, especially erythromycin. I will certainly never forget this patient because I thought she was a classic example of the urethral syndrome; urinary tract tuberculosis was simply not in my differential diagnosis for causes of this syndrome.

Clinical Management of Urethral Syndrome

The clinical management of urethral syndrome is now easier. If the patient is one with documented recurrent bacteriuria, and the urethral syndrome is related to their infections, prophylactic therapy for 6 months to a year will prevent both bacteriuric recurrences and usually the urethral syndrome. If the syndrome persists after several weeks of effective prophylaxis (or even better after 2 or 3 months), careful questioning will usually elicit the history that the urgency and frequency are secondary to infrapubic or suprapubic discomfort (or even pain) when the bladder is full. Moreover, voiding often relieves the infrapubic pain, although it may return a surprisingly short time later before the bladder reaches its functional capacity. Continuous records of voided urine volumes show variable amounts (usually less than 200 ml) but occasionally as much as 400 ml. The urine will be sterile *without evidence of pyuria* except in the very rare patient.

Interstitial Cystitis

We have described the diagnostic cystoscopic findings in early interstitial cystitis.[144] This early diagnosis cannot be made by simple, office cystoscopy under local anesthesia; the bladder will appear normal every time except for a restricted capacity. Under a general or high spinal anesthesia, the bladder will appear normal at first with fine, delicate capillaries in the

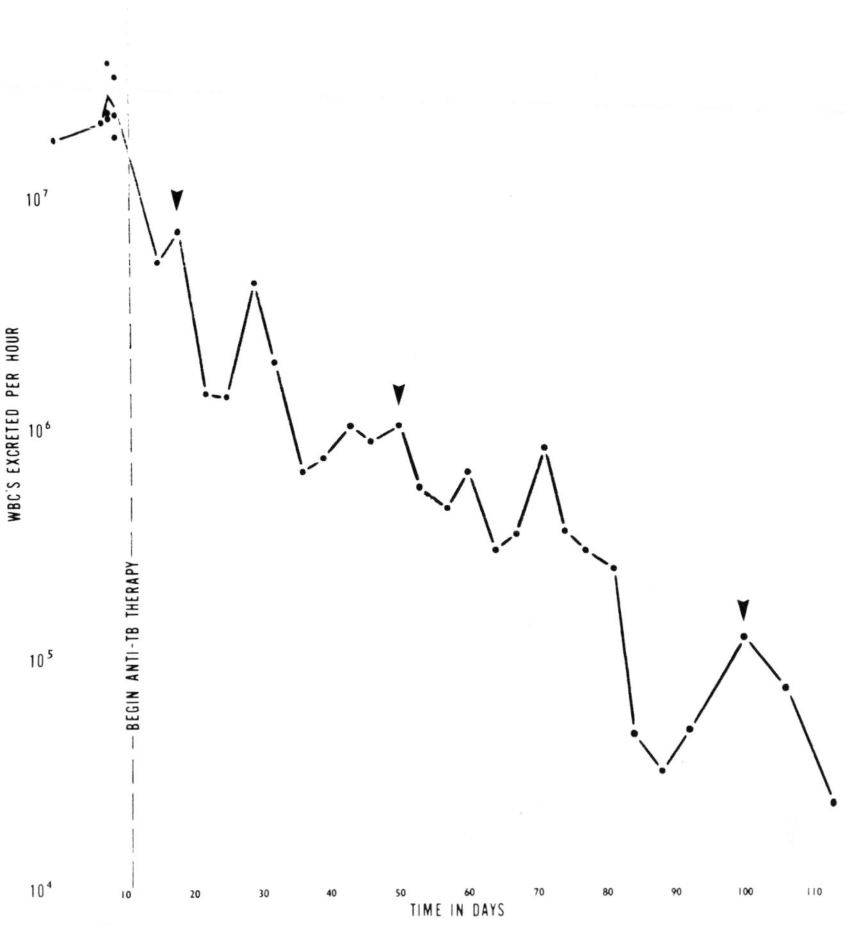

Figure 4.30 The number of white blood cells (WBC) excreted per hour in a 37-year-old, white female with the urethral syndrome. After *Mycobacterium tuberculosis* was proven in the right kidney and bladder, she was begun on triple drug therapy. The centrifuged urine sediment from suprapubic bladder aspirations showed 5–10 wbc/hpf on day 20 (*first arrow*), 1–2 wbc/hpf on day 50 (*second arrow*), and no wbc/hpf on day 100 (*third arrow*).

submucosa during the initial filling at 72 cm H_2O; the maximal bladder capacity will vary from 200 ml to over 1000 ml. The vividly characteristic lesions appear as the bladder is emptied, and thus the cystoscopist must reinspect the bladder after complete emptying, a maneuver I failed to do in my first 20 years of practice. The previously delicate capillaries will now show multiple, smooth, round strawberry-like hemorrhages just off the major capillaries. These spots have been termed "glomerulation" and it is a very fitting description. These glomerulations are not flame-shaped hemorrhages, as seen in the fundi with hypertensive retinopathy, but instead appear like minute strawberries or glomeruli. It is a very dramatic and diagnostic finding and can often be predicted by observing hemorrhagic fluid in the final ounce of irrigating fluid that drains from the bladder following the first overfilling. Sometimes, in addition to these multiple submucosal hemorrhages, larger areas (approaching 1 cm) of confluent hemorrhage can be observed. The so-called Hunner's ulcer occurs in very few patients with this disease, and although also accompanied by glomerulations, it has served more to confuse the diagnosis of interstitial cystitis than to help.

The diagnosis of early interstitial cystitis is important because 70% of women with this disorder can be dramatically helped by the instillation at the time of diagnosis of 1000 ml of 0.4% Chlorpactin WCS 90 (hypochlorous acid).[144] Anesthesia is always required for instillations of this strong oxidizing agent. If reflux is suspected by the cystoscopic appearance of the ureteral orifices, they should be "plugged" by large ureteral catheters before using Chlorpactin WCS 90.

While we see several patients a year with both early interstitial cystisis and recurrent bacteriuria, it is more common to see interstitial cystitis in women who never have had infections, or at least who have not been infected for years. We believe this disease, far more common than generally recognized, is the primary cause of distress in patients who present with intermittent episodes of the urethral syndrome in whom bacteriuric episodes have been excluded. The clinical history that their urgency and frequency are secondary to an uncomfortable bladder immediately prior to voiding (often referred to by the patient as "bladder spasms"), and generally relieved or substantially diminished by voiding, is important and rarely volunteered by the patient.

To be sure, there will be some patients left who have the urethral syndrome without pyuria and without recurrent bacteriuria who do not have interstitial cystitis. There is the occasional patient, especially postmenopausal, who will have a true urethral stenosis (16 Fr or much less) or atrophic vaginitis in whom estrogens will alleviate their lower tract symptoms.

Trigonitis

I hope the label "trigonitis" and "urethrotrigonitis" will soon disappear from our vocabulary of ignorance. The "cobblestone" or "granular appearance" to the trigone and floor of the vesical neck represents normal squamous epithelium in the postpubertal female. It should not be scraped off, resected, or coagulated in the false belief that "trigonitis" is present. The pathologist has encouraged the delusion by reporting biopsy material from these areas as "squamous metaplasia" rather than the normal squamous epithelium which it actually represents. Failure to recognize that vaginal inclusion epithelium covering the trigone and urethra is a normal embryologic development, plus lack of experience in cystoscoping normal women without bladder symptoms, is undoubtedly responsible for the cystoscopic terms "trigonitis" and "granular urethrotrigonitis." The distal third of the vagina, the urethra, and the trigone are all derived from the urogenital sinus, and thus the same squamous epithelium of the vagina usually covers the trigone and floor of the urethra.[145]

A Therapeutic Protocol

We can make a case for the following therapeutic protocol in the investigation of the urethral syndrome. It is far from perfect and, indeed, is certainly experimental in some aspects, especially the ventral urethral meatotomy in those patients who do not have interstitial cystitis. Nevertheless, it represents an organized approach to a difficult problem that will help many patients; unfortunately, in those patients with the urethral syndrome who are not susceptible to bacteriuria, cystoscopy under anesthesia is required to exclude interstitial cystitis, which makes this approach expensive and time-consuming. My approach is as follows:

1. When the patient is first seen with the urethral syndrome, if recurrent bacteriuria cannot be positively excluded from her past history by either documented cultures or urinalyses, then urinary infection can definitely be excluded by placing the patient on 3 months of prophylaxis with trimethoprim-sulfamethoxazole at one half tablet each night. Since this form of prophylaxis will absolutely exclude recurrent bacteriuria,[24] persistence of urethral syndrome symptoms proves that

she is not in the recurrent bacteriuric group of women.

2. Once recurrent bacteriuria is excluded, and the patient remains symptomatic, we cystoscope the patient under general anesthesia to exclude interstitial cystitis. This diagnosis requires full distension of the bladder at 72 cm H_2O pressure and confirmation of gross mucosal hemorrhages *after* the bladder has been emptied from the first overdistension. The bladder must also be lavaged for cytology to exclude the rare patient with *in-situ* carcinoma. If interstitial cystitis is present, we immediately give the first treatment of 0.4% Chlorpactin WCS 90.[144]
3. If interstitial cystitis is absent, *i.e.*, the characteristic mucosal hemorrhages have not occurred, we calibrate the urethra to a 36 Fr sound and perform a simple ventral urethral meatotomy after the technique of Richardson.[142] Because it is important to exclude a secondary infection after either Chlorpactin instillation of the bladder or the ventral urethral meatotomy, we elect to continue prophylactic trimethoprim-sulfamethoxazole for an additional 30 days.
4. If symptoms persist in the absence of interstitial cystitis and the ventral meatotomy, we begin manual application of topical estrogen to the urethral meatus and the vaginal vestibule if the patient is postmenopausal and the vaginal epithelial cells appear to be estrogen deficient.

Lest anyone think I am an advocate of ventral urethral meatotomy, let me hasten to point out that I believe it will prove to be useless. Since meatotomy is harmless, and does have a number of advocates despite the lack of control clinical trials to prove its efficacy, this seems the appropriate place to try it in an investigative protocol.

COAGULASE-NEGATIVE STAPHYLOCOCCAL BACTERIURIA

When urine specimens are obtained by catheter or bladder aspiration, and quantitative cultures performed, it appears that coagulase-negative staphylococci account for 7–26% of urinary infections in women,[146] a frequency that was unrecognized in the early years of quantitating total voided urine specimens. For example, in a study of 278 patients with bacteriuria of pregnancy where the total voided urine specimen was cultured, Elder *et al.*[83] reported coagulase-negative staphylococci in only three patients for an incidence of less than 1%. In the study by McFadyen *et al.*[85] where all urines from pregnant women were obtained by suprapubic bladder aspiration, coagulase-negative staphylococci were found in 8% of 132 patients at their first antenatal visit. Because *Staphylococcus epidermidis* is second only to the *Lactobacillus* as the most common species in the normal introital flora, it is easy to see how coagulase-negative staphylococcal bacteriuria can be missed when the technique for collecting urine relies on the total voided specimen or even the self-caught midstream urine.

Pereira[147] was among the first to call attention to coagulase-negative strains of staphylococci as agents of urinary infections. In 1967, Roberts[148] aspirated the bladders of 40 pregnant women who had staphylococci in their midstream urine in numbers suggestive of bacteriuria. Of the 20 aspirates that were positive for coagulase-negative staphylococci, 14 were micrococci and 6 were staphylococci; of the remaining patients whose aspirates were sterile, 17 of the coagulase-negative staphylococci found in the midstream urine were staphylococci and only 3 were micrococci.

The following year, Mitchell[149] classified 147 strains of coagulase-negative staphylococci isolated in pure growth from urines containing $\geq 10^5$ bacteria/ml. He showed that strains of micrococci subgroup 3 were resistant to novobiocin and that these strains generally came from young women with acute cystitis or pyelonephritis; on the other hand, novobiocin-sensitive strains of coagulase-negative staphylococci came from patients with more chronic, anatomic abnormalities of the urinary tract. Using novobiocin-resistance as synonymous with group 3 micrococci, Maskell,[146] in a very informative study, showed that 7% of urines sent to her lab with a pure growth of $>10^4$

bacteria/ml were due to coagulase-negative staphylococci. The urines with micrococcus subgroup 3 (79% of all coagulase-negative staphylococci) had far more pyuria than the urines which contained novobiocin-sensitive staphylococci, and they occurred almost exclusively in sexually active women between the ages of 16 and 25 years.

Mabeck[150] studied 31 patients with coagulase-negative staphylococci found among 219 bacteriuric women. All 31 were symptomatic, leukocyte excretion was substantially increased in 22 of 22 women in whom it was measured, and urinary concentrating ability was impaired in 19 of these 22 patients. Twenty patients were treated with sulfonamide or ampicillin; all were cured and their pyuria disappeared. Eleven patients were treated with placebo; 10 became sterile within 2 months. Seven of 15 patients showed greater than 25% improvement in urinary concentrating ability when restudied 5–12 months later. In a more detailed report on these same patients, Mabeck[151] noted that 3 of them presented with clinically acute pyelonephritis with fever and flank pain. Intravenous urography was normal in all his patients with coagulase-negative staphylococcal bacteriuria except for a single one with "slight signs of pyelonephritis."[151]

Sellin *et al.*[152] in a prospective study in young women, confirmed that novobiocin-resistant, subgroup-3 micrococci were the most common cause of UTI after *E. coli.* They could not find this organism, however, among the periurethral flora of the normal young woman, and concluded that these infecting micrococci were "selectively pathogenic in the urinary tract," a suggestive conclusion that remains to be confirmed.

Gillespie[153] and the group at the Bristol Royal Infirmary have reported an interesting study on UTI in women attending a clinic for sexually transmitted diseases. Of 103 women under the age of 26 years, coliform bacilli caused 63% of the infections, *Staphylococcus saprophyticus* caused 28%, and *Proteus* 9%. Of 38 women over 26 years, *S. saprophyticus* caused only 5% of all UTI. *S. saprophyticus* caused only two infections in 49 antenatal patients with bacteriuria, aged 26 and 29 years; none of 25 antenatal patients under 26 was infected with *S. saprophyticus.* They found no evidence that the staphylococci were sexually transmitted nor were they (or any of the other bacteriuric strains) related to sexual promiscuity.

Between November 1975 and July 1979 we studied 100 consecutive strains of coagulase-negative staphylococcal bacteriuria encountered in our urologic laboratories, which included outpatient and inpatient urine cultures; the vast majority were outpatient cultures. Only 6 of the 100 strains were novobiocin-resistant. Few of our patients, if any, were young women presenting with their first episodes of UTI.

The more recent papers on this subject follow a new terminology based on the eighth edition of Bergey's Manual.[154] Coagulase-negative, novobiocin-resistant staphylococci isolated from urine specimens are classified as *Staphylococcus saprophyticus* biotype 3.

Williams *et al.*,[155] in a hospital laboratory study, concluded that coagulase-negative staphylococci were infrequent urinary isolates (0.4% of all cultures) in their population and that *S. epidermidis* predominated over *S. saprophyticus.* They drew attention to the difficulties in classifying urinary isolates of coagulase-negative staphylococci, as have Hovelius and Mårdh.[156] The latter authors called attention to the important points that screening tests for bacteriuria—the nitrate reduction test, glucose consumption test, and growth on dip-slides that use MacConkey's agar—will not detect *S. saprophyticus* reliably.

In conclusion, coagulase-negative staphylococci in the urine should probably be divided by biochemical testing[157] and by novobiocin disc sensitivity testing[149] into those that are novobiocin-resistant (which should always be *S. saprophyticus*) and those that are novobiocin-sensitive which will include several staphylococci of which *S. epidermidis* will be the most common. *S. saprophyticus* should be responsible for most staphylococcal outpatient infections in sexually active young women, most of whom will present with acute cystitis but some of whom will have acute pyelonephritis. Pyuria will be present and the infection should be easily cured with a short course of ampicillin, nitrofurantoin, or sulfonamide. If bacterial persistance is suggested by an immediate return of the *S. saprophyticus*, the clinician should not forget that this organism possesses urease and could be associated with a struvite renal stone. In our laboratory, almost all strains of *S. epidermidis* also split urea.

Lastly, quantitative cultures on voided urines may not be reliable unless the bacteriologist has a high index of suspicion for lower colony counts of coagulase-negative staphylococci in pure growth. Half of the urines—both voided and bladder aspirated—contained less than 10^5 bacteria/ml in the report by Hovelius and Mårdh.[156]

Staphylococcus aureus is a rare cause of UTI, accounting for 1% of bacteriuria in hospitalized patients.[158]

ANAEROBIC BACTERIAL INFECTIONS OF THE URINARY TRACT

The anaerobic and aerobic urethral flora in healthy females has been elegantly described and quantitated by Marrie, Harding, and Ronald from Winnipeg.[159] Anaerobes were isolated from 32 to 35 urethral urines; *Bacteroides melaninogenicus* accounted for 46% of these isolates, and *Bacteroides fragilis* group was the next most common isolate. Bartlett *et al.*[137] found peptococci were the most frequent anaerobes in the vagina, but *B. melaninogenicus* was isolated in 8 of 22 women.

It is surprising that more anaerobic UTIs do not occur. Using a positive Gram stain ($\geq 10^5$ bacteria/ml) as the screening technique, Segura *et al.*[160] found 25 out of 5781 urines that had a positive Gram stain with a negative culture. Seventeen of these 25 patients had bladder aspiration and 10 were positive for anaerobes. Compared to the total population, the incidence of anaerobic bacteriuria was about 0.2%. Seven out of 10 of these positive aspirations grew *Bacteroides* species. Urologic disease with surgical and pathologic derangements of normal anatomy was present in 9 of the 10 patients. Alling *et al.*[161] reported anaerobic bacteriuria in 31 of 44 geriatric patients, many of whom had indwelling catheters.

The data, then, on anaerobic bacteria in the urinary tract at this point in time seem to indicate that anaerobes are extremely common and even quite dense on the urethral and vaginal mucosa of normal women. Their role in producing symptoms or disease at these local mucosal sites remains to be proven. As a cause of bacteriuria, anaerobes would seem to be extremely rare and occurring then only in the presence of severe urologic disease. In such instances, however, they may be the responsible organism for serious urologic sepsis and should always be considered when aerobic cultures are sterile.

URINARY INFECTIONS CAUSED BY *Ureaplasma urealyticum*

Ureaplasma urealyticum (T-strain mycoplasma) was first isolated from male patients with nongonococcal urethritis in 1956 by Shepard[162] and Koch's postulates were finally fulfilled by Taylor-Robinson, Csonka, and Prentice[163] in 1977 when they inoculated two different strains of *U. urealyticum*—isolated from men with nongonococcal urethritis—intraurethrally into themselves. While there can be no doubt about *U. urealyticum* causing urethritis in the male, does it cause urinary infection?

The answer is most certainly yes, but we do not know the frequency with which *U. urealyticum* produces urinary infection nor do we know anything about the natural history. It is clearly uncommon. *U. urealyticum* was recovered in 19 of 80 catheterized bladder urines in patients with acute pyelonephritis[164]; urethral swabs prior to catheterization, however, showed *U. urealyticum* in 36 of the 80 patients. When 60 patients with noninfectious urinary tract disease were also catheterized for *U. urealyticum*, 9 were positive but urethral swabs were positive in 24 of the 60 patients.[164] It was apparent to the authors that all of the positive bladder cultures could have been from contamination of the catheter by the presence of *U. urealyticum* in the urethra.

This problem, like the one of anaerobic bacteriuria, can be solved only by suprapubic needle aspiration of the bladder urine. *U. urealyticum* was isolated in 33 of 257 urines (13%) obtained by suprapubic aspiration.[165] In only 15 of these aspirates (6%), however, was *U. urealyticum* recovered in pure culture, unaccompanied by other urinary pathogens.

In March 1978, I saw a 74-year-old lady from Pennsylvania who was referred by Dr. Alexander J. Michie, with urinary frequency, dysuria, urinary incontinence, fatigue, and sterile pyuria. Her symptoms apparently began in late 1977. Dr. Michie aspirated her urine, obtained no growth, and gave the patient a trial of indanyl carbenicillin 0.382 g every 8 hours which greatly relieved her symptoms for a short period. An intravenous urogram was unremarkable in early February 1978 and she was cystoscoped on February 15, 1978. The bladder mucosa was described as markedly injected, slightly edematous, and the submucosal blood vessels were scattered at 0.2- to 0.3-cm intervals over the bladder. The trigone was diffusely injected and edematous, but no submucosal blood vessels were seen in this area. The point of maximum intensity of hyperemia of the bladder was the trigone and especially the inter-ureteric ridge. The ureteral orifices appeared slightly edematous, markedly injected, but effluxed clear urine repeatedly. A cold punch biopsy was taken from the inter-ureteric ridge in the midline of the bladder floor. The biopsy, shown in Figure 4.31, *A* and *B*, shows a severe infiltrate with lymphocytes, plasma cells and some histiocytes. Because of the chronic inflammatory response, schistosomiasis was excluded by a careful search for schistosoma eggs in the urine. Tuberculosis was, of course, excluded by appropriate cultures. A further needle aspiration of the bladder and several voided urines continued to confirm the presence of sterile pyuria.

When I examined her in March 1978, a suprapubic aspiration of the bladder was performed in order to proceed with a sterile pyuria protocol (see section later in this chapter). The centrifuged sediment showed 20–50 glitter cells (polymorphonuclear leukocytes)/hpf; there was no protein in the supernatant urine. Aerobic, anaerobic and L-form cultures were sterile. The culture for *U. urealyticum* grew 1200 colony-forming units/ml of urine.

She was placed on tetracycline 250 mg four times a day for 14 days and returned to Pennsylvania. Follow-up by Dr. Michie revealed immediate improvement in her urinary frequency and return of her physical stamina. Because her urinary frequency did not completely clear until June, Dr. Michie continued her on tetracycline until June 6, 1978. A bladder aspiration showed no *U. urealyticum*, tuberculosis or anaerobes; because of a light growth of *Streptococcus viridans*, however, he elected to continue the tetracycline until July 18, 1978 at which time a urine culture was sterile. On September 6, 1978—7 weeks after cessation of tetracycline therapy—a bladder aspiration showed no WBC, red blood cells (RBC), or casts in the urinary sediment. Culture was sterile. She was voiding five times during the day and zero to one time at night.

In view of the repeated documentation of pyuria, a sterile urine before carbenicillin therapy, the intense inflammatory response of the bladder wall (Figure 4.31, *A* and *B*), the presence of *U. urealyticum* on aspiration before tetracycline therapy, and the failure to reculture *U. urealyticum* after tetracycline therapy argues strongly for the pathogenicity of *U. urealyticum* as the cause of her cystitis. The complete disappearance of her long-standing pyuria probably represents the strongest evidence.

I have documented only one other patient with a pure *U. urealyticum* cystitis. I saw a 21-year-old transplant patient on immunosuppressive therapy who suddenly developed dysuria and sterile pyuria. An aspirated urine grew 44,000 colony forming units/ml of urine for which he received 10 days of tetracycline therapy. His dysuria disappeared almost immediately; bladder aspirations performed at two weeks and three months after completion of tetracy-

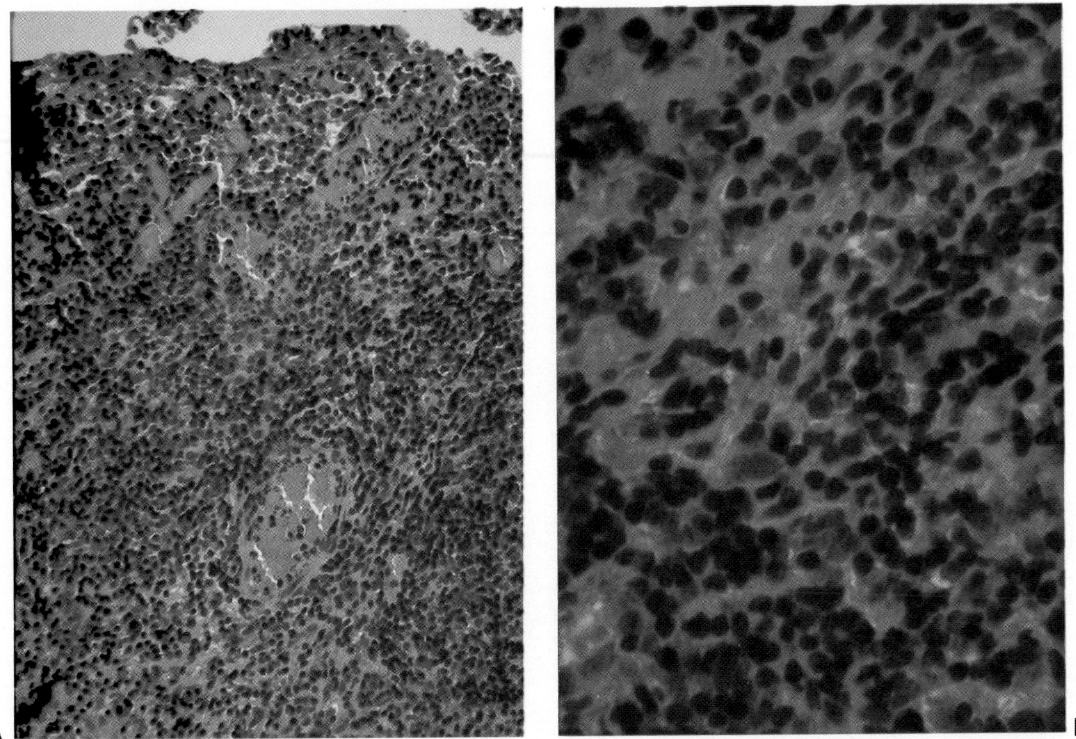

Figure 4.31 *A*, Bladder cup biopsy of a 74-year-old female with *Ureaplasma urealyticum* cystitis (×64). Note the intense infiltrate with lymphocytes, plasma cells, and some histiocytes. Some denuded bladder epithelium is at the top of the microphotograph. *B*, Higher power view (×205) of the chronic lymphocytic reaction. Courtesy of Alexander J. Michie.

cline therapy showed no further *U. urealyticum* on culture, nor were there leukocytes in the spun urine.

ASSESSMENT OF STERILE PYURIA

Sterile pyuria is always a fascinating challenge to the clinician to determine the etiology of the inflammatory response. By "sterile" is meant that routine, aerobic cultures on voided urines are considered negative or insignificant. True pyuria, proven by bladder aspiration, always indicates an inflammatory response somewhere along the uroepithelium of the urinary tract.

Suprapubic needle aspiration of the bladders should be the first discriminating move. If the centrifuged urine contains no leukocytes, the site of the inflammatory reaction is below the internal vesical neck of the bladder in the male or female patient. If the aspirated urine contains leukocytes, even as few as one or two "glitter cells"/hpf in the spun sediment of a hydrated urine, there is an abnormal inflammatory reaction present either in the bladder, ureters, or kidneys; the normal, noninjured urinary tract never has fresh polymorphonuclear cells (glitter cells) on its surface.

If the aspirated urine confirms leukocytes in the bladder, our routine is to culture the aspirate for the usual aerobic and anaerobic bacteria, *Ureaplasma urealyticum*, and for L-form organisms. Despite using this routine for years, we have never had a positive culture for L-form bacteria if the patient was receiving no antibiotics at the time of the suprapubic aspiration.

One-tenth milliliter of urine or more should always be cultured to increase the likelihood of detecting those infections which occur with small numbers of aerobic bacteria, *Candida albicans* or other fungi, as well as anaerobes. One reason for sterile pyuria is the failure to recognize urinary infections with small numbers of pathogenic organisms. If the bladder and/or kidneys are infected with an organism that grows to only 1000 colonies/ml of urine, and the bacteriologic laboratory cultures the urine with a calibrated wire loop which holds 1/1000th of a milliliter, the culture will appear "sterile."

If 0.1 ml of urine is sterile on the aerobic blood agar plates (growing neither bacteria nor fungi), sterile on the anaerobic agar plates, and sterile on the *U. urealyticum* agar and broth, tuberculosis should be excluded by culturing at least three first morning urines for acid-fast bacilli. The physician must constantly remember that any number of pathogenic organisms in the aspirated bladder urine would be highly significant in seeking a cause of the pyuria, and that the 100,000 bacteria/ml as a definition of "significant infection" has no meaning in aspirated bladder urines.

An intravenous urogram, of course, is always indicated in the search for a cause of sterile pyuria. Urinary tract cancers and stones can cause sterile pyuria. Indeed, if the urogram is normal, a voided urine in the male patient or a bladder lavage with saline in the female patient should be sent to cytology to exclude *in-situ* carcinoma. Papillary necrosis from analgesic abuse or diabetes can also cause sterile pyuria.

If all cultures prove to be sterile, and the intravenous urogram is normal, the patient should be cystoscoped to exclude unexpected sources of pyuria such as a foreign body in the bladder undetected in the radiographs. If the urethra and bladder are normal cystoscopically, ureteral urines should be collected after thoroughly washing the bladder; both left and right ureteral urines should be centrifuged and the sediment studied for the presence of leukocytes. Centrifuged renal urines from normal kidneys contain no inflammatory cells, but the ureteral catheter does rub off many renal pelvic epithelial cells into the urine which must not be confused with leukocytes.

The common causes of persistent sterile pyuria found on bladder aspiration are:

1. Aerobic organisms—either Gram-negative or Gram-positive bacteria (*S. saprophyticus*, for example)—that have been interpreted as contaminants in the voided urine cultures because of colony counts less than 100,000/ml of urine
2. Tuberculosis
3. Sterile renal calculi
4. Analgesic abuse nephropathy
5. Urinary tract cancers, especially *in-situ* carcinoma of the bladder
6. *C. albicans*, because of the same misinterpretation as described in number 1 in respect to the aerobic organisms

The less common causes are:

1. *U. urealyticum*
2. Anaerobic bacteria
3. Interstitial cystitis
4. Foreign body

WHEN TO GET AN INTRAVENOUS UROGRAM

Intravenous urograms are critical in the evaluation of patients whose recurrences are due to bacterial persistence in the urinary tract (stones, infected congenital abnormalities, analgesic abuse nephropathy with papillary necrosis, etc.) but they are of almost no value in the 99% of patients with reinfections of the urinary tract. To be sure, the intravenous urogram will identify women with reinfections who have renal scars from pyelonephritis of childhood (as in Figures 4.24 and 4.25), some of whom will have reflux and others not, but since the therapy to prevent infections is the same as in other women with reinfections, the intravenous urogram does not really alter the therapeutic course.

Since many urologists still do not culture urine specimens in their office, and therefore have little opportunity to distinguish bacterial persistence from reinfection as a cause of recurrence, intravenous urograms will continue to be overdone in the large population of women with reinfections of the urinary tract. But even if only the urine sediment is examined, and several months are known to intervene between bacteriuric episodes, bacterial persistence can be excluded and the intravenous urogram will not be helpful.

Mabeck[8] obtained intravenous urograms on 210 of 219 bacteriuric patients referred to him with symptomatic UTI. Renal calculi were found in five cases; "no cases of severe hydronephrosis or hydroureter were found."

William Fair,[166] and his colleagues at Barnes Hospital of Washington University in St. Louis, reviewed the intravenous urograms of 164 consecutive women referred to the Radiology Department because of UTI. In each of these 164 intravenous urograms in which a history of recurrent urinary tract infection was given as the indication for the examination, 144 (88%) were perfectly normal, 11 (6.7%) showed minor anatomic variations and 9 (5.5%) showed positive findings. However, in no patient with a positive intravenous urogram was there a finding that required surgical intervention, nor did the positive finding alter the therapeutic approach. The authors conclude that routine use of the excretory urogram as part of the evaluation of women with a urinary tract infection is "expensive, unrewarding and has little justification." These 164 urograms cost the patients $17,930.

SOME OBSERVATIONS ON "SIGNIFICANT BACTERIURIA"—SUBSTANTIAL LIMITATIONS OF THE 100,000 BACTERIA/ML CONCEPT

I realize it must be clear to most readers that as useful as the $\geq$100,000 bacteria/ml concept has been in epidemiologic studies, there are substantial limitations for the practicing physician who must deal with the individual patient in his practice. I reviewed the theoretical, historical, and observational bases for this concept in Chapter 1; I will not repeat it here except to emphasize that although three consecutive total voided urines with 10^5 or more bacteria/ml have a 95% confidence level (1 out of 20 patients with these counts will not have an infection),[69] these data do not tell the clinician how many of his patients have infection with counts less than 10^5 bacteria/ml.

Suprapubic needle aspiration of the bladder is undoubtedly the ideal way to determine whether or not the urine is infected, and it should be used liberally when there is the slightest question. Thirty-three percent of our bacteriuric women had colony counts less than 10^5 bacteria/ml[96]; although our patients were hydrated prior to bladder aspiration, which might have reduced their bacterial counts, Mabeck's[167] were not and still he found 29% of outpatient women with symptoms of UTI had $<10^5$ bacteria/ml. In our more recent analysis of 145 symptomatic infections in 23 women followed for 15–110 months, 21% of their infections had $<10^5$ bacteria/ml.[9] When McFadyen *et al.*[85] aspirated 2000 pregnant women, 27% of their 132 positive aspirations contained bacteria in colony counts of $<10^5$ bacteria/ml.

Kunz *et al.*,[168] in a very large series of bladder aspirations, found 41% of all culture-positive urines to be $<10^5$ bacteria/ml and 27% were $<10^4$ bacteria/ml. They felt that chemotherapy should be used only in those patients whose infections were proven by bladder aspiration.

All of these data surely indicate that somewhere between 21 and 41% of patients presenting to their physician with urinary infection will have bacterial counts of $<10^5$ bacteria/ml. The problem is clearly substantial and cannot be ignored.

Although a careful examination of the microscopic sediment for the presence of fresh leukocytes in the urine will always add some certainty to the diagnosis in the symptomatic patient, what else can be done—other than bladder aspiration—to increase the clinician's confidence that UTI is present? Carefully collected midstream urines by the nurse, using either our Stanford technique described in Chapter 1 or a similar method described by Hart and Magee[169] but using the toilet or bedpan, is clearly helpful even if troublesome. Pfau and Sacks[170] adopted our technique where the nurse collects the voided urine from the patient on a cystoscopy table; in some excellent studies where all patients had a bladder aspiration before the midstream urine was collected, they compared several different methods of collecting the midstream urine. Without question, the midstream urine collected by the nurse from the patient on the cystoscopy table was far superior to any other technique; their bacterial counts in the voided urine of those patients who had sterile bladder aspirates were not too different from those in Figure 1.7, Chapter 1. Perhaps it should be noted, in addition, that we continue to collect the first voided few milliliters of urine before collecting the midstream specimen. Although this is not practical for most clinicians and adds an additional culture, it increases the confidence limits in deciding whether a low count ($<10^4$ bacteria/ml) represents a bladder infection or urethral contamination of a sterile bladder urine. For example, if the VB_1 is 2000 *E. coli*/ml and the VB_2 50 *E. coli*/ml, the 50 *E. coli* are very likely from the urethra. On the other hand, if the VB_1 and VB_2, collected from the patient on the cystoscopy table, both show 2000 *E. coli*/ml, these *E. coli* are in the bladder and suprapubic aspiration will confirm it.

It should be emphasized that many laboratories reporting quantitative colony counts indicate only the Gram-negative aerobic bacteria, or the Gram-positive organisms if present in pure culture. There is even some merit to this because if *all* the colonies of every species present in the midstream voided urine were counted (lactobacilli, corynebacteria, staphylococci, and streptococci) there would be few midstream urines collected by the patient herself that would not contain $>10^5$ total organisms/ml when the bladder urine is actually sterile. Nevertheless, as I have emphasized in this chapter, this practice of ignoring the normal urethral and introital flora in midstream urine has caused a failure to recognize coagulase-negative staphylococci, β-hemolytic streptococci group B, and other Gram-positive bacteria as infectious agents in symptomatic bacteriuric women.

Lastly, and least desirable because of potential iatrogenic infections, the patient can be catheterized to obtain a less contaminated specimen. I have reviewed Marple's [171] technique and results in Chapter 1, as well as the incidence of catheter-induced infection (Table 1.1). Philpot's[172] excellent study also gives us useful information on the confidence limits of a careful urethral catheterization. He catheterized 50 volunteer normal women; 66% were sterile, 28% contained 1–30 bacteria/ml, and 6% had 30–40 bacteria/ml. *All* the bacteria were counted in 1 ml of urine, and not a single Gram-negative rod or enterococci accounted for the low numbers of contaminating urethral bacteria. If Philpot's or Marple's catheterization technique is used to collect bladder urine from a female, it is clear that 1000 bacteria/ml is a very comfortable confidence limit for separating urinary infection from urethral contamination. As I have said in Chapter 1, if the physician is hesitant to use suprapubic needle aspiration of the bladder, and is confronted with a questionable voided culture, he should catheterize the patient rather than run the risk and expense of treating a nonexistent urinary infection. Hopefully, he will use an excellent catheterization technique, similar to that of Marple[171] or Philpot[172] to increase his confidence limits of detecting a urinary infection. Moreover, he should look at the centrifuged urine sediment of the catheterized urine; if infection is unlikely, he should prophylactically treat the patient for 24 hours with his favorite antimicrobial agent to reduce the chances of an iatrogenic urinary infection.

LACK OF CORRELATION BETWEEN SITE OF INFECTION AND BACTERIAL RECURRENCE WITH CONSECUTIVELY SIMILAR O-SEROGROUPS

Turck *et al.*,[173] using ureteral catheterization to localize the site of infection, reported that 80% of post-treatment recurrences in 29 patients with renal bacteriuria were caused by relapse with the same organism that produced the initial infection; in contrast, 71% of post-treatment recurrences in 25 patients with bladder bacteriuria were caused by reinfection with new organisms. The implication of this study—that the bacteria were persisting in the renal parenchyma in between recurrences in 80% of patients with upper tract infection—was important because persistence of bacteria in the kidney could be recognized by simply identifying two consecutive infections with the same organism ("relapse"). This report, however, did not indicate whether urines were cultured during therapy to insure the presence of a sterile urine or, if they were cultured, what numbers of the original strain of bacteria in the midstream voided urine were acceptable as a definition of cure during therapy. For example, if *any* of the original bacteria were present in the midstream urine, the patient should be classified as a failure of therapy (an unresolved bacteriuria in our classification) rather than a recurrence of bacteriuria. Moreover, the time interval between consecutive recurrences with the same organism was not stated in this paper, although I know the authors intended to mean about a 2-week period.

The important issue here is whether consecutive infections with the same strain really indicate bacterial persistence in the kidney. There are several compelling reasons why this is unlikely. The first reason is that there seems to be no relationship between radiologic abnormalities (excluding stones, congenital anomalies, and papillary necrosis) and the pattern of bacterial recurrence. For example, Guttmann[11] analyzed the pattern of "relapse" and reinfection in relation to radiologic findings; he found that those patients who had pyelonephritic scarring showed a smaller proportion of relapses than those who had normal intravenous urograms. In children, where pyelonephritic scarring and reflux are seen the most often, it has long been recognized that reinfection is equally common in those with renal reflux as in those without.[174] Hence, if bacterial persistence in the kidney (relapse as used by Turck *et al.*[173]) after therapy was truly a clinical problem, we would expect to see it most of all in those patients who have the most serious pyelonephritic scarring; this is clearly not the case.

Second, if bacterial persistence in the kidney is a problem following therapy, then the frequency of bacterial recurrences should be greater in those patients with radiologic abnormalities. In fact, Kunin[175] in children and Guttmann[11] in adults were both unable to show any relationship between the frequency of bacteriuric recurrences after therapy and the presence of radiologic abnormalities.

Third, if bacterial persistence in the kidney is a major problem after therapy, those patients who have five or more recurrences within a specific follow-up period should have more recurrences with the same organism than those patients who have less frequent recurrences. Stated another way, as the number of consecutive recurrences increase in a population under study, the number of reinfections should decline while the "relapses" should increase. Mabeck[8] has analyzed this nicely; with increasing number of recurrences, the relation between treatment failure, relapse, and reinfection remained unchanged (Table 4.38).

Fourth, using fluorescent antibody-coated bacteria in adults to distinguish renal from bladder infection, Forland *et al.*[124] observed the pattern of recurrence in diabetics, while Harris *et al.*[92] observed the post-treatment recurrences in bacteriuria of pregnancy. In the former study, 10 of 15 patients who were initially FA+, recurred with a different species or serotype, eight of which were FA−, three recurred with the same organism, two of which were uncoated and one coated with antibody. In the study by Harris *et al.*[92] on antibody-coated bacteria in pregnant patients with bacteriuria, there were 14 recurrences among 35 FA− bacteriurics; 10 of the 14 were reinfection, not "relapses."

Fifth, Cattell *et al.*[176] also used our technique of ureteral catheterization to localize the site of bacteriuria in 42 patients who were followed for 6 months after therapy.

Table 4.38
Relationship Between the Number of Recurrences and the Pattern of Bacterial Reappearance[a]

Infection No.	No. of Recurrences[b]	Failure[c]	Relapse[d]	Reinfection[e]
		%	%	%
First	27	4	37	59
Second	33	3	24	73
Third	26	4	31	65
Fourth	22	5	31	64
Fifth, and Subsequent	105	10	27	64

[a] Modified from C. E. Mabeck.[8]
[b] No. of recurrences during 5 months of observation.
[c] Failure = persistence of bacteriuria during treatment.
[d] Relapse = recurrence with bacteria of the same serotype and species as found before treatment. Mabeck used the term "recrudescence".
[e] Reinfection = recurrence with a different organism.

They analyzed the response to standard short term therapy of 2 weeks duration; they cultured all patients on the 3rd, 4th, and 5th days of therapy as well as multiple cultures after completion of treatment. Sixteen of the 26 patients who were rendered abacteriuric recurred with the same organism; 8 had upper tract infection and 8 bladder infection. These authors concluded that localization studies were of no predictive value in planning the management of patients with recurrent bacteriuria.

In a recent study where C-reactive protein and other parameters were used to separate acute pyelonephritis from lower tract infection in children,[177] 10 days of therapy in both groups produced an equal number of reinfections—25% and 32%, respectively—and the same number of relapses, 6% and 4%.

The practice of assigning those bacteriurias which recur with the same strain within a 14-day time period as a "relapse" from the kidney assumes that early recurrences are more likely to be of the same strain. I have commented elsewhere in this chapter on how rapidly reinfections can occur (Figure 4.9). We have additional data on this point. In an earlier section of this chapter, the Effect of Nalidixic Acid on Vaginal and Fecal *E. coli*, I presented some data on 54 women who were treated with 4 g a day of nalidixic acid.[43] The urine was *sterilized* in 51 of these women during therapy, including a sterile culture within the 1st week after therapy, but there were 12 women whose bacteriuria recurred with nalidixic acid-sensitive bacteria within the next 3 weeks. Six of these recurrences were of the same serotype as the original bacteriuric strain and 6 were clearly different O-serogroups. The time elapse between the last day of nalidixic acid therapy and the first day the recurrent bacteriuria was detected was 7, 14, 22, 23, 23, and 29 days for those who recurred with the same strain and 12, 12, 15, 15, 24, and 28 days for those with different O-serogroups. One must conclude that the rapidity of bacterial recurrence with the same O-serogroup in women without stones or urinary obstruction cannot be a basis for implying renal persistence in using the term "relapse."

Between 1960 and 1970, our group at Stanford localized several hundred urinary infections before treatment. We soon realized that in the nonobstructed, bacteriuric woman who had neither calculi, papillary necrosis, nor congenital anomalies on intravenous urography, localization of the urinary infection made no difference in our management. We found that upper tract infections were no more difficult to cure with 10 days of appropriate antimicrobial therapy that sterilized the urine than were those infections confined to the bladder.

If our impressions and these data I have reviewed are correct, it does not appear that "relapse" from the kidney is a common cause of bacterial recurrence. In fact, in the absence of renal stones, obstruction, papillary necrosis, and congenital anomalies, I do not believe bacteria persist in the kidney in between bacteriuric recurrences.

The difficulty with the term "relapse," at least in this country, is that it implies bacterial persistence in the kidney. Relapse would be an excellent term if it meant two consecutive bacteriuric infections with the identical strain or serotype regardless of the time elapse between bacteriuric episodes and if it carried no connotation or inference as to where the bacteria persisted during the interval of observation. Precisely because relapse does carry the implication of bacterial persistence in the kidney when the time interval between infections is 2 weeks or less, I think it should not be used or, at the very least, redefined as I have just discussed. Indeed, Mabeck[8] used the term recrudescence to indicate a recurrence with the same species and serotype as present before treatment but he wisely did not imply the interim site of the recrudescent organism. I would like to suggest that when we know an infection has remained in the urinary tract in between two episodes of urinary infection—regardless of how long the interval of a sterile urine—that we use the term bacterial persistence. We can even name the organ where the bacteria are thought to have persisted; for example, bacteria can persist in the kidney in the presence of stones or necrotic papillae, or in the prostate in patients with chronic bacterial prostatitis (see Chapter 7). I believe the term bacterial persistence is the proper expression when the urine has been sterilized but the organisms remain somewhere within the urinary tract.

If the term relapse is to continue to be used, we should use it in the European sense without time limit between recurrences and without implication of where the bacteria resided in between recurrent infections. Lastly, it should be apparent that since introital colonization is the major determinant of recurrent UTI, even if the kidney is shown to be the site of the recurrence with the same O-serogroup that caused the first infection, frequent introital cultures during the 14-day time limit will be required to convince me that the site of bacterial persistence in between infections is not the introitus. The patient shown in Figure 4.7 is an excellent example of continuous introital colonization with the identical O-serogroup (075) which caused three consecutive recurrent infections with the same *E. coli* 075.

REFERENCES

1. Kass, E. H., Savage, W. D., and Santamarina, B. A. G.: The significance of bacteriuria in preventive medicine. In E. H. Kass (Ed.), Progress in Pyelonephritis. Philadelphia, F. A. Davis & Co., 1964, p. 3.
2. Freedman, L. R., Phair, J. P., Seki, M., Hamilton, H. B., Nefzger, M. D., and Hirata, M.: The epidemiology of urinary tract infections in Hiroshima. Yale J. Biol. Med. **37:** 262, 1965.
3. Kunin, C. M., and McCormack, R. C.: An epidemiologic study of bacteriuria and blood pressure among nuns and working women. N. Engl. J. Med. **278:** 635, 1968.
4. Marple, C. D.: The frequency and character of urinary tract infections in an unselected group of women. Ann. Intern. Med. **14:** 2220, 1941.
5. Kass, E. H.: The role of asymptomatic bacteriuria in the pathogenesis of pyelonephritis. In E. L. Quinn and E. H. Kass (Eds.), Biology of Pyelonephritis. Boston. Little, Brown & Co., 1960, p. 399.
6. Gaymans, R., Haverkorn, M. J. Valkenburg, H. A., and Goslings, W. R. O.: A prospective study of urinary-tract infections in a Dutch general practice. Lancet **2:** 674, 1976.
7. Harrison, W. O., Holmes, K. K., Belding, M. E., Wiesner, P. J., and Turck, M.: A prospective evaluation of recurrent urinary tract infection in women. Clin. Res. **22:** 125A, 1974.
8. Mabeck, C. E.: Treatment of uncomplicated urinary tract infection in nonpregnant women. Postgrad. Med. J., **48:** 69, 1972.
9. Kraft, J. K., and Stamey, T. A.: The natural history of symptomatic recurrent bacteriuria in women. Medicine **56:** 55, 1977.
10. Stamey, T. A., Timothy, M., Millar, M., and Mihara, G.: Recurrent urinary infections in adult women. The role of introital enterobacteria. Calif. Med., **115:** 1, 1971.
11. Guttmann, D.: Follow-up of urinary tract infections in domiciliary patients. In Urinary Tract Infection. Chap. 8 Proceedings of the Second National Symposium held in London, 1972, Oxford University Press, 1973, p. 62.

12. Vosti, K. L.: Recurrent urinary tract infections. Prevention by prophylactic antibiotics after sexual intercourse. J. Am. Med. Assoc. **231:** 934, 1975.
13. Gallagher, D. J. A., Montgomerie, J. Z., and North, J. D. K.: Acute infections of the urinary tract and the urethral syndrome in general practice. Br. Med. J., **1:** 622, 1965.
14. O'Grady, F. W., Charlton, C. A. C., Fry, K. I., McSherry, A., and Cattell, W. R.: Natural history of intractable "cystitis" in women referred to a special clinic. In W. Brumfitt and A. W. Asscher (Eds.), Urinary Tract Infection, London, Oxford University Press, 1973, p. 81.
15. Stamey, T. A.: Urinary Infections. Williams & Wilkins, Baltimore, 1972.
16. Stamey, T. A.: The role of introital enterobacteria in recurrent urinary infections. J. Urol., **109:** 467, 1973.
17. Stamey, T. A., and Howell, J. J.: Studies of introital colonization in women with recurrent urinary infections. IV. The role of local vaginal antibodies. J. Urol., **115:** 413, 1976.
18. Stamey, T. A., and Kaufman, M. F.: Studies of introital colonization in women with recurrent urinary infections. II. A comparison of growth in normal vaginal fluid of common versus uncommon serogroups of *Escherichia coli.* J. Urol. **114:** 264, 1975.
19. Stamey, T. A., and Mihara, G.: Studies of introital colonization in women with recurrent urinary infections. V. The inhibitory activity of normal vaginal fluid in *Proteus mirabilis* and *Pseudomonas aeruginosa.* J. Urol., **115:** 416, 1976.
20. Stamey, T. A., and Timothy, M. M.: Studies of introital colonization in women with recurrent urinary infections. I. The role of vaginal pH. J. Urol. **114:** 261, 1975.
21. Stamey, T. A., and Timothy, M. M.: Studies of introital colonization in women with recurrent urinary infections. III. Vaginal glycogen concentrations. J. Urol. **114:** 268, 1975.
22. Bailey, R. R., Roberts, A. P., Gower, P. E., and DeWardener, H. E.: Prevention of urinary-tract infection with low-dose nitrofurantoin. Lancet **2:** 1112, 1971.
23. Kasanen, A., Toivanen, P., Sourander, L., Kaarsalo, E. and Aantaa, S.: Trimethoprim in the treatment and long-term control of urinary tract infection. Scand. J. Infect. Dis. **6:** 91, 1974.
24. Stamey, T. A., Condy, M., and Mihara, G.: Prophylactic efficacy of nitrofurantoin macrocrystals and trimethoprim-sulfamethoxazole in urinary infections. N. Engl. J. Med. **296:** 780, 1977.
25. Grüneberg, R. N., Leigh, D. A., Brumfitt, W.: *Escherichia coli* serotypes in urinary tract infection: studies in domiciliary, antenatal and hospital practice. In F. O'Grady, W. Brumfitt (Eds.), Urinary Tract Infection. p. 68. London, Oxford, Univ. Press, 1968.
26. von Rütte, V. B., and Delnon, I.: Die urethralzytologie und ihre bedeutung zur diagnose hormonal bedingter miktionsstörungen. Praxis **57:** 555, 1968.
27. Stamey, T. A., and Sexton, C. C.: The role of vaginal colonization with Enterobacteriaceae in recurrent urinary infections. J. Urol., **113:** 214, 1975.
28. Schaeffer, A. J., and Stamey, T. A.: Studies of introital colonization in women with recurrent urinary infections. IX. The role of antimicrobial therapy. J. Urol., **118:** 221, 1977.
29. Bollgren I. and Winberg, J.: The periurethral aerobic flora in girls highly susceptible to urinary infections. Acta Paediatr. Scand. **65:** 81, 1976.
30. Lincoln, K., Lidin-Janson, G., and Winberg, J.: Resistant urinary infections resulting from changes in the resistance pattern of fecal flora induced by antibiotics and hospital environment. Br. Med. J. **3:** 305, 1970.
31. Winberg, J., Bergström, T., Lincoln, K., and Lidin-Janson, G.: Treatment trials in urinary tract infection (UTI) with special reference to the effect of antimicrobials on the fecal and periurethral flora. Clin. Nephrol. **1:** 142, 1973.
32. Bergstrom, T., Lincoln, K., Redin, B., and Winberg, J.: Studies or urinary tract infections in infancy and childhood. X. Short or long-term treatment in girls with first or second time urinary tract infections uncomplicated by obstructive urological abnormalities. Acta Paediatr. Scand. **57:** 186, 1968.
33. Grüneberg, R. N., Smellie, J. M., Leaky, A.: Changes in the antibiotic sensitivities of faecal organisms in response to treatment in children with urinary tract infection. In W. Brumfitt and A. W. Asscher (Eds.), Urinary Tract Infection. London, Oxford University Press, 1973, p. 131.
34. Toivanen, A., Kasanen, A., Sundquist, H., and Toivanen, P.: Effect of trimethoprim on the occurrence of drug-resistant coliform bacteria in the faecal flora. Chemotherapy **22:** 97, 1976.
35. Datta, J., Faiers, M. C., and Reeves, D. S. *et al.*: R-factors in *Escherichia coli* in feces after oral chemotherapy in general practice. Lancet **1:** 312, 1971.
36. Hinton, N. A.: The effect of oral tetracycline HCl and doxycycline on the intestinal flora. Curr. Ther. Res. Clin. Exp. **12:** 341, 1970.
37. Ronald, A. R., Jagdis, F. A., Harding, G. K., Hoban, S., Muir, P., and Gurwith, M.: Amoxicillin therapy of acute urinary infections in adults. Antimicrobial Agents and Chemotherapy. **11:** 780, 1977.
38. Sharp, J. L.: The growth of *Candida albicans* during antibiotic therapy. Lancet **1:** 390, 1954.

39. Daikos, G. K., Kontomichalou, P., Bilalis, D., and Pimenidou, L.: Intestinal flora ecology after oral use of antibiotics. Chemotherapy **13:** 146, 1968.
40. Näff, H.: Über die Veränderungen der normalen Darmflora des Menschen durch Bactrim. Pathol. Microbiol. **37:** 1, 1971.
41. Knothe, H.: The effect of a combined preparation of trimethoprim and sulphamethoxazole following short-term and long-term administration on the flora of the human gut. Chemotherapy **18:** 285, 1973.
42. Moorehouse, E. C., and Farrell, W.: Effect of co-trimoxazole on faecal enterobacteria: No emergence of resistant strains. J. Med. Microbiol. **6:** 249, 1973.
43. Stamey, T. A., and Mihara, G.: The effect of nalidixic acid on faecal and vaginal carriage of Enterobacteriaceae in 54 women. In D. van der Waaij and J. Verhoef, (Eds.), New Criteria for Antimicrobial Therapy: Maintenance of Digestive Tract Colonization Resistance. Proceedings of a Symposium. Utrecht, 1979. Excerpta Medica, 1979, p. 234.
44. Stamey, T. A., Bushby, S. R. M. and Bragonje, J.: The concentration of trimethoprim in prostatic fluid: nonionic diffusion or active transport? J. Infect. Dis. **128:**S 686, 1973.
45. Stamey, T. A., and Condy, M.: The diffusion and concentration of trimethoprim in human vaginal fluid. J. Infect. Dis. **131:** 261, 1975.
46. Hoyme, U., Baumueller, A., and Madsen, P. O.: Antibiotics excretion in canine vaginal and urethral secretions. Invest. Urol. **16:** 35, 1978.
47. Hoyme, U., Baumueller, A., and Madsen, P. O.: Rosamicin in urethral and vaginal secretions and tissues in dogs and rats. Antimicrob. Agents and Chemother. **12:** 237, 1977.
48. Grüneberg, R. N., Smellie, J. M., Leaky, A., *et al:* Long-term low-dose cotrimoxazole in prophylaxis of childhood urinary tract infection: bacteriological aspects. Br. Med. J. **2:** 206, 1976.
49. Harding, G. K. M., Ronald, A. R.: A controlled study of antimicrobial prophylaxis of recurrent urinary infection in women. N. Engl. J. Med. **291:** 597, 1974.
50. Bailey, R. R., Roberts, A. P., Gower, P. E., and Stacey, G.: Urinary-tract infection in nonpregnant women. Lancet **2:** 275, 1973.
51. Kasanen, A., Anttila, M., Elfving, R., Kahela, P., Saarimaa, H., Sundquist, H., Tikkanen, R., and Toivanen, P.: Trimethoprim: Pharmacology, antimicrobial activity and clinical use in urinary tract infections. Ann. Clin. Res. **10:** (Suppl. 22): 1, 1978.
52. Ronald, A. R., Harding, G. K. M., Mathias, R., *et al:* Prophylaxis of recurring urinary tract infection in females: a comparison of nitrofurantoin with trimethoprim-sulfamethoxazole. Can. Med. Assoc. J. **112:** Suppl 13, 1975.
53. Smellie, J. M., Grüneberg, R. N., Leakey, A. *et al.:* Long-term low-dose co-trimoxazole in prophylaxis of childhood urinary tract infection: Clinical aspects. Br. Med. J. **2:** 203, 1976.
54. Asscher, A. W., Sussman, M., Waters, W. E., Evans, J. A. S., Campbell, H., Evans, K. T., and Williams, J. E.: The clinical significance of asymptomatic bacteriuria in the nonpregnant woman. J. Infect. Dis. **120:** 17, 1969.
55. MacDonald, R. A., Levitin, H., Mallory, G. K., and Kass, E. H.: Relation between pyelonephritis and bacterial counts in the urine. N. Engl. J. Med. **256:** 915, 1957.
56. Heptinstall, R. H.: The limitations of the pathological diagnosis of chronic pyelonephritis. In D. A. K. Black (Ed.), Renal Disease, Ed. 2, Chap. 14. Philadelphia, F. A. Davis Co., 1967, p. 350.
57. Beeson, P. B.: Urinary tract infection and pyelonephritis. In D. A. K. Black (Ed.), Renal Disease, Ed. 2, Chap. 15. Philadelphia, F. A. Davis & Co., 1967, p. 382.
58. Kimmelstiel, P., Kim, O. J., Beres, J. A., and Wellman, K.: Chronic pyelonephritis. Am. J. Med. **30:** 589, 1961.
59. Kimmelstiel, P.: The nature of chronic pyelonephritis. Geriatrics **19:** 145, 1964.
60. Freedman, L. R.: Chronic pyelonephritis at autopsy. Ann. Intern. Med. **66:** 697, 1967.
61. Angell, M. E., Relman, A. S., and Robbins, S. L.: "Active" chronic pyelonephritis without evidence of bacterial infection. N. Engl. J. Med. **278:** 1303, 1968.
62. Sussman, M., Asscher, A. W., Waters, W. E., Evans, J. A. S., Campbell, H., Evans, K. T., and Williams, J. E.: Asymptomatic significant bacteriuria in the nonpregnant woman. I. Description of a population. Br. Med. J. **1:** 799, 1969.
63. Asscher, A. W., Sussman, M., Waters, W. E., Evans, J. A. S., Campbell, H., Evans, K. T., and Williams, J. E.: Asymptomatic significant bacteriuria in the nonpregnant woman. II. Response to treatment and follow-up. Br. Med. J. **1:** 804, 1969.
64. Kass, E. H., Miall, W. E., and Stuart, K. L.: Relationship of bacteriuria to hypertension: An epidemiological study. J. Clin. Invest. **40:** 1053, 1961.
65. Asscher, A. W., Chick, S., Radford, N. *et al.:* Natural history of asymptomatic bacteriuria (ASB) in non-pregnant women. In W. Brumfitt and A. W. Asscher. (Eds.), Urinary Tract Infection. London, Oxford University Press, 1973, p. 51.
66. Kass, E. H.: Asymptomatic infections of the urinary tract. Trans. Assoc. Amer. Phys. **69:** 56, 1956.
67. Kass, E. H.: The role of asymptomatic bacteri-

uria in the pathogenesis of pyelonephritis. In E. L. Quinn and E. H. Kass (Eds.), Biology of Pyelonephritis. Boston, Little Brown & Co., 1960, p. 399.
68. Miall, W. E., Kass, E. H., Ling, J., and Stuart, K. L.: Factors influencing arterial pressure in the general population in Jamaica. Br. Med. J. **2:** 497, 1962.
69. Savage, W. E., Hajj, S. N., and Kass, E. H.: Demographic and prognostic characteristics of bacteriuria in pregnancy. Medicine **46:** 385, 1967.
70. Pometta, D., Rees, S. B., Younger, D., and Kass, E. H.: Asymptomatic bacteriuria in diabetes mellitus. N. Engl. J. Med. **276:** 1118, 1967.
71. Whalley, P. J., Martin, F. G., and Peters, P. C.: Significance of asymptomatic bacteriuria detected during pregnancy. J. Am. Med. Assoc. **193:** 879, 1965.
72. Johnson, C. W. and Smythe, C. M.: Renal function in patients with chronic bacteriuria: A longitudinal study. South. Med. J. **62:** 81, 1969.
73. Savage, W. E., Hajj, S. N., and Kass, E. H.: Demographic and prognostic characteristics of bacteriuria in pregnancy. Medicine **46:** 385, 1967.
74. Kass, E. H.: Hormones and host resistance to infection. Bacteriol. Rev. **24:** 177, 1960.
75. Kincaid-Smith, P., and Bullen, M.: Bacteriuria in pregnancy. Lancet **1:** 395, 1965.
76. Whalley, P. J.: Bacteriuria in pregnancy. In E. H. Kass (Ed.), Progress in Pyelonephritis. Philadelphia, F. A. Davis Co., 1965, p. 50.
77. Little, P. J.: The incidence of urinary infection in 5000 pregnant women. Lancet **2:** 925, 1966.
78. Whalley, P. J.: Bacteriuria of pregnancy. Am. J. Obstet. Gynecol. **97:** 723, 1967.
79. Wilson, M. G., Hewitt, W. L., and Monzon, O. T.: Effect of bacteriuria on the fetus. N. Engl. J. Med. **274:** 1115, 1966.
80. Condie, A. P., Williams, J. D., Reeves, D. S., and Brumfitt, W.: Complications of bacteriuria in pregnancy. In F. O'Grady and W. Brumfitt (Eds.), Urinary Tract Infection. London, Oxford University Press, 1968, p. 148.
81. Brumfitt, W., Grüneberg, R. N., and Leigh, D. A.: Bacteriuria in pregnancy, with reference to prematurity and long-term effects on the mother. In Symposium on Pyelonephritis. Edinburgh & London, E. & S. Livingstone, 1967, p. 20.
82. Eykyn, S. J., and McFadyen, I. R.: Suprapubic aspiration of urine in pregnancy. In F. O'Grady and W. Brumfitt (Eds.), Urinary Tract Infection. London, Oxford University Press, 1968, p. 141.
83. Elder, H. A., Santamarina, B. A. G., Smith, S., and Kass, E. H.: The natural history of asymptomatic bacteriuria during pregnancy; The effect of tetracycline on the clinical course and the outcome of pregnancy. Am. J. Obstet. Gynecol. **111:** 441, 1971.
84. Turck, M., Goffe, B. S., and Petersdorf, R. G.: Bacteriuria of pregnancy; relation to socioeconomic factors. N. Engl. J. Med. **266:** 857, 1962.
85. McFadyen, I. R., Eykyn, S. J., Gardner, N. H. N., Vanier, T. M., Bennett, A. E., Mayo, M. E., and Lloyd-Davies, R. W.: Bacteriuria in pregnancy. J. Obstet. Gynaecol. Br. Emp. **80:** 385, 1973.
86. Williams, J. D., Reeves, D. S., Brumfitt, W., and Condie, A. P.: The effects of bacteriuria in pregnancy on maternal health. In W. Brumfitt and A. W. Asscher, (Eds.), Urinary Tract Infections. London, Oxford University Press 1973, p. 103.
87. Mortimer, W. C., Mobbs, G. A., Boulton, J., and Roberts, A. P.: The bacterial content of the female urethra in pregnancy. J. Obstet. Gynaecol. Br. Emp. **74:** 579, 1967.
88. Hundley, J. M., Walton, H. J., Hibbitts, J. T., Siegel, I. A., and Brack, C. B.: Physiologic changes occurring in the urinary tract during pregnancy. Am. J. Obstet. Gynecol. **30:** 625, 1935.
89. Fairley, K. F., Bond, A. G., and Adey, F. D.: The site of infection in pregnancy bacteriuria. Lancet **1:** 939, 1966.
90. Gower, P. E., Haswell, B., Sidaway, M. E., and de Wardener, H. E.: Follow-up of 164 patients with bacteriuria of pregnancy. Lancet **1:** 990, 1968.
91. Kaitz, A. L.: Urinary concentrating ability in pregnant women with asymptomatic bacteriuria. J. Clin. Invest. **40:** 1331, 1961.
92. Harris, R. E., Thomas, V. L., and Shelokov, A.: Asymptomatic bacteriuria in pregnancy: Antibody-coated bacteria, renal function, and intrauterine growth retardation. Am. J. Obstet. Gynecol. **126:** 20, 1976.
93. Zinner, S. H., and Kass, E. H.: Long-term (10 to 14 years) follow-up of bacteriuria of pregnancy. N. Engl. J. Med. **285:** 820, 1971.
94. Heidrick, W. P., Mattingly, R. F., and Amberg, J. R.: Vesicoureteral reflux in pregnancy. Obstet. Gynecol. **29:** 571, 1967.
95. Williams, G. L., Davies, D. K. L., Evans, K. T., and Williams, J. E.: Vesicoureteric reflux in patients with bacteriuria in pregnancy. Lancet **2:** 1202, 1968.
96. Stamey, T. A., Govan, D. E., and Palmer, J. M.: The localization and treatment of urinary tract infections: The role of bactericidal urine levels as opposed to serum levels. Medicine **44:** 1, 1965.
97. Vosti, K. L.: Recurrent urinary tract infections. Prevention by prophylactic antibiotics after sexual intercourse. J. Am. Med. Assoc. **231:** 934, 1975.
98. Bran, J. L., Levison, M. E., and Kaye, D.: Entrance of bacteria into the female urinary bladder. N. Engl. J. Med. **286:** 626, 1972.
99. Buckley, R. M., Jr., McGuckin, M., and Mac-

Gregor, R. R.: Urine bacterial counts after sexual intercourse. N. Engl. J. of Med. **298:** 321, 1978.
100. Harding, G., Thompson, L., Preiksaitis, J., Hoban, S., and Ronald, A.: Acquisition of bacteriuria: the role of sexual intercourse. Ann. R. Coll. Physicians Surg. Can. In press, 1980
101. Schechter, H., Leonard, C. D., and Scribner, B. H.: Chronic pyelonephritis as a cause of renal failure in dialysis candidates. Analysis of 173 patients. J. Am. Med. Assoc. **216:** 514, 1971.
102. Murray, T., and Goldberg, M.: Chronic interstitial nephritis: Etiology factors. Ann. Intern. Med. **82:** 453, 1975.
103. Gower, P. E.: A prospective study of patients with radiological pyelonephritis, papillary necrosis and obstructive atrophy. Q. J. Med. **45:** 315, 1976.
104. Asscher, A. W.: The Challenge of Urinary Tract Infection. New York, Academic Press, 1980.
105. Freedman, L. R.: Prolonged observations on a group of patients with acute urinary tract infections. In E. L. Quinn and E. H. Kass (Eds.), Biology of Pyelonephritis. Boston, Little Brown & Co., 1960, p. 345.
106. Pratt, V.: Long term follow-up of patients with urinary tract infection. In J. Vostal and G. Richet (Eds.), Proceedings of 2nd International Congress Nephrology, Basel, S. Karger, 1963, p. 313.
107. Little, P. J., McPherson, L. R., and de Wardener, H. E.: The significance of the long-term antibacterial treatment in chronic pyelonephritis. Lancet **1:** 1186, 1965.
108. Freedman, L. R.: Long term follow-up of urinary infections. In Abstracts of 5th International Congress Nephrology, Mexico. Basel, S. Karger, 1972, p. 25.
109. Asscher, A. W., Chick, S., Radford, N., Waters, W. E., Sussman, M., Evans, J. A. S., McLachlan, M. S. F., and Williams, J. E.: Natural history of asymptomatic bacteriuria (ASB) in non-pregnant women. In W. Brumfitt and A. W. Asscher (Eds.), Urinary Tract Infection. London, Oxford University Press, 1973, p. 51.
110. Bullen, M.: A ten year follow-up study of patients with bacteriuria in pregnancy. In Abstracts of 6th International Congress Nephrology, Florence. Basel, S. Karger, 589, 1975, Abstr. p. 589.
111. Freeman, R. B., Smith, W. M., and Richardson, J. A. *et al.:* Long-term therapy for chronic bacteriuria in men. U. S. Public Health Service Cooperative Study, Ann. Intern. Med. **83:** 133, 1975.
112. Mabeck, C. E.: Studies in urinary tract infections. VI. Significance of clinical symptoms. Acta Med. Scand. **190:** 267, 1971.
113. Parker, J., and Kunin, C.: Pyelonephritis in young women. A 10- to 20-year follow-up. J. Am. Med. Assoc. **224:** 585, 1973.
114. Crabtree, E. G., Prather, G. C., and Prien, E. L.: End results of urinary tract infections associated with pregnancy. Am. J. Obstet. Gynecol. **34:** 405, 1937.
115. Crabtree, E. G., and Prien, E. L.: The nature of renal injury in acute and chronic colon bacillus pyelonephritis in relation to hypertension: A combined clinical and pathological study. J. Urol. **42:** 982, 1939.
116. Crabtree, E. G., and Reid, D.: Pregnancy pyelonephritis in relation to renal damage and hypertension. Am. J. Obstet. Gynecol. **40:** 17, 1940.
117. Bailey, R. R., Little, P. J., and Rolleston, G. L.: Renal damage after acute pyelonephritis. Br. Med. J. **1:** 550, 1969.
118. Davies, A. G., McLachlan, M. S. F., and Asscher, A. W.: Progressive kidney damage after non-obstructive urinary tract infection. Br. Med. J. **4:** 406, 1972.
119. Pfau, A., and Rosenmann, E.: Unilateral chronic pyelonephritis and hypertension: coincidental or causal relationship? Am. J. Med. **65:** 499, 1978.
120. Rocha, H., and Santos, L. C. S.: Relapse of urinary tract infection in the presence of urinary tract calculi: The role of bacteria within the calculi. J. Med. Microbiol. **2:** 372, 1969.
121. Friedland, G. W., and Stamey, T. A.: Recurrent urinary tract infection: With persistent Wolffian duct masquerading as duplicated urethra. Urology **4:** 315, 1974.
122. Leonard, C. D., Cutler, R. E., Johnson, J. T., Striker, G. E., and Turck, M.: Bacteriuria in noninfectious renal disease. Am. J. Med. Sci. **258:** 230, 1969.
123. Arger, P. H., Goldberg, M., Bluth, E. I., and Murray, T.: Analgesic abuse nephropathy. Urology **7:** 123, 1976.
124. Forland, M., Thomas, V., and Shelokov, A.: Urinary tract infections in patients with diabetes mellitus. Studies on antibody coating of bacteria. J. Am. Med. Assoc. **238:** 1924, 1977.
125. Vejlsgaard, R.: Studies on urinary infections in diabetes. IV. Significant bacteriuria in pregnancy in relation to age of onset, duration of diabetes, angiopathy and urological symptoms. Acta Med. Scand. **193:** 337, 1973.
126. Ooi, B. S., Chen, B. T. M., and Yu, M.: Prevalence and site of bacteriuria in diabetes mellitus. Postgrad. Med. J. **50:** 497, 1974.
127. Freiha, F. S., Messing, E. M., and Gross, D. M.: Emphysematous pyelonephritis. J. Contin. Ed. Urol. Digest **18:** 9, 1979.
128. Schainuck, L. I., Fouty, R., and Cutler, R. E.: Emphysematous pyelonephritis. A new case and review of previous observations. Am. J. Med. **44:** 134, 1968.
129. Turman, A. E., and Rutherford, C.: Emphysematous pyelonephritis with perinephric gas. J. Urol. **105:** 165, 1971.

130. Dunn, S. R., De Wolf, W. C., and Gonzales, R.: Emphysematous pyelonephritis: Report of 3 cases treated by nephrectomy. J. Urol. **114:** 348 , 1975.
131. Thorley, J. D., Jones, S. R., and Sanford, J. P.: Perinephric abscess. Medicine **53:** 441, 1974.
132. O'Grady, F. W., Richard, B, McSherry, M. A., O'Farrell, S. M., and Cattell, W. R.: Introital enterobacteria, urinary infection, and the urethral syndrome. Lancet **2:** 1208, 1970.
133. Bruce, A. W., Chadwick, P., Seddon, J. M., and Vancott, G. F.: The significance of perineal pathogens in women. J. Urol. **112:** 808, 1974.
134. Colleen, S., Luttropp, W., Mårdh, P-A., and Ripa, T.: The microbial flora of the urogenital tract in women with symptoms of recurrent urinary tract infection. The non-influence of methenaminehippurate treatment on the indigenous flora. Invest. Urol. **15:** 367, 1978.
135. Maskell, R., Pead, L., and Allen, J.: The puzzle of "urethral syndrome": a possible answer? Lancet **1:** 1058, 1979.
136. Geckler, R. W., Standiford, H. C., Calia, F. M., Kramer, H. C., and Hornick, R. B.: Anaerobic bacteriuria in a male urologic outpatient population. J. Urol. **118:** 800, 1977.
137. Bartlett, J. G., Onderdonk, A. B., Durde, E., Goldstein, C., Anderka, M., Alpert, S., and McCormack, W. M.: Quantitative bacteriology of the vaginal flora. J. Infect. Dis. **136:** 271, 1977.
138. Brooks, D., and Maudar, A.: Pathogenesis of the urethral syndrome in women and its diagnosis in general practice. Lancet **2:** 893, 1972.
139. Gordon, A. M., Hughes, H. E., and Barr, G. T. D.: Bacterial flora in abnormalities of the female genital tract. J. Clin. Pathol. **19:** 429, 1966.
140. Dans, P. E. and Klaus, B.: Dysuria in women. Johns Hopkins Med. J. **138:** 13, 1976.
141. Zufall, R.: Ineffectiveness of treatment of urethral syndrome in women. Urology **12:** 337, 1978.
142. Richardson, F. H.: External urethroplasty in women: technique and clinical evaluation. J. Urol. **101:** 719, 1969.
143. Moore, T., Hira, N. R., and Stirland, R. M.: Differential urethrovesical urinary cell-count. A method of accurate diagnosis of lower-urinary-tract infections in women. Lancet **1:** 626, 1965.
144. Messing, E. M., and Stamey, T. A.: Interstitial cystitis. Early diagnosis, pathology, and treatment. Urology **12:** 381, 1978.
145. Cifuentes, L.: Epithelium of vaginal type in the female trigone: The clinical problem of trigonitis. J. Urol. **57:** 1028, 1947.
146. Maskell, R.: Importance of coagulase-negative staphylococci as pathogens in the urinary tract. Lancet **1:** 1155, 1974.
147. Pereira, A. T.: Coagulase-negative strains of *Staphylococcus* possessing antigen 51 as agents of urinary infection. J. Clin. Pathol. **15:** 252, 1962.
148. Roberts, A. P.: Micrococcaceae from the urinary tract in pregnancy. J. Clin. Pathol. **20:** 631, 1967.
149. Mitchell, R. G.: Classification of *Staphylococcus albus* strains isolated from the urinary tract. J. Clin. Pathol. **21:** 93, 1968.
150. Mabeck, C. E.: Significance of coagulase-negative staphylococcal bacteriuria. Lancet **2:** 1150, 1969.
151. Mabeck, C. E.: Studies in urinary tract infections. II. Urinary tract infection due to coagulase-negative staphylococci. Acta Med. Scand. **186:** 39, 1969.
152. Sellin, M., Cooke, D. I., Gillespie, W. A., Sylvester, D. G. H., and Anderson, J. D.: Micrococcal urinary-tract infections in young women. Lancet **2:** 570, 1975.
153. Gillespie, W. A., Sellin, M. A., Gill, P., Stephens, M., Tuckwell, L. A., and Hilton, A. L.: Urinary tract infection in young women, with special reference to *Staphylococcus saprophyticus*. J. Clin. Pathol. **31:** 348, 1978.
154. Buchanan, R. E., and Gibbons, N. E.: Bergey's Manual of Determinative Bacteriology, Ed. 8, Baltimore, Williams & Wilkins, 1974.
155. Williams, D. N., Lund, M. E., and Blazevic, D. J.: Significance of urinary isolates of coagulase-negative micrococcaceae. J. Clin. Microbiol. **3:** 556, 1976.
156. Hovelius, B., and Mårdh, P-A.: On the diagnosis of coagulase-negative staphylococci with emphasis on *Staphylococcus saprophyticus*. Acta Path. Microbiol. Scand., Sect. B. **85:** 427, 1977.
157. Kloos, W. E., and Schleifer, K. H.: Simplified scheme for routine identification of human *Staphylococcus* species. J. Clin. Microbiol. **1:** 82, 1975.
158. Demuth, P. J., Gerding, D. N., and Crossley, K.: *Staphylococcus aureus* bacteriuria. Arch. Intern. Med. **139:** 78, 1979.
159. Marrie, T. J., Harding, G. K. M., and Ronald, A. R.: Anaerobic and aerobic urethral flora in healthy females. J. Clin. Microbiol. **8:** 67, 1978.
160. Segura, J. W., Kelalis, P. P., Martin, W. J., and Smith, L. H.: Anaerobic bacteria in the urinary tract. Mayo Clin. Proc. **47:** 30, 1972.
161. Alling, B., Brandberg, A., Seeberg, S., and Svanborg, A.: Aerobic and anaerobic microbial flora in the urinary tract of geriatric patients during long-term care. J. Infect. Dis. **127:** 34, 1973.
162. Shepard, M. C.: T-form colonies of pleuropneumonia-like organisms. J. Bacteriol. **71:** 362, 1956.
163. Taylor-Robinson, D., Csonka, G. W., and Prentice, M. J.: Human intraurethral inoculation of ureaplasmas. Q. J. Med. **46:** 309, 1977.

164. Thomsen, A. C.: Occurrence of mycoplasmas in urinary tracts of patients with acute pyelonephritis. J. Clin. Microbiol. **8:** 84, 1978.
165. Bredt, W., Lam, P. S., Fiegel, P., and Höffler, D.: Nachweis von Mykoplasmen im Blasenpunktionsurin. Dtsch. Med. Wochenschr. **99:** 1553, 1974.
166. Fair, W. R., McClennan, B. L., and Jost, R. G.: Are excretory urograms necessary in evaluating women with urinary tract infection? J. Urol. **121:** 313, 1979.
167. Mabeck, C. E.: Studies in urinary tract infections. I. The Diagnosis of bacteriuria in women. Acta. Med. Scand. **186:** 35, 1969.
168. Kunz, H. H., Sieberth, H. G., Freiberg, J., Pulverer, G., and Schneider, F. J.: Zur Bedeutung der blasenpunktion fur den sicheren nachweis einer bakteriurie. Dtsch. Med. Wochenshr. **100:** 2252, 1975.
169. Hart, E. L., Magee, M. J.: Collecting urine specimens. Am. J. Nursing **57:** 1323, 1957.
170. Pfau, A., and Sacks, T. G.: An evaluation of midstream urine cultures in the diagnosis of urinary tract infections in females. Urol. Int. **25:** 326, 1970.
171. Marple, C. D.: The frequency and character of urinary tract infections in an unselected group of women. Ann. Intern. Med. **14:** 2220, 1941.
172. Philpot, V. B., Jr.: The bacterial flora of urine specimens from normal adults. J. Urol. **75: (3):** 562, 1956.
173. Turck, M., Ronald, A. R. and Petersdorf, R. G.: Relapse and reinfection in chronic bacteriuria. II. The correlation between site of infection and pattern of recurrence in chronic bacteriuria. N. Engl. J. Med **278:** 422, 1968.
174. Bergstrom, T., Lincoln, K., Orskov, F., Orskov, I., and Winberg, J.: Studies of urinary tract infections in infancy and childhood. VIII. Reinfection vs. relapse in recurrent urinary tract infections. Evaluation by means of identification of infecting organisms. J. Pediatr. **71:** 13, 1967.
175. Kunin, C. M., Deutscher, R., and Paquin, A. J.: Urinary tract infection in school children: An epidemiologic, clinical and laboratory study. Medicine **43:** 91, 1964.
176. Cattell, W. R., Charlton, C. A. C., McSherry, A., Frey, I. K., and O'Grady, F. W.: The localization of urinary tract infection and its relationship to relapse, reinfection and treatment. London, Oxford University Press, 1973.
177. Wientzen, R. L., McCracken, G. H., Jr., Petruska, M. L., Swinson, S. G., Kaijser, B., and Hanson, L. A.: Localization and therapy of urinary tract infections of childhood. Pediatrics **63:** 467, 1979.

CHAPTER 5

Some Observations on the Pathogenesis of Recurrent Bacteriuria in Women and Children

I review in this chapter much of the data we have obtained over the past 10 years at Stanford in our research efforts to understand the basic cause of recurrent bacteriuria in women. While I will certainly include data from other investigators as well, my major intent is to pull together in one place the chronology of our own research. I realize this chapter may interest the clinical investigator more than the practicing physician, but I believe it serves both groups better by avoiding the reporting of basic research in Chapter 4 where the important clinical issues are presented.

The major and basic question has always been, at least to me, how do the bacteria reach the bladder? I realize that every organ and tissue in the body has both general and specific defense mechanisms against invading bacteria; the bladder must have several, including the powerful one of voiding. I also recognize there must be good reasons why bacteria in the bladder reach the kidney only 50% of the time, as well as why one kidney, rather than both, is infected in one half of all patients who have upper tract involvement (see Chapter 1). But the basic question must always be—how did the bacteria reach the bladder in the first place? For if this step could be prevented, surely the defense mechanisms of the bladder and kidney become academic since they would be unnecessary. To be sure, if all females were continually infected and reinfected in the bladder, then bladder and renal mechanisms of handling the infection would be of first importance; there are, of course, no data to support such a total involvement of all women with recurrent bacteriuria.

An early section of Chapter 4 established the fact that bacteriuria in the female is preceded by colonization of the vaginal introitus with the organism responsible for the infection. It is not surprising, then, that much of the research presented in this chapter relates to the factors responsible for introital colonization by Enterobacteriaceae from the rectal reservoir.

THE RECTAL RESERVOIR: ANTIGENIC DIFFERENCES AMONG *ESCHERICHIA COLI*

Because most urinary infections are caused by *E. coli* that originate from the fecal flora of the lower bowel, and because a relatively few O-serogroups account for most urinary infections (01, 02, 04, 06, 07, 08, 09, 018, 022, and 075), many investigators have searched for pathogenic differences among fecal *E. coli*. The basic question of whether the common O-serogroups that cause urinary infections are "nephropathogenic" or whether they are simply the "prevalent" *E. coli* in the bowel at the time of the bacteriuric episode remains controversial; the term nephropathogenic could be reduced to "uropathogenic" and perhaps finally to "introitopathogenic" if colonization of the introitus is the missing link between the rectal reservoir and urinary infection. Sjöstedt[1] was among the first to show that certain O-groups of *E. coli* possessed considerable toxicity for the mouse, caused skin necrosis, demonstrated hemolysis on solid agar, and showed substantial resistance to phagocytosis and bactericidal activity of human blood.

It is clear that the same O-serogroup of *E. coli* causing a symptomatic urinary infection can be found amongst the fecal flora of the same patient in most instances. For example, Rantz[2] reported an 80% correlation between the common O-serogroup in the urine and those in the stools of the patients with bacteriuria. Grüneberg[3] isolated 10 rectal colonies of *E. coli* from each of 23 patients with acute urinary infection; he found O-group identity between rectal and urinary *E. coli* in 22 of the 23 patients and, in 19 of the 22, over half of the 10 isolated fecal colonies were of the same O-group as the infecting strain in the urine. Many other investigators have arrived at essentially similar conclusions (see Giradet's[4] recent and excellent review). Grüneberg *et al.*[5] also reported that the O-serogroup frequency of *E. coli* in the feces from normal women was the same as that from the urine of infected women (with the exception of *E. coli* 06 which did occur more often in the urine of infected women). Roberts *et al.*[6] in a more recent study, divided their patients into those with symptomatic and asymptomatic infections. In their symptomatic, nonpregnant women, they found *E. coli* of the same O-groups in the urine and feces in 20 of 26 patients (77%), but in only 5 of 25 patients (21%) who had asymptomatic bacteriuria.

Stanford Studies on *Escherichia coli* and *Proteus mirabilis*

In Chapter 4, in the section on the Effect of Nalidixic Acid on Vaginal and Fecal *E. coli*, I presented data on 54 women with urinary tract infection (UTI) treated for 10 days with nalidixic acid. Anal canal cultures were available for O-serogrouping in 50 of these women at the time of the bacteriuria. The bacteriuric strains included 42 *E. coli*, 1 *Citrobacter*, and 7 *P. mirabilis*. The fecal *E. coli* were banked and serogrouped as described in Chapter 1. In 74% of the patients, the same strain causing the UTI was found in the fecal flora; in 40%, the strain was predominant and accounted for >85% of the Enterobacteriaceae. In 18%, it accounted for half of the Enterobacteriaceae in the anal culture, and in 16% it represented less than 33% of the fecal Enterobacteriaceae. The bacteriuric strain could not be found among the fecal bacteria in 13 of the 50 patients (26%), but in 7 of these 13 the bacteriuric strain was found later in anal cultures obtained within the next 30 days, suggesting that a sampling error may have prevented recovery of the bacteriuric strain from the rectum at the time of the bacteriuria. In addition to these 7 patients, 2 more of the 13 carried a self-agglutinating strain of *E. coli* in the rectum at the time of their bacteriuria, thereby preventing O-serogrouping of the *E. coli*. Hence, it is possible that the 74% identity between the bacteriuric and anal strain may have been as high as 92%. It should be noted, however, that 11 of the 37 patients who showed apparent identity could not be serogrouped (nontypable) with the 143 available antisera; apparent identity of the nontypable bacteriuric strain with the rectal *E. coli* was made by finding similar appearing *E. coli* with the same antimicrobial sensitivity pattern which were also nontypable.

The seven patients with *P. mirabilis* UTI are even more interesting in their analysis of anal carriage. All seven of the *P. mirabilis* bacteriurias were accompanied by carriage of the same strain in the fecal flora. The fecal *P. mirabilis* were usually present in numbers of several thousand per ml of transport broth, but still represented less than 50% of the total strains of Enterobacteriaceae present in the anal canal. In contrast, *P. mirabilis* was not detected in the anal flora of the 43 other bacteriuric patients. At first thought, these data suggest that the rectal strains of *P. mirabilis* must have had a pathogenic advantage; we did not examine, however, the fecal flora of 50 matched women who never had urinary infections. It is possible that similar anal cultures exist among control women, as Grüneberg *et al.*[5] have reported is true for *E. coli*. As will be seen shortly, however, Hanson's group at Göteborg have different data, and I am personally uneasy in relying on this single study in adults.[5] There can be no question since the early studies of Rantz[2] and Vosti *et al.*[7] that the bacteriuric strain is readily found among the fecal *E. coli* in the majority of symptomatic women, and that these strains represent relatively few O-serogroups. I wish there were studies available that compared the fecal flora of age-matched patients and controls in the same population; if the common O-serogroups were present more frequently in the fecal flora of patients with UTI, then these O-groups have to be considered as having some advantage both in establishing fecal carriage and in causing UTI. I believe there are no convincing data on this point in women, but the studies of Grüneberg *et al.*[5] were suggestive of greater carriage of common O-groups in bacteriuric women than in the fecal flora of normal women.

The Göteborg Studies

Lars Hansen's group at Göteborg, by dividing their children with urinary infections into those with acute pyelonephritis, acute cystitis, asymptomatic bacteriuria detected by screening surveys (ScBU or screening bacteriuria) and normal controls (fecal flora), have made important contributions to our understanding of antigenic differences among *E. coli*. The most important differences can be summarized as follows:

1. Eighty percent of *E. coli* strains causing acute pyelonephritis in their children belonged to eight of the most common O-serogroups, but such serogroups were found in the fecal flora of only 28% of healthy children.[8] The eight common O-groups were found much less often in the urine from children with ScBU, in part because 45% of all strains were spontaneously agglutinating, indicating that the O-group specificity had been altered.
2. Strains of *E. coli* from patients with acute pyelonephritis and cystitis were more resistant to the bactericidal activity of normal human serum than were the strains from children with ScBU.[9] This difference was largely due to the fact that the common O-groupable bacteria, which make up the majority of symptomatic urinary infections, were more resistant to the bactericidal activity of serum than were the self-agglutinating strains so commonly found in children with ScBU. It is important to note, however, that urine isolates from patients with symptomatic pyelonephritis or cystitis did not differ in sensitivity from their fecal urinary isolates, suggesting that resistance to the bactericidal activity of serum is not a virulence factor of urinary pathogens.
3. The loss of O-antigenic specificity in *E. coli* strains from ScBU patients, combined with their greater serum sensitivity, clearly suggested an alteration of *E. coli* antigenicity in ScBU patients. The finding of the Göteborg group that some asymptomatic, untreated children in time converted their O-groupable *E. coli* to self-agglutinating strains, accompanied by greater serum sensitivity, suggested that urinary antibody might change the surface characteristics of the *E. coli*.[8, 10] These observations add strength to the clinical argument that some patients with *E. coli* ScBU are best left untreated; clearance of the self-agglutinating strain from the urinary tract is likely to be followed by a new *E. coli* with its antigenic O-groupable surface intact and capable of causing symptoms.

Capsular *Escherichia coli* Antigens (K Antigens)

In 1971 Mabeck[11] observed that a particular capsular antigen, labeled K_1, especially when combined with *E. coli* 02, was found more often in strains causing acute pyelonephritis than in those causing cystitis. Glynn *et al.*,[12] in the same year, observed that the K-antigen content was higher in strains causing pyelonephritis than in those causing cystitis. Kaijser,[13] using a more accurate technique for quantifying the K-antigen, confirmed these observations that the K-antigen content of urinary isolates of *E. coli* was greater than that of strains isolated from the feces of schoolgirls. Although McCabe *et al.*[14] confirmed these latter observations in a study of bacteremia in adults, they showed that the amount of K-antigen in blood culture isolates was not significantly greater than that of fecal isolates (even though lower than urinary isolates), and concluded that no correlation could be detected between the K-antigen content of blood culture isolates and the severity and outcome of the bacteremia. Kaijser *et al.*,[13, 15] in a more detailed study, identified ten different K-antigens in children with *E. coli* urinary infections; 50–70% of urinary isolates had only 1 of the 10 K-antigens (K_1 was by far the most common). They found that more K typable strains arose from patients with pyelonephritis (70%) than those with acute cystitis (53%) or ScBU (42%) or from the feces of healthy children (55%).

These findings, like the common O-group antigenic differences in patients with acute pyelonephritis compared to the fecal flora of healthy controls, suggest that K-antigens as well as O-antigens could be virulence factors in determining which *E. coli* strains cause pyelonephritis. Kalmanson *et al.*,[16] however, found no differences in the presence of K-antigens among strains of *E. coli* from upper and lower urinary tract infections in women, and Taylor and Koutsaimanis,[17] using experimental ascending infections in the rat, could not show virulence factors related to bacterial K-antigen or bacterial resistance to serum. Moreover, Hanson *et al.*[18] have pointed out that the K_1 antigen is a poor immunogen, unlike the O-antigens; for example, they found no detectable titers of serum antibody to K_1 antigen in 15 of 17 children with acute pyelonephritis due to K_1 strains of *E. coli.*

Escherichia coli Hemolysis

Hemolysin production by *E. coli* was considered by Dudgeon *et al.*[19] in 1921 to be characteristic of some strains causing urinary infections. McGeachie[20] tested 534 strains of *E. coli* isolated from voided urine for hemolysis; he noted that 5 serologic O-groups (01, 04, 06, 018, and 075) accounted for 72% of all the hemolytic strains isolated (29% of the 534 strains). Hanson *et al.*[21] observed that their *E. coli* strains causing acute pyelonephritis produced hemolysins more often than did fecal strains isolated from healthy children; 55% of bacterial strains from 119 children with acute pyelonephritis, 48% of 109 strains from acute cystitis, 18% of 115 strains from ScBU, and 17% of 709 strains from rectal swabs of normal children produced hemolysis. While the significance of hemolysin production and the potential virulence hemolysis imparts to some *E. coli* stains is unknown, Fried *et al.*[22] showed that a hemolytic *E. coli* (06:H31) commonly caused pyelonephritis in kidneys of mice and rats, but a nonhemolytic mutant of the same *E. coli* did not. Cooke and Ewins[23] reported that hemolytic strains of *E. coli* in the periurethral flora were more likely to be found in subsequent UTI than were nonhemolytic strains in the same flora.

Summary

In summary, antigenic differences among *E. coli* causing pyelonephritis in children, at least in comparison to fecal strains isolated from healthy children, include an increased frequency of *E. coli* common O-groups, an increase in frequency of capsular K_1 antigen as well as larger quantities of K-antigen in general, and an increased likelihood of hemolysin production. Whether these antigenic differences all resided initially with the *E. coli* strain *per se* and therefore contributed to "nephropathogenicity" or whether these differences were induced or selected by the host defense mechanisms is a basic, and largely unanswered question. For example, as will be seen in the next sections of this chapter, the common O-group *E. coli* are more resistant to the bactericidal activity of vaginal fluid than are the uncommon O-groups of *E. coli.* Could the vaginal introitus select out the common O-groups from the rectal reservoir?

INTROITAL COLONIZATION WITH ENTEROBACTERIA IN URINARY TRACT INFECTION-PRONE AND NORMAL WOMEN

If one accepts the data that rectal bacteria represent the ultimate reservoir for most urinary infections, and that colonization of the vaginal introitus precedes bacteriuria,[24] it is clearly important to determine whether UTI-prone female patients are more susceptible to introital colonization with enterobacteria than are normal women who never have urinary infections.

Before presenting our data, as well as the data of other investigators, we should recognize two variables of substantial significance. The first is the selection of representative control subjects; the second is the necessity of making certain that UTI-prone patients have not lost their susceptibility to urinary infections during the period of surveillance. We all know that most patients with recurrent bacteriuria have long periods of sudden remission—often lasting years—and it is reasonable to suspect that the biological defect responsible for susceptibility may not be present during these long remissions. For this reason we have insisted that data on introital colonization—or any other biological measurement of vaginal secretions—include only those studies in between two consecutive bacteriuric episodes. Only in this way can clinicians be certain that the patient has not lost her susceptibility in their search for the basic cause of recurrent bacteriuria. The selection of control volunteers is equally important; they should not be patients attending the hospital or out-patient clinics for any reason, because other diseases may adversely affect the same biologic factors that lead to introital colonization with enterobacteria. For example, the 20% incidence of bacteriuria induced by urethral catheterization of women admitted to a general medical ward[25] is most surely related to a substantial colonization of the urethral mucosa with enterobacteria, especially when compared to a 1% incidence of induced bacteriuria in nonhospitalized normal, young women attending a college.[26] Moreover, as I have shown in Chapter 4, antimicrobial agents like ampicillin can adversely affect the introital flora; volunteers must not have received such drugs, preferably within several months of serving as a normal control. Thus, control volunteers should be healthy, nonhospitalized women who are carefully interviewed as to any history of past UTI, recurrent vaginitis, or antibiotic ingestion. They must also refrain from douching during the study period.

Our data, then, on introital colonization, relate to carefully interviewed control volunteers who agree to the collection of 10 consecutive weekly cultures of their introital mucosa, together with their first voided urethral aliquot of urine (VB_1) and a midstream voided urine (VB_2). The data from UTI-prone women includes all studies in between two consecutive episodes of documented, recurrent bacteriuria. Any patient who took any antimicrobial agent for any reason in between bacteriuric episodes was excluded from the analysis; it is surprising how many times we were forced to exclude patients because of antibiotic ingestion for reasons other than UTI.

Before presenting our published data on introital colonization in normal and UTI-prone women,[27–29] it may be of historical interest to some readers that we recognized in the early 1960s, as soon as we began obtaining introital cultures in all our patients, that women resistant to UTI rarely had Enterobacteriaceae on their introital mucosa. In those years, I saw several hundred women who were candidates for renovascular hypertension, most of whom were not susceptible to UTI, and 80% of whom did not have a single colony of Enterobacteriaceae detectable on their introitus; these early data were presented in a workshop I organized for the National Research Council of the National Academy of Sciences in 1967.[27] I have never forgotten an incident in 1967, while I was spending a sabbatical year with Professor Paul Beeson at the Radcliffe Infirmary in Oxford, England, and where I had discussed these observations at several seminars in Britain during 1967 and 1968, when one of the attending gynecologists walked into my office with 20 blood agar plates. He had streaked onto these agar plates vaginal swabs from 20 normal women in the first trimester of pregnancy; he thought it was incredible that there was not a single *E. coli* colony among the 20 plates! I tell this story only to illustrate how widespread the belief was that cultures of the normal female introitus commonly contained *E. coli*; the basis of this belief probably rest on vaginal cultures from women susceptible to bacteriuria, and the failure to distinguish these from those of healthy, normal women.

Introital Cultures from Normal Volunteers

Our first effort to formally document the introital bacteriology of normal, premenopausal women was published in 1970.[28] Thirty volunteers between the ages of 22 and 49 years were interviewed and cultured one time only; the results of these introital cultures, along with the day of the menstrual cycle and other relevant data, are presented in Table 5.1. Cultures of the first voided few milliliters of urine (VB_1) and the midstream urine (VB_2) are presented in Tables 5.2 and 5.3; 17 of these volunteers were able to void from the usual position on the cystoscopy table, but 13 collected the specimens by voiding from the back edge of the toilet seat.[28] These were about the last studies in which we cleaned the introitus with Betadine solution, followed by copious rinsing with distilled water, before collecting the voided urine samples from the cystocopy table; the introitus was never washed, of course, prior to culturing the introital mucosa. The data in these tables show that only 3 out of 30 patients showed any Enterobacteriaceae on the introital mucosa—550, 120, and 20 *E. coli*/ml of transport saline. Figures 5.1 to 5.3 show graphically the interrelationship of these few *E. coli* to the normal aerobic introital flora. Our second study of the normal introital flora was on 5 volunteers cultured for 10 consecutive weeks[24] which was expanded in 1972 to 10 volunteers.[29] The latter study is reproduced in Table 5.4; the carriage rate of Enterobacteriaceae is clearly higher than the 10% incidence we found when control volunteers were cultured only once. The mean carriage incidence for the 10 subjects in Table 5.4, however, is exactly 20%.

Comparison of Introital Colonization in Normal and Urinary Tract Infection-Prone Women

In 1975, Sexton and I,[30] with the help of the Biostatistics Department at Stanford, analyzed the data from 200 introital cultures on 20 normal volunteers compared to 198 cultures from 9 women in between episodes of recurrent bacteriuria.

All women with recurrent urinary infection were premenopausal out-patients and had documented recurrent episodes of bacteriuria. Cultures were obtained at weekly or biweekly intervals. An occasional patient with longer intervals between bacteriuric episodes had cultures made at triweekly intervals. Vaginal douching was avoided and instrumentation of the urinary tract was never performed. None received antimicrobial agents except for the 5–10 day period of therapy for the bacteriuria. All cultures in this analysis were taken consecutively between episodes of bacteriuria, that is, none was included while the patients were bacteriuric or during the 10-day period they received antimicrobial agents for the bacteriuria. Thus, the data include all cultures beginning with the first one following successful antimicrobial therapy and ending with the final culture before the succeeding infection. The time period and number of cultures between bacteriuric episodes in these 9 patients varied from a minimum of 9 weeks (8 cultures) to a maximum of 62 weeks (20 cultures). The mean interval between bacteriuric episodes for all patients was 30 weeks (15 cultures).

The colonization incidence of *E. coli, enterococci, P. mirabilis, Klebsiella, Enterobacter, Pseudomonas aeruginosa*, as well as the presence of any Gram-negative bacteria, was determined by the ratio of positive cultures to total cultures for each of the 20 control women and the 9 women with recurrent urinary infection. The mean of the 20 proportions for the control women was then compared to the mean for the 9 proportions for the women with infection, using the standard 2-sample t test (Table 5.5).

The numbers of pathogenic bacteria present on the introitus in both groups were analyzed by dividing all cultures into 5 categories: 0, 1–99, 100–999, 1,000–9,999, and 10,000 or more bacteria/ml (Table 5.6).

A comparison was made for both groups as to the duration of consecutive cultures in which the same Enterobacteriaceae or enterococci was found, regardless of numbers, on the introitus. Thus, a single longest consecutive carriage datum was recorded for each woman by showing (1) the total number of weeks the same pathogen was recovered in consecutive cultures and (2) the number of cultures during that interval (Table 5.7).

Table 5.1
Introital Cultures in 30 Control Women[a]

Volunteer	Age	Parity	Oral Contraceptive	Vaginal Vestibule pH	Day of Menstrual Cycle	Bacteria per Milliliter						
						Lactobacillus	Corynebacterium	*Haemophilis vaginalis*	*Staphylococcus epidermidis*	Nonhemolytic streptococcus	*Escherichia coli*	Other
	yr											
E.F.	40	—	Yes	—	22	$>10^4$		10^4				
V.M.	28	4	No	6.0	Postpartum		10^5	10^4				
A.A.	26	1	No	5.5	10		120			350		
M.H.	38	3	Yes	4.5	7	$>10^5$			70			
M.A.	49	0	No	5.0	23–27	10^5			20			$>10^4$ yeast
P.W.	43	2	No	4.5	9		$>10^4$	10^5				
S.C.	25	0	No	5.0	5		10^5		910	1700		
J.G.	35	1	No	5.0	27		$>10^4$					
A.S.	22	0	No	4.5	14	$>10^4$	10^4		300	100		
C.S.	22	0	No	5.0	—	10^4			2000	200	550	
A.K.	32	2	Yes	5.5	19		$>10^5$		2500			
L.L.	25	0	No	5.5	16		$>10^4$		100	20		
L.A.	24	0	No	4.5	13		$>10^5$		70			
M.C.	26	0	No	4.5	26	$>10^5$	120		160	110		
J.S.	24	0	Yes	4.5	6		3610		80	70		
J.H.	27	0	No	4.5	17	$>10^5$	1620		80			
D.O.	27	0	Yes	4.5	10	10^4	850		10			
S.W.	29	0	No	4.5	8	10^5	5000					5000 yeast
D.N.	24	0	No	4.5	20		10^5				120	1980 yeast
N.S.	27	0	Yes	4.5	14	10^4	$>10^4$					
E.G.	27	0	Yes	4.5	2		3500	10^4	80	1240		
Y.L.	38	5	No	4.5	26	10^5	$>10^4$		120			
K.J.	24	0	No	4.5	31		3060		790			
M.R.	23	0	No	4.5	28		$>10^5$					1340 yeast
E.R.	25	0	No	4.5	26	$>10^5$	20			320		
A.O.	25	0	No	4.5	11	$>10^5$				5000		
P.S.	25	0	No	4.5	12	$>10^5$				60	20	
B.A.	23	0	No	4.5	7	$>10^4$	10^4		140	5000		
S.S.	25	0	No	4.5	21	$>10^5$				80		
J.M.	28	0	Yes	4.5	12		10^4		40			10^5 yeast

[a] Reproduced by permission from W. R. Fair, M. M. Timothy, M. A. Millar, and T. A. Stamey, J. Urol. **104:** 426, 1970.[28]

Table 5.2
Urethral Cultures (VB_1) in 30 Control Women[a]

Volunteer	Bacteria per Milliliter						
	Lactobacillus	Coryne-bacterium	*Haemophilis vaginalis*	*Staphylococcus epidermidis*	Nonhemo-lytic strepto-coccus	*Escherichia coli*	Other
E.F.	330						
V.M.[b]		2000					
A.A.[b]		220		20			
M.H.[b]				60			
M.A.[b]	2500	2500					20 yeast
P.W.[b]		710	600				
S.C.[b]		610		180	380		
J.G.[b]		1000		20			
A.S.[b]	10^5	2000		440			
C.S.[b]	10^4			150	120	360	
A.K.[b]		1000		1110	10		
L.L.		4000			60		
L.A.				230			
M.C.	10^4	180		190	300		
J.S.[b]		560		10	10		
J.H.[b]	$>10^4$			310	270		
D.O.	1160	60		20			
S.W.	10^5	2000					5000 yeast
D.N.[b]		250				10	20 yeast 10 *Proteus mirabilis*
N.S.[b]	10^5	10^4					
E.G.		4000	3000	130		10	
Y.L.	10^4	420		30			
K.J.[b]		580		630			
M.R.		80		10	30		70 yeast
E.R.	1500	180			100		
A.O.	10^5			60	1680		
P.S.[b]	2500						
B.A.[b]	5000	60		120	10		
S.S.	5000				1940		
J.M.	2500	560		90	30		2760 yeast

[a] Reproduced by permission from W. R. Fair, M. M. Timothy, M. A. Millar, and T. A. Stamey, J. Urol. **104:** 426, 1970.[28]

[b] Culture obtained on cystoscopy table.

The colonization incidence (mean percent carriage), regardless of bacterial numbers, for Enterobacteriaceae, enterococci, and *P. aeruginosa* is presented in Table 5.5. The probability values that the two populations are different are highly significant for the presence of *E. coli*, enterococci, and for all of the Gram-negative species in Table 5.5 when combined. The lack of significant differences for *P. mirabilis*, *Klebsiella*, *Enterobacter* and *P. aeruginosa* is clearly owing to the small occurrence rate of these organisms in the 398 cultures. *Enterobacter* and *P. aeruginosa* were never found once in 200 control cultures, while they occurred in 5.5 and 1.2%, respectively, in the group with recurrent urinary infection. This, plus the observation that when these organisms (along with *P. mirabilis* and *Klebsiella*) were added to the *E. coli* analysis the *t* test was even more significant than for *E. coli* alone, indicates the potential pathogenicity of carriage despite their less frequent occurrence.

Further analysis of introital carriage with these bacteria as to the actual numbers of

Table 5.3
Midstream Cultures (VB_2) in 30 Control Women[a]

Volunteer	Bacteria per Milliliter						
	Lactobacillus	Corynebacterium	*Haemophilis vaginalis*	*Staphylococcus epidermidis*	Nonhemolytic streptococcus	*Escherichia coli*	Other
E.F.	100						
V.M.[b]		4000	80			20	
A.A.[b]		80		720			
M.H.[b]				20	80		
M.A.[b]	2000						170 yeast
P.W.[b]		3320	100		50	10	
S.C.[b]				20	30		
J.G.[b]		230					
A.S.[b]	10^5	$>10^4$		200			
C.S.[b]	600			20		50	
A.K.[b]		90		70			
L.L.					160		
L.A.		200		50			
M.C.	5000	10		30	30		
J.S.[b]		40		20			
J.H.[b]	3500			10	60		
D.O.	320	350					
S.W.	10^4	650					350 yeast
D.N.[b]		540					
N.S.[b]	1520			10			
E.G.		3900	60	110			
Y.L.	440						
K.J.[b]		400		1500		10	
M.R.				10	130		560 yeast
E.R.	940	50		10			
A.O.	130						
P.S.[b]	40						
B.A.[b]	320	10		20	10		
S.S.				80		10	
J.M.				10			70 yeast

[a] Reproduced by permission from W. R. Fair, M. M. Timothy, M. A. Millar, and T. A. Stamey, J. Urol. **104:** 426, 1970.[28]

[b] Culture obtained on cystoscopy table.

bacteria present is presented in Table 5.6 for *E. coli*, enterococci, and all Gram-negative species combined. These data were derived by simply adding all positive cultures at each count divided by the total cultures in each group rather than averaging the mean of each individual control or patient as was done in Table 5.5. While 76% of the 200 cultures from the 20 control women did not have a single Gram-negative organism detectable on the introitus, only 43% of the total cultures from the women with infection were similarly free of these organisms. Of equal importance is the substantial tendency for the introital colonization of women with recurrent urinary infection to contain much larger numbers of Enterobacteriaceae and enterococci. For example, only 1 of 200 cultures (0.5%) from the control women represented a colonization with 10,000 or more *E. coli*, while 13.6% of all cultures from women with infection were colonized with bacterial numbers of this magnitude. Only in the colonization range of 1–99 bacteria/ml are the percentages even reasonably close, especially for enterococci.

The mean duration of longest consecu-

Table 5.4
Enterobacteria in 10 Normal Volunteers Cultured for 10 Consecutive Weeks[a]

Volunteer (Age in Years) and Site of Culture	*Escherichia coli*[b] per Milliliter of Sample (and Serogroup in Parentheses) at Week:									
	1	2	3	4	5	6	7	8	9	10
1 (22)										
Vaginal vestibule	0	0	2250 (04)	10 (01)	0	0	290 (01)	0	0	880 (01)
			10 (01)							20 (04)
Urethral	0	0	0	0	0	0	10 (01)	0	0	0
Midstream	0	0	0	0	0	0	0	0	0	0
2 (30)										
Vaginal vestibule	0	0	0	0	0	0	0	0	0	0
Urethral	0	0	0	0	0	0	0	0	0	0
Midstream	0	0	0	0	0	0	0	0	0	0
3 (39)										
Vaginal vestibule	0	0	0	0	0	0	0	0	0	0
Urethral	0	0	0	0	0	0	0	0	0	0
Midstream	0	0	0	0	0	0	0	0	0	0
4 (34)										
Vaginal vestibule	0	0	0	0	0	0	0	0	0	0
Urethral	0	0	0	0	0	0	0	0	0	0
Midstream	0	0	0	0	0	0	0	0	0	0
5 (39)[c]										
Vaginal vestibule	0	0	0	30 (06)	0	0	0	0	0	2500 (06)[d]
Urethral	0	0	0	10 (06)	0	90 (06)	0	0	0	100 (06)
Midstream	10 (06)	10 (06)	0	30 (06)	0	130 (06)	0	0	0	50(06)
6 (34)										
Vaginal vestibule	5000 (01)	50 (01)	0	0	0	2500 (01)	0	40 (0132)	20 (01)	1040 (01)
	5000 *Klebsiella*					10 (016)		350 (01)		
Urethral	110 (01)	0	0	0	0	30 (01)	0	0	0	0
	220 *Klebisella*									
Midstream	30 (01)	0	0	0	0	0	0	0	0	0
	30 *Klebsiella*									
7 (26)[e]										
Vaginal vestibule	0	110	60	0	10	20	0	0	0	0
Urethral	10	500	40	0	20	40	100	0	80	160
Midstream	10	130	30	0	10	10	0	20	0	0
8 (28)										
Vaginal vestibule	0	0	0	0	0	0	0	0	0	0

Urethral	0	0	0	0	0	0	0	0	0
Midstream	0	0	0	0	0	0	0	0	0
9 (18)									
Vaginal vestibule	0	30 (025)	0	0	0	10 (NT)[f]	0	0	0
Urethral	0	710 (025)	750 (025) 40 (NT)	30 (025)	0	10 (NT)	30 (NT)	0	0
Midstream	0	30 (025)	0	0	0	0	0	0	0
10 (43)									
Vaginal vestibule	0	0	0	10 (NT)	0	0	40 *Klebsiella*	0	0
Urethral	0	0	0	0	0	0	0	0	0
Midstream	0	0	0	0	0	0	0	0	0

[a] Reproduced by permission from T. A. Stamey, Urinary Infections, Williams & Wilkins, Baltimore, 1972.[29]

[b] No gram-negative enterobacteria, other than *E. coli*, was ever isolated from these cultures except for the *Klebsiella* during the 1st week in patient 6, the 8th week in patient 10, and the *Proteus mirabilis* in patient 7.

[c] Volunteer 5 could never void from the cystoscopy table and had to collect her own voided specimens; this accounts for the negative introital cultures but contaminated, low count voided specimens.

[d] April 1, 15 days following 10th week culture, there were no *E. coli* on the introitus; a rectal culture showed the predominant serogroup was *E. coli* 010.

[e] All colony counts shown in this volunteer were *P. mirabilis*.

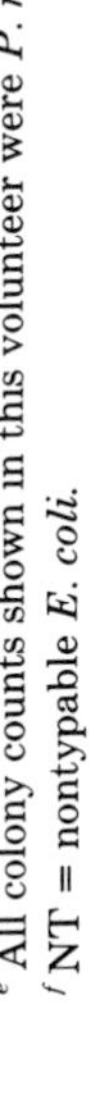

[f] NT = nontypable *E. coli*.

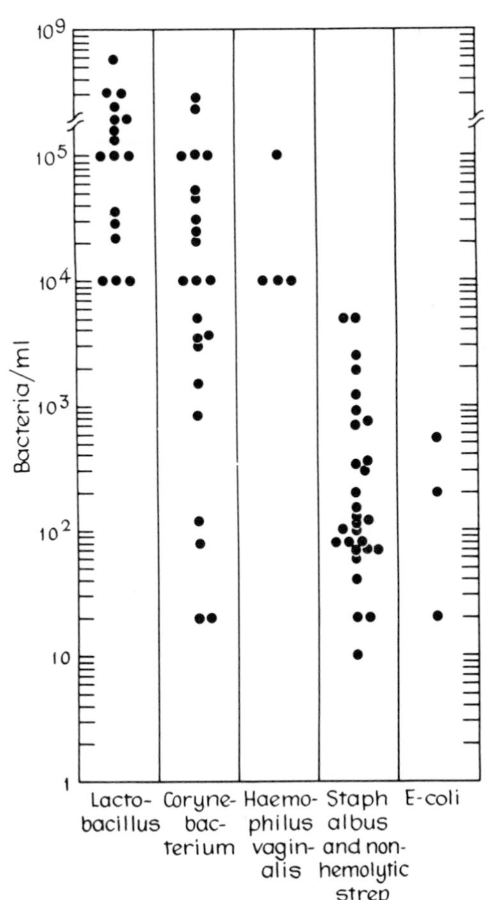

Figure 5.1 Introital cultures in 30 control women.

tive carriage in which the same organism was cultured in successive cultures is presented in Table 5.7. Because the controls were cultured at weekly intervals, the longest time of consecutive carriage and the number of cultures are always the same. Because the time between bacteriuric occurrences in women with recurrent urinary infection was usually months, cultures were obtained often at 2 or 3 weekly intervals, accounting for the uneven numbers between weeks and cultures in the group with recurrent infection.

We concluded that women susceptible to recurrent urinary infection are far more likely to carry Enterobacteriaceae and enterococci on the introital mucosa of the

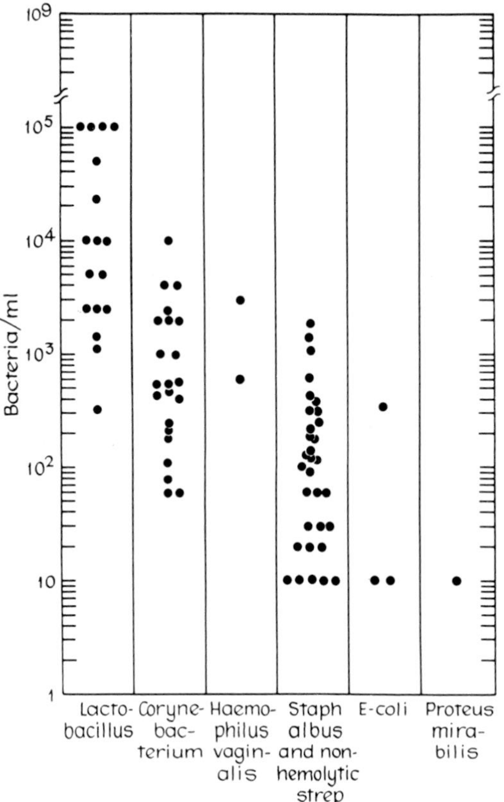

Figure 5.2 Urethral cultures (VB_1) in 30 control women.

vagina than control women of similar age and endocrine status who never have urinary infections. Moreover, this carriage is characterized by larger numbers and more prolonged carriage of these bacteria in UTI-prone women.

The Question of Antimicrobial Therapy in Relation to Introital Carriage

We have always realized that, in comparing our UTI-prone women to normal volunteers, the control volunteers did not have 5–10 days of antimicrobial therapy before starting their 10 consecutive weeks of cultures. If a short course of antimicrobial therapy in our patients really influenced introital carriage, it seemed reasonable that it should do so within the first 30 days after completion of therapy. Accordingly, Schaeffer and I[31] expanded the number of patients and controls. We analyzed the data on the patients by dividing the interval between bacteriuric episodes into two periods as shown in Figure 5.4.

The control group consisted of 31 premenopausal, nonhospitalized volunteers from whom cultures were obtained weekly for about 10 weeks (range 5–13). All were healthy women without apparent disease. Each volunteer was carefully interviewed to ensure that (1) she never had a history of urinary infection, (2) she had not received antibiotics in the past months, and (3) there would be no douching or antibiotic ingestion during the study.

The patients included all women seen in the urology clinic with documented recur-

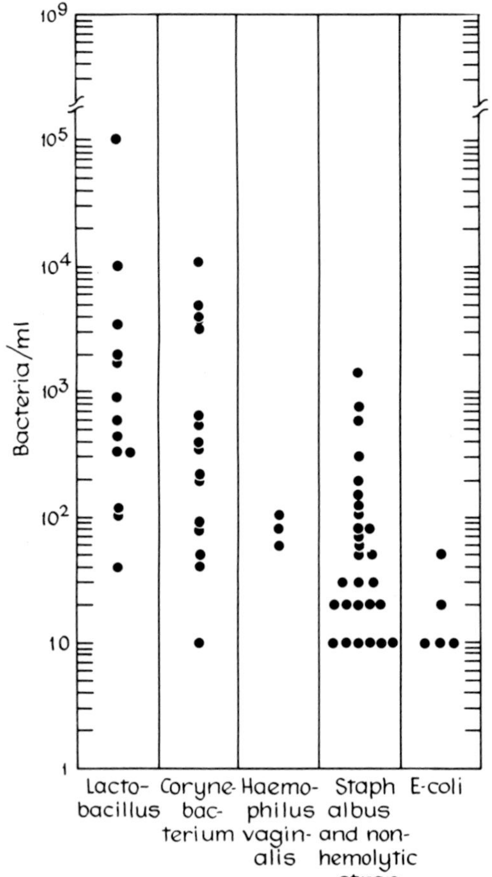

Figure 5.3 Midstream cultures (VB_2) in 30 control women.

Table 5.5
Mean Percent Carriage Incidence of Enterobacteriaceae, Enterococci and *Pseudomonas aeruginosa* in 20 Control Women (200 Introital Cultures) Resistant to Urinary Infections is Compared to the Mean Percent Carriage in 9 Women (198 Cultures) with Recurrent Urinary Infections[a]

Bacteria	Normal Controls	Recurrent Infections	*P* Value
	% carriage[b]	*% carriage*[b]	
Escherichia coli	22.5 ± 18.9	53.5 ± 27.3	0.001
Enterococci	16.5 ± 21.6	47.0 ± 33.3	0.003
Proteus mirabilis	3.0 ± 9.8	11.6 ± 17.5	0.08
Klebsiella	2.0 ± 4.1	8.9 ± 9.7	0.02
Enterobacter	0.0	5.5 ± 12.6	0.09
P. aeruginosa	0.0	1.2 ± 2.8	0.10
Any Gram-negative carriage of above species	24.0 ± 19.0	56.1 ± 12.6	0.0003

[a] Reproduced by permission from T. A. Stamey and C. C. Sexton, J. Urol. **113:** 214, 1975.[30]
[b] Plus or minus 1 standard deviation.

rent urinary infections who (1) were premenopausal, (2) received no incidental antibiotics, and (3) three or more cultures were obtained between episodes of bacteriuria. The women were treated with a 7-10 day course of one of the following: cephalexin, cephaloglycin, nalidixic acid, nitrofurantoin, oxytetracycline, penicillin, sulfamethizole, or sulfisoxazole. Vaginal douching and instrumentation of the urinary tract were avoided. All cultures were obtained consecutively between episodes of bacteriuria, that is, none was included while the patients were bacteriuric or for the 10-day period they received antimicrobial therapy for the bacteriuria. The data include all cultures, beginning with the first one after the completion of successful antimicrobial therapy and ending with the last culture before the succeeding infection. Cultures were made from most patients at weekly or biweekly intervals. A longer interval (4–5 weeks) occasionally occurred in patients followed 6–12 months. The time period and number of cultures between bacteriuric episodes in these 14 patients (22 symptomatic bacteriuric episodes) varied from a minimum of 6 weeks (3 cultures) to 62 weeks (20 cultures). The mean interval between bacteriuric episodes was 23 weeks (12 cultures).

The interval between bacteriuric episodes was divided into two periods to assess the impact of antibiotics on subsequent vaginal introital cultures. The first period (A) included all cultures in the 30-day period after completion of therapy and the second (B) included all subsequent cultures until the next episode of bacteriuria (Figure 5.4).

The colonization rate of *E. coli*, Enterobacteriaceae other than *E. coli*, enterococci, and any Gram-negative bacteria was determined by the ratio of positive cultures to total cultures for periods A and B in each of the 14 patients and for each of the 31 controls. The mean of the ratios in period A was compared to the mean of the ratios in period B, using the standard paired *t* test. The mean of the ratios in period B also was compared to the mean for the 31 controls using the 2-sample *t* test.

The numerical distribution of the bacteria present on the vaginal vestibule was analyzed by dividing all cultures into five categories; 0, 10–100, 110–1,000, 1,010–10,000, and greater than 10,000 bacteria/ml.

The mean density of introital carriage of *E. coli*, Enterobacteriaceae other than *E. coli*, enterococci, and any Gram-negative bacteria was determined for each control and patient in the following manner. The five categories of bacterial counts were assigned code numbers 0 through 4. For each individual the number of cultures per category was multiplied by the code number of the category. The sum of these products was then divided by the total number of cultures. The mean of the 14 ratios in period

Table 5.6
Numbers of *Escherichia coli*, Enterococci and any Gram-negatives (*E. coli*, *Proteus mirabilis*, Klebsiella, Enterobacter and *Pseudomonas aeruginosa*) Present on Vaginal Introitus in 200 Control Cultures Compared to 198 Cultures from Women with Recurrent Urinary Infections

Bacteria per Milliliter	Normal Controls	Recurrent Infections
	% cultures	*% cultures*
E. coli:		
0	77.5	44.9
1–99	13.0	17.8
100–999	4.0	10.1
1,000–9,999	5.0	13.6
10,000 or more	0.5	13.6
Enterococci:		
0	83.5	52.0
1–99	6.0	5.6
100–999	6.5	9.6
1,000–9,999	4.0	20.2
10,000 or more	0	12.6
Any Gram-negatives[b]:		
0	76.0	43.4
1–99	15.5	18.2
100–999	3.0	10.6
1,000–9,999	5.0	13.6
10,000 or more	0.5	14.2

[a] Reproduced by permission from T. A. Stamey and C. C. Sexton, J. Urol. **113:** 214, 1975.[30]

[b] Only the gram-negative organism in highest concentration (when 2 or more were present) is counted in this analysis.

A was compared to the mean of the ratios in period B by the 1-sample *t* test. The mean of the 31 ratios for the control women was then compared to the 14 ratios in period B using the 2-sample *t* test.

The colonization rate (mean percentage carriage of any number of bacteria) for *E. coli*, Enterobacteriaceae other than *E. coli*, enterococci, and any Gram-negative bacteria is presented in Table 5.8. There is no significant difference between the colonization rates during the first 30 days after administration of an antibiotic and the rate after 30 days. There is a high degree of probability ($P = <0.005$) that the normal population is different from the recurrent infection population for the presence of *E. coli*, enterococci, and all Gram-negative species combined (Enterobacteriaceae and *P. aeruginosa*). The lack of a significant difference for Enterobacteriaceae other than *E. coli—P. mirabilis, Klebsiella* and *Enterobacter*—may be a result of their infrequent occurrence.

The percentage distribution (number of cultures in each count divided by the total number of cultures) is presented in Table 5.9. There is no appreciable difference between periods A and B. While 80% of the control cultures did not have a single Gram-negative organism on the introitus, only 40% of the cultures from patients were similarly free. Of equal importance is the tendency for the bacteria to be present in higher counts. Ten percent of the cultures from patients had more than 10,000 Gram-negative rods, as compared to less than 1% of the control cultures.

The density of introital carriage, which incorporates the mean culture rate of introital carriage and the numbers of bacteria per culture, is expressed as the mean of the individual ratios in each category (Table 5.10). A low rate of carriage and the occurrence of the organisms in small numbers are reflected in the low (0.09–0.35) mean density for the four bacterial categories analyzed in control women. The mean densities for women with recurrent urinary infections were significantly higher, reflecting a more frequent and heavier vaginal colonization pattern. Of equal importance is the observation that the antibiotics used to treat the urinary infections did not significantly alter the vaginal colonization patterns when the cultures from the period within the first 30 days after administration

Table 5.7
Mean Duration of Longest Consecutive Carriage for *Escherichia coli*, Enterococci and Any Gram-negatives[a]

Bacteria	Normal Controls	Recurrent Infections
	wk/cultures	*wk/cultures*
E. coli	1.8/1.8	7.8/5.1
Enterococci	2.0/2.0	7.9/5.0
Any Gram-negatives	1.8/1.8	7.9/5.2

[a] Reproduced by permission from T. A. Stamey and C. C. Sexton, J. Urol. **113:** 214, 1975.[30]

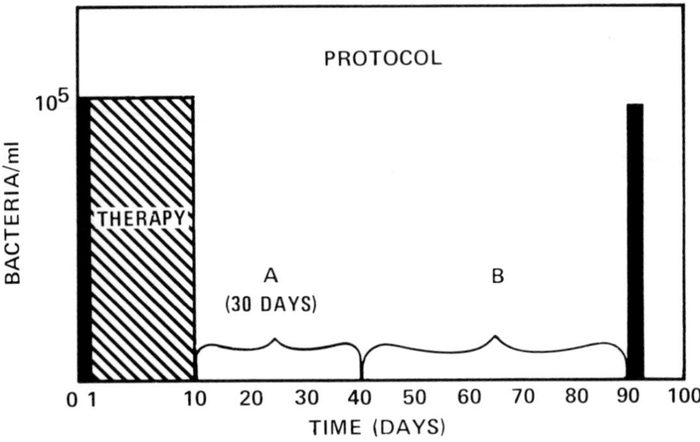

Figure 5.4 Protocol for analyzing the influence of antimicrobial therapy on introital carriage in the first 30 days after the completion of 10 days of therapy (*A*) compared to the remainder of the days until the next bacteriuric episode (*B*).

Table 5.8
Mean Percentage Carriage Incidence[a]

Bacteria	Control[b] (31 Women—416 Cultures)	Recurrent Infection[b] (14 Women—254 Cultures)		A *vs.* B	ΔC *vs.* B
	C	A	B	*P* Value	
Escherichia coli	20 ± 4	58 ± 9	51 ± 10	0.05	<.001
Enterobacteriaceae other than *E. coli*	6 ± 2	17 ± 7	20 ± 8	NS[c]	NS
Enterococci	17 ± 3	53 ± 10	49 ± 11	NS	<.001
Any gram-negatives (Enterobacteriaceae or Pseudomonas)	23 ± 4	58 ± 10	52 ± 10	NS	<.005

[a] Reproduced by permission from A. J. Schaeffer and T. A. Stamey, J. Urol. **118:** 221, 1977.[31]

[b] A—cultures obtained within first 30 days after antibiotic therapy for urinary infection. B—cultures obtained 31 or more days after antibiotic therapy for urinary infection. C—controls. Values given are plus or minus 1 standard deviation.

[c] NS = not significant.

of the antibiotic were compared to the succeeding cultures.

Other Investigations

O'Grady et al.[32] obtained introital, urethral, and deep vaginal swabs from 158 "control" women, most of whom were attending hospital clinics and many of whom may have been on antibiotics for disorders unrelated to urinary infections. These swabs were directly streaked onto agar plates; some colonies of Enterobacteriaceae were found in 58%, and 5 or more colonies were found in 23% of the subjects. I would hope this surprisingly high carriage rate is related to (1) attendance at medical and surgical clinics; (2) antibiotic ingestion, especially ampicillin (see Chapter 4); and (3) possibly an older group of postmenopausal women (ages are not given).

Cox and his colleagues[33, 34] recovered Gram-negative bacilli from the urethra in 54% of UTI-prone women and in 27% of healthy women. Controls in this study also were women seen in the hospital, some had dysuria, and 10% had *Aerobacter aerogenes* on their urethra.[33]

Bailey *et al.*[35] examined 524 women attending a "well woman clinic" for a cervical smear examination; urethral and vaginal swabs were plated directly (as in O'Grady's study) and reported positive only if 5 or more colonies of Enterobacteriaceae were

Table 5.9
Numerical Distribution of Enterobacteriaceae and Enterococci[a]

Bacteria per Milliliter	Control[b] (416 Cultures)	Recurrent Infections[b] (254 Cultures)	
	C	A	B
Escherichia coli			
0	83.4	39.5	47.2
10–100	10.1	27.6	12.9
110–1,000	4.8	10.5	10.7
1,010–10,000	1.4	14.5	18.5
>10,000	0.3	7.9	10.7
Enterobacteriaceae other than *E. coli*:			
0	94.7	77.6	81.0
10–100	3.1	5.3	8.4
110–1,000	1.7	9.2	7.3
1,010–10,000	0.5	5.3	2.8
>10,000	0.0	2.6	0.5
Enterococci:			
0	84.1	48.7	49.4
10–100	6.7	2.6	7.9
110–1,000	7.5	17.1	11.2
1,010–10,000	1.7	27.6	26.4
>10,000	0.0	4.0	5.1
Any Gram-negative[c]:			
0	79.8	38.2	42.7
10–100	12.3	26.3	15.7
110–1,000	6.5	10.5	11.8
1,010–10,000	1.2	14.5	19.1
>10,000	0.2	10.5	10.7

[a] Reproduced by permission from A. J. Schaeffer and T. A. Stamey, J. Urol. **118:** 221, 1977.[31]

[b] A—cultures obtained within first 30 days after antibiotic therapy for urinary infection. B—cultures obtained 31 or more days after antibiotic therapy for urinary infection.

[c] Only the gram-negative organism in highest concentration (when 2 or more were present) is counted in this analysis.

present per agar plate. Fifteen percent of the premenopausal, nonbacteriuric "well women" had positive introital cultures compared to 23% of postmenopausal women attending the same clinic. Unfortunately, at least to compare with our method of reporting any colonies present, we are not told how many cultures had <5 colonies of enterobacteria per agar plate.

In contrast to these studies, Pfau and Sacks[36] cultured the introitus, urethra and midvagina in 100 healthy, premenopausal women who were neither attending clinics nor taking antibiotics; only 7 of the 100 introital cultures contained Enterobacteriaceae. These authors used our technique of placing the swabs into 5 ml of transport medium (Chapter 1) but wisely compared it to the direct plate streaking technique used by O'Grady[32] and Bailey[35]; in general, the bacterial numbers per ml of transport broth far exceeded the number of colonies per agar plate from direct streaking of the swab. Two out of 30 paired studies, however, failed to show agreement; in both instances, small numbers of bacteria (70 and 16 colonies per plate) present with the direct plating technique were not found in the cultures from the transport fluid. The authors do not note which swab of the introitus was taken first in these duplicate experiments. It is possible the first swab could remove the surface bacteria, especially if present in small numbers.

Marsh *et al.*[37] examined introital swabs in 83 patients in relation to their subsequent history of developing bacteriuria. Apparently introital cultures were rarely obtained because they expressed their data on bacteriuria in relation to the first introital swab or to growth of *E. coli* in the first two swabs. There are no indications of the time that elapsed between these swabs and the occurrence of bacteriuria. I trust it is clear from the data in Chapter 4 and this chapter that many introital swabs are required to establish the relationship between introital colonization and the occurrence of bacteriuria.

The failure of other investigators to confirm our observations can be attributed, in part, to their limited search based on a few vaginal cultures to distinguish between susceptible and nonsusceptible populations. For example, Cattell and associates[38] limited their observations to 6 weekly cultures beginning 6 weeks after the last bacteriuric episode. Indeed, it is not clear from this investigation whether the patients even had a further episode of bacteriuria. Precisely because of the tendency of patients with recurrent bacteriuria to undergo long periods of remission, usually with reversion of enterobacterial colonization of the vagina

Table 5.10
Mean Density of Introital Carriage[a]

Bacteria	Control[b] (31 Women—416 Cultures)	Recurrent Infections[b] (14 Women—254 Cultures)		A *vs.* B	C *vs.* B
	C	A	B	*P* Value	
Escherichia coli	0.30 ± 0.07	1.22 ± .29	1.09 ± .29	Not sign.	<0.001
Enterobacteriaceae other than *E. coli*	0.09 ± 0.03	0.39 ± .16	0.30 ± .10	Not sign.	0.02
Enterococci	0.28 ± 0.06	1.46 ± .29	1.24 ± .31	Not sign.	<0.001
Any Gram-negatives (Enterobacteriaceae or Pseudomonas)	0.35 ± 0.07	1.27 ± .29	1.20 ± .28	Not sign.	<0.001

[a] Reproduced by permission from A. J. Schaeffer and T. A. Stamey, J. Urol. **118:** 221, 1977.[31]

[b] A—cultures obtained within first 30 days after antibiotic therapy for urinary infection. B—cultures obtained 31 or more days after antibiotic therapy for urinary infection. C—controls. Values given are plus or minus 1 standard deviation.

$$\text{Density} = \frac{\text{Sum of products of number of cultures per category} \times \text{category number}}{\text{Number of cultures}}\text{; see text.}$$

Category—0, 10–100, 110–1,000, 1,010–10,000 and more than 10,000.
Category number—0, 1, 2, 3 and 4.

to normal, we analyzed all vaginal cultures between two consecutive episodes of bacteriuria.

Part of the difficulty, too, is the understandable desire to separate UTI-prone women from normal women by a single introital culture. I hope it is apparent from clinical examples like K.S. (Figures 4.5 and 4.6 in Chapter 4) as well as the data in Table 5.9 that these two populations cannot be separated on the basis of a single culture. In Table 5.9, for example, 40% (38.2–42.7%) of all introital cultures from UTI-prone patients did not contain one single colony of Enterobacteriaceae or pseudomonas; on the other hand, 20% of all cultures from normal, premenopausal women contained at least some Gram-negative bacteria, even though over one-half of these positive cultures contained only 10–100 bacteria/ml of transport broth.

Bollgren and Winberg[39] have studied the periurethral aerobic bacterial flora in healthy boys and girls. Similar to our premenopausal women, they found that, after the age of 5 years, *E. coli* and enterococci are very rare in the healthy child. They confirmed our studies[29] that voided urine samples from healthy school girls contain very few Gram-negative bacteria, even when collected without preceding cleansing and even when the first-voided few milliliters of urine is cultured separately. They collected VB_1 and VB_2 urine samples from 72 healthy school girls 8–16 years old; 90% of these samples contained no *E. coli* or enterococci, and only 2 girls had more than 1000 *E. coli*/ml of urine.

Bollgren and her associates[40] have recently compared the periurethral aerobic microflora in pregnant women to that in nonpregnant women attending a family planning clinic. They were especially interested in Group B-streptococci (see Table 4.33 in section on Bacteriuria of Pregnancy, Chapter 4), enterococci, and Enterobacteriaceae. Group B-streptococci were isolated in 34 of 88 nonpregnant women (39%); interestingly, the carrier rate was 56% in the first week of the menstrual cycle but only 27% later in the cycle ($P < 0.05$). Enterobacteriaceae were isolated from 17 of 72 pregnant women (24%) and from 14 of 88 nonpregnant women (16%); their culture technique of pressing gelatin to a 1-cm square surface area would certainly detect small numbers of bacteria. Periurethral carriage of enterococci, 98% of which were *Streptococcus faecalis*, occurred in 42% of the pregnant women, of whom 24% were heavily colonized; in contrast, only 18% of the nonpregnant women were colonized with enterococci and only one of these 88 women was heavily colonized (1%). These data, therefore, on carriage of Enterobacteriaceae (16%) and enterococci (18%) in the periurethral area of nonpregnant women are virtually identical to the carriage rate in our introital cultures from healthy volunteers (20% and 16%, respectively, Table 5.9).

Pérez-Miravete and Jaramillo[41] determined the incidence of *E. coli* isolation from the anterior vagina in high, medium, and low socioeconomic groups in Mexico City; the percent with positive cultures—16.5, 9.7, and 13.1, respectively—was not significantly different among the three groups. These isolation rates are comparable to ours, Pfau and Sacks,[36] and Bollgren and associates.[40]

Other interesting studies on vaginal microbiology include the careful one by Morris and Morris[42] who studied 291 nonpregnant women attending a family planning clinic, 75% of whom were between the ages 20 and 35 years. Culture plates were swab inoculated. *E. coli* were isolated in 5.8% and proteus in 2.7%; *E. coli* was isolated more often in the first half of the menstrual cycle (8.6%) than during the second half (4.3%). Only 2 of the 291 women had increased leukocytes in their vaginal secretion; both of these had *Trichomonas vaginalis*. *S. faecalis* occurred in 10% of the women. β-Hemolytic streptococci occurred in 11%; Lancefield's Group B occurred twice as often as Group D. There was a similarity of the vaginal flora irrespective of whether vaginal tampons or oral contraceptives were used.

Hite *et al.*[43] recovered *E. coli* in 3.3% of 61 vaginal vault cultures from normal prenatal women. Isolation rates increased only to 9.6% in 73 patients with trichomoniasis. Eleven percent of 45 pathological postpartum uteri cultured *E. coli*.

Lock *et al.*[44] using a glass cylinder passed to the midvagina of 75, unmarried, healthy student nurses between the ages of 17 and 25 years, recovered *E. coli* from only 1 of the 75 volunteers!

Our data, and all of the last five reports, seem to clearly indicate that colonization of the vagina or the introitus with *E. coli* in the normal, healthy woman is uncommon; it is surely less than that which occurs in UTI-prone women.

ENTEROBACTERIAL SURVIVAL ON THE VAGINAL MUCOSA

We were convinced from our studies (Tables 5.1–5.10), even if others were not, that colonization of the introital mucosa with Enterobacteriaceae in UTI-prone females was the key to understanding, and perhaps ultimately preventing, recurrent bacteriuria. We believe the data in Tables 5.5–5.10 indicate that Enterobacteriaceae and enterococci colonize the vaginal introitus of the susceptible women with greater frequency than occurs in women resistant to urinary infections; moreover, this enterobacterial colonization seems to occur with a greater density of bacteria (Table 5.10) which persist for longer periods of time (Table 5.7) than we observed in healthy, normal women.

The major question we faced in 1970 was what were the biologic factors that might promote growth of enterobacteria in the vagina or on the introital mucosa? We thought that the factors determining bacterial survival on the vaginal mucosal surface might be broadly divided into: (1) factors affecting bacterial growth rates, (2) microbial interference by the indigenous flora, and (3) host defense mechanisms such as phagocytosis, antibody, etc.

Factors Affecting Bacterial Growth Rates

Enterobacterial Growth in Normal Vaginal Fluid

What happens when *E. coli* from the anal canal reach the introital mucosa of the vagina? What happens when *E. coli* from the male urethra or prostate are deposited within the vaginal canal at the time of ejaculation?

Of the two ways to study this question, *in vivo* by placing *E. coli* in the vagina and determining the characteristics of their survival, or *in vitro* by removing the vaginal fluid from the subject and adding *E. coli* in the laboratory, the latter method offered far greater freedom for both the investigator and the patient. Kaufman and I[45] performed the following experiments.

Vaginal secretions from normal premenopausal women who denied any history of urinary infections were used in this study. No volunteer received antibiotics. Although sexually active these women abstained for at least 24 hours before each collection of vaginal fluids and visits during menstruation were avoided. Specimens were collected with the subject in the lithotomy position by irrigating the vagina through a No. 16F plastic catheter with 50 ml sterile distilled water. The fluid was lyophilized and stored at minus 20°C.

In preliminary experiments pooled vaginal fluid was reconstituted with sterile distilled water at dilutions of 6, 12, 24, 48, and 96 ml. The pH of the 6-ml reconstitution was invariably less than 4.3, and that of the larger dilutions was slightly higher. The pH was adjusted to 6.5 with 0.1 normal and 0.01 normal sodium hydroxide with a Beckman pH meter. Aliquots (3-ml) of pH-adjusted fluid at each dilution were inoculated with 0.1 ml *E. coli* 04 to produce a final concentration of 100–1000 bacteria/ml. Subcultures of 0.1-ml aliquots onto blood agar were obtained at 0, 2, 4, 6, and 24 hours after incubation at 37°C. Appropriate controls of inoculated soy broth adjusted to pH 6.5 as well as uninoculated vaginal fluids also were incubated. These experiments were repeated 4 times on vaginal fluid from four different pools with similar results in each study. Changes in pH during incubation were minimal. As seen in Figures 5.5 and 5.6, the *E. coli* 04 was able to grow at pH 6.5 in all reconstituted dilutions from 6 to 96 ml, although growth only approached that of soy broth in the least diluted specimen. The 12-ml dilution, because of volume requirements, was used in all subsequent studies.

Two basic sets of experiments were performed. In the first, 8 common O-groups of *E. coli* (04, 06, 07, 016, 018, 023, 050, and 075), isolated from patients with urinary infections, were compared to 7 uncommon O-groups (010, 013, 015, 038, 062, 0115, and 0132). Except for 0115, obtained from the Communicable Disease Center in Atlanta, Georgia, the uncommon serogroups were isolated from rectal cultures of our own patients and none had caused a urinary infection. All serogroups were inoculated into 12-ml dilutions of lyophilized vaginal secretions divided into aliquots that had been adjusted to pH of 4.0, 4.2, 4.4, 4.6, 4.8, and 5.0. The 8 common O-groups were run twice (16 experiments), 5 of the uncommon groups were run twice and 2 were run once (12 experiments). Subcultures, size of inoculum and measurements of pH during in-

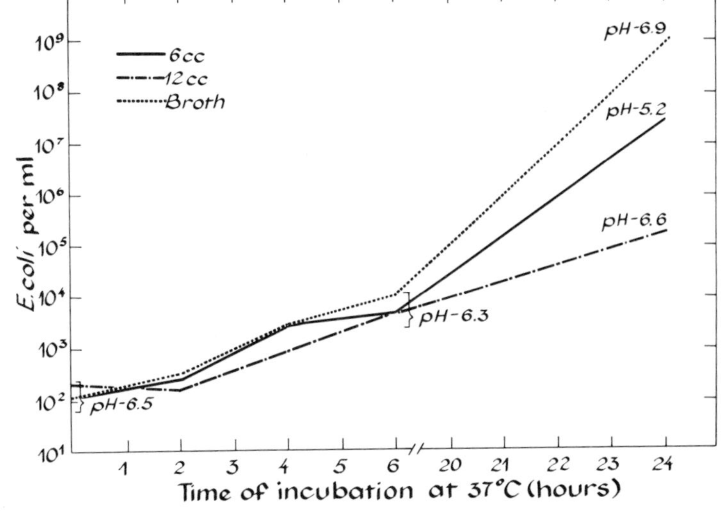

Figure 5.5 Growth of *Escherichia coli* 04 in normal vaginal fluid diluted to 6 and 12 ml volumes and adjusted to pH 6.5. Growth is compared to that in soy broth adjusted to same pH. (Reproduced by permission from T. A. Stamey and M. F. Kaufman, J. Urol. **114:** 264, 1975.[45])

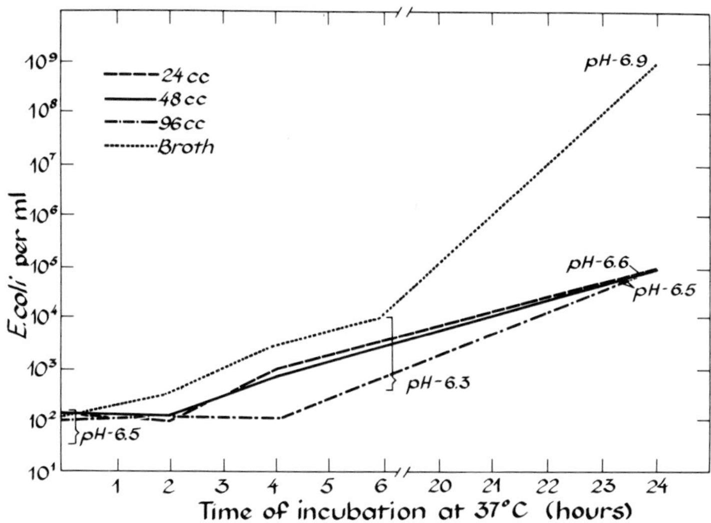

Figure 5.6 Growth of *Escherichia coli* 04 in normal vaginal fluid diluted to 24, 48, and 96 ml volumes and adjusted to pH 6.5. Growth is compared to that in soy broth adjusted to same pH. (Reproduced by permission from T. A. Stamey and M. F. Kaufman, J. Urol. **114:** 264, 1975.[45])

cubation were the same as in the initial dilution experiments in Figures 5.5 and 5.6. Uncommon O-groups were always run simultaneously with common O-groups in separate aliquots of the same vaginal fluid. Growth in vaginal fluid was defined as that pH level at which there was at least a 1 logarithm increase in the number of bacteria above the original inoculum, provided the pH remained within the range of the study (4.0–5.0).

Experiments with 8 Common and 7 Uncommon O-Groups of *E. coli* Inoculated into Vaginal Fluid at 0.2 pH Increments between 4.0 and 5.0. None of the 16 experiments with the common O-groups of *E. coli* or the 12 experiments with uncommon O-groups showed growth at pH 4.0 (Table 5.11). In fact, the 24-hour subcultures at pH 4.0 were sterile except for an *E. coli* 07 and a 075, both showing a 90% kill of the original inoculum. As seen in Table 5.11, 94% of the common O-groups grew at pH 5.0, whereas only 58% of the uncommon O-groups grew at this pH. Of the 16 experiments with common O-groups at pH 4.6, 11 showed growth (69%) compared to only 3 of 12 (25%) of the uncommon O-groups.

From this first set of experiments at 0.2 pH increments, it was apparent that potential growth differences could be measured in vaginal fluid adjusted to pH 4.3, 4.6, and 4.9 with subcultures at 0.6–9 and 24 hours after incubation. For the second set of experiments, pooled vaginal fluid from 12 normal volunteers was used. Common and uncommon O-groups of *E. coli* were inoculated in parallel aliquots for each experimental run. The 10 common O-groups of *E. coli* were 01, 02, 04, 06, 07, 08, 011, 022, 025, and 075. Except for the 01, 02, and 025, which were obtained from the Communicable Disease Center, all others were isolates from patients with urinary infections. The 10 uncommon groups of *E. coli* were selected at random from O-groups never reported as a cause of urinary infection; these O-groups, 034, 043, 053, 063, 0103, 0104, 0116, 0130, 0142, and 0143, were all obtained from the Communicable Disease Center collection. All groups were studied at least 3 times, totaling 35 experiments for the common O-groups and 34 for the uncommon. Growth was compared also in vaginal fluid that was (1) Millipore-filtered (0.20 μ) and (2) boiled for 30 minutes at 100°C. In the presentation of results the natural and filtered secretions are considered as one group, while the data from the boiled secretions are reported separately. For statistical analysis (Wilcoxon 2-sample test), all experiments are combined and tested for significance.

Growth of 10 Common Versus 10 Uncommon O-groups of *E. coli* in Normal

Table 5.11
Growth of 8 Common and 7 Uncommon *Escherichia coli* Serogroups in Vaginal Secretions[a]

pH	Common		Uncommon	
	no.	%	*no.*	%
4.0	0/16	(0)	0/12	(0)
4.2	3/16	(19)	1/12	(8)
4.4	6/16	(37)	1/12	(8)
4.6	11/16	(69)	3/12	(25)
4.8	13/16	(82)	5/12	(42)
5.0	15/16	(94)	7/12	(58)

[a] Reproduced by permission from T. A. Stamey and M. F. Kaufman, J. Urol. **114:** 264, 1975.[45]

Table 5.12
Growth of 10 Common and 10 Uncommon Serogroups in Natural and Filtered Vaginal Secretions[a]

pH	*Escherichia coli* Showing Growth	
	Common	Uncommon
	%	%
4.3	40	20
4.6	80	40
4.9	90	60

[a] Reproduced by permission from T. A. Stamey and M. F. Kaufam, J. Urol. **114:** 264, 1975.[45]

Vaginal Fluid Adjusted to pH Values of 4.3, 4.6, and 4.9. Growth of the common O-groups in natural and filtered vaginal fluid is compared to growth of the uncommon O-groups in Table 5.12. Of the common O-groups 80% were able to grow at pH 4.6 compared to only 40% of the uncommon O-groups. Serogroups 06, 08, 011, and 075 were able to grow at pH 4.3, whereas only two of the uncommon groups grew at the lowest pH.

Growth of both O-groups in boiled vaginal fluid is compared in Table 5.13. Differences in growth are equally apparent except the uncommon O-groups are even more inhibited since 6 of the 10 uncommon O-groups did not grow even at pH 4.9.

When all experiments were combined, whether vaginal fluid was used as collected, filtered or boiled, there were 35 runs with the common serogroups and 34 with the uncommon *E. coli* (Table 5.14). Differences in growth between the two populations of *E. coli* are statistically significant at each pH level (*P* less than 0.01). For example 60% of the common O-groups were able to grow in vaginal fluid at pH 4.6 and only 17.5% of the uncommon O-groups grew at this pH.

Because *P. mirabilis* and *P. aeruginosa* are uncommon causes of bacteriuria, Mihara and I[46] used the same technique to study the inhibitory effect of normal vaginal fluid inoculated with these two urinary pathogens. Fourteen isolates of *P. aeruginosa* and 10 of *P. mirabilis* from patients with bacteriuria were grown overnight in tryptose broth and diluted with distilled water to give a final inoculum of 100–1000 bacteria/ml in the reconstituted vaginal fluid. Then 0.1-ml bacterial suspension was added to 1.5 ml of each pH-adjusted aliquot of vaginal fluid and subcultures of 0.1 ml were made at 0, 6, and 24 hours during incubation at 36°C. Tubes of uninoculated vaginal fluid (negative control), as well as 1.5-ml tubes of tryptose broth inoculated with 0.1 ml bacterial suspension (positive

Table 5.13
Growth of 10 Common and 10 Uncommon Serogroups in Boiled Vaginal Secretions[a]

pH	*Escherichia coli* Showing Growth	
	Common	Uncommon
	%	%
4.3	30	10
4.6	70	10
4.9	80	40

[a] Reproduced by permission from T. A. Stamey and M. F. Kaufman, J. Urol. **114:** 264, 1975.[45]

Table 5.14
Growth of 10 Common and 10 Uncommon Serogroups in Vaginal Secretions (All Experiments Combined)[a]

pH	*Escherichia coli* Showing Growth			
	Common		Uncommon	
	no.	%	*no.*	%
4.3	11/35	(32)	4/34	(12)
4.6	21/35	(69)	6/34	(18)
4.9	25/35	(72)	15/34	(44)
		$P < 0.01$		

[a] Reproduced by permission from T. A. Stamey and M. F. Kaufman, J. Urol. **114:** 264, 1975.[45]

Table 5.15
Effect of pH Adjusted Vaginal Fluid on 10 Strains of *Proteus mirabilis*[a]

Bacteria after incubation	pH 4.3	pH 4.6	pH 4.9
Dead	10	9	8
Viable[b]	—	1	2
Growth[c]	—	—	—
Totals	10	10	10

[a] Reproduced by permission from T. A. Stamey and G. Mihara, J. Urol. **115:** 416, 1976.[46]

[b] Ten to less than 1 log increase above initial inoculum.

[c] At least 1 log increase above initial inoculum.

control) were included with each incubation. The pH was measured on randomly selected tubes to ensure a stable pH during incubation. Colony counts at 0 and 24 hours were compared. Growth was defined as an increase of 1 log or more in numbers of bacteria, viable as the presence at 24 hours of bacteria (10 or more per ml) but showing less than a log increase, and bacterial death as a sterile culture on subculture at 24 hours.

Survival figures for *P. mirabilis* at each pH are shown in Table 5.15 and for *P. aeruginosa* in Table 5.16. Neither organism survived a pH of 4.3 in vaginal fluid. Nine of 10 strains of *P. mirabilis* and 12 of 14 of *P. aeruginosa* were killed at pH 4.6. Viability and growth of *P. aeruginosa* at pH 4.9 was substantial, while *P. mirabilis* was still sharply inhibited at this pH.

These studies show that pH-adjusted vaginal fluid is much more inhibitory to *P. mirabilis* and *P. aeruginosa* than to the common serogroup strains of *E. coli*, and may offer one explanation (among several) of why those organisms are less frequent causes of bacteriuria in the female patient.

These studies establish that normal vaginal fluid supports growth of enterobacteria when the pH is raised. Vaginal fluid is known to contain glycogen, lactic acid, glucose, maltose, maltotriose, maltotetreose, and several amino acids,[47–49] clearly giving it the potential of a minimal growth medium. Whether the inhibitory effect on enterobacteria at the lower pH is caused by hydrogen ion concentration alone or by a change in biologic ionization of organic acids or some other inhibitory substance is unknown. However, it is interesting that human vaginal fluid does not contain an antimicrobial factor such as we have described in prostatic fluid where the antibacterial activity is bactericidal and active over a wide range of pH.[50]

One possible explanation for the greater resistance of the common O-group *E. coli* to a lower vaginal pH could be previous adaptation to the vaginal environment since these *E. coli* were selected from women with bacteriuria (except for the 01, 02, and 025 obtained from the Communicable Disease Center). Because of this possibility, additional common O-groups of *E. coli* were isolated from the rectal flora of 10 male volunteers and growth again was compared to uncommon O-groups in normal vaginal fluid. The results were no different from the data reported herein; 20% of the uncommon O-groups grew at pH 4.3, while 50% of the common *E. coli* grew at this pH.

Thus, it appears that one reason uncommon O-groups rarely cause urinary infections is their greater susceptibility to the inhibitory action of vaginal fluid at a pH between 4.0 and 5.0. Another reason, of course, is their less frequent occurrence in the bowel flora.[8]

pH of the Introital Mucosa

Bacterial growth rates of *E. coli* and other enterobacteria are influenced by the hydrogen ion concentration of the fluid to

Table 5.16
Effect of pH Adjusted Vaginal Fluid on 14 Strains of *Pseudomonas aeruginosa*[a]

Bacteria after Incubation	pH 4.3	pH 4.6	pH 4.9
Dead	14	12	4
Viable[b]	—	2	3
Growth[c]	—	—	7
Totals	14	14	14

[a] Reproduced by permission from T. A. Stamey and G. Mihara, J. Urol. **115:** 416, 1976.[46]

[b] Ten to less than 1 log increase above initial inoculum.

[c] At least 1 log increase above initial inoculum.

which they are exposed. We looked at the relationship between surface pH of the vaginal introitus and the presence of *E. coli*, *P. mirabilis*, and enterococci.[51]

We examined 800 vaginal cultures from 169 women between 18 and 81 years old, including 88 cultures from 8 women who had never had urinary infections. Of these 800 cultures, 363 were from 24 women who were more closely followed for recurrent infections. The remaining 137 women were seen at the urologic out-patient unit with a variety of conditions, including urinary incontinence, calculous disease, and urinary infections. All vaginal cultures were included regardless of whether the patient had bacteriuria at the time of the culture.

A sterile surface electrode (Instrumentation Laboratories, Model 14043) attached to a radiometer digital pH meter was placed on the mucosal surface of the vaginal vestibule at the level of the hymenal ring at the 3 and 9 o'clock positions. The mean of the two recordings, which rarely differed by more than 0.2 pH units, was used for this analysis. After the introital pH was recorded a quantitative culture of the same surface area was obtained.

The mean pH of all 800 measurements was 4.9 with a range of 3.7–7.5. When the pH was plotted against the numbers of bacteria cultured, either individually or collectively, a complete scattergram was obtained without any relationship between the two variables.

Because 93.5% of all introital cultures from normal, healthy women contain 100 or less *E. coli*/ml of transport broth (Table 5.9), we decided to look at only those cultures which were likely to be pathological (*i.e.*, >100 bacteria/ml).

The data in Table 5.17 show the percentage of all cultures at each pH that contained more than 100 bacteria/ml of *E. coli*, *P. mirabilis*, and enterococci on the vaginal introitus. For *E. coli* and *P. mirabilis* there is a substantial increase in bacterial carriage above a pH of 4.4. Accordingly, Figures 5.7–5.9 indicate the number of cultures with ≤100 and >100 bacteria/ml that occurred at a pH of ≤4.4 and a pH of >4.4. The difference in vaginal carriage within these pH divisions, using a chi-square analysis, is highly significant for all three bacteria ($P < 0.005$).

Whereas these data show that vaginal carriage of *E. coli*, *P. mirabilis*, and enterococci at more than 100 bacteria/ml is more often associated with an introital pH of more than 4.4, carriage of this magnitude clearly occurs at a pH of ≤4.4 (Table 5.17). Moreover, a high vaginal pH can occur without pathogenic introital carriage. Indeed, if all vaginal carriage, regardless of the number of organisms, is plotted against the pH of each sample, a scattergram is obtained. Thus, we conclude that while there is no direct relationship between pH and vaginal colonization with enterobacteria, it is clear that carriage with more

Table 5.17
Percentage of Cultures with More than 100 *Escherichia coli*, *Proteus mirabilis* and Enterococci (per ml) in Relation to Introital pH[a]

pH	No. Samples	Percentage of Cultures with >100 Bacteria/ml		
		E. coli	*P. mirabilis*	Enterococci
3.8	3	0.0	0.0	0.0
3.9	22	9.0	4.5	13.6
4.0	21	4.8	0.0	14.3
4.1	53	17.0	7.5	20.7
4.2	58	13.8	0.0	24.1
4.3	58	12.0	1.9	20.7
4.4	83	20.5	8.5	30.1
4.5	51	47.0	11.7	31.3
4.6	39	33.3	7.7	35.9
4.7	55	32.7	7.3	32.7
4.8	37	40.5	10.5	40.5
4.9	26	38.4	19.2	30.8
5.0	32	31.2	3.1	31.2
5.1	15	33.3	13.3	53.3
5.2	21	42.9	9.5	47.6
5.3	28	42.8	14.3	50.0
5.4	19	57.9	10.4	57.9
5.5	24	41.7	12.5	58.3
5.6	15	33.3	6.7	40.0
5.7	17	58.8	11.6	35.3
5.8	14	35.7	21.4	42.9
5.9	11	54.5	27.3	27.3
6.0	14	50.0	14.3	14.3
>6.0	84	27.1	21.6	31.2

[a] Reproduced by permission from T. A. Stamey and M. M. Timothy, J. Urol. **114:** 261, 1975.[51]

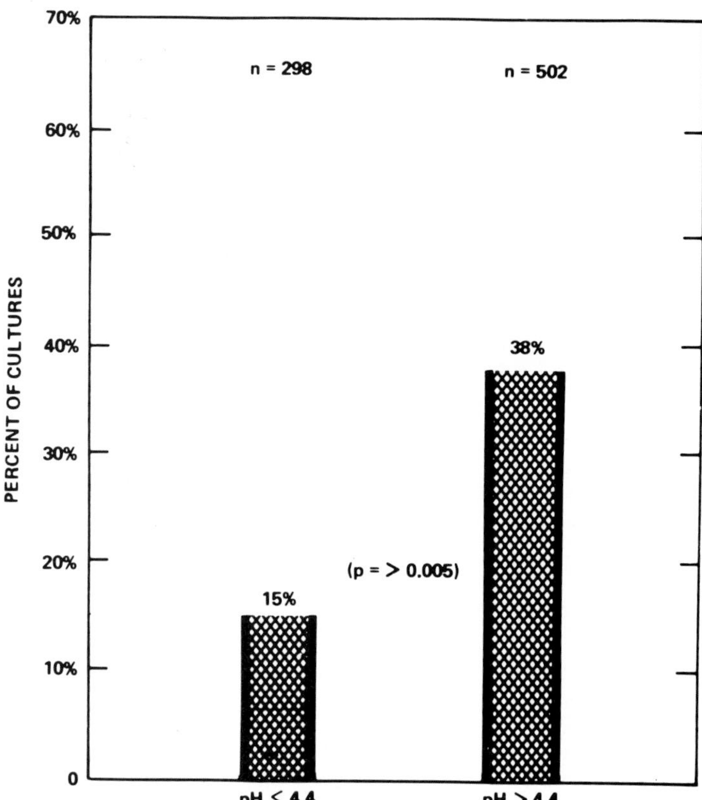

Figure 5.7 Percentage of introital cultures showing more than 100 *Eschericia coli*/ml at an introital pH of ≤4.4 and >4.4. (Reproduced by permission from T. A. Stamey and M. M. Timothy, J. Urol. **114:** 261, 1975.[51])

than 100 bacteria/ml is often associated with a pH of >4.4. One of the reasons that carriage with ≤100 bacteria/ml may occur on the introitus at a pH ≤4.4 probably relates to the transient nature of the colonization, that is these fecal organisms could have reached the introitus only minutes or hours before the culture and do not necessarily represent a real colonization in the true sense of bacterial persistence. If introital pH is a significant defense mechanism in accounting for the biologic difference in introital colonization between women susceptible and not susceptible to urinary infections, it is more difficult to explain the absence of enterobacterial colonization in those samples with a higher pH. Indeed, two of our control premenopausal subjects who have never had urinary infections and who are either never colonized with enterobacteria or only transiently colonized with ≤100 bacteria/ml have a consistently high introital pH (5.5–6.0).

The literature before 1955 is contradictory on the relation of vaginal pH and bacterial flora; there is an excellent review by Lang.[52] In general, cultures were not quantitated, the emphasis was on Döderlein's bacillus, studies were limited to the upper vagina and pH was determined by indicator dyes or paper. More recent investigations emphasize vaginal discharge, especially trichomonas and monilia.[53] There are no previous reports relating vaginal pH to the carriage of enterobacteria in patients without vaginal discharge who are susceptible to urinary infection. In our earlier longitudinal studies on individual patients,[24] we reported no difference in introital pH between controls and women susceptible to urinary infections but pH was measured with litmus paper.

In a later study on vaginal glycogen,[54] we measured introital pH with the digital radiometer in controls and patients without regard to introital colonization with enter-

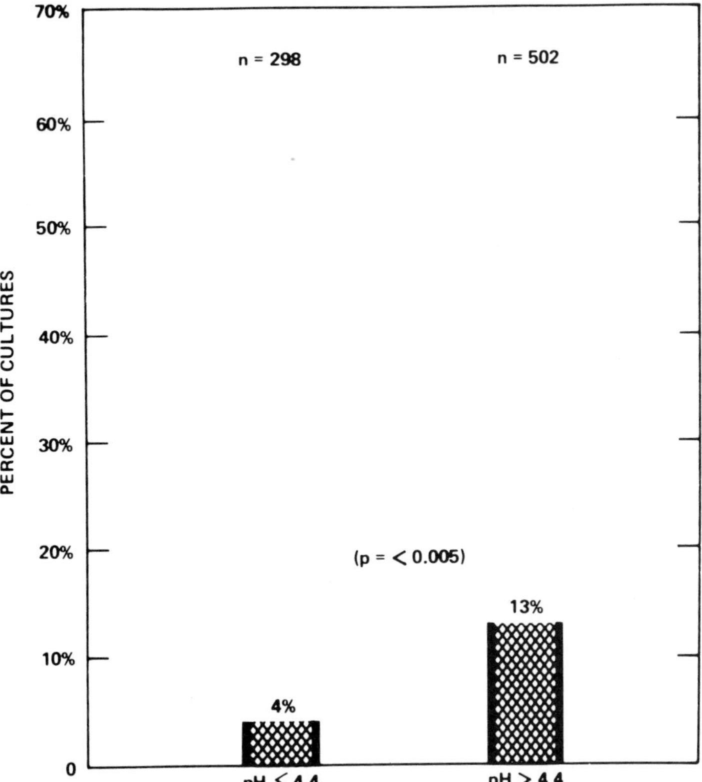

Figure 5.8 Percentage of introital cultures showing more than 100 *Proteus mirabilis*/ml at an introital pH of ≤4.4 and >4.4. (Reproduced by permission from T. A. Stamey and M. M. Timothy, J. Urol. **114:** 261, 1975.[51])

obacteria. As seen in Table 5.18, 90 measurements from 10 premenopausal, healthy volunteers (pH 4.4 ± 0.3) were no different than 226 measurements in 12 premenopausal patients with recurrent bacteriuria (4.5 ± 0.5).

I conclude from these studies that pH of the introital mucosa *per se* does not determine susceptibility to urinary infections. The higher pH in women colonized with >100 enterobacteria/ml may be secondary to the bacteria.

Vaginal Glycogen

Although lactobacilli are unable to use human vaginal glycogen in their metabolism,[55] several enzymes for glycogenolysis have been identified in human cervical epithelium[56] and α-amylase is present in cervical mucus.[57] Once glycogen is debranched to glucose-1-phosphate, the major nucleotide fractions required for glycolysis to lactic acid have been identified in the vaginal mucosa of the rabbit, undergoing substantial reduction after castration and increasing with estrogen therapy.[58]

Thus, just in case glycogen was playing a significant role in bacterial metabolism, Timothy and I[54] thought we should measure glycogen in vaginal secretions of UTI-prone patients and healthy controls.

During a 6-month period 12 premenopausal women with documented recurrent urinary infections were followed with frequent clinic visits. Six normal premenopausal women who denied a history of bacteriuria and who were free from vaginitis made weekly visits for 10 consecutive weeks. At each visit quantitative cultures of the introital mucosa were made followed by surface electrode recordings of the introital pH. A soft plastic catheter was then inserted into the midvagina and 50 ml sterile distilled water was gently injected and withdrawn in a syringe. The syringe was emptied into a sterile vial and the content was lyophilized.

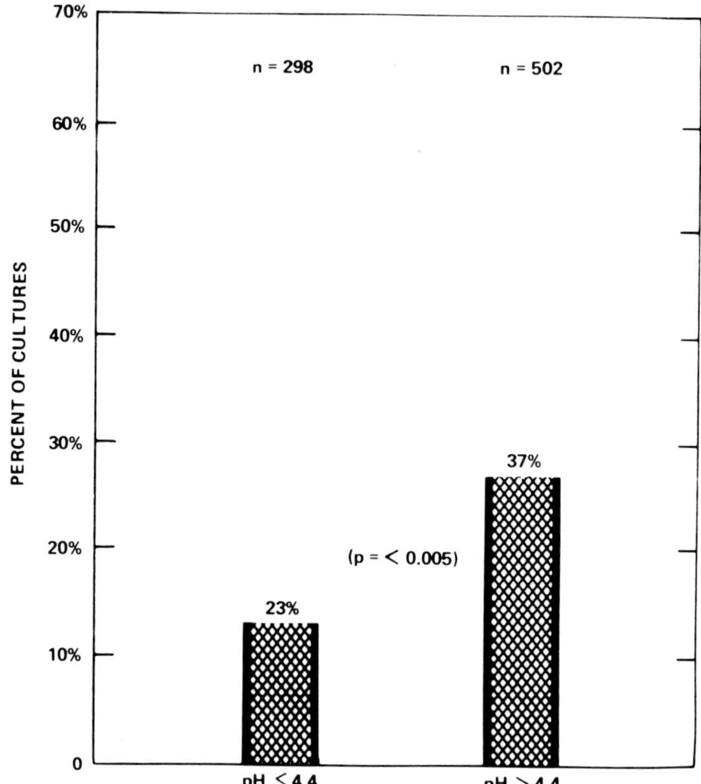

Figure 5.9 Percentage of introital cultures showing more than 100 enterococci/ml at an introital pH of ≤4.4 and >4.4. (Reproduced by permission from T. A. Stamey and M. M. Timothy, J. Urol. **114:** 261, 1975.[51])

Table 5.18
pH of Introital Mucosa in Premenopausal, Healthy Controls and Urinary Tract Infection-Prone Women

Subjects	No. of Women	No. of Determinations	pH ± S.D.[a]	
Controls	10	90	4.4 ± 0.3	P = >0.05
Patients	12	226	4.5 ± 0.5	

[a] S.D. = 1 standard deviation.

The lyophilized material was reconstituted to 10 ml with sterile distilled water. Sodium and potassium concentrations were determined by flame photometry. Glycogen content was measured in 1 ml reconstitution, using the method of Seifter and associates.[59]

Glycogen content was measured in 37 collections from the control volunteers and 96 samples from the infection group. Sodium and potassium determinations were made in a larger number of samples. Student's t test was used to analyze statistical differences between the groups.

The data are presented in Table 5.19. There was no statistical difference in vaginal glycogen content between the two groups. If anything, glycogen concentration was higher in the vaginal fluid from women susceptible to recurrent urinary infections but a greater disparity in standard deviation also occurred. The concentration of potassium was the same in both groups. Interestingly, sodium content was higher (P <0.01) in the women with recurrent infections.

The relationship between glycogen content and pH of the introitus is seen in Table

Table 5.19
Concentration of Glycogen, Sodium and Potassium in Human Vaginal Fluid of Women with Recurrent Urinary Infections Compared to Normal Control Volunteers[a]

	Glycogen		Potassium		Sodium	
	Controls	Patients	Controls	Patients	Controls	Patients
	μg/ml		*mEq/L*		*mEq/L*	
No. samples	37	96	45	114	45	112
Mean	440	564	1.4	1.4	4.5	6.3
Standard deviation	±432	±669	±0.6	±0.8	±1.8	±4.5
	t = 1.039		t = 0		t = 264	
	P = >0.05				*P* = <0.01	

[a] Reproduced by permission from T. A. Stomey and M. M. Timothy, J. Urol. **114:** 268, 1975.[54]

Table 5.20
Relationship of Introital pH to Vaginal Glycogen content[a]

Controls (37)			Patients (92)		
Mean Glycogen Concentration	No. with <4.4 pH	No. with ≥4.4 pH	Mean Glycogen Concentration	No. with <4.4 pH	No. with ≥4.4 pH
μg/ml			*μg/ml*		
>440	14	0	>564	25	3
<440	12	11	<564	34	30

[a] Reproduced by permission from T. A. Stamey and M. M. Timothy, J. Urol. **114:** 268, 1975.[54]

5.20. The distribution of all samples with a pH <4.4 or ≥4.4 in relation to the mean glycogen concentration of controls (440 μg/ml) and patients (564 μg/ml) is shown. While high and low glycogen concentrations were found at an introital pH >4.4, a higher pH was nearly always associated with low vaginal concentrations.

In a previous study we measured the sodium and potassium concentrations of natural vaginal fluid by direct micropipetting followed by the 50-ml wash of the vagina with distilled water.[60] We showed that this method of washing the vagina to collect fluid recovers about 1 ml. pure vaginal fluid. Thus, the glycogen concentrations in undiluted vaginal fluid, as well as the sodium and potassium concentrations, are 10 times those shown in Table 5.19 (a 10-ml reconstitution of the lyophilized material was used for analysis). It is known that the normal vagina produces about 6 g/day of aqueous material with reabsorption of 4.5 g/day,[61] and that cotton swabbing of the vaginal walls produces about 1 g of aqueous material.[62]

Although the method we used for collecting vaginal fluid is clearly semiquantitative, the standard deviation of potassium and sodium in the normal controls does not suggest large variations in the amount of vaginal fluid collected with each 50-ml wash. The larger variation in glycogen content of vaginal fluid is difficult to understand unless it represents a natural biologic variation. Gregoire and associates[63] measured vaginal tissue glycogen from biopsies in patients undergoing a gynecological operation. They also used the method of Seifter and associates for chemical analysis and reported a surprising constancy of vaginal wall glycogen in all patients regardless of menstrual cycle phase or even whether the patient was premenopausal or postmenopausal. Their data suggest higher glycogen content near the vaginal outlet rather than deep within the vaginal canal. Our control patients were similar to the women with recurrent urinary infections in age and birth control measures. We have analyzed the variation of vaginal glycogen in our subjects in respect to three periods of the menstrual cycle. In agreement with the tissue studies by Gregoire and associates[63] and the enzyme analyses by Fienberg and Cohen,[56] we could show no correlation with vaginal glycogen and the various phases of the endocrine cycle but no patient had daily collections throughout the cycle to truly test this hypothesis. It is interesting that our patients with a higher introital pH had smaller concentrations of glycogen (Table 5.20).

We have no explanation for the differences between the two groups in sodium concentration of vaginal fluid. However, these differences were so impressive in a few patients that we thought at one time we could detect biologic susceptibility to urinary infections by simply determining the sodium concentration of vaginal fluid.

These studies indicate that, using these methods to collect and assay vaginal glycogen, susceptibility to introital colonization and recurrent urinary infections in women is not caused by failure of glycogen synthesis nor is it likely owing to a defect in glycogenolysis.

Estrogen

In our original studies, Papanicolaou's stains were made of both vaginal smears and 1.0 ml of the VB_1 urine passed through a 0.45 μ membrane filter. The karyopyknotic index, representing the percentage of squamous epithelial cells with a pyknotic nucleus, was calculated for both control, healthy volunteers[28] and UTI-prone patients.[24] No difference in this crude index of estrogen activity could be detected in the two groups.

These patients and controls were premenopausal; we have not studied this index in postmenopausal women. I would, however, like to note one interesting postmenopausal, healthy control subject whom I studied in some detail and who agreed to take oral estrogen after our preliminary observations. She was a 57-year-old, black woman who had never had urinary infections and had been in good health all her life; an abdominal hysterectomy without oophorectomy was done in 1950 at the age of 34 years. She volunteered for 10 consecutive weeks of introital cultures and urine specimens. In Figure 5.10, one can observe the introital cultures, the introital pH, and the number of leukocytes/ml of transport broth from the introital swab culture. We were impressed with the high introital pH (between 7 and 8) and the constant presence of enterobacteria, mainly *Klebsiella* and *P. mirabilis* at every culture, even though they were present in small numbers for the most part. Several of the leukocyte counts on the introitus seemed elevated (see section below on vaginal leukocytes) but the variation was great. She agreed to take 0.30 mg of conjugated estrogens each day for 13 weeks. Figure 5.10 shows the dramatic fall in introital pH from 7.5 to 4.0, and its surprising persistence at the 5.3 level 2 years after discontinuing the estrogen. These studies in Figure 5.10 were carried out between 1973 and 1975 and, in April and May of 1979, she was restudied on five occasions; all of her introital pH values were between 5.2 and 5.5, and she was continually colonized with both *E. coli* and *P. mirabilis* in substantial numbers at every culture (3 of the 5 introital cultures showed *E. coli* greater than 1000 bacteria/ml). The only time in her life she has ever taken any form of estrogen is shown in Figure 5.10. Why the hydrogen ion concentration should remain 100-fold increased over her pre-estrogen values 6 years after stopping the estrogen remains a mystery. Weinstein and Howard[64] also observed this phenomenon after 3 weekly injections of estrogen, but their follow-up extended only 6 months.

The introital cultures and vaginal leukocytes in Figure 5.10 are also interesting. These longitudinal studies suggest both a decline in vaginal leukocytes and a greater frequency of cultures devoid of enterobacteria during the period of estrogen therapy.

Microbial Interference by the Indigenous Flora

Bacterial colonization of mucosal surfaces is determined in part by interrelationships between the colonizing bacteria and the bacterial flora already present on the surface.[65–67] Do variations in the normal vaginal flora alter the susceptibility of this mucosal surface to colonization by Enterobacteriaceae or enterococci from the fecal reservoir? Fowler, Latta, and I[68] undertook a statistical analysis of the vaginal flora of normal women resistant to urinary infection and women with recurrent urinary infection in an attempt to identify interrelationships between the normal vaginal flora and colonization by Enterobacteriaceae or enterococci.

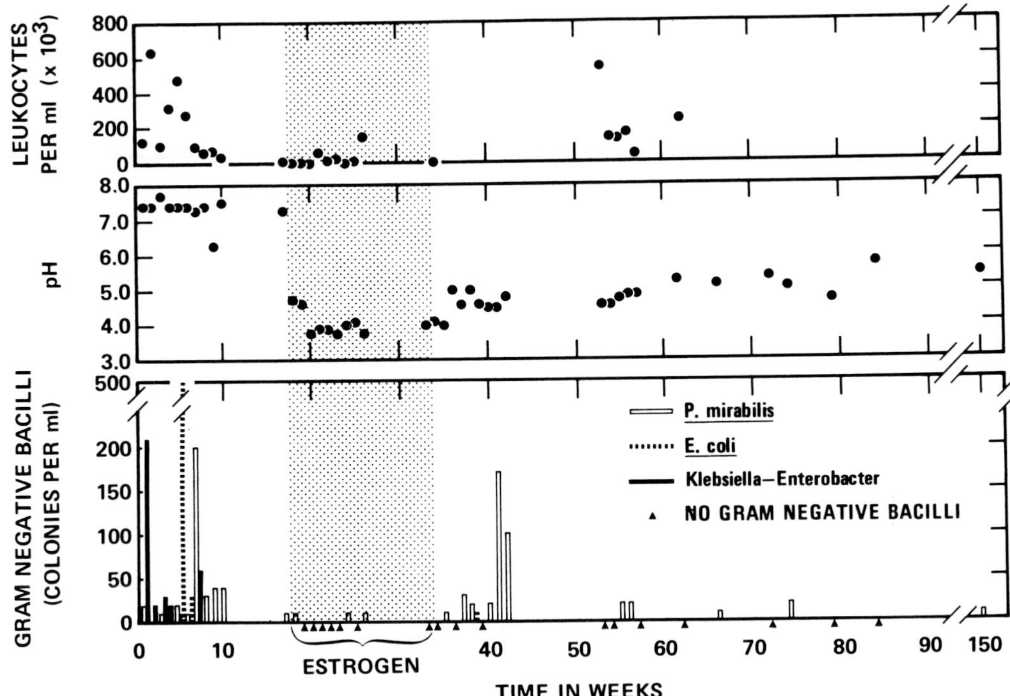

Figure 5.10 Vaginal leukocytes, introital pH, and introital cultures (top to bottom) in a 57-year old, black female patient before, during, and after a 13-week course of 0.30 mg of conjugated estrogen each day. Note the dramatic fall in introital pH from 7.5 to 4.0 and the apparent diminution in vaginal leukocytes and introital carriage of enterobacteria. Six years after her last dose of estrogen, her introital pH remains between 5.2 and 5.5, a 100-fold increase in H+ concentration compared to the pre-estrogen values.

Quantitative cultures of the vaginal introitus obtained before the collection of voided urine, as well as bacterial identification, were performed by techniques described in Chapter 1. The control group consisted of 10 premenopausal, nonhospitalized random volunteers with no history of urinary infection who received no antibiotics before or during the study. Each control woman was cultured at weekly intervals for 10 consecutive weeks.

Eleven premenopausal women with documented recurrent bacteriuria comprised the infection group. None was taking antimicrobial agents immediately prior to or at the time of culture. Cultures were obtained from these subjects weekly or biweekly between episodes of bacteriuria. Five to 12 cultures were obtained from each subject, for a total of 97 cultures. Neither control subjects nor patients douched during the study.

The colonization incidence, regardless of the number, of any Enterobacteriaceae or enterococci expressed as percent of total cultures was tabulated for each group and compared using a 2-sample t test. The colonization incidence, regardless of the number of any identifiable nonpathogenic aerobic organism, was tabulated for each subject and each group. The colonization incidence of each nonpathogenic organism was compared for the control and infection groups, using a 2-sample t test, and the correlation coefficient of the colonization incidence of each of the five most common nonpathogenic organisms and the colonization incidence of any Enterobacteriaceae or enterococci were calculated for each group and tested for significance. Last, the data were analyzed in an effort to uncover associations between the occurrence of nonpathogenic organisms and Enterobacteriaceae or enterococci in individual cultures from each subject. For each of the five most common nonpathogenic organisms four values were tabulated for each woman in both groups: (1) M_{11} equals the number of cultures that yielded the nonpathogenic organism and Enterobacteriaceae or enterococci, (2) M_{12} equals the number of cultures that yielded the nonpathogenic organism but no Enterobacteriaceae or enterococci, (3) M_{21} equals the number of cultures that did not yield the nonpathogenic organism but did grow Enterobacteriaceae or enterococci, and (4) M_{22} equals the number of cultures that did not yield the nonpathogenic organism, or Enterobacteriaceae or enterococci.

We used these values to calculate a measure of association between the nonpathogenic organism and Enterobacteriaceae or enterococci for each woman. The measure used was log $[(M_{11} + 0.5)\ (M_{22} + 0.5)\ (M_{12} + 0.5)\ (M_{21} + 0.5)]$. This is the log of a modified odds ratio. If any of four events occurred, (1) M_{11} equals M_{12} equals 0, (2) M_{11} equals M_{21} equals 0, (3) M_{22} equals M_{12} equals 0, and (4) M_{22} equals M_{21} equals 0, then there was no information on the association in that particular woman and no measure was calculated for her.

Under the null hypothesis of no association between the nonpathogenic organism and Enterobacteriaceae or enterococci these measures should be distributed symmetrically about zero. For each of the 5 nonpathogenic organisms in the control and patient groups the measures were subjected to 1-sample t test to measure for a mean of zero.

Group Analyses. The mean colonization incidence and its standard deviation of any Enterobacteriaceae or enterococci were 75 ± 9% for the infection group and 41 ± 8% for the control group. This difference is statistically significant ($P = 0.01$). In addition, the infection group had carriage by quantitatively greater numbers of these organisms.

The mean colonization incidence and its standard deviation of the nonpathogenic vaginal organisms for the infection and control groups are summarized in Table 5.21. The difference in colonization incidence between the two groups for each of the organisms is not statistically significant except for γ-hemolytic streptococcus, which was present more frequently in introital cultures from the control group ($P = 0.002$).

Table 5.21
Mean Colonization Incidence of Nonpathogenic Vaginal Organisms (Percentage of Total Cultures)[a]

	Control Group	Infection Group
	%	%
Lactobacilli	80 ± 10	62 ± 10
Staphylococcus epidermidis	72 ± 6	64 ± 9
Corynebacteria	43 ± 10	35 ± 7
Candida species	22 ± 10	29 ± 12
γ-hemolytic streptococcus	32 ± 6	9 ± 4[b]
β-hemolytic streptococcus	12 ± 8	21 ± 9
α-hemolytic streptococcus	12 ± 6	9 ± 4

[a] Reproduced by permission from J. E. Fowler, R. Latta, and T. A. Stamey, J. Urol. **118:** 296, 1977.[68]
[b] $P = 0.002$.

The sample correlation coefficients of the colonization incidence of the nonpathogenic organisms and the colonization incidence of Enterobacteriaceae or enterococci for each group are tabulated in Table 5.22. Taken by themselves two of the P values for the sample correlation coefficients appear to be of borderline significance. Since we have made several tests of the hypothesis in the study these may be just spurious significant results.

Individual Culture Analyses. Table 5.23 shows the mean measure of association between each of five nonpathogenic organisms and Enterobacteriaceae or enterococci for the two groups. The number of women upon which a measure was available also is shown. The P value for lactobacilli in the infection group and *Staphylococcus epidermidis* and γ-hemolytic streptococcus in the control group implies that the occurrence of these organisms and Enterobacteriaceae or enterococci are not independent. This may be a spurious significant result since we are testing several things simultaneously. The power of this analysis to detect a significant association is reduced by the fact that in many cases no measure of association was available.

Table 5.22
Sample Correlation Coefficients of Colonization Incidence of Each Non-Pathogenic Organism and Colonization Incidence of Enterobacteriaceae or Enterococci

	Control Group	Infection Group
Lactobacilli	−0.53	−0.12
Staphylococcus epidermidis	0.34	−0.01
Corynebacteria	0.65[b]	0.01
Candida species	−0.62[c]	−0.29
γ-hemolytic streptococcus	0.16	0.09

[a] Reproduced by permission from J. E. Fowler, R. Latta, and T. A. Stamey, J. Urol. **118:** 296, 1977.[68]
[b] $P = 0.04$.
[c] $P = 0.06$.

The aforementioned analyses considered the colonization incidence of Enterobacteriaceae or enterococci and the nonpathogenic organisms, regardless of number. The individual culture data also were analyzed in a quantitative manner to determine whether heavy colonization (greater than 10^3 colonies/ml) by the nonpathogenic organisms was associated with limited colonization (< 100 colonies/ml) by Enterobacteriaceae or enterococci, or whether limited colonization by the nonpathogenic organisms was associated with heavy colonization by Enterobacteriaceae or enterococci. The analysis failed to demonstrate any significant correlations. Indeed, heavy colonization by Enterobacteriaceae or enterococci rarely occurred in the absence of heavy colonization by at least 1 of the 5 most common nonpathogenic organisms.

It also should be noted that although the aforementioned analyses compared the culture incidence of nonpathogenic organisms to that of Enterobacteriaceae or enterococci, nearly identical relationships were obtained when enterococci were excluded from the analysis and only Enterobacteriaceae were considered.

Indigenous microorganisms have been demonstrated to limit the colonization of pathogenic bacteria in the upper respiratory and gastrointestinal tracts.[65–67] *T. vaginalis* has been associated with a significant reduction in the growth of lactobacilli and an increase in the growth of other organisms (nonhemolytic aerobic streptococcus, *Haemophilis vaginalis* and *Mycoplasma* species) on the vaginal mucosa.[69] Although this alteration of the vaginal flora is likely secondary to, and not the cause of the trichomonal infestation, similar interrelationships between vaginal colonization by urinary pathogens and the normal vaginal flora have not been explored previously.

The nonpathogenic vaginal flora is a fluctuating bacterial population, often changing between weekly cultures. However, the overall culture incidence of the nonpathogenic organisms is relatively constant. The culture incidence of nonpathogenic organisms listed in Table 5.21 is similar to that found by other investigators.[42, 70, 71]

The culture incidence of the aerobic nonpathogenic vaginal organisms, except for γ-hemolytic streptococcus, is not significantly different between the infection and control groups. Furthermore, no strongly significant correlations could be demonstrated between the vaginal colonization by Enterobacteriaceae or enterococci and colonization by the common nonpathogenic organisms, when compared for each group or when compared for individual cultures. Although γ-hemolytic streptococcus was cultured more frequently in the control group ($P = 0.002$) the relative infrequency with which this organism was cultured and the lack of correlation between colonization by γ-hemolytic streptococcus and Enterobacteriaceae or enterococci in the patient and control groups suggest that this difference is of no clinical significance.

The susceptibility of the vaginal introitus to colonization by Enterobacteriaceae and enterococci in women with recurrent urinary infection cannot be explained by interrelations between these urinary pathogens and the normal vaginal flora.

I recognize that the statistical analyses in this section are complex, which is why Dr. R. Latta—a biostatistician—is co-author on the original paper with Dr. Fowler and myself.[68] For my part, I have a simpler explanation as to why microbial interference by lactobacilli, *S. epidermidis*, and corynebac-

Table 5.23
Measure of Association Between Occurrence in Individual Cultures of Each Nonpathogenic Organism and of Enterobacteriaceae or Enterococci[a]

	No. Women Yielding Measure of Association	Mean and Standard Deviation
	Infection Group	
Lactobacilli	7	−1.0 ± 0.5[b]
Staphylococcus epidermidis	6	0.6 ± 0.9
Corynebacteria	8	−0.3 ± 0.3
γ-hemolytic streptococcus	4	−0.9 ± 1.0
Candida species	4	−0.5 ± 0.2
	Control Group	
Lactobacilli	5	−0.9 ± 0.7
Staphylococcus epidermidis	6	1.4 ± 0.4[c]
Corynebacteria	6	0.2 ± 0.6
γ-hemolytic streptococcus	8	−1.5 ± 0.6[d]
Candida species	2	−0.3 ± 1.0

[a] Reproduced by permission from J. E. Fowler, R. Latta, and T. A. Stamey, J. Urol. **118:** 296, 1977.[68]
[b] $P = 0.07$.
[c] $P = 0.02$.
[d] $P = 0.03$.

teria is not an effective mechanism in preventing introital colonization with enterobacteria. In Chapter 4, in the section Prophylactic Prevention of Recurrent Bacteriuria, I pointed out that after months of prophylaxis with TMP-SMX—during which time the introital flora is normal without a single colony of enterobacteria (see Figures 4.14 and 4.15)—56% of our patients recolonize with enterobacteria and develop an UTI within 3 months of stopping prophylaxis (Table 4.30). If the presence of a normal introital flora is an effective defense mechanism, it seems to me that colonization with enterobacteria should not recur after months of being absent on prophylaxis.

Bacteriocins

Last, we have screened the vaginal flora of healthy controls for bactericidal or inhibitory activity against *E. coli.* Bacteriocins are bactericidal proteins produced by one organism which inhibit or destroy other bacteria. Fredericq's[72] overlay technique was used to screen the normal flora for inhibitory activity against *E. coli.* Different strains of *E. coli* were poured as an agar overlay on to the surface colonies of the normal vaginal flora. Reincubation of the plates failed to show any inhibition of the six strains of *E. coli* tested.

We then screened individual colonies of lactobacilli and corynebacteria for bacteriocin production against *E. coli*, without any significant success. We did find one colony of corynebacteria that showed a strong inhibition of *E. coli* (Figure 5.11), but the concentration of the corynebacteria in the agar stab was so enormous that the experiment surely has no *in vivo* meaning.

In general, the search for bacteriocin production against *E. coli* by the normal introital flora proved to be a futile effort, at least in our hands.

Host Defense Mechanisms

Phagocytosis—Analysis of Vaginal Leukocytes

It is probably important to know whether colonization of the vaginal introitus with enterobacteria is accompanied by an inflammatory response on the mucosa. Mihara and I[73] examined this question.

The vaginal vestibule was swabbed with a pair of cotton applicator sticks in the area of the hymenal membrane and placed in 5

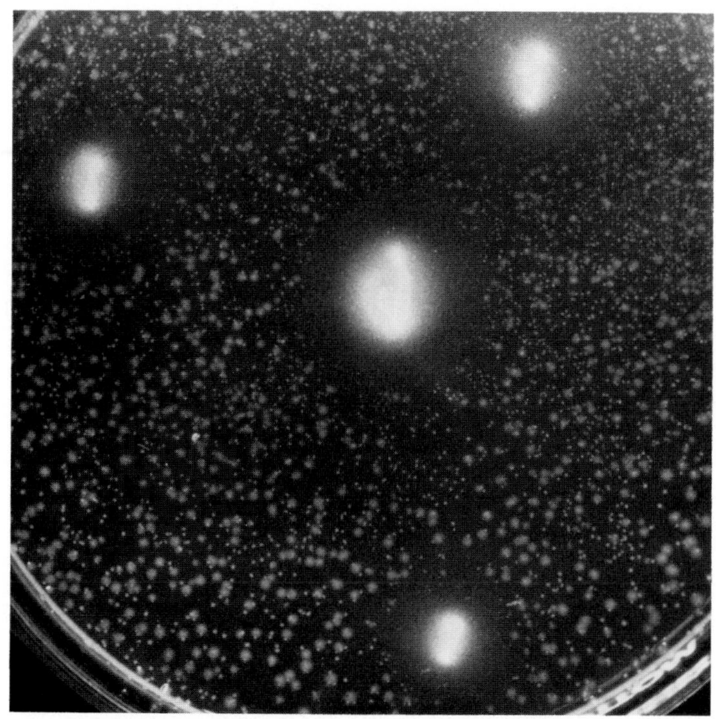

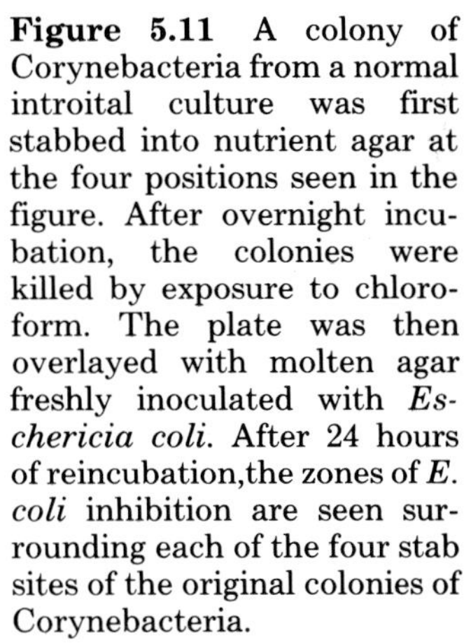

Figure 5.11 A colony of Corynebacteria from a normal introital culture was first stabbed into nutrient agar at the four positions seen in the figure. After overnight incubation, the colonies were killed by exposure to chloroform. The plate was then overlayed with molten agar freshly inoculated with *Escherichia coli.* After 24 hours of reincubation,the zones of *E. coli* inhibition are seen surrounding each of the four stab sites of the original colonies of Corynebacteria.

ml Earle's transport fluid. The sticks were discarded after mixing on a laboratory vibrator. The perineum was not cleansed before or after the collection and vaginal douching was avoided by all subjects. Segmented leukocytes in the transport fluid were enumerated with a Fuchs-Rosenthal counting chamber and recorded as the number per ml transport fluid.

We obtained 93 specimens from 27 women followed for recurrent bacteriuria and 251 specimens from 26 volunteers who had never had urinary infections. All cell counts on any patient within 2 weeks after a bacteriuric episode were excluded.

Because the volunteers were studied with weekly collections for 10 consecutive weeks, leukocytes on the vaginal introitus were analyzed also in relation to the day of the menstrual cycle.

The leukocyte counts varied from 0 to greater than 1,000,000/ml transport fluid in both groups. The number of specimens at each count is shown in Figure 5.12. The mean for the patients, $1.03 \times 10^5 \pm 4.9 \times 10^5$ cells/ml, was not significantly different ($P > 0.6$) from the mean for the controls, $8.0 \times 10^4 \pm 1.7 \times 10^5$/ml.

If the leukocyte counts in the patients and the controls are divided into those cultures containing more than 100 Enterobacteriaceae (31 specimens) and those in whom not a single colony was detected (255 specimens) the mean leukocyte counts were $6.4 \times 10^4 \pm 1.0 \times 10^5$ cells/ml and $8.7 \times 10^4 \pm 3.3 \times 10^5$, respectively. The differences are not significant ($P > 0.9$).

Most leukocytes were polymorphonuclear. Eight of the 93 collections from patients and 25 of the 226 samples from controls showed 50% or more of the leukocytes to be mononuclear.

Data were available on 21 premenopausal controls with regular menstrual cycles in whom serial, weekly cultures could be accurately related to each segment of the endocrine cycle. Of the 21 controls 9 showed a constant leukocyte count at all segments of the endocrine cycle (Figure 5.13*A*), 5 peaked toward the end of the cycle or between days 23–30 (Figure 5.13*B*), 3 showed the highest counts between days 10–20, 1 at

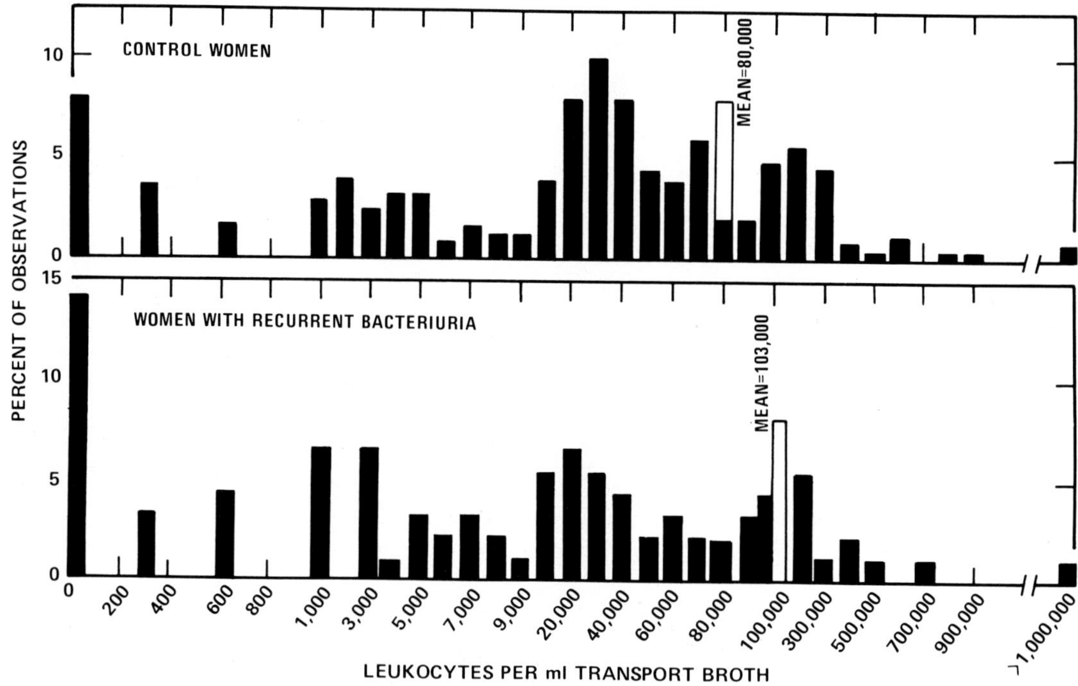

Figure 5.12 Segmented leukocytes on vaginal vestibule in 93 collections from 27 patients with recurrent bacteriuria compared to 251 specimens from 26 control women resistant to urinary infections. (Reproduced by permission from T. A. Stamey and G. Mihara, J. Urol. **116:** 72,1976.[73])

5 days and the remaining 3 were quite variable, often showing double peaks.

We have emphasized in all our observations that colonization of the vaginal vestibule with Enterobacteriaceae, even with large numbers, is not accompanied by visual evidence of inflammation. Indeed, it is impossible to distinguish by careful inspection those vestibules that have no Enterobacteriaceae and those that are heavily colonized with fecal bacteria; they all appear the same. These clinical observations are supported by the data here, which fail to show that enterobacterial colonization is accompanied by a segmented leukocyte response by the vaginal epithelium. Antibody and non-antibody mediated opsonizing activity has been demonstrated in vaginal fluid when mixed with human peripheral blood leukocytes and Enterobacteriaceae.[74] Despite this *in vitro* demonstration there appears to be no significant local leukocyte response *in vivo* to the presence of Enterobacteriaceae on the mucosa of the vaginal introitus.

The high white blood counts in the two control patients of more than 1,000,000/ml (Figure 5.12) could not be explained by vaginal bacteriology. Although one carried *Ureaplasma urealyticum*, five other controls were also regular carriers with a mean introital white blood count of less than 10,000 cells/ml. Since 10% of normal women will carry yeast on the vaginal mucosa without overt evidence of vaginitis, we examined the white blood counts in these samples as well. The mean white blood count was less than 13,000 cells/ml, substantially less than the mean of the entire control group (80,000).

The opportunity to look at the relationship of vaginal leukocytes to the various phases of the menstrual cycle in 21 premenopausal women failed to confirm the clinical impression that leukocytes are most frequent during or just prior to the men-

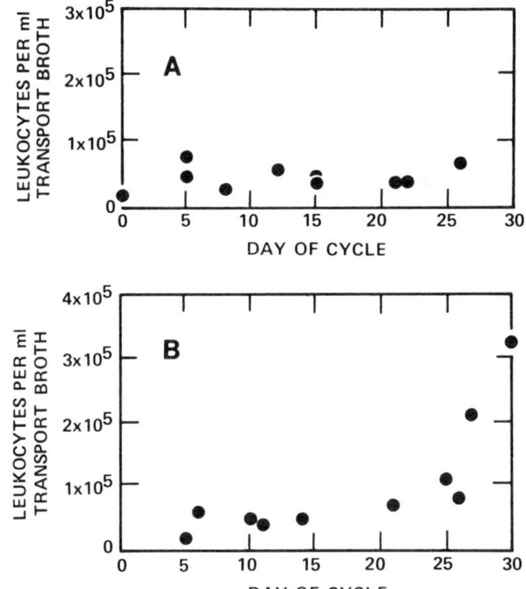

Figure 5.13 Representative examples. *A*, constant vaginal leukocyte excretion in relation to menstrual cycle. *B*, apparent 3-fold increase in vaginal leukocytes between 25 and 30 days. (Reproduced by permission from T. A. Stamey and G. Mihara, J. Urol. **116:** 72, 1976.[73])

strual period. Nine controls showed no variation throughout the endocrine cycle, 5 excreted the highest numbers between days 23 and 30 and the remaining 7 peaked at different periods.

Without question our introital swab technique is very semiquantitative in measuring vaginal leukocytes, but there seems to be no difference between healthy controls and UTI-prone patients.

Serum Antibody Responses to *Escherichia coli* Urinary Infection

The clinical assessment of antibody responses in patients has two purposes: (1) the determination of antibody response as a diagnostic index, and (2) assessment of the protective effect of antibody. Because serologic antibody responses might influence enterobacterial survival on the vaginal mucosa, I review some of the data on serum antibody and *E. coli* UTI here.

I discussed in Chapter 1 the immune response of urinary antibody in urinary infections, especially the data on antibody-coated bacteria in the urine. It appears from these data that the urinary tract may mount a significant immune response in the urine without a detectable antibody response in the serum; Harris *et al.*[75] found that only 25% of asymptomatic, pregnant patients with fluorescent antibody-positive (FA+) bacteriuria had serum antibody titers above the normal control serums. Thus, if a serologic immune response is to be used diagnostically, it is clear that antibody-coating of bacteria in the urine is a much more sensitive indicator of an immune response to urinary infection. Using a radioimmunoassay based on ^{125}I-tagged anti-human immunoglobulin, Sanford and associates[76] found an elevated serum antibody titer in only 49% of patients with pyelonephritis and FA+ bacteria in their urine. This is in contrast to bacterial prostatitis where serum antibodies are not only useful in diagnosis, but are especially helpful in assessing bacteriologic persistence following chemotherapy (see Chapter 7).

Some of the difficulty in determining serum antibody responses to urinary infection is methodologic. Since the total amount of serum antibody is almost never increased in urinary infections, simply quantitating the amount of IgM, IgG, or IgA by Mancini single, radial immunodiffusion plates[77] is useless. Antigen-specific antibody, however, can be increased substantially without any detectable change in the total amount of serum antibody. Early studies used hemagglutination and bacterial agglutination techniques to measure antigen-specific antibody, techniques which showed increases in O-antibody in patients with acute pyelonephritis[78–80]; we know now, however, that both indirect hemagglutination and direct bacterial agglutination techniques measure mainly IgM antibodies, although some IgG antibody is included in direct bacterial agglutination methods.[81, 82] Moreover, it was soon shown that upper urinary tract infections, as proven by localization bacteriologic studies, in the absence of symptomatic pyelonephritis, occurred without elevated levels of serum agglutination titers. As Girardet has pointed out, reasons for these conflicting results include differences in immunologic technology,[82–86] inhomogeneous patient groups, lack of an absolute standard clinical diagnosis in both the establishment of bacteriuria and the separation of upper from lower tract infections, and variable immunogenic capacity from one antigen to another, perhaps even including from one serotype to another.[4] Perhaps the best studies are again from the Göteborg group where Jodal and associates found that the serum antibodies were diagnostically valuable if both the IgM and IgG agglutinin titers were determined along with the evolution of the changes in the titers; in a study of 94 girls with symptomatic urinary infections, 89% of the patients with pyelonephritis showed diagnostically significant changes in contrast to 5% of the cystitis patients.[87] It is important to emphasize that these serum titer changes are in symptomatic, upper tract infected patients where the diagnosis is largely apparent and that these techniques are not useful in asymptomatic urinary infections of the upper tract.

What is needed if the serologic response to *E. coli* urinary infections is to be adequately characterized, is to follow patients with acute pyelonephritis, patients with recurrent symptomatic lower tract infections, patients whose bacteriuria is detected by screening for bacteriuria (ScBU), and patients who persist with asymptomatic bacteriuria following a symptomatic episode, with quantitative measurements of antigen-specific antibody to IgM, IgG and IgA. Such studies require either an enzyme-linked immunoabsorbentassay (ELISA),[88] a solid phase radioimmunoassay (SPRIA)[89] (see discussion of SPRIA in this chapter and Chapter 7), or the indirect immunofluorescent assay of antibody-coated bacteria, the latter of which is particularly cumbersome because of the serial dilutions of serum required for immunofluorescence titers. Not only will the patients have to be carefully selected and placed in homogeneous groups, but they will have to be followed for many months, and through more than one infection if the serologic response to urinary infections is to be characterized adequately. Unfortunately, I have a suspicion that the effort—and these assays require considerable effort—will not be worth the information. In addition, local urinary antibody (as reviewed in Chapter 1) has already proven to be of more diagnostic value in adults, and local cervicovaginal antibody (as reviewed in this chapter) may be of far more practical importance in terms of pathogenesis of urinary infections.

Even though acute pyelonephritis is usually accompanied by an increase in levels of O-antibody in the serum (IgM) and acute cystitis is not,[78, 79] other techniques unaffected by differences in immunoglobulin class have shown an increase in serum antibody in some patients with acute cystitis.[86] As a further complication to the interpretation of low serum antibody levels, Jodal *et al.*[90] have shown fluctuations in levels of serum antibodies in normal individuals which possibly relate to antibody responses to intestinal *E. coli.*

Fortunately, however, some of the urgency in characterizing *E. coli* antibodies in serum has been eased by Kaijser *et al.*[91] who observed that when specific antisera to *E. coli* O-antigen was used to study renal tissue from children undergoing surgery for pyelonephritic scarring, O-antigen could be found in only 1 of the 12 patients; IgG and IgA-containing plasma cells were observed 10 times and IgM-containing cells, 6 times.

Hanson and his colleagues[18] have summarized their interesting observations on serum antibodies to K-antigens. They reported that antibodies to K-antigens of *E. coli* were more protective than the O-antibodies in ascending pyelonephritis in rats. On the other hand, they found K-antibodies in children with acute pyelonephritis due to *E. coli* in only 2 of 17 children even though they all formed large amounts of O-antibodies in the serum. Because the K-antigen is tolerogenic in animals, and may be in humans, they have proposed that secretory IgA antibodies to the K-antigen may be easier to induce in the urine, presumably by direct bladder inoculation. It would seem, then, that these excellent immunologic investigators, who have done so much to characterize the humoral antibody response to urinary infections, may also believe that further characterization of the serologic immune system in urinary infections is unwarranted, at least at this time. In their most recent analysis with Wientzen *et al.*,[92] they used C-reactive protein (CRP+) as indicative of pyelonephritis in children; interestingly, serum antibody titers (IgG, IgA, and IgM) to the K_1-antigen, using the ELISA technique, were lower in patients with CRP+ urinary infections than in those who were CRP negative.

So complex is the antigen-antibody reaction in the serum of patients with UTI, that a clinically useful synthesis—either in terms of a practical diagnostic test or protective immunization—is far from accomplished in late 1979. Indeed, in terms of the latter possibility, it is sobering to realize that Miller and associates[93] have shown that cyclophosphamide-treated rats, which cannot produce antibacterial antibody, are able to eliminate bacteria more readily from the infected kidney than untreated animals can with a normal humoral immune response!

Vaginal Lysozyme

Govers and Girard[74] found lysozyme in 46 of 55 vaginal secretions in patients attending an obstetrical and gynecologic clinic; in 45% of the 46 secretions, the level of lysozyme exceeded that of normal human serum (5–10 ng/ml). They further observed that both lysozyme and complement were capable of enhancing phagocytosis. The role of lysozyme or complement in enterobacterial colonization of the vaginal mucosa is unknown.

BACTERIAL ADHERENCE TO VAGINAL EPITHELIAL CELLS

In July 1974, Jackson Fowler and I began our study of enterobacterial adherence to vaginal epithelial cells. We did this partly out of frustration over our failure to find any differences between UTI-prone and healthy women in the factors that determine bacterial growth rates on mucosal surfaces; we wondered if *E. coli* in UTI-prone women were simply sticking better to vaginal epithelial cells of susceptible patients. We were also impressed with the accumulating literature of the early 1970s on bacterial adherence to mucosal surfaces in diseases of the intestinal, respiratory and pharyngeal tracts.[94–101]

When we began these studies in 1974, we had no difficulty in showing strong adherence between lactobacilli and *S. epidermidis* when these indigenous bacteria were added to washed vaginal epithelial cells in a 1:1 ratio (Figure 5.14, *A–C*). The *E. coli* proved to be a substantial problem. Indeed, so different was the avidity between *E. coli* and vaginal epithelial cells that we almost discontinued the experiments; it was a great credit to Fowler's persistence that he finally succeeded in showing that *E. coli* had to be added to epithelial cells in a ratio of 1000:1 in order for *E. coli* to attach to vaginal epithelial cells. We presented these data (and the manuscript) before the American Society of Genitourinary Surgeons in March 1976, although for reasons best known to them, it was not published until April 1977.[102]

The technique we used is as follows: With the subject in the dorsal lithotomy position the vagina was irrigated with 100 ml normal saline, and superficial mucous and epithelial cells were scraped gently from the lateral vagina just proximal to the hymenal ring and discarded. The area was rescraped with a fresh applicator stick and the desquamated cells were suspended in 50 ml normal saline. The cells were refrigerated at 10°C and all experiments were begun within 6 hours of collecting the cells.

The cells were recovered from suspension by centrifugation at 3000 revolutions per minute for 5 minutes and resuspended in phosphate buffered saline (PBS) (pH 6.4). Adherent bacteria and mucus were washed from the cells by mixing the suspension on a Vortex mixer for 15 seconds. Vaginal cells were recovered by centrifugation and the entire process was repeated 4 times.

A portion of the final cell suspension was dried, heat fixed on a microscope slide and Gram stained. Cell suspensions free of adherent bacteria, when examined with oil

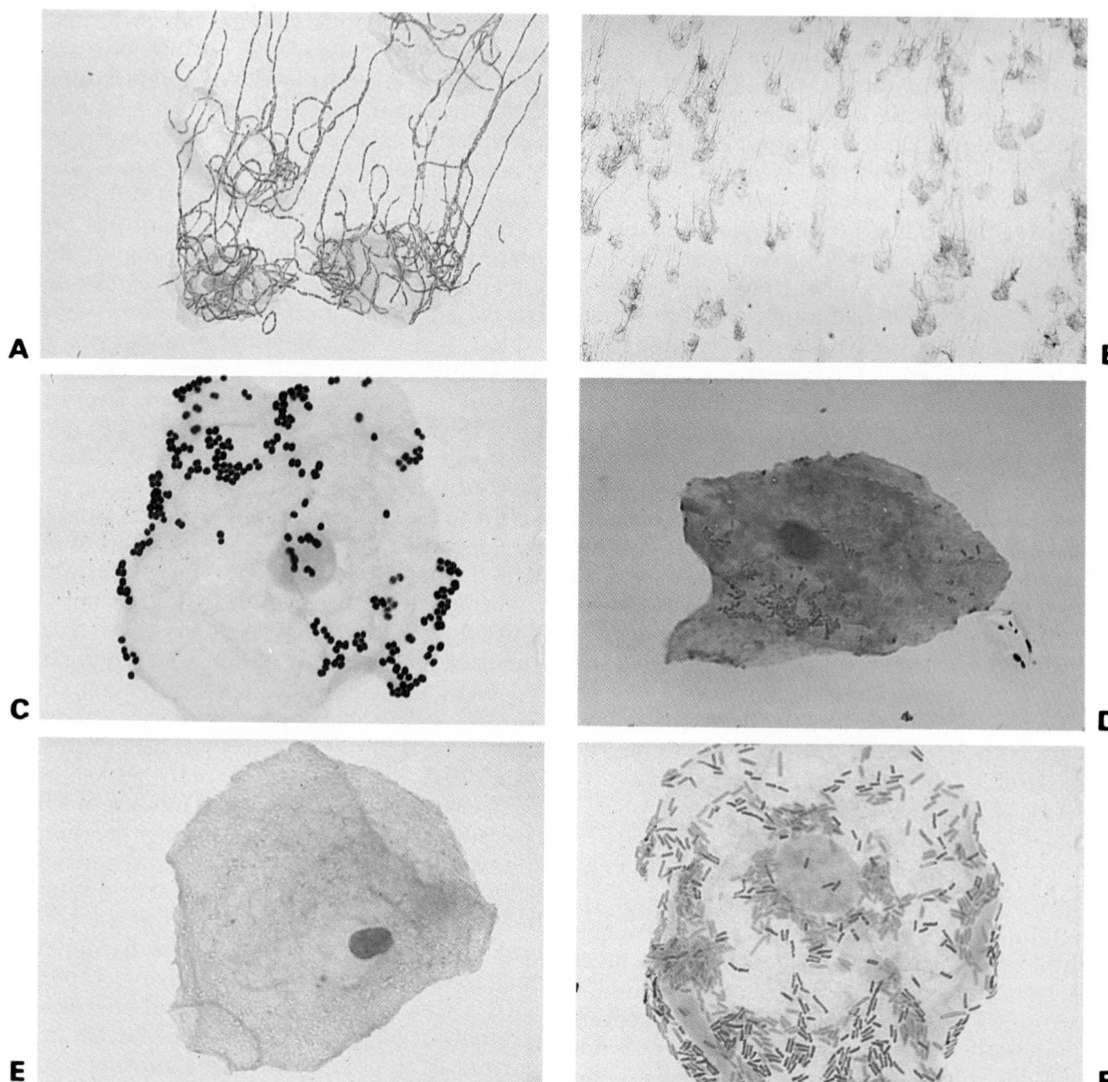

Figure 5.14 Bacteria isolated from the introitus of women were incubated with washed human epithelial cells from the vaginal mucosa. (*A*) Human lactobacilli added to washed vaginal epithelial cells at high power magnification. (*B*) Low power view of lactobacilli adherent to washed epithelial cells. (*C*) *Staphylococcus epidermidis* adherent to human vaginal cells. (*D*) Unwashed, vaginal epithelial cell stained with safranin, showing adherent indigenous bacteria. (*E*) Vaginal epithelial cell after washing (see text). (*F*) *Escherichia coli* added to washed, vaginal epithelial cells at a ratio of 10^8 *E. coli* to 10^5 vaginal cells.

emersion light microscopy (×1000), were used for the study and were standardized to a concentration of 10^4–10^5 cells/ml with a hemocytometer. Superficial vaginal epithelial cells usually have several to hundreds of Gram-positive or Gram-negative rods and cocci adherent to them (Figure 5.14*D*). Vaginal cell suspensions obtained from 11 of 31 patients and 9 of 29 control women were unacceptable for study owing to an inability to wash the cells free of adherent bacteria. Only cell suspensions free of adherent bacteria were accepted for study (Figure 5.14*E*). Quantitative aerobic cultures of the vaginal introitus of the rejected subjects revealed bacterial flora similar to that cultured from the introitus of subjects whose vaginal cells were washed free of bacteria. None of the rejected subjects had clinical evidence of vaginal infection.

Eighteen different O-serogroups of *E. coli* were isolated: 10 O-serogroups that commonly cause urinary infection were isolated from the urine of infected patients seen in the urology clinic and 8 O-serogroups that rarely cause infection were isolated from fecal *E. coli.* Each O-group was banked on multiple trypticase soy agar slants and sealed until used. A suspension of each O-group was obtained from an 18-hour growth in 10 ml Mueller-Hinton culture broth. The bacteria were washed twice in PBS before use. The final concentration was 10^8–10^9 bacteria/ml as determined by quantitative cultures.

For each study 1 ml of 10^4–10^5 washed vaginal epithelial cells/ml PBS and 1 ml of a twice-washed bacterial suspension were mixed together and incubated in a shaker water bath (37°C) for 30 minutes. After incubation the vaginal cell-bacterial suspension was added to 5 ml PBS and centrifuged at 3000 rpm for 2 minutes. The supernatant, which contained free bacteria, was discarded, the recovered epithelial cells were resuspended in 5 ml PBS and the process was repeated. The epithelial cells were then suspended in 40 ml PBS and filtered with gentle suction over a 14 μm Millipore dermalon filter, allowing passage of any residual free bacteria while retaining the epithelial cells on its surface. After filtering, a glass microscope slide was pressed gently against the filter, lifting off the retained epithelial cells. This cell preparation was then air dried, heat fixed and stained for 2 minutes with safranin. Each bacterial suspension was recultured to verify that only a pure suspension of bacteria was used.

The final cell preparation was then examined with oil immersion light microscopy (×1000). The resultant preparation consisted only of vaginal epithelial cells and bacteria adherent to them. No free bacteria were present. The number of bacteria adherent to each of the first 50 epithelial cells visualized was counted. Only bacteria that were actually in contact with the cell surface were counted and epithelial cells that overlapped other cells were excluded from evaluation. The mean number of bacteria per cell and the standard error of the mean were calculated for each preparation.

Adherence of Lactobacilli to Vaginal Cells

So avidly do lactobacilli attach to washed vaginal epithelial cells, as shown in Figure 5.14, *A* and *B*, that we were unable to quantitate the degree of attachment. Figure 5.14, *A* and *B*, however, makes it easy to understand why the *Lactobacillus* is the dominant indigenous organism of the vaginal flora.

Adherence of *Staphylococcus epidermidis* to Vaginal Cells

A suspension of *S. epidermidis* (10^6–10^7 bacteria/ml) was incubated with a vaginal epithelial cell suspension from each of seven different control subjects. The mean number of adherent *S. epidermidis* per cell in cell preparations derived from seven different control subjects is summarized in Table 5.24. A representative vaginal cell with adherent *S. epidermidis* as viewed under the light microscope with oil immersion (×1000) is shown in Figure 5.14*C*. The

Table 5.24
Mean Number of Adherent *Staphylococcus Epidermidis* per Cell[a]

Control Subject	Mean Bacteria/Cell[b]
1	71.1 ± 7.2
2	59.9 ± 7.5
3	54.9 ± 8.7
4	50.2 ± 6.6
5	48.9 ± 6.9
6	34.2 ± 5.0
7	31.0 ± 4.1
Mean = 50.0 ± 14.0	

[a] Reproduced with permission from J. E. Fowler and T. A. Stamey, J. Urol. **117:** 472, 1977.[102]

[b] Plus or minus standard error of mean.

mean bacteria per cell score of these seven subjects was 50.0 ± 14.0.

The concentration of *S. epidermidis* needed to demonstrate adherence in this model was 100-fold less than that necessary to demonstrate adhesion by *E. coli*. In preliminary work using concentrations of *E. coli* comparable to that of *S. epidermidis* (10^6–10^7 bacteria/ml) no adhesion could be demonstrated.

Adherence of Different O-serogroups of *Escherichia coli* to Vaginal Cells

Vaginal epithelial cells were pooled from five subjects in the patient group. A suspension of each *E. coli* serogroup (10^8–10^9 bacteria/ml) was prepared and incubated with a portion of the pooled vaginal epithelial cells. A representative cell with adherent *E. coli* is shown in Figure 5.14*F*.

The mean number of adherent bacteria per cell for each of 18 different *E. coli* O-serogroups is summarized in Table 5.25. It is apparent that the tendency for different O-groups of *E. coli* to adhere to pooled vaginal cells *in vitro* varies greatly. The mean bacterial adherence for the common serogroups, 23.1, was greater than that for the uncommon O-groups, 9.4 ($P > 0.1$). The relative adherence of each *E. coli* serogroup in this study was compared to preliminary work in which adherence of the same serogroups was measured using a 4-hour incubation time. The correlation was statistically significant (P = 0.01), using Spearman's rank correlation coefficient, indicating reproducibility of the experimental technique. It is important to recognize that all of the common O-serogroups in Table 5.25 had caused bacteriuria, despite some of them showing almost no attachment capacity.

Although the *E. coli* O-groups that commonly cause urinary infection show greater adherence as a group than the O-groups that rarely cause infection, this difference is not statistically significant ($P > 0.1$). Furthermore, the common O-groups were all isolated from the urine of infected patients while the uncommon O-groups were isolated from anal cultures. Therefore, the relative virulence of the *E. coli* in each group may be different. As will be shown in the sections that follow, this variation in bacterial adherence is due mainly to bacterial pili.

Adherence of *Escherichia coli* 06 to Vaginal Cells of Patients and Control Subjects

Twenty adult women with a history of at least three documented urinary infections were followed in our urologic clinic with frequent quantitative cultures of the vaginal introitus, and the first-voided and mid stream urine. Most patients had frequent colonization of the vaginal introitus with large numbers of Gram-negative bacteria and enterococci, and all had been treated either with prophylactic antibiotics for recurrent urinary infection prior to the study or were under antibiotic therapy at the time of study. The mean age of these patients was 35.7 years, with a range of 19–66 years. Seventeen patients were premenopausal, 7 used birth-control pills, 2 had intrauterine devices, and 3 had had hysterectomies and were taking replacement estrogens.

The control group consisted of 20 volunteer women with no history of urinary or vaginal infection. Several quantitative cultures of the vaginal introitus, as well as the first-voided and midstream urine, were obtained from each volunteer to verify the absence of bacteriuria. The mean age of the control subjects was 29.2 years, with a range of 22–50 years. Nineteen control women were premenopausal, 7 used birth-control pills, 4 had intrauterine devices, and 1 had had a hysterectomy and was taking replacement estrogens.

Individual suspensions of vaginal epithelial cells from each of 20 patients and control women were incubated with a suspension of *E. coli* 06 (10^8–10^9 bacteria/ml). The mean number of adherent *E. coli* 06 per cell for each of 20 patients and 20 control subjects is summarized in Table 5.26 and Figure 5.15. A representative vaginal cell with adherent *E. coli* as viewed under the light microscope with oil immersion (×1000) is shown in Figure 5.14*F*.

Table 5.25
Mean Number of Adherent Bacteria per Cell for 18 Different *Escherichia Coli* O-Serogroups[a]

Common Serogroups[b]		Uncommon Serogroups[c]	
O-Serogroups	Mean Bacteria/Cell[d]	O-Serogroups	Mean Bacteria/Cell[d]
06	49.9 ± 4.5	0128	26.1 ± 3.2
023	46.5 ± 5.3	0125	16.5 ± 1.7
050	38.9 ± 4.5	0115	11.5 ± 1.6
02	36.9 ± 3.8	0138	8.9 ± 1.5
01	25.6 ± 2.9	0135	6.1 ± 1.2
04	13.1 ± 1.5	077	3.1 ± 0.8
07	9.4 ± 0.9	0127	2.0 ± 0.4
08	6.8 ± 0.9	0111	1.0 ± 0.4
075	3.4 ± 0.5		
018	0.54 ± 0.2		
Mean = 23.1 ± 18.8[e]		Mean = 9.4 ± 8.5[e]	
$P > 0.1$			

[a] Reproduced by permission from J. E. Fowler and T. A. Stamey, J. Urol. **117:** 472, 1977.[102]
[b] O-groups isolated from infected urine.
[c] O-groups isolated from feces.
[d] Plus or minus standard error of mean.
[e] Standard deviation.

The mean score of adherent bacteria per cell was 42.6 ± 25.5 in the patient group and 19.4 ± 9.4 in the control group. The difference between the mean bacteria per cell score for the two groups is highly significant: with Student's *t* test the 2-sided *P* = < 0.001.

The degree of bacterial adherence for each subject in the patient and control groups was correlated with the age of the subject, the day of the menstrual cycle on which the cells were obtained, the presence or absence of enterobacteria in the introital culture at the time of cell sampling, the use of birth-control pills or intrauterine devices and whether the patient had had a hysterectomy. In addition, the patient group was analyzed with regard to the use of antimicrobial agents at the time of cell sampling. None of these variables correlated with the degree of bacterial adhesion for the patients or controls.

The most intriguing observation from these adherence studies is that a single *E. coli* species adheres to the vaginal cells of patients with frequent urinary infection to a greater degree than to the cells of controls. The difference in mean bacterial adherence between the two groups, although statistically significant, was not correlated with an *in vivo* study of bacterial adhesion. However, Liljemark and Gibbons,[97] using a similar *in vitro* method to evaluate streptococcal adherence to human cheek cells, have shown close correlation between the *in vitro* analysis and an *in vivo* study in which streptococcal adherence to the cheek surface in the mouth was measured.

If our current understanding of the process of bacterial colonization of mucosal surfaces in general, and of the vaginal introitus in particular, is accurate, it seems fair to conclude that microbial adherence to the vaginal mucosa is important in the organism's ability to colonize the surface. Furthermore, it would appear that the adhesive ability of a microbe is determined in part by the surface characteristics of the vaginal mucosa. The vaginal mucosa of women with recurrent urinary infection may allow more avid adherence of enterobacteria than that of normal women, thus promoting more frequent and quantitatively greater colonization by enterobacteria.

These studies have been confirmed by two different groups, both investigating children. Kållenius and Winberg[103] compared the adherence of periurethral epithe-

Table 5.26
Mean Number of Adherent *Escherichia coli* 06 per Cell for Patients and Controls[a]

Patient	Mean Bacteria/Cell[b]	Control	Mean Bacteria/Cell[b]
1	89.2 ± 10.3	1	50.4 ± 5.3
2	86.2 ± 9.3	2	30.3 ± 3.6
3	76.7 ± 7.1	3	28.3 ± 3.5
4	67.6 ± 7.5	4	23.8 ± 2.9
5	67.5 ± 5.7	5	23.0 ± 3.3
6	59.3 ± 7.7	6	21.2 ± 1.8
7	58.8 ± 4.4	7	20.8 ± 3.0
8	52.6 ± 5.3	8	18.8 ± 2.8
9	43.8 ± 4.5	9	18.2 ± 3.1
10	38.8 ± 3.6	10	18.2 ± 2.0
11	33.2 ± 3.9	11	18.1 ± 1.9
12	32.6 ± 4.4	12	18.0 ± 1.9
13	27.7 ± 3.2	13	15.0 ± 3.0
14	25.1 ± 2.9	14	15.0 ± 2.3
15	20.6 ± 3.3	15	14.8 ± 2.9
16	20.1 ± 2.8	16	13.5 ± 1.7
17	18.0 ± 2.6	17	12.2 ± 2.2
18	14.8 ± 1.8	18	10.6 ± 1.6
19	12.9 ± 2.4	19	8.6 ± 1.4
20	7.0 ± 1.2	20	8.1 ± 1.6
	Mean = 42.6 ± 25.5[c]		Mean = 19.4 ± 9.4[c]
		$P < 0.001$	

[a] Reproduced by permission from J. E. Fowler and T. A. Stamey, J. Urol. **117:** 472, 1977.[102]
[b] Plus or minus standard error of mean.
[c] Standard deviation.

lial cells from 20 patients and 20 controls to an *E. coli* 075; their figure showing the spread of the mean number of adherent bacteria per cell in UTI-prone girls and healthy controls is virtually superimposable on our Figure 5.15. Svanborg-Edén, Jodal, and Pettersson[104] at Göteborg compared the attachment of the infecting strain of *E. coli* in 96 children with recurrent UTI to 109 children without a history of UTI; voided uroepithelial cells were used from each donor for attachment studies, and both patients and controls were compared to a reference standard comprised of epithelial cells from one nonbacteriuric donor. Patients and controls were age-matched. Epithelial cells from the UTI-prone children had a greater avidity for *E. coli* than did the epithelial cells from the healthy children.

Kållenius, Möllby, and Winberg[105] have made an important observation which I have reproduced with their permission in Figure 5.16. All investigators have recognized that when the number of epithelial cells is kept constant, increasing the number of bacteria at the time of incubation increases the number of organisms that attach to the cells. What Figure 5.16 says, however, is that increasing the number of *E. coli* enhances the differences in attachment between patient and control cells.

While this observation should serve as a caution to other investigators who study bacterial attachment to uroepithelial cells, I wonder if it does not also have some biological significance. Could it mean, for example, that susceptibility is related to an increase in the number of attachment sites on the epithelial cells of UTI-prone females? If so, what could cause an increase in the number of receptor sites?

Electron Microscopy of *Escherichia coli* Adherence to Vaginal Cells

Cell preparations of several patients and control women were placed in glutaraldehyde immediately after the vaginal cells

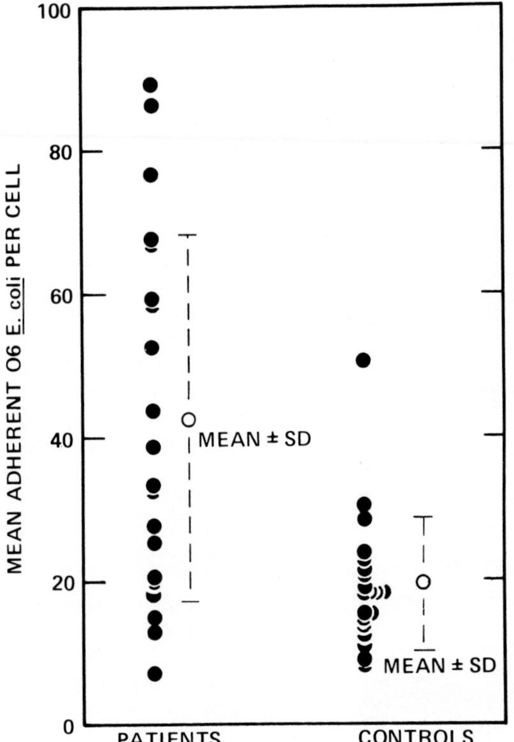

Figure 5.15 Mean adherent *Escherichia coli* 06 per cell for vaginal cells from each patient and control subject. (Reproduced by permission from J. E. Fowler and T. A. Stamey, J. Urol. **117:** 472,1977.[102])

with adherent *E. coli* 06 were lifted from the dermalon filter and examined with scanning electron microscopy. In addition, the vaginal cell-bacterial suspensions of several patients and control subjects were taken after incubation but before filtering and suspended in glutaraldehyde for examination with transmission electron microscopy.

Examination of the vaginal cells (Figure 5.17*A*) with scanning and transmission electron microscopy provided little insight into the nature of bacterial adhesion and cells from patient and control subjects looked similar. The vaginal epithelial cells have faceted surfaces with desmosomal ridges that bond adjacent epithelial cells (Figure 5.17, *C* and *E*). The *E. coli* adherent to the epithelial cells appear to attach to the desmosomal ridges. The quantity and appearance of the desmosomal ridges were similar in the cells examined from the patient and control groups.

Figure 5.17*B* demonstrates the hemidesmosomes of a single cell and Figure 5.17*D* shows the opposing hemidesmosomes of two adjacent vaginal epithelial cells. Glutaraldehyde-fixed, epithelial cell-bacterial suspensions from patients and controls were examined after staining with the colloidal iron method to evaluate the neuraminic acid content of the vaginal cell surface (Figure 5.17*F*). No defects in the colloidal iron distribution were demonstrated at the point of bacterial attachment.

Bacterial Adherence as a Measure of Urinary Pathogenicity

In the first section of this chapter I reviewed some of the antigenic differences

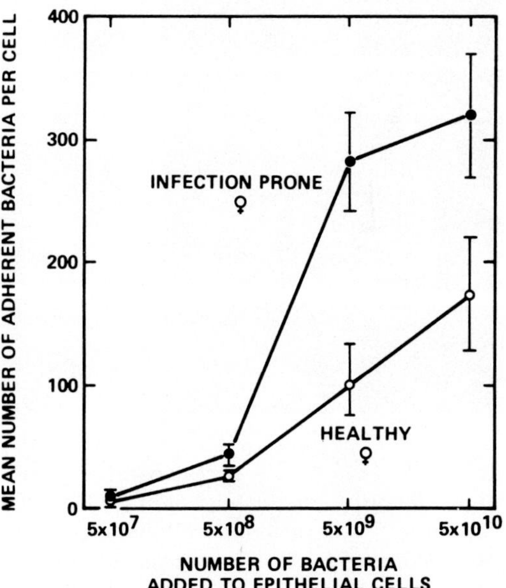

Figure 5.16 Three healthy, control women and three urinary tract infection-prone patients were each studied on 24 separate occasions. Each point represents the distribution of the means of the three individuals in each group. (Reproduced by permission from G. Kållenius, R. Möllby and G. Winberg.)

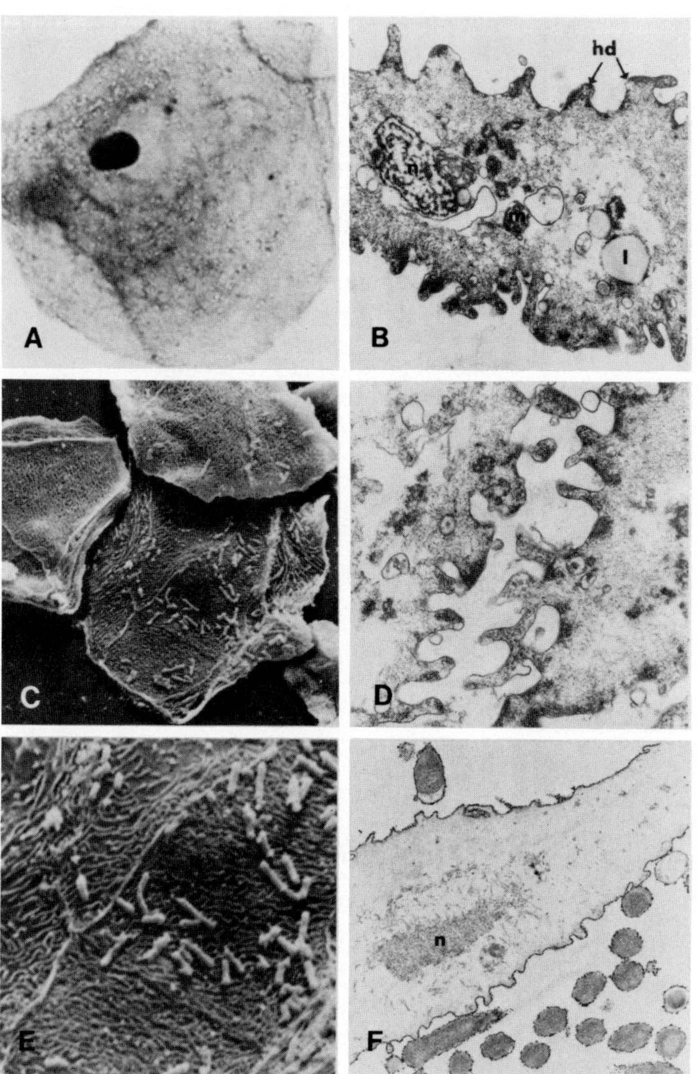

Figure 5.17 *A*, washed vaginal cell free of indigenous bacteria, ×1,000. *B*, vaginal cell: pyknotic nucleus, *n*; mitochondria, *m*; lipid, *l*; hemidesmosomes, *hd*. Transmission electron microscopy, ×5,000. *C*, vaginal cells with adherent *E. coli*. Scanning electron microscopy, ×2,000. *D*, vaginal cells. Transmission electron microscopy, ×11,000. *E*, vaginal cell with adherent *E. coli*. Scanning electron microscopy, ×6,000. *F*, vaginal cells and *E. coli* stained by colloidal iron method. Transmission electron microscopy, ×2,000. (Reproduced by permission from J. E. Fowler and T. A. Stamey, J. Urol. **117:** 472, 1977.[102])

among *E. coli* in the rectal reservoir that might account for pathogenicity. Bacterial attachment to epithelial cells is almost an ideal property to account for pathogenicity. Because we had patients who had been followed closely in and out of bacteriuric episodes, with frequent sampling of their rectal and introital bacterial flora, Fowler and I[106] thought our material was ideally suited to study this important question. We studied 37 strains of *E. coli* isolated from anal and midstream urine cultures of 13 women with frequent reinfections of the lower urinary tract. Each woman had been followed with weekly to monthly cultures of the anal canal, vaginal introitus, first voided and midstream urine by methods described in Chapter 1. Each isolate was banked on trypticase soy agar slants until studied. All isolates were obtained in the absence of antimicrobial therapy. Of the 37 strains of *E. coli*, representing 9 different O-serogroups, 18 were obtained from the midstream urine during 18 bacteriuric episodes in the 13 patients. The remaining 19 strains (14 different O-serogroups) were isolated from anal cultures of the patients, none having caused bacteriuria or colonized

Table 5.27
Mean Number of Adherent *Escherichia coli* per Vaginal Cell[a]

Vesical *E. coli*		Anal *E. coli*	
O-Serogroup	Mean bacteria/cell[b]	O-Serogroup	Mean bacteria/cell[b]
018	139.7 ± 9.5	018	161.1 ± 7.7
SA	104.1 ± 7.7	0113	131.5 ± 8.9
NT	99.7 ± 10.9	06	69.1 ± 7.8
018	92.0 ± 9.7	040	59.3 ± 7.5
06	81.2 ± 6.6	0124	38.2 ± 6.7
075	68.3 ± 8.3	03	37.9 ± 5.3
06	45.4 ± 4.1	0147	34.6 ± 4.6
NT	24.2 ± 3.0	SA	29.8 ± 3.0
013	23.2 ± 3.0	06	24.6 ± 4.5
025	20.7 ± 3.5	011	19.1 ± 2.9
01	17.5 ± 3.2	NT	16.1 ± 3.0
SA	17.2 ± 2.6	051	12.8 ± 2.1
NT	13.2 ± 2.1	NT	8.5 ± 1.3
023	12.4 ± 2.0	NT	8.5 ± 1.4
SA	10.6 ± 1.2	01	7.7 ± 1.1
NT	10.3 ± 2.3	0127	5.8 ± 1.2
06	6.9 ± 0.9	050	3.1 ± 1.4
01	0.0 ± 0.0	NT	1.9 ± 0.3
		NT	1.4 ± 0.3
Mean ± standard deviation = 43.7 ± 42.3		Mean ± standard deviation = 35.3 ± 43.8	

[a] Reproduced by permission from J. E. Fowler and T. A. Stamey, J. Urol. **120:** 315, 1978.[106]

[b] Plus or minus standard error of mean.

the vaginal vestibule and most being only transiently detected in the fecal cultures.

Eight strains of *P. mirabilis* were obtained from renal pelvic stones in 8 additional patients at the time of nephrolithotomy. Each crushed stone culture yielded only 1 strain of *P. mirabilis*, which was banked on trypticase soy agar slants until studied. Thus, in contrast to the *E. coli* isolates that were obtained from symptomatic patients who probably had lower tract bacteriuria, these 8 strains of *P. mirabilis* were clearly pathogenic for the kidney. They were compared to 10 anal isolates of *P. mirabilis* from the 13 patients with recurrent *E. coli* infections. These anal isolates of *P. mirabilis*, like the *E. coli* anal strains, had never colonized the vaginal introitus.

Vaginal epithelial cells were collected from two normal volunteer women. Vaginal cells used for evaluation of *E. coli* adherence were obtained from one volunteer, while those used to study *P. mirabilis* adherence were collected from the second volunteer.

Reproducibility of these studies was assessed by repeating the adherence experiments with 9 *E. coli* and 8 *P. mirabilis* strains. Vaginal cells from the same donor were used in both studies but collected on different occasions.

The adhesive properties of the 37 different *E. coli* strains expressed as the mean number of adherent bacteria per vaginal cell is summarized in Table 5.27 and Figure 5.18. The mean number of adherent bacteria per cell for the 19 strains that caused transient anal colonization was 35.3, with a standard deviation of 43.8. The mean number of adherent bacteria per cell for the 18 strains isolated from infected urine (vesical *E. coli*) was 43.7, with a standard deviation of 42.3. There is no statistical difference between the mean adherence values for the anal and vesical isolates, $P = 0.56$ using a 2-sided Student t test.

The adhesive properties of 18 different *P. mirabilis* strains are shown in Table 5.28 and Figure 5.18. The mean number of adherent bacteria per cell for the 10 anal isolates was 66.5, with a standard deviation of 51.9. The mean number of adherent bac-

Table 5.28
Mean Number of Adherent *Proteus Mirabilis* per Vaginal Cell[a]

Renal *P. mirabilis*	Anal *P. mirabilis*
Mean bacteria/cell[b]	Mean bacteria/cell[b]
129.8 ± 13.2	147.0 ± 9.8
114.9 ± 8.0	144.4 ± 7.9
104.2 ± 8.9	97.8 ± 8.7
79.1 ± 7.8	71.0 ± 6.0
72.0 ± 7.4	69.8 ± 8.5
45.8 ± 6.9	65.9 ± 6.5
21.9 ± 4.1	40.1 ± 6.6
18.9 ± 4.0	23.0 ± 3.4
	4.3 ± 1.9
	1.8 ± 0.5
Mean ± standard deviation = 73.3 ± 41.9	Mean ± standard deviation = 66.5 ± 51.9

[a] Reproduced by permission from J. E. Fowler and T. A. Stamey, J. Urol. **120:** 315, 1978.[106]

[b] Plus or minus standard error of mean.

Table 5.29
Reproducibility of Measure of Bacterial Adherence[a]

	Initial Measure of Adherence	Repeat Measure of Adherence
	Mean bacteria/cell[b]	Mean bacteria/cell[b]
	Escherichia coli	
O-Serogroup		
0113	131.5 ± 8.9	124.3 ± 8.5
SA	104.1 ± 7.7	98.8 ± 7.9
013	23.2 ± 3.0	9.4 ± 1.5
011	19.1 ± 2.9	86.9 ± 7.6
NT	10.3 ± 2.3	12.8 ± 3.2
01	7.7 ± 1.1	10.6 ± 1.5
06	6.9 ± 0.9	16.1 ± 2.1
0127	5.8 ± 1.2	21.6 ± 2.4
NT	1.4 ± 0.3	10.1 ± 1.5
	Proteus mirabilis	
	147.0 ± 9.8	122.4 ± 11.8
	114.9 ± 8.0	182.7 ± 6.2
	104.2 ± 8.9	151.2 ± 12.8
	23.0 ± 3.4	53.6 ± 10.1
	21.9 ± 4.1	35.8 ± 6.9
	18.9 ± 4.0	18.4 ± 5.5
	4.3 ± 1.9	11.0 ± 4.8
	1.8 ± 0.5	2.2 ± 0.4

[a] Reproduced by permission from J. E. Fowler and T. A. Stamey, J. Urol. **120:** 315, 1978.[106]

[b] Plus or minus standard error of mean.

teria per cell for the 8 strains cultured from infected renal calculi was 73.3, with a standard deviation of 41.9. Again, no statistical difference is demonstrated between the adhesive properties of the *P. mirabilis* strains of anal and renal pelvic origin, $P = 0.77$ using a 2-sided Student *t* test.

The adhesive properties of the 37 *E. coli* strains as a group (mean adherent bacteria per cell equals 39.4) were compared to those of the 18 *P. mirabilis* strains (mean adherent bacteria per cell equals 69.5). The difference in adhesive properties between these 2 species of bacteria showed weak significance, $P = 0.021$ using a 2-sided Student *t* test.

Finally, the reproducibility of this *in vitro* measure of bacterial adherence is shown in Table 5.29 and Figure 5.19. Despite variation in numbers of adherent bacteria per cell in each preparation, a close correlation is found between the initial and repeat determinations of adhesive properties of the 17 bacterial strains studied. The probability of concordance, $(\tau + 1)/2$ (τ = Kendall's rank correlation coefficient), equaled 0.82. Figure 5.19 clearly shows that bacterial strains displaying avid or limited adherence on the initial determination adhered to a similar degree on the repeat determination. All repeat experiments were done without any knowledge of the specific sample that was counted under the microscope.

Bacterial colonization of four mucosal surfaces are important in the pathogenesis of urinary infection in female subjects. These surfaces include the mucosa of the rectum, the vaginal introitus (including the external urethra), the bladder and the upper urinary tract (ureter and renal pelves).

The vaginal introitus may represent the most important mucosal surface in the pathogenesis of urinary infection in female subjects since colonization of this surface precedes the development of bacteriuria. We have demonstrated that bacteria adhere tenaciously to vaginal cells *in vivo* and that *E. coli* adhere more avidly *in vitro* to the vaginal cells of women with frequent urinary infection than to vaginal cells of normal control women (Table 5.26 and Figure 5.15), indicating the importance of bacterial adherence in the colonization of this surface. Mårdh and Weström[107] have investigated the adhesive properties of bacterial species that cause infections of the female genital tract using an *in vitro* method similar to that described herein. Bacterial species associated with infection of the lower genital tract, *Neisseria gonorrhoeae*, group B streptococci, and *Corynebacterium vaginale*, were shown to adhere to vaginal cells more than nonpathogenic vaginal flora.

However, our data fail to establish a correlation between the adhesive properties of an *E. coli* strain and the affinity of that strain to colonize the vaginal introitus. Each of the bacteriuric *E. coli* isolates colonized the vagina for varying intervals before or during the bacteriuric episode, while none of the anal *E. coli* was ever cultured from the vaginal introitus (Table 5.27). The adhesive properties of the bacteriuric *E. coli* did not differ significantly from the adhesive properties of the anal *E. coli*.

Bacterial adherence to the vesical mucosa may be important in the development

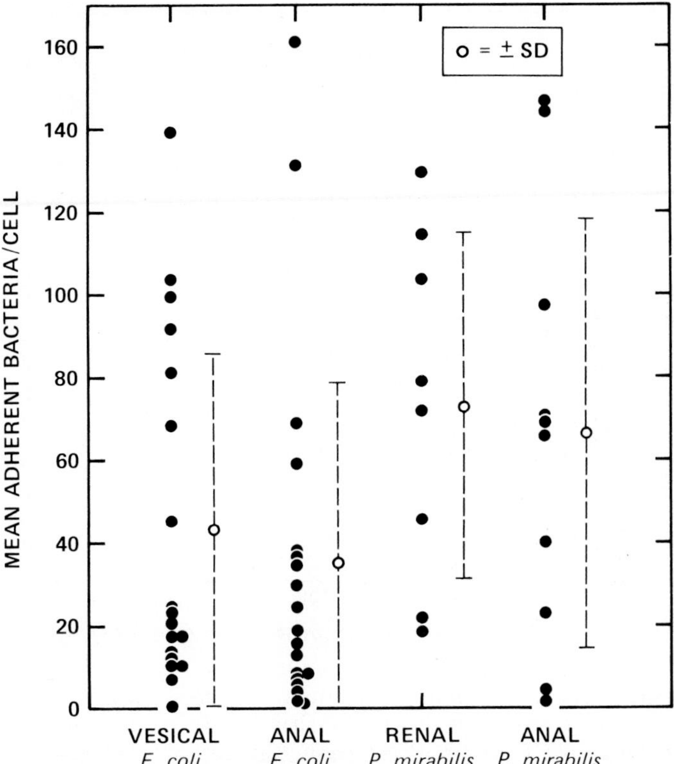

Figure 5.18 Mean bacterial adherence per vaginal epithelial cell for vesical and anal *Escherichia coli* and renal and anal *Proteus mirabilis*. (Reproduced by permission from J. E. Fowler and T. A. Stamey, J. Urol. **120:** 315, 1978.[106])

of bacteriuria. Norden and associates[108] have shown with the guinea pig model that approximately 0.1% of intravesical bacteria remain adherent to the vesical mucosa after voiding.[108] More recent investigations have suggested that a surface mucoprotein prevents bacterial attachment to the bladder mucosa, implying that prevention of this bacterial adherence is a primary defense mechanism of the bladder.[109] Thus, one might assume that the capacity of a bacterial strain to colonize the bladder is related to its ability to adhere to the vesical mucosa. However, these data fail to substantiate this assumption since the adherence properties of the bacteriuric *E. coli* did not differ from that of the anal *E. coli*.

The propensity of bacterial species to adhere to a mucosal surface may promote colonization of the ureters and renal pelves by retrograde infection from the bladder. It has been shown in the rat model that during the course of experimental pyelonephritis bacteria adhere to the renal pelvic epithelium before the establishment of intrarenal infection.[110] Svanborg-Edén *et al.*[111] have found that *E. coli* isolated from the urine of patients with clinical pyelonephritis and cystitis attach with greater affinity to voided epithelial cells than do *E. coli* isolated from patients with asymptomatic bacteriuria. However, the data presented herein do not reveal differences in the adhesive properties of *P. mirabilis* strains of upper urinary tract origin and anal *P. mirabilis* strains, which have never caused bacteriuric episodes. The contrast between the clinical virulence of these two groups of *P. mirabilis* strains cannot be overstated. The *P. mirabilis* isolated from stone cultures may represent the most tenacious organisms to colonize the urinary tract since considerable longevity of renal pelvic colonization must be required for alkalization of the renal pelvic urine and subsequent precipitation of $MgNH_4PO_4$.

It is of interest that the adhesive properties of *E. coli* differed little from that of *P. mirabilis*. Cotran and associates[112] have observed that *P. mirabilis* seemed to have

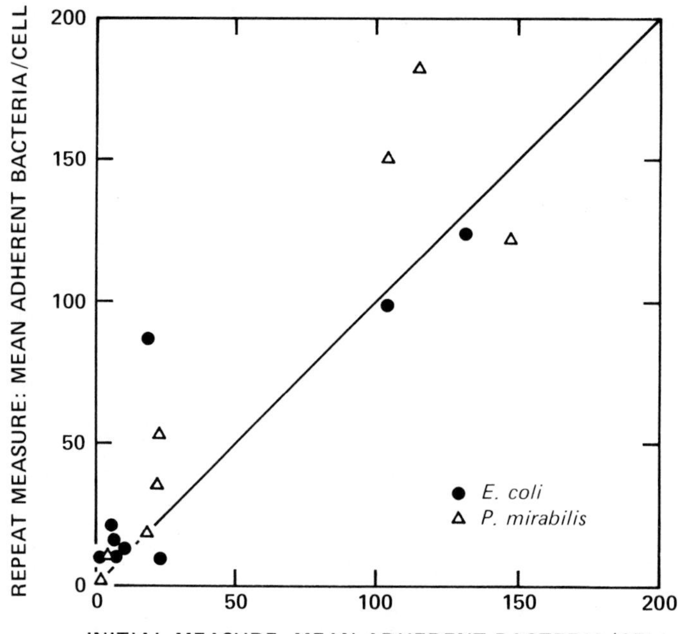

Figure 5.19 Comparison of initial and repeat measurement of bacterial adherence. (Reproduced by permission from J. E. Fowler and T. A. Stamey, J. Urol. **120:** 315, 1978.[106])

greater renal pathogenicity than *E. coli* in studies of retrograde pyelonephritis in the rat. Our data would suggest that this variability in virulence between the two bacterial species is unrelated to their adhesive properties.

This report reconfirms our previous findings that different strains of *E. coli* adhere to vaginal cells with varying affinity and demonstrates marked variability in the capacity of different *P. mirabilis* strains to adhere to vaginal cells. Moreover, the data suggest that the ability of an *E. coli* strain to adhere is unrelated to the O-serogroup since strains with the same O-antigen showed great variability in adhesive properties.

The reproducibility of this *in vitro* measure of bacterial adherence and the close correlation between similar *in vitro* and *in vivo* measures reported by others suggest that these data are an accurate measure of bacterial adherence to squamous cells.[113] The standardized culture techniques and frequency of longitudinal cultures in the patient population have provided a convincing assessment of the clinical urinary virulence of the bacteria studied. However, one might argue that these data cannot be applied to estimates of bacterial adherence to transitional cell epithelium. While no data are available to compare the relative adherence of a bacterial strain to squamous and transitional mucosal cells, colonization of the squamous vaginal epithelium remains the most important event in the pathogenesis of bacteriuria in the female subject.

In summary, the adhesive properties of a bacterial strain from the fecal reservoir is shown to be unrelated to the urinary virulence of the strain. However, bacterial adhesion seems to be important in colonization of the vaginal introitus and urinary conduits. It seems that a variability in the vaginal biology of the host that allows more avid adherence of enterobacteria, regardless of the adhesive properties of the bacteria itself, is the predominant factor mediating bacterial adherence to the vaginal mucosa.[102]

Role of Bacterial Pili (Fimbriae) as a Cause of Variation in Bacterial Adherence among Different O-Groups of *Escherichia coli*

Between July 1, 1977, and June 30, 1978, Drs. David Lark and Darrell Cornelius—

during their residency rotation in the urologic laboratories—accomplished a number of interesting experiments on bacterial adherence to vaginal epithelial cells. The reader will recall that Fowler and I [102] had to discard about one-third of our epithelial cells from both patients and controls because of residual bacteria attached to the cells after four simple washings and centrifugations in phosphate buffered saline (PBS) (pH 6.4). Kållenius and Winberg[103] had to discard a proportion of their periurethral cells as well. We made two major changes in the technique of washing and counting the epithelial cells: (1) the original cell suspension, after the initial centrifugation, was washed with large volumes of PBS over a Nucleopore filter; washing and centrifugation was done only after incubation with the bacteria rather than use a micropore filter, and (2) after consultation with our Department of Biostatistics, a better method of recording the number of bacteria attached to each epithelial cell was instituted. Because these modifications were important, the details are reproduced here for the use of other investigators before presenting our data on the role of pili in bacterial adherence.

The vaginal epithelial cell suspension was centrifuged at 900 × *g* for 10 minutes and the supernatant discarded. The epithelial cells were filtered through a Nucleopore dermalon 12 μm filter, using 300 ml of PBS to wash and agitate the cells. The epithelial cells were gently scraped from the filter with a rubber paddle and the process repeated a second time. The cells were finally resuspended in sterile PBS, and a portion of the cells heat-fixed on a glass slide and stained with safranin for the presence of adhering bacteria. In 66 samples from 20 subjects, only 1.8% of 2650 cells counted had more than 4 bacteria per epithelial cell; 87% of all cells had no detectable bacteria per epithelial cell. The concentration of vaginal cells used in the adherence studies which follow was 10^5–10^6 epithelial cells/ml. The *E. coli* were grown on blood agar plates overnight, cultured for 16–18 hours in 4 ml of Mueller-Hinton broth, harvested by centrifugation at 500 × *g* for 5 minutes, and resuspended in 2 ml of acetate buffer at pH 4.5 which produced a bacterial concentration of approximately 10^8–10^9 bacteria/ml.

Bacteria and epithelial cells were combined in a 1:1 volume ratio in 1–2 ml aliquots in siliconized test tubes and placed on a shaker water bath at 37°C for 60 minutes. After incubation, 5 ml of acetate buffer was added, the suspension centrifuged at 250 × *g* for 10 minutes, the supernatant discarded, and the bacteria resuspended for three additional washes. After the fourth wash, an aliquot of the cell suspension was placed on a glass slide, air dried, heat fixed, and stained with safranin for 2 minutes. The number of bacteria adherent to each of the first 40 cells visualized were counted in a systematic fashion. The bacteria per cell were recorded according to the following groups: 0–9, 10–19, 20–29, 30–39, 40–49, 50–99, 100–149, and greater than 150, and were given the rank of 1, 2, 3, 4, 5, 6, 7, and 8, respectively. The mean rank and standard deviation were recorded for each preparation, using the logarithm of the geometric mean.

A review of Table 5.25 confirms the large variation in bacterial adherence among *E. coli* isolated from bacteriuric patients as well as among uncommon O-groups rarely involved in UTI; Table 5.27 shows again the substantial variation in adherence among another 18 strains of *E. coli* that had caused bacteriuria as well as an equal variation among anal *E. coli* that had never caused urinary infections. In many respects, this striking variation from minimal adherence to maximal adherence, among strains of apparently equal pathogenecity, is one of the most uncomfortable observations in all adherence data.

Ten strains of *E. coli* from the bacteriuric (vesical) strains in Table 5.27 were selected so that 5 represented the high adhering strains and 5 were low adhering *E. coli*. The same selection was used for the anal *E. coli*, 5 high and 5 low adhering strains. Adherence of these 20 strains was determined with vaginal epithelial cells from healthy volunteer women. Hemagglutination of guinea pig erythrocytes for each strain of *E. coli* was determined simultaneously from the same Mueller-Hinton broth used to grow the organisms for the adherence work. As seen in Table 5.30, the high adhering *E. coli* caused substantial hemagglutination of guinea pig erythrocytes, while the low adhering *E. coli* did not. Since bacterial pili are known to agglutinate guinea pig erythrocytes,[114] piliation probably explains the variation observed in bacterial adherence.

It is recognized that broth-to-broth transfers of bacteria enhance attachment, whereas agar-to-agar transfers inhibit attachment.[114] In Table 5.31, the *E. coli* 018(a) was grown in Mueller-Hinton broth for 6 days with three 48-hour broth transfers, while *E. coli* 018(b) was grown on nutrient-poor agar for 8 days with four 48-hour transfers. Both the *E. coli* 018(a) and 018(b) were studied on three different occasions with vaginal epithelial cells from three different control volunteers. The broth-to-broth transfers show high bacterial adherence, accompanied by high hemagglutination guinea pig red cell titers, while the *E. coli* 018(b) grown in agar-to-agar transfers show negligible bacterial adherence to epithelial cells and virtually no hemagglutination.

While the hemagglutination experiments were convincing that the variation we were observing in *E. coli* adherence was due to bacterial pili, the following study utilizing rabbit antipili antisera seems more specific. Pure pili were obtained by blending an *E. coli* 018, and separating the pili from the bacterial cell wall by centrifugation at pH 4.0 at 4°C.[115] The pili were precipitated with 0.1 M magnesium chloride, the protein concentrated and measured, and confirmed by electron microscopy studies to consist of pure pili. Rabbits were injected with 50-μg amounts of the protein precipitate at weekly intervals for 4 weeks and the antisera recovered. One milliliter of rabbit antipili antisera was combined with 1 ml of 10^9 washed *E coli* 018, the bacteria separated from the antisera, and resuspended in acetate buffer. In Table 5.32, the bacteria treated with the antipili antibody substantially reduced adherence in 5 experiments. When the *E. coli* 018 were treated with control rabbit antisera obtained before injection of the pili, there was minimal reduction in maximal adherence.

Additional experiments confirming the presence of Type I pili showed that D-mannose and α-methyl D-mannoside blocked bacterial adherence when added to the incubation mixtures of bacterial and epithelial cells[116]; D-glucose, D-fructose, D-lactose, L-mannose, D-galactose, and D-sucrose all failed to inhibit bacterial attachment.

Pili have been shown to mediate bacterial attachment and virulence in other circumstances, including gonococci of colony Types 1 and 2,[117] *Shigella flexneri* and attachment to human intestinal epithelial cells,[116] the K88 and K99 protein antigens of *E. coli* in intestinal diarrhea of piglets,[118] and in several experimental animals including proteus pyelonephritis in rats[110] and the adherence of *E. coli* K12 to monkey kidney cells.[119]

Svanborg-Edén and Hansson[120] have presented excellent evidence that pili are probably the main mediators of *E. coli* attachment to human urinary tract epithelial cells; their electron microscopic studies are especially striking.

I began this section with my concern over the wide variation in bacterial adherence among *E. coli* O-serogroups of apparently

Table 5.30
Relationship of High and Low Adhering *Escherichia coli* to Hemagglutination of Guinea Pig Erythrocytes

Source and No. of Strains of *E. coli*	Mean Adherence Bacteria/Cell	Mean Hemagglutination Titer[a]
Bacteriuric high adhering 5	103	6.0
Bacteriuric low adhering 5	8	0.4
Anal high adhering 5	91	3.0
Anal low adhering 5	4	0.8

[a] Reciprocal of dilution.

Table 5.31
Broth-to-Broth (a) and Agar-to-Agar (b) Transfers of an *Escherichia coli* 018 Before Measuring Adherence and Hemagglutination

Control Subjects	*E. coli* 018(a)		*E. coli* 018(b)	
	Bacteria/Cell	Hemagglutination	Bacteria/Cell	Hemagglutination
1	79	6.0	3	0.0
2	106	8.0	2	1.0
3	103	8.0	3	0.0

equal pathogenecity. While this variation can probably be accounted for, at least in part, by differences in bacterial pili, the data from Svanborg-Edén and her colleagues[121] that the variation in *E. coli* adherence to human urinary tract epithelial cells cannot be accounted for by differences in K antigen is unique; as these authors noted however, 94% of their *E. coli* with K12 capsular antigen adhered well. They also concluded that O-groups 1, 2, 4, 6, 7, 16, 18, and 75 had higher proportion of adhering strains than did those of the remaining O-groups.[121] This observation is not apparent in our Tables 5.25 and 5.27, but their study compared 328 typable, 53 nontypable, and 74 self-agglutinating strains of *E. coli*—numbers we cannot compete with.

Some *In Vitro* Determinants of Bacterial Adherence to Vaginal Epithelial Cells

While pili appear to be the major determinant of differences in bacterial adherence, several *in vitro* conditions influence the number of bacteria that attach per epithelial cell.

Variation in Bacterial Adherence to Epithelial Cells from the Same Subject on Different Days

Forty-six studies were performed on 18 subjects with the same *E. coli* 018. The mean number of bacteria per epithelial cell was 93.3 ± 18 for a coefficient of variation (CV) of 19%. One of these subjects was studied on 9 different occasions (83.2 ± 31; CV = 37%); a second subject was studied on 8 different days (74 ± 14; CV = 19%).

Svanborg-Edén, Eriksson, and Hanson[122] found similar variations (16–19%) on the same subject studied on 8 different days. Schaeffer *et al.*,[123] however, using bacteria labeled with [^{3}H]uridine, reported a striking day-to-day variation in the receptivity of the same epithelial cells, a variation he attributed to different phases of the menstrual cycle with greater adherence occurring in the first 14 days.

Influence of *Escherichia coli* Concentration on Bacterial Adherence

If the number of vaginal cells is maintained constant at 10^5/ml, and the number of bacteria increased from 10^5–10^8/ml, bacterial attachment increases from 4.5 to 74.5 bacteria per epithelial cell.

Svanborg-Edén *et al.*[122] showed that there was less adherence during the logarithmic growth phase than after termination of this rapid growth phase, a finding in keeping with stimulation of pili during the stationary phase after growth has ceased. They also noted that adherence increased over incubation periods of up to 180 minutes when epithelial cells and bacteria were added together; most of the increase occurred in 1 hour, which is probably the most satisfactory incubation time to use.

Schaeffer's technique of [^{3}H]uridine-labeled bacteria, however, which does not remove the indigenous bacteria from the cells, showed that maximal adherence occurs within 1 minute with a gradual decline of radioactivity over the next 30 minutes to a stationary level.

Superficial *vs.* Deep Vaginal Cells

In four experiments, *E. coli* were found to adhere equally well to the superficial and deep layers of vaginal epithelial cells. In seven experiments, trypan blue stains

Table 5.32
Bacterial Adherence of *Escherichia coli* Before and After Exposure to Rabbit Antipili Antibody

Antipili Antibody	No. of Determinations	Log of Geometric Mean (±S.D.)	Bacteria/Cell	Student *t*-Test
–	5	1.92 ± 0.11	83.2	$P < 0.001$
+	5	1.21 ± 0.14	16.2	

showed no difference in the number of resident bacteria adherent to viable *versus* dead vaginal epithelial cells.

Influence of pH

Using control vaginal epithelial cells from six subjects, but changing the pH of the buffer at which the bacteria and epithelial cells were suspended, bacterial attachment was twice as great at pH 4.5 as at pH 6.4 (Table 5.33).

The viable bacterial count was not influenced by suspending the bacteria in PBS buffer at 6.4 compared to acetate buffer of pH 4.5; this was true whether the bacteria were incubated at 37°C for 30 minutes or 4 hours.

Mårdh and Weström[107] showed a similar dependency of the gonococcus on pH in its adherence to vaginal epithelial cells. Apparently, maximal adherence of *E. coli* to uroepithelial cells in the voided urine occurs at pH 6.0,[122] although Schaeffer *et al.*[123] also found maximal adherence at pH 4.0.

Effect of Washing Bacteria

In seven studies on a highly piliated *E. coli*, bacterial adherence to control vaginal cells was compared with washing the bacteria twice with PBS to no washing of the bacteria before incubation with the vaginal cells. As seen in Table 5.34, washing the bacteria has a profound effect on adherence, presumably from knocking off pili. Svanborg-Edén *et al.*[122] showed a similar effect from washing.

Effect of Banking *Escherichia coli* on Agar Slants for Long Periods before Adherence Studies

A substantial number of bacteriuric strains of *E. coli* were studied that had been banked for varying intervals of time from day 0 to 15 months. These data suggest (Table 5.35) that bacterial attachment to epithelial cells is influenced by the length of time the organisms have been banked prior to attachment experiments. These data are particularly important in population studies where bacteria may have been banked for several years.

Attachment of Bacteria Taken Directly from Urine

If bacteria are taken directly from infected urine, rather than grown in broth, and mixed with control vaginal epithelial cells, the degree of adherence depends in part on whether the bacteria are coated with antibody from the urinary tract. As seen below in Table 5.36, the degree of adherence was twice as great with non-antibody-coated bacteria as in those which were fluorescent antibody positive.

It is important to note, however, that attachment to epithelial cells is never as great when bacteria are taken directly from urine as when they are grown in broth prior to attachment studies. As can be seen in Table 5.36, the standard method of processing bacteria for *in vitro* attachment studies—urine to agar to broth—produces 3 times the number of bacteria attached to human vaginal cells (55/cell) as occurs when non-antibody-coated bacteria are taken directly from urine and exposed to human epithelial cells (17.9/cell). These observations suggest some caution in the transfer of *in vitro* studies to *in vivo* pathogenesis, *i.e.*, growth of bacteria in nutrient laboratory media clearly increases the degree of piliation disproportionately to what may exist at mucosal surfaces in the body.

Some Additional Studies and Comments on Bacterial Adherence to Squamous Epithelial Cells

Mårdh, Colleen, and Hovelius,[124] who also used voided, human uroepithelial cells,

Table 5.33
Influence of pH on Incubation of *Escherichia coli* and Vaginal Cells

pH	No. of Determinations	Log of Geometric mean	Bacteria/Cell	Student *t* Test
4.5	31	1.414 ± 0.396	25.9	P <0.001
6.4	31	1.058 ± 0.300	11.4	

looked at the adherence of different bacterial species in a few experiments; *S. faecalis* and *Staphylococcus saprophyticus* adhered better than *S. epidermidis*. These authors also reported some data on bacterial adherence using male uroepithelial cells in comparison to female cells.

Techniques have been reported for measuring bacterial attachment to whole tissues rather than detached epithelial cells. Attachment of enteropathogenic *E. coli* to the mucosa of human fetal small intestine has been reported[125] as well as segments of ureter turned inside out (everted) which have been used to measure the release of bacteria from the mucosal surface.[126]

One cannot close a section on bacterial adherence to human epithelial cells without a few comments on the mannose receptor sites on the epithelial cells. Duguid and Gillies[116] were the first to recognize these receptors in 1957; they showed that these receptor sites for *E. coli* could be blocked by D-mannose. Recognition of these mannose specific sites on the surface of epithelial cells is potentially important because, if they could be successfully blocked, bacterial adherence presumably could be prevented. Ofek *et al.*[127] described a dose-response relationship between D-mannose and the inhibition of *E. coli* adherence to human buccal epithelial cells. Svanborg-Edén *et al.*,[120] however, could not inhibit *E. coli* attachment to voided uroepithelial cells by D-mannose, although they could prevent adherence to buccal mucosal cell. Schaeffer *et al.*,[123] on the other hand, obtained almost complete inhibition, in their assay of adherence, with α-D-mannose[123]; we obtained similar results with either D-mannose or α-methyl D-mannoside, but no other sugars would block *E. coli* adherence to vaginal epithelial cells. Ofek *et al.*[127] also showed that the inhibition of bacterial adherence by D-mannose was reversible by simply washing the epithelial cells; moreover, the addition of D-mannose to epithelial cells, to which *E. coli* were preattached, caused rapid displacement of the organism from the epithelial cell while other sugars failed to displace the *E. coli*. It is also interesting that D-mannose could be bound by concanavalin-A which inhibited attachment of *E. coli* to buccal cells but not streptococcal attachment. Hence, the D-mannose receptor sites seem specific for *E. coli*. Type 1 pili usually correlate with mannose-sensitive agglutination of guinea pig erythrocytes (*i.e.*, agglutination can be inhibited by D-mannose). Kållenius and Möllby,[128] however, have described an *E. coli* 075 isolated from a patient with acute pyelonephritis that adheres avidly to periurethral cells, agglutinates guinea pig erythrocytes poorly but human erythrocytes strongly, and D-mannose is ineffective in preventing hemagglutination of either erythrocytes or the adhesive ability of the *E. coli* 075. This observation clearly means that not all *E. coli* causing UTI will be blocked by manipulating the mannose receptor sites, even if this were feasible; indeed, Duguid and Gillies[116] noted that hemagglutination could not be blocked by D-mannose in 50% of *E. coli* strains causing urinary infections.

Lastly, the data of Svanborg-Edén and her colleagues[121] at Göteborg are convincing that strains of *E. coli* isolated from children with acute pyelonephritis and cystitis adhere to urinary epithelial cells more avidly than do strains isolated from patients with asymptomatic bacteriuria detected during screening surveys, and, that the latter strains are more sensitive to the serum bactericidal activity than are the strains causing acute UTI symptoms. It seems reasonable that the bacterial cell wall has been modified in these asymptomatic infections of long standing duration (presumably by local antibody), and the observation that 40% of such strains are self-

Table 5.34
Effect of Washing Bacteria Before Incubation

Escherichia coli	No. of Determinations	Log of Geometric mean	Bacteria/Cell	Student *t* Test
Piliated (0 wash)	7	1.814 ± 0.252	65.2	$P < 0.001$
Piliated (2× wash)	7	1.220 ± 0.112	16.7	

agglutinating is surely indicative of that modification.

What surprises me about their data is that *E. coli* selected from the rectal flora of healthy children shows such a low order of bacterial adherence. To be sure, only 41 of 120 *E. coli* strains (34%) belonged to O-groups 1, 2, 4, 6, 7, 16, 18, 25, and 75 which caused 80% of all *E. coli* infections in acute pyelonephritis, but even this 34% of these common O-groups isolated from the rectums of healthy children showed minimal adherence; only 7 of the 41 strains showed any adherence at all. If the rectal reservoir bears any similarity to the infected strains that cause acute UTI, I am at a loss to explain these data. Moreover, our data in Tables 5.27 and 5.28 in adult women failed to show any difference in adherence between nonbacteriuric strains isolated from the rectum and strains that cause symptomatic UTI. I suppose the fecal flora from children could be different from adult women in respect to bacterial adherence as well as the occurrence of common O-serogroups, but I find this difficult to believe.

The other explanation, of course, which I expect the Göteborg investigators prefer, is that normal children do not become susceptible to UTI until they colonize their intestinal tract with common O-serogroups with an increased capability of bacterial adherence. But where is the reservoir of these common O-groups with increased adherence and why are not all children exposed to these bacteria?

Is there another possible explanation? Is it possible that these rectal *E. coli* with few common O-groups and low adherence strains described in normal healthy children by the Göteborg group are selected and changed by the introital mucosa to those characteristics exhibited by *E. coli* in symptomatic UTI? I have presented data in women that the common O-groups are more likely to survive than the uncommon ones in normal human vaginal fluid and it is not inconceivable that bacterial piliation could increase by virtue of colonizing the introital and vaginal mucosa. The problem with this latter explanation, of course, is to explain why then the common O-groups are easily found in the fecal flora once a patient has an acute symptomatic UTI; one possibility, as unattractive as it is, could be that once bacteriuria is established with a common O-group that adheres well, the act of voiding in the female recolonizes the anus and rectum with the infecting organism.

Perhaps it is as Freter[129] pointed out in 1978, "A pathogen must be able to (1) survive in the environment, (2) attach to and multiple on the body surface, (3) spread within the body, (4) resist numerous defense mechanisms of mammalian tissue, and (5) produce a toxin or interfer with the host's physiology in some other way. If only one of these links is missing the chain will be broken. The bacterium's progress will stop, and it will not be able to cause disease."

ROLE OF CERVICOVAGINAL ANTIBODY IN ENTEROBACTERIAL COLONIZATION OF THE INTROITAL MUCOSA

Introduction and Early Studies

When we realized that *E. coli* attached more readily to vaginal epithelial cells from women susceptible to UTI than to similar cells from healthy, control women[102] (see Table 5.26, and Figure 5.15), we knew that local surface antibody could also be important in determining bacterial adherence.[100, 101]

We had, however, already looked at local vaginal antibody in UTI-prone and healthy women.[130] Immunoglobulins IgG and IgA were determined in 94 collections of vaginal

Table 5.35
Effect of Banking *Escherichia coli* from Bacteriuric Site for Long Periods of Time

Banked	No. of Determinations	Log of Geometric mean (±S.D.)	Bacteria/Cell
mo			
0	28	1.74 ± 0.25	55.0
1–3	22	1.68 ± 0.25	47.6
4–8	16	1.51 ± 0.39	32.2
9–14	19	1.45 ± 0.30	28.2
15	26	1.29 ± 0.28	18.6

fluid from 10 patients before, during, and after 17 episodes of bacteriuria. The results were compared to 49 collections from 6 volunteer controls who had never had bacteriuria. The mean IgG concentration in patients (48 ± 54 mg/100 ml) was no different from controls (50 ± 33 mg/100 ml). IgA concentrations were 2.6 ± 2.1 and 2.6 ± 2.4 mg/100 ml, respectively. Bacterial agglutination titers in vaginal fluid to *E. coli* colonizing the introitus of the patients were no different (7.7 ± 9.8, reciprocal tube titer) than the titers to the predominant *E. coli* cultured from the anal canal of the controls (9.7 ± 5.0). Longitudinal studies in patients were especially disappointing in that they failed to show any relationship between vaginal colonization with changing serotypes of *E. coli* and agglutination titers in vaginal fluid. Moreover, bacterial agglutination titers to an *E. coli* OX9, a rare *E. coli* unlikely to have occurred in patients or controls, were no different (11.3 ± 6.8, controls; 8.3 ± 6.1, patients) than the titers of the pathogenic *E. coli.*

Because these agglutination titers, even when factored by the total amount of IgG or IgA, seemed to represent low, nonspecific agglutination to *E. coli* O-antigens, and because bacterial agglutination titers were probably more specific for IgM than IgG, we were essentially frustrated with these measurements of secondary antibody-antigen reactions.

Indirect Immunofluorescent Technique of Measuring Antigen-Specific Antibody

The indirect immunofluorescent technique of measuring serum antibody titers, as described by Thomas *et al.*[131] seemed ideal for measuring antigen-specific antibody in cervicovaginal fluid.

Using indirect immunofluorescence with fluorescein-conjugated antisera to human immunoglobulins, we have asked the following questions: (1) Is introital carriage with Enterobacteriaceae in women susceptible to bacteriuria related to the absence of specific cervicovaginal antibody (CVA)? (2) Is absence of introital carriage in women resistant to bacteriuria related to the presence of CVA against their predominant fecal *E. coli*? (3) We have been intrigued by an earlier observation that 10–20% of bacteriuric women have no viable bacteria on the introitus at a time when millions of bacteria are voided across the vaginal vestibule.[24] Is bacteriuria associated with specific CVA against the infecting organism in the urinary tract? (4) Is antibody present in cervicovaginal fluid (CVF) against the normal indigenous flora, lactobacilli and *S. epidermidis*? (5) How much CVA is present (in relation to serum antibody), what type is present (IgG, IgA, or IgM), and how long does it last? (6) Is local antibody present in the vagina in the absence of the cervix and uterus?

Ten premenopausal and three hysterectomized adult female volunteers who had never experienced urinary infections were selected as controls. An average of 3 weekly collections of CVF were obtained from each control; introital and anal canal swabs for culture were obtained at each visit. The predominant anal *E. coli* was isolated and serotyped. If introital Enterobacteriaceae were present, which is unusual, they were stored also. CVF was collected as a 50-ml distilled water wash of the cervix and vagina. The sample was filtered through a Nalgene 0.2 μ filter, frozen, lyophilized, and

Table 5.36
Attachment of FA+ and FA− *Escherichia coli* Taken Directly from Urine Compared to Standard Culture Technique[a]

Patients	No. of Determinations	FA	Log of Geometric Mean (±S.D.)	Bacteria/Cell	Student t Test
9	9	+	0.90 ± 0.17	7.9	$P < 0.01$
17	17	−	1.25 ± 0.31	17.9	
26	35		1.65 ± 0.39	55.0[b]	

[a] FA = fluorescent antibody.
[b] *E. coli* passed from urine to agar to broth before adherence studies.

later reconstituted to 1 ml as previously described[60]; the 1-ml reconstitution approximates the Na and K concentration of natural vaginal fluid.

Fifty-one premenopausal, 1 postmenopausal, and 11 hysterectomized female patients with recurrent bacteriuria were selected as the patient group. Longitudinal studies on some patients included collections while they were bacteriuric as well as during and after therapy. Cultures of the vaginal introitus and midstream voided specimen as well as the diagnosis of bacteriuria were accomplished as described in Chapter 1. Fecal cultures were obtained by rotating a moistened swab stick in the anal canal until yellow with fecal material; the swab stick was placed in 5 ml of Earle's broth, vibrated with a vortex mixer, and the broth streaked onto appropriate agar plates.

Fluorescein-conjugated horse antiserum to human globulin was obtained from Roboz Surgical Instrument Company, Washington, D.C. Fluoresceinconjugated monospecific antisera (goat) to human IgA, IgG, and IgM were obtained from Microbiological Associates, Bethesda, Maryland.

Quantitation of immunoglobulins was performed by low and ultra low level radial immunodiffusion Endoplates obtained from Kallestad Laboratories, Chaska, Minnesota.

Detection of Antibody-Coated Bacteria

Antibody coating of bacteria was assessed in CVF by the indirect immunofluorescence technique of measuring serum antibody titer as described by Thomas *et al.*[131]. The method is illustrated in Figures 5.20 and 5.21.

Approximately 10 colonies from an 18-hour blood plate subculture of the organisms to be tested were harvested and suspended in phosphate buffered saline. The suspension was diluted to a reading of 50% transmission at 590 mμ with a 1-cm light path. This dilution represented greater than 2×10^8 bacteria/ml and usually resulted in at least 200 bacteria per high powered field that remained on a glass slide after the washing procedures were completed. A volume of approximately 30 μl was spread thinly on precleaned microscope slides, air dried, and fixed in acetone for 10 minutes. Slides were then washed twice in phosphate buffered saline for 4 minutes, air dried, and the bacteria ringed with a glass marking pen. The ringed area was flooded with approximately 30 μl of the reconstituted 1 ml of CVF, incubated at 37°C for 30 minutes, washed twice, air dried and treated with approximately 30 μl of a 1:5 dilution of the appropriate fluoresceinconjugated antihuman globulin. After incubation at 37°C for 30 minutes the slides were again washed twice and air dried; one drop of Bacto-FA mounting fluid was applied and a coverslip affixed. The slides were kept in a light tight box at 10°C until examined for fluorescence, usually on the same day, with a Leitz microscope containing a 200 watt mercury lamp and appropriate filters for fluorescein fluorescence.

The intensity of fluorescence was recorded as negative or positive with arbitrary gradations of 1+ to 4+. Appropriate controls of bacteria unexposed to CVF were used to measure nonspecific fluorescence.

Two-fold serial dilutions of CVF were made in sterile distilled water (1:2 through 1:256) to estimate the amount of fluorescent

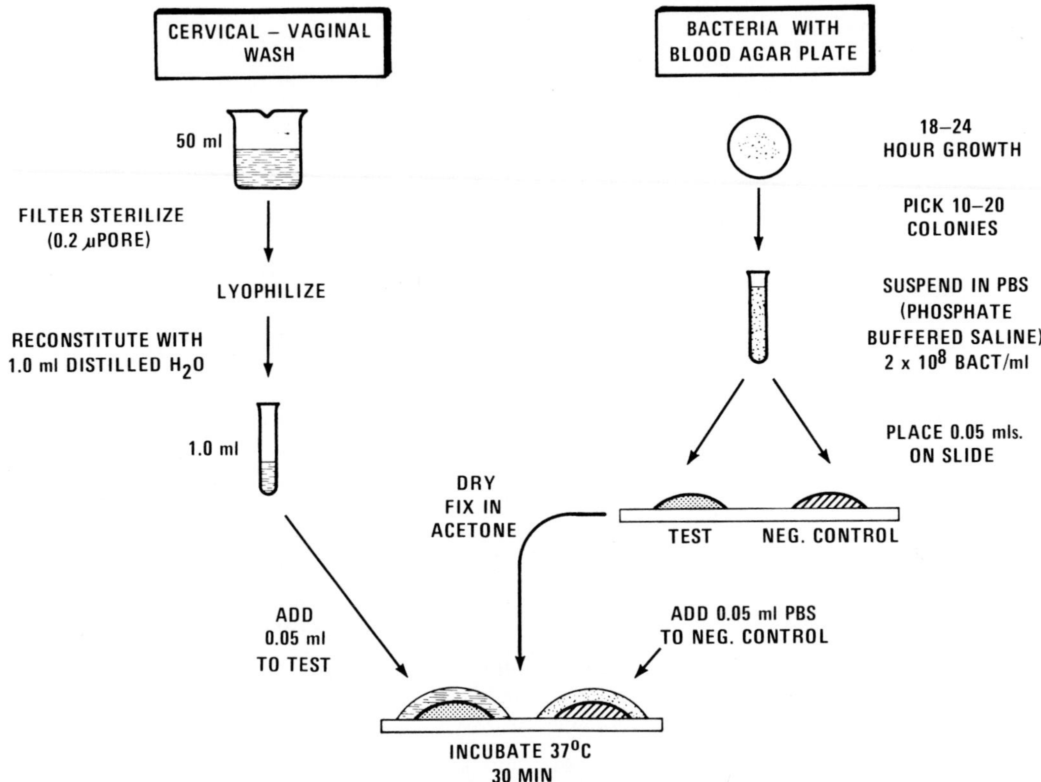

Figure 5.20 Indirect immunofluorescence technique: preparation of antigen and antibody.

antibody. The lowest intensity (1+) of fluorescence was considered positive for fluorescent antibody (FA).

Fluorescent Antibody Results in Controls and Urinary Tract Infection-Prone Women

In 13 control volunteers, studied 36 times, the predominant fecal *E. coli* was coated with CVA (FA+) 78% of the time after exposure to CVF (Table 5.37). A representative, healthy volunteer is shown in Figure 5.22.

In contrast, in 23 patients with enterobacterial introital carriage who were not bacteriuric, antibody-coating occurred in only 27% of 37 collections (Table 5.37). Longitudinal studies on a representative patient are presented in Figure 5.23. That failure to coat with CVA in 73% of these 37 determinations was unrelated to some biochemical change in the colonizing organism *after* it had reached the introitus was shown by similar lack of fluorescence when the same serotype on the introitus was isolated from the feces and exposed to CVF.

When bacteriuric patients, with and without introital carriage of the urinary infecting strain, were studied for specific CVA against the bacteriuric strain, the percent of FA+ strains in those patients without introital colonization was twice that of those whose bacteriuric organisms persisted on the introitus (Table 5.38). Indeed, the rate of FA+ strains in the former group was the same as control volunteers tested against their predominant fecal *E. coli* (Table 5.37).

Longitudinal studies on a particularly instructive patient are presented in Figure 5.24. A 22-year-old, unmarried, white female with recurrent bacteriuria was followed closely throughout 1976 during which time she experienced four episodes of symptomatic bacteriuria. Each of the four uri-

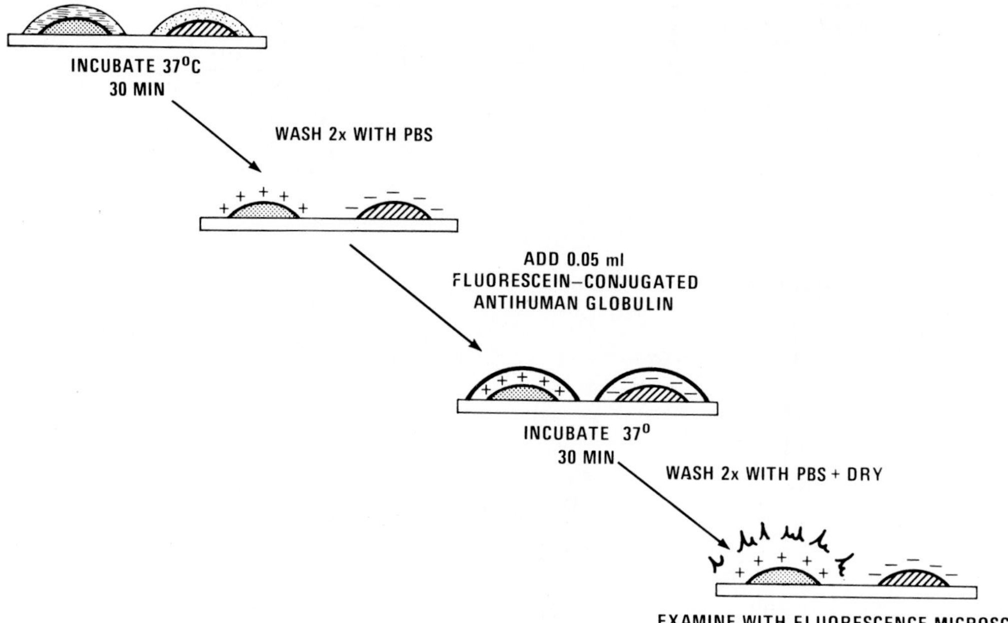

Figure 5.21 Indirect immunofluorescence technique: processing of antigen, antibody, and antihuman globulin.

nary tract infections were FA negative, an indication that the bacteriuria was confined to the bladder.[131] An intravenous urogram was normal and she was never instrumented. Each urinary infection was treated with a 7- to 10-day course of nalidixic acid, which promptly sterilized the urine until the next episode of bacteriuria several weeks or months later. The longitudinal studies in Figure 5.24 are noteworthy in four respects. First, introital colonization with *E. coli*, *Klebsiella*, and *Enterobacter* between episodes of bacteriuria always occurred in the absence of CVF antibody with one exception (300 *E. coli* SA on 6/10). Second, absence of introital colonization between episodes of bacteriuria, always occurred in the presence of CVF antibody to either the predominant fecal strain (5/18, 11/19) or to the preceding bacteriuric strain (5/4, 8/18). No fecal *E. coli* were present on 8/18 during the 9th day of nalidixic acid therapy, a common occurrence during therapy with nalidixic acid[132]; the fecal *E. coli* on 5/4 unfortunately were not saved for CVA studies. Third, 2 of the 4 bacteriuric episodes occurred without a single organism of the bacteriuric strain (or any other Enterobacteriaceae) on the introitus and a third had only 20 *E. coli* 07 per ml at the time of the bacteriuria (2/23); in each instance there was 3+ FA in CVF against the bacteriuric strain. The remaining bacteriuric episode (4/12), an *E. coli* 07, occurred with heavy introital colonization of *E. coli* SA; neither antibody to this introital rough strain (*E. coli* SA) nor the bacteriuric strain of *E. coli* 07 was detectable in the CVF. It is likely that the self-agglutinating introital strain was an *E. coli* 07. Fourth, the CVF studies on 7/29 are of particular interest. The introitus was heavily colonized with *Klebsiella* and *Enterobacter*, both of which were FA negative in CVF, 12 days before an *E. coli* 07 bacteriuria (8/10). On 7/29, the anal culture contained large numbers of an *E. coli* SA and non-typable *E coli*, neither of which were cultured from the introitus, and the CVF was FA+ to both strains. Of equal interest, there was no CVF antibody to the *E. coli* 07 which infected the bladder 12 days later, suggesting that in-

Table 5.37
Comparison of Antibody-Coated Bacteria After Exposure to Cervicovaginal Fluid of Normal Volunteers and Women Susceptible to Bacteriuria with Introital Carriage of Enterobacteriaceae[a]

Subjects	No. of Subjects	No. of Determinations	No. of FA+[b]	Percentage Determination FA+	Percentage Subjects FA+
Control women[c]	13	36	28	78	77
Susceptible women[d]	23	37	9	27	26

[a] Reproduced by permission from T. A. Stamey, N. Wehner, G. Mihara, and M. Condy, Medicine (Baltimore) **57:** 47, 1978[134].
[b] FA = fluorescent antibody.
[c] Predominent fecal. E. *coli* used for bacteria.
[d] Introital Enterobacteriaceae used for bacteria.

troital colonization with this 07 was an immunologic possibility during the succeeding 12 day interval. The bacteriologic and immunologic course of this patient strongly suggest the controlling influence of local vaginal antibody in determining introital colonization and subsequent bacteriuria. It should be noted that she received 100 mg of nitrofurantoin macrocrystals each night as prophylaxis between 6/10/76 and 12/17/76 in an attempt to prevent bacteriuria. One month after stopping prophylaxis she was reinfected with Enterobacter, preceded by heavy introital colonization with the same organism.

Tuttle and his colleagues[169] in South Carolina investigated girls from 2–10 years of age with recurrent UTI and compared their vaginal antibody to enuretic girls of the same age who were resistant to UTI; they found a strong correlation between UTI and reduced levels of vaginal antibody.

Specific Immunoglobulins Coating the Fluorescent Antibody Positive Strains

Using monospecific antisera (goat) to human IgA, IgG, and IgM, all FA+ strains in Tables 5.37 and 5.38 were investigated as to the type of antibody coating the bacteria (Table 5.39). While IgA was the most common, IgG was almost as prominent. Moreover, IgM fluorescence was not infrequent.

If the total percentage of IgA, IgG and IgM coating in Table 5.39 is considered in relation to 50 separate strains of Enterobacteriaceae (Table 5.40), the combination of IgA-IgG-IgM and IgA-IgG is the most common. Of those few strains coated with a single immunoglobulin, IgA is the most common.

Total immunoglobulins, determined by radial immunodiffusion, demonstrated no statistically significant difference between patients and controls in IgA or IgG (Table 5.41), as we have also shown in a previous study.[130] IgM was rarely detectable by immunodiffusion. Sensitivity of the radial immunodiffusion plates was 5.0 mg/dl for IgM, 1.9 mg/dl for IgA, and 1.1 mg/dl for IgG. More important, there was no relationship between total immunoglobulins as measured by radial immunodiffusion and the presence or absence of fluorescent antibody. With IgM, for example, there were 44 FA+ specimens but IgM was undetectable by radial immunodiffusion in 43. In 53 FA+ CVF for IgA, 15 showed undetectable levels by immunodiffusion. In 53 FA+ fluids for IgG, only one had undetectable amounts of IgG by radial immunodiffusion. On the other hand, in 41 CVF which were FA negative for antihuman immunoglobulins, measurable levels of IgG by radial immunodiffusion were present in 11, IgA in one and both IgA and IgG in one.

The specific immunoglobulins coating the bacteria in human CVF are of considerable immunologic interest because clinical inspection of the introitus colonized with Enterobacteriaceae fails to show any evidence of inflammatory reaction.[24] Indeed, quantitation of leukocytes on the introital mucosa in colonized patients and normal controls has shown no difference in

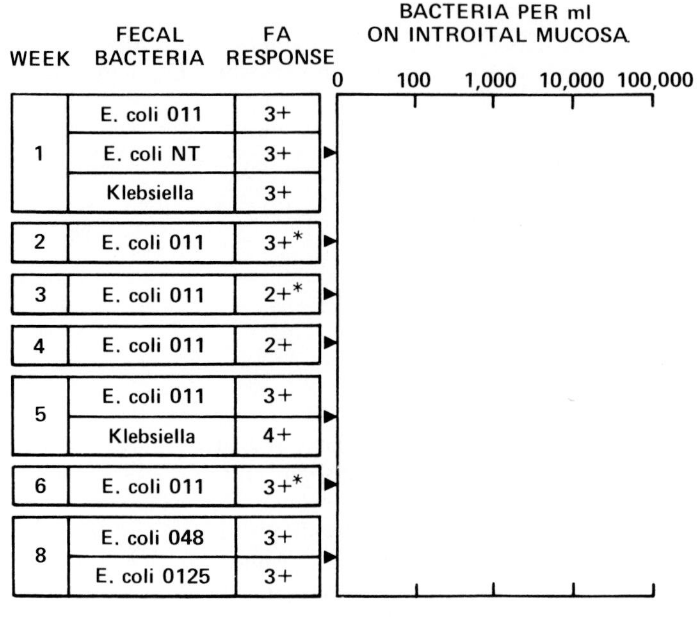

Figure 5.22 A 31-year-old white female volunteer who had never experienced urinary tract infections. Enterobacteriaceae were never cultured from the vaginal introitus. The predominant strains from the fecal flora always coated with fluorescent antibody (FA) when exposed to her cervicovaginal fluid. Cervicovaginal antibody was undetectable (FA–) to *Escherichia coli* 0X9 and 0103, rare O-serogroups she was unlikely to have encountered. NT = nontypable strain of *E. coli*. 011, 048, etc. = O-serogroups of *E. coli*. 2+ to 4+ = intensity of fluorescent antibody. Reproduced by permission from T. A. Stamey, N. Wehner, G. Mihara, and M. Condy, Medicine (Baltimore) **57:** 47, 1978[134].

numbers of leukocytes (Figure 5.12). Hence, the CVA measured in this study is probably unrelated to any inflammatory exudate from the serum. Secretory IgA (SIgA) was not measured because antiserum to the secretory component was not available but without question, total IgA (especially the dimeric form of SIgA) was underestimated (Table 5.41), perhaps by a factor of three as suggested by Vaerman and Férin[133]; Govers and Girard,[74] who had SIgA in their radial immunodiffusion plates and who used the same technique as we have of collecting CVF, found 14 mg/dl of SIgA, a value close to the control subjects in Table 5.41 if IgA is increased 3-fold. Nevertheless, it is clear that IgG and to a lesser extent IgM were equally important in contributing to specific antibody-coating of Enterobacteriaceae in CVF (Table 5.39).

Vaginal fluid could be diluted very little (<1:64) in controls and patients and maintain fluorescence of the bacteria. In all cases studied, serum titers exceeded cervicovaginal titers. IgA fluorescence was of special interest but all ratios of cervicovaginal titers to serum titers were much less than 1.0. Representative studies are presented in Table 5.42.

Specificity of Cervicovaginal Antibody for Different Antigens of Enterobacteriaceae

In our original paper in 1978,[134] we noted that *E. coli* of O-groups OX9 and 0103 rarely showed antibody coating when exposed to CVA (Figure 5.22). Since these rare O-groups were unlikely to have colonized the rectum of our volunteer controls, we considered that CVA might be fairly specific and show little cross-reactivity with other O-group antigens of *E. coli*. Our choice of OX9 and 0103 O-groups proved to be an unfortunate one. Lark, Cornelius, and I studied this question in some detail. CVF was collected on 48 occasions from 3 healthy controls and on 77 occasions from 8 premenopausal UTI-prone women; both patients and controls were different from those studied in Tables 5.37–5.42 because they were later entries into our study group.

As seen in Table 5.43, 85% of the CVF specimens from control volunteers showed antibody against the predominant rectal *E. coli* of the volunteer. Similar specificity,

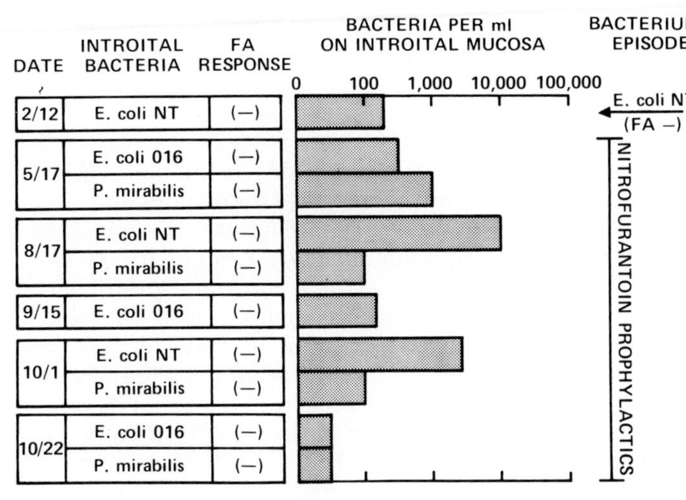

Figure 5.23 A 66-year-old white female patient with recurrent bacteriuria caused by *Proteus mirabilis*, enterococci, and *Escherichia coli* in the previous 10 months. Following the *E. coli* NT bacteriuria, she was placed on nightly nitrofurantoin prophylaxis. Introital colonization was continuously present with *E. coli* and *P. mirabilis*, despite a normal vaginal mucosal pH of 4.5. Fecal carriage with the same organisms cultured from the introitus was always present. Fluorescent antibody to these strains of Enterobacteriaceae was never detectable in her vaginal fluid. At the time of her *E. coli* NT bacteriuria, both the bacteriuric and introital strain were FA− after exposure to vaginal antibody. NT = nontypable strains of *E. coli*. FA(−) = absence of fluorescent antibody after exposure to vaginal fluid. Reproduced by permission from T. A. Stamey, N. Wehner, G. Mihara, and M. Condy, Medicine (Baltimore) **57:** 47, 1978[134].

however, was shown for the common *E. coli* antigens (075, 06, and 04), for the uncommon *E. coli* antigens (0139, 0124, 0103, and 01028), and for the galactose-deficient J_5 mutant of *E coli* 0111 (this mutant, obtained from A. Braude, lacks the "O" side chains of the smooth parent strain and presents the central R core of lipopolysaccharide for antibody-antigen reactivity). As also seen in Table 5.43, less than 50% of the CVF collected from susceptible, premenopausal patients contained CVA against these bacterial antigens, while control volunteers showed antibody in 85–95% of the studies. These data indicate that CVF contains antibody with broad cross-reactivity to the *E. coli* O-group antigens as well as to core lipopolysaccharide. It is interesting that cross-reactivity to *E. coli* OX9 occurred in less than one-third of the CVF from control volunteers.

Salivary Fluid Studies in Patients Who Lack Cervicovaginal Antibody

Salivary fluid was obtained from these 8 patients in Table 5.43 on 18 different occasions. In every instance there was salivary antibody directed against the *E. coli* even though CVA was absent. Precautions were taken to remove or destroy the mucin in salivary fluid before the antibody studies. A total of 12 patients and 4 volunteers have been studied on 31 occasions; all have shown salivary antibody against *E. coli*. We conclude that the lack of CVA in susceptible patients is not a generalized immunological deficiency and may be restricted to CVF.

Cervicovaginal Antibody and IgG Concentration in Patients with Substantial Introital Colonization with Enterobacteria

Table 5.38
Comparison of Antibody-Coated Bacteria After Exposure to Cervicovaginal Fluid of Bacteriuric Women With and Without Introital Carriage of Infecting Strain[a]

Subjects	No. of Subjects	No. of Determinations	No. of FA+	Percentage Determinations FA+	Percentage Subjects FA+
With introital carriage	20	25	11	44	40
Without introital carriage	9	14	12	86	78

[a] Reproduced by permission from T. A. Stamey, N. Wehner, G. Mihara, and M. Condy, Medicine (Baltimore) **57:** 47, 1978[134].

[b] FA = fluorescent antibody.

What little colonization of the introitus with *E. coli* that occurs in healthy controls, occurs mostly in bacterial numbers less than 100 organisms/ml of transport broth (Tables 5.6 and 5.9). Because of this observation, a case can be made for looking at a subset of susceptible patients whose cultures of the vaginal introitus show >100 Enterobacteriaceae/ml of transport broth.

As seen in Table 5.44, 98% of 46 collections from 4 control women were positive for CVA antibody against the volunteer's fecal *E. coli*; their CVF contained 20.4 ± 21.9 mg/100 ml of IgG. Only 13 of 47 collections from 13 patients colonized vaginally with >100 *E. coli*/ml showed specific CVA against the introital *E. coli*; their CVF showed only 2.1 ± 3.9 mg/100 ml of IgG. These data suggest that patients who have heavier introital colonization with *E. coli* not only lack specific CVA in their CVF, but also have diminished total IgG in comparison to control volunteers.

Cervicovaginal Antibody and the Normal Introital Flora

Lactobacilli were isolated from introital cultures of 8 control volunteers in 28 experiments. Neither lactobacilli nor *S. epidermidis* (7 experiments, 4 control subjects) ever demonstrated fluorescent antibody.

Potential Causes of Reduced Cervicovaginal Antibody in Urinary Tract Infection-Prone Patients with Enterobacterial Colonization of the Introital Mucosa

Some of the more obvious reasons for reduced CVA include (1) antigen-antibody complexing of the available CVA, (2) failure to produce local CVA, or (3) inactivation of CVA by means other than antigen-antibody complexing. Whatever the reason, including antigen-antibody complexing of available CVA by the colonizing Enterobacteriaceae organisms *per se*, it is difficult to ignore the absence of CVA in colonized UTI-prone women as an important permissive factor in recurrent bacteriuria.

Most of our patients with introital colonization with Enterobacteriaceae are also colonized throughout the vaginal canal (Table 5.45). In these studies, after first collecting the introital culture, the vaginal speculum was carefully opened about mid-vagina and advanced in such a way that the cervix and vaginal vault were not touched by the blades of the speculum before collecting the deep vaginal culture. This similarity of uncontaminated deep vaginal cultures with the introital cultures speaks for a biologic cause of pathogenic colonization that is present throughout the vagina rather than limited to the introital area.

Current work in our urologic laboratories at Stanford is based on efforts to understand the reason for reduced CVA in UTI-prone patients with colonization of their introitus with Enterobacteriaceae. Antigen-antibody complexing is clearly a good possibility, as can be seen best in Figure 5.24 where heavy introital colonization coincides with absence of CVA and absence of introital colonization coincides with presence of CVA. CVA could also be inactivated by proteolytic enzymes in vaginal fluid or by bacterial proteases.[135] If antibody complexing and proteolytic inactivation can be excluded, local vaginal vaccination with formalin-treated, whole *E. coli* should be tried as the simpliest way to exclude the possi-

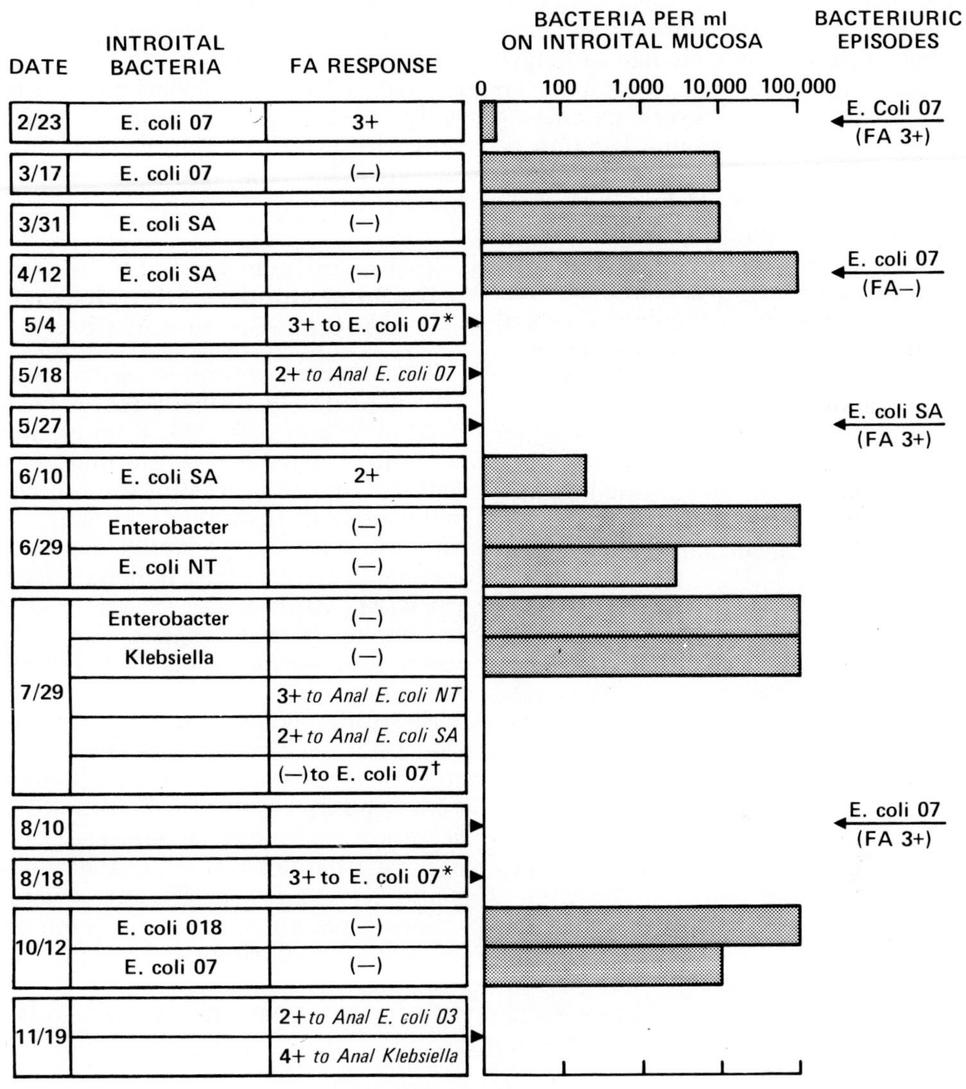

Figure 5.24 Bacteriologic and immunologic course of a 22-year-old white female patient with recurrent bacteriuria followed from February to November 1976. See text for details. All FA data relate to exposure of introital, bacteriuric, or fecal strains to cervicovaginal fluid. SA = self-agglutinating (rough) strain of *Escherichia coli*. NT = nontypable strain of *E. coli*. FA(−) = absence of fluorescent antibody-coated bacteria. FA+ = intensity (2+ to 4+) of fluorescent antibody-coated bacteria. Reproduced by permission from T. A. Stamey, N. Wehner, G. Mihara, and M. Condy, Medicine (Baltimore) **57:** 47, 1978[134].

bility of failure to produce local antibody. Failure to produce antibody at the cervicovaginal surface is unlikely due to failure of enterobacterial antigen as an immunogen at the intestinal level (Peyer's patches)[136] for two reasons: (1) the same O-group *E. coli* that cause urinary infection is usually the predominant intestinal *E. coli*, and (2) our finding that antigen-specific antibody to *E. coli* is present in salivary fluid of patients who lack CVA would indicate that intestinal stimulation of immunocytes and their subsequent migration to other mucosal secretory sites appears intact. In terms of stimulating local vaginal antibody by vaccination, Strauss stimulated vaginal antibody to *Salmonella typhosa* by local application of soluble antigen soaked into a tampon and inserted into the vagina for 3 days.[137] Vaginal agglutinin titers (1:100 to 1:200) were present by the third day of exposure to the antigen, remained at this level until the fourth week, and declined thereafter. Since the agglutinin titers in this early but classic study probably measured IgM with little IgG, the response of cervicovaginal IgG and IgA is, of course, unknown.

Table 5.39
Percent IgA, IgG, and IgM in Fluorescent Antibody Positive Controls and Patients[a]

Subjects	IgA	IgG	IgM
Controls	69	72	45
Susceptible women[b]	78	67	22
Bacteriuric women with introital carriage	90	60	35
Bacteriuric women without introital carriage	100	93	53

[a] Reproduced by permission from T. A. Stamey, N. Wehner, G. Mihara, and M. Condy, Medicine (Baltimore) **57:** 47, 1978[134].

[b] With introital carriage of Enterobacteriaceae.

Zollinger Technique of Solid Phase Radioimmunoassay for Measuring Antigen-Specific Antibody

The indirect method of immunofluorescent detection of antibody-coated bacteria, used in Tables 5.37–5.44, is fairly cumbersome for vaginal and serum dilution work and it is too subjective in the presence of small amounts of antibody. Because of this limitation, we have adapted the Zollinger technique of solid phase radioimmunoassay (SPRIA), which measures serum antibody to meningococcal antigens,[89] to measure vaginal and serum antibodies to Enterobacteriaceae.

Shortliffe, Wehner and I[138] have found the Zollinger technique to be eminently suitable for measuring antigen-specific antibodies in serum, prostatic fluid, and vaginal secretions to Enterobacteriaceae. Because of the extraordinary usefulness of this technique, and its low coefficient of variation (8%), we present here a brief summary of our minor modifications.

Since the introital mucosa of women susceptible to urinary infections is colonized

Table 5.40
Distribution of IgA, IgG, and IgM Among 50 Strains of Enterobacteriaceae Exposed to Cervicovaginal Fluid[a]

	Percentage of Controls	Percentage of Non-Bacteriuric with Carriage	Percentage of Bacteriuric with Carriage	Percentage of Bacteriuric without Carriage
IgA, IgG, IgM	37	25	18	33
IgA and IgG	26	38	46	33
IgA and IgM	11	0	9	0
IgG and IgM	5	0	0	0
IgA (only)	5	25	18	33
IgG (only)	11	12	0	0
IgM (only)	5	0	9	0
	$n = 19$	$n = 8$	$n = 11$	$n = 12$

[a] Reproduced by permission from T. A. Stamey, N. Wehner, G. Mihara, and M. Condy, Medicine (Baltimore) **57:** 47, 1978[134].

Table 5.41
Total IgA and IgG in Fluorescent Antibody Positive Vaginal Fluids[a]

Subjects	IgA	IgG	IgA/IgG
	mg/dl ± S.D.	*mg/dl ± S.D.*	
Controls	4.7 ± 6.9	29.2 ± 32.3	0.16
Susceptible women[b]	2.3 ± 1.8	12.0 ± 10.1	0.19
Bacteriuric women with introital carriage	1.4 ± 1.7	20.1 ± 22.8	0.07
Bacteriuric women without introital carriage	3.4 ± 4.3	25.4 ± 19.9	0.13

[a] Reproduced by permission from T. A. Stamey, N. Wehner, G. Mihara, and M. Condy, Medicine (Baltimore) **57:** 47, 1978[134].

[b] With introital carriage of Enterobacteriaceae.

Table 5.42
Representative Fluorescent Antibody Positive Cervicovaginal Fluid and Serum Titers[a]

Subjects	Antihuman Immunoglobulin		IgA	
	Vaginal fluid	Serum	Vaginal fluid	Serum
Controls				
1	1:16	1:64	1:0	1:16
2	1:0	1:8		
3	1:16			
4	1:32			
5			1:0	1:16
6	1:0	1:32	1:2	1:32
7	1:2	1:64	1:2	1:128
8	1:2	1:16	1:0	1:64
Bacteriuric without introital carriage			1:4	1:16

[a] Reproduced by permission from T. A. Stamey, N. Wehner, G. Mihara, and M. Condy, Medicine (Baltimore) **57:** 47, 1978[134].

with whole Enterobacteriaceae, and since we have shown a broad cross-reactivity of CVA to enterobacterial antigens, we think it is probably better to use whole bacterial antigen rather than a purified or even sonified antigen. The Zollinger assay is performed in disposable polyvinyl "U" microtiter plates. Twenty-five microliters of bacterial antigen is added first to the plastic well, incubated for 1 hour to bind the antigen to the well, and the antigen solution removed by aspiration; the wells are then washed and incubated with 100 μl of 1% bovine serum albumin to fill unoccupied binding sites on the plastic wall. After aspirating the filler and washing the plate several times with phosphate buffered saline (PBS), 2-fold dilutions of the unknown antibody fluid (vaginal, serum, or salivary in our studies) are placed in the wells and allowed to bind during overnight incubation at room temperature. After several PBS washes, iodinated (^{125}I) anti-immunoglobulin (anti-IgG or anti-IgA in our studies) is placed in each well and incubated in a humidity chamber at room temperature for 12–16 hours. The excess unbound radiolabeled anti-antibody is removed by washing the plate several times with PBS, and then dried. The wells are cut and placed individually into counting tubes for the gamma counter. Controls for each run include a control serum of normal antibody content and a filler control of bovine serum albumin to determine nonspecific binding. All titrations are performed in duplicate.

We have determined the optimum binding concentration of whole fixed bacteria and found that 0.5% formalin fixation for 18 hours represents the best concentration of formalin. Varying concentrations of bacteria from 4.5×10^6/ml to 2.35×10^9/ml, determined with a Coulter counter (30 μ aperture), were tested for optimum binding parameters. Maximum binding occurred between 1.47×10^8/ml to 2.35×10^9/ml. At this concentration, binding of formalin-fixed bacteria showed no significant difference from that of unfixed whole bacteria. With formalin fixation, lower counts, such as 4.5×10^6/ml to 7.3×10^7/ml, exhibited only 25 to 75 per cent of maximum binding. Hence, our antigens are Coulter counted, whole formalin-fixed bacteria at a concentration of 10^9–10^{10} bacteria/ml resuspended in PBS. All broth and wash solutions are triple filtered through a 0.2 μ Nalgene filter to prevent particulate contamination.

Commercial antiserums were obtained from Bio-Rad Laboratories, the sodium azide preservative removed, and the antiserums iodinated by the lactoperoxidase method of Marchalonis.[139] The specific activity is 300–1000 counts per minute (cpm)/ng which is further diluted to contain about 20 ng of active antibody/25 μl. The rabbit anti-human IgA (prepared from colostrum) is specific for α-chain as well as the secretory piece. It does not react with IgG or IgM. The rabbit anti-human IgG is specific for the γ-chain and does not cross-react with IgA or IgM. Appropriate absorption experiments in our laboratory have demonstrated this specificity.

Total immunoglobulin is measured from the same dilutions of the test fluid used to measure antigen-specific antibody. Instead of placing the bacterial antigen in the plastic wells in the technique just described, unlabeled anti-human IgG or IgA is substituted for the bacterial antigen. Zollinger has found that serial dilutions of serum Ig standards produce a linear curve (cpm bound *vs.* Ig concentration) over the range from 5 to 150 ng antibody/ml.[140] Therefore, dilutions of a control serum can be used as a standard curve to reference the antigen-specific antibody as well as the total antibody. The dilution of CVF that gives a specific number of predetermined counts per minute is compared to the corresponding dilution of the control serum; dilutions of both control serum and the unknown test solution must be parallel when the ^{125}I cpm is plotted against the logarithm of the dilutions. The two numbers on the curves intercepted by the predetermined cpm are used to compute a ratio which represents a measure of the antigen-specific activity of the test solution compared to the control (see Figure 7.9, Chapter 7). This measure of specific antibody is then expressed as activity per ng per dl of total IgA or IgG. By referencing antigen-specific antibody

Table 5.43
Specificity of Enterobacteriaceae Associated Antibody[a]

Study Group	Predominant Rectal *Escherichia coli*		Common *E. coli* (075,06,04)		Uncommon *E. coli* (0139,0124, 0103,128)		J_5 Mutant	
	No. FA+/ No. CVF	%	No. FA+/ No. CVF	%	No. FA+/ No. CVF	%	No. FA+/ No. CVF	%
Control volunteer	41/48	85	20/21	95	12/13	92	12/13	92
Premenopausal patients	30/77	39	20/45	44	15/31	48	21/43	49

[a] FA = fluorescent antibody; CVF = cervicovaginal fluid.

Table 5.44
Cervicovaginal Antibody and IgG Concentration in Patients with >100 Enterobacteriaceae in Their Introital Cultures

Subjects	No. of Subjects	No. of Samples	No. of FA+	Percentage of Samples FA+	IgG
					mg/100 ml
Control volunteers	4	46	45	98	20.4 ± 21.9
Susceptible patients[a]	13	47	6	13	2.1 ± 3.9

[a] Introitus colonized with >100 Enterobacteriaceae per ml of transport broth.

Table 5.45
Comparison of Enterobacteriaceae and Enterococci on the Introital Mucosa and in Cervical Os

Organism	Introital Concentration Higher than Cervical	Similar Concentration in Introital and Cervical Cultures[a]	Introital Concentration Lower than Cervical
Enterobacteriaceae (47 cultures)	13	30	4
Enterococci (44 cultures)	12	27	5

[a] Difference in number of colonies per ml was less than 10-fold.

activity to total antibody in the same SPRIA system, collection errors in dilution of vaginal fluid will hopefully be minimized.

Using this technique, antibody to *E. coli* in normal vaginal fluid was determined by both the SPRIA and the indirect fluorescent antibody-coating technique. The vaginal fluid was serially diluted at 2-fold dilutions between 1:2 and 1:1024. Fluorescent antibody coating was 3+ at a dilution of 1:2 and SPRIA (IgG) counts were 10,000 cpm. At a vaginal dilution of 1:32, fluorescent antibody coating of bacteria could no longer be detected but the SPRIA counts were 1,000/minute above background. The cpm for the SPRIA method continued to decline in a straight line between 1,000 cpm and 250 cpm above background at vaginal dilutions between 32 and 512. From these comparisons, we believe the SPRIA is 32 times more sensitive than the fluorescent antibody-coating technique, an increase in sensitivity which represents a substantial advantage in the study of vaginal fluid where smaller amounts of specific antibody are present.

As observed in Chapter 7, this technique has been extraordinarily useful in detecting high titers of antigen-specific IgG in the serum when bacterial agglutination titers are high normal or even low; moreover, it has allowed us to detect and follow very high titers of secretory IgA in the prostatic fluid of patients with chronic bacterial prostatitis due to *E. coli.*

Other Studies of Cervicovaginal Antibody in Relation to Our Observations

If the total percentage of IgA, IgG, and IgM coating in Table 5.39 is considered in relation to 50 separate strains of Enterobacteriaceae (Table 5.40), the combination of IgA-IgG-IgM and IgA-IgG is the most common. Of those few strains coated with a single immunoglobulin, IgA is the most common. However, if highly significant amounts of SIgA (secretory IgA) directed against *E. coli* were present in CVF, the 2-fold dilutional titers in Table 5.42 should have been higher. It is probable that the SIgA system in CVF of the human, at least to Enterobacteriaceae, is no more important than IgG and perhaps IgM. Because IgM has not been consistently reported as a significant immunoglobulin in CVF, we rechecked the purity of our conjugated goat antisera to human IgM and found only a single band on immunoelectrophoresis corresponding to human IgM. Moreover, the data in Table 5.40 do not suggest contamination of IgM with antisera to IgA or IgG. Vaerman and Férin[133] have pointed out that except for published reports using *Candida albicans*[141, 142] and an inactivated poliomyelitis virus[143] as antigens, there is little evidence to support the local synthesis of IgA in the human female genital tract; Vaerman and Férin, in fact, were unable to demonstrate local antibody synthesis in human volunteers when feritin and bovine serum albumin were repeatedly applied to the cervical mucosa. O'Reilly *et al.*[144] have shown SIgA response to *N. gonorrhoeae* in titers of 1:32 or less.

If IgG and perhaps IgM are as important as IgA in influencing enterobacterial colonization of the introitus, what is the source of these cervicovaginal immunoglobulins and how are they influenced by the occurrence of bacteriuria? Possible sources include local immunocytes anywhere in the genital tract, transudation from the systemic circulation especially at the time of menstruation, and secretions from the endometrium, uterine tubes and vagina. Elstein[145] observed a 20–50-fold variation in the concentration of immunoglobulins in cervical mucus during the menstrual cycle of healthy volunteers; at midcycle, immunoglobulins could not be detected, but appeared during the secretory phase shortly after ovulation, becoming prominent during the luteal phase and diminishing early in the proliferative phase of the next cycle. Schumacher[146] has shown that this cyclical variation is particularly characteristic of IgG in CVF. Rebello *et al.*[147] histologically examined 58 surgically removed uteri; they reported IgA-containing lymphoid cells in the endocervix of all specimens, IgM immunocytes in 81%, and IgG cells in 55%; the mean population density of immunocytes in 35 premenopausal cervices was 92, 30, and 11 immunocytes per square millimeter, respectively. Except for the endocervix, immunocytes appear to be rare in the remainder of the genital tract. On the other hand, stromal, basement membrane, intercellular, and luminal IgG is reported as the predominant immunoglobulin in histologic studies of the endometrium and uterine tubes.[147, 148] Thus, it appears that the major source of IgA is local immunocytes in the endocervix while IgG is primarily derived from the endometrium during the secretory phase and during menstruation. Quantitation of immunoglobulins in cervicovaginal secretions, in all studies[8, 130, 149, 150] but one,[141] show that IgG is present in greater concentration than IgA. IgM in CVF is presumably derived from the immunocytes of the endocervix and certainly the serum during menstruation.

Our observation of specific antibody to Enterobacteriaceae in vaginal fluid of hysterectomized women is of some immunologic interest. Vaerman and Férin[133] point out that the vaginal wall, with its stratified squamous epithelium as opposed to the classic longitudinal cells of mucoglandular mucosae known to secrete IgA, is "almost incompatible" with local antibody secretion. Nevertheless, Waldman *et al.*[141] had 3 completely hysterectomizd women in their 131 subjects in whom they measured immunoglobulins in CVF and they reported IgA, IgG, and IgM antibodies in these 3 vaginal secretions. Immunofluorescence studies on biopsy specimens are inconclusive, perhaps because very few specimens have been studied. Tourville,[148] Lippes,[151] and Vaerman[133] could find no IgA or IgM plasma cells beneath the vaginal epithelium whereas Lai A Fat *et al.*[152] reported IgA and IgG immunocytes. Vargas-Linares *et al.*[153] observed increased concentrations of IgG and IgA in CVF after the menopause and reported that plasma cells in the vaginal mucosa also increase after the menopause. Our data are clear that local vaginal antibody is present in CVF of completely hysterectomized women. The three hysterectomized control volunteers, plus two others recently studied, all showed FA coating when their fecal *E. coli* were exposed to their vaginal fluid. In the 11 hysterectomized patients with recurrent bacteriuria, studied on 18 separate occasions, vaginal antibodies to their colonizing introital *E. coli* were present 22% of the time when they were not bacteriuric and 56% of the time when they were bacteriuric. In the nine instances of bacteriuria, introital carriage of the bacteriuric strain was always present. Although the numbers are too small, when vaginal antibody was present, IgA coated the bacteria every time, IgG 71%, and IgM 14% of the time. Further studies are obviously indicated in hysterectomized women to determine the source of these local antibodies in a stratified squamous epithelium. Posthysterectomy estrogen supplements should be avoided since there is some evidence that estrogens reduce both cervical and vaginal antibody.[153]

It is possible that bacteriuria, in view of the low titers of specific antibody as measured by immunofluorescence in our studies, boost cervicovaginal antibody titers through serum transudation of immunoglobulins. Upper urinary tract bacteriuria, with its primary serum antibody titers of ≥256,[131] could clearly contribute to CVA by transudation, but even bladder infections with titers <256 might raise serum antibody within the 1:16 or 1:32 primary antibody titers found in CVF. Such a mechanism would be consistent with the report by Ogra and Ogra that inactivated poliomyelitis vaccine injected intramuscularly produced a delayed appearance of IgG in cervicovaginal secretions which was correlated with the highest IgG antibody titers in serum; when the poliomyelitis vaccine was placed locally in the vagina and separately in the uterus, IgA occurred in the former and only IgG in the latter secretions.[143]

It is clear that the amount of specific antibody coating the bacteria in our studies is not large (Table 5.42) and appears to have little relationship to the total amount of immunoglobulin (as measured by radial immunodiffusion) present in cervicovaginal secretions. It is of interest that the titers of SIgA to *N. gonorrhoeae* in cervicovaginal secretions were never higher than 1:32 (uninfected controls < 1:2), as reported by O'Reilly *et al.*[144] The duration of the antibody response following an episode of bacteriuria is also of interest. Too few patients have had longitudinal studies so far, but these early studies suggest that CVA following bacteriuria in the presence of continuing susceptibility does not last longer than a few weeks. In Figure 5.24, for example, CVA to the *E. coli* 07 bacteriuric strain on 2/23 and 8/10 could not be detected 3 and 8 weeks later, respectively.

IgG and IgM in CVF could prevent introital colonization with Enterobacteriaceae by complement mediated bacteriolysis or enhanced phagocytosis. While IgA antibodies (especially the polymeric form of SIgA) can agglutinate particulate antigens, activate complement by the alternate pathway, and perhaps cause bacteriolysis in the presence of activated complement and lysozyme,[154, 155] the interest in SIgA lies more with preventing bacterial adherence to mucosal surfaces.[100, 101] The studies reported here implicate a role for CVA in preventing enterobacterial colonization of the introital mucosa; moreover, our observation that lactobacilli and *S. epidermidis*, normal indigenous vaginal flora, do not elicit antibody coating when exposed to cervicovaginal fluid, is in keeping with the potential role of local SIgA in preventing bacterial adherence. Nevertheless, CVA is unlikely to be the only determinant of bacterial adherence to introital mucosal cells of the vagina. I have shown in Figure 5.15 and Table 5.26 how an *E. coli* 06, when exposed to washed mucosal cells from the vaginal wall of 20 normal women resistant to urinary infections and 20 women susceptible to urinary infections, adhered much better to vaginal cells from the group susceptible to bacteriuria ($P < 0.001$).[102] Since the *E. coli* 06 was obtained from subculture, and therefore uncoated with CVA, it is unlikely that SIgA or any other immunoglobulin accounted for bacterial adherence in those two groups. It is true that the secretory component on epithelial cells can serve as a receptor for polymeric Ig,[156] but most of the secretory cells in the vagina must be within the endocervix. Thus, while cervicovaginal antibody seems to be an important influence in introital colonization and clearly offers some therapeutic possibilities in preventing recurrent bacteriuria, it is not the only mechanism involved. Other possibilities, besides the mannose epithelial cell receptors I have already reviewed, include biochemical mediators of cell membrane adherence as shown by Springer *et al.*[157] in the attachment of Gram-negative endotoxin to lipopolysaccharide in the surface membrane of human erythrocytes.

Effect of Hysterectomy on Colonization of the Introitus—An Experimental Study

We have developed an experimental model in the rabbit to study vaginal biology in relation to *E. coli* colonization.[158] The rabbit is an excellent model because the intestinal tract is usually free of coliform bacteria[159]; the vaginal vestibule can be inoculated with a specific strain of *E. coli* without fear of subsequent extraneous fecal contamination. The mucosal clearance of *E. coli* from the vaginal vestibule was studied in sham-operated, oophorectomized, and hysterectomized rabbits. In addition, systemic IgM antibody titers were determined in the rabbit to ascertain the immunologic impact of oral, vaginal, and intravenous inoculation of *E. coli*.

New Zealand White female rabbits

weighing 2.5–4 kg were used throughout. The rabbits were fed water and Purina rabbit chow which was free of antibiotics.

All cultures were obtained from the vaginal vestibule with a calcium aginate swab (Wilson Diagnostics, Inc.) which had been wet with Earle's balanced salt solution. An assistant held the rabbits in the prone position while a hemostat was clamped to the hair on the ventral surface of the vestibule and a sterile nasal speculum was inserted. A culture was obtained by rotating the swab on the internal surface of the introital ring. The swab was streaked immediately on an eosin-methylene blue plate which was then incubated for 24 hours at 37°C. All results were reported as colonies of *E. coli* per plate.

Inoculation. *E. coli* (serogroup 06) was grown overnight in trypticase soy broth at 37°C. The sites of inoculation were: intravenous: six control (unoperated) rabbits received a single injection of 1 ml of *E. coli* (10^7) bacteria; oral: six control rabbits received 1 ml of *E. coli* in their drinking water twice a day for 14 days; introital: five sham-operated, six oophorectomized, and five hysterectomized rabbits were inoculated 6 weeks after surgery with 1 ml of *E. coli* on the mucosal surface of the introitus. The inoculum was delivered by gravity from a sterile pipette and allowed to run into the distal vestibule. Four of the hysterectomized rabbits were reinoculated vaginally 69 days after their initial inoculation.

Hemagglutination Titers. Passive hemagglutination titers were performed as described by Neter.[160] Sheep red blood cells (SRBC), which had been washed with Difco hemagglutination buffer (HA buffer), were used as carriers of the *E. coli* 06 antigen. The antigens were attached to the SRBC by suspending 2 ml of packed SRBC in 20 ml of antigen and incubating at 37°C for 60 minutes. The SRBC were then washed three times in HA buffer and suspended in buffered saline to a concentration of 2.5%. The test serum was heated at 56°C for 30 minutes and diluted 1:10 with HA buffer. SRBC suspension, 0.05 ml, was added to 0.5 ml of 2-fold serial dilutions of the test serums. The hemagglutination reactions were carried out in glass tubes at 37°C for 1 hour and were read after standing at room temperature overnight. Uncoated SRBC in serum and antigen-coated SRBC in HA buffer were included as controls.

The results were based on the hemagglutination patterns of the sedimented SRBC and the titers are expressed as the reciprocal of number of positive 2-fold serial dilutions of the serum.

Five rabbits underwent a sham operation in which a transverse incision was made in the anterior wall of the proximal vagina and closed without removal of any tissue. Six rabbits had bilateral oophorectomies. Five rabbits had hysterectomies, with removal of both uteri and a 1-cm cuff of vaginal tissue.

Midline abdominal incisions and 4-0 chromic catgut were used in all operations; vaginal incisions were closed with a double layer, extramucosal running suture.

Introital Carriage after Primary Inoculation. All of the rabbits were free of Gram-negative bacteria before inoculation (Figure 5.25). After inoculation, introital cultures were taken at 1- to 2-day intervals for the 1st week and then every 3–7 days until two consecutive cultures were sterile.

Sham-Operated Rabbits. Three of the sham-operated rabbits had sterile introital cultures on Day 3. The remaining two rabbits had low counts of *E. coli* in the introitus through Day 7 but subsequent cultures were sterile.

Oophorectomized Rabbits. Four of the six oophorectomized rabbits had sterile introital cultures on the 3rd day after inoculation. The remaining two rabbits had sterile introital cultures on Day 7.

Hysterectomized rabbits. Introital carriage of *E. coli* was present in the five hysterectomized rabbits for a minimum of 20 days and two of the rabbits (nos. 4 and 5) had positive cultures on the 42nd day. Although the introital carriage was generally in the range of 100–5000 colonies per plate, on several occasions colony counts fell to zero, only to rise again on subsequent cultures.

Systemic Antibody Response to Pri-

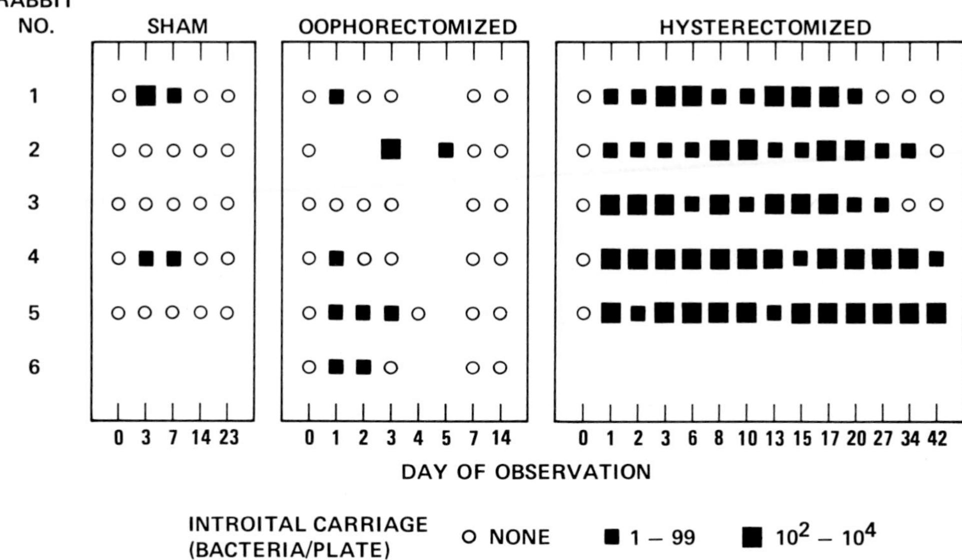

Figure 5.25 Comparison between introital carriage in five sham-operated, six oophorectomized, and five hysterectomized rabbits 6 weeks after surgery. The introital mucosa was inoculated with 10^7 *Escherichia coli* (06). Sham-operated rabbits cleared *E. coli* within 7 days. Clearance was unaffected by oophorectomy. Hysterectomy, however, substantially prolonged the period of *E. coli* colonization. (Reproduced by permission from A. J. Schaeffer and T. A. Stamey, Invest. Urol. **14:** 10, 1976.[158])

mary Inoculation. The course of the anti-O antibody response after oral, intravenous, and introital inoculation is presented in Table 5.46. The mean anti-O titer to oral inoculation did not exceed 5 despite continuous feeding of *E. coli* and, in many instances, heavy colonization of the anal flora. After a single intravenous injection of 10^7 *E. coli*, a rapid anti-O agglutination response was recorded with a peak mean titer of 1877 reached on Day 7. Introital inoculation produced a more gradual response with a peak titer of 86 on Day 14.

Introital Carriage and Antibody Response to Secondary Inoculation. Introital inoculation with 10^7 *E. coli* was repeated in four hysterectomized rabbits 69 days after the initial introital inoculation (Table 5.47). The vaginal mucosa was free of *E. coli* in three rabbits by Day 3 and in all rabbits by Day 7. An antibody response was found in all control titers (mean: 166) and subsequent titers showed little fluctuation over the following 14 days.

These data indicate that the mucosa of the vaginal vestibule of the normal rabbit rapidly clears *E. coli* within 7 days and that clearance is unaffected by oophorectomy. Hysterectomy, however, substantially prolongs the period of *E. coli* colonization. Every clinician has observed patients whose problems with urinary infection either began or became much worse after hysterectomy. The experimental observations reported here suggest that hysterectomy, although not oophorectomy, may enhance colonization of the vaginal vestibule with *E. coli* and thereby increase the patient's susceptibility to bacteriuria.

Rapid clearing of the second introital inoculation in hysterectomized rabbits which initially had heavy, prolonged carriage suggests a secondary immunologic response by the vaginal epithelium.

It is of interest that although the pH of the vaginal vestibule in the sham-operated, oophorectomized, and hysterectomized rabbits was 7–7.5, a range quite favorable to growth of *E. coli*, only the hysterectomized animals exhibited persistent introital carriage.

URINARY ANTIBODY

Although a number of references in the preceding section relate to secretory IgA (SIgA), I would like to close this chapter with a few references to some interesting work on urinary antibody. The literature on SIgA is immense and little purpose would be served to review even the high points of this exciting immunologic field. The interested reader is referred to the recent presentation by Hanson and Brandtzaeg[161] on mucosal defense systems and the 1975 review by Holmgren and Smith[162] on the immunological aspects of urinary tract infections.

Sohl Åkerlund *et al.*[163] have measured the antibody responses in urine and serum in 13 girls with pyelonephritis and 7 with cystitis. Using the ELISA technique, they characterized the IgG, IgA, SIgA, and IgM in both serum and urine to the infecting O-antigen of *E. coli*. All four antibodies, including SIgA, were elevated in the serum of patients with pyelonephritis when compared to the serum of patients with cystitis; IgG was the most diagnostically high titer. In the urine, IgG, IgA and SIgA were elevated in the patients with acute pyelonephritis. SIgA antibodies appeared in the urine from some patients with pyelonephritis before the antibodies could be detected in the serum.

In patients with screening bacteriuria, Jodal *et al.*[164] reported that secretory component-containing IgA antibodies to *E. coli* were often found in the urine in the absence of detectable serum IgA antibodies.

IgG and IgM antibodies protect the host through agglutination, complement activation, and stimulation of phagocytosis. Since SIgA is inefficient in these functions, what role does it play in the urinary tract?

Svanborg-Edén and Svennerholm[165] have shown that the adhesion of *E. coli* to human uroepithelial cells was inhibited by commercial gammaglobulin and by isolated IgG and secretory IgA fractions of urine from patients with acute pyelonephritis. It is interesting that absorption of antibodies directed against the O-antigen substantially reduced the anti-adhesive effect of all antibody preparations used in their studies, but elimination of antibodies to the K-antigen had a minimal effect in preventing the anti-adhesive effect of antibody. Thus, it would appear that urinary antibody to the K-antigen is not protective in terms of preventing bacterial adherence to uroepithelium, while O-antigen antibodies are clearly protective. Lastly, it should be noted that IgG antibody is very effective in preventing bacterial adherence to urothelial cells and that this effect is by no means limited to SIgA.

Uehling and associates[166] found that bladder immunization was more effective than subcutaneous immunization in preventing bacterial adherence to the urothelium of the rat bladder.

Pazin and Braude[167] showed over 10 years ago that type-specific immobilizing antibodies to *P. mirabilis* occurred in both the serum and urine during the course of retrograde experimental pyelonephritis in rats. The highest immobilizing titers were found in the 7S fractions of sera and were therefore thought to represent IgG in both the serum and the urine.

Silverblatt,[110] using an ascending model

Table 5.46
Passive Hemagglutination Titers in Serums after Oral, Introital, or Intravenous Inoculation

Route of Inoculation	Passive Hemagglutination Titer (Mean ± S.E.) at Day:				
	0	3	7	14	21
Oral (n = 6)	0 ± 0	2 ± 1.3	3.3 ± 1.1	5.0 ± 1.0	3.0 ± 1.2
Introital (n = 3)	0.67 ± 0.66	6.7 ± 4.8	28 ± 18	86 ± 85	5.3 ± 1.3
Intravenous (n = 6)	0.33 ± 0.33	22 ± 4.3	1877 ± 170	1024 ± 229	

[a] Reproduced by permission from A. J. Schaeffer and T. A. Stamey, Invest. Urol. **14:** 10, 1976.[158]

Table 5.47
Introital Carriage and Serum Antibody Response to Secondary Inoculation in Hysterectomized Rabbits

	Day 69[b]	Day 72	Day 76	Day 83
Rabbit 1				
Introital culture[c]	0	0	0	0
Serum titer[d]	8	16	4	64
Rabbit 2				
Introital culture	0	0	0	0
Serum titer	512	512	256	512
Rabbit 3				
Introital culture	0	0	0	0
Serum titer	16	32	8	16
Rabbit 4				
Introital culture	0	200	0	0
Serum titer	128	128	32	128

[a] Reproduced by permission from A. J. Schaeffer and T. A. Stamey, Invest. Urol. **14:** 10, 1976.[158]
[b] Introital culture and serum titer 69 days after initial inoculation and before second inoculation.
[c] Bacteria per plate.
[d] Titer = reciprocal of passive hemagglutination titer.

of *P. mirabilis* infection in rats, has demonstrated the presence of pili on the wall of the infecting organism and adhesion of the pili to the renal pelvic epithelial wall. More recently, using *E. coli* and a transiently ligated-ureter method of ascending infection, he has shown that immunization of rats with purified *E. coli* pili afforded substantial protection from pyelonephritis; moreover, shared pili antigens with different O, K and H antigens were equally protective with passive immunization.[168]

REFERENCES

1. Sjöstedt, S.: Pathogenicity of certain serological types of *E. coli.* Their mouse toxicity, hemolytic power, capacity for skin necrosis and resistance to phagaocytosis and bactericidal faculties of human blood. Acta Pathol. Microbiol. Scand. Suppl. 58, 1946.
2. Rantz, L. A.: Serological grouping of *E. coli.* Study in urinary tract infection. Arch. Intern. Med. **109:** 37, 1962.
3. Grüneberg, R. N.: Relationship of infecting urinary organism to the faecal flora in patients with symptomatic urinary infection. Lancet **2:** 766, 1969.
4. Girardet, P.: Twenty years of research on urinary tract infections in children; progress and problems. Adv. Intern. Med. Pediatr. **42:** 133, 1979.
5. Grüneberg, R.N., Leigh, D. A., and Brumfitt, W.: *Escherichia coli* serotypes in urinary tract infection; studies in domiciliary, anternatal and hospital practice. In F. O'Grady and W. Brumfitt (Eds.), Urinary Tract Infection. New York, Oxford University Press, 1968, p. 68.
6. Roberts, A. P., Linton, J. D., Waterman, A. M., Gower, P. E., and Koutsaimanis, K. G.: Urinary and faecal "*Escherichia coli*" O-sero-groups in symptomatic urinary-tract infection and asymptomatic bacteriuria. J. Med. Microbiol. **8:** 311, 1975.
7. Vosti, K. L., Goldberg, L. M., Monto, A. S., and Rantz, L. A.: Host parasite interaction in patients with infections due to *Escherichia coli*; I. The serogrouping of *E. coli* from intestinal and extraintestinal sources. J. Clin. Invest. **43:** 2377, 1964.
8. Lindberg, U., Hanson, L. A., Jodal, U., Lidin-Janson, G., Lincoln, K., and Olling, S.: Asymptomatic bacteriuria in schoolgirls; II. Differences in *Escherichia coli* causing asymptomatic and symptomatic bacteriuria. Acta Paediatr. Scand. **64:** 432, 1975.
9. Olling, S., Hanson, L. A., Holmgren, J., Jodal, U., Lincoln, K., and Lindberg, U.: The bactericidal effect of normal human serum on *E. coli* strains from normals and from patients with urinary tract infections. Infection **1:** 24, 1973.
10. Lidin-Janson, G., Hanson, L. A., Kaijser, B., Lincoln, K., Lindberg, J., Olling, S., and Wedel, H.: Comparison of *Escherichia coli* from bacteriuric patients with those from feces of healthy schoolchildren. J. Infect. Dis. **136:** 346, 1977.
11. Mabeck, C. E., Orskov, F., and Orskov, I.: *Escherichia coli* serotypes and renal involvement in urinary-tract infection. Lancet **1:** 1312, 1971.
12. Glynn, A. A., Brumfitt, W., and Howard, C. J.: K antigens of *Escherichia coli* and renal involve-

ment in urinary-tract infections. Lancet **1:** 514, 1971.

13. Kaijser, B.: Immunology of *Escherichia coli*; K antigen and its relation to urinary tract infection. J. Infect. Dis. **127:** 670, 1973.
14. McCabe, W. R., Carling, P. C., Bruins, S., and Greely, A.: The relation of K-antigen to virulence of *Escherichia coli*. J. Infect. Dis. **131:** 6, 1975.
15. Kaijser, B., Hanson, L. A., Jodal, U., Lidin-Janson, G., and Robbin, J. B.: Frequency of *E. coli* K antigens in urinary tract infections in children. Lancet **1:** 663, 1977.
16. Kalmanson, G. M., Harwick, H. J., Turck, M., and Guze, L. B.: Urinary-tract infection: localisation and virulence of *Escherichia coli*. Lancet **1:** 134, 1975.
17. Taylor, P. W., and Koutsaimanis, K. G.: Experimental *Escherichia coli* urinary infection in the rat. Kidney Int. **8:** 233, 1975.
18. Hanson, L. A., Ahlstedt, S., Fasth, A., Jodal, U., Kaijser, B., Larsson, P., Lindberg, U., Olling, S., Sohl-Akerlund, A., and Svanborg-Edén, C.: Antigens of *Escherichia coli*, human immune response, and the pathogenesis of urinary tract infections. J. Infect. Dis. (Suppl.) **136:** S144, 1977.
19. Dudgeon, L. S., Wordley, E., and Bawtree, F.: On *Bacillus coli* infection of the urinary tract, especially in relation to haemolytic organisms. J. Hyg. **20:** 137, 1921.
20. McGeachie, J.: Hemolysis by urinary Escherichia coli. Am. J. Clin. Pathol. **45:** 222, 1966.
21. Hanson, L. A., Lincoln, K., Lidin-Janson, G., Jodal, U., and Lindberg, U.: Personal communication, July 26, 1979.
22. Fried, F. A., Vermeulen, C. W., Ginsburg, M. J., and Cone, C. M.: Etiology of pyelonephritis; further evidence associating the production of experimental pyelonephritis with hemolysis in *Escherichia coli*. J. Urol. **106:** 351, 1971.
23. Cooke, E. M., and Ewins, S. P.: Properties of strains of *Escherichia coli* isolated from a variety of sources. J. Med. Microbiol. **8:** 107, 1975.
24. Stamey, T. A., Timothy, M., Millar, M., and Mihara, G.: Recurrent urinary infections in adult women. The role of introital enterobacteria. Calif. Med. **115:** 1, 1971.
25. Thiel, G., and Spuhler, O.: Urinary tract infection by catheter and the so-called infectious (episomal) resistance. Schweiz. Med. Wochenschr. **95:** 1155, 1965.
26. Turck, M., Goffe, B., and Petersdorf, R. G.: the urethral catheter and urinary tract infection. J. Urol. **88:** 834, 1962.
27. Stamey, T. A.: Workshop summary and comment. In T. A. Stamey, F. Hinman, Jr., and J. P. Sanford (Eds.), Urinary Infections in the Male; Proceedings of a Workshop. Washington, D.C., National Research Council, National Academy of Sciences, 1967.
28. Fair, W. R., Timothy, M. M., Millar, M. A., and Stamey, T. A.: Bacteriologic and hormonal observations of the urethra and vaginal vestibule in normal, premenopausal women. J. Urol. **104:** 426, 1970.
29. Stamey, T. A.: Urinary Infections. Baltimore, Williams & Wilkins, 1972.
30. Stamey, T. A., and Sexton, C. C.: The role of vaginal colonization with Enterobacteriaceae in recurrent urinary infections. J. Urol. **113:** 214, 1975.
31. Schaeffer, A. J., and Stamey, T. A.: Studies of introital colonization in women with recurrent urinary infections; IX. The role of antimicrobial therapy. J. Urol. **118:** 221, 1977.
32. O'Grady, F. W., McSherry, M. A., Richards, B., O'Farrell, S. M., and Cattell, W. R.: Introital enterobacteria, urinary infection, and the urethral syndrome. Lancet **2:** 1208, 1970.
33. Cox, C. E.: The urethra and its relationship to urinary tract infection; the flora of the normal female urethra. South. Med. J. **59:** 621, 1966.
34. Cox, C. E., Lacy, S. S., and Hinman, F., Jr.: The urethra and its relationship to urinary tract infection; II. The urethral flora of the female with recurrent urinary infection. J. Urol. **99:** 632, 1968.
35. Bailey, R. R., Roberts, A. P., Gower, P. E., and Stacey, G.: Urinary tract infection in non-pregnant women. Lancet **2:** 275, 1973.
36. Pfau, A., and Sacks, T.: The bacterial flora of the vaginal vestibule, urethra and vagina in the normal premenopausal woman. J. Urol. **118:** 292, 1977.
37. Marsh, F. P., Murray, M., and Panchamia, P.: The relationship between bacterial cultures of the vaginal introitus and urinary infection. Br. J. Urol. **44:** 368, 1972.
38. Cattell, W. R., McSherry, M. A., Northeast, A., Powell, E., Brooks, H. J. L., and O'Grady, F.: Periurethral enterobacterial carriage in pathogenesis of recurrent urinary infection. Br. Med. J. **4:** 136, 1974.
39. Bollgren, I., and Winberg, J.: The periurethral aerobic bacterial flora in healthy boys and girls. Acta Paediatr. Scand. **65:** 74, 1976.
40. Bollgren, I., Vaclavinkova, V., Hurvell, B., and Bergqvist, G.: Periurethral aerobic microflora of pregnant and non-pregnant women. Br. Med. J. **1:** 1314, 1978.
41. Perez-Miravete, A., and Jaramillo H.: Studies on vaginal flora; 1. Frequency and significance of *Escherichia coli* isolated from the vagina. Am. J. Obstet. Gynecol. **80:** 80, 1960.
42. Morris, C. A., and Morris, D. F.: "Normal" vaginal microbiology of women of childbearing age in

relation to the use of oral contraceptives and vaginal tampons. J. Clin. Pathol. **20:** 636, 1967.
43. Hite, K. E., Hesseltine, H. C., and Goldstein, L.: A study of the bacterial flora of the normal and pathologic vagina and uterus. Am. J. Obstet. Gynecol. **53:** 233, 1947.
44. Lock, F. R., Yow, M. D., Griffith, M. I., and Stout, C.: Bacteriology of the vagina in 75 normal young adults. Surg. Gynecol. Obstet. **87:** 410, 1948.
45. Stamey, T. A., and Kaufman, M. F.: Studies of introital colonization in women with recurrent urinary infections; II. A comparison of growth in normal vaginal fluid of common versus uncommon serogroups of *Escherichia coli*. J. Urol. **114:** 264, 1975.
46. Stamey, T. A., and Mihara, G.: Studies of introital colonization in women with recurrent urinary infections; V. The inhibitory activity of normal vaginal fluid on *Proteus mirabilis* and *Pseudomonas aeruginosa*. J. Urol. **115:** 416, 1976.
47. Hunter, C. A., Jr. and Nicholas, H. J.: A study of vaginal acids. Am. J. Obstet. Gynecol. **78:** 282, 1959.
48. Sumawong, V., Gregoire, A. T., Johnson, W. D., and Rakoff, A. E.: Identification of carbohydrates in the vaginal fluid of normal females. Fertil. Steril. **13:** 270, 1962.
49. Gregoire, A. T.: Carbohydrates of human vaginal tissue. Nature **198:** 996, 1963.
50. Stamey, T. A., Fair, W. R., Timothy, M. M., and Chung, H. K.: Antibacterial nature of prostatic fluid. Nature **218:** 444, 1968.
51. Stamey, T. A., and Timothy, M. M.: Studies of introital colonization in women with recurrent urinary infections; I. The role of vaginal pH. J. Urol. **114:** 261, 1975.
52. Lang, W. R.: Vaginal acidity and pH. A review. Obstet. Gynecol, Surv. **10:** 546, 1955.
53. Cohen, L.: Influence of pH on vaginal discharges. Br. J. Vener. Dis. **45:** 241, 1969.
54. Stamey, T. A., and Timothy, M. M.: Studies of introital colonization in women with recurrent urinary infections; III. Vaginal glycogen concentrations. J. Urol. **114:** 268, 1975.
55. Stewart-Tull, D. E.: Evidence that vaginal lactobacilli do not ferment glycogen. Am. J. Obstet. Gynecol. **88:** 676, 1964.
56. Fienberg, R., and Cohen, R. B.: Enzymes of glycogen metabolism in the squamous epithelium of the cervix. A histochemical study. Obstet. Gynecol. **31:** 608, 1968.
57. Gregoire, A. T., Rankin, J., Johnson, W. D. Rakoff, A. E. Adams, A.: α-Amylase content in cervical mucus of females receiving sequential, nonsequential, or no contraceptive therapy. Fertil. Steril. **18:** 836, 1967.
58. Bengtsson, L. P., Deutsch, A., and Nilsson, R.: The effect of oestrogen on the acid-soluble nucleotide content of the rabbit vagina. Acta Obstet. Gynecol. Scand. **43:** 369, 1964.
59. Seifter, S., Dayton, S., Novic, B., and Muntwyler, E.: Estimation of glycogen with the anthrone reagent. Arch. Biochem. **25:** 191, 1950.
60. Stamey, T. A., and Condy, M.: The diffusion and concentration of trimethoprim in human vaginal fluid. J. Infect. Dis. **131:** 261, 1975.
61. Odeblad, E.: Intracavity circulation of aqueous material in the human vagina. Acta Obstet. Gynecol. Scand. **43:** 360, 1964.
62. Stone, A., and Gamble, C. J.: The quantity of vaginal fluid. Am. J. Obstet. Gynecol. **78:** 279, 1959.
63. Gregoire, A. T., Kandil, O., and Ledger, W. J.: The glycogen content of human vaginal epithelial tissue. Fertil. Steril. **22:** 64, 1971.
64. Weinstein, L., and Howard, J. H.: The effect of estrogenic hormone on the H-ion concentration and the bacterial content of the human vagina, with special reference to the Döderlein bacillus. Am. J. Obstet. Gynecol. **37:** 698, 1939.
65. Savage, D. C.: Survival on mucosal epithelia, epithelial penetration and growth in tissues of pathogenic bacteria. In: Society for General Microbiology, Symposium No. 22. New York; Oxford University Press, 1972, pp. 25–57.
66. Sprunt, K., and Redman, W.: Evidence suggesting importance of role of interbacterial inhibition in maintaining balance of normal flora. Ann. Intern. Med. **68:** 579, 1968.
67. Sprunt, K., Leidy, G. A., and Redman, W.: Prevention of bacterial overgrowth. J. Infect. Dis. **123:** 1, 1971.
68. Fowler, J. E., Latta, R., and Stamey, T. A.: Studies of introital colonization in women with recurrent urinary infections; VIII. The role of bacterial interference. J. Urol. **118:** 296, 1977.
69. Gordon, A. M., Hughes, H. E., and Barr, G. T. D.: Bacterial flora in abnormalities of the female genital tract. J. Clin. Pathol. **19:** 429, 1966.
70. Bartlett, J. G., Onderdonk, A. B., Drude, E., Goldstein, C., Anderka, M., Alpert, S., and McCormack, W. M.: Quantitative bacteriology of the vaginal flora. J. Infect. Dis. **136:** 271, 1977.
71. Marrie, T. J., Harding, G. K. M., and Ronald, A. R.: Anaerobic and aerobic urethral flora in healthy females. J. Clin. Microbiol. **8:** 67, 1978.
72. Fredericq, P.: Diagnostic bacteriologique des bacilles intestinaux pathogénes par recherche de leur sensibilité a divers antibiotiques. C. R. Soc. Biol. (Paris) **140:** 1133, 1946.
73. Stamey, T. A., and Mihara, G.: Studies of introital colonization in women with recurrent urinary infection; VI. Analysis of segmented leukocytes

on the vaginal vestibule in relation to enterobacterial colonization. J. Urol. **116:** 72, 1976.

74. Govers, J., and Girard, J. P.: Some immunological properties of human cervical and vaginal secretions. Gynecol. Invest. **3:** 184, 1972.
75. Harris, R. E., Thomas, V. L., and Shelokov, A.: Asymptomatic bacteriuria in pregnancy; antibody-coated bacteria, renal function, and intrauterine growth retardation. Am. J. Obstet. Gynecol. **126:** 20, 1976.
76. Sanford, B. A., Thomas, V. L., Forland, M., Carson, S. and Shelokov, A.: Immune response in urinary tract infection determined by radioimmunoassay and immunofluorescence; serum antibody levels against infecting bacterium and Enterobacteriaceae common antigen. J. Clin. Microbiol. **8:** 575, 1978.
77. Mancini, G., Carbonara, A. O., and Heremans, J. F.: Immunochemical quantitation of antigens by single radial immunodiffusion. Immunochemistry **2:** 235, 1965.
78. Winberg, J., Andersen, H. J., Hanson, L. A. and Lincoln, K.: Studies of urinary tract infections in infancy and childhood; I. Antibody response in different types of urinary tract infections caused by coliform bacteria. Br. Med. J. **2:** 524, 1963.
79. Percival, A., Brumfitt, W., and de Louvois, J.: Serum-antibody levels as an indication of clinically inapparent pyelonephritis. Lancet **2:** 1027, 1964.
80. Vosti, K. L., Monto, A. S., and Rantz, L. A.: Host-parasite interaction in patients with infections due to *Escherichia coli*; II. Serologic response of the host. J. Lab. Clin. Med. **66:** 613, 1965.
81. Benedict, A. A.: Immunology: Sensitivity of passive haemagglutination for assay of 7S and 19S antibodies in primary rabbit anti-bovine serum albumin sera. Nature **206:** 1368, 1965.
82. Ahlstedt, S., Jodal, U., Hanson, L. A., and Holmgren, J.: Quantitation of *Escherichia coli* O antibodies by direct and indirect agglutination in comparison with a radioimmunoassay. Int. Arch. Allergy Appl. Immunol. **48:** 445, 1975.
83. Fairley, K. F., Grounds, A. D. Carson, N. E., Laird, E. C., Gutch, R. C., McCallum, P. H. G., Leighton, P., Sleeman, R. L., and O'Keefe, C. M.: Site of infection in acute urinary-tract infection in general practice. Lancet **2:** 615, 1971.
84. Clark, H., Ronald, A. R., and Turck, M.: Serum antibody response in renal versus bladder bacteriuria. J. Infect. Dis. **123:** 539, 1971.
85. Lindberg, U., Jodal, U., Hanson, L. A., and Kaijser, B.: Asymptomatic bacteriuria in schoolgirls; IV. Difficulties of level diagnosis and the possible relation to the character of infecting bacteria. Acta Paediatr. Scand. **64:** 574, 1975.
86. Ahlstedt, S., Jodal, U., and Hanson, L. A.: Amount and avidity of antibody to *Escherichia coli* O antigen measured with the ammonium sulphate precipitation technique in children with urinary tract infections. Int. Arch. Allergy Appl. Immunol. **49:** 615, 1975.
87. Jodal U.: The immune response to urinary tract infections in childhood; I. Serological diagnosis of primary symptomatic infection in girls by indirect hemagglutination. Acta Paediatr. Scand. **64:** 96, 1975.
88. Engvall, E., and Perlmann, P.: Enzyme-linked immunosorbent assay, ELISA; III. Quantitation of specific antibodies by enzyme-labelled anti-immuno-globulin in antigen-coated tubes. J. Immunol. **109:** 129, 1972.
89. Zollinger, W. D., Dalrymple, J. M., and Artenstein, M. S.: Analysis of parameters affecting the solid phase radioimmunoassay quantitation of antibody to meningococcal antigens. J. Immunol. **117:** 1788, 1976.
90. Jodal, U., Ahlstedt, S., Hanson, L. A., Janson-Lidin, G., and Akerlund, A. S.: Intestinal stimulation of the serum antibody response against *Escherichia coli* 083 antigen in healthy adults. Int. Arch. Allergy Appl. Immunol. **53:** 481, 1977.
91. Kaijser, B., Hagberg, S., Hanson, L. A., and Olling, S.: A search for *Escherichia coli* antigens in kidneys from children with urinary tract infection by means of immunofluorescence. Pediatr. Res. **8:** 935, 1974.
92. Wientzen, R. L., McCracken, G. H., Petruska, M. L., Swinson, S. G., Kaijser, B., and Hanson, L. A.: Localization and therapy of urinary tract infections of childhood. Pediatrics **63:** 467, 1979.
93. Miller, T. E., Burnham, S., and North, J. D. K.: Immunological enhancement in the pathogenesis of pyelonephritis. Clin. Exp. Immunol. **24:** 336, 1976.
94. Savage, D. C.: Survival on mucosal epithelia, epithelial penetration and growth in tissues of pathogenic bacteria. In: Society for General Microbiology, Symposium No. 22. New York: Oxford University Press, 1972, pp. 25–57.
95. Ellen, R. P., and Gibbons, R. J.: M protein-associated adherence of *Streptococcus pyogenes* to epithelial surfaces: prerequisite for virulence. Infect. Immun. **5:** 826, 1972.
96. Gibbons, R. J., and van Houte, J.: Selective bacterial adherence to oral epithelial surfaces and its role as an ecological determinant. Infect. Immun. **3:** 567, 1971.
97. Liljemark, W. F., and Gibbons, R. J.: Proportional distribution and relative adherence of *Streptococcus miteor (mitis)* on various surfaces in the human oral cavity. Infect. Immun. **6:** 852, 1972.
98. Liljemark, W. F., and Gibbons, R. J.: Ability of *Veillonella* and *Neisseria* species to attach to oral surfaces and their proportions present indigenously. Infect. Immun. **4:** 264, 1971.

99. Bertschinger, H. U., Moon, H. W., and Whipp, S. C.: Association of *Escherichia coli* with the small intestinal epithelium; I. Comparison of enteropathogenic and nonenteropathogenic porcine strains in pigs. Infect. Immun. **5:** 595, 1972.
100. Williams, R. C., and Gibbons, R. J.: Inhibition of bacterial adherence by secretory immunoglobin A; a mechanism of antigen disposal. Science **177:** 697, 1972.
101. Fubara, E. S., and Freter, R.: Protection against enteric bacterial infection by secretory IgA antibodies. J. Immunol. **111:** 395, 1973.
102. Fowler, J. E., and Stamey, T. A.: Studies of introital colonization in women with recurrent urinary infections; VII. The role of bacterial adherence. J. Urol. **117:** 472, 1977.
103. Kållenius, G., and Winberg, J.: Bacterial adherence to periurethral epithelial cells in girls prone to urinary-tract infections. Lancet **2:** 540, 1978.
104. Svanborg-Edén, C., Jodal, U., and Pettersson, H.: Personal communication, 1979.
105. Kållenius, G., Möllby, R., and Winberg, G.: Personal communication, 1979.
106. Fowler, J. E., and Stamey, T. A.: Studies of introital colonization in women with recurrent urinary infections; X. Adhesive properties of *Escherichia coli* and *Proteus mirabilis*. Lack of correlation with urinary pathogenicity. J. Urol. **120:** 315, 1978.
107. Mårdh, P. A., and Weström, L.: Adherence of bacteria to vaginal epithelial cells. Infect. Immun. **13:** 661, 1976.
108. Norden, C. W, Green, G. M., and Kass, E. H.: Antibacterial mechanisms of the urinary bladder. J. Clin. Invest. **47:** 2689, 1968.
109. Shrom, S. H., Parsons, C. L., and Mulholland, S. G.: Role of urothelial surface mucoprotein in intrinsic bladder defense. Urology **9:** 526, 1977.
110. Silverblatt, F. J.: Host-parasite interaction in the rat renal pelvis: a possible role for pili in the pathogenesis of pyelonephritis. J. Exp. Med. **140:** 1696, 1974.
111. Svanborg-Edén, C., Hanson, L. A., Jodal, U., Lindberg, U., and Akerlund, A. S.: Variable adherence to normal human urinary tract epithelial cells of *Eschericia coli* strains associated with various forms of urinary-tract infection. Lancet **2:** 490, 1976.
112. Cotran, R. S., Vivaldi, E., Zangwill, D. P., and Kass, E. H.: Retrograde Proteus pyelonephritis in rats. Bacteriologic, pathogenic and fluorescent-antibody studies. Am. J. Pathol. **43:** 1, 1963.
113. Gibbons, R. J., and van Houte, J.: Selective bacterial adherence to oral epithelial surfaces and its role as an ecological determinant. Infect. Immun. **3:** 567, 1971.
114. Duguid, I. P., Smith, I. W., Dempster, G., and Edmunds, P. N.: Non-flagellar filamentous appendages ("fimbriae") and haemagglutinating activity in *Bacterium coli.* J. Pathol. Bacteriol. **70:** 335, 1955.
115. Brinton, C. C.: The structure, function, synthesis and genetic control of bacterial pili and a molecular model for DNA and RNA transport in gram negative bacteria. Trans. N.Y. Acad. Sci. **27:** 1003, 1965.
116. Duguid, J. P., and Gillies, R. R.: Fimbriae and adhesive properties in dysentery bacilli. J. Pathol. Bacteriol. **74:** 397, 1957.
117. Kellogg, D. S., Jr., Peacock, W. L., Jr., Deacon W. E., Brown, L., and Pirkle, C. J.: *Neisseria gonorrhoeae*; I. Virulence genetically linked to clonal variation. J. Bacteriol. **85:** 1274, 1963.
118. Jones, G. W, and Rutter, J. M.: Role of the K88 antigen in the pathogenesis of neonatal diarrhea caused by *Escherichia coli* in piglets. Infect. Immun. **6:** 918, 1972.
119. Salit, I. E., and Gotschlich, E. C.: Type I *Escherichia coli* pili; characterization of binding to monkey cells. J. Exp. Med. **146:** 1182, 1977.
120. Svanborg-Edén, C., and Hansson, H. A.: *Escherichia coli* pili as possible mediators of attachment to human urinary tract epithelial cells. Infect. Immun. **21:** 229, 1978.
121. Svanborg-Edén, C., Eriksson, B., Hanson, L. A., Jodal, U., Kaijser, B., Lidin Janson, G. Lindberg, U., and Olling, S.: Adhesion to normal human uro-epithelial cells of *Escherichia coli* from children with various forms of urinary tract infection. J. Pediatr. **93:** 398, 1978.
122. Svanborg-Edén, C., Eriksson, B., and Hanson, L. A.: Adhesion of *Escherichia coli* to human uroepithelial cells *in vitro*. Infect. Immun. **18:** 767, 1977.
123. Schaeffer, A. J., Amundsen, S. K., and Schmidt, L. N.: Adherence of *Escherichia coli* to human urinary tract epithelial cells. Infect. Immun. **24:** 753, 1979.
124. Mårdh, P. A., Colleen, S., and Hovelius, B.: Attachment of bacteria to exfoliated cells from the urogenital tract. Invest. Urol. **16:** 322, 1979.
125. McNeish, A. S., Fleming, J., Turner, P., and Evans, N.: Mucosal adherence of human enteropathogenic *Escherichia coli.* Lancet **2:** 946, 1975.
126. Kivisto, A-K., Vasenius, H., Lindberg, L-A., and Sandholm, M.: A functional in vitro test for measuring the adhesion of *E. coli* on the urinary tract epithelium. Invest. Urol. **15:** 412, 1978.
127. Ofek, I., Mirelman, D., and Sharon, N.: Adherence of *Escherichia coli* to human mucosal cells mediated by mannose receptors. Nature **265:** 623, 1977.
128. Kållenius G., and Möllby, R.: Adhesion of *E. coli* to human periurethral cells correlated to mannose resistant agglutination of human erythrocytes. FEBS Lett. **5:** 295, 1979.

129. Freter, R.: Possible effects of foreign DNA on pathogenic potential and intestinal proliferation of E. coli. J. Infect. Dis. **137:** 624, 1978.
130. Stamey, T. A., and Howell, J. J.: Studies of introital colonization in women with recurrent urinary infections; IV. the role of local vaginal antibodies. J. Urol. **115:** 413, 1976.
131. Thomas, V., Shelokov, A., and Forland, M.: Antibody-coated bacteria in the urine and the site of urinary-tract infection. N. Engl. J. Med. **290:** 588, 1974.
132. Stamey, T. A., and Bragonje, J.: Resistance to nalidixic acid: A misconception due to underdosage. J.A.M.A. **236:** 1857, 1976.
133. Vaerman, J. P., and Férin, J.: Local immunological response in the vagina, cervix and endometrium. Acta Endocrinol. (Suppl.) **78** (194)**:** 281, 1975.
134. Stamey, T. A. Wehner, N., Mihara, G., and Condy, M.: The immunologic basis of recurrent bacteriuria; role of cervicovaginal antibody in enterobacterial colonization of the introital mucosa. Medicine (Baltimore) **57:** 47, 1978.
135. Plaut, A. G.: Microbial IgA proteases N. Eng. J. Med. **298:** 1459, 1978.
136. Rowley, D.: The problems of oral immunisation. Aust. J. Exp. Biol. Med. Sci. **55:** 1, 1977.
137. Strauss, E. K.: Occurrence of antibody in human vaginal mucus. Proc. Soc. Exp. Biol. Med. **106:** 617, 1961.
138. Shortliffe, L., Wehner, N., and Stamey, T. A.: The use of a Solid phase radioimmunoassay and formalin-fixed whole bacterial antigen in the detection of antigen-specific immunoglobulin in human prostatic fluid. Submitted to J. Clin. Invest. 1980.
139. Marchalonis, J. J.: An enzymic method for the trace iodination of immunoglobulins and other proteins. Biochem. J. **113:** 299, 1969.
140. Zollinger, W. D.: Personal communication, Nov. 3, 1978.
141. Waldman, R. H., Cruz, J. M., and Rowe, D. S.: Immunoglobulin levels and antibody to Candida albicans in human cervicovaginal secretions. Clin. Exp. Immunol. **10:** 427, 1972.
142. Waldman, R. H. Cruz, J. M., and Rowe, D. S.: Intravaginal immunization of humans with Candida albicans. J. Immunol. **109:** 662, 1972.
143. Ogra, P. L., and Ogra, S. S.: Local antibody response to poliovaccine in the human female genital tract. J. Immunol. **110:** 1307, 1973.
144. O'Reilly, R. J., Lee, L., and Welch, B. G.: Secretory IgA antibody responses to *Neisseria gonorrhoeae* in the genital secretions of infected females. J. Infect. Dis. **133:** 113, 1976.
145. Elstein, M.: The proteins of cervical mucus and the influence of progestagens. J. Obstet. Gynaecol. Br. Commonw. **77:** 443, 1970.
146. Schumacher, G. F. B.: Soluble proteins of human cervical mucus. In M. Elstein, K. S. Moghissi, and R. Borth (Eds.), Cervical Mucus in Human Reproduction, Geneva, World Health Organization Colloquium, 1972, p. 93.
147. Rebello, R., Green, F. H. Y., and Fox, H.: A study of the secretory immune system of the female genital tract. Br. J. Obstet. Gynaecol. **82:** 812, 1975.
148. Tourville, D. R., Ogra, S. S., Lippes, J., and Tomasi, T. B., Jr.: The human female reproductive tract: Immunohistological localization of γA, γG, γM, secretory "piece," and lactoferrin. Am. J. Obstet. Gynecol. **108:** 1102, 1970.
149. Chipperfield, E. J., and Evans, B. A.: Effect of local infection and oral contraception on immunoglobulin levels in the cervical mucus. Infect. Immun. **11:** 215, 1975.
150. Hulka, J. F., and Omran, K. F.: The uterine cervix as a potential local antibody secretor. Am. J. Obstet. Gynecol. **104:** 440, 1969.
151. Lippes, J., Ogra, S., Tomasi, T. B., and Tourville, D. R.: Immunohistological localization of γG, γA, γM secretory piece and lactoferrin in the human female genital tract. Contraception **1:** 163, 1970.
152. Lai A Fat, R. F. M., Cormane R. H., and Van Furth, R.: An immunohistopathological study on the synthesis of immunoglobulins and complement in normal and pathological skin and the adjacent mucous membranes. Br. J. Dermatol. **90:** 123, 1974.
153. Vargas-Linares, C. E. Roig de, Domenech, V. Balaguer de and Pérez-Elizalde, R.: Immunoglobulins of vaginal fluid in postmemopausal women. Acta Physiol. Lat. Am. **21:** 263, 1971.
154. Adinolfi, M., Glynn, A. A., Lindsay, M., and Milne, C M.: Serological properties of γA antibodies to *Escherichia coli* present in human colostrum. Immunology **10:** 517, 1966.
155. Vaerman, P. P.: Comparative immunochemistry of IgA. In J. B. G. Kwapinski (Ed.), Research in Immunochemistry and Immunobiology, Vol. 3. Baltimore, University Park Press, 1973, p. 91.
156. Crago, S. S., Kulhavy, R., Prince, S. J., and Mestecky, J.: Secretory component on epithelial cells is a surface receptor for polymeric immunoglobulins. J. Exp. Med. **147:** 1832, 1978.
157. Springer, G. F., Adye, J. C., Bezkorovainy, A., and Murthy, J. R.: Functional aspects and nature of the lipopolysaccharide-receptor of human erythrocytes. J. Infect. Dis. **128:** S202, 1973.
158. Schaeffer, A. J., and Stamey, T. A.: The effect of hysterectomy on colonization of the vaginal vestibule with *Escherichia coli.* Invest. Urol. **14:** 10, 1976.
159. Braude, A. I., Douglas, H., and Jones, J.: Experimental production of lethal *Escherichia coli*

bacteremia of pelvic origin. J. Bacteriol. **98:** 979, 1969.

160. Neter, E.: Bacterial hemagglutination and hemolysis. Bacteriol. Rev. **20:** 166, 1956.
161. Hanson, L. A., and Brandtzaeg, P.: Mucosal defense systems. In E. R. Stiehm and V. A. Fulginiti (Eds.), Immunologic Disorders in Infants and Children, Ed. 2. Philadelphia, W. B. Saunders, 1979.
162. Holmgren, J., and Smith, J. W.: Immunological aspects of urinary tract infections. Progr. Allergy **18:** 289, 1975.
163. Sohl Åkerlund, A., Ahlstedt, S., Hanson, L. Å., and Jodal, U.: Antibody responses in urine and serum against *Escherichia coli* O antigen in childhood urinary tract infection. Acta. Pathol. Microbiol. Scand. Sect. C **87:** 29, 1979.
164. Jodal, U., Ahlstedt, S., Carlsson, B., Hanson, L. A., Lindberg, U., and Sohl, A.: Local antibodies in childhood urinary tract infection; a preliminary study. Int. Arch. Allergy Appl. Immunol. **47:** 537, 1974.
165. Svanborg-Edén, C., and Svennerholm, A.-M.: Secretory IgA and IgG antibodies prevent adhesions of *E. coli* to human urinary tract epithelial cells. Infect. Immun. 1980. In press.
166. Uehling, D. T., Mizutani, K., and Balish, E.: Effect of immunization on bacterial adherence to urothelium. Invest. Urol. **16:** 145, 1978.
167. Pazin, G. J., and Braude, A. I.: Immobilizing antibodies in pyelonephritis. J. Immunol. **102:** 1454, 1969.
168. Silverblatt, F. J.: Antipili antibody protects rats against ascending urinary tract infection. Clin. Res. **27:** 43A, 1979.
169. Tuttle, J. P., Jr., Sarvas, H., and Koistinen: The role of vaginal immunoglobulin A in girls with recurrent urinary tract infections. J. Urol. **120:** 742, 1978.

ADDENDUM

Since the preparation of this chapter, Kunin *et al.* have reported on the "Periurethral bacterial flora in women" (J.A.M.A., **243:** 134, 1980) in which they could not confirm more "periurethral" colonization in UTI-prone women than occurred in healthy, control volunteers. They did not culture, however, either the introital or the periurethral mucosa, but relied instead on bacteria from these surface areas to contaminate the midstream voided urine, urines which were self-collected by sexually active women on first arising in the morning. The difficulty with this methodology is that we have seen many women whose introital mucosa is devoid of aerobic Gram-negative bacteria, but whose voided urine contains *E. coli* or *P. mirabilis*; these bacteria can be demonstrated to originate from the hairs of the labia majora. In addition, Kunin relied on dip-slide cultures, a method which cannot detect bacteria at levels <200/ml. They present no data to correlate proven introital carriage with numbers of bacteria in the voided urine; it is likely that substantial introital colonization can occur with less than 200 *E. coli*/ml in the voided urine. Their paper is useful in showing how often Enterobacteriaceae can reside somewhere on the perineum in all sexually active women, but their conclusions as to periurethral bacteria are clearly speculative.

CHAPTER 6

Urinary Infections in Infancy and Childhood

THE NEWBORN

General Characteristics

SAUER,[1] in 1925, reported 15 cases of "neonatal pyelitis"; 13 of the 15 were boys. He called attention to several earlier papers in the foreign literature that had also noted a preponderance of males over females. Sauer observed that the most frequent findings were anorexia, diarrhea, vomiting, pallor, and even cyanosis; that recovery was usually complete in 6 weeks; and that pyuria as well as traces of albumin continued for weeks after the symptoms had subsided. Treatment was limited to diuresis and alkalinization of the urine; the efficacy of alkalinization was greatly debated in the discussion that followed his paper.

Ten years later, Craig[2] presented a detailed clinical analysis of urinary infections in 61 newborns and compared their urinary findings with those from healthy infants. He emphasized that (1) large numbers of bacteria were found in the catheterized urine specimens of the sick infants, but pyuria was variable (three seriously ill babies had no pus cells on repeated examinations); (2) in some cases symptoms occurred before the appearance of abnormalities in the urine; (3) fever, although 102°F or more in 50% of the cases, was often absent; (4) recovery was complete in those discharged from the hospital, and their subsequent general health was unimpaired; and (5) in the fatal cases, autopsy studies showed involvement of the cortex and rarely the pelvis of the kidney.

James[3] noted that failure to gain weight, loss of weight, apathy, and anorexia were the common symptoms which led to the finding of urinary infection in 32 infants between the ages of 6 and 12 days.

Detailed information on urinary infections in the newborn is available from the careful studies of Winberg and his group[4, 5] at Göteborg. Their analysis[5] of 80 consecutive cases with neonatal infection represents the most comprehensive study published on this subject. With their permission, I have summarized the significant aspects of this work. Obstructive malformations were proven in only three patients and suspected in two; all were males. Obstructive abnormalities, according to these authors, constitute only about 6% of urinary infections in the newborn.

An analysis of the remaining 75 cases reveals the following:

1. There were 54 boys and 21 girls.
2. An abnormal weight loss during the first few days of life, often associated with a characteristic gray color of the skin which sometimes deepened to cyanosis, was the most characteristic feature.*
3. Six patients had meningitis; another 5 without meningitis had generalized convulsions; and still another 12 had symptoms of probable cerebral origin. A pleocytosis of the spinal fluid was found in several patients even though the fluid was sterile. Abdominal distension not due to the bladder was present in 12 patients. Fever was usually absent in the youngest patients (30/46) but generally present (20/29) in the babies who presented later between the 11th and 30th day of life.
4. A blood urea nitrogen of 25 mg/100 ml or more was transiently present in 13 of 57 patients; James[3] also observed marked elevations in 5 out of 17 patients, all values returning to normal a few weeks later.
5. The bacteria responsible for these 75 infections may reflect the hospital environment. Gram-positive infections occurred mainly in girls. Spontaneous disappearance of bacteria before treatment occurred in nine patients, four girls and five boys, all of whom had pyuria. Forty-six of 57 strains of *Escherichia coli* were serogrouped (Table 6.1); 68% belonged to one of the eight common O-groups (01, 2, 4, 6, 7, 8, 18, and 75). *E. coli* 04 serogroup occurred 11 times and *E. coli* 02 occurred 7 times in the 46 strains, a distribution the authors considered similar to that found in older girls seen with their first or second infections.
6. Eleven patients had definite symptoms one to several days before the bacteriuria became signficant, an observation also commented upon by Craig.[2] This finding, among others, led both authors to consider strongly a hematogenous origin of the urinary infection. Blood cultures were positive in one-third of those cultured in the Göteborg study.[5]

* Jaundice and hepatomegaly have been reported also as the primary presentation of urinary infections in newborns.[6] Azotemia is common in this group.

Table 6.1
Bacterial Species Responsible for Urinary Infection in 75 Newborns[5]

Species	Boys	Girls
Escherichia coli	45	12
Klebsiella	5	3
Alcaligenes faecalis	0	1
Enterococci	0	2
α-Streptococci	0	1
Staphylococcus epidermidis	1	0
Haemophilus vaginalis	0	1
E. coli + Enterococci	2	1
Unknown	1	0
Total	54	21

7. Of 36 patients studied for serum antibodies against the infecting strain, only 1 had an increased agglutination titer. The authors interpreted this failure to develop antibody, as well as the absence of temperature in most of their patients, as a manifestation of endotoxinemia. They pointed out that endotoxin might also explain the circulatory disturbances (the gray, cyanotic appearance), the signs of central nervous system irritability, and the loss of weight.

A high frequency of maternal urinary infection was demonstrated in this study, as had been shown previously by Patrick.[7] The authors questioned whether an immunologic interference between transmitted maternal antibodies and the infant's defense mechanism should be considered.

8. Six of the 75 patients died, 5 of them with meningitis. An intravenous urogram was performed in 60 of the surviving 69 patients (47 males and 13 females). *None showed obstruction.* The intravenous urogram was repeated in 30 patients 6 months or later after the first infection; progressive scarring occurred in 3.

Voiding cystourethrograms were done in 47 patients, 38 boys and 9 girls, shortly after the acute infection. Ureteral reflux was present in about 50% of cases, filling the calyces in 17 of the 21 refluxing patients; however, the reflux disappeared spontaneously on follow-up studies although it persisted for 2 years or more in a few instances.

Because the reflux usually disappeared spontaneously on follow-up studies, because recurrent infections (26%) did not correlate with the presence or absence of reflux, and because Winberg and his associates[5] considered these infections to be hematogenous in origin, they concluded that the reflux was probably secondary to the infection.

9. The recurrence rate of urinary infection was 29% in the males and 17% in the females (average for both groups was 26%). There was a higher recurrence rate among those patients whose infection began between the 10th and 30th day of life (11/29) than in those who presented during the first 10 days of life (7/40). Fourteen of these 18 patients had their first recurrence within 2 months of the original infection; there were no recurrences after the age of 18 months. Despite the early nature of the recurrence, reinfection was common while relapse was rare, long term therapy was not superior to short term, and severe generalized symptoms suggestive of septicemia did not characterize the recurrences.

Littlewood[8] analyzed the clinical presentation and course of 66 infants with urinary tract infection (UTI) in the first month of life. Boys were more affected than girls, the overall mortality was 11%, and further infection occurred in 37% of girls and 10% of boys.

The dire symptomatology of the septicemic infant with urinary infection in the 1st days of life clearly places this medical problem in the hands of the pediatrician, if not, indeed, in the hands of those who specialize in serious illnesses of the newborn. I have, nonetheless, presented the data of the Göteborg group[5] in detail because these urinary infections in newborns must be seriously considered in the natural history of urinary infections.

If infections in infancy account for some of the gross morphologic damage seen in kidneys of children and adults, we should try more often to obtain hospital nursery records. Urinary infections in the newborn are so severe and life-threatening because of the accompanying septicemia that nursery records should be helpful.

Except for the preponderance of males and the probability of hematogenous spread to the kidney in the newborn, as opposed to the ascending urinary route in older girls and women, there are far more similarities than differences when urinary infections in the newborn are compared to those in older children. These similarities seem important: the intravenous urogram is usually normal; ureteral reflux is common, renal scars occur only occasionally; and congenital obstructions are rare. The serogroups of *E. coli* that cause urinary infections belong to the same common O-groups. Recurrences tend to occur early and fail to correlate with the presence or absence of reflux; reinfection is more common than recurrence with the same organism; and long term therapy with sulfonamides is no better than short term.

Asymptomatic Bacteriuria in the Newborn

The foregoing characteristics relate to sick newborns with urinary infection. How often does asymptomatic bacteriuria occur in the newborn? Of all studies on the incidence of asymptomatic bacteriuria, assessment in the newborn is the most difficult because of extreme perineal contamination. But within these limitations, the incidence of asymptomatic neonatal infections is presented in Table 6.2 (I am indebted to Dr. J. Winberg for this compilation). Although different collection techniques were used in each study, and results should be evaluated on the basis of the validity of the methodology in each report, the average incidence from the five investigators shows that bacteriuria is 10 times as common in male neonates as in females.

As will be seen later in this chapter, the data on natural history from the last 8 years of clinical investigation indicate that it is the infant who is at the greatest risk of developing renal scarring from UTI and not the school age girl. For this reason, the detection of asymptomatic bacteriuria with screening bacteriuria surveys (ScBU), if it is ever indicated at any time of life, may be justified in the newborn and infant under 2 years of age. Randolph and his associates[13] developed an excellent home screening technique for the detection of UTI in infancy. They processed 870 specimens during the screening of 165 infants; UTI was detected in five girls and one boy (3.6% of the study population) ages 3–18 months, but two of the infant girls entered the study on the day of diagnosis with recurrent fever, foul urine, and diaper rash. It can be argued that these two children should be omitted because their parents sought medical help for their UTI and it would have been detected without the screening survey; if so, the incidence of ScBU is 2.5% in this age group. The urologic follow-up of these six infants was complete with intravenous urograms (IVUs), voiding cystourethrograms (VCUs), and cystoscopy. All six infants had normal IVUs, five of the six had grade II reflux up undilated ureters on the VCU, and the five who refluxed had incompetent-appearing ureteral orifices which were laterally displaced in three of the infant girls. All responded to antimicrobial therapy and were placed on long term trimethoprim-sulfamethoxazole (TMP-SMX) in a prophylactic single dose at bedtime for 6 months to 1 year; no further infections occurred. Reflux disappeared on repeat VCUs 4 to 6 months after the initial diagnosis, renal growth was normal on IVUs, and no renal scars were detectable on IVUs repeated 1 year after the start of therapy. It is obvious that this is a carefully performed study that offers an acceptable technique for the screening of large numbers of infants in the home. It is probably not inexpensive since three home cultures are required. More important than expense, however, will be the need in a future study to treat only half the patients randomly (as has been done with school children) to determine (1) would the untreated children have ultimately sought medical help anyway because of UTI symptoms and (2) in long term follow-ups, is there any difference between treated and untreated infants in terms of renal morbidity and scarring.

Kunin *et al.*[14] successfully used a nitrite dip-strip on three consecutive first morning specimens in a home screening program on

Table 6.2
Incidence of Urinary Infection in Five Surveys of Healthy Newborns

Study	Males		Females	
	Surveyed	Infected	Surveyed	Infected
Lincoln and Winberg, 1964[4]	298	8	286	0
McCarthy and Pryles, 1963[9]	100	1	100	1
O'Brien *et al.*, 1968[10]	579	1	421	0
O'Doherty, 1968[11]	410	9	420	0
Littlewood *et al.*, 1969[12]	309	7	291	1
Total	1696	26	1518	2
Percent infected	1.5%		0.13%	

3- to 5-year-old girls. Twenty-one of 26 bacteriuric girls detected from the screening survey were cultured at 3-month intervals with both the nitrite dip-strip and the Uricult dip-slide agar technique.[15] Their data suggested that the nitrite dip-strip test, even when administered on three first morning specimens, would miss 15–20% of girls with bacteriuria due to Gram-negative infections and 5% due to Gram-positive infections.

The Randolph study[13] used an agar surface technique for culturing the urine at home.

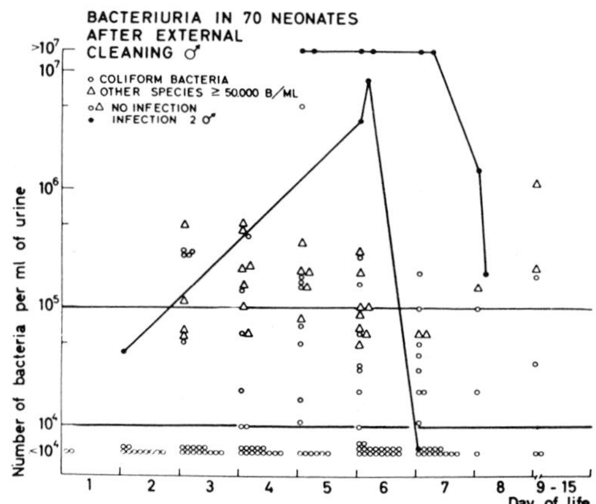

Figure 6.1 Bacterial counts in 123 urine specimens from 70 males during the first 15 days of life; external genital cleaning with soap and water. For each urine sample the coliform count is indicated by one *circle*. Other species are indicated by *triangles* when the count was 50,000 or more bacteria/ml. A bacterial count of 100,000 or more bacteria/ml of urine was found in 43 specimens from 24 boys. Only in two patients was the bacteriuria accompanied by leukocyturia. (Reproduced by permission from K. Lincoln and J. Winberg, Acta Paediatr. Scand. **53:** 307, 1964.[4])

Relationship to Perineal Contamination.

Bergström, Larson, Lincoln, and Winberg,[5] as well as Craig[2] and Sauer[1] consider the hematogenous route as the most likely source of renal infection in the newborn. The high incidence of general sepsis, the appearance of symptoms before the presence of bacteriuria in some cases, and the finding at autopsy[2, 16] of cortical infection in the presence of a normal renal pelvis are all strongly suggestive of the hematogeneous rather than the ascending route. But why then are boys more susceptible than girls? In considering this question, I think some earlier studies of Lincoln and Winberg[4] in the neonate are interesting. Their work on the bacterial flora of the male prepuce and the vaginal vestibule can be interpreted as showing a greater exposure of the male urethra to contaminating fecal bacteria than occurs with the female urethra. I believe these data are surprising and deserve more attention; they are reproduced in Figures 6.1–6.4. After external cleaning of both genital tracts and surrounding skin with soap and water, the area was dried with sterile gauze, and glass containers were attached to collect voided specimens. Of 70 normal neonate boys, randomly selected, 24 had 10^5 or more bacteria/ml of urine (Figure 6.1). Of 70 normal girls, only 5 had 10^5 or more bacteria/ml (Figure 6.2). Urine cultures were then obtained from 228 neonate boys after extensive irrigation of the preputial sack. The sack was injected twice with a lukewarm solution of 5% soap in 10-ml amounts; the preputium was massaged; and the whole genital tract was cleaned thoroughly. The preputial sack was then irrigated four times with 10 ml of sterile water, and the entire genital tract was washed with water and finally dried with gauze. A corresponding irrigation and cleaning was done in 216 neonate girls. Despite all this cleaning and repeated irrigation of the preputial sack, the degree of bacterial contamination, including both coliform bacteria and other species, is greater in the males (Figure 6.3) than in the females (Figure 6.4). Only 4 of 216 neonate girls had 10^5 or more bacteria/ml (Figure 6.4) while 19 of 228 boys had at least 10^5 bacteria/ml (Figure 6.3). Six boys and one girl were thought to be infected because of the accompanying leukocyturia. These six neonate boys, however, were asymptomatic and clearly different from the usual septicemic group of sick newborns. Nevertheless, the preputial contamination in the uncircumcised neonate is so impressive that, when compared with the vulval contamination in the female, one cannot help but wonder if it is related to the greater incidence of neonatal pyelonephritis in males. All of the boy babies in Sweden go uncircumcised so there is no way to test this hypothesis in the Göteborg material. Interestingly, James[3] noted that all of his male infants with urinary infections were uncircumcised. Enterobacteria could ascend up the urethra of the male and still reach the kidney by a hematogenous route. Most of the authors quoted here,[1, 2, 5] however, believe that the intestine is the source of the septicemia, but only because colonization of the gut occurs in the first few days of life at about the same time as the urinary infection. But if *E. coli* reach the blood stream directly from the intestinal mucosa, why do they do so more readily in male than female newborns?

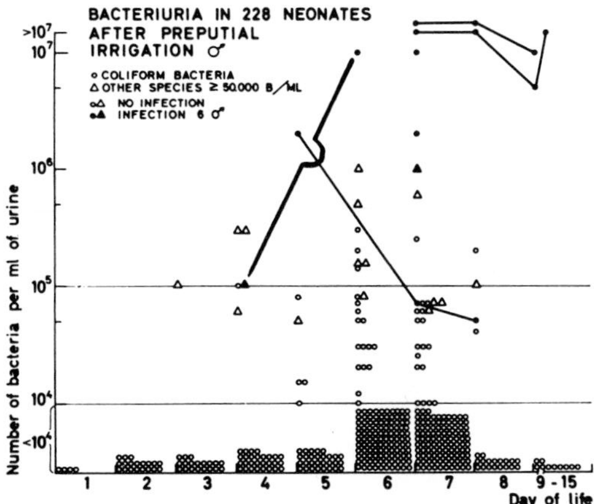

Figure 6.3 Bacterial counts in 394 specimens from 228 males during the first 15 days of life; external genital cleaning and preputial irrigation with soap and water. A bacterial count of 100,000 bacteria/ml or more was found in 27 specimens from 19 boys. In six boys bacteriuria was accompanied by leukocyturia. (Reproduced by permission from K. Lincoln and J. Winberg, Acta Paediatr. Scand. **53:** 307, 1964.[4])

URINARY INFECTIONS IN CHILDREN

The epidemiologic studies of Kunin and his associates in Charlottesville, Virginia,[17–21] and the clinical investigations of Winberg and his group in Göteborg, Sweden,[22–26] together represent a remarkable series of papers. Kunin screened thousands of asymptomatic school children for bacteriuria and, along with the late Albert Paquin, Professor of Urology at Charlottesville, evaluated the urologic status of those children found to be infected. Winberg's subjects, by contrast, were often symptomatic and were referred to a university hospital which served as the only referral center for children in a large city; thus, patients were often seen with first or second infections, early in the course of their disease. Both groups obtained IVUs and VCUs on bacteriuric patients, and their treatment regimens were surprisingly similar. The duration of therapy was short (about 10 days); each group insisted on a sterile urine while the patient was on therapy.

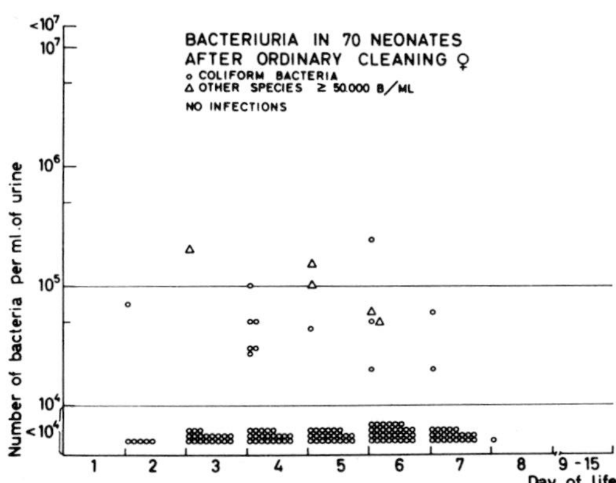

Figure 6.2 Bacterial counts in 132 specimens from 70 females during the first 8 days of life; external genital cleaning with soap and water. A bacterial count of 100,000 or more bacteria/ml of urine was found in five specimens from five girls, none accompanied by leukocyturia. (Reproduced by permission from K. Lincoln and J. Winberg, Acta Paediatr. Scand. **53:** 307, 1964.[4])

Sex Incidence

Except for the newborn and the infant under one year of age, infections in children occur mainly in girls. In Kunin's initial survey of school children,[17] only two instances of bacteriuria were detected among 7731 males (a 0.026% prevalence rate). Meadow *et al.*,[27] admittedly using different screening

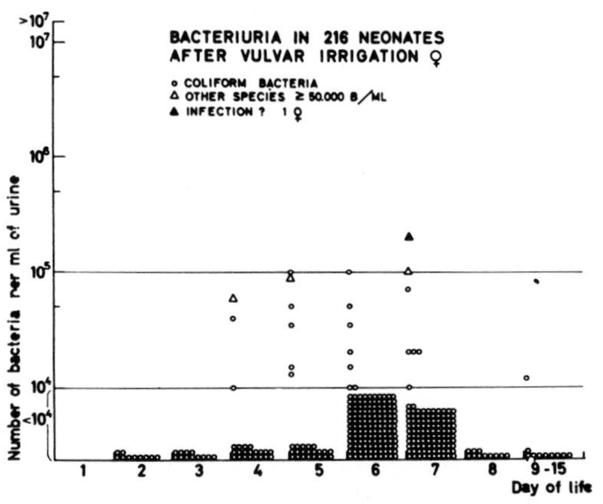

Figure 6.4 Bacterial counts in 335 specimens from 216 females during the first 15 days of life; external genital cleaning and vulvar irrigation with soap and water. A bacterial count of 100,000 bacteria/ml or more was found in four specimens from four girls, only in one accompanied by leukocyturia. (Reproduced by permission from K. Lincoln and J. Winberg, Acta Paediatr. Scand. **53:** 307, 1964.[4])

methods, found no instances of bacteriuria among 1096 schoolboys, but 10 cases among 1026 school girls (a 1% prevalence). In Meadow's population study, 99.8% of pupil participation was achieved.

Bergström[28] has analyzed the sex differences in 419 girls and 104 boys as to the age of onset between the second month and 16 years.

Age Incidence and Other Demographic Data

Although Kunin[17, 20] reported the same frequency of infection, about 1%, in schoolgirls of 5–9, 10–14, 15–19, and 20–24 years of age, this apparent constancy in the prevalence of urinary infection should be interpreted with caution. In fact, some consideration should be given to the possibility that urinary infections are most prevalent in the early years of life and thereafter decline during school years until the period of sexual activity begins sometime after puberty. Several papers based on admissions to pediatric hospital services clearly show a greater incidence in the first years of life. Smellie *et al.*[29] showed that the age distribution at the onset of symptomatology and presentation to the hospital in 200 children was highest in the 1st year of life and thereafter steadily declined between ages 1 and 12. Stansfield[30] reported similar data. This declining incidence is best observed in the studies of Bergström *et al.*[26] in 279 girls aged 2 months to 16 years. All girls presented with either their first or second urinary infections; a few patients were excluded from Bergström's analysis who had obstruction, stones, and radiographically demonstrable renal parenchymal reduction. Newborns, too, were excluded below 2 months of age because the authors considered their infections to be hematogenous rather than ascending. Figure 6.5, from their data,[26] documents the predominance of younger patients within the group below 1 year of age (even though newborns are excluded); the progressive decline of new infections with increasing age is clearly seen.

Winberg and his co-workers[31] have presented a classic and unique monograph entitled "Epidemiology of Symptomatic Urinary Tract Infection in Childhood". Because of the unusual referral nature of their

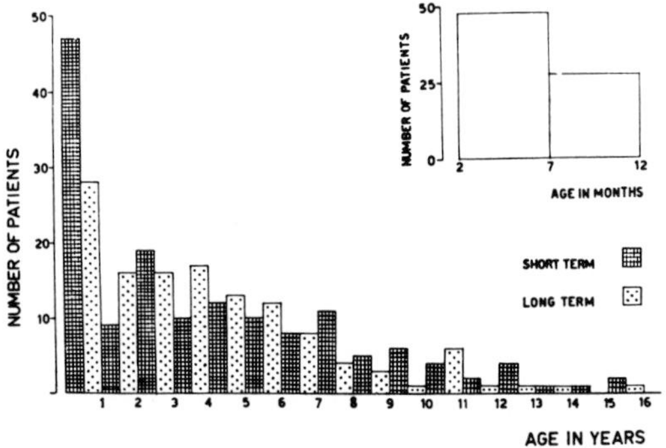

Figure 6.5 Age distribution of 279 girls with uncomplicated urinary infections presenting with their first or second urinary infection. Newborn infants less than 2 months old are excluded from the analysis. "Short term" and "long term" refer to whether they received 10 days or 60 days of sulfisoxazole therapy. The predominance of patients in the earliest years of life and the progressive decline in new infections in the older age groups are clearly apparent. (Reproduced by permission from T. Bergström *et al.*, Acta Paediatr. Scand. **57:** 186, 1968.[26])

material, they were able to calculate the aggregate morbidity risk for boys up to 11 years to develop an UTI as 1.1% and the aggregate risk for girls 3%. The morbidity risk of developing an UTI appeared to decrease more rapidly in the 1st year of life in boys than in girls so that, during the 2nd year of life, the average number of new cases per month was 3.2 for girls and 0.25 for boys (13 times greater for girls than boys).

Symptomatic children, 14 years old and under, presenting in a general practice setting over a 4-year interval showed 7.7/1000 girls at risk per year and 3.8/1000 boys at risk per year.[32] Of 794 boys 14 years and under, 12 presented with infections during the 4-year period (1.5%); of 838 girls, 26 presented with bacteriuria (3.1%). These data appear to confirm Winberg's[31] calculations almost exactly.

The early data of Kunin[17] suggested that the prevalence of bacteriuria in schoolgirls 5–9 years of age was 0.7%, falling to 0.5% in the 10- to 14-year age group. In a later series,[20] he reported no difference in these two age groups in white schoolgirls but a substantial drop with increasing age in Negro schoolgirls as follows: 0.7% prevalence in ages 5–9 and 0.3% at ages 10–14. In the paper by Meadow *et al.*,[27] 1.7% of the girls in the 5- to 7-year age group were bacteriuric, 0.9% in the 8- to 10-year age group, and only 0.6% in the girls 11–16 years old. DeLuca *et al.*[33] also commented on the decrease in incidence after the age of 7. Even in children with urinary infection undergoing surgical correction of reflux, Williams and Eckstein[34] reported that of 276 operated cases 25% showed their first evidence of disease in the 1st year of life; about 50% of their cases developed urinary infections before they were 3 years old. Admittedly, all of these percentages, including Kunin's[17] are based on small numbers of bacteriuric cases.

The Newcastle group,[35] however, screened 13,464 school girls aged 4–18 years. While the overall prevalence was 1.9%, in girls aged 4–6 years it was 1.4%, in girls aged 7–11 years it was 2.5%, and in girls aged 12–18 years it was 1.6%, which the authors considered a statistically significant rise and fall.

The Newcastle study[35] included only 278 girls age 4 (1.08% incidence of bacteriuria), but Köhler *et al.*[36] reported a survey of 1606 4-year-old children; the incidence of bacteriuria was 0.8% among the girls and 0% among the boys. Thus, the 1% or so of bacteriuric school girls at age 6 does not appear to come from a falling incidence of substantially higher rates in younger children.

Kunin's data[21] showed that 0.32% of school girls acquire bacteriuria each year; his prediction from these data that 5% of girls should be bacteriuric by the time they complete high school (about age 18 years) is surely incorrect, which must mean that as many girls cease having recurrent bacteriuria as those who acquire bacteriuria for the first time (0.32%/year). The prevalence of bacteriuria in teenagers is really no greater than among school children. For example, the prevalence in 16-, 17-, and 18-year-olds in the Newcastle study[35] was 0.98–1.54%. Heale screened 2435 girls just beginning university in Australia (W. F. Heale, personal communication, of April 17, 1973); 37 had $>10^5$ bacteria/ml in their midstream voided culture, but on bladder aspiration only 29 were infected (1.2% prevalence rate).

Girardet[37] has reviewed at least 15 epidemiologic surveys in school children published between 1964 and 1976. I admit that it is difficult to be certain of a definite change in the prevalence rate of asymptomatic bacteriuria detected on screening surveys between the ages 4 and 18; the real incidence probably lies between 1 and 2%. It is clear, however, that the incidence of symptomatic infections on first presentation is highest in the first year of life and declines steadily as shown in Figure 6.5. These differing statistics serve as a reminder that we must constantly separate studies on children whose bacteriuria brings them to their physician from those whose bacteriuria is detected during screening surveys (ScBU). Among recent studies, the interested reader could do no better than to read the Winberg paper[31] on symptomatic infections and contrast it with the Newcastle findings[35] in children with ScBU.

In summary, it would appear that the prevalence of bacteriuria in screening surveys in children between the ages of 4 and 18 is 1–2% and that there is no basis for a rising prevalence rate with increasing age. In contrast to screening surveys, the risk of a boy developing a symptomatic UTI during the first 11 years of life is 1.1% and 3% for girls; if newborns in the first month are excluded, the risk is 0.7% for boys and 2.8% for girls. In terms of general practice statistics, 7.7/1000 girls are at risk per year compared to 3.8/1000 boys aged 14 years or less.

Symptomatology

In the Newcastle study[35] of 254 girls with ScBU, 76% had some symptoms on questioning; 39% admitted to urgency, 31% to abdominal pain, and 30% had nocturnal enuresis. Only 13.4% (34 girls) had previously been diagnosed as having an UTI. Thus, "asymptomatic" bacteriuria detected during screening surveys in children is very similar to that in adults (Chapter 4): for most subjects, their bacteriuria is really not asymptomatic. The Newcastle[35] figure of 76% is very similar to the 75% found by Savage, *et al.*[38] as well as the 66% found by Kunin.[39]

In symptomatic infections that bring the patient to the physician, almost all infants over 30 days old present with fever in both girls and boys which Winberg's group[31] believe is an indication of renal involvement in this age group. Dysuria and frequency are much more common than in patients with ScBU, but Meadow has pointed out how common urinary symptoms are in the absence of UTI.[40] Heale, Weldon, and Hewstone[41] presented some interesting date on 789 children presenting over a 17-week period to a large general pediatric clinic with symptoms compatible with an UTI. Fourteen and three-tenths percent of patients with specific urinary symptoms and 4.4% with nonspecific symptoms were infected; it is clear that most children presenting with symptoms compatible with an UTI did not have an UTI. UTI was present in 33% who presented with any combination (two or more) of urinary frequency, dysuria, and loin pain, but was present in only 9% of children who had only one of these three classic symptoms. Infection was present in a third of the patients with a recent onset of enuresis, but in only 4% of those with chronic wetting.

Bacteriologic Findings

In symptomatic infections, Winberg *et al.*[31] have presented some interesting and important differences in the bacteriology of first infections. In the neonates, *E. coli* is less common in the females than males (see Table 6.1) and *Klebsiella-Enterobacter* is more common in neonates than in older children. The most important finding, confirmed by numerous investigators, is that *Proteus* infections were as frequent as *E. coli* infections in boys over the age of 1 year, and that *Staphylococcus epidermidis* accounted for one-third of all infections in girls above the age of 10 years. As will be seen in a later section, these differences reflect the different urethral and introital flora of the growing child.

I have discussed in detail in Chapter 5 the O-serogroup differences among *E. coli* in children with symptomatic UTI compared to those with ScBU. *E. coli* was the responsible organism in 92% of the 254 girls with ScBU in the Newcastle study[35]; *Klebsiella* caused 13 infections and *Proteus mirabilis* 3 infections.

Renal Scarring

In symptomatic infections, renal scarring was present in 13% of 156 boys but in only 4.5% of 440 girls followed from their first known UTI[31]; the scarring was progressive in 22 (58%) of the 38 patients (1/4 of the boys and 3/4 of the girls) despite early diagnosis, successful treatment, and thorough follow-up with treatment of recurrences. In our Stanford series[42, 43] of all girls, 17 of 40 kidneys (43%) with clubbing and scarring developed or increased clubbing or scarring while the patients were being treated medically; 16 of 24 kidneys (67%) previously clubbed and scarred showed progression of clubbing and scarring following successful correction of vesicoureteral reflux (VUR). These data from the Stanford series strongly suggest that progressive scarring occurred only after acute episodes of pyelonephritis and that about 2 years is required for a scar to develop radiologically following a clinical episode of acute pyelonephritis; this observation is important in interpreting the Christchurch studies to be presented in the section on vesico-ureteral reflux.

In contrast to Winberg's study[31] on symptomatic girls followed from their first known UTI and who showed 4.5% scarring, renal scarring in girls with ScBU varies between 13 and 20 percent.[35, 38, 39, 44] It is probably not by accident that the incidence of renal scarring in adult patients with ScBU is about the same.[45, 46] In the general practice study of Brooks and Houston,[32] only 2/26 girls had renal scarring (8%).

In the Newcastle series[35] of girls 4–18 years old with ScBU, there was no evidence that the severity of the scarring increased with age—which was one of the main objects of the study, and one of the important conclusions. In fact, although scarring occurred in 39 of the 254 girls (15%), the prevalence in relation to the total population was 0.29%; severe renal scarring was present in only 0.05% of the total population. As the authors imply, is it worth screening 2000 children to detect 1 with serious renal scarring?

Renal scarring in the Newcastle study[35] was unrelated to symptoms. Radiologically, scarring related statistically to reflux (18/39 had both reflux and scars), to duplication (7/39), to hydroureter (5/39), and to a single saccule on the filling phase of the VCU (5/39). No reflux was detectable at the time of the VCU, however, in 21/39 girls with scarring.

In the Cardiff-Oxford Bacteriuria Study Group,[47] 1.8% (294) of 16,800 school girls, aged 5–12, had bacteriuria. Two hundred eight girls had IVUs and VCUs when initially detected and 4 years later at follow-up. One hundred ten were treated and 98 were not; 15% of the treated group were bacteriuric compared to 45% of the untreated group at the end of the study. Forty-four patients (21%) has scarred kidneys (31 unilateral, 13 bilateral). New and/or deepening scars were found in 12 of the 44 girls (27%) who initially showed scarred kidneys; 6 were in the treated and 6 in the nontreated group, but the 3 girls with new scars were all in the untreated group. All those that had no scars at the start of the study, developed no scars during the 4 years of follow-up, regardless of whether they were in the treated or nontreated group; 77% of the treated girls had infection for less than 2 years whereas only 38% of the untreated girls were bacteriuric for less than that time. The risk factors for renal scarring from this study appear to be (1) the presence of pre-existing scars, (2) persistent infection, and (3) VUR; all 12 girls who developed further scarring had ureteral reflux on the initial VCU and should be compared to the overall prevalence of reflux in 34% of the 208 girls in the study.

The informative prospective studies by Savage and associates[48] at Dundee, Scotland, Lindberg and his colleagues[49] at Göteborg, and the analysis of the Cardiff-Oxford Study Group by Verrier-Jones *et al.*[50] all confirm that radiologic evidence of new renal scarring in children over 4 years of age is a relatively minor problem and unlikely to be influenced by a public health approach to detection and treatment by the medical profession.

All of these studies make it fairly clear that most renal scarring develops before the age of 4 years, and that most of it is due to VUR and infection.

Vesicoureteral Reflux—Grade, Prevalence, and Relation to Renal Scarring

The degree of VUR is most simply divided into three grades: grade I represents reflux into the ureters but not into the renal pelvis (Figure 6.6); in grade II reflux, the contrast extends to the renal pelvis and calyces without significant dilatation of the calyces (Figure 6.7); and in grade III reflux, there is dilatation and often distortion of the renal calyces (Figure 6.8). There are

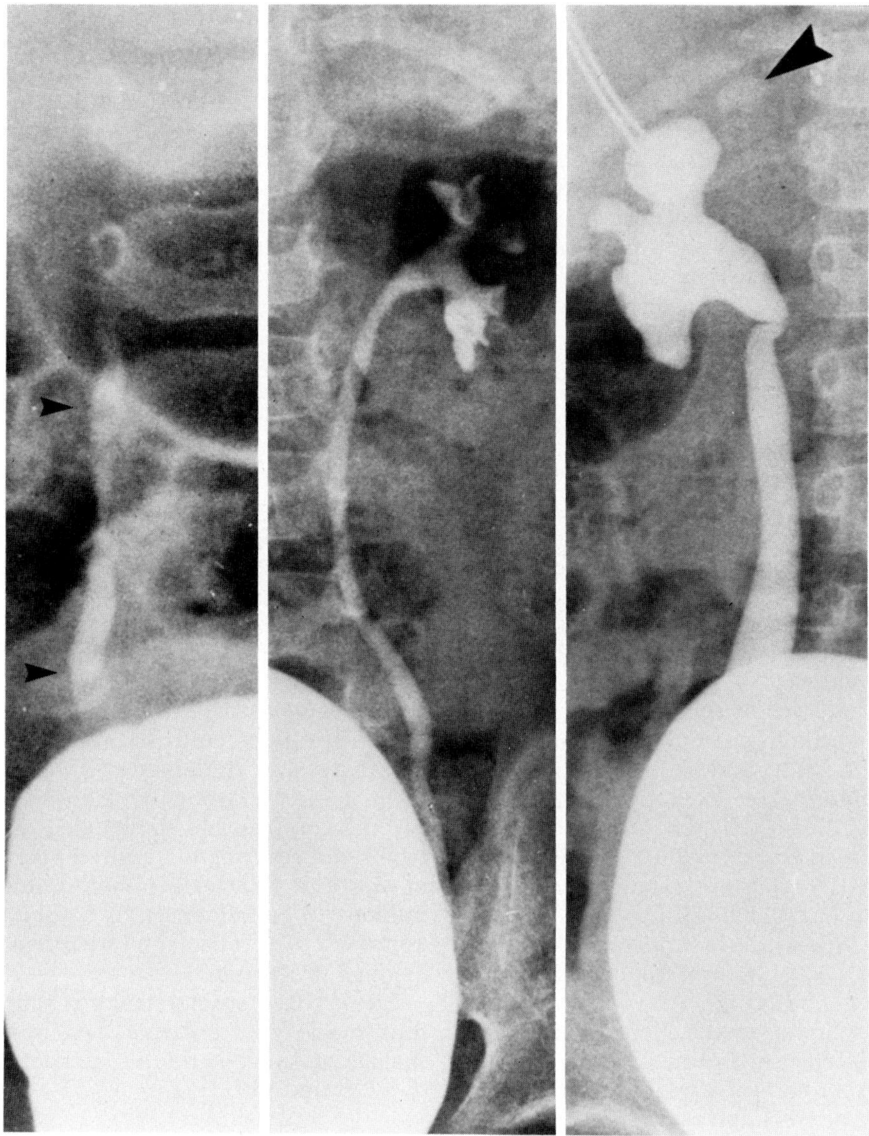

Figure 6.6 (*left*) Example of grade I reflux extending into the right ureter (*arrows*) but not into the kidney or renal pelvis.
Figure 6.7 (*center*) Example of grade II reflux extending into the kidney and calyces without producing calyceal dilatation or distortion.
Figure 6.8 (*right*) Example of grade III reflux extending to the kidney with gross calyceal dilatation and distortion. The *arrow* marks a faint shadow of intrarenal reflux.

many different classifications and variations of the three grades presented here; for example, megaloureters, ureteral tortuosity, or absence of ureteral peristalsis are considered a fourth grade by some authors and, from the surgical viewpoint, this distinction is undoubtedly important because it is this group that is the most difficult to repair. Intrarenal reflux, which will be considered later in this chapter, could be an important subsection to grades II and III, but it occurs infrequently and is limited to children under 4 years of age. Taking everything into consideration, the three grades of VUR presented in Figures 6.6–6.8 represent the best basis for discussion in this chapter.

In Kunin's[18] report on 3057 school children, 19% of those bacteriuric showed reflux on VCU. The Newcastle study[35] found reflux in 15% of girls without renal scarring and 46% of those with scarring; the overall prevalence rate was 21%. In the Cardiff-Oxford Bacteriuria Study Group,[47] 34% of the 208 bacteriuric girls showed reflux at entry into the study. Twenty-eight percent showed reflux in the study by Savage *et al.*[48] and 21% in the screening survey of Lindberg, *et al.*[49] Thus, in all these screening surveys for asymptomatic bacteriuria, the prevalence of reflux varied between 19 and 34%.

VUR in symptomatic patients presenting to their general physician appears to be no different in prevalence than in children with ScBU. Thirty-two percent of bacteriuric girls between the age of 1 and 16 years showed reflux in Winberg's study[31] while 34% of children referred to Smellie[51] had reflux. Children referred to urologists, of course, will have an even higher incidence of reflux, depending upon their type of practice.

In general, the more severe grades of reflux are associated with renal scars, particularly in infancy.[52, 53] In the Christchurch series,[52, 53] Rolleston divided the reflux into gross, moderate, and slight, which approximates our grades III, II, and I in Figures 6.6–6.8. Of the 130 refluxing ureters in the 175 infants investigated, 32 showed gross reflux and accounted for 26 of 29 renal scars among the 130 kidneys. As seen in Figure 6.9, scars were present in only 3 of 74 ureters with moderate reflux and in none of 24 ureters with slight reflux. On re-examining 54 kidneys by intravenous urography 6 months to 5 years later, all kidneys that showed progressive renal damage were among the grossly refluxing ureters (Figure 6.10); none of the ureters with moderate reflux showed progressive scarring. It is important to recognize that 11 of the 13 kidneys with gross reflux which showed progressive renal scarring also had recurrent UTI; moreover, since 2 years may be required for an episode of acute pyelonephritis to fully develop into a radiologic scar,[42] it is possible if not highly probable that the two patients who developed progressive renal damage in the presence of sterile urine did so from their initial UTI that caused the radiologic evaluation in the first place. Thus, although I cannot agree with the authors' conclusion that sterile reflux in grossly dilated ureters is a cause of progressive renal damage, this careful radiologic analysis of UTI in infants under 1 year old is a much needed and splendid contribution to our understanding of urinary infections in infants.

DEGREE OF REFLUX vs RENAL SCARS

GROSS	– 32	→	26/32
MODERATE	– 74	→	3/74
SLIGHT	– 24	→	0/24
	130 URETERS		

Figure 6.9 The relationship of renal scars to the degree of ureteral reflux in 130 kidneys from 175 infants under 1 year of age with UTI.[53] Reflux was bilateral in 44 and unilateral in 42 of the 86 infants with reflux. There were 91 males and 84 females with UTI; both bilateral and unilateral reflux were about equally distributed among males and females.

RE-EXAMINATION OF 54 URETERS BY I.V.P.
(6 MONTHS – 5 YEARS LATER)

DEGREE OF REFLUX vs PROGRESSIVE DAMAGE

GROSS – 17 → 13/17
("RECURRING INFECTION")
MODERATE – 34 → 0/34
SLIGHT – 3 → 0/3
54 URETERS

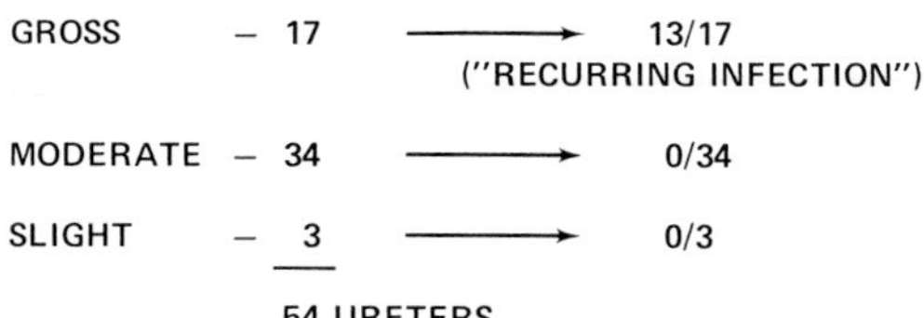

Figure 6.10 When the intravenous urogram was repeated months to years later, only those kidneys with gross ureteral reflux showed progression of renal scarring. Eleven of the 13 kidneys with progressive damage had recurring infections between the two radiologic evaluations[53]

Winberg *et al.*[31] also found a higher rate

of VUR in infants than in older children; they reported an incidence of 57% for girls between 3 and 12 months of age, and 30% for boys between the 2nd and 12th month compared to 18% in older boys 2–16 years of age (Table 6.3). Reflux occurred in 49% of the 175 infants in the Christchurch series.[53]

The Newcastle study[35] also reported a relationship between the more severe grades of ureteral reflux and renal scarring, although 21 of their 39 girls with renal scars had no reflux. It is reasonable that the older the child the more likely the reflux that produced the scar has either disappeared or possibly reduced in severity. It is one of the contributions of the Christchurch study[53] that most of the renal scarring occurring in infancy appears to be associated with gross reflux; perhaps what we see later in life as grade I or II reflux with renal scarring was all grade III during infancy when the scarring probably occurred. Vermillion and Heale[54] showed in children over 14 years with renal scarring and no reflux that the ureteral orifice at cystoscopy was quite abnormal and suggested VUR.

Our group at Stanford[42] found 3 renal scars out of 100 nonrefluxing ureters in children with UTI, 6 scars out of 26 ureters (23%) with grade I reflux, 17 scars out of 34 ureters (50%) with grade II reflux, and 36 scars out of 47 ureters (77%) with grade III reflux (Figure 6.11); the difference in renal scarring between the higher grades of reflux and the lower grades was obviously statistically significant ($P < 0.001$).

Table 6.3
Prevalence of Vesicoureteral Reflux (VUR) in Infants and Children Presenting with First Symptomatic Urinary Tract Infection[a]

Patient Group	Percent with VUR	Number with VUR
Neonates	47	47
Males		
2nd–12th month	30	52
2nd–16th year	18	34
Females		
3rd–12 month	57	14
2nd–16th year	32	41

[a] Reproduced by permission from J. Winberg *et al.*, Acta. Paediatr. Scand. (Suppl.) **252:** 3, 1974.[31]

Renal Growth

The effect of bacteriuria, with or without VUR, on the kidney can be assessed radiologically not only by the presence of renal scarring but by growth of the kidney. Hodson[55, 56] has described the radiologic parameters of renal growth in the normal child.

Several studies have shown that the 3-5 mm annual growth-rate of the normal kidney is impaired in some children with scarred kidneys, VUR, and recurrent episodes of UTI.[47–49] Although the Cardiff-Oxford study detected no difference in treated and nontreated children in terms of renal

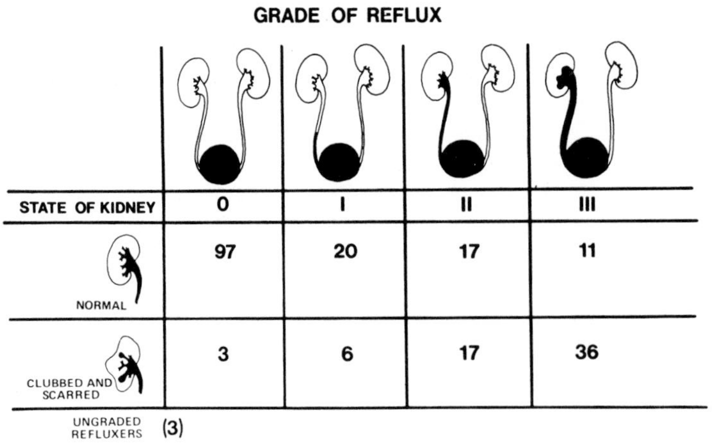

GRADE OF REFLUX

STATE OF KIDNEY	0	I	II	III
NORMAL	97	20	17	11
CLUBBED AND SCARRED	3	6	17	36
UNGRADED REFLUXERS (3)				

Figure 6.11 The relationship between the grade of reflux and the presence or absence of renal clubbing and scarring in the Stanford series. (Reproduced by permission from R. A. Filly *et al.*, West. J. of Med. **121:** 374, 1974.[42])

growth, Edwards *et al.*,[57] using long term prophylaxis, found normal renal growth in 74% of 19 scarred kidneys.

Winberg *et al.*[58] has recently examined renal growth after neonatal pyelonephritis in patients who did not develop focal scarring. He found significant growth retardation 4 years after the original infection. Surprisingly, the majority of patients had only a single infection, 60% of the kidneys showed no reflux and only 5% had grade III reflux. These authors suggest that focal scarring and growth impairment are two different consequences of renal infection, a conclusion that Asscher and Chick[59] also reached when they found that the intravesical infection of 10^6 heat-killed *E. coli* into the rat bladder produced impairment of kidney growth without renal scarring.

Recurrent Urinary Tract Infections

Recurrences in Symptomatic Children Presenting to a Physician

The frequency of recurrences and the duration of remissions are determined, in part, by the age of the patient at first presentation and the sex. In male and female neonates, the recurrence rate in the 1st year of life is 26%; the rate is about the same (18%) for infant boys falling ill in the first year of life.[31] In both of these groups, recurrent UTI one year after the first infection was rare.

In boys older than 1 year at the time of their first infection, 32% will have recurrences on follow-up, most of them in the first few months; as already noted, *P. mirabilis* will be as common as *E. coli*.[31]

In the female infant, Randolf *et al.*[60] reported a 10-year follow-up on 29 infants falling ill at a median age of 9 months. Nine of the 29 (31%) recurred within 18 months, but there were no recurrences after the age of 3 years.

In girls other than neonates, the recurrence rate after the initial infection is 40–42%.[31, 61] As with adult women (see Chapter 4), recurrences tend to be early rather than late. In Winberg's material, about two-thirds of all recurrences in girls under 11 years were within 12 months of the first infection, with 54% of these appearing during the first 3 months. Only 8% had their first recurrence more than 4 years after the primary infection. The interval between the primary infection and the first recurrence was not a measure of the risk of subsequent recurrence, but the risk of a recurrence clearly increases with the number of preceding infections. I have reproduced the data of Winberg *et al.*[31] in Figure 6.12 which shows how much more at risk a girl is for further infections once she has had her first one, and how much that risk grows with subsequent recurrences.

Cohen observed that in girls 2–14 years of age, reinfections gradually decreased from a 42% recurrence rate 6 months after the initial infection to a 1% rate after 6 years.[61]

Lastly, it is important to recognize the

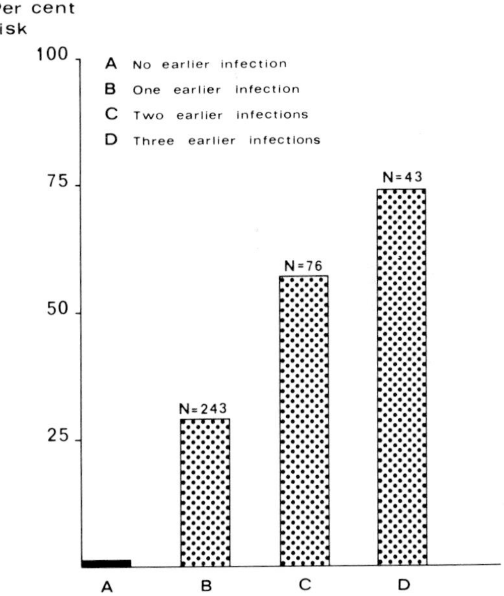

Figure 6.12 Risk of recurrence within 1 year after preceding infection. Recurrence rate within 1 year of a preceding infection related to the number of earlier infections. (*A*) Approximate risk of a 30-day-old healthy girl to have an infection before 11 years of age. (*B*) Observed risk in 243 girls with one earlier infection. (*C*) Observed risk in 76 patients with two earlier infections. (*D*) Observed risk in 43 patients with three earlier infections. (Reproduced by permission from J. Winberg *et al.*, Acta Paediatr. Scand. (Suppl.) **252:** 1, 1974.[31])

following additional facts about recurrent UTI in symptomatic children presenting to their primary physicians or to urologist[31]:

1. One-third of the recurrences will be asymptomatic. Table 6.4 shows the nature of the recurrences in the 279 infants and children presented in Figure 6.5; most of the febrile recurrences were in infants.
2. There is no relationship between ureteral reflex and susceptibility to UTI, at least in grades I and II reflux, and probably not in grade III.
3. There is no correlation between risk of recurrence and age of the girl or site of infection (bladder or kidney).

Recurrences in Girls with Screening Bacteriuria

The frequency of recurrent bacteriuria in girls with ScBU after therapy depends on (1) the rate of spontaneous cure and reinfection, (2) the duration of follow-up, and perhaps (3) the duration and type of antibacterial therapy. For these reasons, it is difficult to assess the rate of recurrent bacteriuria in these girls with ScBU, but it is clearly greater than the recurrence rate in symptomatic girls presenting to their physician (40–42%). For example, Kunin[20] reported a 60% recurrence rate within 1 year of a short course of therapy, which is substantially greater than Bergström's[26] 36% in the 279 symptomatic girls shown in Table 6.4.

Table 6.4
Recurrences in 279 Infants and Children with First or Second-Time Infections[a]

	Number	Percent
Total	279	(100)
No recurrence	179	(64)
Total number of recurrences	100	(36)
Asymptomatic recurrences	37	(13)
Symptomatic recurrences	63	(23)
Febrile	46	
Afebrile, micturition symptoms	14	
Afebrile, anorexia, abdominal pain, etc.	3	

[a] Adapted from T. Bergström *et al.*, Acta Paediatr. Scand. **57:** 186, 1968.[26]

In the more recent clinical trials of Savage *et al.*,[48] 29 girls with ScBU were treated initially for 3 months or 6 months depending on whether the IVU and VCU were normal (3 months) or abnormal (6 months). Twenty-four percent recurred with their bacteriuria in 6 months, 48% in 12 months, and 74% at 2 years. Only 21% remained free of infection from the initial treatment. In comparison to the control group of 32 untreated patients, 84% were bacteriuric at 2 years which was no different from the 74% bacteriuric schoolgirls in the treatment group at 2 years. It is obvious that, like the treatment trials in adult women with ScBU (see Chapter 4), noncontinuous therapy seems to make little difference in the ultimate outcome of schoolgirls with ScBU.

Epidemiologic studies, in terms of therapy, can be difficult and even misleading. In the Cardiff-Oxford study,[47] for example, 110 girls with ScBU were initially treated for 7–14 days with appropriate antibacterial therapy; recurrences, however, were later treated with low-dosage maintenance therapy and it is not stated how many girls at the end of 4 years were on maintenance therapy at the time of the final cultures. The authors found that only 17 of the 110 girls (15%) were infected at 4 years which surely reflects continuing antimicrobial therapy in many of them. Fifteen percent is far too low a figure in comparison to the data of Kunin,[20] Savage *et al.*,[48] and Lindberg *et al.*[49] It is interesting that 45% of the 98 girls in the control, untreated group were infected at the end of the 4-year study, implying that 55% were spontaneously cured, which is also probably much too high. This study points out that epidemiologic investigations are difficult to control when it comes to therapy; the authors recognized that eight of the control girls required treatment for symptomatic UTI, and undoubtedly others received antibiotics for other purposes than their urinary infection.

Additional Observations from the Controlled Treatment Trials of Girls with Screening Bacteriuria

Despite all the treatment problems in the Cardiff-Oxford study,[47] 77% of the treated girls were free from infection for at least half of the 4-year follow-up, while only 38% of the untreated controls were similarly free from infection. Even with this difference, treatment had no effect on emergence of symptoms, disappearance of VUR, kidney growth, or progression of renal scars.

In the Dundee study,[48] renal growth was better in the treated girls with normal radiology than in the control, untreated subjects, but therapy made no significant difference in those girls with abnormal radiology.

In both the Dundee[48] and the Cardiff-Oxford[47] reports, it is surprising how asymptomatic the untreated girls with ScBU were in the 4 years they were followed. Only 8% of both the treated and untreated girls in the Cardiff-Oxford study were reported to have symptoms during the 4 years, but this must surely relate to serious symptoms requiring therapy; the Newcastle[35] study, among others, established that 76% of girls with ScBU had some symptoms at the time of diagnosis.

The study by Lindberg *et al.*[49] in their controlled treatment trial of schoolgirls with ScBU, showed that 30% of their 31 untreated girls spontaneously lost their bacteriuria during the 3 years of follow-up: three during the 1st year, two during the 2nd year, and four during the 3rd year. After 3 years, 47% were still bacteriuric which was not significantly different from their treatment group (52%). Normal kidney growth, however, was seen in all girls with radiologically normal urinary tracts—treated and untreated—as long as they remained asymptomatic. This study by Lindberg and associates appears to be a very careful one in which antibacterial therapy for purposes other than the patient's UTI was carefully monitored.

Reinfection or "Relapse"

Over 90% of recurrent infections in girls are reinfections with different serogroups of *E. coli* rather than relapses with the same organisms.[20, 25, 62] Indeed, the Göteborg studies[31] demonstrated that 11 out of 12 recurrent infections, occurring within 60 hours of completing a 10-day course of therapy that sterilized the urine, were actually different bacteria and not relapses. The presence of urologic abnormalities did not influence the rate of recurrence,[20, 31] and reinfection (rather than relapse) was just as common in children with reflux as in those without.[25, 31, 63]

Bergström *et al.*[26] also demonstrated that 60 days of successful antimicrobial therapy is no better than 10 days in preventing recurrent infections. In fact, 60 days of sulfonamide therapy simply produced more asymptomatic recurrent infections (and sulfonamide resistant bacteria) than occurred following 10 days of treatment. With repeated recurrent infections, the distribution of bacterial species in Kunin's[20] investigations showed a small increase in *Proteus*, *Pseudomonas*, enterococcus, and *Staphylococcus*, but *E. coli* remained the most common species.

In the Virginia schoolgirls, studied six times over a period of 7 years after entering school, new infections occurred at the rate of 0.32% per year[21]; thus, the *cumulative* rate of bacteriuria over the first 7 years of school was 2.9% although 1% only were bacteriuric at any single survey. Of considerable interest is Kunin's[21] conclusion that, since the 0.32% rate of emergence of new cases of bacteriuria is linear with time, all girls between age 6 and 13 are at equal risk for acquiring bacteriuria. It is of interest that if the 36 girls with Gram-negative bacteria in their VB_1 (voided bladder one) urine (perineal) specimens, (see Table 6.6) are plotted in terms of age versus degree of Gram-negative colonization, the number of enteric Gram-negative bacteria are randomly distributed in relation to the age of the girl. That is, perineal colonization with Gram-negative bacteria in girls between ages 5 to 12 is not related to the age of the patient collecting the specimen.

Of more importance are Kunin's[21] data which suggest that each course of therapy provides long term remission for 20–25% of white and about 40% of Negro girls. His 5-year follow-up studies on 65 white and 18 Negro girls, showing the percentage remaining who had recurrent bacteriuria after each course of short term treatment, are reproduced in Figure 6.13. These stud-

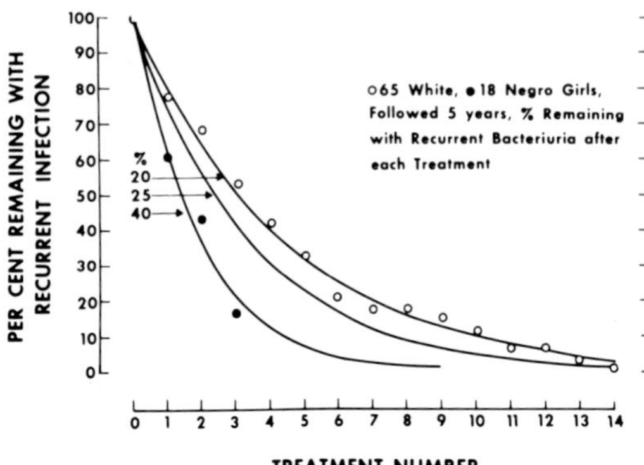

Figure 6.13 Theoretical rates of extraction of girls into remission at rates of 20, 25, and 40% for each treatment. The observed percentage remaining in the population that required further treatment is superimposed on the theoretical projections for white and Negro girls followed for 5 years. (Reproduced by permission from C. M. Kunin, N. Engl. J. Med. **282:** 1443, 1970.[64])

ies are important and have been confirmed by us at Stanford.[65] As will be emphasized in the next section on vesical neck "obstructions" and antireflux operations, since short term therapy alone provides long term remission for 20–25% of white girls—regardless of the number of preceding recurrences—then surgical procedures that allegedly prevent recurrence of urinary infections will have to be checked against a closely matched control group of nonsurgically treated patients. It should also be noted that Kunin's[64] studies were in girls with ScBU while our confirmation of his observation is from girls with symptomatic UTI presenting to our urologic outpatient unit.

Bacteriologic Flora of the Introitus and Periurethral Area of the Healthy Child

In Chapter 4, I presented our evidence that (1) urinary infections in adult women are preceded by the establishment of significant numbers of enterobacteria on the introital mucosa and that (2) normal women have only transient colonies of enterobacteria in small numbers on the introitus. In early 1970, it was clear that more information was needed on the bacterial flora of the healthy female child. Accordingly, Dr. T. L. Ho, a urologic resident in our program at Stanford, and I teamed up with Drs. J. I. Ball, B. Harvey, and C. Vogl, who hold clinical University appointments and who practice pediatrics in an office adjacent to Stanford University. We decided to culture all girls who were seen in their office for a routine annual precamp or preschool physical examination.[66] Without any preceding perineal or introital cleansing whatsoever, the office nurse had each girl hold a wide-mouth, 2-ounce, sterile plastic container near the labia; each child initiated voiding from the routine sitting position on a standard toilet seat. The first 30 ml or so to cross the urethra and labia were collected in the first container, which was labeled VB_1. The girl was then given a second container and, after reinitiating voiding, a late midstream specimen was collected (VB_2). It is important to emphasize that the perineum was not washed before the collection of these cultures. Thus, the bacterial counts represent the bacteriologic flora on the urethra, vaginal introitus, labia, and perhaps even the perirectal area in very young girls. All specimens were immediately refrigerated and cultured as outlined in Chapter 1. Of 117 girls, ages 30 months to 15 years (average, 8 years), who attended the office for a routine physical examination, 12 were found to have an overt past history or office record evidence of a urinary infection earlier in life. The bacteriologic flora in the VB_1 cultures of these 12 girls are presented in Table 6.5. L.O. and L.H. were bacteriuric with $> 10^5$ *E. coli* and *Aerobacter aerogenes*, respectively, in their VB_2 (midstream) specimens as well as in their VB_1 aliquots. Six of the 12 had no Gram-negative bacteria in their VB_1 (perineal) aliquots of urine.

Of the 105 remaining girls who had neither a past history nor laboratory documentation of urinary infections, 66% did not contain a single Gram-negative pathogen in their VB_1 urines and 80% contained none in their VB_2 specimens. The number of colonies and type of bacteria cultured in the 34% (36 girls) who had Gram-negative

Table 6.5
Perineal Urine Cultures (VB_1) in 12 of 117 Healthy Girls Who Had an Overt Past History or Laboratory Evidence of a Urinary Infection Earlier in Life

Patient	Age	Culture
	yr	
K.R.	6	*Escherichia coli* 5000
		Proteus mirabilis 10
L.O.	8	*E. coli* $>10^5$
L.H.	6	*Aerobacter aerogenes* $>10^5$
N.C.	8	*E. coli* 560
		Staphylococcus epidermidis 110
		Streptococcus faecalis 50
		Diphtheroids 3000
O.R.	8	*E. coli* 10
		S. epidermidis 10^3
		γ-Streptococcus 10^3
		Diphtheroids $<10^4$
J.S.	8	*E. coli* 10
		S. epidermidis 50
		S. faecalis 10^3
		Diphtheroids 250
L.S.	11	Diphtheroids 2000
		S. faecalis 50
L.M.	9	*γ-Streptococcus* 10^3
		Diphtheroids 20
D.D.	10	*S. epidermidis* 260
		γ-Streptococcus 50
J.G.	5	Culture negative
S.E.	10	*S. epidermidis* 40
L.K.	7	*S. epidermidis*80

bacteria in their VB_1 urine are presented in Table 6.6. We were able to obtain repeat cultures on several of these children, and these data are also shown in Table 6.6. We have divided these results in Table 6.6 into five groups: group I = >5000 bacteria/ml, group II = 1000–5000 bacteria/ml, group III = 100–999 bacteria/ml, group IV = 11–99 bacteria/ml, and group V = 1–10 bacteria/ml.

Thus, of the 105 girls, 36 had some Gram-negative bacteria in their perineal area. But of these 36, only 14 had 100 or more colonies/ml of urine, and only 4 had >5000/ml. When the method of collecting the first voided few milliliters is considered, together with the absence of any perineal washing and the age of the child, I am impressed with how few enteric pathogens are present on the perineum of the normal girl. Indeed, the observation that 66% of the girls cultured did not contain a single Gram-negative enterobacteria is almost unbelievable.

Bollgren and Winberg[67] were the first to study the periurethral aerobic bacterial flora in healthy boys and girls systematically in detail. A quantitative sampling of the periurethral flora was accomplished by pressing a 1-cm^2 area of gelatin over the periurethral area of girls and counting the bacteria attached to the gelatin; boys were cultured by preputial irrigation with phosphate buffer. Three hundred ninety-four girls and 305 boys were cultured from birth to 16 years. During the first few weeks of life, a "massive aerobic bacterial flora" was present in the periurethral area of both sexes, including *E. coli*, enterococci, and staphylococci. Colonization with *E. coli* and enterococci diminished in the first year of life and became rare after the age of 5 years. In boys, *E. coli* was predominant in the first 7 months of life, but above this age *Proteus* and *E. coli* were equally common. *P. mirabilis* was the most common species; *Proteus morganii* was almost as frequent. In girls, *E. coli* predominated throughout the study, but colonization began to diminish in the second 6 months of life and disappeared about age 5 years. During the first 6 months of life, *Klebsiella-Enterobacter* was common and often dense in girls, undoubtedly accounting for the frequency of *Klebsiella* infection in early life. Bollgren and Winberg[67] also obtained VB_1 and VB_2 urines from girls above 5 years without any preceding cleaning; 90% of the urines were free from *E. coli* and enterococci. In VB_1 urines from 66 boys, only three contained any detectable colonies of Enterobacteriaceae and only four contained enterococci. Lastly, this excellent study was interesting in that few Gram-negative species tended to coexist together in the periurethral area; only 1 out of 123 girls and none of the boys had as many as three Gram-negative species present simultaneously.

The periurethral anaerobic microflora in healthy girls has also been studied by Bollgren and her associates[68] in Stockholm; they studied 18 premenarcheal girls, 5–14

Table 6.6
Analysis of Perineal Bacterial Flora in 36 of 105 VB_1 Cultures That Contained Gram-Negative Bacteria

Subject and Age, in Years	Initial Culture	Repeat Culture
I. Culture containing >5000 Gram-negative bacteria/ml of urine in VB_1 specimens		
P.G., 10	*Escherichia coli* >10^5	
	Proteus mirabilis 10	
D.H., 6	*E. coli* >10^5	*E. coli* 10
	E. coli Intermedia >10^5	*E. coli Int.* 0
	Klebsiella 0	*Klebsiella* 30
	Enterobacter 0	*Enterobacter* 40
L.A.,[a] 7	*E. coli* >10^5	*E. coli* 10
	Klebsiella 10^4	*Klebsiella* 10
	Sreptococcus faecalis 0	*S. faecalis* 160
	E. coli Int. 0	*E. coli Int.* 10
A.B.,[a] 8	*E. coli* 50	*E. coli* 10
	P. mirabilis 5000	*P. mirabilis* 180
	Proteus morgani 0	*P. morgani* 60
II. Culture containing 1000–5000 Gram-negative bacteria/ml of urine in VB_1 specimens		
L.D., 4	*P. mirabilis* 3000	*P. mirabilis* 0
	Klebsiella 0	*Klebsiella* 1000
A.A., 10	*E. coli* 3000	
	S. faecalis 20	
K.T., 5	*E. coli* 1000	*E. coli* 0
A.R., 10	*E. coli* 3000	
III. Culture containing 100–999 colonies of Gram-negative bacteria/ml in VB_1 specimens		
K.J., 9	*E. coli* 200	*E. coli* 20
N.G., 7	*E. coli* 130	
	S. faecalis 50	
L.U., 5	*Flavobacterium* 100	
S.S., 5	*E. coli* 350	*E. coli* 20
M.H., 7	*E. coli* 440	
N.W., 9	*E. coli* 580	*E. coli* 50
	S. faecalis 1500	*S. faecalis* 0
	Pseudomonas 0	*Pseudomonas* 1950
IV. Culture containing 11–99 colonies/ml of Gram-negative bacteria in VB_1 specimens		
S.K., 7	*Pseudomonas* 10	
	Achromobacter 20	
C.K., 5	*Achromobacter* 20	
S.E., 12	*E. coli* 50	
C.R., 6	*E. coli* 20	
	S. faecalis 2000	
L.G., 9	*E. coli* 40	*E. coli* 30
	Klebsiella 0	*Klebsiella* 20
E.H., 5	*E. coli* 20	
B.U.,[a] 9	*E. coli* 20	*E. coli* 0
S.A., 12	*E. coli* 60	
B.M., 10	*E. coli* 60	
C.P., 5	*Achromobacter* 70	
K.P., 4	*E. coli* 50	
J.R., 8	*E. coli* 30	
V. Culture containing 1-10 colonies of Gram-negative bacteria per ml in VB_1 specimens		
L.S., 12	*E. coli* 10	
K.K., 9	*E. coli* 10	
E.S., 10	*E. coli* 10	
N.F., 11	*E. coli* 10	
	S. faecalis 1000	
C.B., 6	*E. coli* 10	
C.M., 5	*E. coli* 10	
K.S., 7	*E. coli* 10	
D.B., 8	*E. coli* 10	
	Klebsiella 10	
	E. coli Int. 20	
A.H., 12	*Aerobacter aerogenes* 10	
A.A., 7	*E. coli* 10	

[a] On antibiotic at time of culture.

years of age. Obligate anaerobic bacteria made up 95 ± 5.8% of the total colony forming units per cm^2 of periurethral area. On average, 7 different anaerobic and 2.7 different aerobic strains were identified per specimen; anaerobic Gram-positive cocci and Gram-positive rods predominated. The majority of bacteria isolated from the periurethral area included peptococci, peptostreptococci, bifidobacteria, and eubacteria. The mean total colony forming units per cm^2 of periurethral area was 1.4×10^6.

I have reviewed in Chapters 4 and 5 the data on colonization of the introitus and periurethral area with Enterobacteriaceae in women and children susceptible to recurrent UTI and the relationship of this colonization to recurrent bacteriuria; these data will not be repeated here in this chapter.

Long Term Follow-Up Studies

Lindblad and Ekengren[69] found progressive renal disease in 19% of girls hospitalized for pyelonephritis during the 1940s who were reinvestigated 15–25 years later.

Gillenwater, Harrison, and Kunin[70] obtained 9–18 year follow-ups on 60 bacteriuric schoolgirls originally detected in Kunin's[17] earlier epidemiologic surveys; they were matched with 38 nonbacteriuric controls from the same classroom rosters who had never shown bacteriuria during the serial surveys at school. Urines were cultured at 6-month intervals in both groups between 1972 and 1977. Each episode of bacteriuria was treated 10–14 days with appropriate therapy. Blood pressure was measured yearly, IVUs and VCUs were obtained at least once on all subjects, the urethra was calibrated with bougie à boules at the time of cystography, and most subjects had at least two 24-hour creatinine clearances.

Blood pressures were normal in patients and controls. Serum creatinine was higher in patients (0.88 ± 0.24 mg%) than controls (0.76 ± 0.15 mg%) which was significantly different ($P < 0.004$) but did not exceed the normal range in any individual. Measurements of creatinine and inulin clearance showed only one patient with an inulin clearance below 85 ml/min; this patient had an atrophic kidney and an inulin clearance of 67 ml/min. Urethral diameter measured by bougie à boule was normal in all subjects, both patients and controls.

The radiologic changes, as always, are important, because in the absence of blood pressure and substantial changes in renal function, the IVU is the only examination that gives the investigator or student a feel for just how serious the renal disease really is. The only radiologic abnormality among the 38 controls was a single renal calculus in one individual. Although IVUs were not done at the initial screening on six patients, at follow-up five were normal and one had a renal scar. IVUs and VCUs were normal on follow-up in 34 of 60 patients (56.6%); renal scars or caliectasis were present in 16 (27%), including 2 patients with atrophic pyelonephritis. Radiologic disease in the remaining 10 patients at the final IVUs, except for one subject with sponge kidney and calcinosis, was related to VUR which was either surgically corrected, persisted as slight reflux, or disappeared. Although renal scarring and caliectasis are not separated in this analysis, 9 of 40 patients with IVUs known to be normal originally, developed "scars or caliectasis"; we also do not know the severity of the scarring but presumably it was not severe.

The morbidity for 6 of these 60 patients must have been substantial because 5 had their reflux corrected by surgery and 2 required nephrectomy. In all six instances, however, the radiologic abnormalities were detected at the initial examinations. We do not know the grade of the reflux that was corrected.

The morbidity of the bacteriuric schoolgirls in terms of hospital admissions and episodes of UTI, including bacteriuria of pregnancy, is clearly higher–as would be expected–than among the control girls. Even so, it is interesting that one-fourth of the controls were bacteriuric at pregnancy, and that 37.5% of controls had one or more episodes of bacteriuria between 1969 and 1977; 2.6% of controls had five or more bacteriuric episodes. One conclusion from this study might have been that urinary tract infections appear to reach epidemic proportions in the state of Virginia! Although the numbers are small and statistically insignificant, premature infants weighing less than 2500 grams occurred 4 times more often among controls than patients.

In summary, this important follow-up emphasizes the morbidity from recurrent bacteriuria and the clinical episodes of pyelonephritis which occurred in 25% of schoolgirls whose bacteriuria was originally detected by screening surveys. It must be emphasized that these infections were treated only with short courses of therapy; as I have indicated in Chapter 4, virtually *all* of the clinical morbidity can be stopped *completely* by continuous prophylaxis, regardless of reflux or the presence of renal scars. Some of the new scarring and caliectasis in this study, if not all of it, might have been prevented by prophylaxis.

Moreover, the morbidity in this study seems excessive when compared to the control schoolgirls left untreated in the bacteriuric surveys at Dundee,[48] Cardiff-Oxford,[47] and at Göteborg.[49] Indeed, I have commented in the preceding section how minimal the symptoms were in the untreated girls with ScBU; in the Cardiff-Oxford study, only 8% of 98 girls followed for 4 years required treatment for symptoms of UTI. How do we account for these differences? For one thing, we are not told in the Gillenwater[70] follow-up whether the few cases with high morbidity, including those with atrophic pyelonephritis or enough reflux to require surgical reimplantation, were among those children at the time of the original screening survey who were already seeing their own physician for recurrent bacteriuria. This makes a substantial difference because, to the extent that these patients fall into that symptomatic group, they really are not children whose disease is detected by screening surveys. In the Newcastle study,[35] for example, 13.4% of bacteriuric girls were known to be previously bacteriuric and should not count in screening surveys. Savage carefully excluded the 6 patients detected in his study who had a past history of UTI,[48] and I cannot tell about the Cardiff-Oxford study.[47] I believe this to be an important question because considerable surgery was performed in the Gillenwater[70] study, unlike the other three reported follow-ups, and this suggests that the populations may be different.

This study does show that 70% of bacteriuric children detected on screening surveys are susceptible to further infections later in life and about the same proportion will experience bacteriuria at one or more of their pregnancies. Since all of the serious reflux—and presumably the severe evidence of pyelonephritis—was detectable at the first IVU in this study, the major premise that most of the significant renal damage that occurs from UTI in children occurs before the age of 4 years seems unaltered by this study. Nor would anyone argue over the utility of detecting these 10% or so of young children with UTI who are at serious renal risk and increased morbidity. What remains to be seen is how many would be detected by symptomatic presentation to their physician and whether the course of their disease can be altered by treatment, either medically or surgically.

Hypertension and Renal Scarring

Although none of the patients in the Gillenwater *et al.*[70] follow-up developed hypertension, nor did any in the Cardiff-Oxford study,[47] including the 12 with renal scars, there are some patients with renal scarring who do. Andersen *et al.*[71] reported four children (ages 9–13) seen over a 11-year period at Göteborg who had severe hypertension, asymmetric renal scarring, sterile urine, and high serum antibody titers to *E. coli* 08. Three of the four had episodes of overt pyelonephritis in their earlier childhood; their published radiologic figures are typical of renal scarring and atrophy from childhood pyelonephritis. These patients need to be pointed out because all the screening surveys with long term follow-ups are showing little or no relationship between UTI and hypertension; we must not forget the exceptions because these children are seriously ill from their hypertension. The section later in this chapter on the *Ask-Upmark* kidney relates to the same problem of hypertension and atrophic kidneys.

Vesical Neck "Obstruction," Vesicoureteral Reflux, and "Distal Urethral Stenosis"

The literature on each of these three subjects is voluminous. I will discuss each briefly, primarily in the context of the female child with recurrent urinary infections who has a nonobstructive intravenous urogram, with or without evidence of localized calyceal dilatation, cortical scarring, or mild dilatation of the ureter. Consideration of children with megaloureters, from whatever cause, is beyond the scope of this chapter.

I have placed all three of these "obstructive" conditions together because a historical perspective, beginning with vesical neck "obstruction", is helpful.

Vesical Neck "Obstruction"

Interest in the etiology of urinary infections grew logarithmically in the early 1950s, largely due to the pioneering efforts of Marple (1941),[72] Barr and Rantz (1948),[73] Sanford *et al.* (1956)[74] and Kass (1956),[75] who placed the diagnosis on an objective, quantitative basis. It was therefore inevitable that urinary infections in children would occupy an important part of the American literature. In North America, as opposed to Europe and especially Sweden, most of the publications on children have appeared in the urologic literature; for this reason, much of the opinion and practice in this country—even among pediatricians—has been determined by urologists. Conditioned by his training, the urologist looked for obstruction from the very beginning. Since the most common obstruction in urologic experience is benign prostatic hyperplasia, it is perhaps understandable that the emphasis on etiology in little girls was first ascribed to vesical neck "obstruction"—despite the fact that the vast majority of men with prostatic obstruction and significant residual urine present with sterile urine prior to instrumentation.[76] Thus, much of the urologic literature between 1950 and 1965 emphasized the vesical neck as the cause of urinary infections in female children. For example, as late as 1964, Marshall[77] wrote that in children with persistent or recurring urinary infections, "over 90% are obstructive in nature" and that "nearly half of the recognizable obstructions in children are at the bladder neck." Murphy felt that 41 out of a consecutive series of 141 children with urinary infections were caused by obstruction at the bladder neck, while Hendren reported 200 operations on the vesical neck in a period of 4 years![78] Further experience, however, probably determined largely by the failure of corrective surgery at the vesical neck to prevent recurrent infections, as well as by the failure to find the hallmarks of obstruction—trabeculation, residual urine, and radiologic or physiologic evidence of obstruction—led many observers to question the vesical neck as an etiologic factor. Fortunately, Harrow, Sloane, and Witus[79] published in 1967 in the *Journal of Urology* a paper entitled "A Critical Examination of Bladder Neck Obstruction in Children." After reviewing 52 major references and carefully considering the opposing points of view, they observed the lack of evidence for a diagnosis of obstruction in cineradiographic studies, in bladder-urethral pressure measurements, in the presence of residual urine or trabeculation, and, finally, in the lack of a characteristic cystoscopic appearance at the vesical neck. They concluded that, out of 217 cases of urinary infection in their pediatric practice, true bladder obstruction could be diagnosed in only 3 instances, an experience with which many centers, including our own, would agree. The credit for the final "nail in the coffin" of bladder neck obstruction must go to Shopfner.[80] Before any urologist or pediatrician considers bladder neck obstruction based on roentgenological evidence of "contracture" or narrowing at the vesical neck, trabeculation, or residual urine, he should carefully consider Shopfner's excellent paper. Winberg[31] has commented even in 1974 that "narrowing" of the bladder neck on VCU was common in males below the age of 1 year, that the frequency decreased with increasing age, and that in longitudinally followed cases the "narrowing" tended to disappear spontaneously.

It is not important that so many urologic authorities who enthusiastically wrote and endorsed vesical neck obstruction 10 years ago were wrong, because one-half of what all of us believe today to be true will most certainly be shown one day to be incorrect—including the material in this book.

But surely from the point of history alone, should not many of those who so strongly believe today that ureteral reflux or distal urethral stenosis is the basis for childhood urinary infections recall the recent enthusiasm for correcting vesical neck "obstruction"? Indeed, it is of interest that several authorities and staunch advocates of ureteral reflux as the primary cause of urinary infections today believed with equal conviction less than a decade ago that the vesical neck was the major cause.

Vesicoureteral Reflux

Any student interested in the ureterovesical junction should begin by studying the classic paper of Tanagho and Pugh,[81] "The Anatomy and Function of the Ureterovesical Junction." After examining 20 ureterovesical junctions by dissection and 5 by serial histologic sections, Tanagho and Pugh concluded that the longitudinal muscle fibers of the roof of the intravesical segment of the ureter sweep around the ureteral orifice to join the fibers in the floor of the ureter to form the superficial trigonal muscle. By demonstrating muscular continuity of the ureter with the trigone, as well as the continuation of Waldeyer's sheath from around the extravesical and intramural ureter into the middle layer of the trigone, they tied the function of the ureterovesical junction firmly to the development of the trigonal muscles. Tanagho and Pugh also reviewed the many contributions of others who have investigated the ureterovesical junction. The essential features, then, of a normal ureterovesical junction are a delicate, slit-like orifice in a ureter that has a long submucosal intravesical segment (ratio of length of submucosal tunnel to the diameter of the orifice averages 6 or 7 to 1) and whose muscular layers (longitudinal and Waldeyer's sheath) insert into and are continuous with the trigone.

Is Vesicoureteral Reflux Normal? From a number of studies on children without evidence of urinary tract disease, it is apparent that ureteral reflux is uncommon in older children and infants who do not have urinary infection. Köllermann and Ludwig,[82] however, reported that 30% of 102 urologically normal children showed reflux on VCUs; all cases except one that showed reflux were under 3 years of age (Figure 6.14). Thus, is it possible, as Köllermann and Ludwig contended, that reflux *is a normal event* in one-third of children under 3 years of age? The 330 normal children collected by McGovern *et al.*[83] from a review of the literature in 1960, including their own "26 children under the age of 14 years," showed an incidence of reflux of only 2%. But it is important that, except for the paper by Iannaccone and Panzironi[84] almost all of these children were probably over 3 years of age, making it difficult to dispute Köllermann and Ludwig's conclusion. The paper by Lich *et al.*[85] who obtained cystograms on 26 newborns (sex not stated) in the first 48 hours of life, as well as the cystograms reported by Peters *et al.*[86] in premature infants, might at first seem to exclude reflux as a normal event in the early period of life. Lenaghan and Cussen's[87] studies, however, are interesting and may be relevant to this question of normal reflux during early development. Many of the lower species, especially the rat and rabbit, normally reflux in a majority of animals. The adult dog, however, has a normal ratio of intravesical tunnel to ureteral diameter of 6:1[88] and does not reflux except in rare instances (<5%). Despite these data in the adult dog, Lenaghan and Cussen[87] showed that 80% of pups refluxed at 2 months of age and that 50% refluxed between 2 and 4 months; only 5% refluxed at the age of 6 months. These studies mean that, in one animal which has a ureterovesical junction similar to that of man, early reflux during development is normal. The studies by Lich *et al.*[85] and Peters *et al.*[86] showing no reflux in newborn and premature infants would seem to make man different from the dog, except for an important observation: the newborn pup does not reflux until about 3 weeks of age![89]

Roberts has shown that VUR in the primate monkey is common during the first year of life.[90, 91] When present at birth, VUR gradually disappears with time in a pattern very similar to Figure 6.14 in humans[91]; almost all monkeys cease to reflux by 36

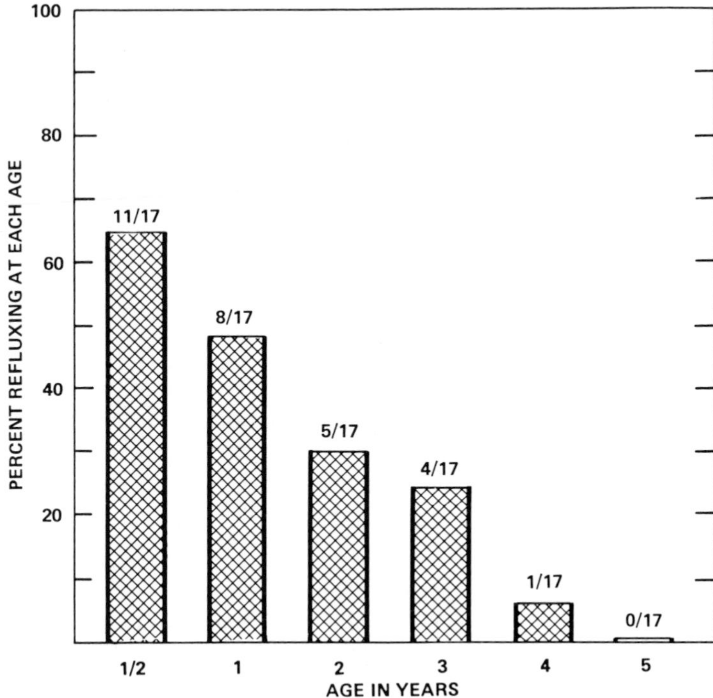

Figure 6.14 Percent of normal children demonstrating reflux between ages 6 months and 5 years. Cystourethrograms on 102 urologically normal children (boys and girls). Seventeen were studied at each age group. The declining incidence with age is clearly seen; only one child over 3 years of age refluxed. (Adapted from Köllermann and Ludwig.[82])

months of age, and there is no difference between males and females (as also found by Köllerman and Ludwig[82]).

These data in monkeys appear very similar to Köllerman and Ludwig's[82] study in young children. It is true that Köllerman and Ludwig's study has been criticized because the bladders were filled manually using a syringe which could cause high intravesical pressures. While this criticism has some validity, it cannot explain the decline in reflux with increasing age (Figure 6.14). Thus, even if high intravesical pressures were used in the Köllerman and Ludwig study, it is clear that the younger boys and girls have a less competent ureterovesical junction than children over the age of 4 years—which is, I believe, what maturation is all about.

In view of the Köllermann and Ludwig[82] investigation, Lenaghan's[87] observations on puppies, and Roberts' work with primates,[90, 91] and especially the probability that few normal children, especially girls, between the ages of 2 months and 3 years have had cystograms, it is reasonable to me that some transient reflux may be a part of normal development in completely healthy children. After all, the ureterovesical junction, as shown by Tanagho and Pugh,[81] is an elaborate neuromuscular structure intimately related to the function of the trigone.

A child does not walk when it is born; why should a complicated structure like the ureterovesical junction function as competently as an adult's in the early months of life? In truth, the question is not really important, but unfortunately there are those who view all vesicoureteral reflux as a sign of a primary defect that requires surgical correction. It is these individuals who should consider Köllermann and Ludwig's observations in children, Lenaghan's[87] studies in puppies, and Roberts'[90, 91] work in primates.

Comparison of Vesicoureteral Reflux in Children and Adults with Urinary Tract Infections. Although ureteral reflux is rare in older children (>3 years) without evidence of urinary tract disease, it is extremely common in girls who present with recurrent urinary infections. Depending somewhat on the method of doing the cystogram and undoubtedly depending on whether the cystogram is performed in the presence of untreated bacteriuria, incidence figures vary from 19% of asymptomatic schoolgirls in Kunin's series[18] to 55% in Govan and Palmer's report.[92] Smellie[51] found reflux in 34% of children referred to her because of urinary infections; in her series, cystography was performed soon after the infections were eradicated. These, and many other excellent studies, clearly establish that ureteral reflux is extraordinarily common in girls with recurrent urinary infections.

On the other hand, ureteral reflux is not common in adult women with recurrent infections. Baker and his associates[93] reported their data on 588 consecutive children and 210 consecutive adult patients studied cystographically for VUR at their initial urologic evaluation. Seventy-one percent of the children examined and 74% of the adults had a history of urinary infection; of these, 30% of the pediatric group and 5.7% of the adult group showed reflux. Of the patients with bacteriuria at the time of the cystogram, 45% of the children and 10% of the adults had reflux. When the percentage of children in each age group showing reflux was plotted against the age of the group under study, reflux was found in 70% of all children under 1 year of age, in 50% of children 1 year old, and thereafter gradually declined to the adult level of 5% (Figure 6.15). Since these data suggest that 80% of children with reflux will not show reflux in adulthood, the authors were careful to point out that neither demise from renal disease nor surgical correction can account for the apparent reversal of reflux in their population.

Heidrick, Mattingly, and Amberg[94] obtained single film cystograms during voiding in 200 patients randomly chosen in the last trimester of pregnancy. Catheterized urines were carefully obtained for culture at the time of cystogram. A group of 121 additional patients had a cineradiographic study of the entire act of voiding within the first 30 hours postpartum. Of the 321 patients, 9 (2.8%) showed VUR while 20 (6.2%) were bacteriuric. Of the nine patients

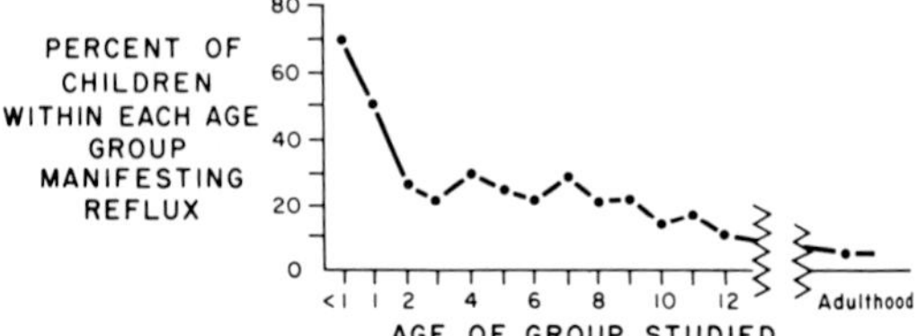

Figure 6.15 The percentage of children showing reflux within each age group (vertical scale) is plotted against the age of each group studied. These data are derived from a study of 588 consecutive children under 13 years old; the single point for adulthood (>12 years old) is based on 210 consecutive adult patients. Seventy-one percent of the children and 74% of the adults had a history of urinary infections. (Reproduced by permission from R. Baker *et al.*, J. Urol. **95:** 27, 1966.[93])

showing VUR, only one was infected, but three had a previously documented episode of acute pyelonephritis. There was, however, "conspicuous absence of radiographic changes consistent with chronic pyelonephritis in all cases of reflux."

Williams, Davies, Evans, and Williams[45] in a most thorough study, investigated, 4–6 months after delivery, 100 of 115 women who had proven coliform bacteriuria during pregnancy. No patient was treated after delivery. Four to 6 months following delivery, residual urine, urine culture, IVU, and VCU were performed on all 100 patients. Thirty-two patients were infected and 68 were sterile; there was no difference in residual urine between the two groups, and the "majority had residual volumes of less than 10 ml." VUR was found in 21 patients (21%), and coliform bacteriuria was present in 13 of these 21 (62%).

Is Vesicoureteral Reflux Caused by Obstruction? The increasing use of the image intensifier and television fluoroscopy in cystourethrography in the 1950s and early 1960s emphasized the high incidence of ureteral reflux in children with urinary tract disease. It was only natural that bladder neck obstruction would be considered a primary cause for ureteral reflux.

Stephens and Lenaghan[95] first questioned this practice and presented some compelling evidence to the contrary. They pointed out the lack of radiographic evidence for bladder neck or urethral obstruction in children with VUR who had VCUs. More importantly, they measured the bladder and urethral pressures synchronously during filling and voiding in three groups of children: (1) those with normal urinary tracts (21 patients), (2) those with definite proven urethral obstruction (24 patients, mainly with prostatic valves), and (3) those with idiopathic VUR (25 patients). There was no difference in the filling or voiding pressures between the normal children and the idiopathic VUR group. Only the children with proven urethral obstruction showed high bladder pressures. Even in this group, the authors could observe no correlation between the degree of obstruction and the presence of reflux; *i.e.*, the highest vesical pressures were often associated with either no reflux or unilateral reflux. Moreover, in Stephens' series[96] of prostatic valves in children, surely the worst obstruction encountered in pediatric urology, only one-third showed reflux. Thus, since reflux was not related *per se* to severe proven urethral obstruction, in the words of Stephens and Lenaghan,[95] "it is still less likely to be caused by hypothetical unproven obstructions of the bladder neck." As further evidence that pure obstruction is a rare cause of ureteral reflux, Morielo *et al.*,[97] using an excellent radiographic technique, obtained cystograms on 100 men with bladder neck obstruction; 79 had benign prostatic hyperplasia, 11 had bladder contracture, and 10 had prostatic carcinoma. Reflux, ranging from a "trickle of dye" to a "complete pyeloureterogram," was demonstrated in only 13 of the 100 men, and 9 of the 13 were infected at the time of the cystogram. Their two published examples of reflux to the kidney show minimal dilatation of the collecting system. It is clear that classic prostatic obstruction is rarely associated with even minimal reflux.

Two final studies should be presented. Zatz[98] measured the voiding pressures, intra-abdominal pressures, and maximal urinary flow rates in conjunction with cineradiography in 30 of our girls at Stanford with recurrent urinary infections. There was no detectable difference in bladder function between the 15 girls who refluxed and the 15 who did not, thereby excluding an obstructive factor as the cause of reflux. The majority of children showed no evidence of outlet obstruction, but in the few that did, the obstruction was not located at the vesical neck. Zatz also emphasized the lack of correlation between the findings at cystoscopy or on VCU (the radiologic configuration) with the physiologic evaluation of the condition of the outlet.

The last study which emphasizes that reflux is rarely, if ever, caused by obstruction at the bladder outlet is the work by Lenaghan and Cussen[87] on puppies. After observing that virtually all puppies reflux at 1 month of age, but only 5% at 6 months, Lenaghan and Cussen ingeniously superimposed severe urethral obstruction on refluxing puppies. In no instance did the superimposed obstruction prevent or even delay the spontaneous cessation of reflux.

Does Sterile Reflux Cause Renal Damage? This is the least controversial question of all to answer. The evidence shows that primary reflux, in the absence of urinary infection, does not produce progressive renal deterioration. All of us have had the experience of seeing the healthy adult patient in whom reflux was an unexpected finding, such as in a preoperative cystogram to measure urethral angles for stress incontinence in an older female. The best documented single case report, however, is that of Sargent,[99] who described a 36-year-old man with bilateral reflux and a "gaping right ureteral orifice" documented at age 14; there was no evidence of renal damage. He was seen again 23 years later because of symptoms of "chronic prostatitis." A complete urologic examination confirmed bilateral reflux, gaping ureteral orifices, and sterile urine without "the slightest change in the entire urinary tract on urographic examination."

Stephens and Lanaghan[95] followed 34 patients with reflux for 5–10 years, studying renal function by repeated urography (including measurements of the thickness of renal parenchyma), concentration tests, and blood urea concentrations. Nineteen of the 34 patients were cured of their infections by antibiotics and a triple-voiding regimen; no deterioration of renal function occurred in these patients, and reflux gradually ceased in many of them.

Perhaps the most convincing study is that of Fritjofsson and Sundin from Göteborg.[100] They studied renal function in nine patients with unilateral, iatrogenic reflux and compared the refluxing kidney to the contralateral, nonrefluxing kidney for a period of 1–11 years. Six patients had no urinary infection during the years of follow-up and no change occurred in any parameter of renal function, including glomerular filtration rate, renal plasma flow, and the extraction of *p*-aminohippurate. Three patients had repeated episodes of urinary infection and showed deterioration on the refluxing side; one of these three, however, also showed evidence of chronic pyelonephritis in the contralateral kidney as well where micturition cystography had failed to demonstrate reflux.

The most convincing study of sterile reflux in children is that of Heale and Ferguson.[101] They followed 34 boys with gross, grade III, reflux for 10 years. Fifty-one kidneys were involved. No scars developed in 12 normal kidneys and 26 scarred kidneys in the presence of sterile urine, but scars did develop in 6 kidneys associated with infection. In three patients, renal function deteriorated during the teenage years in the presence of sterile urine and tumultuous bilateral reflux; all three of these patients, however, had thin rim cortical kidneys when they first presented with symptoms.

From these studies, and in the absence of any evidence to the contrary, the practicing physician can safely conclude that reflux in the presence of a sterile urinary tract does not harm the kidneys.

Vesicoureteral Reflux in Female Children with Recurrent Urinary Infections: Surgical Correction or Medical Maintenance of a Sterile Urine? This, of course, is the major problem. I would like to reemphasize that I am not concerned here with the intravenous urographic finding of grossly dilated and tortuous megaureters; these present special problems, not only in the question of proper surgical management but also as to the question of etiology. For example, they are sometimes seen in children in whom infection is only transient and not a major problem. Stephens and Lenaghan[95] believe that these large ureters represent a primary developmental anomaly and that the reflux is not the cause of the dilatation. These cases constitute only a small fraction of the 50% of symptomatic girls with urinary infections who have radiographically demonstrable reflux.

Medical Treatment. Before considering the reported results of antireflux surgery, certain facts seem well established. First, reflux in the presence of infections is an indisputable cause of pyelonephritis and scarring in children. Williams and Eckstein[34] found renal scarring in 31% of their series of 276 children with reflux. Smellie and Normand[102] reported that 38 of 130 cases (29%) had pyelonephritic scars; the radiologic abnormalities found on intravenous urography and voiding cystography in these 130 children are reproduced in Table 6.7. I have already reviewed the prevalence and grade of VUR in relation to renal scarring in both children who present with symptomatic infections and those who are detected by screening surveys.

Table 6.7
Urinary Tract Abnormalities Associated with Reflux in 130 Children
Thirty-one males; 99 females.[a]

Condition	Number	Percent
Abnormal IVU or cystogram	62	(48)
Chronic pyelonephritis	38	(29)
Double kidney ± ureter	10	
Hydronephrosis	7	
Horseshoe kidney	1	
Renal calculus	1	
Ectopic kidney	1	
Urethrocele	1	
Bladder diverticulum	3	
"Corkscrew" urethra	3	
No other abnormality of IVU or cystogram	68	(52)

[a] Adapted from J. M. Smellie and I. C. S. Normand: Urinary Tract Infection. London, Oxford University Press, 1968, p. 123[102]

Second, it is equally indisputable that reflux disappears in a significant number of these children when a sterile urine is continuously maintained for months or years. Several investigators have established this point. Stephens and Lenaghan[95] followed 34 patients (59 refluxing ureters) for 5–10 years; reflux spontaneously ceased in 19, decreased in 17, and remained unchanged in 23. They related these differences to the control of infection. Smellie and Normand[102] performed serial cystograms on 100 refluxing ureters in children on continuous antimicrobial therapy; reflux disappeared in 42 of these ureters, but subsequently returned in 5 of the 42. Twenty-four of the 100 ureters showed no reflux on two successive cystograms. In an earlier publication, reproduced in Figure 6.16, Smellie[51] showed that all grades of reflux tended to improve with control of the infection except when reflux was associated with severe dilatation of the ureter and renal pelvis. In their latest analysis,[57] the group at University College Hospital in London has shown that reflux disappeared spontaneously in 71% of children and from 79% of affected ureters during long term prophylaxis. This occurred at any age and was unrelated to infancy or puberty. Reflux disappeared from 85% of ureters of normal calibre but from only 41% of dilated ureters. The period of follow-up reported in this informative study was 7–15 years.[57] Penn and Breidahl[103] followed 47 children with 63 refluxing ureters for periods of 1–5 years (70% were followed for 3 or more years). Reflux spontaneously ceased in one-third of the ureters, and, again, these ureters were in patients who had the least problem with infection. Howerton and Lich[104] reported their observations in 1963 on 1000 consecutive voiding vesicourethrograms in 558 patients. Of 130 patients with ureteral reflux, 32 showed no reflux after 3 months of successful medical therapy. I have already referred to the excellent study by Rolleston, Shannon, and Utley[53] in 175 consecutive infants with UTI investigated at Christchurch. Their classification of reflux was similar to that in Figures 6.6–6.8. The relationship between the grade of reflux and

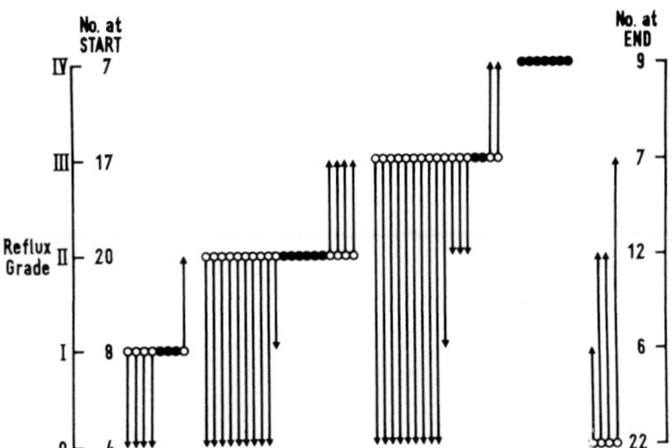

Figure 6.16 The progress of reflux in 56 ureters (34 children) followed for 1–9 years. Each circle represents a ureter; the *filled circles* remained unchanged, but the *open circles* moved in the direction indicated by the *arrow*. Reflux was graded as follows: grade I, reflux into the lower ureter, not extending above the pelvic brim; grade II, reflux up to the kidney on micturition; grade III, reflux in a normal-sized ureter up to the kidney both at rest and on micturition; and grade IV, reflux extending up to the kidney with dilatation of the renal pelvis and ureter. The number of ureters in each grade at the start of therapy (left-hand vertical scale) is compared to the number in each grade at the end of therapy (right-hand vertical scale). Thus, there were 17 ureters with grade III reflux at the beginning of treatment but only 7 in this grade at the time of this report; only 2 of the original 17 advanced to grade IV and 2 (*filled circles*) remained unchanged. (Reproduced by permission from J. M. Smellie, J. R. Coll. Phys. **1:** 189, 1967.[51])

renal scars on presentation (Figure 6.9) and the progression of renal damage (Figure 6.10) has already been presented in this chapter. VCUs were repeated in 28 infants, comprising 35 of the original ureters. As seen in Figure 6.17, reflux had spontaneously ceased in 19 of the 35 ureters (54%); 18 of these 19 occurred in children with moderate (grade II) reflux while only 1 occured in an infant with gross reflux. In Edwards *et al.*[57] study, however, with much longer follow-ups and during long term prophylaxis, 41% of these grossly dilated ureters ceased refluxing.

In the Cardiff-Oxford study,[47] reflux disappeared completely in 33 of 81 ureters (41%) and was reduced in severity in another 17 (21%) during the 4-year follow-up.

DEGREE OF REFLUX vs DISAPPEARANCE OF REFLUX

GROSS	– 8	→	1/8
MODERATE	– 27	→	18/27
	35 URETERS		

Figure 6.17 Re-examination of 35 ureters by cystogram 6 months to 5 years later. VCUs were repeated in 28 children of the original 175 infants in the Christchurch series.[53] These VCUs comprised 35 of the original 130 refluxing ureters. Reflux disappeared in 18 of the 27 ureters with moderate (grade 2) reflux (67%), but in only one of the 8 ureters with gross reflux (13%).

Of the 12 ureters with grade III reflux, VUR disappeared in only 2 (17%). It was particularly interesting that disappearance of reflux occurred with equal frequency in treated and control groups and appeared unrelated to the duration of bacteriuria over the 4-year interval.

In the 24 of 78 schoolgirls who refluxed in Lindberg's study,[49] VUR disappeared in 12 of the 30 refluxing ureters (40%) during the 3-year follow-up. VUR changed from grade II to grade I in 6 ureters, was unchanged in 10, and increased from grade I to grade II in 2 ureters. Disappearance of VUR or a change from grade II to grade I was much more common in girls with unscarred kidneys than in those with renal scarring, even though at the time of initial detection of VUR the degree of reflux did not differ between the groups with and without parenchymal changes.[105]

Lenaghan observed spontaneous cessation of reflux in 42% of 35 boys and 67 girls.[106]

Stephens[107] observed 101 children with reflux from 5–15 years; he excluded those with duplication of the ureter, urethral obstruction, paraureteral diverticula and neurogenic bladders. Reflux ceased spontaneously in 68% of normal calibre and 33% of dilated ureters. Renal scarring correlated with infection and reflux.

It seems fair to conclude from these carefully documented reports that at least one-third of ureteral reflux in children with urinary infection will cease in a reasonably short period of time, certainly within a year or two, with no other therapy than control of the urinary infection. With long term prophylaxis, however, VUR ceased in 71% of children.[57] Even those ureters with grade 4 dilatation by Smellie's[57] classification showed disappearance of VUR in 41% after 7–15 years of follow-up.

Surgical Treatment. The difficulty with evaluating the results of surgical therapy lies not in the question of whether the reflux can be corrected, because the Leadbetter-Politano technique of tunneling the ureter[108] has an 80–90% success rate with many urologists. As with many surgical operations today, the first and basic question is not whether the surgical procedure is technically feasible, but *whether or not a technically successful operation influences the course of the disease.* Since even a casual review of the literature shows that reflux in children is mainly of importance in the presence of infection, those who advocate antireflux operations must show either a significant improvement in renal function or a decreased susceptibility to urinary infections. Renal function, however, is difficult to measure serially in children, it requires ureteral catheterization studies in unilateral reflux, and interpretation of any result is complicated by hypertrophy of renal parenchyma that is unaffected by infection. For these reasons, there are no data available on changes in renal function following antireflux operations. Orikasa *et al.*[109] have suggested that renal growth be used as a functional measure in following kidneys with grade 3 reflux; they present a convincing case for failure of some of these kidneys to grow. In the presence of UTI or even a past episode of pyelonephritis, the recent studies of Winberg *et al.*[58] must be considered carefully before attributing the failure to grow to the presence of VUR. Indeed, Wikstad *et al.*[110] followed renal growth in 8 girls with grade 3 reflux for 3–6 years; they found a positive correlation between the reduction of renal parenchyma, which occurred in all girls, and the number of episodes of pyelonephritis. Since renal function data are not available, do successful antireflux operations prevent recurrence of urinary infection? To answer this question requires only serial cultures in an operated and nonoperated group of reasonably matched controls. Despite hundreds of these operations in the past 18 years, there are few published data to answer this question, largely owing to the historical reticence of the urologist to do urine cultures. In one of the few papers with bacteriologic data, Govan and Palmer[92] compared 62 children with urinary infections; 31 had reflux and successful antireflux procedures while 31 showed no reflux and had only urethral dilatation. Seventy-one percent of those without reflux had recurrence of urinary infection within 12 months, while 58% of the previously refluxing children recurred by 1 year. Although the numbers are somewhat confusing in this report, the major difficulty is that the control children were not similar to the refluxing group. Nevertheless, this paper does establish that over half of the children with successful antireflux operations will have recurrence of bacteriuria in the first 12 months after surgery. Indeed, we pointed out in 1965[111] that surgical correction of ureteral reflux in a female child with recurrent urinary infection did not prevent recurrence of the infection and that earlier publications reporting "surgical correction of reflux . . . sterilizes the urine"[112] were questionable. Huland, Scherf, and Köllermann[113] from Hamburg, Germany have allowed me to reproduce their careful study on UTI before and after successful reimplantation of refluxing ureters; it is obvious in Figure 6.18 that surgical correction of ureteral reflux did not prevent reinfection of the urinary tract. Govan and Palmer[92] contended that surgical correction of reflux reduced the incidence of clinical episodes of pyelonephritis from 79% preoperatively to 7% postoperatively. But without a matched series of controls, it is possible—indeed highly

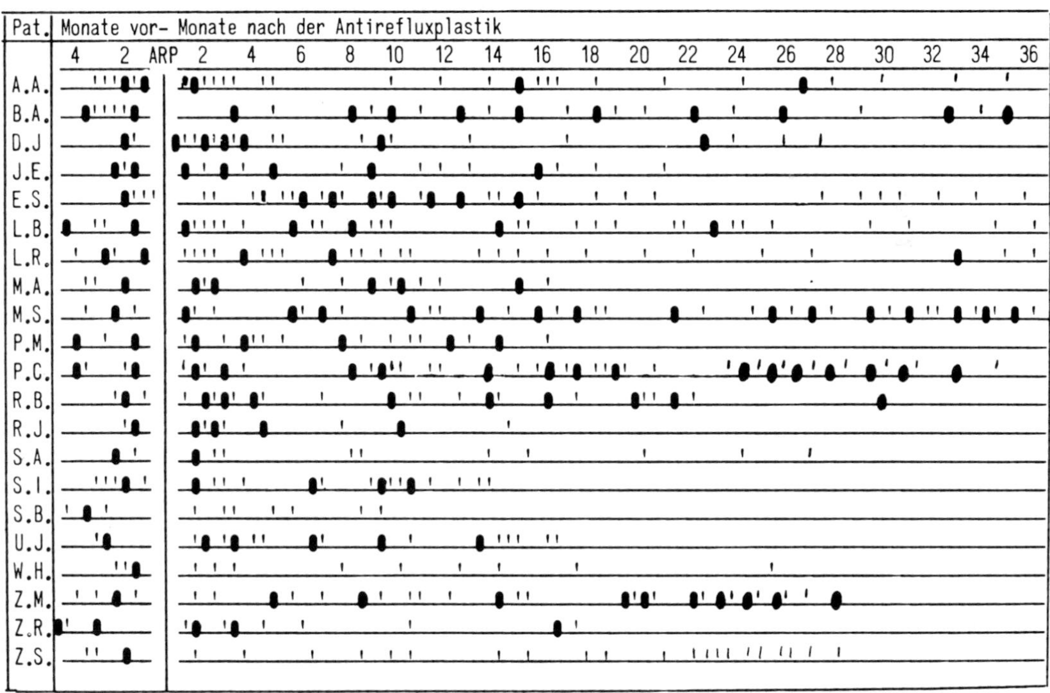

Figure 6.18 Urine cultures before and after ureteral reimplantation for vesicoureteral reflux in 21 females (mean age, 12 years). Voiding cystourethrograms after surgery showed persistent reflux in patients S.B. and W.H., two of the only three patients whose recurrent infections ceased. All other patients continued to have reinfections after the successful antireflux surgery. Each infection was treated for 10 days only. (Reproduced by permission from H. Huland, *et al.*, Urologe, A **17:** 282, 1978.[113])

likely—that postoperative antimicrobial management and family awareness of the problem were far superior to the period before surgery.

In 1975, Govan *et al.*[43] summarized the Stanford experience in managing children with UTI and VUR. They divided all patients who had received only short term therapy for each infection, and who had been followed for at least 1 year, into three groups: (1) 42 girls with VUR who were treated only with antimicrobial therapy; (2) 61 girls with VUR whose ureters were surgically reimplanted; and (3) 66 nonrefluxing girls with recurrent UTI. The percent remaining with recurrent infections after each treatment is plotted on the vertical axis of Figure 6.19 and the number of treatments on the horizontal axis. As can be readily seen, recurrent infections were the same in all three groups; surgical correction of VUR did not change the susceptibility of the child to recurrent UTI. The rate at which girls go into remission after each treatment in Figure 6.19 is essentially the same as Kunin[64] found for short term medical treatment—about 20% (see Figure 6.13). I know of no figure or table in the infection literature that indicates more strongly than Figure 6.19 that the basic cause of recurrent UTI in females must be biological; it certainly is not surgical.

Hendren[114] has published his 10-year experience in which he maintains that 73% of 409 children (807 ureters) were free of urinary infection following reimplantation of their ureters. Excluding cases less than 6 months postoperative, he reported "91% of the overall group are now off therapy and free of infection." Although Hendren stated that "all children were followed with monthly cultures with colony counts," he did not define a "positive culture" or describe how the cultures were obtained. Since a "high proportion [of his patients] represented problem cases referred often from a considerable distance," the methodology of collecting, culturing, and interpreting the urine cultures must have varied widely, and probably negated much of the bacteriologic data.

Intrarenal Reflux. If contrast agent is injected with sufficient force during retrograde pyelograms performed at the time of cystoscopy, the contrast agent will pass from the calyces into the renal tubules (pyelotubular backflow); the cortex drained by the papillus is usually filled in a broad,

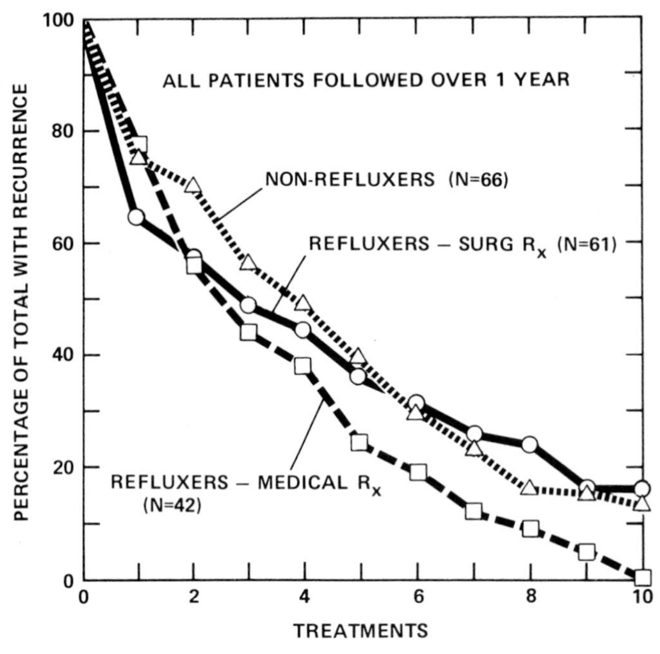

Figure 6.19 Urinary tract infection in girls. Extraction percentage following each infection. Results of short-term antibacterial therapy in three groups of children with recurrent bacteriuria: 66 without ureteral reflux, 42 with ureteral reflux treated with medical therapy alone, 61 with reflux corrected surgically. Results as plotted indicate similar cure rate in each of three groups after each treatment of an infection.

wedge-shaped area extending to the renal capsule (Figure 6.20). Hodson, who had earlier in 1960 with Edwards called attention to the relationship between renal scarring in children and VUR,[115] was able to obstruct the bladder neck of pigs and produce intrarenal reflux (IRR) and scarring at abnormally high bladder pressures[116]; most of the IRR occurred at bladder pressures greater than 35 mm Hg (normal voiding pressures for the pig were 15–30 mm Hg). At these high pressures, the ureterovesical junction decompensated, the ureters became dilated and aperistaltic, and the high bladder pressure was freely communicated to the renal calyces thereby producing the IRR.

Ransley and Risdon[117-119] showed that the anatomy of the renal papillae determined the presence or absence of IRR in infants, children and pigs. Renal papillae are either simple or compound papillae (Figure 6.21). In simple papillae, the openings of the papillary ducts are slit-like so that when intracalyceal pressure rises from obstruction or high pressure reflux, these slit-like openings are forced shut and no IRR occurs. In compound papillae, however, the papillary duct openings are circular which cannot close when the intracalyceal pressure rises. On further study, it was found that the openings of the renal tubules at the tips of the compound papillae were either convex (type 1), concave (type 2), or deeply concave (type 3); the degree of concavity appeared to determine the ease with which IRR occurred. They showed that relatively low pressures caused intrarenal reflux in type 3 and some type 2 papillae; high pressure forced the type 1 compound papillus from a convex into a concave position which then admitted reflux into the renal tubules. My colleague and friend, Professor Gerald Friedland at Stanford University, has compiled the research information of Ransley and Risdon[119] into a single, comprehensive figure which he has kindly allowed me to reproduce as Figure 6.22. The representation of the changes in the openings of the ducts of Bellini in relation to the type of compound papillus is detailed but accurate.

It is clinically important that compound calyces are mainly found in the upper and lower pole calyces, which is exactly where most of the renal scarring occurs in children. It is also interesting clinically that these investigators were unable to produce renal scars or calyceal clubbing in young growing pigs with IRR regardless of the pressure at which the IRR occurred; when bacteriuria was present, however, with the IRR, acute pyelonephritis occurred with subsequent typical scar formation.

Tamminen and Kaprio[120] examined 20 cadavers in children from premature infants to 10 years of age; they found that the size of the papillary orifices were the same in small kidneys (4–17 g) as they were in large kidneys (30–110 g), which means they are relatively larger and closer together in small kidneys. They also found that 25% of all papillae were concave ("nonconvex"); 50% were located in the upper pole and 30% in the lower pole. In only one-third of the kidneys were all the papillae convex and presumably nonrefluxing.

Funston and Cremin[121] monitored intrarenal pressure and performed retrogrades in 100 normal necropsy kidneys from infants and children under 12 years old. One hundred percent of compound calyces showed IRR at 20 mm Hg, while only 6.3% of simple calyces refluxed at this pressure. At 50 mm Hg, 100% of all simple calyces could be made to reflux. It is interesting to compare these pressures to the intravesical pressures developed by the obstructed bladder of the pig in Hodson's studies.[116]

Perhaps the most important aspect of this simple but intriguing study by Funston and Cremin[121] is their demonstration that the pressure at which IRR occurs in infants under 1 year is proportional to their age; neonates less than 30 days old showed IRR at 2 mm Hg, and the pressure gradually rose with each succeeding month of infancy until at 12 months of age 20 mm Hg was required to cause IRR in all children (for the compound calyces).

When one considers these pressure studies in fresh cadaver kidneys[121] and the constant size of the openings of the ducts of Bellini whether the kidneys weigh 5 g or

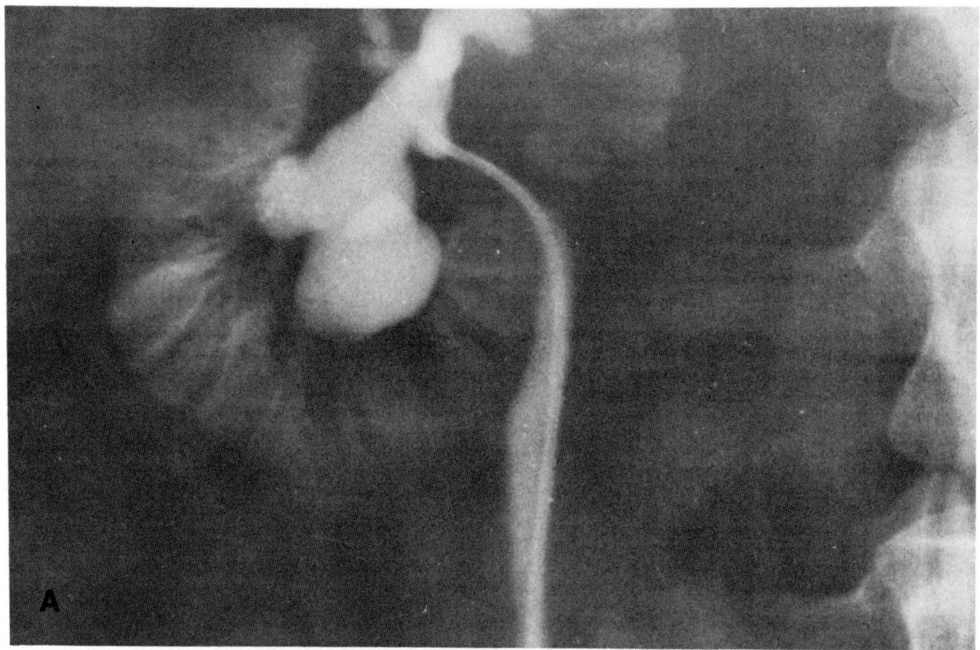

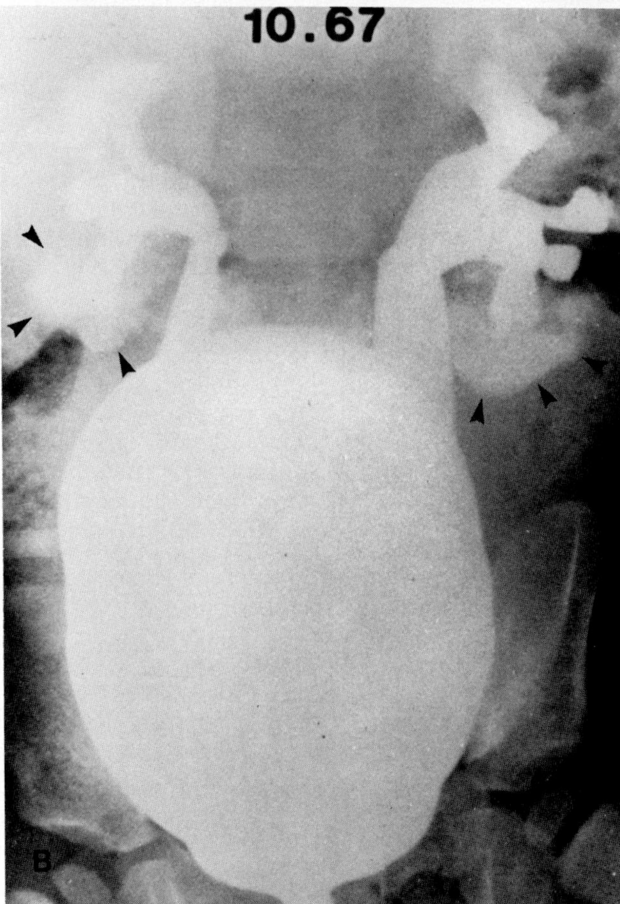

Figure 6.20 (*A*) Intratubular renal reflux in a right retrograde urogram. The streaking of contrast through the renal tubules is particularly well seen. (*B*) A voiding cystourethrogram in a 4-year-old girl seen at Stanford in October 1967. Notice the gross intrarenal reflux at both lower poles (*arrows*); it is also present in the upper pole calyces but is too faint to be seen well. By January 1969, renal scars had developed in all four areas of intrarenal reflux. (Reproduced by permission from R. A. Filly *et al.* West. J. Med. **121:** 374, 1974.[42])

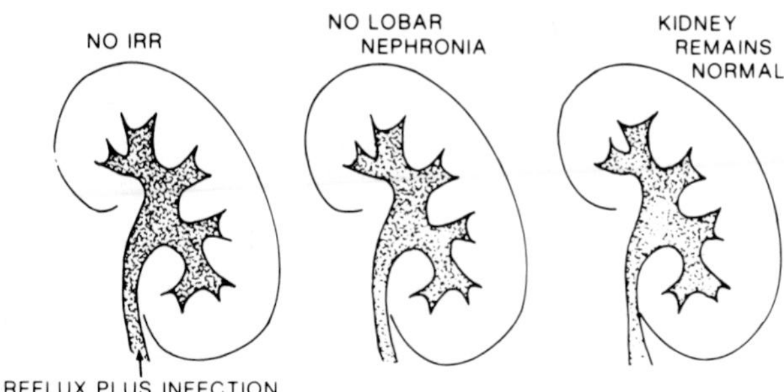

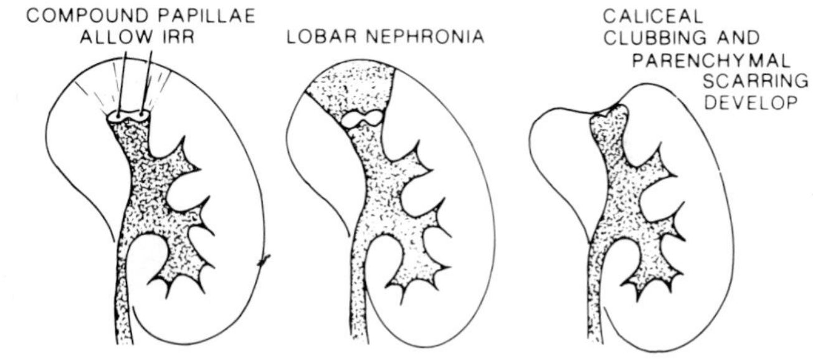

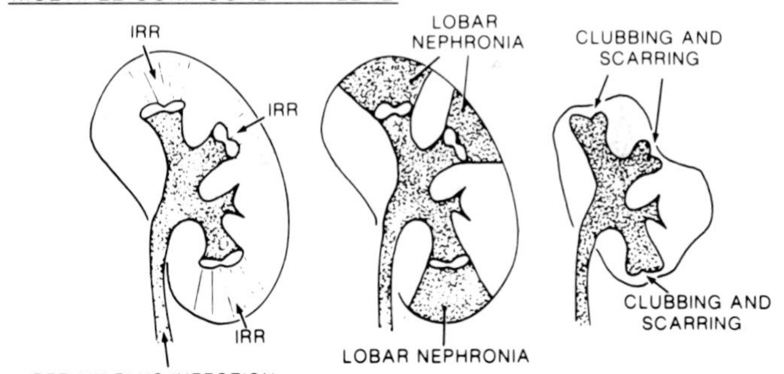

Figure 6.21 *IRR* = intrarenal reflux; *lobar nephronia* = bacterial inflammation of a renal lobe (the area drained by a calyx). Thirty percent of human kidneys contain only simple papillae. Fifty percent of nonconvex, potentially refluxing papillae are located in the upper pole and 30% in the lower pole of the human kidney (see text). (Reproduced by permission from R. A. Filly *et al.*, West. J. Med. **121:** 374, 1974.[42])

100 g,[120] it is little wonder that much of the renal scarring occurs in infants with UTI under 1 year.

How common is IRR in children? Rolleston, Maling, and Hodson[122] reviewed the Christchurch VCUs and found 16 instances of IRR in 386 patients who had VUR (4%); in terms of refluxing kidneys, rather than patients, there were 20 with IRR out of 564 ureters (3.5%). An important observation is that all instances of IRR occurred in children under the age of 4 years, and 10 of the 16 patients were under 1 year of age. Of the 241 patients with reflux under 4 years of age, the 16 children with IRR represent 6.6% of the total who refluxed.

If my mathematics are correct, the number of children with IRR is as follows: if 1% of children under 4 years of age have bacteriuria, if 30% of the bacteriuric children have reflux, and if 6% of those who reflux have IRR, then $0.01 \times 0.30 \times 0.06 = 1.8 \times 10^{-4}$, or 1 in 5555 children under 4 will have IRR. It is clearly not a problem of public health magnitude.

Duplication of the Ureters. Several investigators[31, 35, 105] have commented on the apparently unexpected incidence of ure-

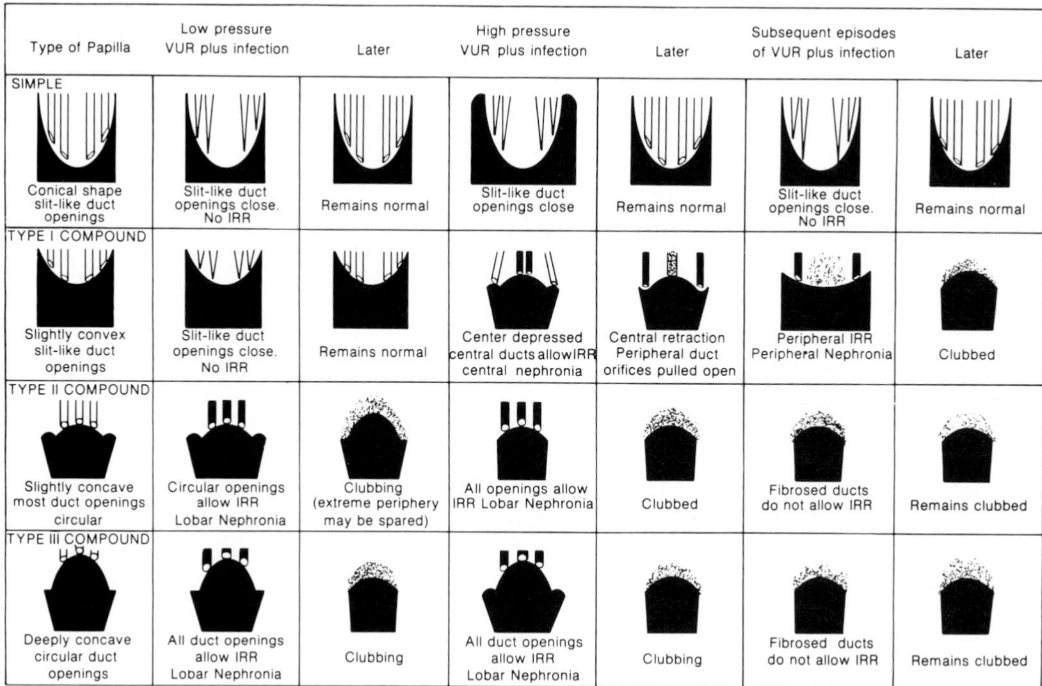

Figure 6.22 The theoretical relationship of the type of papilla with low or high pressure vesicoureteral reflux (VUR) in relation to intrarenal reflux based on the studies of Ransley and Risdon.[119] In this diagram, courtesy of Dr. Gerald Friedland, Stanford University, the response of the four types of renal papillae in the presence of vesicoureteral reflux and infection is nicely demonstrated. The reader should initially follow the behavior of the four types of renal papillae in the presence of vesicoureteral reflux and infection by following the diagram from top to bottom. In the *left-most column*, the papillae vary from a convex shape in which the papillary duct openings are slit-like, to a less convex shape, to a progressively more concave shape, in which the papillary duct openings become progressively more circular as well. Reading the diagram horizontally, however, will show what happens to each type papilla, given the presence of VUR plus infection. The simple papilla (*first row*) will under no circumstance allow intrarenal reflux (IRR). Type I compound papilla (*second row*) will not allow IRR in the presence of low-pressure VUR; in the presence of high-pressure VUR, however, the center of the papilla may be depressed, allowing IRR through the central ducts, which may then retract as they scar, and pull peripheral duct orifices open. Further VUR may lead to IRR through these peripheral ducts, so that the entire process may be progressive. With both types II and III compound papillae (*third and fourth rows*), the circular duct openings will allow IRR in the presence of VUR at any pressure, leading to clubbing and scarring, in the presence of infection.

teral duplication in children with UTI. In the Lindberg[105] series it occurred in 4.3%, and in the Newcastle study[35] 6.3%, with which there was a statistically significant association with reflux and scarring. Interestingly, most of the association in the Newcastle study was not with complete duplication, but rather bifid renal pelves which makes the association difficult to understand. Winberg has an excellent discussion of duplication in his analysis of UTI in symptomatic children.[31]

Familial Reflux. De Vargas *et al.*[123] reported a 10–20 times increase in the expected incidence of VUR in siblings and parents of children with UTI. Bailey and Wallace[124] at Christchurch investigated the immediate family of 42 patients with "reflux nephropathy"; in 12 families they found 1 or more affected members. In a separate study, they found a weak association ($P < 0.05$) between reflux nephropathy (RN) in patients with renal failure and the HLA-B 12 genetic marker in comparison to other causes of renal failure. RN, a term apparently originated simultaneously by Bailey and Heale, is best defined as VUR with renal caliectasis and thinning of the renal cortex.

Heale *et al.*[125] studied the family members of 15 children and adults among 213 patients with RN in whom a casual enquiry revealed some familial history relating to urinary tract disease. There were 175 relations to these 15 patients and all had IVUs(!); VCUs were obtained in those who showed renal scarring or a confirmed history of urinary infection. Scars with reflux were found in 21 subjects, scars without reflux in 17, reflux alone in 5, and other urinary tract abnormalities in 24; an autosomal dominant inheritance with variable clinical expression was suggested in 12 of the 15 families. It is clear from this study that investigation of families with a history of urinary tract disease will uncover substantial renal scarring.

The literature of the past decade now contains many references to the familial occurrence of VUR, most of which can be obtained from the more recent ones of the last 4 years.[126–132] In the recent follow-up by Gillenwater *et al.*,[70] UTI occurred in 7 of the offspring from 60 patients with childhood UTI but in none of the children of the controls.

Vesicoureteral Reflux as a Cause of End-Stage Renal Failure. One of the strongest arguments that sterile VUR may be harmful to the kidney has always been a small group of patients who present in renal failure with contracted kidneys, VUR of varying grades, and no discernible history of UTI. The data of Heale *et al.*[125] gives us the best idea of the numbers involved in terms of those who present with sterile VUR from their large series of patients with RN at Christchurch. Of 213 infants, children, and adults with RN seen in the Radiology Department at Christchurch Public Hospital, 20 either presented with or ultimately developed renal failure (10%), a figure that easily approximates the percent of renal scars detected on screening surveys that appear radiologically serious (one-sixth of the scars in the Newcastle study[35] were considered "severe"; only 1 of the 12 children with parenchymal reduction in Lindberg's series[49] had severe bilateral scarring; one cannot assess in the Cardiff-Oxford study[47] how substantial the renal scarring was in the 13 of the 44 who had bilateral disease; and there were apparently no serious cases of bilateral pyelonephritis in the small series of 3 children with scarring reported by Savage *et al.*[133] Of these 20 patients with renal failure, however, 9 came from the only 18 patients in the 213 with RN who had "sterile" RN. Thus, there is clearly a disproportionate number of patients who present with sterile RN (sterile on presentation and no discernible history of UTI) who are in renal failure; these patients, of course, usually present late in the course of their disease.

Heale and Ferguson[101] observed the effect of prolonged gross reflux on 51 kidneys in 34 boys followed for at least 10 years. No scars developed with sterile reflux in 12 normal kidneys and 26 scarred kidneys. Scars did develop in six kidneys associated with UTI. In three boys, however, renal function deteriorated during the teenage period in association with sterile and "tumultuous bilateral reflux"; in these three boys, all had bilateral thin rim kidneys at the time of initial presentation. These authors, from a study of 342 children with renal scarring from a population of 1000 with VUR, believe that a significant number of children with reflux are born with congenital renal disease (whether from intrauterine reflux damage or not); they base this belief on the clinical observation of the severity of the renal disease on first presentation in infancy and the paucity of infection morbidity to account for the degree of renal disease, even though there was a recorded urinary infection or a history of infection immediately prior to presentation in 326 of the 342 children (95%) with renal scarring.[101] Of 79 affected kidneys with a mean age at presentation of 11 weeks, 25 already showed a thin rim of renal cortex and extreme caliectasis similar to that usually associated with obstructive uropathy; Heale and Ferguson[101] believe this disease is congenital rather than acquired, and they make a good case for it.

Salvatierra and Tanagho[134] examined 32 patients (mean age 21.2 years) presenting with end-stage renal failure who had bilateral, low pressure VUR; 22 had experienced recurrent UTI, but 10 were sterile and had no history of UTI. It is these latter 10 patients that create the classic dilemma of whether sterile reflux causes renal disease or not. Clearly, however, they could come from the "thin rim" kidneys observed by Heale and Ferguson[101] in infancy because, although a few of these infants die in childhood or earlier, most do not and many show some renal growth on short term follow-ups of a few years.

It would be useful to know the grade of reflux from VCUs in the 32 patients reported by Salvatierra and Tanagho[134] because one would expect all to have a grade III reflux since this is the group that shows most of the renal damage in infancy; unfortunately, this information is not available, but it is my impression from examining similar cases that the ureters rarely show extreme tortuosity and that the pelvis and calyces are often dilated only in proportion to the severe renal cortical atrophy.

Huland *et al.*[135] followed-up on their transplant patients in Hamburg, Germany who had nonobstructive ureteral reflux at the time of presentation with end-stage renal failure and drew different conclusions from the San Francisco group.[134] Because the Hamburg group[135] transplanted local patients who had lived in the city all their lives, they had access to their records virtually from birth to transplantation. Patients who seemed to have sterile reflux at the time of renal transplantation all had histories or documentation of substantial morbidity from UTI at some time in their life.

It is interesting in another reported series[136] that of 180 consecutive patients with end-stage renal failure, 10.5% (19 patients) had VUR which was *equally* distributed between patients with proven glomerulonephritis and chronic pyelonephritis; indeed, these authors suggested that a uremic dysfunction of the bladder might cause incompetence of the uretero-vesical junction and they presented some soft evidence to support their concern.[137] The Miami group[138] also obtained VCUs on 50 consecutive patients presenting for transplantation; 30%, 7 males and 8 females, had VUR.

In concluding this section on end-stage renal failure, some general statistics on the seriousness of UTI and RN may be helpful. The problem can be approached from two viewpoints, (1) how many patients with renal failure have end–stage pyelonephritis (which is the easier question), or (2) how many patients with UTI and RN progress to renal failure. The Renal Transplant Registry for 1975 lists 13% of all transplants (15,921) as caused by chronic pyelonephritis; the San Francisco group[134] listed 10% of 965 transplants as due to chronic pyelonephritis. In pediatric transplants, however, chronic pyelonephritis naturally accounts for a larger percentage of those transplanted; 6 of 25 cases reported by Potter *et al.*[139] were girls with chronic pyelonephritis (24%). These authors estimated that about 1250 new cases of end-stage renal disease occur each year in the United States in children, or about 300 cases of girls with pyelonephritis. It is not known how representative their 6 of 25 cases with chronic pyelonephritis is of the general transplant statistics.

How many patients with UTI and RN might progress to renal failure? These data can be estimated by taking the 1–2% prevalence rate of bacteriuria in girls under 12, estimating the percent who have renal scarring (15–20%), and taking 10% of that group as *perhaps* showing serious scarring: $0.015 \times 0.175 \times 0.10 = 2.63 \times 10^{-4}$ or about 1 in 4000 girls under 12 years of age. Considering all the estimates, this figure is surprisingly close to the number of children under 4 years of age who should have IRR (1 in 5555 children as I estimated in the earlier section on IRR). Both of these figures, of course, are substantially greater than the estimated 300 girls transplanted each year in the United States for chronic pyelonephritis. It is clear that much of the renal disease represented by these two estimates of either severe pyelonephritic scarring or IRR in grossly dilated ureters of children under 4 years of age does not carry a serious prognosis in most cases. From my interpretation of the reports in the literature on renal scarring detected on screening surveys, I think the estimate I made that 10% of renal scarring found on surveys is serious is grossly overestimated.

Asscher,[140] based on the data from the Dundee[48] and Cardiff-Oxford[47] studies of the number of girls whose renal scarring progressed over the 4 years, and taking a 2% prevalence rate of bacteriuria in schoolgirls, estimated that 1 in every 1000 schoolgirls should experience progressive renal damage. This estimate, of course, is even further from the mark than mine, but both emphasize that neither serious bilateral scarring detected in schoolgirls during screening surveys nor progression of renal scarring over a 4-year period, in any way accounts for the very few patients with chronic pyelonephritis who go on to renal failure.

Ask-Upmark Kidney. The Ask-Upmark kidney has been commonly thought to represent a congenital dysplastic kidney.[141-143] Johnston and Mix,[144] however, reported an infant with VUR and recurrent UTI who had all the hallmarks of the Ask-Upmark kidney, and they seriously questioned, as have others like Robert Heptinstall for instance, whether the Ask-Upmark kidney was not another example of pyelonephritic atrophy. Aranc and Bernstein[145] may have settled the issue by adding 17 cases of their own to the 169 reported in the literature. Of the 82 children in the literature, 77% are girls; 69% of the 87 adults are women. They note that 58% of the girls and 50% of the boys who had a VCU showed reflux. Ninety-five percent of the children were hypertensive, which is how our single case from Stanford was detected.[146] In their own series of 17 patients, end-stage renal disease was present in seven, five of whom had bilateral Ask-Upmark kidneys and two of whom had a solitary kidney; five of these seven patients were girls, four of whom were hypertensive. More importantly, Aranc and Bernstein[145] could find evidence for congenital dysplasia in only 2 of the 17 kidneys. Their study is convincing that the Ask-Upmark kidney, considered to be a segmental hypoplastic kidney by many, is a variation of pyelonephritic atrophy in patients with reflux and recurrent UTI.

"Distal Urethral Stenosis"

Introduced by Lyon and Smith in 1963,[147] distal urethral stenosis refers to a ring of resistance observed in the distal one-third of the urethra of female children when a bougie à boule (which has an acorn-like tip) is withdrawn from the bladder neck to the urethral meatus. They observed this "stenosis" in 70% of 100 girls with "recurrent or chronic urinary tract infections." The diameter of the ring varied in caliber from 12 F to 26 F. There was no characteristic radiographic appearance seen on voiding cystourethrography, and neither clinical severity of the infection nor response to rupture (dilatation) of the ring was proportional to the caliber of the stenosis. With rupture of the ring, Lyon and Tanagho[148] reported that 80% of female children were cured of lower urinary tract infections and 60% cured of upper tract infections. Cure was defined as an asymptomatic child whose urine was microscopically free of leukocytes and bacteria and who had a normal voiding pattern and rate of urine flow; antimicrobial therapy, either short or long term, was not described in their paper, and cultures were not obtained.

Graham *et al.*[149] compared the bougie calibration of the distal urethra in 191 girls with urinary infections to that of 76 normal female children. They found the distal urethral ring averaged 14 F in normal controls and was slightly larger (16 F) in the infected children. They concluded that other factors must be responsible for urinary infections in female children.

Shopfner,[150] studying 287 female children, including 53 normal girls and 198 with urinary infection, measured the caliber of the urethral meatus, the area of the "distal urethral stenosis," and the midurethra during full voiding at the time of cystourethrography. There was no pathologic correlation among any of these diameters along the urethra, including the presence of vesicoureteral reflux or bladder trabeculation.

Whitaker and Johnston[151] compared the shape of the urethra to synchronous measurements of urethral resistance during voiding cystourethrography in 60 females (7 controls, 23 with recurrent urinary infections with radiographically normal upper tracts, and 30 with vesicoureteral reflux). A cylinder shape to the urethra was present in 28 patients; the other shapes—fusiform, arrowhead, cone, wine-glass, and string—were not particularly associated with any one of the three clinical groups studied. In the cylinder, fusiform, arrowhead, and cone-shaped urethras, the resistance was less than 0.07 mm Hg/ml^2/second (the upper limit of normal resistance). Although the wine glass and string-shaped urethras showed resistance measurements greater than 0.07 mm Hg/ml^2/second, in four of the seven patients the urethral narrowing and elevated resistance were due to voluntarily controlled micturition and not to organic abnormality of the urethra.

Gillenwater *et al.*[70] measured the urethra with bougie à boules in their 60 women followed from childhood with recurrent UTI; they found no difference in urethral calibration between their 60 patients and 38 age-matched controls.

Although these studies suggest that neither urethral meatal stenosis nor "distal urethral stenosis" is a major factor in the cause of urinary infections in children, one report needs to be confirmed. Halverstadt and Leadbetter,[152] disappointed in their results from urethral dilatation of Lyon's distal ring, adopted the technique of cold cutting the entire urethra using the Otis urethrotome. They used the technique of Keitzer and Benavent[153] even though Keitzer and Benavent considered that their operation was for obstruction at the bladder neck (50% of their children were operated upon for enuresis*). Halverstadt and Leadbetter, however, felt that they were relieving urethral obstruction, apparently at the level of the distal ring. The importance of their investigation is that it was a prospective study, with carefully defined bacteriologic methodology, and a control group of patients apparently similar to the two treatment groups. They compared the recurrence rate of urinary infection at 6, 12, and 18 months in 21 patients treated with drugs alone for 3 months (group I), in 28 patients treated with urethrotomy and 2 weeks of drugs (group II), and in 58 patients treated with urethrotomy plus 3 months of drugs (group III). Seventy-one percent failed in the first group, 41% in the second, but only 10% in the third group. This study represents a valiant effort to control three different treatment regimens, but there is no assurance in their report that the drug therapy was initially successful (achieved a sterile urine) *equally* in all three groups. Furthermore, the practice of taking failures out of groups I and II and placing them immediately in group III is highly questionable because the children in group III then received two treatment regimens one after the other whereas group I did not. This difference alone may have contributed to the better results in group III. Despite these concerns, this study is an excellent effort in the urologic literature at attempting to answer whether a specific surgical procedure influences the course of urinary infections. After all, if a urethrotomy and 3 months of antimicrobial therapy cure 90% of girls with urinary infections at 18 months follow-up, we should all get on the bandwagon.

Fair and his associates[65] here at Stanford reviewed the infection history of 29 girls who had urethral dilation according to the technique of Lyon and Tanagho.[148] The 29 girls were followed for an average of 36 months each before dilation and for an average of 27 months after dilation. Each child averaged one UTI every 5.8 months before and one every 5.5 months after dilation; there were a total of 180 infections before and 143 after dilation among the 29 children. The authors concluded that urethral dilation in girls with recurrent UTI does not alter the rate of recurrent infections.

Kaplan and associates[154] compared dila-

* I have reviewed the lack of evidence for bladder neck obstruction in children with recurrent infections and there must be even less evidence to support bladder neck obstruction as a cause of enuresis.

tion, urethrotomy, and medication alone and reported no differences in cure rates. They were apparently unable to confirm Halverstadt and Leadbetter's work.[152]

Hendry and his colleagues[155] compared medication alone to urethral dilation plus medication and found no difference between the two regimens.

During a recent visit to Hamburg, Germany, Dr. Köllermann showed me some convincing data on 39 females from age 6 to 40 years (mean age 14.5 years) who had an internal urethrotomy for recurrent UTI. It is clear in Figure 6.23 that the urethrotomy did not alter the course of their recurrent infections.

Need for Closely Matched Controls and Careful Bacteriology in Evaluation of Surgical Procedures Performed to Prevent Recurrent Urinary Infections

No one can read the surgical literature of the past 28 years on urinary infections in girls without feeling sorry for the many children who have had unwarranted surgical procedures to prevent urinary infections. Bladder neck resections, both open and transurethral, have too often been done for a few milliliters of residual urine, a mild trabeculation, a subjective impression of rigidity at the bladder neck during urethroscopy, or a "contracture" appearance at the vesical neck during voiding cystourethrography. If these children had been matched with similar cases, equally treated with successful (sterile urine on therapy) antimicrobial therapy, and each group followed at monthly intervals with careful bacteriologic cultures, hundreds of operations would not have had to be done before the urologic community recognized the poor results. Much of the difficulty is due to the historical teaching that obstruction predisposes to urinary infection, which it probably does not—a fact that I will review in Chapter 9. Perhaps, also, we have failed to appreciate that the bacteriuria *per se* may be responsible for some of the cystoscopic and radiographic findings.

Whatever the reason, needless operations could be avoided if patients undergoing surgery for recurrent urinary infections are simply matched with similar patients who are treated conservatively. There is an urgent need for this approach in children undergoing antireflux operations; there was an urgent need 10 years ago. Since sterile reflux does not cause renal damage,[100] and since even moderate degrees of reflux (complete pyeloureterogram with moderate dilatation) are not destructive to renal parenchyma in the absence of infection,[95, 101–104] there is as much moral reason for treating these patients conservatively as there is for operative intervention. It is possible that antireflux surgery may change the natural history of urinary infections, but there is no published evidence to support this conviction; we need to know the truth, and it is surely incumbent upon the urologist to prove the efficacy of his surgery. It is not enough to say, as some have said, that "at least no harm has been done." These operations have been performed to prevent the recurrence of urinary infections. Either they do or they do not, and matched, simultaneously treated controls should give the answer. The study by Govan *et al.*[43] in 1975 (see Figure 6.19) clearly shows that correction of VUR does not influence the occurrence of bacteriuria.

Kunin's data,[64] reproduced in Figure 6.13, should make all observers cautious: 10 days of successful antimicrobial therapy in any group of children with established recurrences will provide long term remission for 20% of the group, almost regardless of the number of past infections. Antireflux operations are never done without simultaneous antimicrobial therapy for varying periods after surgery. Moreover, the type and quality of therapy (intramuscular antibiotics, better sensitivity testing, etc.) are likely to be more accurate, more potent, and better controlled during the hospitalization which accompanies the antireflux surgery than during earlier attempts on an outpatient basis. Furthermore, the data in Chapter 4 on recurrent infections in adult women are also convincing that the natural history of many females, without any instrumentation whatsoever, is to suddenly cease their frequency of recurrences and experience a long remission between infections. These observations make it mandatory that equal numbers of children, with the same degree

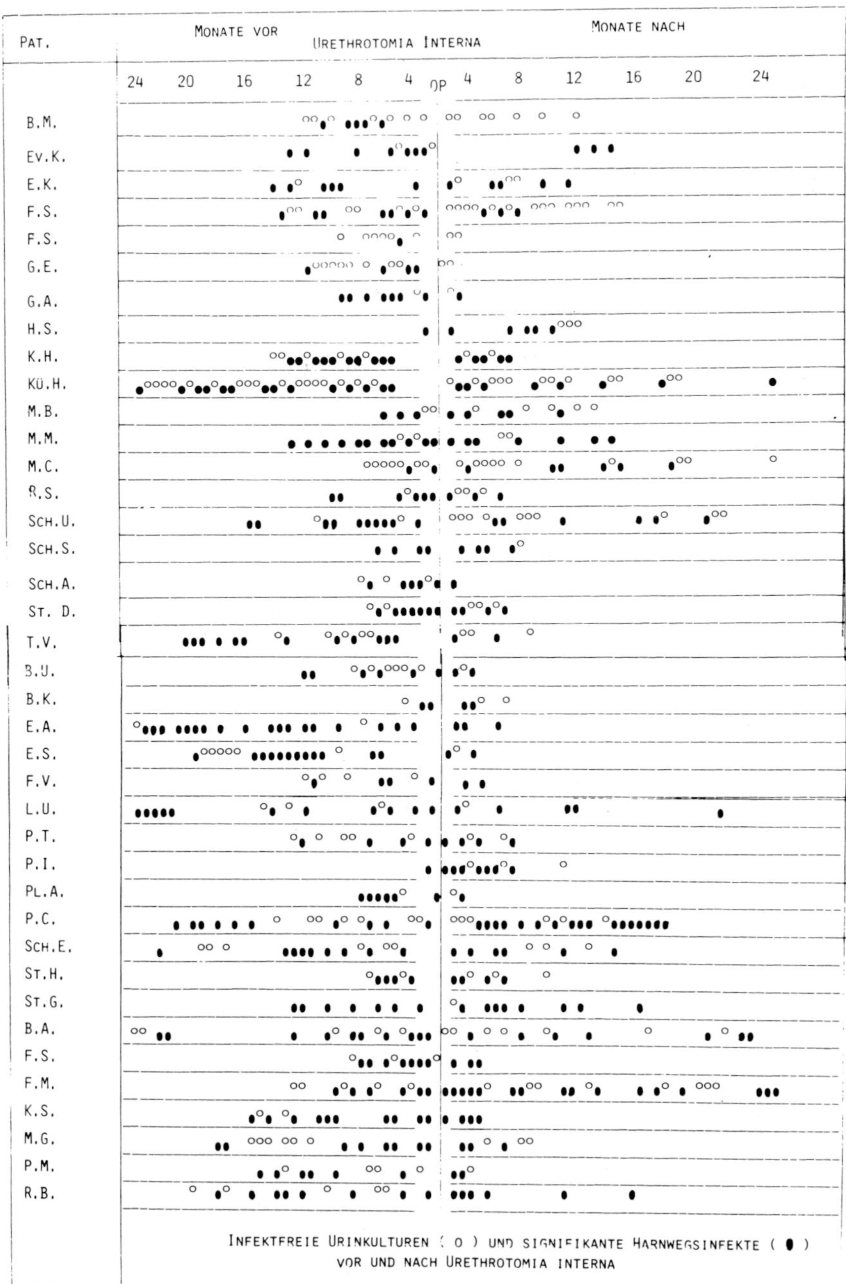

Figure 6.23 Urine cultures before and after internal urethrotomy for recurrent urinary infection in female children. The *open circles* indicate the infection-free cultures and the *black circles* those cultures with significant bacteriuria. The time period includes the intervals 24 months before and 24 months after urethrotomy. Each infection episode was treated for 10 days with appropriate antimicrobial therapy. (Reproduced by permission from Köllermann and Busch, University of Hamburg, Germany.)

of reflux and a reasonably similar past history of clinical episodes, be treated nonoperatively with the identical care and intensity that accompanies surgical procedures.

Relationship of Bacteriuria to Functional Abnormalities of the Bladder and Ureterovesical Junction in Children with Urinary Infections

If reflux were the basic cause of susceptibility to urinary infections, then surely the recurrence rate after initial sterilization and cure of specific infections in children should be significantly greater in those who reflux. In fact, however, three separate studies, one in newborns and two in female children, have shown no difference in the recurrence rates. Bergström *et al.*[25] followed 20 girls aged 6 months to 12 years, through 102 infections; neither the number of recurrences nor the interval between infections distinguished the 10 refluxing children from the 10 who did not reflux. Winberg *et al.*[63] expanded these data to an analysis of 55 girls in 1970. Kunin, Deutscher, and Paquin,[20] comparing schoolgirls with and without urologic abnormalities, could find no difference between the two groups in the time required for the first recurrence of their urinary infection. Bergström *et al.*[5] found no correlation with reflux in the 26% of their newborns whose infections recurred by the 18th month of life. These four papers, plus Govan and Palmer's[92] documentation that over half of the children with successful antireflux operations will have a recurrence of bacteriuria in the first 12 months after surgery, plus the 1975 report by Govan and his associates at Stanford,[43] make the hypothesis that urinary infections are caused by reflux untenable.

It is more likely that the urinary infection contributes to the reflux. To be sure, a neurogenic bladder with a sacule in the region of the ureterovesical junction would be expected to reflux in the absence of infection.[156] Congenital abnormalities like ureteral duplication, diverticula, and ureterocele that weaken the normal course and insertion of the ureter into the trigone would be expected also to reflux in the absence of infection, although infection is still the major danger in nonobstructive ureteral duplication and diverticula. But primary idiopathic reflux in children with urinary infections comprises the largest number of cases,[34] and it is here that a good argument can be made that infection contributes to the reflux.

We know that local bladder edema around the intravesical ureter clearly produces reflux. Auer and Seager,[157] injecting as little as 0.5 ml of saline in the mucosa of the dog's bladder, observed instantaneous reflux at the moment of infiltration, even at low vesical pressures. The clinical counterpart of this experiment is probably the reflux seen in some patients only during the period of the active infection. For example, S.W., a 33-year-old, white female was seen in 1969 for recurrent urinary infections. She had experienced several acute infections each year for 3 or 4 years. An IVU was not remarkable and cystoscopy was normal. Her infections were characterized by urgency, hourly frequency, dysuria, and occasional hematuria. The first recurrence under our observation was an *E. coli*; ureteral catheterization studies on March 25, 1969 proved both renal urines were infected, the right greater than the left ($>10^5$ *E coli*/ml in four consecutive cultures). She was started on 500 mg of oral penicillin-G every 6 hours at the end of the localization study, and a midstream culture on April 1, 1969 was sterile. A VCU on April 8, 1969, on the last day of oral penicillin-G therapy, showed no reflux (Figure 6.24), and a normal appearing urethra; there was no residual urine either at the time of catheterization for the cystogram or on the postvoiding x-ray film, and the catheterized bladder urine was sterile. She was asymptomatic, off therapy, from March 25, 1969 to June 6, 1969 when acute symptoms recurred and *P. mirabilis* was cultured in $>10^5$/ml of urine; six intervening cultures of the midstream urine had been free of infection. A repeat VCU on June 6, 1969, while bacteriuric with *P. mirabilis*, showed reflux up the undilated right ureter to the level of the fifth lumbar vertebra (see Figure 6.25). Again, no residual urine was present at the time of

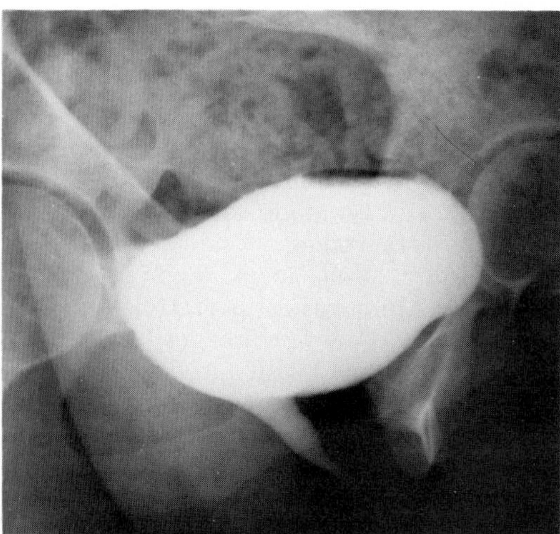

Figure 6.24 Voiding cystourethrogram on S.W., a 33-year-old, white female with recurrent urinary infections, performed 14 days after an *Escherichia coli* bacteriuria that had involved both kidneys, especially the right. The urine was sterile at the time of the cystogram. There is no reflux.

catheterization or on the postvoiding x-ray film. It is interesting that the radiographic configuration of the urethra on the uninfected cystogram (Figure 6.24) is identical to the one at the time of *P. mirabilis* bacteriuria (Figure 6.25).

But more importantly, we know that reflux can persist after the bacteriuria has cleared and still disappear with further passage of time. For example, all of Smellie's[102] initial cystograms were performed after eradication of the infection. Thus, in the absence of acute edema from infection, reflux was present in 34% of her cases and yet disappeared in one-third of these on subsequent follow-up (Figure 6.16). These observations suggest that reflux is caused not only by acute bacteriuria (Figures 6.24 and 6.25), but also by chronic changes that gradually revert to normal in the absence of infections and the passage of time. Interesting data on the disappearance of reflux have come from the controlled treatment trials of patients with ScBU. In the Cardiff-Oxford trial,[47] reflux disappeared or reduced in severity as often in the untreated children as in those who received therapy. In the long term prophylactic trial of Edwards *et al.*[57] reflux disappeared just as often in children who had a recurrence of urinary infection as in those who had no further infection, but one presumes the recurrences were of short duration. These data clearly suggest that reflux tends to disappear irrespective of bacteriuria.

A number of observers have commented upon the shortened intravesical tunnel and wide-appearing trigone in refluxing ureters. Lowell King, Professor of Urology at Northwestern University, has just presented data (personal communication) to show that spontaneous disappearance of reflux in children is related to the degree of reflux, the diameter of the ureteral orifice, and the length of the intravesical submucosal tunnel. Vermillion and Heale[54] evaluated 134 ureteral orifices (94% were in females) in subjects over the age of 12 who had nonobstructive pyelonephritis. Ninety-seven orifices occurred with renal scarring and 45 had demonstrable VUR. Of those orifices associated with renal scarring but no VUR, 79% had cystoscopic abnormalities that suggested reflux must have occurred in the past. This is an important study.

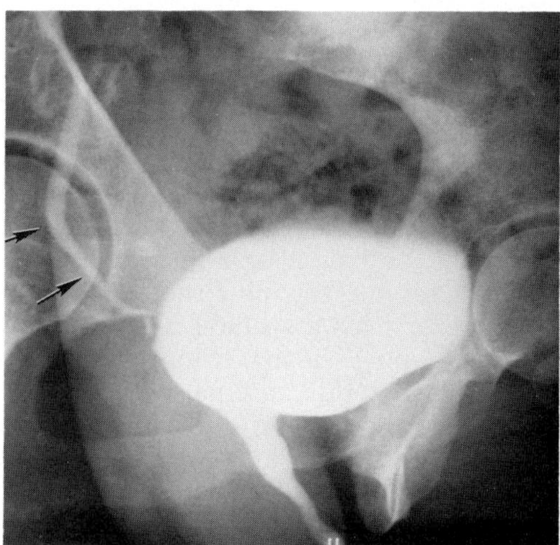

Figure 6.25 Voiding cystourethrogram on the same patient as in Figure 6.24, but performed 2 months later, at the time of a *Proteus mirabilis* bacteriuria. The *arrows* indicate the reflux up the right ureter. Observe that the urethral configuration is the same on both studies.

It is not uncommon to observe an abnormally large bladder in many of these children with chronic urinary infections, an appearance that gave rise to the term "megacystis syndrome."[158] Campbell[159] has reported that maximal bladder capacity in normal female children is about 5 ml/pound of body weight whereas similar children with chronic urinary infection average 10 ml/pound.

Since reflux is rare in adults (about 5%) even though 50% have upper tract infection at the time of their bacteriuria,[111] the possibility of greater susceptibility of the ureterovesical junction in childhood to shortening of the tunnel in the presence of chronic ureteral infection would have to be related to other factors—such as chronic infection occurring during maturation and growth of the ureter in early life. Experiments are needed to test this possibility because, as I have already reviewed in detail, most urinary infections and reflux begin in the first 3 years of life. The model of normally occurring transient reflux in pups, used by Lenaghan and Cussen[87] to prove that severe obstruction did not interfere with spontaneous cessation of reflux, would seem to be ideal. Unilateral, chronic renal infection could be established in pups 1 month old, followed by observations on the persistence of reflux and measurements on the intravesical ureter.

Kjellberg, Ericsson, and Rudhe[160] in their splendid book, *The Lower Urinary Tract in Childhood*, reported their observations in 1957 on a consecutive series of 290 children with "non-obstructive urinary tract infection." Their analysis of these children, including the 35% who refluxed, led them to conclude: "Infection was unquestionably the factor chiefly responsible for development of vesicoureteral reflux, and was perhaps the only one of decisive importance." As I have emphasized, the controlled treatment trial of the Cardiff-Oxford study,[47] and the long-term prophylactic trial of Edwards *et al.*[57] may soften this conclusion somewhat. On the other hand, epidemiologic protocols are never very clear in terms of treatment trials and this is the weakest part of the Cardiff-Oxford effort. In the study by Edwards and his associates, we are not told anything about the duration or severity of the bacteriuric recurrences and perhaps they should not be overemphasized in trying to understand the cause of VUR.

In 1963, Howerton and Lich,[104] correlating the clinical and radiographic findings in 1000 consecutive voiding cystourethrograms, had this to say: "In our 558 patients reflux did not occur in a single instance with obstruction unless concomitant infection was present. Posterior urethral valves were present in seven cases but only three of these demonstrated reflux. Severe and long-standing vesical infection had been present in each instance." They also pointed out that reflux and urinary infection had an identical ratio in the female and male child (9:1), an observation also apparent in Kjellberg's book.[160] Howerton and Lich[104] were among the first to emphasize that "infection is the inciting agent in the development of ureteral reflux."

In a review of an enormous series of cystourethrograms and IVUs in 3,505 infants and children, Shopfner[161] concluded also that the basic cause of reflux is urinary infection and that no proof exists that VUR either causes or propagates urinary infection. Although Shopfner's paper is as casual about establishing the validity of urine culture data as Hendren's,[114] his paper[161] does contain some unique data on the relationship of reflux to renal size and atrophy.

Two valiant experimental efforts at establishing the effect of chronic urinary infection on the bladder and ureterovesical junction should be mentioned. In 1962, Jeffs and Allen[88] suggested that the megaureter megacystis syndrome, including the shortening of the intravesical ureter, might be due to infection, but their studies on 10 dogs were clearly inconclusive. They did establish from measurements in 50 normal dogs that the ratio of ureteral diameter to intravesical ureter was about 1:6 at all dog weights.

Kaveggia, King, Grana, and Idriss[162] believed that pyelonephritis might cause ureteral reflux from chronic ureteral infection. They established a chronic infection in nine dogs by injecting bacteria through a nephrostomy tube in one kidney. All nine dogs developed reflux on the infected side within 1–5 months; in two dogs bilateral reflux occurred. Four different organisms seemed equally capable of producing reflux. Six dogs with nephrostomy tubes failed to develop chronic infection, and reflux did not occur in these animals.

A Recommendation for Treatment

Urinary Infections in Male Children

After eradication of the infection, an IVU should be obtained. With good radiology, and 1 ml of 50% Hypaque/pound of body weight as the dose of intravenous contrast solution (including a 1-minute film for optimal visualization of the renal cortex to detect scarring), an excellent evaluation of the bladder as well as the kidneys can be obtained. After the bladder has filled during the renal excretion of the contrast agent, a steep oblique x-ray film should be obtained during voiding to exclude lower tract obstruction due to prostatic valves or congenital stricture. If a male child has no obstruction to the upper tracts, reasonably delicate ureters, and no evidence for prostatic valves or stricture on the voiding x-ray film, it is pointless to obtain a cystogram and even more pointless to cystoscope the child. Minor degrees of reflux, such as that caused by ureteral duplication, should not be treated surgically, and all attention should be concentrated on keeping the urinary tract sterile.

If the IVU shows obstruction to the upper tracts, or gross dilatation of the ureters, or a dilated prostatic fossa with valves, then a complete urologic evaluation, including voiding cystourethrography and often cystoscopy, is indicated. Surgery will usually be required.

Urinary Infections in Female Children

More specific principles of therapy are presented in Chapter 10 which are equally applicable to children and adults; here I would like to discuss a broader picture of management in relation to the morbidity of recurrences and the radiologic findings on the IVU and the VCU.

The Easy Decision. Several careful studies reviewed in this chapter are in agreement that if renal scarring is absent on the IVU, the kidney should grow normally without renal scarring almost irrespective of whether asymptomatic bacteriuria is present or not and also irrespective of the grade of reflux. For this reason, I consider the IVU, with an early 1-minute film for the nephrogram phase to evaluate the cortical thickness and renal outline, to be the most valuable study of all in decision making for the child with UTI and potential RN; I fully realize that substantial reflux can occur in the presence of reasonably normal-appearing ureters, but this is not common and does not alter the clinical considerations if the kidneys are normal without scarring or thinning of the renal cortex.

If the IVU is normal and the girl is asymptomatic, should she be treated? In general, I think so, although I have discussed in this chapter the Göteborg data that *E. coli* tend to become antigenically altered, and therefore less symptomatic with the passage of time, so that the physician does run the risk of replacing an asymptomatic infection with a symptomatic one, and even an episode of clinical pyelonephritis if the child has VUR. Nevertheless, as the Newcastle data[35] show, 76% of these girls will have mild urinary symptoms: 39% had urgency, 31% had abdominal pain, and 30% enuresis. In addition to getting rid of mild irritating symptoms, there is also a small danger of renal scarring if clinically acute pyelonephritis occurs, especially in the child under 4 years of age. It is clear that any child with *P. mirabilis* should be treated (Chapter 8). Because of these considerations, I treat recurrent bacteriuria in the child; if they have 2 or more infections in a 6-month period (see Chapter 4 on natural history), I treat for 3–5 days with full-dosage therapy and follow this with single, low-dosage, nightly prophylaxis. I keep the dosage as low as possible commensurate with the prevention of bacteriuria; it does not have to be one-third the full dosage regimen as suggested in much of the pediatric literature. For how long? As outlined in Chapter 4, we use prophylaxis for 6 months to 1 year, depending on the morbidity and frequency of past infections, but then it should be stopped to see if the current period of high susceptibility has passed. At the first sign of a symptomatic recurrence, the patient obtains a home-caught urine for culture, and immediately restarts antimicrobial therapy without waiting to see a physician. In practice, this is a very satisfactory regimen which eliminates the risk of potential renal scarring or growth failure of the kidney from acute pyelonephritis. It allows the physician to repeatedly test to see if susceptibility to UTI has ceased, at least for a time, without subjecting the patient to undue morbidity.

The More Difficult Decision. If the IVU shows one or two mild renal scars, and especially if they are confined to one kidney as most will be, provided the ureters show little or no tortuosity, I see no reason to obtain a VCU and the patient can be handled as outlined in the section above. The younger the child the more likely there will definitely be grade I or grade II reflux (Figures 6.6 and 6.7). If the symptomatic morbidity, especially chills and fever, has been substantial, I would probably proceed with a VCU to detect the occasional patient who will have grade III reflux (Figure 6.8), but it is unlikely the VCU will change my decision for long term prophylaxis and to await the spontaneous cessation of reflux. Environmental and social disturbance where either the child or the mother cannot be relied upon for prophylaxis and follow-up is an indication for surgical reimplantation of the ureters.

The Very Difficult Decision. If there is much more than minimal renal scarring on the IVU, or if the ureter appears dilated and tortuous on the IVU, then a VCU is indicated to decide upon the severity of the reflux. If grade III or worse reflux is present, the decision between conservative long term prophylaxis and reimplantation of the dilated ureter is a difficult one indeed.

It has been made more difficult by the 1977 report from the group at University College Hospital that prophylaxis for periods of 7–15 years is associated with disappearance of reflux in 41% of these dilated ureters.[57] My own dilemma in facing these problems has always been as follows: since reimplantation of the ureters will not cause recurrent bacteriuria to cease (Figure 6.19), and since I have felt that bacteriuria in general should be treated in these children, I am confronted with the necessity of prophylactic therapy even if I reimplant the ureters. Since I must treat the patient with prophylaxis anyway, and if 85% of reflux disappears from nondilated and 41% from dilated ureters[57] treated conservatively, it is very difficult to know who should be reimplanted and who should not.

I do know that I have seen several tragic patients whose large ureters were reimplanted in the presence of minimal renal scarring and who now need renal transplantation because of obstructive complications following ureteral reimplantation into the bladder; how much better off these children were with their large refluxing ureters and good kidneys.

I do not question that successful antireflux surgery in infants and young children with renal scarring and gross reflux up tortuous ureters—admittedly the most difficult cases to correct—combined with careful bacteriologic follow-up, offers the best chance of restoring these urinary tracts. These difficult patients must be referred to urologic surgeons with experience in reimplantation of these grossly dilated ureters. Two excellent monographs on the operative management of the megaureter have been published by Hendren,[163, 164] who clearly is an accomplished surgeon at these reimplantations.

It should be obvious that what is really needed is better medicine in terms of office management and control of these recurrent infections, whether done by the pediatrician or the urologist. What is the point of detecting urinary infections in children by screening surveys if the level of medical practice devoted to following and treating their bacteriuric recurrences is too poor to influence the course of the disease? I have reviewed in Chapter I the current alternatives for determining the bacteriologic status of the urine. More importantly, I have shown in Chapter 4 that the surgeon and physician now have some powerful prophylactic, antimicrobial regimens at their disposal which offer almost complete efficacy. The more severe the reflux and the worse the renal scarring, the more closely the child must be followed bacteriologically, whether reimplanted or not.

Finally, whatever office method is used, it must be recognized that these urinary infections in infancy and childhood can be serious. Beginning with children hospitalized for urinary infections associated with fever above 100.4°F and who had "nonobstructive urinary tracts" on intravenous urography, Lindblad and Ekengren[69] were able to obtain 15- to 24-year follow-ups on 58 women. On radiologic examination, 19% showed progressive reductions in renal mass while the remaining 80% either were normal or had no progression. Those who showed progressive reduction in renal mass had early and late histories of multiple recurrences of their infections. Reinvestigation of 18 boys showed no evidence of disease or recurrences. For some as yet unexplained reason, most infections cease in boys after the age of 4.[101]

REFERENCES

1. Sauer, L. W.: Neonatal pyelitis. J. Am. Med. Assoc. **85:** 327, 1925.
2. Craig, W. S.: Urinary disorders occurring in the neonatal period. Arch. Dis. Child. **10:** 337, 1935.
3. James, U.: Urinary infection in the newborn. Lancet **2:** 1001, 1959.
4. Lincoln, K., and Winberg, J.: Studies of urinary tract infections in infancy and childhood. II. Quantitative estimation of bacteriuria in unselected neonates with special reference to the occurrence of asymptomatic infections. Acta Paediatr. Scand. **53:** 307, 1964.
5. Bergström, T., Larson, H., Lincoln, K., and Winberg, J.: Studies of urinary tract infections in infancy and childhood. XIII. Eighty (80) consecutive cases with neonatal infection. J. Pediatr. **80:** 858, 1972.
6. Seeler, R. A., and Hahn, K.: Jaundice in urinary tract infection in infancy. Am. J. Dis. Child. **118:** 553, 1969.
7. Patrick, M. J.: Influence of maternal renal infection on the foetus and infant. Arch. Dis. Child. **42:** 208, 1967.
8. Littlewood, J. M.: 66 Infants with urinary tract infection in first month of life. Arch. Dis. Child. **47:** 218, 1972.
9. McCarthy, J. M., and Pryles, C. V.: Clean voided and catheter neonatal urine specimens. Am. J. Dis. Child. **106:** 473, 1963.
10. O'Brien, N. G., Carroll, R., Donovan, D. E., and Dundon, S. P.: Bacteriuria and leucocyte excretion in the newborn. J. Ir. Med. Assoc. **61:** 267, 1968.
11. O'Doherty, N.: Urinary tract infection in the neonatal period and later infancy. In F. O'Grady and W. Brumfitt (Eds.), Urinary Tract Infection. London, Oxford University Press, 1968, p. 113.
12. Littlewood, J. M., Kite, P., and Kite, B. A.: Incidence of neonatal urinary tract infection. Arch. Dis. Child. **44:** 617, 1969.
13. Randolph, M. F., Woods, S. E., Hodson, C. J., and Klauber, G. T.: Home screening for the detection of urinary tract infection in infancy. Am. J. Dis. Child. **133:** 713, 1979.
14. Kunin, C. M., DeGroot, J. E., Uehling, D., and Ramgopal, V.: Detection of urinary tract infections in 3- to 5-year-old girls by mothers using a nitrite indicator strip. Pediatrics **57:** 829, 1976.
15. Kunin, C. M., and DeGroot, J. E.: Sensitivity of a nitrite indicator strip method in detecting bacteriuria in preschool girls. Pediatrics **60:** 244, 1977.
16. Porter, K. A., and Giles, H. McC.: A pathological study of five cases of pyelonephritis in the newborn. Arch. Dis. Child. **31:** 303, 1956.
17. Kunin, C. M., Zacha, E., and Paquin, A. J.: Urinary tract infections in school children. I. Prevalence of bacteriuria and associated urologic findings. N. Engl. J. Med. **266:** 1287, 1962.
18. Kunin, C. M., Southall, I., and Paquin, A. J.: Epidemiology of urinary tract infection: A pilot study of 3057 school children. N. Engl. J. Med. **263:** 817, 1960.
19. Kunin, C. M., and Halmagyi, N. E.: Urinary tract infections in school children. II. Characterization of invading organisms. N. Engl. J. Med. **226:** 1297, 1962.
20. Kunin, C. M., Deutscher, R., and Paquin, A. J.: Urinary tract infection in school children: An epidemiologic, clinical and laboratory study. Medicine **43:** 91, 1964.
21. Kunin, C. M.: Emergence of bacteriuria, proteinuria, and symptomatic urinary tract infections among a population of school girls followed for 7 years. Pediatrics **41:** 968, 1968.
22. Andersen, H. J., Hanson, L. A., Lincoln, K., Ørskov, F., Ørskov, I., and Winberg, J.: Studies of urinary tract infections in infancy and childhood. IV. Relation of the coli antibody titre to clinical picture and to serological type of the infecting *Escherichia coli* in acute, uncomplicated urinary tract infections. Acta Paediatr. Scand. **54:** 247, 1965.
23. Andersen, H. J., Lincoln, K., Ørskov, F., Ørskov, I., and Winberg, J.: Studies of urinary tract infec-

tions in infancy and childhood. V. A comparison of the coli antibody titer in pyelonephritis measured by means of homologous urinary and fecal *E. coli* antigens. J. Pediatr. **67:** 1073, 1965.

24. Andersen, H. J., Bergström, T., Lincoln, K., Ørskov, F., Ørskov, I., and Winberg, J.: Studies of urinary tract infections in infancy and childhood. VI. Determination of coli antibody titers in the diagnosis of acute urinary tract infections lacking the usual urinary findings. J. Pediatr. **67:** 1080, 1965.
25. Bergström, T., Lincoln, K., Ørskov, F., Ørskov, I., and Winberg, J.: Studies of urinary tract infections in infancy and childhood. VIII. Reinfection vs. relapse in recurrent urinary tract infections. Evaluation by means of identification of infecting organisms. J. Pediatr. **71:** 13, 1967.
26. Bergström, T., Lincoln, K., Redin, B., and Winberg, J.: Studies of urinary tract infections in infancy and childhood. X. Short or long-term treatment in girls with first or second-time urinary tract infections uncomplicated by obstructive urological abnormalities. Acta Paediatr. Scand. **57:** 186, 1968.
27. Meadow, S. R., White, R. H. R., and Johnston, N. M.: Prevalence of symptomless urinary tract disease in Birmingham schoolchildren. I. Pyuria and bacteriuria. Br. Med. J. **3:** 81, 1969.
28. Bergstrom, T.: Sex differences in childhood urinary tract infections. Arch. Dis. Child. **47:** 227, 1972.
29. Smellie, J. M., Hodson, C. J., Edwards, D., and Normand, I. C. S.: Clinical and radiological features of urinary infection in childhood. Br. Med. J. **2:** 1222, 1964.
30. Stansfeld, J. M.: Clinical observations relating to incidence and aetiology of urinary tract infections in children. Br. Med. J. **1:** 631, 1966.
31. Winberg, J., Andersen, H. J., Bergström, T., Jacobsson, B., Larson, H., and Lincoln, K.: Epidemiology of symptomatic urinary tract infection in childhood. Acta Paediatr. Sand. (Suppl.) **252:** 3, 1974.
32. Brooks, D., and Houston, I. B.: Symptomatic urinary infection in childhood: Presention during a four-year study in general practice and significance and outcome at seven years. J. Roy. Coll. Gen. Prac. **27:** 678, 1977.
33. DeLuca, F. G., Fisher, J. H., and Swenson, O.: Review of recurrent urinary tract infections in infancy and early childhood. N. Engl. J. Med. **268:** 75, 1963.
34. Williams, D. I., and Eckstein, H. B.: Surgical treatment of reflux in children. Br. J. Urol. **37:** 13, 1965.
35. Newcastle Asymptomatic Bacteriuria Research Group: Asymptomatic bacteriuria in schoolchildren in Newcastle-upon-Tyne. Arch. Dis. Child. **50:** 90, 1975.
36. Köhler, L., Fritz, H., and Scherstén, B.: Health control of four-year old children. Acta Paediatr. Scand. **61:** 289, 1972.
37. Girardet, P.: Twenty years of research on urinary tract infections in children: Progress and problems. Adv. Int. Med. Peds. **42:** 133, 1979.
38. Savage, D. C. L., Wilson, M. I., McHardy, M., Dewar, D. A. E., and Fee, W. M.: Covert bacteriuria of childhood: A clinical and epidemiological study. Arch. Dis. Child. **48:** 8, 1973.
39. Kunin, C. M.: A ten-year study of bacteriuria in schoolgirls: Final report of bacteriologic, urologic, and epidemiologic findings. J. Infect. Dis. **122:** 382, 1970.
40. Meadow, R.: Disorders of micturition, abnormalities of urine, and urinary tract infection. Br. Med. J. **1:** 1200, 1976.
41. Heale, W. F., Weldon, A. P., and Hewstone, A. S.: Reflux nephropathy presentation of urinary infection in childhood. Med. J. Aust. **1:** 1138, 1973.
42. Filly, R. A., Friedland, G. W., Govan, D. E., and Fair, W. R.: Urinary tract infections in children. Part II—Roentgenologic Aspects. West. J. Med. **121:** 374, 1974.
43. Govan, D. E., Friedland, G. W., Fair, W. R., and Filly, R. A.: Management of children with urinary tract infections: The Stanford experience. Urology, **6:** 273, 1975.
44. Asscher, A. W., Verrier-Jones, R., Sussman, M., McLachlan, M. S. F., Meller, S., Harrison, S., Johnston, H. H., Sleight, G., and Fletcher, E.: Screening for asymptomatic urinary tract infection in schoolgirls. A two-centre feasibility study. Lancet **2:** 1, 1973.
45. Williams, G. L., Davies, D. K. L., Evans, K. T., and Williams, J. E.: Vesicoureteric reflux in patients with bacteriuria in pregnancy. Lancet **2:** 1202, 1968.
46. Sussman, M., Asscher, A. W., Waters, W. E., Evans, J. A. S., Campbell, H., Evans, K. T., and Williams, J. E.: Asymptomatic significant bacteriuria in the non-pregnant woman. I. Description of a population. Br. Med. J. **1:** 799, 1969.
47. Asscher, A. W., Fletcher, E. W. L., Johnston, H. H., Ledingham, J. G. G., McLachlan, M. S. F., Mayon-White, R. T., Meller, S. T., Sleight, G., Smith, E. H., Smith, J. C., Sussman, M., Verrier-Jones, E. R., and Williams, L. A.: (Cardiff-Oxford Bacteriuria Study Group): Sequelae of covert bacteriuria in school girls. A four-year follow-up study. Lancet **2:** 889, 1978.
48. Savage, D. C. L., Adler, K., Howie, G., and Wilson, M. I.: Controlled trial of therapy in covert bacteriuria of childhood. Lancet **1:** 358, 1975.
49. Lindberg, U., Claësson, I., Hanson, L. A., and Jodal, U.: Asymptomatic bacteriuria in schoolgirls. VIII. Clinical course during a 3-year follow-up. J. Pediatr. **92:** 194, 1978.

50. Verrier-Jones, E. R., Meller, S. T., McLachlan, M. S. F., Sussman, M., Asscher, A. W., Mayon-White, R. T., Ledingham, J. G. G., Smith, J. C., Fletcher, E. W. L., Smith, E. H., Johnston, H. H., and Sleight, G.: Treatment of bacteriuria in schoolgirls. Kidney Int. **8:** 5, 1975.
51. Smellie, J. M.: Medical aspects of urinary infection in children. J. R. Coll. Phys. **1:** 189, 1967.
52. Rolleston, G. L.: The significance and management of vesico-ureteric reflux in infancy. II. Radiological aspects. In P. Kincaid-Smith and K. F. Fairley (Eds.), Renal Infection and Renal Scarring. Melbourne, Australia, Mercedes Publishing, 1970, p. 246.
53. Rolleston, G. L., Shannon, F. T., and Utley, W. L. F.: Relationship of infantile vesicoureteric reflux to renal damage. Br. Med. J. **1:** 460, 1970.
54. Vermillion, C.D., and Heale, W. F.: Position and configuration of the ureteral orifice and its relationship to renal scarring in adults. J. Urol. **109:** 579, 1973.
55. Hodson, C. J., Drewe, J. A., Karn, M. N., and King, A.: Renal size in normal children. A radiographic study during life. Arch. Dis. Child. **37:** 616, 1962.
56. Hodson, C. J., Davies, Z., and Prescod, A.: Renal parenchymal radiographic measurement in infants and children. Pediatr. Radiol. **3:** 16, 1975.
57. Edwards, D., Normand, I. C. S., Prescod, N., and Smellie, J. M.: Disappearance of vesico ureteric reflux during long-term prophylaxis of urinary tract infection in children. Br. Med. J. **2:** 285, 1977.
58. Winberg, J., Claësson, I., Jacobsson, B., Jodal, U., and Peterson, H.: Renal growth after acute pyelonephritis in childhood. An epidemiological approach. In J. Hodson and P. Kincaid-Smith (Eds.), Reflux Nephropathy, New York, Masson Publishing, 1979, p. 309.
59. Asscher, A. W., and Chick, S.: Increased susceptibility of the kidney to ascending *Escherichia coli* infection following unilateral nephrectomy. Br. J. Urol. **44:** 202, 1972.
60. Randolph, M. F., Morris, K. E., and Gould, E. B.: The first urinary tract infection in the female infant. Prevalence, recurrence, and prognosis: a 10-year study in private practice. J. Pediatr. **86:** 342, 1975.
61. Cohen, M.: Urinary tract infections in children.I. Females aged 2 through 14, first two infections. Pediatrics **50:** 271, 1972.
62. Smellie, J. M., Katz, G., and Grüneberg, R. N.: Controlled trial of prophylactic treatment in childhood urinary tract infection. Lancet, **2:** 175, 1978.
63. Winberg, J., Larson, H., and Bergström, T.: Comparison of the natural history of urinary infection in children with and without vesico-ureteric reflux. In P. Kincaid-Smith and K. F. Fairley, (Eds.), Renal Infection and Renal Scarring. Melbourne, Australia, Mercedes Publishing, 1970, p. 293.
64. Kunin, C. M.: The natural history of recurrent bacteriuria in schoolgirls. N. Engl. J. Med. **282:** 1443, 1970.
65. Fair, W. R., Govan, D. E., Friedland, G. W., and Filly, R. A.: Urinary tract infections in children. Part I—young girls with nonrefluxing ureters. West. J. Med. **121:** 366, 1974.
66. Stamey, T. A.: Urinary Infections. Baltimore, Williams & Wilkins, 1972.
67. Bollgren, I., and Winberg, J.: The periurethral aerobic bacterial flora in healthy boys and girls. Acta Paediatr. Scand. **65:** 74, 1976.
68. Bollgren, I., Källenius, G., Nord, E.-E., and Winberg J.: The periurethral anaerobic microflora of healthy girls. In press, 1979.
69. Lindblad, B. S., and Ekengren, K.: The long term prognosis of non-obstructive urinary tract infection in infancy and childhood after the advent of sulfonamides. Acta Paediatr. Scand. **58:** 25, 1969.
70. Gillenwater, J. Y., Harrison, R. B., and Kunin, C. M.: Natural history of bacteriuria in schoolgirls: A long-term case control study. N. Engl. J. Med. **301:** 396, 1979.
71. Andersen, H. J., Jacobsson, B., Larsson, H., and Winberg, J.: Hypertension, asymmetric renal parenchymal defect, sterile urine, and high *E. coli* antibody titre. Br. Med. J. **3:** 14, 1973.
72. Marple, C. D.: The frequency and character of urinary tract infections in an unselected group of women. Ann. Intern. Med. **14:** 2220, 1941.
73. Barr, R. H., and Rantz, L. A.: The incidence of unsuspected urinary tract infection in a selected group of ambulatory women. Calif. Med. **68:** 437, 1948.
74. Sanford, J. P., Favour, C. B. Mao, F. H., and Harrison, J. H.: Evaluation of the "positive" urine culture. Am. J. Med. **20:** 88, 1956.
75. Kass, E. H.: Asymptomatic infections of the urinary tract. Trans. Assoc. Am. Phys. **69:** 56, 1956.
76. Hasner, E.: Prostatic urinary infection. Acta Chir. Scand. Suppl. **285:** 1, 1962.
77. Marshall, V. F.: Management of the child with urinary infection. N. Y. State J. Med. **64:** 733, 1964.
78. Spence, H. M., Murphy, J. J., McGovern, J. H., Hendren, W. H., and Pryles, C. V.: Urinary tract infections in infants and children. J. Urol. **91:** 623, 1964.
79. Harrow, B. R., Sloane, J. A., and Witus, W. S.: A critical examination of bladder neck obstruction in children. J. Urol. **98:** 613, 1967.
80. Shopfner, C. E.: Roentgenological evaluation of bladder neck obstruction. Am. J. Roentgenol. **100:** 162, 1967.
81. Tanagho, E. A., and Pugh, R. C. B.: The anatomy and function of the ureterovesical junction. Br. J. Urol. **32:** 151, 1963.
82. Köllerman, M. W., and Ludwig, H.: Uber den

vesico-ureteralen Reflux beim normalen Kind im Säuglings-und Kleinkindalter. Z. Kinderheilk. **100:** 185, 1967.

83. McGovern, J. H., Marshall, V. F., and Paquin, A. J.: Vesicoureteral regurgitation in children. J. Urol. **83:** 122, 1960.
84. Iannaccone, G., and Panzironi, P. E.: Ureteral reflux in normal infants. Acta Radiol. **44:** 451, 1955.
85. Lich, R., Jr., Howerton, L. W., Jr., Goode, L. S., and Davis, L. A.: The ureterovesical junction of the newborn,. J. Urol. **92:** 436, 1964.
86. Peters, P. C., Johnson, D. E., and Jackson, J. H., Jr.: The incidence of vesicoureteral reflux in the premature child. J. Urol. **97:** 259, 1967.
87. Lenaghan, D., and Cussen, L. J.: Vesicoureteral reflux in pups. Invest. Urol. **5:** 449, 1968.
88. Jeffs, R. D., and Allen, M. S.: The relationship between ureterovesical reflux and infection. J. Urol. **88:** 691, 1962.
89. Christie, B. A.: Incidence and etiology of vesicoureteral reflux in apparently normal dogs. Invest. Urol. **9:** 184, 1971.
90. Roberts, J. A.: Vesicoureteral reflux in the primate. Invest. Urol. **12:** 88, 1974.
91. Roberts, J. A., and Riopelle, A. J.: Vesicoureteral reflux in the primate. II. Maturation of the ureterovesical junction. Pediatrics **59:** 566, 1977.
92. Govan, D. E., and Palmer, J. M.: Urinary tract infection in children—The influence of successful antireflux operations in morbidity from infection. Pediatrics **44:** 677, 1969.
93. Baker, R., Maxted, W., Maylath, J., and Shuman, I.: Relation of age, sex and infection to reflux: Data indicating high spontaneous cure rate in pediatric patients. J. Urol. **95:** 27, 1966.
94. Heidrick, W. P., Mattingly, R. F., and Amberg, J. R.: Vesicoureteral reflux in pregnancy. Obstet. Gynecol. **29:** 571, 1967.
95. Stephens, F. D., and Lenaghan, D.: The anatomical basis and dynamics of vesicoureteral reflux. J. Urol. **87:** 669, 1962.
96. Stephens, F. D.: Congential Malformations of the Rectum, Anus and Genitourinary Tracts. Edinburgh, E. & S. Livingstone, Ltd., 1963, p. 145.
97. Morillo, M. M., Orandi, A., Fernandes, M., and Draper, J. W.: Vesicoureteral reflux in male adults with bladder neck obstruction. J. Urol. **89:** 389, 1963.
98. Zatz, L. M.: Combined physiologic and radiologic studies of bladder function in female children with recurrent urinary tract infections. Invest. Urol. **3:** 278, 1965.
99. Sargent, J. W.: Bilateral ureteral reflux observed in a patient over a 23-year period: Case report. J. Urol. **91:** 650, 1964.
100. Fritjofsson, A., and Sundin, T.: Studies of renal function in vesico-ureteric reflux. Br. J. Urol. **38:** 445, 1966.
101. Heale, W. F., and Ferguson, R. S.: The pathogenesis of renal scarring in children. In E. H. Kass and W. Brumfitt, (Eds.), Infections of the Urinary Tract. Chicago, University of Chicago Press, 1978, p. 201.
102. Smellie, J. M., and Normand, I. C. S.: Experience of follow-up of children with urinary tract infection. In F. O'Grady and W. Brumfitt (Eds.), Urinary Tract Infection. London, Oxford University Press, 1968, p. 123.
103. Penn, I. A., and Breidahl, P. D.: Ureteric reflux and renal damage. Aust. N. Z. J. Surg. **37:** 163, 1967.
104. Howerton, L. W., and Lich, R., Jr.: The cause and correction of ureteral reflux. J. Urol. **89:** 672, 1963.
105. Lindberg, U., Claësson, I., Hanson, L. A., and Jodal, U.: Asymptomatic bacteriuria in schoolgirls. I. Clinical and laboratory findings. Acta Paediatr. Scand. **64:** 425, 1975.
106. Lenaghan, D., Whitaker, J. G., Jensen, F., Stephens, F. D.: The natural history of reflux and long-term effects of reflux on the kidney. J. Urol. **115:** 728, 1976.
107. Stephens, F. D.: Preliminary follow-up study of 101 children with reflux treated conservatively. In P. Kincaid-Smith and K. R. Fairley, (Eds.), Renal Infection and Renal Scarring. Melbourne, Australia, Mercedes Publishing, 1970, p. 283.
108. Politano, V. A., and Leadbetter, W. F.: An operative technique for correction of vesicoureteral reflux. J. Urol. **79:** 932, 1958.
109. Orikasa, S., Takamura, T., Inada, F., and Tsuji, I.: Effect of vesicoureteral reflux on renal growth. J. Urol. **119:** 25, 1978.
110. Wikstad, I., Aperia, A., Broberger, O., and Ekengren, K.: Vesicoureteric reflux and pyelonephritis. Long time effect on area of renal parenchyma. Acta Radiol. Diagn. **20:** 252, 1979.
111. Stamey, T. A., Govan, D. E., and Palmer, J. M.: The localization and treatment of urinary tract infections: The role of bactericidal urine levels as opposed to serum levels. Medicine **44:** 1, 1965.
112. Hutch, J. A., Miller, E. R., and Hinman, F., Jr.: Vesicoureteral reflux: Role in pyelonephritis. Am. J. Med. **34:** 338, 1963.
113. Huland, H., Scherf, H., and Köllerman, M. W.: Zur Infektanfälligkeit des harntraktes nach erfolgreicher anti-refluxplastik (I). Urologe A **17:** 282, 1978.
114. Hendren, W. H.: A ten year experience with ureteral reimplantation in children. In P. Kincaid-Smith and K. F. Fairley (Eds.), Renal Infection and Renal Scarring, Proceedings of an International Symposium on Pyelonephritis, Vesicoureteric Reflux and Renal Papillary Necrosis. Melbourne, Australia, Mercedes Publishing, 1971, p. 269.
115. Hodson, C. J., and Edwards, D.: Chronic pyelonephritis and vesicoureteral reflux.Clin. Radiol. **11:** 219, 1960.

116. Hodson, C. J., Maling, T. M. J., McManamon, P. J., and Lewis, M. G.: The Pathogenesis of Reflux Nephropathy. (Chronic Atrophic Pyelonephritis). Br. J. Radiol. **Suppl. 13**, 1975.
117. Ransley, P. G., and Risdon, R. A.: Renal papillae and intrarenal reflux in the pig. Lancet **2:** 1114, 1974.
118. Ransley, P. G., and Risdon, R. A.: Renal papillary morphology in infants and young children. Urol. Res. **3:** 111, 1975.
119. Ransley, P. G., and Risdon, R. A.: Reflux and Renal Scarring. Br. J. Radiol. **Suppl. 14,** 1978.
120. Tamminen, T. E., and Kaprio, E. A.: The relation of the shape of renal papillae and of collecting duct openings to intrarenal reflux. Br. J. Urol. **49:** 345, 1977.
121. Funston, M., and Cremin, B. J.: Intrarenal reflux—papillary morphology and pressure relationships in children's necropsy kidneys. Br. J. Radiol. **51:** 665, 1978.
122. Rolleston, G. L., Maling, T. M., and Hodson, C. J.: Intrarenal reflux and the scarred kidney. Arch. Dis. Child. **49:** 531, 1974.
123. de Vargas, A.: A familial study of vesico-ureteric reflux. J. Med. Genet. **15:** 85, 1978.
124. Bailey, R. R., and Wallace, M.: HLA-B_{12} as a genetic marker for vesicoureteric reflux? Br. Med. J. **1:** 48, 1978.
125. Heale, W. F., Shannon, F. T., Utley, W. L. F., and Rolleston, G. L.: Familial and hereditary reflux nephropathy. In J. Hodson and P. Kincaid-Smith (Eds.), Reflux Nephropathy. New York, Masson Publishing, 1979, p. 48.
126. Frye, R. N., Patel, H. R., and Parsons, V.: Familial renal tract abnormalities and cortical scarring. Nephron **12:** 188, 1974.
127. Brendin, H. C., Winchester, P., McGovern, J. H., and Degnan, M.: Family study of vesicoureteral reflux. J. Urol. **113:** 623, 1975.
128. Fried, K., Yuval, E., Eidelman, A., and Beer, S.: Familial primary vesicoureteral reflux. Clin. Genet. **7:** 144, 1975.
129. Lewy, P. R., and Belman, A. B.: Familial occurrence of nonobstructive, noninfectious vesicoureteral reflux with renal scarring. J. Pediatr. **86:** 851, 1975.
130. Middleton, G. W., Howard, S. S., and Gillenwater, J. Y.: Sex-linked familial reflux. J. Urol. **114:** 36, 1975.
131. Dwoskin, J. Y.: Sibling uropathology. J. Urol. **115:** 726, 1976.
132. Mogg, R. A.: Familial and adult reflux. In National Foundation (Eds.), Birth Defects: original article series, volume 13. New York, Alan R. Liss, 1977 p. 365.
133. Savage, D. C. L., Wilson, M. I., Ross, E. M., and Fee, W. M.: Asymptomatic bacteriuria in girl entrants to Dundee primary schools. Brit. Med. J. **3:** 75, 1969.
134. Salvatierra, O., and Tanagho, E. A.: Reflux as a cause of end-stage kidney disease: Report of 32 cases. J. Urol. **117:** 441, 1977.
135. Huland, H., Buchardt, P., Köllermann, M., and Augustin, J.: Vesicoureteral reflux in end-stage renal disease. J. Urol. **121:** 10, 1979.
136. Mosconi, C. E. V., Ianhez, L. E., Borrelli, M., Sabbaga, E., and Campos-Friere, J. G.: Vesicoureteral reflux in patients in end-stage chronic renal failure. Urol. Int. **30:** 357, 1975.
137. Mosconi, C. E. V., Ianhez, L. E., Borrelli, M., Sabbaga, E., and Campos-Friere, J. G.: Bladder dysfunction in uremic patients. Acta Urol. Belg. **42:** 418, 1974.
138. Bakshandeh, K., Lynne, C., and Carrion, H.: Vesicoureteral reflux and end-stage renal disease. J. Urol. **116:** 557, 1976.
139. Potter, D., Belzer, F. O., Rames, L., Holliday, M. A., Kountz, S. A., and Najarian, J. S.: The treatment of chronic uremia in childhood. I. Transplantation. Pediatrics **45:** 432, 1970.
140. Asscher, A. W.: Covert bacteriuria—peril or partnership? Br. Med. J. **1:** 1649, 1978.
141. Ask-Upmark, E.: Uber juvenile maligne nephrosklerose und ihr verhaltnis zu storungen in der nierenentwicklung. Acta Pathol. Microbiol. Scand. **6:** 383, 1921.
142. Habib, R., Courtecuisse, V., Ehrensperger, J., and Royer, P.: Hypoplasia segmentaire du rein avec hypertension arterielle chez l'enfant. Ann. Pediatr. **12:** 262, 1965.
143. Benz, G., Willich, E., and Scharer, K.: Segmental renal hypoplasia in childhood. Paediatr. Radiol. **5:** 86, 1976.
144. Johnston, J. H., and Mix, L. W.: The Ask-Upmark kidney: A form of ascending pyelonephritis? Br. J. Urol. **48:** 393, 1976.
145. Arant, BS, Jr., Sotelo-Avila, Co., and Bernstein, J.: Segmental "hypoplasia" of the kidney (Ask-Upmark). J. Pediatr., **95:** 931, 1979.
146. Meares, E. M. J. Jr., and Gross, D. M. Hypertension owing to unilateral renal hypoplasia. J. Urol. **108:** 197, 1972.
147. Lyon, R. P., and Smith, D. R.: Distal urethral stenosis. J. Urol. **89:** 414, 1963.
148. Lyon, R. P., and Tanagho, E. A.: Distal urethral stenosis in litte girls. J. Urol. **93:** 379, 1965.
149. Graham, J. B., King, L. R., Kropp, K. A., and Uehling, D. T.: The significance of distal urethral narrowing in young girls. J. Urol. **97:** 1045, 1967.
150. Shopfner, C. E.: Roentgen evaluation of distal urethral obstruction. Radiology **88:** 222, 1967.
151. Whitaker, J., and Johnston, G. S.: Correlation of urethral resistance and shape in girls. Radiology **91:** 757, 1968.
152. Halverstadt, D. B., and Leadbetter, G. W., Jr.: Internal urethrotomy and recurrent urinary tract infection in female children. I. Results in the management of infection. J. Urol. **100:** 297, 1968.

153. Keitzer, W. A., and Benavent, C.: Bladder neck obstruction in children. J. Urol. **89:** 384, 1963.
154. Kaplan, G., Sammons, T. A., and King, L.: A blind comparison of dilatation, urethrostomy and medication alone in the treatment of urinary tract infection in girls. J. Urol. **109:** 917, 1973.
155. Hendry, W. F., Stanton, S. L., and Williams, D. I.: Recurrent urinary infections in girls; Effects of urethral dilation. Br. J. Urol. **45:** 72, 1973.
156. Hutch, J. A.: Vesicoureteral reflux in the paraplegic; cause and correction. J. Urol. **68:** 457, 1952.
157. Auer, J., and Seager, L. D.: Experimental local bladder edema causing urine reflux into ureter and kidney. Proc. Soc. Exp. Biol. Med. **35:** 361, 1936.
158. Paquin, A. J., Jr., Marshall, V. F., and McGovern, J. H.: The megacystic syndrome. J. Urol. **83:** 634, 1960.
159. Campbell, W. A.: Functional abnormalities of the bladder in children: Characteristics of chronic cystitis and chronic urethritis. J. Urol. **104:** 926, 1970.
160. Kjellberg, S. R., Ericsson, N. O., and Rudhe, U.: The lower urinary tract in childhood. Chicago, Yearbook Publishers, 1957, p. 182.
161. Shopfner, C. E.: Vesicoureteral reflux, five year re-evaluation. Radiology **95:** 637, 1970.
162. Kaveggia, L., King, L. R., Grana, L., and Idriss, F. S.: Pyelonephritis: A cause of vesicoureteral reflux? J. Urol. **95:** 158, 1966.
163. Hendren, W. H.: Megaureter. In W. T. Mustard, M. M. Ravitch, W. H. Snyder, K. J. Welch, and C. D. Benson (Eds.), Pediatric Surgery. Chicago, Yearbook Medical Publishers, 1969, p. 1142.
164. Hendren, W. H.: Functional restoration of decompensated ureters in children. Am. J. Surg. **119:** 477, 1970.

CHAPTER 7

Urinary Infections in Males

INTRODUCTION

In epidemiologic surveys, asymptomatic urinary infections in males are rare. Freedman,[1] in a study of 1234 males in Hiroshima, Japan, found no positive cultures in persons under the age of 49, but 0.6% had bacteriuria between ages 50 and 59, 1.5% in the next decade, and 3.6% above age 70. Miall *et al.*,[2] in Jamaican population studies, found only 3 of 700 men had bacteriuria. Two of these had recently undergone prostatectomy. Kunin[3] cultured 7731 boys and young men (1116 were university students, ages 15–29). Only two cases of infection were found, both in boys, one 13 and the other 14 years old; and both had normal intravenous urograms.

Thus, infections are rare in younger age groups. Because urinary infections in males, at least in the absence of surgical manipulation such as prostatectomy or indwelling catheters, tend to be very symptomatic and require specific therapy, it is probable that population surveys underestimate the prevalence of this disease. Moreover, it is too easy to assign all urinary infections in the male to instrumentation of the urinary tract. Any practicing physician who cultures the urine and takes a history recognizes the spontaneous appearance of documented urinary infections in males.

Despite a large experience of seeing many adult males of all ages with recurrent urinary infections, we see so few with their first infection that we cannot present data relating to the pathogenesis of their initial infection. In older men who are instrumented for prostatic symptoms, their infections are often clearly iatrogenic. This is equally true of some younger men who require Foley catheter drainage following extensive surgical procedures. Excluding these obvious causes of initial infections, we see several men each year in the 30- to 50-year age group in whom the first infection was not associated with instrumentation or hospitalization. These latter patients are referred after they have had repeated recurrences; for this reason, we lack data on bacteriologic localization studies at the time of their initial infection.

Given an adult male patient, however, who has recurrent urinary infections, the site of bacterial persistence—and, therefore, the cause of the recurrent infection—can be shown, by appropriate bacteriologic studies, most often to be in the prostatic fluid. Even if the upper urinary tract is involved with pyelonephritic scars, obstructive disease, or even infection stones (Chapter 8), we have surgically corrected more than one upper tract only to have the infection recur and then find that persistence of the bacteria in prostatic fluid was the basic problem from the beginning.

The reader of this chapter is encouraged to review the techniques and methodology in Chapter 1 that relate to localization of infection in the lower tract of the male; these techniques are of critical importance in the interpretation of the following pages.

PROSTATITIS

The diagnosis of bacterial prostatitis is often made by the clinician, but this is rarely accompanied by objective evidence.

Indeed, the available data have been so poor that some authors question the existence of bacterial prostatitis as a disease entity.[4, 5] The term "prostatitis," unfortunately, is all too often a wastebasket of clinical ignorance, used to describe any condition associated with prostatic inflammation or prostatic symptoms. In this context, "prostatitis" is most commonly diagnosed in patients who have no history or evidence of bladder infection, despite the presence of perineal aching, low back pain, or urinary discomfort.

Classification of Prostatitis

In 1978, Drs. Drach, Meares, Fair, and myself[6] presented a classification with definitions that has some merit and should improve communication. We divided "prostatitis" into four categories that have both diagnostic and therapeutic implications:

Acute Bacterial Prostatitis
Chronic Bacterial Prostatitis
"Nonbacterial" Prostatitis
Prostatodynia

In Table 7.1 I have summarized the distinguishing characteristics of each group. Observe that the first three categories cannot be distinguished by inflammatory cells in the expressed prostatic secretion (EPS); they all have evidence of purulence, including white blood cells (WBC), clumps of WBC, and large macrophages laden with cholesterol particles (Figure 7.1). These macrophages actually occur in all sizes from

Table 7.1
Clinical Classification of "Prostatitis"

Condition	Evidence of Inflammation (EPS)[a]	Culture Positive (EPS)	Culture Positive (Bladder)	Common Etiologic Bacteria	Rectal Exam (Prostate)	Percent Cure With Antimicrobials	Antimicrobial of Choice	Other Drugs
Acute bacterial prostatitis	+	+	+[b]	Enterobacteriaceae	Abnormal	100	Aminoglycoside	
Chronic bacterial prostatitis	+	+	+[c]	Enterobacteriaceae	Normal	~50	TMP-SMX[d]	
"Nonbacterial" prostatitis	+	0	0	?	Normal	0		
Prostatodynia	0	0	0	0	Normal	0		Phenoxybenzamine

[a] EPS = Expressed prostatic secretion.
[b] Acute bacterial prostatitis is nearly always accompanied by bladder infection.
[c] Characterized by recurrent bacteriuria, at varying intervals up to several months, after stopping antimicrobial therapy.
[d] TMP-SMX = trimethoprim-sulfamethoxazole.

that of a WBC to ones several times the diameter of a WBC; they appear brown under the low power field (green granules under the high power field (hpf)) and show the typical maltese crosses of cholesterol deposits if the substage light is polarized.

Since prostatodynia is characterized by an uninflamed EPS, the definition of a normal EPS is important in terms of WBC. There is obviously some disagreement as to how many WBCs in EPS are normal, but I believe more than 12/hpf is statistically abnormal and indicative of an inflammatory process in the prostate provided urethral inflammation is absent. Blacklock[7] examined 52 normal naval volunteers, 17–55 years old (only nine over 40 years old), and reported that 70% had no WBC/hpf, 18% had less than 5/hpf, 6% had 5–10 WBC/hpf, and only 6% had greater than 10 WBC/hpf. Pfau *et al.*[8] in a study of the pH of EPS in health and disease, examined 28 men (mean age, 34 years) considered to be free of prostatic disease; except for one individual with necrospermia, all others had "no or few white cells per hpf." Although convenient, examination of EPS under a coverslip is semiquantitative at best; a better technique is to dilute prostatic fluid in isotonic solution and count the WBCs in a Fuchs-Rosenthal chamber per mm^3. Dr. Rodney Anderson at Stanford has studied 20 normal men (mean age, 35 years, range 21–73 years) after 72 hours of ejaculatory abstinence: the total WBC count was 887 ± 111/mm^3. Assuming that the volume of EPS that usually fits snugly under a 22-mm-square coverslip is 0.02 ml, and that there are 2025 hpf under a coverslip, 95% of all normal men (2½ standard deviations above the mean of 887/mm^3) should have less than 11.5 WBC/hpf. Anderson and Weller's careful study has been published in the J. Urol. **121:** 292, 1979.[127] Thus, on the basis of these limited data, and being unaware of any other, the diagnosis of inflammatory disease of the prostate should have a 95% chance of certainty in the presence of 12 or more WBC/hpf. Jameson,[9] however, has shown that a normal basal level of 4–10 WBC/hpf can treble up to 72 hours after ejaculation.

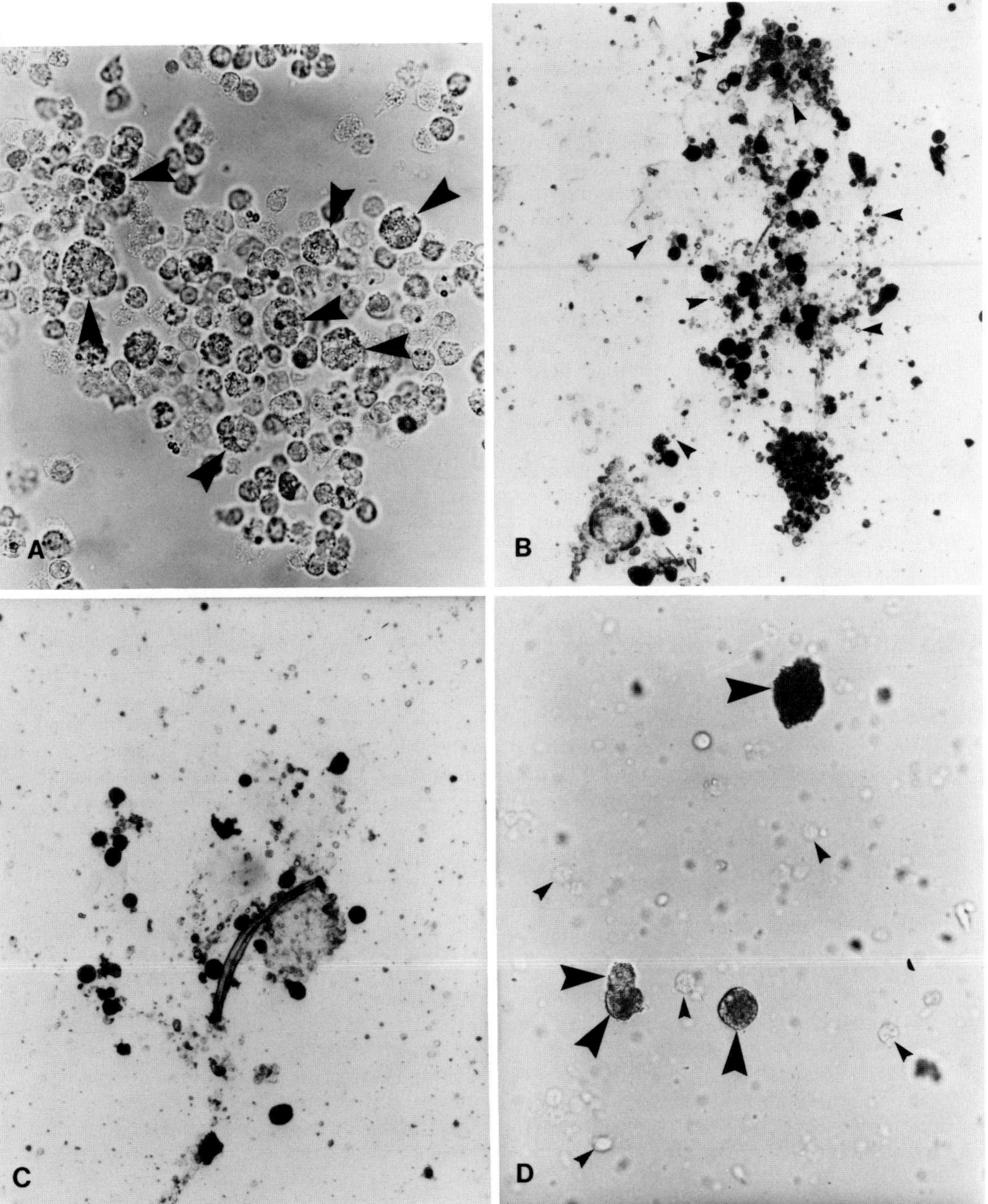

Figure 7.1 *A*, Expressed prostatic secretion (EPS) from a 45-year-old patient with recent onset of acute bacterial prostatitis (*Escherichia coli*). Note large, early oval fat macrophages (indicated by *large arrows*) that are 2–4 times the size of the polymorphonuclear leukocytes (×570 magnification, unstained). *B*, Same patient, but EPS obtained 1 month later. Under the low power field of the microscope (×100), the oval fat macrophages appear dark brown and are sometimes called "oval brown bodies." The leukocytes are much less in number but can be seen faintly in the background. Doubly-refractile, free fat droplets are marked with *arrows*. *C*, Same EPS as seen in *Part B* but a different field (×100). *D*, Same EPS as seen in *Parts B* and *C*, but observed under the high power field of the microscope (×570). The leukocytes (*small arrows*) are slightly out of focus. The four *large arrows* mark the oval fat macrophages; the uppermost one shows doubly-refractile fat droplets on the edges.

Note in Table 7.1 that bacterial prostatitis, both acute and chronic, are caused by Enterobacteriaceae (and sometimes *Pseudomonas* as well as enterococci) and that they are invariably associated with bacteriuria (bladder and sometimes renal infection). In acute bacterial prostatitis, the urine is infected by the time the patient is seen by the physician, but in chronic bacterial prostatitis months may elapse after discontinuing antimicrobial therapy before the bacteria which persist in the prostate infect the bladder and produce symptoms in the patient.

The physician should note that while the prostate is usually abnormal (swollen, tender, hot) to palpation in acute bacterial prostatitis, it is not abnormal to palpation in the remaining three categories of "prostatitis."

"Nonbacterial" prostatitis is placed in quotation marks because it is possible that the inflammation is caused by some, as yet, unproven bacteria, such as *Chlamydia* or *Mycoplasma*. It could be viral or even an autoimmune reaction. The fact is we do not know the agent causing the inflammation and for this reason treatment is most unsatisfactory. Antimicrobial agents are not helpful and should not be prescribed.

Clinical examples, with further comments on each of the clinical categories, are presented in the following pages.

Acute Bacterial Prostatitis

Acute bacterial prostatitis is easy to recognize because its presentation as an acute bacterial infection in an organ that is normally uninfected is very similar to that of acute pyelonephritis. Early symptoms include malaise, myalgia, and fever which usually occur before the onset of localizing bladder or prostatic symptoms. Indeed, the patient often thinks he has the "flu," but the rapid development of urinary frequency, dysuria, and obstructive voiding quickly dispels any doubts as to the site of the infection. The fever is often 39–40°C, a substantial leukocytosis is present, and the urine invariably becomes infected soon after the presentation of the initial symptoms. On rectal examination, the prostate can be tense and exquisitely tender, while in rare cases examined very early in their presentation, the prostate may not be so dramatic on palpation. The following patient is an excellent example of acute bacterial prostatitis.

H.H., a 49-year-old Caucasian man, was first seen on November 28, 1962. He was asymptomatic but 4 weeks previously had experienced dysuria with discomfort in the perineum, low back area, and lower abdomen; his discomfort was aggravated during defecation. He had had shaking chills, with fever as high as 102°F, and was given an unknown medication for 6 days; all symptoms subsided. In 1960, he had a single episode of dysuria and frequency which had also been treated successfully with medication. Physical examination revealed some induration at the base of the right lobe of the prostate. The segmented cultures on 11/28/62 showed no Gram-negative organisms. He was instructed to return for repeat cultures but failed to do so. On 5/23/63, he returned with complaints of fever (101°F), chilly sensations, urinary frequency, and dysuria. On rectal examination, the prostate was tender and slightly irregular, but probably unchanged from the previous examination. His WBC was 12,300 with 79% segmented leukocytes. The cultures on 5/23 and 5/24/63 (Table 7.2) showed an infected prostate. The midstream culture (VB_2) on 5/23/63 demonstrated a fall in the urethral count from 4200 to 23 *Escherichia coli*/ml. The postprostatic massage specimen contained greater than 100,000 *E. coli*/ml (Table 7.2). The following morning the bladder was aspirated prior to collection of the voided specimens. Virtually the same pattern was present, *i.e.*, extremely high numbers of bacteria originating in the prostate. At this time, however, the prostatic infection had reached the bladder (aspiration showed 3600 *E. coli*/ml). The bladder infection on 5/24 was related either to the prostatic massage on 5/23 or more probably represented the natural history of an infected prostate. Immediately following the cultures on 5/24, the patient was started on oxytetracycline, 500 mg by mouth every 6 hours for 12 days. Tube dilution sensitivi-

Table 7.2
Acute Bacterial Prostatitis in H.H., a 49-year-old, Caucasian Man

Date	Days on (+) or off (−) Drug	Drug	VB1[a]	VB2	VB3	Organism Type	Organism Sensitivity
			bacteria/ml[b]				
11/28/62	−21	Unknown medication	0	0	0		
5/23/63	−7 mo		4200	23	100,000	*Escherichia coli*	Oxytet (5 μg/ml)
5/24/63	−7 mo		5340	4500[c]	187,000	*E. coli*	
5/27/63	+3	Oxytet (500 mg q 6 hr)	0	0	0		
5/29/63	+5	Oxytet	0	0	0		
6/5/63	+12	Oxytet	0	0	0		
6/11/63	−6	Oxytet	0	0	0		
6/25/63	−14	Oxytet	0	0	0		
8/27/63	−2½ mo		0	0	0		
12/3/63	−6 mo		4000	513	456	*E. coli*	
1/28/64	−8 mo		10	0	0	*E. coli*	
1/19/65	−20 mo		513	19	30	*E. coli*	
5/4/65	−24 mo			0			
7/27/65	−26 mo		228	41	151	*E. coli*	
11/14/67	−54 mo		0	0	0[d]		
6/21/71	−97 mo		0	0	0[d]		
12/18/78	−15 yrs		0	0	0[d]		

[a] VB_1 = First voided 5–10 ml of urine from urethral meatus; VB_2 = Midstream aliquot of urine; VB_3 = First voided 5–10 ml of urine from urethral meatus after prostatic massage; Oxytet = Oxytetracycline.
[b] Small counts of Gram-positive organisms are not included in the table.
[c] Suprapubic bladder aspiration revealed 3600 *E. coli*/ml on April 24, 1963.
[d] Expressed prostatic secretion (EPS) was also sterile.

ties showed that a concentration of 1 μg/ml of oxytetracycline had no effect on the *E. coli*, whereas 5 μg/ml was bactericidal. Cultures on 5/27 and 5/29/63 and 6/5/63 were during antibiotic therapy; the remainder of the cultures were after therapy (Table 7.2). The patient became afebrile 24 hours after starting therapy; some urgency and frequency remained for an additional 48 hours. An intravenous urogram showed normal upper tracts; there was no residual urine after voiding. Several small prostatic calculi were plainly visible. He remained asymptomatic during the next 8 years of follow-up. Segmented cultures in June, 1971 showed no Gram-negative bacteria in any of the specimens. A plain film x-ray of his prostatic area showed the prostatic calculi to be unchanged. In view of our observation that the sexual partners of women with recurrent bacteriuria carry the same pathogenic bacteria on the male urethra as the female carries on her introitus, it is of interest that the wife of H.H. had recurrent cystitis for 15 years. This observation possibly explains the transient appearance of *E. coli* on his urethra in late 1963 and in 1964 and 1965. Indeed, it may explain the two episodes of acute bacterial prostatitis. He was seen for interview on 12/18/78. Urologically, he had remained in good health in the intervening 6 years. His cultures were sterile for *E. coli* and his EPS contained no WBCs or oval fat macrophages. His VB_1 culture grew 1000 α-streptococci/ml, his VB_2 was sterile, his EPS grew 1000 α-streptococci and 120 *Staphylococcus epidermidis*, and his VB_3 was sterile. A plain film X-ray of his pelvis showed no change in the prostatic calculi.

Patients such as H.H. (Table 7.2) who have acute bacterial prostatitis often respond dramatically to therapy with antimicrobial agents that normally do not diffuse from plasma into prostatic fluid. Perhaps, as in acute meningitis, the intense, diffuse inflammatory reaction of acute bacterial prostatitis allows the passage of antimicrobial agents from plasma into prostatic ducts. An appropriate antibiotic should be given to this patient in doses that achieve bactericidal concentrations of the drug in the blood (if possible). The aminoglycosides are the first choice if parenteral therapy is to be used, while trimethoprim-sulfamethoxazole (TMP-SMX) is first choice if the patient is to be treated as an outpatient. General supportive measures, such as adequate hydration, analgesics, antipyretics, bed rest, and stool softeners should also be employed. Urethral instrumentation should be avoided. If acute urinary retention occurs, suprapubic needle aspiration of the bladder is safer and more comfortable for the patient than urethral catheterization. When prolonged bladder drainage is required, a suprapubic catheter (punch cystostomy) causes fewer complications than a urethral catheter (see Chapter 10, Figure 10.13).

Difference between Acute and Chronic Bacterial Prostatitis. Our concern in this chapter will be primarily with those adults who have relapsing urinary infections caused by small numbers of bacteria in the prostatic fluid. These patients with chronic bacterial prostatitis usually have lower urinary symptoms from their bladder infection, sometimes associated with chills and fever, but their prostates are not remarkable by either rectal or cystoscopic examination. This is in contrast to the adult, usually young, who has chills and fever with varying urinary symptomatology, but a hard, irregular, exquisitely tender prostate, and who responds rapidly to most antibacterial agents; this patient has acute bacterial prostatitis. Except for the absence of overt irregularity, as usually seen with acute bacterial prostatitis, patient H.H. (Table 7.2) is quite representative. It is difficult to understand why antibacterial therapy seems so successful in acute bacterial prostatitis. Since the prostate is often hard and grossly distorted, even raising a suspicion of carcinoma by palpation, the interstitial tissue of the gland must be grossly involved; if so, plasma levels of antibacterial agents might be expected to be effective, as in patient H.H. But how are the bacteria cleared so readily from the prostatic fluid? Perhaps the prostatic epithelium, in the presence of gross inflammatory distortion, no longer serves as an antibacterial barrier between the plasma and the prostatic fluid. Or perhaps the normal bactericidal activity of prostatic fluid kills the bacteria in the prostatic fluid once the interstitial inflammation is controlled by the antibacterial drug. Whatever the mechanism, it is clear that acute and chronic bacterial prostatitis are two different therapeutic problems.

Acute bacterial prostatitis can be dramatic in its clinical manifestations, associated with large numbers of bacteria in the EPS or VB_3, easy to diagnose on physical examination, readily treated, and usually self-limiting (patient H.H.); we have seen, however, some patients who had chronic, asymptomatic prostatic infection in between acute episodes.

Chronic bacterial prostatitis, by contrast, is a subtle disease with small numbers of bacteria in the prostatic fluid, impossible to diagnose on physical or cystoscopic examination, and very difficult to eradicate with antibacterial therapy.

Prostatic Abscess. An acute abscess of the prostate is probably related to acute bacterial prostatitis. In modern society with reasonably good medical care, prostatic abscess is a rare complication of bacterial prostatitis unless antimicrobial host defenses are compromised as in patients with diabetes or patients on immunosuppressive drug therapy. Pai and Bhat[10] in 1972 reported on 24 patients with an abscess of the prostate, and Dajani and O'Flynn described 25 cases in 1968[11]; 70% were caused by *E. coli.* Systemic antimicrobial therapy should be instituted immediately with either aminoglycosides or TMP-SMX. If the prostate is fluctuant on rectal examination, perineal or transurethral drainage should be performed as soon as possible. If the prostate is rock hard, suggesting cancer of the prostate, the patient should be treated as an acute bacterial prostatitis; several months are sometimes required before the prostate softens to a normal consistency on rectal examination.

Granulomatous Prostatitis. In the absence of tuberculosis and rare mycotic infections of the prostate, granulomatous prostatitis is almost always a histologic stage of resolving acute bacterial prostatitis. It is usually detected as a hard lobe or area of the prostate, suspicious of carcinoma, but it nearly always follows a urinary infection in which the prostate is acutely involved. Indeed, Kelalis *et al.*[12] found bacteriuria in 65% of their 70 patients at the time of biopsy; clinical findings of a severe lower urinary tract infection of short duration were present in 83%. Except for excluding carcinoma of the prostate, and recognizing that a granulomatous tissue reaction is not unusual in patients with resolving acute bacterial prostatitis, no special therapy is warranted. These patients should be followed bacteriologically like any other patient with acute bacterial prostatitis.

A good clinical example of granulomatous prostatitis is that of a 57-year-old white man whom I first saw in August 1966, 4 weeks after the acute onset of severe malaise, urinary frequency, dysuria, and shaking chills with fever to 104°F. His urine was described as loaded with WBCs and contained 300 mg% proteins. He was treated with 1.0 g of sulfisoxazole every 6 hours for 7 days; he felt better within 8 hours of starting therapy. Unfortunately, a urine culture was not obtained. A the time I saw him 4 weeks later, he felt well except for some diminution in the size and force of his urinary stream, and he described one episode of initial and terminal hematuria 4 days before. On physical examination, the prostate was smooth, no enlarged, but stony hard in the right lobe and abnormally firm in the left lobe; the median furrow was palpable, the lateral sulci were empty, and the base of the bladder was soft. His urine contained 100 or more WBCs and 1–5 bacilli/hpf; the midstream urine grew $> 10^5$ *E. coli*/ml which were highly sensitive to nitrofurantoin (50 μg/ml), penicillin-G (100 μg/ml), ampicillin (5 μg/ml), and nalidixic acid (10 μg/ml). He was treated for 7 days with 2 g/day of nalidixic acid, and all subsequent cultures were sterile. An intravenous urogram showed minimal intravesical prostate. A serum acid phosphatase was normal. When examined biweekly over the next 3 months, the right lobe of the prostate remained very hard, although it seemed somewhat smaller. On 12/21/66, several needle biopsies of both lobes were obtained perineally under general anesthesia; cystourethroscopy was normal. The biopsies from both lobes showed extensive infiltration with plasma cells and lymphocytes, accompanied by giant cells and epithelioid cells; acid-fast and fungus stains were negative. Three different pathologists considered the histologic changes typical of granulomatous prostatitis. The patient had no further urinary infections and the indurated prostate gradually resolved. In 1978, 12 years after his acute urinary infection and granulomatous prostatitis, I saw him again with symptoms of hesitancy, decreased stream, urgency, and urinary frequency, and a 4-month history of recurrent *E. coli* urinary infections, well controlled on TMP-SMX therapy. On rectal examination, the prostate was symmetrically enlarged and firm, but not hard. Cystourethroscopy showed the prostatic urethra to be occluded by irregular nodules of prostatic tissue; 31 g of prostate was resected, most of which showed infiltrating columns and sheets of cells of adenocarcinoma of the prostate. There was no evidence of chronic inflammation in any of the tissue sections.

Chronic Bacterial Prostatitis

Several investigators have indicated the fallacy of diagnosing bacterial prostatitis by the number of leukocytes in the prostatic secretion.[4, 13, 14] The use of prostatic needle biopsy for tissue culture is equally ineffective[15]; the low yield of valid cultures with this technique is not surprising since the infection may be focal. Furthermore, the needle biopsy for culture is random, small, easily contaminated from the perineum, and almost impossible to quantitate bacteriologically. The difficulty with diagnosing bacterial prostatitis by histologic examination is similar to the problem of diagnosing pyelonephritis; too many diseases other than bacterial infection produce an inflammatory reaction to injury.

In 1965, we presented a technique designed to distinguish urethral from prostatic infection in the male.[16] This method was based on quantitative bacterial counts of the voided urine partitioned into 10-ml segments of urethral (first voided), bladder (midstream), and prostatic (postprostatic massage) specimens. From these studies we mistakenly concluded that chronic bacterial prostatitis was exceedingly rare. With additional experience, the technique was modified to include a quantitative culture of pure prostatic secretion (in addition to the 10-ml sample of urine obtained after prostatic massage). This modification proved to be important; it led to the diagnosis of chronic bacterial prostatitis in a greater number of patients and to the recognition that bacteria could persist in prostatic fluid in much smaller numbers than we suspected in 1965. In fact, our experience would indicate that chronic bacterial prostatitis, characterized by small numbers of bacteria in prostatic secretion, is the most common cause of recurrent bladder infection in the male patient with normal intravenous urograms. Even in patients with upper tract evidence of infection, persistence in the prostatic fluid must be considered after the upper tracts are sorted out.

It is important to recognize that every patient we have ever seen with chronic bacterial prostatitis with persistence of Enterobacteriaceae or *Pseudomonas* in the EPS has recurrent bacteriuria; indeed, in the absence of documentation of bacteriuria, the diagnosis of chronic bacterial prostatitis is higly unlikely. Moreover, in between episodes of bladder infection, whether on or off antimicrobial therapy, these patients are asymptomatic despite bacterial persistence in the EPS and despite gross purulence of their prostatic fluid. In other words, patients with chronic bacterial prostatitis are symptomatic only when the prostatic bacteria reach the bladder and cause cystitis; to be sure, an occasional patient is asymptomatic with his bacteriuria but most are not.

Before presenting several diagnostic patterns, the reader is encouraged again to review the section in the first chapter on the technique of segmenting the voided urine into urethral (VB_1), midstream (VB_2), EPS, and the first voided few milliliters after prostatic massage (VB_3). The basic bacteriologic problem has always been to culture prostatic fluid in such a way that the contribution of urethral bacteria to prostatic fluid is recognized. It is probably fair to comment that 98% of all "positive" cultures in EPS reported in the literature actually represent urethral contamination of an otherwise sterile prostatic fluid. The practice of culturing the midstream urine followed by collection of EPS is based on the fallacy that all the urethral bacteria are washed away by the sterile bladder urine. This error can be demonstrated in any patient with urethral bacteria by simply comparing an initial VB_1 to a repeat urethral aliquot of urine (another VB_1) a few minutes after he has stopped voiding. Observe in Table 7.3 that if the VB_1 had not been collected on 4/30/63 the VB_3 would be considered excellent evidence of prostatic infection. The collection 2 weeks later clearly shows the same accumulation of *Proteus morganii* in the second VB_1 when prostatic massage was not performed. The critical culture on 4/30/63 is the VB_1 because it indicates the magnitude of urethral bacteria that can be expected when a sterile bladder urine opens the closed urethral

Table 7.3
Urethral Reaccumulation of Bacteria in Chronic Urethral Infection (W.M., age 38)

4/30/63		5/14/63	
Source	*Proteus morganii*	Source	*Proteus morganii*
	bacteria/ml		*bacteria/ml*
SPA[a]	0	SPA	0
VB_1	16,000	VB_1	3,600
VB_2	60	VB_2	67
Prostatic massage		Pause 3–5 min	
VB_3	1,440	VB_1	1,260

[a] SPA = suprapubic needle aspiration of the bladder; VB_1 = first voided 5–10 ml of urine from urethral meatus; VB_2 = midstream aliquot of urine; VB_3 = first voided 5–10 ml of urine from urethral meatus after prostatic massage.

canal, whether prostatic massage is performed or not; clearly, in this collection, all of the bacteria obtained in the VB_3 after prostatic massage can be accounted for by the density of urethral colonization. Stated in another way, any time bacteria are recovered in the EPS or VB_3 after prostatic massage they must not be accounted for by the addition of urethral bacteria.

Despite the diagnostic advantage of the EPS culture over the VB_3 in those patients who have bacterial persistence in small numbers in prostatic fluid (as emphasized in Chapter 1), there are some theoretical disadvantages to the EPS culture that can be misleading. The basic problem is that the VB_1 serves as a true control for the VB_3 but not for the EPS. That is, a sterile voided bladder urine opens the urethral canal before (VB_1) and after (VB_3) prostatic massage and the fluid volume and flow characteristics are nearly similar for both cultures. On the other hand, there really is no true control for EPS since it represents a small viscous volume that must travel more slowly through the urethra and nearly always hangs in the fossa navicularis before falling free into the collection tube. For example, it is not uncommon to see corynebacteria (diphtheroids) present in segmented cultures as follows: VB_1, 5000/ml; VB_2, 10/ml; EPS, 100,000/ml; VB_3, 2000/ml. Are we to interpret this as indicative of a corynebacterial prostatitis? I doubt it. It is possible that the EPS picks up far more urethral bacteria than the VB_3 or VB_1. Technical considerations such as these may account, at least in part, for Drach's[17] finding of many patients with Gram-positive bacterial prostatitis.

Because chronic bacteriae prostatitis is either curable or completely controllable and because its diagnosis and behavior is firmly established, several clinical examples with long-term observations are presented.

Clinical Examples: Diagnostic and Therapeutic Techniques.

Diagnostic Cultures on Antimicrobial Therapy. Example 1. T.E.L., a 60-year-old white man, had a febrile urinary infection in January 1966 which responded to antibiotic therapy. Thereafter, each time therapy was stopped, bacteriuria recurred with essentially asymptomatic *E. coli* urinary infections. Excretory urography was normal, endoscopy revealed mild trilobar intrusion, the prostatic ducts appeared uninflamed, and the bladder wall was smooth. Bacteriologic localization at cystoscopy on 9/11/67 was performed according to the techiques in Chapter 1. The following counts of *E. coli* were obtained per milliliter of urine: CB (catheterized bladder) = 100,000, WB (washed bladder) = 1,000, RK_1 = 10, RK_2 = 40, RK_3 = 40, RK_4 = 20, and RK_5 = 20. LK_1 through LK_5 were sterile (RK, right kidney; LK left kidney). This localization study suggested that small numbers of *E. coli* were present in the right kidney. Following cystoscopy, 500 mg of ampicillin were given by mouth every 6 hours for 10 days. Prostatic localization cultures were obtained after 4 and 6 days of ampicillin therapy, after which the patient was maintained on a low dosage of nitrofurantoin for 2 years (Table 7.4).

TMP-SMX became available to us in 1971, and the patient was treated for 14 days at full dosage therapy, 160 mg of TMP and 800 mg of SMX twice daily. The two cultures while on TMP-SMX showed bacterial persistence of an *E. coli* 011, but the next two cultures at 14 and 41 days off therapy were surprisingly sterile, almost suggesting that the prostatic massage on the final day of TMP-SMX therapy manually emptied the prostate of the last 011 *E. coli* (Table 7.4). Seventy days after the course of TMP-SMX, he noticed nocturia and mild dysuria; cultures showed $>10^5$ *E. coli* but an 075 serotype. During the next 4 years, he was seen on 33 occasions with segmented cultures at each visit. Except for a 3-month trial of full dosage TMP-SMX in mid-1972, the *E. coli* 075 was cultured from his EPS or VB_3 at every visit. This *E. coli* was very sensitive to all antimicrobial agents and except for the 3 months of TMP-SMX in 1972, nitrofurantoin or nitrofurantoin macrocrystals 100 mg twice daily maintained a sterile urine. Bacteriuria with the *E. coli* 075 occurred repeatedly within 7–30 days of discontinuing therapy during the years 1971–1975. For 18 months, during

Table 7.4
Chronic Bacterial Prostatitis (T.E.L.)

Date	Days on (+) or off (−) Drug	Source				Organism
		VB_1[a]	VB_2	EPS	VB_3	
			bacteria/ml			
9/11/67	−43 NA		100,000			*Escherichia. coli*
9/14/67	+4 Amp	10	0	1,300	40	*E. coli*
9/17/67	+6 Amp	10	0	1,900	30	*E. coli*
9/10/68	+41 Nitrofur	30	0	100,000	1,000	*E. coli*
4/1/69	−5 Nitrofur	50,000	50,000	50,000	50,000	*E. coli*
4/23/69	+23 Nitrofur	0	0	410	70	*E. coli*
4/23/71	+25 mo Nitrofur	1,000	0	1,700	240	*E. coli* 011
4/30/71	+7 TMP-SMX	0	0	140	50	*E. coli* 011
5/7/71	+14 TMP-SMX	0	0	100	10	*E. coli* 011
5/20/71	−14 TMP-SMX	0	0	0	0	
6/16/71	−41 TMP-SMX	0	0	0	0	
7/15/71	−70 TMP-SMX		100,000			*E. coli* 075
1971–75	+ Nitrofur		VB_3 or EPS always positive			*E. coli* 075
6/17/76	−7 TMP-SMX		100,000			*E. coli*
2/9/79	−1 year TMP-SMX		0			

[a] VB_1 = first voided 5–10 ml of urine from urethral meatus; VB_2 = midstream aliquot of urine; VB_3 = first voided 5–10 ml of urine from urethral meatus after prostatic massage; EPS = expressed prostatic secretion; TMP-SMX = trimethoprim-sulfamethoxazole (Septra); Amp = ampicillin; Nitrofur = nitrofurantoin (Furadantin); NA = nalidixic acid (NegGram).

1975 and 1976, his midstream urine remained sterile on one tablet daily of TMP-SMX, but his bacteriuria recurred within 7 days of stopping the TMP-SMX (June 1976, Table 7.4). After this culture, he was lost to follow-up but apparently restarted the TMP-SMX for about 1 year and then stopped therapy completely. In January 1979 he was contacted by telephone for a follow-up. He said he was asymptomatic, 72 years old, and had stopped all antimicrobial agents about a year before. A dip-slide agar culture was obtained by mail in February 1979, and it contained only small numbers of Gram-positive bacteria (!).

Comment. Because the bacterial counts of the VB_1 and VB_3 cultures were so similar on 9/14 and 9/15/67, the EPS culture was valuable in establishing the diagnosis of *E. coli* prostatitis. The VB_3 of 9/10/68 was diagnostic of bacterial prostatitis without knowledge of the EPS bacterial count; 1000 *E. coli*/ml in the VB_3 cannot be accounted for by the 30 bacteria/ml washed from the urethra in the VB_1 culture.

Example 2. I.A., a 58-year-old white man, was found to have an asymptomatic urinary tract infection in 1963. From 1963 until June 1966 the patient received numerous courses of antibiotic therapy but none was successful in permanently eradicating the bacteriuria. Excretory urography revealed delicate upper tracts and no prostatic calculi. Catheterization showed no residual urine. The prostate was palpably and endoscopically normal. When the patient was first seen on 1/16/67, the bladder urine was heavily infected with *Klebsiella*. Cystoscopic localization studies showed that the right renal urine was infected (bacterial counts were several thousand per milliliter in serial specimens). During the ensuing 2 years, many diagnostic prostatic localization cultures were obtained while the patient was taking a variety of antimicrobial drugs. None of these regimens have cleared the prostatic infection or prevented the recurrence of bladder bacteriuria when therapy was stopped (Table 7.5). A report from his local urologist in January 1979 indicated the patient (now 71 years old) was doing well without infections but required one tablet per day of TMP-SMX to keep his urine sterile from the *Klebsiella* prostatitis, a drug he has received continuously since October, 1974.

Table 7.5
Chronic Bacterial Prostatisis (I.A.)[a]

Date	Days on (+) or off (−) Drug	Bacteria				Organism
		VB_1[b]	VB_2	EPS	VB_3	
		bacteria/ml				
1/16/67	−180 Pen-G		100,000			*Klebsiella*
3/28/67	+7 Kana	50	0	2,300	30	*Klebsiella*
4/18/67	−18 Kana		100,000			*Klebsiella*
5/2/67	+14 Sulf	250	0	100,000	8,000	*Klebsiella*
6/27/67	+21 NA	0	0	10,000	1,000	*Klebsiella*
7/11/67	−14 NA		100,000			*Klebsiella*

[a] Reproduced by permission from T. A. Stamey *et al.*, J. Urol. **103:** 187, 1970.[18]

[b] VB_1 = first voided 5–10 ml of urine from urethral meatus; VB_2 = midstream aliquot of urine; VB_3 = first voided 5–10 ml of urine from urethral meatus after prostatic massage; EPS = expressed prostatic secretion; Pen-G = penicillin-G; Kana = kanamycin; Sulf = sulfonamide; NA = nalidixic acid.

Comment. These bacteriologic patterns are obviously diagnostic. When first seen, the patient had taken no antibacterial drugs for a period of 6 months. Initial localization showed infection in the right kidney. Had prostatic cultures not been obtained while the bladder urine was sterile on therapy, this infection could easily have been misdiagnosed as chronic pyelonephritis.

Example 3. J.J.T., a 51-year-old white man, had a febrile urinary infection due to *Klebsiella* in April 1965. In the ensuing year he had five recurrences, and each time the midstream urine yielded 100,000 *Klebsiella*/ml. Following long term nalidixic acid therapy, the midstream urine eventually remained sterile without medication for more than a month. The patient remained asymptomatic and was not seen again for 15 months. On 9/8/67, fever, chills, urgency, dysuria, and frequency developed. Excretory urography was normal. The prostate was tender, boggy, and enlarged 10–15 g (Table 7.6).

Comment. Following sterilization of the bladder infection, the cultures on 9/11 and 10/16/67 and 2/14/68 clearly showed the prostate to be the source of the *Klebsiella*. Two weeks of nitrofurantoin, 210 days of nalidixic acid, and 10 days of kanamycin all failed to clear the *Klebsiella* from the prostatic fluid. Of particular interest is the absence of bladder infection in the presence of 10,000 *Klebsiella*/ml of EPS 3 months after kanamycin therapy (Table 7.6). This suggests that some patients may harbor their prostatic bacteria for long periods between bladder infections. Because of similarity of the VB_1 and VB_3 counts, the culture on 9/24/68 again illustrates the importance of the EPS culture in differentiating between chronic infection of the urethra and prostate.

Sometime between 9/24/68 and 4/29/71, this patient became free of recurrent urinary infection. His medical records at a Veterans Administration Hospital are unclear as to what happened; he was not operated upon. Multiple urinalyses between 1971 and 1978 show no cells in the urinary sediment when he was followed for cardiopulmonary disease. Was he a spontaneous cure? It is unfortunate the medical records are inadequate, because further antimicrobial administration may have occurred and possible served as a therapeutic cure.

Diagnostic Cultures in the Absence of Expressed Prostatic Secretion; Cure by Transurethral Prostatectomy. Example 1. C.G.H., a 50-year-old white man, had two episodes of urinary infection in early 1968 associated with chills, fever, dysuria, frequency, acute urinary retention, and 100,000 *E. coli*/ml of bladder urine. A left epididymitis accompanied the second episode. Both infections were treated successfully with kanamycin, but the *E. coli* bacteriuria recurred within 10 days of stopping therapy. In the 6 months prior to seeing us on 11/25/68, the patient had six severe infections, all with *E. coli*. Continuous ni-

Table 7.6
Chronic Bacterial Prostatitis (J.J.T.)[a]

Date	Days on (+) or off (−) Drug	Source				Organism
		VB_1[b]	VB_2	EPS	VB_3	
		bacteria/ml				
4/19/65	1st infection		100,000			*Klebsiella*
9/8/67	−480 NA		100,000			*Klebsiella*
9/11/67	+3 Nitrofur	50	0	100,000		*Klebsiella*
10/16/67	+35 NA	10	0	10,000		*Klebsiella*
2/14/68	−90 Kana	0	0	10,000		*Klebsiella*
9/24/68	+210 NA	2500	1,000	100,000	3,000	*Klebsiella*
4/29/71	See text		0			

[a] Reproduced by permission from T. A. Stamey *et al.* J. Urol. **103:** 187, 1970.[18]

[b] VB_1 = first voided 5–10 ml of urine from urethral meatus; VB_2 = midstream aliquot of urine; VB_3 = first voided 5–10 ml of urine from urethral meatus after prostatic massage; EPS = expressed prostatic secretion; Nitrofur = nitrofurantoin; NA = nalidixic acid; Kana = kanamycin.

trofurantoin therapy prevented symptomatic episodes. On admission, the prostate gland was slightly enlarged (about 10 g) but was neither firm nor tender. An excretory urogram was normal except for multiple, small prostatic calculi (Figure 7.2). Endoscopy showed slight trilobar intrusion. After we obtained cultures diagnostic of chronic bacterial prostatitis (Table 7.7), a transurethral resection of the prostate was performed on 12/10/68. The method described in Chapter 1 was used to culture quantitatively a portion of both the prostatic tissue and the stones. The tissue contained *E. coli*, but the stones were sterile. A postoperative x-ray indicated no residual calculi.

Comment. The bacteriologic patterns on 11/28/68 and 12/1/68 during nitrofurantoin therapy probably represent the most reliable of all diagnostic patterns of prostatitis; *i.e.*, there were no *E. coli* in any urine segment prior to prostatic massage (Table 7.7).

Example 2. E.S., a 41-year-old Caucasian male, had his first urinary infection in 1943 at the age of 18; his symptoms were urinary frequency, dysuria, nocturia, perineal pain, chills, and fever, but he did not have flank pain or renal tenderness. Acute prostatitis was diagnosed, and he responded to a few days of sulfonamide therapy. He was asymptomatic until 1955, and again in 1960, when similar episodes occurred; both responded to short courses of sulfonamide therapy. The fourth urinary infection occurred in January 1964; initially the infection responded to sulfonamides, but it recurred within 3 weeks of stopping the medication. Several different antibacterial agents were tried in the ensuing 6 months, but each failed to cure the infection permanently. With each episode, the symptoms were generally severe, and quite similar to those of the first infection. In the summer of 1964, the patient was referred to a urologist who diagnosed chronic prostatitis. An excretory urogram and cystoscopy were both normal. Despite frequent prostatic massages, a variety of antibiotics, sitz baths, and even intraurethral antibiotic instillations, he continued to relapse symptomatically each time a drug was stopped. Several catheterizations showed no residual urine.

When initially seen at Stanford University Hospital on 2/1/66, the patient was asymptomatic but he had stopped oral penicillin-G only 2 days before. Physical examination revealed a healthy, robust male; the prostate was smooth, symmetrical, of normal consistency without tenderness, and enlarged by perhaps 10 g. Urinalysis was normal. Segmented urine cultures were sterile (Table 7.8).

On 2/8/66 (9 days off antibiotic) he was asymptomatic, although the urine cultures showed large numbers of *E. coli* in all three samples (Table 7.5). He was not treated because cystoscopy was scheduled for the following day. At cystoscopy, minimal tri-

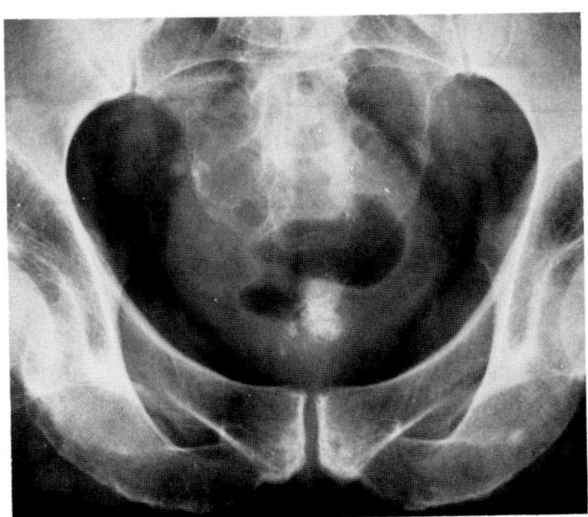

Figure 7.2 Plain film of pelvis shows multiple, small prostatic calculi in patient C.G.H. The opaque mass above the symphysis pubis represents prostatic calculi and not calcification of the coccyx.

lobar prostatic intrusion without occlusion was noted; the urethra and bladder looked normal. Bacteriologic localization of the infection showed that both renal urines were sterile, and that the infection was clearly localized to the lower urinary tract (Table 7.8). Tube dilution sensitivities of the *E. coli* showed that ampicillin was bactericidal at 5 μg/ml; he was started on ampicillin, 250 mg by mouth four times daily, at the conclusion of the cystoscopy.

He remained asymptomatic with sterile cultures while on ampicillin. Each time ampicillin was stopped (2/21, 3/5, and 3/16/66), *E. coli* appeared in the bladder urine by the 6th or 7th day (Table 7.8). Cultures on 3/10, 3/14, and 3/22/66 suggested that the prostate was the source of the *E. coli* (Table 7.8). To further substantiate an *E. coli* prostatitis, the patient was placed on nitrofurantoin, 100 mg by mouth four times daily; tube dilution sensitivities showed nitrofurantoin was bactericidal at 50 μg/ml. All three cultures on nitrofurantoin therapy demonstrated *E. coli* in the prostatic cultures while the urethral and midstream aliquots were sterile (Table 7.8).

Tube dilution sensitivities again showed that ampicillin was bactericidal at 5 μg/ml. On 4/5/66, ampicillin was restarted at a dosage of 1000 mg by mouth every 6 hours. Despite sterile urines during therapy, *E. coli* were cultured from the prostatic fluid on the 2nd day after stopping ampicillin, and the bladder was heavily infected by the 6th day (Table 7.8). Colistin methane sulfonate (Coly-Mycin), 75 mg intramuscularly every 12 hours was injected for 7 days. Within 10 days of stopping therapy, the bladder was again infected with *E. coli*.

The data in Table 7.8 show that *E. coli* were demonstrated in the prostatic secretion on the 1st day of sulfomethyl colistin therapy, on the 3rd day of ampicillin at 250 mg every 6 hours and throughout nitrofurantoin therapy—all at a time when the urethral and midstream aliquots were sterile.

Ampicillin was restarted and, on 5/25/66, an uncomplicated transurethral prostatectomy was accomplished. The CB urine prior to resection was sterile. A few small, brownish, prostatic calculi were uncovered near the apex; a single area of thick, yellowish, toothpaste material was resected in the area of the calculi. Microscopic examination of the resected prostate was not remarkable except for focal periacinar aggregates of lymphocytes and plasma cells. About one-half of the prostatic fragments were ground in a tissue blender and cultured; no bacteria were recovered. This failure to grow *E. coli* may have been caused by the ampicillin serum levels, the serumcidal activity of the emulsified tissue, or a combination of both. It is also possible that the infected part of the prostate was not in the sample chosen for culture. The Foley catheter was removed on the 3rd postoperative day; the patient was discharged on ampicillin, 500 mg by mouth every 6 hours, for 2 weeks. The ampicillin was stopped 6/10/66; he has remained well without any urinary symptoms. All urine cultures have failed to grow *E. coli* or any other pathogenic bacteria (Table 7.8), including cultures 10 months after the transurethral prostatectomy. Moreover, a letter from the patient in July 1971, 4 years after the last culture in Table 7.8, revealed that he had been healthy during the intervening 4 years.

Bacterial Persistence in Prostatic Fluid and Recurrence of Bacteriuria. L.P., a 63-

Table 7.7
Chronic Bacterial Prostatitis (C.G.H.)[a]

Date	Days on (+) or off (−) Drug	Source			Organism
		VB_1[b]	VB_2	VB_3	
			bacteria/ml		
11/25/68	−7 Oxytet		100,000		*Escherichia coli*
11/28/68	+3 Nitrofur	0	0	200	*E. coli*
12/1/68	+6 Nitrofur	0	0	2000	*E. coli*
12/3/68	+8 Nitrofur	100	20	200	*E. coli*
12/10/68	Transurethral prostatectomy				
1/10/69	+45 Nitrofur		0		
2/7/69	−28 Nitrofur		0		
3/7/69	−60 Nitrofur	80	0	0	Proteus mirabilis
4/2/69	−90 Nitrofur	0	0	0	

[a] Reproduced by permission from T. A. Stamey *et al.*, J. Urol. **103:** 187, 1970.[18]
[b] VB_1 = first voided 5–10 ml of urine from urethral meatus; VB_2 = midstream aliquot of urine; VB_3 = first voided 5–10 ml of urine from urethral meatus after prostatic massage; EPS = expressed prostatic secretion; Nitrofur = nitrofurantoin; Oxytet = oxytetracyline.

year-old Caucasian man first noted the onset of chills, fever, low back pain, urinary urgency and frequency, dysuria, and nocturia in 1961. He was thought to have prostatitis; his symptoms cleared with sulfonamide therapy. During the following months, his symptoms recurred each time antibiotics were stopped. In 1962, he was referred to a local urologist, who described the prostate as small, benign, and nonocclusive cystoscopically. An excretory urogram and a cystogram were normal. Fifty to 100 ml of residual urine were found on several catheterizations. A urine culture showed 100,000 *E. coli*/ml. The *E. coli* recurred each time medication was stopped despite numerous courses of various antibiotics. In February, 1963, a transurethral resection of the prostate was performed in a last effort to clear the infection. Eleven grams of tissue were removed; a diagnosis of benign prostatic hyperplasia and chronic prostatitis was made from the tissue sections. Despite absence of postoperative residual urine, a normal cystogram and urethrogram, the patient continued to recur with symptomatic *E. coli* urinary infections. Because of this, he was placed on a continuous regimen of oral penicillin-G.

He was first seen at Stanford University Hospital on 5/24/66; he had no symptoms, but the penicillin-G had been stopped only 2 days previously. Physical examination was not remarkable; the prostate was small, smooth, and non-tender. Urine cultures on admission grew 8000 *E. coli* in all three aliquots. By the time of cystoscopy the following day, he was having perineal pain and urinary urgency. Localization studies at cystoscopy showed 100,000 *E. coli*/ml of bladder urine, but both ureteral urines were sterile (Table 7.9). The urethra appeared normal, the prostatic fossa was well resected with no residual tissue, and the bladder was normal except for a single, small, wide mouth diverticulum above the right ureteral orifice. Retrograde pyelograms were delicate; pelvic tomograms revealed no prostatic calculi.

Tube dilution sensitivities indicated that nalidixic acid was bactericidal for the *E. coli* at 2 μg/ml. Immediately following cystoscopy, he was started on 1.0 g of nalidixic acid by mouth every 6 hours but, for diagnostic purposes, the drug was stopped after 4 g. Cultures on the 1st day of nalidixic acid therapy suggested the prostate as the focus of infection. Repeat cultures the next day were sterile; unfortunately, the EPS was not cultured. He was not cultured the following day (5/28/66) and by the next day it was too late: the *E. coli* were back in the bladder in large numbers—indeed, he was symptomatic (Table 7.9). On 5/30/66, cultures at 11:00 AM, just prior to starting 1.0 g of nalidixic acid every 6 hours grew

Table 7.8
Chronic Bacterial Prostatitis (E.S.)[a]

Date	Days on (+) or off (−) Drug	Drug	Dose	VB1[b]	VB2	VB3	Organism	
							Type	Sensitivity
			mg q 6 hr		*bacteria/ml*[c]			
2/1/66	−2	Pen-G	500	0	0	0		
2/8/66	−9	Pen-G		100,000	100,000	100,000	*Escherichia coli*	Amp (5)[d]
2/9/66	Cytoscopy and localization[e]				CB 100,000 WB 100		*E. coli*	
2/15/66	+6	Amp	250	0	0	0		
2/28/66	−7	Amp		7,000	8,000	8,000	*E. coli*	
3/1/66	Rx Amp.		250, for 5 days					
3/7/66	−2	Amp		0	0	0		
3/8/66	−3	Amp		0	0	0		
3/9/66	−4	Amp		0	0	0		
3/10/66	−5	Amp		0	0	50	*E. coli*	
3/11/66	−6	Amp		10,000	10,000	10,000	*E. coli*	
3/14/66	+3	Amp	250	0	0	50	*E. coli*	
3/22/66	−6	Amp		0	0	70	*E. coli*	
3/23/66	−7	Amp		100,000	100,000	100,000	*E. coli*	Nitrofur (50)
3/28/66	+5	Nitrofur	100	0	0	10	*E. coli*	
4/1/66	+9	Nitrofur		0	0	300	*E. coli*	
4/5/66	+13	Nitrofur		0	0	20	*E. coli*	
4/7/66	+2	Amp	1000	0	0	0		
4/12/66	+7	Amp		0	0	0		
4/14/66	−2	Amp		0	0	20	*E. coli*	
4/18/66	−6	Amp		100,000	100,000	100,000	*E. coli*	
4/20/66	+1	Colistin	150 mg qd	0	0	1,250	*E. coli*	
4/28/66	−2	Colistin		0	0	0		
5/3/66	−9	Colistin		0	0	0		
5/4/66	−10	Colistin		8,000	8,000	10,000	E. coli	Colistin (5)
5/4/66	Rx Amp.		500, continuously					
5/25/66	Transurethral prostatectomy[f]							
6/7/66	+13	Amp	500	0	0			
6/14/66	−3	Amp		0	0	0		
6/28/66	−17	Amp		0	0	0		
7/12/66	−31	Amp		0	0	0		
8/9/66	−2 mo			0	0	0		
10/4/66	−4 mo			0	0	0		
7/11/66	−10 mo			0	0	0		

[a] Reproduced by permission from E. M. Meares and T. A. Stamey, Invest. Urol. **5:** 492, 1968.[19]

[b] VB_1 = first voided 5–10 ml of urine from urethral meatus; VB_2 = midstream aliquot of urine; VB_3 = first voided 5–10 ml of urine from urethral meatus after prostatic massage; EPS = expressed prostatic secretion.; Pen-G = penicillin-G; Amp = ampicillin; Nitrofur = nitrofurantoin; Colistin = colistin methane sulfonate. Solid transverse line divides longitudinal cultures into major periods of significance.

[c] Small counts of Gram-positive organisms (*Staphylococcus epidermidis*, streptococci, diphtheroids) are not included in the table.

[d] Numbers in parentheses are bactericidal concentrations in micrograms per milliliter. The value for nitrofurantoin does not represent the *minimal* bactericidal concentration of the antibacterial agent required to kill the bacteria. It is a single tube dilution sensitivity checked at the estimated average urinary concentration of the drug and found to be bactericidal. Thus, the minimal bactericidal concentration may be less than this concentration.

[e] CB = catheterized bladder urine; WB = washed bladder (after 3000-ml sterile water irrigation); LK_1 to LK_4, serial catheterized left kidney urines, and RK_1 to RK_4, serial catheterized right kidney urines, each had 0 colonies/ml.

[f] CB, sterile (on ampicillin during surgery); ground prostatic tissue, sterile.

100,000 *E. coli* in all three aliquots. Repeat cultures at 5, 7, and 11 hours after the start of therapy showed a sterile urethra and midstream aliquots, while the prostatic sample (VB_3) was diagnostic of *E. coli* in the prostatic fluid (Table 7.9).

The patient was then discharged on nalidixic acid therapy and returned to his local urologist for follow-up. During the next 5 months, each time the drug was stopped, he relapsed with 100,000 *E. coli* in the bladder urine within 3–5 days.

Upon readmission to Stanford on 10/9/66, segmented cultures again confirmed small numbers of *E. coli* in the prostatic fluid. Within 48 hours of stopping nalidixic acid, the bladder became heavily infected—a pattern almost identical to the recurrence 5 months before (Table 7.9).

In preparation for an attempt at transurethral resection of the infected prostatic tissue, nitrofurantoin was started on 10/12/66, 100 mg every 6 hours; tube dilutions showed 50 μg/ml were bactericidal to the *E. coli*. Twenty-four hours later he was cystoscoped prior to transurethral biopsy; the catheterized urine grew 20 *E. coli*/ml. Inspection of the prostate showed a completely resected prostatic fossa with a thickened capsule and normal appearing mucosa. Several thin fragments of tissue from the floor of the prostatic fossa were removed with the resectoscope. One-half of the prostatic biopsies were ground in a tissue blender following four transfers through 5 ml each of sterile saline (Fig. 7.3). The fourth wash grew 10 *E. coli*/ml prior to blending the tissue; the ground tissue grew 900 *E. coli*/ml of saline. The remaining one-half of the resected tissue was submitted for microscopic examination. The sections revealed chronic inflammatory changes in focal areas.

The postoperative days were uncomplicated; the catheter was removed on the 2nd day. He was discharged asymptomatic on nalidixic acid (500 mg by mouth every 6 hours), with instructions to stop medication in 11 days and to return for culture on the 14th day. Cultures on 11/1/66 indicated an early recurrence of the *E. coli*; by 11/2/66, he was so symptomatic that nalidixic acid was restarted by telephone without first obtaining a culture. Because of the lack of residual prostatic tissue amenable to transurethal resection, the patient was offered the alternatives of either a total prostatectomy or nalidixic acid, 250 mg morning and night. He chose the latter alternative because of sexual considerations. On this regimen he remained symptom-free with sterile midstream urines.

The nalidixic acid was reduced by his family physician to 250 mg once a day sometime in 1968 and discontinued in January 1970. He remained free of symptoms; three urinalyses (but no cultures) by his physician in 1970 showed only a rare WBC. He returned to Stanford for a follow-up culture on 10/14/71, 20 months after stopping the nalidixic acid. Urine cultures showed he was bacteriuric with the same *E. coli* 06 present in earlier cultures (Table 7.9), an *E. coli* that was still sensitive to 2 μg/ml of nalidixic acid and 10 μg/ml of nitrofurantoin. His bladder urine was easily sterilized with nitrofurantoin and remained so on 100 mg twice a day (12/2/71). The bacteriologic course of this patient illustrates the necessity of continuous therapy if the urine is to remain sterile and the almost inevitability of relapse from the prostate when therapy is stopped.

Bacterial Persistence in Prostatic Fluid and Recurrence of Bacteriuria Despite Retropubic Prostatectomy. Two patients presented earlier were cured of their bacterial prostatitis by transurethral surgery because the focus of infection was successfully resected. The following case history shows that open prostatic surgery with enucleation of a large adenoma need not include the site of bacterial persistence.

J.S., a 69-year-old Caucasian man, who appeared at least 10–15 years younger than his stated age, had a transurethral prostatectomy in 1953 for obstructive symptoms. He was referred to Stanford in late December of 1967 because of recurrent hematuria, and a bladder mass found on intravenous urography (Figure 7.4). His midstream urine contained many leukcoytes, red blood cells (RBC), and 100,000 *Enterobacter*/ml of urine. Cystoscopy and ureteral cathe-

Table 7.9
Chronic Bacterial Prostatitis (L.P.)[a]

Date	Days on (+) or off (−) Drug	Drug	Dose	VB_1[b]	VB_2	VB_3	Organism Type	Organism Sensitivity	O-Serogroup
			mg q 6 hr		*bacteria/ml*[c]				
5/24/66	−2	Pen-G	500	8,000	8,000	8,200	*Escherichia coli*		
5/25/66	Cystoscopy and localization[d]			CB 100,000			*E. coli*	NA (2)[e]	06
				WB 1,200					
				LK_1 10	LK_3 0				
				LK_2 10	LK_4 0				
				RK_1 70	RK_3 0				
				RK_2 40	RK_4 0				
5/26/66	+1	NA	1000	0	0	10	*E. coli*		
5/27/66	−1	NA		0	0	0			
5/29/66	−3	NA		10,000	10,000	10,000	*E. coli*		
5/30/66									
11 AM		NA		100,000	100,000	100,000	*E. coli*		
2 PM	−3 hr	NA	1000	30	10	40	*E. coli*		
4 PM	+5 hr			0	0	10	*E. coli*		
6 PM	+7 hr			0	0	400	*E. coli*		
10 PM	+ 11 hr			0	0	120	*E. coli*		
5/31/66	Discharged on nalidixic acid, 500 mg q 6 hr, to be followed by his local physician; infection flared when drug was stopped; urine sterilized each time nalidixic acid was restarted.								
10/9/66	+4 mo	NA		10	0	180	*E. coli*		06
10/10/66	−1	NA		0	0	30	*E. coli*		
10/11/66	−2	NA		100,000	100,000	100,000	*E. coli*		06
10/12/66	+1	Nitrofur	100	Transurethral prostatectomy[f]			*E. coli*		06
				CB 20			*E. coli*		
				4th wash, 10			*E. coli*		
				Ground prostatic tissue, 900			*E. coli*		
10/13/66	+1	NA	500	Foley catheter aspiration, 10			*E. coli*		
11/1/66	−3	NA		1,000	900	1,100	*E. coli*		
10/14/71	−20 mo	NA		100,000	100,000	100,000	*E. coli*		06
12/2/71	+21	Nitrofur	100 mg q 12 hr	0	0	0			

[a] Adapted by permission from E. M. Meares and T. A. Stamey, Invest. Urol. **5:** 492, 1968.[19]

[b] VB_1 = first voided 5–10 ml of urine from urethral meatus; VB_2 = midstream aliquot of urine; VB_3 = first voided 5–10 ml of urine from urethral meatus after prostatic massage; Pen-G = penicillin-G; Nitrofur = nitrofurantoin; NA = nalidixic acid.

[c] Small counts of Gram-positive organisms (*Staphylococcus epidermidis*, streptococci, diphtheroids) are not included in the table.

[d] Numbers in parentheses are bactericidal concentrations in micrograms per milliliter. The value for nitrofurantoin does not represent the *minimal* bactericidal concentration of the antibacterial agent required to kill the bacteria. It is a single tube dilution sensitivity checked at the estimated average urinary concentration of the drug and found to be bactericidal. Thus, the minimal bactericidal concentration may be less than this concentration.

[e] CB = catheterized bladder urine; WB = washed bladder (after 3000-ml sterile water irrigation); LK_1 to LK_4, serial catheterized left kidney urines, and RK_1 to RK_4, serial catheterized right kidney urines, each had 0 colonies/ml.

[f] CB, sterile (on ampicillin during surgery); ground prostatic tissue, sterile.

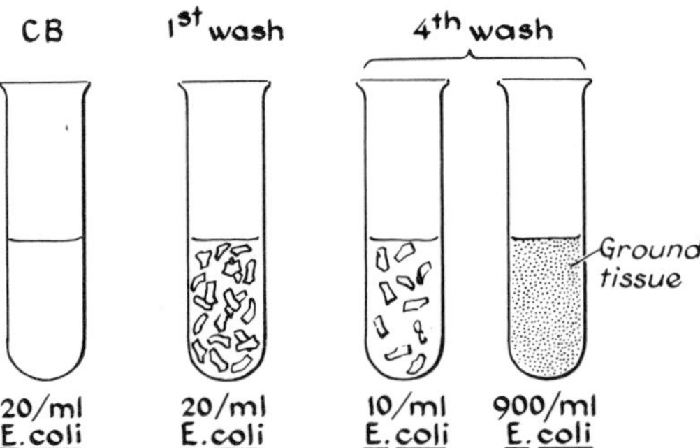

Figure 7.3 Chronic bacterial prostatitis L.P. (63-year-old white man). Method of culturing prostatic tissue chips from L.P. (Table 7.9). The catheterized bladder urine (CB) before beginning the transurethral resection contained 20 *Escherichia coli*/ml. Successive washings of the prostatic chips in sterile saline yielded 10 *E. coli*/ml in the fourth wash. When the tissue chips in the fourth tube of saline were ground with a tissue blender, the bacterial count increased from 10 to 900 *E. coli*/ml.

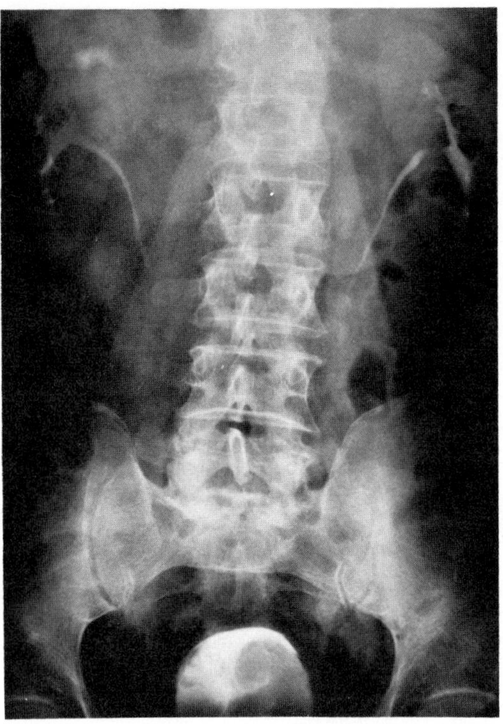

Figure 7.4 Intravenous urogram on J.S. The large intravesical prostate can be seen in the bladder. The right upper calyx appears distorted in comparison with the calyces of the left kidney; the right renal urine grew large numbers of *Enterobacter* (Table 7.10a).

terization on 1/5/68 showed that the bladder mass was intravesical prostate and that the *Enterobacter* was present in the right renal urine in large numbers (Table 7.10a). Nalidixic acid was bactericidal in tube dilutions at 10–20 μg/ml. After the localization study, he was treated with colistin methane sulfonate (Coly-Mycin) for 24 hours, which sterilized the urine (Table 7.10b). Between the 6th and 16th of January, he received 4 g/day of nalidixic acid. The urine was sterile 14 days after stopping the nalidixic acid, but 5 days later he had a massive bladder hemorrhage requiring an emergency retropubic prostatectomy. At surgery, a 145-g prostate was easily enucleated; he received nitrofurantoin postoperatively for 4 weeks. As can be seen in Table 7.10b, however, 32 days after discontinuing the nitrofurantoin, he was again infected with *Enterobacter*. A variety of antimicrobial agents between 4/9/68 and 9/10/68 produced a sterile urine, but *Enterobacter* always recurred each time therapy was stopped. In September of 1968 he began a continuous regimen of 250 mg of nalidixic acid morning and night. On this schedule, he maintained a sterile bladder urine, but most localization cultures were diagnostic of bacterial persistence in the prostatic fluid (Table 7.10b). An x-ray film of the pelvis showed no prostatic calculi to account for the persistence of the *Enterobacter* (Figure 7.5). After more than 576 days of continuous therapy, cessation of nalidixic acid was promptly followed by bacteriuria 7 days later accompanied by dysuria and frequency. Nalidixic acid was restarted, his symptoms disappeared, and the bladder urine became sterile. He will continue indefinitely on 250 mg of nalidixic acid twice a day. Tube dilution sensitivities of the *Enterobacter* to nalidixic acid were performed eight times between December 1967 and April 1970; 10–20 μg/ml were always bactericidal, thereby excluding resistance as the cause of bacterial persistence.

Surgical Cure of Bacterial Persistence in Prostatic Fluid by Radical Perineal

Table 7.10
a. Chronic Bacterial Prostatitis (J.S.): Localization data, 1/5/68

Bladder = > 100,000/ml *Enterobacter*; wash bladder = 1,800/ml *Enterobacter*. $LK_1 - LK_4$ = serial cultures on consecutive aliquots of left renal urine. $RK_1 - RK_4$ = serial cultures, right renal urine. Observe the high counts of *Enterobacter* in the right renal urine; the right upper calyx in the intravenous urogram (Figure 7.4) appears distorted in comparison with the calyces of the left kidney.

Left kidney	Right kidney
LK_1 = 80	RK_1 = >10,000
LK_2 = 1,000	RK_2 = >10,000
LK_3 = 60	RK_3 = >10,000
LK_4 = 0	RK_4 = >10,000

b. Chronic Bacterial Prostatitis (J.S.): Bacteriologic Course

Date	Days on (+) or off (−) Therapy	VB_1[a]	VB_2	VB_3	Organism
			bacteria/ml		
1/6/68	+1 Colistin		0		
1/6/68			NA, 4 g/day, for 10 days		
1/16/68	+10 NA	0	0		
2/1/68	−10 NA	0	0		
2/7/68	Retropubic prostatectomy; treated with Nitrofur for 4 wk				
3/12/68	−4 Nitrofur		0		
4/9/68	−32 Nitrofur		$>10^5$		*Enterobacter*
4/9/68 to 9/10/68:	RX with Pen-G, sulfonamides, and Colistin, always relapsed with *Enterobacter*				
9/10/68	Started NA, 2 g/day for 10 days, then 250 mg AM and PM				
10/1/68	+21 NA	0	0	40	*Enterobacter*
10/29/68	+50 NA	10	0	120	*Enterobacter*
1/28/69	+142 NA	20	10	190	*Enterobacter*
4/15/69	+202 NA	410	90	340	*Enterobacter*
7/22/69	+310 NA	0	0	230	*Enterobacter*
10/30/69	+408 NA	110	10	10,000	*Enterobacter*
1/15/70	+492 NA	20	0	230	*Enterobacter*
4/2/70	+576 NA	0	0	60	*Enterobacter*
4/24/70	−7 NA	$>10^5$	$>10^5$	$>10^5$	*Enterobacter*
4/24/70		NA, 2 g/day × 5 days; then 250 mg AM and PM			
5/7/70	+14 NA	0	0	10	*Enterobacter*
7/9/70	+74 NA		0		
9/17/70	+140 NA	40	30	110	*Enterobacter*

[a] VB_1 = first voided 5–10 ml of urine from urethral meatus; VB_2 = midstream aliquot of urine; VB_3 = first voided 5–10 ml of urine from urethral meatus after prostatic massage; Pen-G = penicillin-G; Nitrofur = nitrofurantoin; Colistin = colistin methane sulfonate; NA = nalidixic acid.

Prostatectomy; the Etiologic Relationship between Prostatic Bacteria and Renal Infection. W.D., a 57-year-old Caucasian man, was first seen at Stanford University Hospital on 1/7/65 with a 1-year history of intermittent bouts of chills, fever, nausea, dysuria, urinary urgency and frequency, and low back pain. His symptoms were controlled with antibiotics, especially oxytetracycline, but recurred when drugs were stopped. He had passed about 18 urinary calculi in the past 40 years. Previous surgery included a left ureterolithotomy in 1955, a right ureterolithotomy in 1960, and a left ureterolithotomy in 1961, with postoperative ureteral stricture and subsequent left nephrectomy. Physical examination revealed an indurated left epididymis and a diffusely firm, non-nodular prostate enlarged by about 30 g. Laboratory data included a serum creatinine of 1.8 mg/100 ml, a blood urea nitrogen (BUN) of 22 mg/100 ml, a normal serum acid phosphatase, and a serum calcium of 9.5 mg/100 ml (average

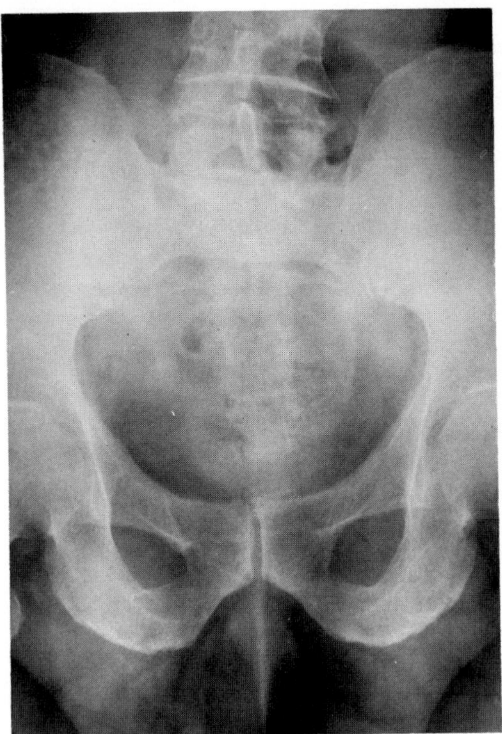

Figure 7.5 An x-ray film of the pelvis in J.S. made 2 years after the retropubic prostatectomy in February 1968. There are no visible prostatic calculi to account for the persistence of the *Enterobacter* in the patient's prostatic fluid.

of three determinations). Excretory urography showed multiple prostatic calculi, and a small opaque calculus in the lower calyx of an otherwise normal solitary right kidney. The right ureter and bladder were unremarkable; there was no significant residual urine after voiding.

A midstream urine culture grew 240 *Pseudomonas*/ml upon hospital admission (he was taking oxytetracycline). Medication was stopped, and 4 days later a suprapubic needle aspiration of the bladder grew 10,000 colonies of *E. coli* and *Pseudomonas* (Table 7.11a). He was cystoscoped the next day; bacteriologic localization techniques for both kidney and prostate (Chapter 1) were used. The data in Table 7.11a show that small numbers of *E. coli* and *Pseudomonas* were present in the right kidney and also suggest that both organisms were present in the prostate. Before leaving the cystoscopy room, the patient was given 150 mg intramuscularly of colistin methane sulfonate followed by 75 mg every 12 hours for 7 days. With a sterile urine and free of symptoms, he was discharged on oxytetracycline, 250 mg by mouth twice daily, to control the *Pseudomonas*; tube dilution sensitivities showed that 100 μg/ml of oxytetracycline were bactericidal.

During the ensuing 10 months, the patient remained asymptomatic on the oxytetracycline maintenance; he worked in his business and played golf twice a week. Cultures in March and October 1965, on oxytetracycline, showed persistence of the *Pseudomonas* in the midstream urine although the bacterial count was low (Table 7.11a). He was admitted, however, on 11/19/65 with right flank pain, microhematuria, and nausea, but no fever. A midstream urine culture grew 1600 *Pseudomonas*/ml (he was on oxytetracycline). An excretory urogram showed moderate right hydroureteronephrosis above the calculus, which was now located in the right midureter. He remained afebrile with minimal pain; the oxytetracycline was increased to 250 mg by mouth every 6 hours. On this regimen the midstream urine grew only 2 colonies of *Pseudomonas* per ml on 11/21/65 (Table 7.11a). After 3 days of conservative management, the stone had not moved; on 11/22/65, a right ureterolithotomy was performed without complication. The calculus was washed four times with sterile saline and crushed with a sterile mortar and pestle; a saline suspension of the ground stone grew 100,000 colonies of both *E. coli* (predominant) and *Pseudomonas* (Table 7.11a). Since the first treatment with colistin may have failed because of the bacteria within the renal calculus, a second trial of 10 days of therapy at a dosage of 75 mg intramuscularly every 12 hours was started postoperatively. He was asymptomatic with a sterile urine upon discharge on 12/4/65. After 13 days without medication, he developed chills, malaise, fever, and dysuria. The midstream culture grew 5,000 *Pseudomonas*/ml (Table 7.11a); unfortunately, neither a VB_3 nor an EPS was obtained. He was treated with 4 days of colistin to control his symptoms and then was discharged on a maintenance dosage of 250 mg of oxytetracycline twice daily. This time the midstream urine remained sterile, even when the dosage was reduced to 125 mg twice daily in May 1966. Efforts to prove that the *Pseudomonas* were in the prostate were unsuccessful except for one culture on 3/22/66.

After 9 months of repeatedly sterile cultures, the oxytetracycline was stopped on 10/5/66. Within 5 days he was symptomatic for the first time since 12/17/65; to our surprise, segmented urine cultures revealed a heavy growth of *E. coli* and not *Pseudomonas* (Table 7.11a). With this relapse, cystoscopic localization studies showed that neither the right kidney nor the left ureteral stump represented the site of the infection (Table 7.11a). On physical examination a firm nodule was palpable in the right prostatic lobe; a transperineal needle biopsy of the prostate was positive for a well differentiated adenocarcinoma. At the completion of cystoscopy and needle biopsy of the prostate, a single 150-mg dose of colistin was given intramuscularly; 4 hours later the urine was sterile. Because of the *E. coli* tube dilution sensitivities to nalidixic acid, the patient was started on 500 mg by mouth every 6 hours. Subsequent cultures showed no *E. coli* but did show reappearance of the *Pseudomonas* (Table 7.11a). He was then placed on 125 mg of oxytetracycline twice daily by mouth until he could return for a radical prostatectomy.

He was readmitted on 3/5/67; he had been asymptomatic on the low dose of oxytetracycline, and the urine was sterile. Acid and alkaline phosphatases were normal, a bone survey was negative for metastasis, and an excretory urogram was normal except for prostatic calculi and the surgically absent left kidney. Colistin methane sulfonate, 75 mg intramuscularly every 12 hours, was begun on 3/7/67; the following day a radical perineal prostatovesiculectomy was performed. At the time of surgery several large prostatic calculi were recovered; these were washed with four transfers into 5 ml of sterile saline and then crushed in the 5 ml of the fourth wash (Chapter 1). The fourth saline wash of the stones (prior to crushing) showed only 60 colonies of *E. coli* and *Pseudomonas*/ml, whereas the ground stone grew 10,000 colonies. The prostatic tissue was cultured in two different areas: the periurethral inner prostate and the compressed, outer prostate near the area of the stones. The tissue cultures were washed by the same method as the stones, but ground with a tissue blender. The periurethral inner prostate grew no bacteria, but the biopsy of the outer prostate showed both *Pseudomonas* and *E. coli* (Table 7.11a).

Microscopic examination of the surgical specimen showed the adenocarcinoma was well differentiated; although perineural invasion was present, invasion of the seminal vesicles was absent. Focal areas of inflammation were present in the prostate but not in the seminal vesicles; both intraacinar and periacinar aggregations of neutrophilic polymorphonuclear leukocytes and plasma cells were seen.

Ten days after surgery the catheter was removed and the colistin was stopped. The patient was discharged with excellent urinary control; he was asymptomatic without antibacterial agents. Twenty-one days after stopping the colistin, he was still asymptomatic; the midstream urine was sterile, and there were a few colonies of *E. coli* in the urethra but of a different O-serogroup than before (Table 7.11b). He remained free of symptoms and off all antibacterial drugs; follow-up culture on 11/11/67 was sterile and confirmed a cure of his previously chronic urinary infection. Except for a few colonies of *P. morganii* on the urethra in January 1968, all cultures in 1968, 1969, 1970, 1971, and 1972 contained only a few colonies of diphtheroids, *S. epidermidis*, and *Streptococcus faecalis* on the urethral mucosa (Table 7.11a). He was seen at yearly intervals from 1972 until his death in 1978 from a coronary infarction. His urine was never infected and his VB_1 always free from Enterobacteriaceae. The O-serogroup data in Table 7.11b confirm the constant presence of the same *E. coli* 06 during the 27 months of observation prior to the radical prostatectomy.

Antibacterial Cure of Chronic Bacterial Prostatitis; the Importance of Expressed Prostatic Secretions in Detecting Persist-

Table 7.11
a. Chronic Bacterial Prostatitis (W.D.)

Date	Days on (+) or off (−) Drug	Drug	Dose	VB_1[a]	VB_2	VB_3	Organism	
							Type	Sensitivity
			mg q12 h	*bacteria/ml*[b]				
1/7/65	+2	Oxytet	250		240		*Pseudomonas*	Oxytet (100)[c]
1/10/65	−3	Oxytet			900		*Pseudo*[d]	
1/11/65	−4	Oxytet		Suprapubic bladder aspiration, 10,000			*Pseudo*	Colistin (20)[c]
							Escherichia coli	Colistin (20)[c]
1/12/65	Cystoscopy with renal and prostatic localization			CB 7,020			*Pseudo, E. coli*	
				WB_1 77			*Pseudo*	
				WB_2 11			*Pseudo*	
				WB_3 2,460			*E. coli, Pseudo*	
				RK_1 228[e]			*Pseudo, E. coli*	
				RK_2 179			*Pseudo, E. coli*	
				RK_3 167			*Pseudo, E. coli*	
				RK_4 160			*Pseudo, E. coli*	
1/13/65	+2	Colistin	75		0			
1/18/65	+7	Colistin			0			
3/2/65	+41	Oxytet	250		5		*Pseudo*	
10/5/65	+258	Oxytet		1,398	1,696	2,858	*Pseudo, E. coli*	
10/8/65	−3	Oxytet		10,000	10,000		*Pseudo*	
11/19/65	+39	Oxytet			1,600		*Pseudo*	Oxytet (100)[c]
11/21/65	+2	Oxytet	250 (q 6 h)		2		*Pseudo*	
11/22/65	Right ureterolithotomy			4th wash, ureteral stone, 100,000			*Pseudo*	
	+1	Colistin	75	Ground stone culture, 100,000			*E. coli, Pseudo*	
12/4/65	+13	Colistin			0			
12/17/65	−13	Colistin		10,000	5,000		*Pseudo*	Colistin (20)[c]
12/18/65		Rx Colistin	75					
12/22/65	+4	Colistin		0	0			
2/1/66	+42	Oxytet	250	0	0			
3/22/66	+92	Oxytet		0	0	10	*Pseudo*	
4/23/66	+124	Oxytet		0	0	0		
5/16/66	+13	Oxytet	125	0	0	0		
9/13/66	+146	Oxytet		0	0	0		
10/9/66	−5	Oxytet		100,000	100,000	100,000	*E. coli*	Colistin (20)

10/10/66	Cystoscopy with localization, including left ureteral stump irrigation			CB 100,000 WB 10 RK$_1$ 10 LU$_1$ 20[f] LU$_2$ 10			*E. coli*	NA (10)
10/10/66	+4 hr	Colistin	150 (one dose)		0			
10/15/66	+5	NA	500 (q 6 h)	3,000	2,000	3,500	*Pseudo*	Oxytet (100)
3/5/67	+147	Oxytet	125		0			
3/8/67	Radical perineal prostatovesiculectomy			4th wash, prostatic stone, 60			*E. coli, Pseudo*	
				Ground stone culture, 10,000			*E. coli, Pseudo*	
	+1	Colistin	150 mg	4th wash, inner prostatic tissue, sterile				
				Ground inner prostatic tissue, sterile				
				4th wash, outer prostatic tissue, sterile				
				Ground outer prostatic tissue, 500			*E. coli, Pseudo*	
3/9/67		Rx Colistin	75		0			
3/20/67	−2 mo	Colistin			0			
4/14/67	−21 mo	Colistin		30	0		*E. coli* (different serogroup)	
7/11/67	−4 mo			0	0			
11/11/67	−8 mo			0	30			
1/9/68	−10 mo			190	0		*Proteus morganii*	
7/23/68	−16 mo			0	0			
12/10/68	−21 mo			0	0			
6/10/69	−27 mo			0	0			
12/4/69	−33 mo			0	0			
6/4/70	−39 mo			0	0			
6/4/71	−51 mo			0	0			
1/20/72	−58 mo			0				

Table 7.11, *Continued*

b. Chronic Bacterial Prostatitis (W.D.): *E. coli* O-serogroups during a 27-month interval

Date	Occasion	Specimen Cultured	*E. coli* Serotype
1/11/65	Initial admission	Suprapubic needle bladder aspiration	06
11/22/65	Ureterolithotomy	Ground ureteral calculus	06
10/10/66	Cystoscopic localization	Catheterized bladder	06
3/8/67	Prostatovesiculectomy	Ground prostatic calculus	06
3/8/67	Prostatovesiculectomy	Ground prostatic tissue	06
4/14/67	Clinic visit	Urethral (VB_1)	083

[a] VB_1 = first voided 5–10 ml of urine from urethral meatus; VB_2 = midstream aliquot of urine; VB_3 = first voided 5–10 ml of urine from urethral meatus after prostatic massage; Oxytet = oxytetracycline; WB_1 = initial washed bladder culture; WB_2 = repeat washed bladder culture prior to prostatic massage; WB_3 = washed bladder culture after postprostatic massage (see Chapter 1); Colistin = colistin methane sulfonate; NA = nalidixic acid CB = catheterized bladder urine. Solid transverse line divides longitudinal cultures into major periods of significance.

[b] Small counts of Gram-positive organisms are not included in the table.

[c] This value does not represent the minimal bactericidal concentration of the antibacterial agent required to kill the bacteria. It is a single tube dilution sensitivity checked at the estimated average urinary concentration of the drug and found to be bactericidal. Thus, the minimal bactericidal concentration may be less than this concentration.

[d] *Pseudo* = *Pseudomonas*; if two organisms are present, the predominant one is listed first.

[e] RK_2, RK_3, and RK_4 were each 0 colonies/ml. [f] LU, serial left ureteral stump irrigation cultures. LU_3 and LU_4 were each 0 colonies/ml.

ence of Prostatic Bacteria. S.T., a 57-year-old Caucasian man, was initially seen in the Medical Clinic at Stanford University Hospital in July 1966, with a 6-year history of rheumatoid arthritis. Routine urinalysis showed bacteriuria, and a midstream urine culture grew greater than 100,000 *E. coli*/ml. He was referred untreated to the Division of Urology on 7/28/66.

His urinary symptoms first began in 1960; they were limited to intermittent hesitancy, a slight decrease in the force of his stream, and occasional low back pain associated with malodorous urine. He had not experienced chills, fever, dysuria, nocturia, or hematuria, and he denied previous urologic investigation or treatment.

Physical examination revealed normal external genitalia and a symmetrically enlarged (15-g excess size), slightly boggy, nontender prostate without nodules. An excretory urogram was normal with no evidence of renal or prostatic calculi; no significant residual urine was noted. Midstream urinalysis showed no proteinuria, rare white blood cells (WBC) in the spun sediment, but numerous bacilli. Urine cultures grew 100,000 *E. coli* in the VB_1, VB_2, and VB_3 segments (Table 7.12). Tube dilution sensitivities showed that penicillin-G was bactericidal to the *E. coli* at 100 μg/ml, ampicillin at 5 μg/ml, and nalidixic acid at 10 μg/ml. The patient was treated first for 10 days with penicillin-G in a dosage of 500 mg by mouth every 6 hours; cultures on 8/4/66 (the 7th day of penicillin therapy) suggested that the prostate was the source of the infection (Table 7.12). Further cultures on 8/15, 8/18, and 8/25/66, after stopping the penicillin, proved the prostate was the source of the *E. coli*; without the EPS culture on 8/15 and 8/18, the two VB_3 cultures would have been misleading.

By 8/25/66, the patient noted the onset of generalized arthralgia and low back pain; the segmented cultures showed a substantial increase in numbers of *E. coli* in the prostate, although the midstream urine was sterile. Sensitivities again showed nalidixic acid was bactericidal for this *E. coli* at 10 μg/ml; accordingly, he was started on nalidixic acid, 1.0 g by mouth every 6 hours.

Table 7.12
Chronic Bacterial Prostatitis (S.T.)

Date	Days on (+) or off (−) Drug	Drug	Dose	VB_1[a]	VB_2	EPS	VB_3	Organism	
								Type	Sensitivity
			mg q 6 h		*bacteria/ml*[b]				
7/28/66				100,000	100,000		100,000	*Escherichia coli*	Pen-G (100)[c]
8/4/66	+7	Pen-G	500	100	70		6,500	*E. coli*	
8/15/66	−7	Pen-G		0	0	70	0	*E. coli*	
8/18/66	−10	Pen-G		0	0	120	0	*E. coli*	
8/25/66	−17	Pen-G		0	0	10,000	600	*E. coli*	Pen-G (100)[c] NA (5)
8/25/66		Rx NA	1000 (for 2 weeks); then 500 (for 2 weeks)						
9/1/66	+7	NA	1000	0	0	0	0		
9/8/66	+14	NA		0	0	0	0		
9/15/66	+21	NA	500	0	0	0	0		
9/22/66	−3	NA		0	0	0	0		
9/29/66	−10	NA		0	0	0	0		
10/6/66	−17	NA		0	0	0	0		
10/20/66	−31	NA		100,000	100,000	100,000	100,000	*E. coli*	NA (5)
11/3/66	−45	NA			100,000			*E. coli*	
11/4/66			Reaction to *SMX* after four doses; drug stopped						
11/21/66	−17	SMX		100,000	100,000			*E. coli*	Amp (5)
12/1/66		Rx Amp	500 (for 14 days); then 250 (for 21 days)						
12/8/66	+7	Amp	500	0	0		0		
12/15/66	+14	Amp		0	0	10	0	*E. coli*	
12/22/66	+21	Amp	250	0	0	1,500	120	*E. coli*	Amp (5) Kana (20)
12/29/66	+28	Amp		0	0	7,000	10	*E. coli*	Amp (5)
1/5/67	+35	Amp		0	0	900	220	*E. coli*	Amp (5)
1/12/67	−7	Amp		0	0	4,000	120	*E. coli*	Amp (5)
1/23/67	−18	Amp		100,000	100,000			*E. coli*	Kana (20)
1/27/67	+5	Kana	500 mg q 12 h	0	0	0	0		
9/13/67	−8 mo	Kana		0	0	0	0		
4/9/68	−15 mo			0	0		0		
7/2/68	−18 mo			0	0	0	0		
9/10/68	−20 mo			0	0		0		
10/21/69	−33 mo			0	0	0	0		

[a] VB_1 = first voided 5–10 ml of urine from urethral meatus; VB_2 = midstream aliquot of urine; VB_3 = first voided 5-10 ml of urine from urethral meatus after prostatic massage; EPS = expressed prostatic secretion; SMX = sulfamethoxazole (Gantanol); Pen-G = penicillin-G; Amp = ampicillin; NA = nalidixic acid (NegGram); Kana = kanamycin (Kantrex). Solid transverse line divides longitudinal cultures into major periods of significance.

[b] Small counts of Gram-positive organisms are not included in the table.

[c] This value does not represent the *minimal* bactericidal concentration of the antibacterial agent required to kill the bacteria. It is a single tube dilution sensitivity checked at the estimated average urinary concentration of the drug and found to be bactericidal. Thus, the minimal bactericidal concentration may be less than this concentration.

After 14 days of therapy at 1.0 g every 6 hours, he was continued for an additional 2 weeks at 500 mg every 6 hours. Throughout this month of therapy, repeated urine and prostatic cultures revealed no growth of *E. coli*. Furthermore, cultures obtained every week for 3 weeks after stopping the nalidixic acid also failed to grow *E. coli*.

On 10/20/66, 5 weeks after stopping nalidixic acid, 100,000 *E. coli* were cultured in all aliquots. Despite this infection he was asymptomatic. Unfortunately, these *E. coli* were not serogrouped to distinguish bacterial persistence from reinfection; the tube dilution sensitivities showed the same bactericidal end points as the *E. coli* present in August. On 11/3/66, he was started on a course of sulfamethoxazole (Gantanol), 1.0 g three times daily. After 4 g of this drug, he developed a generalized skin rash, the medication was stopped, and he was treated with antihistamines.

Three weeks later, after the rash was gone, the bladder urine was still heavily infected with *E. coli*. Since tube dilutions showed ampicillin was bactericidal at 5 μg/ml, 500 mg every 6 hours was started on 11/21/66; after 14 days the dosage was reduced to 250 mg every 6 hours for an additional 21 days. While the patient was on ampicillin, segmented cultures showed the same pattern previously seen with penicillin-G, *i.e.,* sterile urethral and midstream urines, but persistent *E. coli* in the prostatic fluid still sensitive to ampicillin at 5 μg/ml. Within 3 weeks of stopping the ampicillin, the midstream culture was again heavily infected with an *E. coli* sensitive to ampicillin at 5 μg/ml. Tube dilution sensitivities had shown that kanamycin was bactericidal at 20 μg/ml. The patient was given 5 days of kanamycin (500 mg intramuscularly twice daily), and all cultures were sterile by the 5th day (Table 7.12). He was not seen again for 8 months, but during this interim he was completely asymptomatic and had received no antibacterial drugs. Cultures on 9/13/67, 8 months after the kanamycin therapy, showed an apparent cure of his chronic bacterial prostatitis (Table 7.12). Follow-up cultures in April 1968, July 1968, September 1968, and October, 1969 confirmed the absence of infection 33 months after his final treatment with 5 days of kanamycin therapy. His EPS had 8–10 WBC/hpf.

Prostatic Calculi as a Source of Bacterial Persistence in the Prostate R.F., a 33-year-old, white Caucasian male who was first seen at Stanford University Hospital on 5/13/71. In June 1970, he first observed perineal discomfort described as a "warm swelling," particularly noticeable after sitting or riding in a car. Shortly thereafter, he had his first of six episodes of chills, fever (to 104°F on one occasion), right flank discomfort, urinary frequency, urgency, and nocturia. Antimicrobial therapy, consisting of either ampicillin, penicillin-G, tetracycline, or sulfonamide, promptly relieved his symptoms; relapse, however, occurred each time about 2 weeks after stopping therapy. With each episode, a midstream pyuria was reported but cultures were not obtained until he was hospitalized with a particularly severe recurrence in April, 1971. *Pseudomonas aeruginosa,* $>10^5$/ml of urine was cultured at the April admission, and he was treated for 10 days with gentamicin. His urine promptly became sterile; cytoscopy was reported to be normal. A cystogram showed no reflux, and an intravenous urogram was unremarkable except for a small calcification seen above the symphysis pubis (Figure 7.6). Cultures on 5/13/71 when R.F. was first seen in our outpatient unit, were clearly diagnostic of *P. aeruginosa* in the prostatic fluid (Table 7.13); at the time of these cultures, he had received no antibiotics for 25 days.

He was admitted to Stanford University Hospital on 5/23/71, where repeat cultures confirmed a sterile bladder urine, but persistent *P. aeruginosa* in the prostatic fluid (Table 7.13). On 5/23/71, prior to catheterization for a voiding cystourethrogram, a VB_1 and a VB_2 culture were obtained just before the patient produced a complete ejaculate for culture. As seen in Table 7.13, the numbers of *P. aeruginsa* in the seminal plasma were similar to those in his expressed prostatic fluid. The voiding cystourethrogram (Figure 7.7) indicated tht the calcifications (*double arrows*) were be-

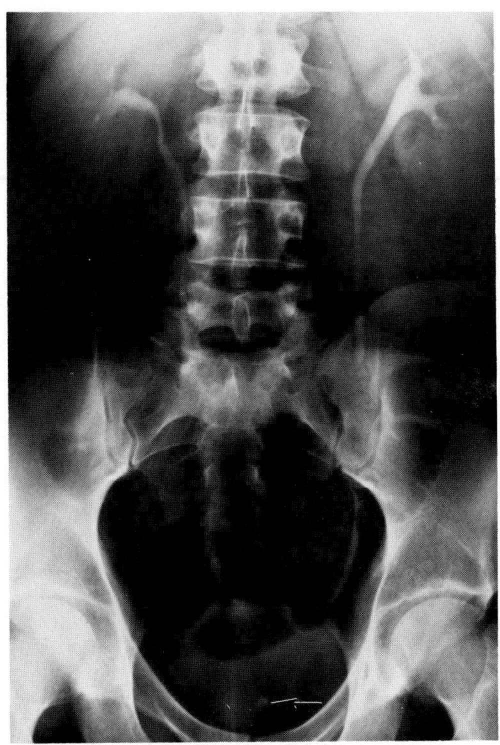

Figure 7.6 An intravenous urogram on R.F., a 33-year-old man with *Pseudomonas aeruginosa* in his prostatic fluid and a history of six episodes of chills, fever, right flank pain, dysuria, and frequency. The upper tracts were not remarkable, but a single calcification is seen just above the symphysis pubis slightly to the left of the midline.

low the vesical neck and posterior to the prostatic urethra (*single arrow*).

Prior to transurethral resection the following day, both vasa were exposed in the scrotum and small polyethelene tubes were passed toward the seminal vesicles. Unfortunately, the vasa could be cannulated for only 4 cm on each side, preventing aspiration of seminal vesicle fluid for direct culture. Injection with contrast suggested an anatomical distortion of the left seminal vesicle (Figure 7.8), on the same side of the midline as the prostatic calcification (*single arrow*). Close inspection, however, of Figure 7.8 shows the ejaculatory ducts to lie at some distance from the calcifications. Injection of increasing volumes of contrast solution into the left vas served only to fill the bladder rather than the ampulla of the left vas and seminal vesicle. On rectal examination, some induration was present in the area of the left seminal vesicle.

The bladder and prostatic urethra were entirely normal at cystoscopy; there was no intraurethral prostatic tissue and no sign of inflammation along the prostatic urethra. Transurethral resection was begun along the left floor and lateral wall of the prostatic urethra. By the third sweep of the resecting loop, the stones were uncovered just in front of the verumontanum, not more than 2 or 3 mm deep from the urethral mucosa, and certainly superficial to the ejaculatory ducts. The resection was completed, removing all the calculi (proven by x-ray films taken on the table) and about 6 g of prostatic tissue. Cultures of the stones showed large numbers of *P. aeruginosa* within the calculi, but we were unable to culture a single organism from the prostatic tissue, including pieces immediately adjacent to the calculi (Table 7.13). Analysis of the stone showed 96% tricalcium phosphate deposited over a nucleus of microcrystalline hydroxyl apatite. Microscopic study of the tissue sections showed both acute and chronic inflammation in some areas, but 80% of the sections showed normal prostatic glands and fibromuscular tissue.

At the end of the resection he was started on gentamicin, 40 mg every 8 hours. The minimal inhibitory concentration (MIC) of gentamicin for this strain of *P. aeruginosa* was 0.22 μg/ml. The bladder urine was sterile on 5/28/71 at the time of removing the Foley catheter, and he was discharged 3 days later. On the day of discharge, which was the 5th and last day of gentamicin therapy, the VB_1 and VB_2 were sterile, but the VB_3—obtained after gentle massage of the prostate—showed 90 colonies of *P. aeruginosa*/ml (Table 7.13). Seventeen days later he was seen in the out-patient unit for follow-up cultures. He had moderate dysuria and frequency, pyuria, and 10^4 *P. aeruginosa*/ml in his bladder urine (Table 7.13). Tetracycline was started on 6/17/71 (MIC = 1.6 μg/ml). One week later, he was essentially asymptomatic, his blad-

Table 7.13
R.F., a 33-year-old, Caucasian Man with *Pseudomonas* Bacterial Prostatitis and Probable Seminal Vesiculitis

Date	Days on (+) or off (−) Drug	VB_1[a]		VB_2		EPS		VB_3	
					bacteria/ml[b]				
4/8/71				*Pseudomonas aeruginosa*	>100,000				
4/16/71	+8 Gentamicin				0				
5/13/71	−25 Gentamicin	*P. aeruginosa* *Streptococcus faecalis*	500 30	*P. aeruginosa*	80	*P. aeruginosa*	5,000	*P. aeruginosa*	10,000
5/23/71	−35 Gentamicin	*P. aeruginosa* *S. faecalis* *Staphylococcus epidermidis*	300 30 110	*P. aeruginosa*	300	*P. aeruginosa* *S. faecalis* *S. epidermidis*	10,000 120 50	*P. aeruginosa* *S. faecalis* *S. epidermidis*	1,000 40 30
5/25/71	−37 Gentamicin	*P. aeruginosa*	20	*P. aeruginosa*	30	Ejaculate: *P. aeruginosa* *S. epidermidis* *α-Streptococcus* Diphtheroids	 10,000 130 3,000 <10,000		
5/26/71	−38 Gentamicin	Right vas Left vas Deep prostatic tissue Superficial prostatic tissue	sterile						
		Prostatic stone Wash 1 ..... *P. aeruginosa* 600 Wash 4 ..... *P. aeruginosa* 20 Crushed stone . *P. aeruginosa* 2,000							
5/28/71	+2 Gentamicin 40 mg q 8 hr			Foley catheter aspiration = 0					
5/31/71	+5 Gentamicin 40 mg q 8 hr		0		0			*P. aeruginosa*	90
6/17/71	−17 Gentamicin	*P. aeruginosa* *γ-Streptococcus*	10,000 1,000	*P. aeruginosa*	10,000				
6/24/71	+7 Tetracycline 250 mg q 6 hr		0		0	*P. aeruginosa*	$<10^4$	*P. aeruginosa*	6,000

9/16/71	+60	Tetracycline 250 mg q 12 hr	*P. aeruginosa*	10^3	*P. aeruginosa*	60	*P. aeruginosa*	10^4	*P. aeruginosa*	500
			α-*Streptococcus*	10^4	α-*Streptococcus*	80	α-*Streptococcus*	4,000	α-*Streptococcus*	2,000
			S. epidermidis	180			*S. epidermidis*	70	*S. epidermidis*	190
12/2/71	+137	Tetracycline 250 mg q 12 hr	*P. aeruginosa*	60	*P. aeruginosa*	30	*P. aeruginosa*	5,600	*P. aeruginosa*	130
									S. epidermidis	10

[a] VB_1 = first voided 5–10 ml of urine from urethral meatus; VB_2 = midstream aliquot of urine; VB_3 = first voided 5–10 ml of urine from urethral meatus after prostatic massage; EPS = expressed prostatic secretion.

[b] Small counts of Gram-positive organisms are not included in the table.

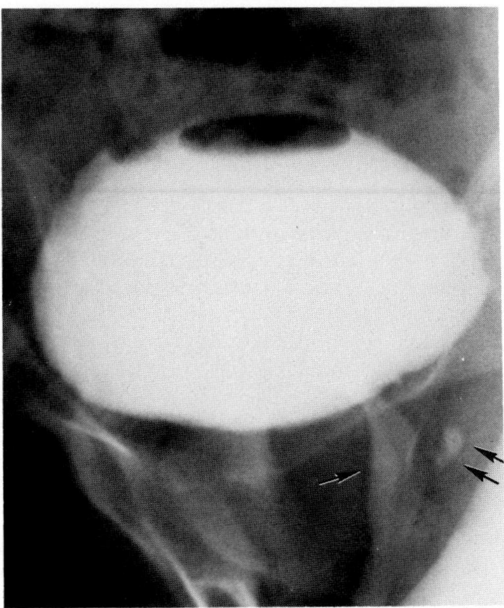

Figure 7.7 Voiding cystourethrogram on R.F., showing that the calcification (*double arrow*) is well below the vesical neck of the bladder and posterior to the prostatic urethra (*single arrow*) near the verumontanum. This study clearly showed that the site of calcification was in the prostate.

der urine was sterile, but *P. aeruginosa* could be cultured from his prostatic fluid. He was maintained on 250 mg of tetracycline morning and evening. When seen on 9/16/71 and 12/2/71, his bladder urine was uninfected and he felt in excellent health; *P. aeruginosa* was easily cultured from his prostate on both visits (Table 7.13). His white cell blood count and differential were normal; his sedimentation rate was 5 mm/hour.

In April 1972, he was switched from tetracycline:HCl to full dosage minocycline:HCl, 100 mg twice daily, for 8 months. Despite prolonged, full-dosage therapy, monthly cultures always grew 10^4–10^5 *P. aeruginosa* in the EPS while the VB_1 contained less than 10^3 and the VB_2 less than 10^2 *Pseudomonas*. Symptomatic bacteriuria always occurred when minocycline was stopped. He was maintained on one tablet of minocycline daily until June 1974, when he was switched back to tetracycline:HCl,

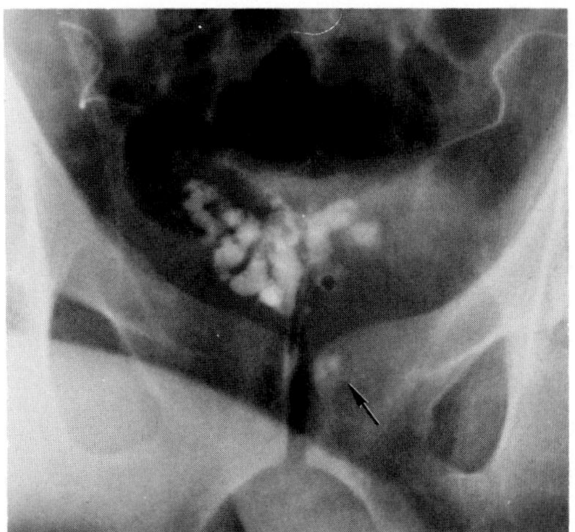

Figure 7.8 Bilateral seminal vesiculogram performed just prior to transurethral resection of the prostatic calculi in patient R.F. The left seminal vesicle is anatomically distorted and the ampulla of the left vas cannot be seen; further contrast injection down the left vas filled only the bladder rather than further distending the left seminal vesicle. The calcification in the prostate (*arrow*) is separate from and to the left of the ejaculatory ducts.

250 mg twice daily. Plain x-ray films of the pelvis in 1972, 1974, and 1975 showed a small opacity to the right of the symphysis pubis which suggested a single prostatic calculus. In January 1976, after 48 hours of gentamicin therapy, a second transurethral resection of the prostate, accompanied by perineal and transurethral injection of the prostate with 80 mg of gentamicin, was done followed by several days of parenteral gentamicin. Despite these efforts, and the finding by x-ray that the prostatic calculus was removed, symptomatic *Pseudomonas* bacteriuria returned a few days after discharge from the hospital. Prostatic tissue cultures at the time of the prostatic resection were sterile. He was maintained on tetracycline:HCl, 250 mg twice daily, throughout 1976 and 1977; the bladder urine remained sterile, but his EPS always grew *Pseudomonas* in large numbers, usually 100,000/ml of EPS. His general health has remained excellent and he continues to work hard as a farmer.

We are concerned, and confused, about the appearance of the left seminal vesicle (Figure 7.8). The failure to grow bacteria from his prostatic chips in 1971 is difficult to understand unless the ground prostatic tissue killed the bacteria during incubation of the cultures. Since Huggins and Bear[20] have shown that most prostatic stones form in the larger ducts as they proceed toward the verumontanum, it is possible that we resected the stones in the ducts without removing the more peripherally located glands that contain the *Pseudomonas*. If he has an accompanying seminal vesiculitis due to the *Pseudomonas*, it is indisputable from the prostatic massage cultures as well as the location and results of the stone cultures that the prostate is also involved.

Despite the lack of answers to these important questions, this patient serves as a reminder that spontaneous urinary infections do occur in young men in the absence of instrumentation, that the prostate is the site of persistence, that prostatic calculi can, in some instances, contain the infecting organisms, and that tetracyline is a marvelous antimicrobial agent for bladder prophylaxis when *P. aeruginosa* infects the prostate.

Bacterial Persistence Despite "Sterile" Expressed Prostatic Secretion; Usefulness of Serum Antibody Titers. J.H., a 47-year-old, Caucasian man had a vagotomy and pyloroplasty for peptic ulcer disease in 1961 when he was 37 years old. Following surgery, he required a Foley catheter for 5 days, from which he developed a urinary infection. Because of repeated recurrences, characterized by dysuria, hesitancy, frequency, and perineal and low back discomfort, he received sulfonamides almost continuously for the next 3 years. Intravenous urograms in 1964 were said to be normal. Between 1964 and 1967 he was treated alternately with nitrofurantoin, methenamine, and prostatic massage every 1–2 weeks.

Seven days prior to his initial visit at Stanford in October 1967, he had taken nalidixic acid for 3 days but stopped because of abdominal cramps and diarrhea. When first seen on 10/17/67 (Table 7.14), he had only 1780 *E. coli* in his midstream urine, suggesting his usual bladder bacteriuria had not recurred at that time (especially in view of the VB_1 count). Shortly following this initial visit, however, he developed a right epididymitis and was treated with oral penicillin-G. When seen again on the 16th day of penicillin-G therapy, the bladder urine was not infected and the VB_3 cultures were not diagnostic of bacterial prostatitis. An *E. coli* bacteriuria occurred by the 7th day after stopping oral penicillin-G (11/28/67). Not until EPS cultures were obtained on 12/30/67 and 2/1/68, both off medication, was the site of bacterial persistence identified as the prostate. An intravenous urogram showed a few scattered prostatic calcifications that were linearly oriented in the area of the prostatic ducts near the verumontanum. The kidneys were normal.

He was admitted to Stanford University Hospital, started on intravenous polymyxin-B sulfate therapy, and cultures were obtained every day; on the 2nd, 3rd, 5th, and 8th day of therapy they were diagnostic of bacterial persistence in the prostatic fluid (Table 7.14). The intravenous administration of 3 mg/kg/24 hours, divided into 8-hour dosages given over a 40-minute period, increased his serum creatinine from 0.8 mg/100 ml to only 1.3 mg/100 ml. By the 4th and 5th day after discontinuing therapy, *E. coli* were easily culturable from the prostatic fluid and 17 days later his bacteriuria had recurred. Tube dilution sensitivities to polymyxin-B sulfate showed bactericidal activity at < 0.5 μg/ml against his *E. coli* (Table 7.14).

For the next 34 months, his bladder urine was kept sterile with oral penicillin-G despite numerous diagnostic cultures that proved persistence of *E. coli* in the prostatic fluid (Table 7.14). Several cultures were also suggestive of a *P. morganii* accompanying the *E. coli* in his prostatic fluid (5/21/68, 7/17/69, 1/13/70), but the bacterial counts were very small and other cultures (4/9/68) were equally suggestive of the urethra as the site of the *P. morganii.* After 35 months of oral penicillin-G, the *E. coli* were found in the bladder urine. These *E. coli* were still sensitive to penicillin-G (MIC = 16 μg/ml); it is not known if he omitted his penicillin-G during these cultures in preparation for TMP therapy.

The penicillin-G was stopped and he was treated for 14 days with a combination of TMP and SMX, a drug that will be discussed later in this chapter. As seen in Table 7.14, the *E. coli* causing his bacteriuria on 2/23/71 and persisting in his prostatic fluid on the 7th day of TMP therapy was a serogroup 06. Seven days later on the last day of TMP therapy, and for 133 days after completing therapy, six consecutive cultures (including EPS) failed to grow a single Gram-negative organism. The agglutination titer in his blood serum to his *E. coli* 06 was 1:640 on 2/23/71 and 3/2/71 and remained at this level until 5/25/71 when it decreased by only one tube to 1:320. His serum titer on 7/20/71 was still 1:320, 133 days after completion of therapy. Seven days later he presented with acute bacterial prostatitis and bacteriuria due to his *E. coli* 06. He had fever, chills, dysuria, obstructive voiding, and a tender, swollen, hard prostate. His serum agglutination titer to the *E. coli* 06 was >1:2560. After 7 days of cephalexin, he was placed again on chronic penicillin-G therapy. The *E. coli* present in his prostatic fluid on 8/17/71, 10/12/71, 10/26/71, and 12/16/71 was a new serogroup, 075. These observations that the serum titer to his *E. coli* 06 never returned to normal (1:160 or less) suggest persistence of the *E. coli* despite 133 days of negative cultures; this persistence is apparently confirmed by culturing the same 06 serogroup as the responsible organism for his acute bacterial prostatitis and bacteriuria. The O-agglutination titer in his serum to the *E. coli* 075 first detected on 8/17/71 was 1:640 but, surprisingly, all of his earlier sera from 2/23/71 to 10/12/71 showed the same high titer. Serum titers on 12/16/71 showed 1:1,280 for the *E. coli* 075 and a persistent 1:640 for the original *E. coli* 06. These observations suggest that both the *E. coli* 06 and the *E. coli* 075 have been continuously present in his prostate despite the periods of negative cultures. The *Enterobacter* cultured on 8/3/71 is probably urethral or foreskin in origin; this

Table 7.14
Bacteriologic Course of J.H., a 47-year-old, Caucasian Man with Chronic Bacterial Prostatitis due to *Escherichia coli*

Date	Days on (+) or off (−) Drug		VB_1[a]	VB_2	EPS	VB_3	Organism	Serum Antibody
				bacteria/ml				*serotype/titer*
10/17/67	−4	NA	10,000	1,780			*E. coli*	
11/9/67	+16	Pen-G 250 mg q.i.d.	1,000	220		20	*Proteus morganii*	
			10,000	10		10	*E. coli*	
11/28/67	−7	Pen-G	100,000	100,000		100,000	*E. coli*	
			1,000	1,000		1,000	*P. morganii*	
12/7/67	−3	Methenamine mandelate	10,000	1,000		1,400	*E. coli*	
12/26/67	−3	Nitrofur	1,200	3,200		760	*E. coli*	
12/30/67	−7	Nitrofur	60	20	2,000	40	*E. coli*	
2/1/68	−9	Nitrofur	520	280	10,000	3,280	*E. coli*	
2/2/68	+1	Poly-B sulf 150 mg/24 hr	1,670	10		2,200	*E. coli*	
2/3/68	+2	Poly-B sulf 150 mg/24 hr	1,740	30	1,950	360	*E. coli*	
2/4/68	+3	Poly-B sulf 150 mg/24 hr	10	0	1,320	10	*E. coli*	
2/5/68	+4	Poly-B sulf 150 mg/24 hr	0	0	0	0		
2/6/68	+5	Poly-B sulf 150 mg/24 hr	0	0	80	10	*E. coli*	
2/8/68	+7	Poly-B sulf 225 mg/24 hr	0	0	0	0		
2/9/68	+8	Poly-B sulf 225 mg/24 hr	0	0	10	0	*E. coli*	
2/11/68	+10	Poly-B sulf 225 mg/24 hr	0	0	0	0		
2/12/68	−1	Poly-B sulf	0	0	0	0		
2/13/68	−2	Poly-B sulf	0	0	0	0		
2/14/68	−3	Poly-B sulf	0	0	0	0		
2/15/68	−4	Poly-B sulf	0	0	90	70	*E. coli*	
2/16/68	−5	Poly-B sulf	0	0	470	440	*E. coli*	
2/27/68	−17	Poly-B sulf	100,000	100,000	100,000	100,000	*E. coli*	
4/9/68	+1	mo Pen-G 500 mg t.i.d.	0	0	90		*E. coli*	
			280	0	100		*P. morganii*	
5/21/68	+6	wk Pen-G 500 mg t.i.d.	0	0	70	0	*P. morganii*	
			50	0	90	20	*E. coli*	
7/16/68	+3.5	mo Pen-G 500 mg b.i.d.	800	0	500	60	*E. coli*	
			1,800	0	5,000	650	*P. morganii*	
9/19/68	+5.5	mo Pen-G 500 mg b.i.d.			10,000		*E. coli*	
12/26/68	+9	mo Pen-G 500 mg b.i.d.	50	10	10,000	950	*E. coli*	
3/20/69	+13	mo Pen-G 500 mg b.i.d.	0	0	0	0		
7/17/69	+17	mo Pen-G 500 mg b.i.d.	20	0	10,000	180	*E. coli*	
			0	0	40	0	*P. morganii*	
1/13/70	+23	mo Pen-G 500 mg b.i.d.	20	0	460	0	*E. coli*	

			0	0	20	0	*P. morganii*	
7/14/70	+29	mo Pen-G 500 mg b.i.d.	20	0	0	10	*P. morganii*	
			0	0	600	0	*E. coli*	
1/12/71	+34	mo Pen-G 500 mg b.i.d.	10	10	6,000	140	*E. coli*	
2/9/71	+35	mo Pen-G 500 mg b.i.d.?	100,000	100,000			*E. coli*	
2/22/71	+36	mo Pen-G 500 mg b.i.d.?	100,000	100,000	100,000	100,000	*E. coli* 06	
2/23/71	−1	Pen-G	100,000	100,000	100,000	100,000	*E. coli*	06/1:640; 075/1:640
3/2/71	+7	TMP 160 mg SMX 800 mg } b.i.d.	0	0	110	0	*E. coli*	06/1:640; 075/1:640
3/9/71	+14	TMP 160 mg SMX 800 mg } b.i.d.	0	0	0	0		
3/30/71	−21	TMP SMX	0	0	0	0		
4/27/71	−48	TMP SMX	0	0	0	0		
5/25/71	−77	TMP SMX	0	0	0	0		06/1:320
6/22/71	−105	TMP SMX	0	0	0	0		
7/20/71	−133	TMP SMX	0	0	0	0		06/1:320
7/27/71[c]	−140	TMP SMX	100,000	100,000			*E. coli* 06	06/1:2,560
8/3/71	+7	cephalexin 500 mg q 6 hr	40	10	30	160	*Enterobacter*	
8/17/71	+14	Pen-G 500 mg t.i.d.	10	0	120	0	*E. coli* 075	075/1:640
9/14/71	+42	Pen-G 500 mg t.i.d.	0	0	0	0		
10/12/71	+70	Pen-G 500 mg t.i.d.	100	0	1,000	10	*E. coli* 075	075/1:640
10/26/71	+84	Pen-G 500 mg t.i.d.	10	0	40	0	*E. coli* 075	
12/16/71	+135	Pen-G 500 mg t.i.d.	0	0	70	330	*E. coli* 075	075/1:1,280; 06/1:640
			0	0	80	150	*P. morganii*	

[a] VB_1 = first voided 5–10 ml of urine from urethral meatus; VB_2 = midstream aliquot of urine; VB_3 = first voided 5–10 ml of urine from urethral meatus after prostatic massage; EPS = expressed prostatic secretion; Pen-G = penicillin-G; Nitrofur = nitrofurantoin; NA = nalidixic acid; Poly-B sulf = Polymyxin-B sulfate; TMP = trimethoprim; SMX = sulfamethoxazole.

[b] Small amounts of Gram-positive organisms are not included in the table.

[c] Acute bacterial prostatitis. See text.

patient is uncircumcised and despite careful cleaning of the glans after retraction of the foreskin, contaminating organisms in the distal end of the urethra can never be excluded.

This patient was followed from December 1971 (end of Table 7.14) until April 1975. He was maintained on penicillin-G, 500 μg twice daily, during those years, except for a 3-month course of full dosage TMP-SMX. Seven days after stopping the TMP-SMX, he had dysuria, perineal pain, low grade fever, and $> 10^5$ *E. coli* 06 in his VB_2 urine. He has remained on penicillin-G since that time and is asymptomatic. A repeat x-ray of his pelvis in June 1973, showed no change in the prostatic calcifications noted in late 1967.

Some Important Observations Based Upon These Clinical Examples. These clinical studies, chosen in part from our previous reports,[18,19] are representative of our experience with chronic bacterial prostatitis. No diagnostic test is clinically helpful unless its results are reasonably reproducible. The bacteriologic data presented here demonstrate the usefulness of these culture techniques. Furthermore, these clinical examples, together with other similar patients, have convinced us that the diagnosis of chronic bacterial prostatitis is a bacteriologic diagnosis; it cannot be made on the basis of rectal examination of the prostate or by the cystoscopic appearance of the prostate, urethra, or bladder. Several observations from these data deserve further comment.

Errors in Culture Methodology. Although the bacteriologic cultures are reproducible, it must be remembered that the site of bacterial persistence within the prostate is focal rather than diffuse. For this reason, every prostatic massage will not be equally effective in producing fluid from the infected ducts or glands. More than one set of cultures may be required to establish the diagnosis. If large numbers of bacteria from the prostate are on the urethra, and if the bacterial count is low in the prostatic fluid, then it may appear, incorrectly, as if the urethra is the primary source. Antibacterial therapy with nitrofurantoin or penicillin-G is very useful in these instances to clear the urethra but leave the prostatic bacteria unaffected.

As emphasized in Chapter 1, if the patient is uncircumcised, and if there is the slightest contamination of the urethral meatus by the foreskin prior to collection of the EPS or VB_3, thousands of contaminating pathogens can suddenly appear in the prostatic cultures. In recent years, I have learned to tape the foreskin back on the shaft of the penis before cleaning the glans. In the uncircumcised patient, a sterile, wet, cotton swab stick, rotated in a circular motion between the glans penis and the overlying foreskin, and then placed in 5 ml of saline, is often useful to quantitate the surface bacteria in this area.

The diagnostic value of a direct culture of the EPS in order to avoid the 1:100 or 1:1000 dilution of the prostatic bacteria inherent in the VB_3 culture has been emphasized in Chapter 1. There are numerous instances in these clinical examples where a sterile VB_3 could not be relied upon as indicative of a sterile prostatic fluid. Nevertheless, Tables 7.4 and 7.5 show at least one set of cultures where the EPS count was unnecessary to establish the diagnosis, and all the localizing data in Tables 7.7, 7.8, 7.9, 7.10, and 7.11 are based on VB_1, VB_2, and VB_3 cultures only, without obtaining EPS.

One last potential error in these cultures has been mentioned but should be emphasized. If the bacterial count in the EPS is compared directly to the VB_1 aliquot, the greater viscosity and smaller volume of the EPS, especially if a drop of the EPS "hangs" at the urethral meatus before falling free into the culture tube, may result in considerable contamination by bacteria at the urethral meatus. We have particularly observed this phenomenon with diphtheroids and *S. epidermidis.*

Use of Antibacterial Therapy as a Diagnostic Tool. In many patients, cultures obtained while on therapy were diagnostic: in Table 7.8, 3/14/66 (on ampicillin), all three cultures on nitrofurantoin, and 4/20/66 (the 1st day of colistin therapy) were all diagnostic; in Table 7.12, almost all cultures on ampicillin and penicillin-G were diagnostic; and in Tables 7.9 and 7.10, almost every culture on nalidixic acid indicated a bacterial prostatitis. Table 7.9 also illustrates the usefulness of cultures obtained at 2-hour intervals after the start of therapy. For diagnostic cultures during therapy, oral penicillin-G and nitrofurantoin are the best drugs because of their high urinary and low plasma concentrations. For *Pseudomonas* prostatitis, tetracycline is the only reasonable choice for diagnostic and prophylactic purposes.

The presence of antibacterial drug concentrations in the VB_3 urine, which exceed by many times the minimal inhibitory concentration of the bacteria from prostatic fluid, does not seem to inhibit bacterial growth on the surface plates; all these clinical examples show numerous instances of a sterile VB_1 and VB_2 but positive cultures from the VB_3 urine. Furthermore, the bacterial counts in the VB_3 urines of patient S.T. in Table 7.12, were about the same with and without ampicillin in the urine, (1/5 and 1/12/67). On the other hand, it is good practice to surface streak reasonably soon any VB_3 or EPS cultures that contain significant concentrations of antibacterial agents under no circumstances must these two aliquots be left at room temperature.

Time Interval of Relapse from Prostate to Bladder. The time required for bacteria in the prostatic fluid to reach the bladder urine varied from 48 hours (in Table 7.9) to >90 days (in Table 7.6). In Table 7.8, the relapse times were 7, 6, and 7 days after stopping ampicillin and 10 days after colistin. In Table 7.11 it was not recognized until late in the illness that infection in the prostate was the primary disease; thus, although VB_3 data are lacking, Table 7.11, bacteriuria occurred repeatedly between the 4th and 7th days after stopping oxytetracycline. In Table 7.12, bladder bacteriuria occurred 8–18 days after ampicillin and 18–31 days after nalidixic acid. The ampicillin recurrence (1/23/67) is interesting because the urine on 1/12/67, had remained sterile for 7 days in the presence of numerous *E. coli* in the prostate. The recurrence pattern in Table 7.9 deserves particular attention. Each time the antibacterial agent was stopped, bladder bacteriuria was present in 48 hours, and the patient was symptomatic the following day. In fact, the bacteriuria appeared so rapidly that we could not localize the infection in the absence of therapy. This short recurrence time was undoubtedly caused by the previous complete resection of the prostatic fossa and vesical neck; bladder urine was probably in continuous contact with the prostatic fossa.

Chronic Bacterial Prostatitis as a Source of Renal Infection. Whereas the localization studies at cystoscopy showed the renal urines in Tables 7.8 and 7.9 were sterile despite several years of recurrent infections, W. D., a 57-year-old man in Table 7.11, had already lost his left kidney from recurrent stones and infection. The right kidney contained a small stone in the lower calyx, and both *Pseudomonas* and *E. coli* were cultured from the right renal urine. Although the prostatic localization studies at cystoscopy (see Chapter 1 for methodology) suggested that the same bacteria were in the prostatic fluid (WB_2 and WB_3 cultures in Table 7.11), this information was overlooked largely because of his subsequent renal history. When the stone was removed from his partially obstructed ureter on 11/22/65, it was not surprising that the same *E. coli* and *Pseudomonas* were cultured from the stone. Upon removal of the stone containing the *E. coli* and *Pseudomonas*, we expected to cure him of his recurrent infections. To our disappointment, he developed the same symptoms of chills, fever, nausea, dysuria, and frequency about 12 days after stopping the colistin (Table 7.11, 12/17/65). Had he been cystoscoped and localized with this first recurrence after the ureterolithotomy, we would undoubtedly have found a sterile renal urine and would have been months ahead in arriving at the proper diagnosis of bacterial prostatitis. Instead, we assumed the diagnosis was chronic pyelonephritis and placed him again on a maintenance dose of oxytetracycline. After 9 months of a sterile urine (with one very suggestive culture on 3/22/66, that *Pseudomonas* were in the prostate), medication was stopped to see if a cure had been achieved. To our surprise, he became infected for the first time with *E. coli* but with the same symptoms as before. This time localization studies confirmed that the kidney and the opposite ureteral stump were not the source of the infection. Maintenance therapy with nalidixic acid for the *E. coli* soon produced a recurrence with the *Pseudomonas*. It was then clear that both *Pseudomonas* and *E. coli* were present in the prostate, as we should have suspected at the first cystoscopic localization on 1/12/65. With the appearance of prostatic adenocarcinoma, we had two reasons to suggest a radical prostatectomy. At the time of surgery, bacteriologic studies on both the prostatic calculi and prostatic tissue showed *Pseudomonas* and *E. coli* in high counts at a time when the bladder urine was sterile from colistin therapy (Table 7.11). The identity of the *E. coli* as an 06 serogroup in the original cystoscopic localization on 1/12/65, in the ureteral calculus removed on 11/22/65, and in the prostatic calculi and tissue on 3/8/67 (Table 7.11b) certainly suggest that an original prostatic infection could have been the source of all his urinary tract disease.

The patients in Tables 7.5 and 7.10 had proven unilateral renal infections that accompanied their bladder bacteriuria, and J.S. in Table 7.10 probably had a diseased right upper calyx from his infection (Fig 7.4). Cystoscopic localization in Table 7.4 suggested a right ureteral bacteriuria. The remainder of the patients (Tables 7.6, 7.7, 7.12) were not localized prior to therapy. It is clear from these studies that renal infections in the male can be secondary to persistence in the prostate. Interestingly, Friedlander and Braude[21] have shown that pyelonephritis is much more severe in male rats than females, and that this difference is due to bacterial prostatitis in the male rat.

Effectiveness of Low Dosage Antimicrobial Therapy in Preventing Bladder Bacteriuria. Whereas transurethral resection may cure some patients when antibiotics have failed (Tables 7.7 and 7.8), complete removal of every infected focus will not be possible in all patients (Tables 7.9 and 7.10). When these latter patients, for reasons of sexual activity or other personal preference, choose not to have a total prostatectomy (which cured patient W.D. in Table 7.11), it is important to realize how little antibacterial drug is required to keep them symptom-free and their bladder urines sterile. Most patients with chronic bacterial prostatitis become symptomatic only when the bladder is infected. In Table 7.11, the bladder urine remained sterile for 9 months with only 125 mg of oxytetracycline twice a day; the urinary levels of oxytetracycline were bactericidal to both the *E. coli* and the *Pseudomonas*. When a surgical cure of patient L.P., Table 7.9, was not feasible, he remained asymptomatic with a sterile bladder urine on only 250 mg of nalidixic acid twice a day; 2 μg/ml of nalidixic acid were bactericidal for his *E. coli*. Thus, bacterial seeding of the bladder urine by a few bacteria from the prostatic fluid can be controlled effectively with unusually small amounts of the proper antibacterial agent. It is only fair that this alternative to potential surgical cure be offered to every patient.

Anatomical Difficulty with Simple Prostatectomy. The major reason simple prostatectomy (transurethral or retropubic will not remove the site of infection in most patients is that the bacteria probably reside in the true "outer" prostate rather than in the periurethral glands that cause benign prostatic hyperplasia. As McNeal[22] has so clearly emphasized, the ducts from the true prostate (McNeal's central and peripheral zones) empty at the verumontanum; indeed, the ducts from the peripheral zone glands that comprise the bulk of the true prostate actually empty *distal* to the verumontanum. It is unlikely that transurethral resections will be complete in this area, and open enucleations never include the true prostate.

Despite these formidable problems, Smart and Jenkins[23] advocate transurethral prostatectomy for "chronic prostatitis"; they reported 72% of 32 patients were "rendered asymptomatic" and 19% improved by surgery. There is no documentation of recurrent bacteriuria in any patient and not a single localizing culture either pre- or postoperatively is presented; apparently five patients had "recognized urinary pathogens" in their EPS but no data are presented to exclude an urethral origin of these bacteria. Even the surgical tissue cultures are uninterpretable because they were placed in broth which will not distinguish between a few bacteria as contaminants and thousands of bacteria as a true infection. Whatever Drs. Smart and Jenkins operated upon, it is clear that few if any patients had chronic bacterial prostatitis. Unfortunately, Silber[24] in a recent book on transurethral resection, has based an entire chapter *("Chronic Prostatitis and Radical Transurethral Resection of the Prostate (TURP)")* on Smart and Jenkins'[23] paper. Silber[24] reports 11 of 11 patients (100%!) with chronic bacterial prostatitis cured of their infection by a radical TURP; no pre- or postoperative localizing bacteriologic data are given to support these claims.

In a later and more careful analysis of patients with chronic bacterial prostatitis (even though the authors still include unquantitated, tissue positive broth cultures at the time of TURP), Smart, Jenkins, and Lloyd[25] report that only 50% of their patients with "pathogenic bacterial prostatitis" are asymptomatic on follow-up, a figure probably not statistically different from our own 33% cure rate.

Role of Prostatic Calculi in Chronic Bacterial Prostatitis. Most prostatic calculi are not associated with prostatic infection. Small, brown, 1-mm-or-less prostatic calculi (tricalcium phosphate) are frequently found at the time of transurethral resection in patients who have never had urinary infections. Fox found that 14% of 3510 men had prostatic calculi radiologically visible on plain x-ray films of the pelvis.[26] Even prostates with multiple, large stones, covering the prostatic area on the x-ray film, are often uninfected. For example, H.R., a 63-year-old, white, Caucasian man, was seen in consultation for prostatic calculi discovered during an x-ray examination for symptoms of a gastric ulcer (Fig. 7.8.1). He had never had urinary tract symptoms, his intravenous urogram was normal, and segmented cultures showed the following: VB_1 = 30 *S. epidermidis* and *Streptococcus viridans*/ml, VB_2 = 10 *S. viridans*/ml, and the VB_3 was sterile. A drop of prostatic fluid showed 4–6 WBC/hpf and 1–3 fresh RBC.

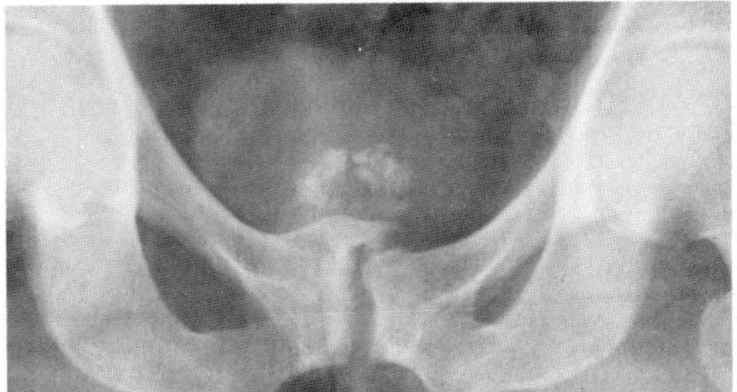

Figure 7.8.1 An x-ray film of the pelvis in H.R., a 63-year-old, Caucasian man, showing prostatic calculi that were discovered during the course of an upper bowel examination. He had never had urinary tract symptoms, and his prostatic fluid was sterile.

Nevertheless, prostatic calcifications may be associated with bacterial prostatitis, as demonstrated in W.D., Table 7.11 where the crushed stones, as well as the outer, true prostate, (but not the inner, periurethral prostate) grew large numbers of *Pseudomonas* and *E. coli.*

An equally convincing case, also representing an example of the spontaneous onset of bacterial prostatitis with recurrent urinary infections in a young man, is that of R.F., a 33-year-old man whose culture data were presented in Table 7.13. Since the ground prostatic tissue was sterile, while the crushed stone grew *P. aeruginosa* in numbers 100 times greater than the fourth saline wash of the stone, there can be little question that his prostatic calculi contained *Pseudomonas*. Meares[27] has reported this patient along with two others from Stanford whose prostatic calculi were infected with *E. coli*. Interestingly, while one of the two was tricalcium phosphate (Whitlockite) as in R.F., the third infected prostatic stone was 98% Brushite and only 2% Whitlockite. Eykyn *et al.*[28] have also reported on prostatic calculi as a source of recurrent bacteriuria. Much could be learned about prostatic calculi and bacterial prostatitis; for interested readers, the classic paper on prostatic calculi is by Huggins and Bear,[20] while the monograph by M.J.V. Smith[29] on prostatic corpora amylacea is equally important.

Usefulness of Serum Antibody Titers in Diagnosis of Bacterial Prostatitis and in Assessment of Both Bacterial Persistence and Eradication. The failure of serum antibody titers to fall to normal in patient J.H. (Table 7.14) probably indicated the persistence of the *E. coli* 06 in his prostatic fluid despite 4 months of a sterile EPS following 2 weeks of therapy with TMP-SMX.

M.E.O., a 45-year-old white man was first seen at Stanford on 3/15/73 with a 6-year history of recurrent urinary infections. As seen in Table 7.15, the first two cultures on 3/15/73 and 3/22/73 localized an *E. coli* 04 to his prostate. Bacterial agglutination titers in his serum[30] on the 36th and 57th day of a 3-month course of full dosage TMP-SMX showed persistence of serum antibodies to his *E. coli* 04 at 1:1280 dilution. Five weeks later, at the end of therapy, serum antibodies began to fall and returned to normal levels by the end of the year. He continued to do well until November 1974 (16 months after completion of TMP-SMX therapy) when he was admitted to his local hospital with fever, dysuria, and acute retention requiring catheterization. His urine was not cultured, but his prostate was hard and tender and he was successfully treated with ampicillin. An intravenous urogram was normal and cystoscopy was unremarkable except for benign prostatic hyperplasia. His prostate softened within a few weeks and he was well for the next 4 years until 12/15/78 when he suddenly presented with acute bacterial prostatitis. When seen at Stanford on 12/18/78, on tetracycline therapy, localization cultures showed a sterile VB_1 and VB_2 but 10,000 self-agglutinating *E. coli* in his EPS. This patient dem-

Table 7.15
Bacteriologic course of M.E.O., a 45-year-old white man with chronic bacterial prostatitis, cured by TMP-SMX,[a] and accompanied by decreasing serum antibody titers.

Date	Days on (+) or off (−) Drug	VB_1	VB_2	EPS	VB_3	Organism	Serum Antibody Titer
				Bacteria/ml[b]			
1967–73	Six year history of recurrent UTI's treated elsewhere						
3-15-73	+2 Amp.	140	30	3000	410	*Escherichia coli* 04	
3-22-73	+9 Amp.	0	0	100	0	*E. coli* 04	
3-27-73	−5 Amp.	2500	3000	5000	1500	*E. coli* 04	
4-3-73	−12 Amp.	20	10	100	20	*E. coli* 04	1:1280
4-17-73	+14 Amp.	0	0	0	0		
5-9-73	+36 TMP-SMX	0	0	0	0		1:1280
5-30-73	+57 TMP-SMX	0	0	0	0		1:1280
7-5-73	+93 TMP-SMX	0	0	0	0		1:640
8-15-73	−41 TMP-SMX	0	0	0	0		1:640
9-19-73	−76 TMP-SMX	0	0	0	0		1:320
10-18-73	−95 TMP-SMX	0	0	0	0		
11-15-73	−123 TMP-SMX	0	0	0	0		
1-16-74	−196 TMP-SMX	0	0	0	0		1:160
11/74	−16 months	Acute Bacterial Prostatitis					
12-15-78	−4 years		>10^5			*E. coli* SA	
12-18-78	+3 tetracycline	0	0	1000	5000	*E. coli* SA	
12-29-78	+11 TMP-SMX	0	0	0	0		
1-26-79	+39 TMP-SMX	0	0	0	0		

[a] TMP-SMX = trimethoprim-sulfamethoxazole; EPS = expressed prostatic secretion; Amp = ampicillin; VB_1 = first voided 5–10 ml of urine from urethral meatus; VB_2 = midstream aliquot of urine; VB_3 = first voided 5–10 ml of urine from urethral meatus after prostatic massage; SA = Self-agglutinating bacteria.

[b] Includes Gram-negative bacteria only. Urethral Gram-positive organisms are deleted.

onstrates the value of observing a decline in elevated serum antibody titers, especially when contrasted with the persistence of antibody titers in J.H. (Table 7.14). While it is true that he had two episodes of acute bacterial prostatitis in November 1974 and December 1978, 16 and 65 months after cure of his chronic bacterial prostatitis due to an *E. coli* 04, I have already indicated that acute bacterial prostatitis is usually a self-limiting disease and proved to be so in his case; note that the episode in November 1974 was easily cured with a short course of ampicillin whereas ampicillin had failed to eradicate the *E. coli* 04 from his prostate in March 1973. Why, however, does he continue to be susceptible to acute bacterial prostatitis?

The value of elevated serum antibody titers in the diagnosis of chronic bacterial prostatitis has been nicely documented by Meares.[31] He found low bacterial agglutination titers (median 1:20) in control men using their own fecal *E. coli*, low titers in men whose urethra was colonized with *E. coli* (median 1:10), and higher titers in men with chronic bacterial prostatitis (median 1:640). Four men with chronic bacterial prostatitis, however, had very low titers and are excluded from the median analysis of 1:640. Meares[32] also reported the longitudinal changes in bacterial agglutination titers in 22 men treated with TMP-SMX.

Because bacterial agglutination titers measure mainly IgM, and not IgG or IgA, in 1978 we switched to a more sensitive technique of indirect solid phase radioimmunoassay developed by Zollinger and his colleagues[33] in 1976. The diagnostic potential of this antibody assay (IgG, IgA, IgM) is shown by the following consultation. In September 1978, I saw T.C., a 55-year-old white man with recurrent *E. coli* urinary infections since 1962. He would have two to three episodes each year of dysuria, frequency, and fever whenever he stopped nitrofurantoin, 50 mg twice daily. A 12-week course of TMP-SMX at full dosage was completed in December 1975 and he remained well until April 1976 when his *E. coli* infection returned. He responded to TMP-SMX and was maintained on one tablet per day from that time onward. An excretory urogram with voiding films showed normal kidneys, a residual urine of about 30 ml, and numerous prostatic calculi. My surgical intern examined the patient first and was unable to obtain prostatic fluid; the VB_1 grew 100 *S. epidermidis*/ml, the VB_2 was sterile, and the VB_3 had 10 *S. epidermidis*/ml. I examined the patient about 30 minutes later, found a smooth, but slightly enlarged prostate that was not indurated, and several drops of prostatic fluid were obtained. Microscopically, the EPS showed 15 WBC/hpf, 12 RBC/hpf, and occasional oval fat macrophages under the low power examination. One-tenth of a milliliter of EPS was cultured and grew *two* colonies of *E. coli* (20/ml) the next day. Note that if 1/100 or 1/1000 of a milliliter of EPS was cultured, we could not have detected these two colonies. But were they contaminants? Fortunately, he was circumcised, but I had not obtained the VB_1, VB_2, and VB_3 at the same collection sequence as the EPS. Serum was obtained from the patient, the *E. coli* was serotyped and found to be an *E. coli* 04, and his serum antibodies were determined against his *E. coli* 04 using my own serum as a control (Figure 7.9); Zollinger's[33] solid phase radioimmunoassay was used. Note that the patient has about 100 times more serum antibody against the *E. coli* 04 than I have in my serum, *i.e.*, at I^{125} antihuman IgG counts of 6000/min., the patient's serum had to be diluted 100 times more than mine. This much antibody against the *E. coli* 04 clearly indicates that the two colonies recovered from the culture of only 0.1 ml of his EPS were not contaminants but, instead, pathogenic bacteria which persist in his prostate and cause a very substantial production of serum antibodies against the causative organism. The diagnostic and therapeutic usefulness of this technique is surely evident. Our modification of the Zollinger[33] solid phase radioimmunoassay is presented in Chapter 5.

Immunoglobulins, of course, are also present in prostatic secretion.[34–36] Although Gray, *et al.*[36] have looked at the amount of total immunoglobulin in prostatic fluid of

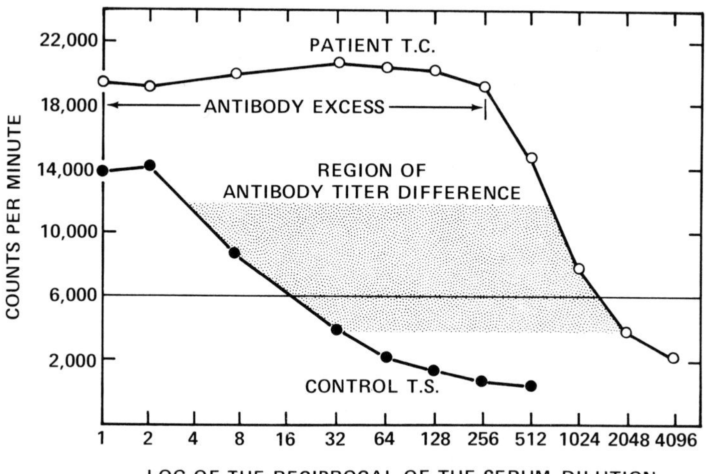

Figure 7.9 Solid phase radioimmunoassay of serum antibodies against *Escherichia coli* 04 antigen in patient with chronic bacterial prostatitis compared to a control.

normal controls and in patients with bacterial prostatitis,* there are no reported studies on specific antibody titers in prostatic fluid directed against the infecting organism. Because local antibody may be more important, and perhaps more diagnostic with higher titers, measurements of specific antibody locally produced in prostatic secretion are clearly important. Since the Zollinger[33] technique is ideally suited for this purpose, we have begun these studies. Dr. Linda Shortliffe, Nancy Wehner, and I have shown that antigen-specific secretory IgA in EPS is several hundred times greater than the IgA response in serum in patients with bacterial prostatitis, leaving no doubt that the source of the prostatic IgA is a local immune response. The immunologic response in the serum is mainly IgG in chronic bacterial prostatitis. The report by Riedasch *et al.*[37] on the presence of antibody-coated bacteria in the ejaculate is uninterpretable because the authors did not localize the infection to the prostate, did not separate nonbacterial from bacterial prostatitis, and used 100,000 bacteria/ml of ejaculate as "significant."

"Nonbacterial" Prostatitis

"Nonbacterial" prostatitis, as noted in Table 7.1, is characterized by evidence of inflammation in the EPS, the absence of localizing cultures to the prostate (including Gram-positive organisms), and the fact that bacteriuria never occurs. These men may have a variety of pelvic symptoms, including perineal pain, suprapubic or infrapubic aching, testicular, loin or inguinal discomfort, frequency and sometimes dysuria, but almost never a urethral discharge. Indeed, the presence of a urethral discharge should place these patients into the urethritis category rather than prostatitis. In some patients, ejaculatory complaints are present. In others, a low back or sacral pain may accompany their perineal discomfort, a discomfort that is often aggravated by activity, including sitting for long periods, but relieved on lying down. On physical examination, the prostate is within the normal range on palpation. We have seen an occasional patient who is completely asymptomatic and whose EPS, loaded with WBCs, was discovered accidentally.

Treatment of the symptomatic patient with "nonbacterial" prostatitis is extremely unsatisfactory because we do not know the cause of the inflammatory response in the prostate. Until we do, treatment is likely to remain unsatisfactory. Two or three prostatic massages, a confession to the patient of our ignorance, and a lot of reassurance as to the benigness of the process and its ultimate symptomatic resolution, is about as good as one can do. Antimicrobial agents should not be prescribed since they are not

* In a personal communication with Prof. N. J. Blacklock on January 10, 1979, he kindly informed me that approximately half of their 48 cases[36] had either acute or chronic bacterial prostatitis and the other half nonbacterial prostatitis with purulent EPS.

only ineffective and a waste of money, but serve to strengthen the patient's concern that an infectious process is present.

While it is true that such infectious agents as highly fastidious anaerobic bacteria or *Chlamydia* and possibly *Ureaplasma urealyticum* (T-strain mycoplasma) have not been excluded completely as a cause of the inflammation in the EPS, the interested physician should keep the following clinical observation in mind: why is it that patients with proven, uncurable chronic bacterial prostatitis carry Enterobacteriaceae (and even *Pseudomonas* as in Table 7.13) in their prostate for years and *never* have a single pelvic or ejaculatory complaint as long as the bacteria remain confined to their prostate? When their bladder becomes infected, to be sure, they do have symptoms of a lower urinary tract infection, but while taking prophylactic medicine to prevent a bladder infection, they have none of the pelvic complaints characteristic of "nonbacterial" prostatitis. While I applaud every effort to find an infectious agent as the cause of "nonbacterial" prostatitis, the organism, finally isolated, will have to have far greater antigenicity in terms of causing pain and discomfort than does *E. coli*, *Klebsiella*, *Proteus*, and *Pseudomonas*. Because of this single, but I think significant, clinical observation, it is more appealing to me to look for an abnormal biochemical mediator of inflammation in the prostate than to look for an infectious process. As a start, Dr. Robert Andonian (a resident urologist in our Stanford program) has found some intriguing evidence that prostaglandins in the seminal fluid may be substantially elevated in these patients, especially during their symptomatic periods. While much more data are needed, my point is that we must not exclude biochemical, noninfectious mediators of prostatic inflammation while we continue to search for an infectious etiology.

S. Colleen and P.-A. Mårdh, a urologist and microbiologist at the University Hospital in Lund, Sweden, have studied 78 patients with what they term "nonacute prostatitis" and compared the findings to 20 normal males.[38–40] Extensive and careful microbiologic cultures were done, including *Neisseria gonorrhoeae*, *Corynebacterium vaginale*, T-mycoplasma and *Mycoplasma hominis*, *Trichomonas vaginalis*, *Candida albicans*, anaerobic bacteria, and even viruses. Their technique of collecting samples was markedly different from ours; the urethral and prostatic massage specimens were collected with cotton-tipped swabs (with a midstream voided urine in between) and followed 2–4 hours later by collection of the ejaculate for culture. Since males are rarely circumcised in Sweden, it is interesting that the preputium was retracted and the meatus cleaned only with a "sterile, dry dressing" prior to the urethral and prostatic swab cultures. The authors concluded that "cultures of the expressed prostatic fluids and the samples of semen gave no information of the occurrence of bacteria over and above that obtainable from examination of the urethral specimens." Since this technique of swab cultures does not provide for a quantitative distinction between urethral and prostatic origin of the organism (as the VB_1 and VB_3 does), it is difficult to know what these studies actually mean in terms of urethral or prostatic origin of the bacteria. Moreover, while their classification of "nonacute prostatitis" may include predominantly patients with "nonbacterial prostatitis" (Table 7.1), it does not exclude those with chronic bacterial prostatitis and certainly contains some with prostatodynia (21 of 68 patients in whom EPS was obtained at the first examination had less than 15 WBC/hpf). Indeed, most of these latter patients with little evidence of somatic disease showed signs of personality disturbances and defects in sex identification.[40] Finally, a urethral discharge, especially in the morning, was reported by 42% of the patient group, perhaps explaining why 33% of the patients had complement-fixing antibodies in their serum to *Chlamydia* (compared to 5% of the controls) and why tetracycline was better than placebo in alleviating symptoms. This study emphasizes the need for a reliable technique to separate bacteria originating from the urethra from those originating in the prostate; I believe our VB_1-VB_2-EPS-VB_3 method is substantially superior to the Lund[38–40] techniques although it is more difficult and time-consuming to do. The microbiologic value of the Lund[38–40] studies rests with their finding of few bacteriologic differences between their patients and controls since their technique of collecting samples could not distinguish between urethral and prostatic infection. Moreover, the value of these studies is somewhat limited by the potential inclusion of a few patients with chronic bacterial prostatitis and a number of men with prostatodynia under the author's classification of "nonacute prostatitis"; in short, their patients are not a pure group of "nonbacterial prostatitis" as defined in Table 7.1.

The best study that excludes anaerobic bacteria as a cause of "nonbacterial" prostatitis is by Nielsen and Justesen,[41] and the most convincing investigation that excludes viruses, especially herpes virus type 2, is by Gordon *et al.*[42] The latter authors also failed to culture *Chlamydia* in a single one of their 50 patients. In a very recent report, Mårdh *et al.*[43] did not isolate *Chlamydia* from the urethra or prostate of men with prostatitis.

Before proceeding to the last group (prostatodynia) in our classification of prostatitis, it is important to recognize that occasional patients with interstitial cystitis can be mistaken for "nonbacterial" prostatitis. Since the diagnosis of interstitial cystitis can be made only under spinal or general anesthesia and by careful reinspection of the bladder *after* overdistention,[44] the physician should be aware of this potential confusion in diagnosis. Lastly, carcinoma-in-situ of the bladder can produce pelvic symptoms which can occasionally mimic prostatic symptoms; it should be excluded by cytologic examination of the voided urine or saline lavage of the bladder at the time of cystoscopy.

Prostatodynia

There remains a group of patients with a variety of pelvic, ejaculatory, and urinary complaints in whom the EPS appears normal without evidence of inflammatory disease. In these patients, and especially in those whose ejaculatory complaints are accompanied by hesitancy of urination and a slow stream, phenoxybenzamine (10 mg at night) can be surprisingly successful. The following clinical example illustrates this syndrome of prostatodynia ("prostate pain"); it is especially instructive because both the patient (an infectious disease physician) and the referring urologist thought the diagnosis was chronic bacterial prostatitis.

The patient was a 40-year-old infectious disease physician first seen at Stanford in February 1978. In 1963 he had one episode of "lower tract irritation" with frequency and dysuria; cultures were negative but his symptoms were sufficiently severe enough to warrant an intravenous urogram, which was normal. His symptoms spontaneously subsided and he had no further medical problems until March 1977, when he developed suprapubic discomfort, urinary hesitancy, perineal pressure, and pain with initiation of voiding, and some dribbling of a few milliliters at the end of urination. He had no nocturia, dysuria during voiding, chills, or fever. Urinalysis was negative, the prostate was described as small but "congested," and the EPS reportedly grew 5 *E. coli*/ml on culture. Biweekly prostatic massages helped his symptoms at first but gradually failed. In June 1977, he was treated with full dosage TMP-SMX for 3 weeks but his symptoms returned once the massages were stopped. Enterococci were cultured from his EPS and he was restarted on TMP-SMX 160/00 mg, as a single daily dose, combined with prostatic massage. On 11/22/77 all medication and prostatic massages were stopped.

When seen at Stanford in February 1978, his complaints were suprapubic pain, perineal fullness, hesitancy of urination, and slight postvoid dribbling. Segmented voided cultures (Table 7.16) showed urethral *S. epidermidis*, enterococci, and α-streptococci without localization to the EPS or VB_3. The EPS showed 2–3 WBC/hpf, no clumps, no oval fat macrophages, and plenty of normal lecithin granules. The prostate was small and unremarkable; the left lobe was softer than the right.

The patient was placed on 10 mg phenoxybenzamine at bedtime with instructions to increase the dosage to two

Table 7.16
Segmented Localization Studies in a 40-year-old Male with Prostatodynia

Date	Mo on (+) or off (−) Therapy	VB_1[a]	VB_2	EPS	VB_3	Organism
			Bacteria/ml			
Feb 1978	− 3 mo TMP-SMX	100	60	170	70	Enterococci
		1000	40	1000	500	α-Streptococci
		120	70	200	120	Staphylococcus epidermidis

[a] VB_1 = first voided 5–10 ml of urine from urethral meatus; VB_2 = midstream aliquot of urine; VB_3 = first voided 5–10 ml of urine from urethral meatus after prostatic massage; EPS = expressed prostatic secretion. (Note that all of the bacteria in the EPS and VB_3 can be accounted for by urethral contamination.) TMP-SMX = trimethoprim-sulfamethoxazole.

or three times a day if necessary. He was asked to return in 1 month, to bring a bacteriologic record of his past cultures, and to also bring a first voided VB_1 and VB_2 urine from his wife. The phenoxybenzamine at a 10 mg/day dosage dramatically and completely relieved all his symptoms; he lost his suprapubic and perineal discomfort, his urinary hesitancy, observed a large increase in the size and force of his stream, and his postvoid dribbling had practically disappeared.

When I first examined him in February 1978, I did not believe he had chronic bacterial prostatitis because of two observations: he had never had bacteriuria and he did not have inflammatory cells in his EPS. Nevertheless, I was perplexed by the report from his referring urologist, and from the physician-patient, himself, who had personally carried his urine specimens to the bacteriology laboratory, that *E. coli* and enterococcus had been cultured from the EPS. I have reproduced these cultures in Table 7.17 because they are instructive. Observe that they do *not* localize the *E. coli* (4/11, 4/15, 12/22/77) or the enterococci (8/18, 9/6, 11/1, 11/22/77) to the prostate because a VB_1 urethral culture was not obtained to exclude urethral colonization as the source of the enterococci and *E. coli*. What was the source of the *E. coli* and enterococcus that must have colonized his urethra? His wife. Because she had had cystitis some years before, I asked the patient bring in her VB_1 and VB_2 without perineal cleaning in order to determine the colonizing bacteria on her vaginal introitus. Her VB_1 grew 8000 *E. coli* and 5000 enterococci/ml of urine along with lactobacilli, diptheroids and *S. epidermidis*; indeed, her VB_2 contained 1000 *E. coli* and 200 enterococci/ml of voided urine (with lactobacilli and *S. epidermidis*). The importance of these observations is that an astute, infectious disease physician-patient and a careful urologist did not realize that you cannot interpret a postvoid EPS culture without a VB_1 to exclude the urethra as the source of the bacteria in the prostatic fluid. Unfortunately, this practice is widespread and much of the literature on prostatitis is uninterpretable because of the same error.

The patient stopped his phenoxybenzamine after 3 months, and his symptoms gradually returned. He restarted the same regimen in June 1978, with complete relief of his symptoms, but by November and December of 1978 the patient observed that 30 mg/day of phenoxybenzamine was required to keep him asymptomatic. Because of this, he was cystoscoped in February 1979. The bladder, prostate and urethra were absolutely normal.

Although this patient had no ejaculatory symptoms accompanying his urinary and pelvic complaints, other patients with prostatodynia do and they can be dramatically helped with phenoxybenzamine. Most are helped with a single, nightly dose of 10 mg. Those who take more usually develop retrograde ejaculation which they should be warned about. Urine flow rates before and after phenoxybenzamine can be helpful as objective parameters of phenoxybenzamine efficacy, but a happy, relieved patient is the best yardstick.

As we gain more experience with this classification of prostatitis (Table 7.1), it may be that those patients with prostato-

Table 7.17
Localization Studies Performed at an Outside Hospital on a 40-year-old, White Man with Prostatodynia

Date	Days on (+) or off (−) Therapy	VB_1[a]	VB_2	EPS
4/11/77	− many months			5 *Escherichia coli* 10 Lactobacilli
4/12/77	− many months		NG	
4/15/77	− many months		1000 *E. coli*	Light growth *E. coli*
7/12/77	+12 TMP-SMX			NG
8/18/77	−28 TMP-SMX		NG	Light growth enterococci
8/30/77	+13 TMP-SMX		NG	
9/6/77	+20 TMP-SMX			Light growth enterococci
9/9/77	+23 TMP-SMX	3000 Enterococci/ml	NG	NG
11/1/77	+44 TMP-SMX			Light growth enterococci Light growth *Staphylococcus epidermidis*
11/8/77	+51 TMP-SMX	Rare enterococcus	NG	Rare enterococcus
11/22/77	+65 TMP-SMX			Rare enterococcus Rare *S. epidermidis*
12/22/77	−30 TMP-SMX		NG	1000 *S. epidermidis* 1000 Gram-negative rods

[a] VB_1 = first voided 5–10 ml of urine from urethral meatus; VB_2 = midstream aliquot of urine; EPS = expressed prostatic secretion; NG = no growth. All cultures were apparently performed with a bacteriologic loop containing 1/1000 ml by volume. Sometimes, however, all the EPS was cultured. The culture from 12/22/77 represented a single colony from a loop culture. TMP-SMX = trimethoprim-sulfamethoxazole.

dynia who respond best to phenoxybenzamine will be those with objective evidence of adrenergic overactivity at the internal vesical neck (urinary flow problems) or at the seminal vesicles (ejaculatory complaints). For those patients with prostatodynia who do not have symptoms suggestive of adrenergic overactivity and/or who do not respond to phenoxybenzamine, psychiatric counseling should be seriously pursued. We should not forget the Lund[40] study where those patients without evidence of somatic prostatic disease (absence of inflammation in the EPS) had signs of serious personality disturbances and defects in sex identification.

Some Observations on Antibacterial Therapy of Chronic Bacterial Prostatitis

As we began to recognize and to more fully appreciate this disease of chronic bacterial prostatitis in the early 1960s, several therapeutic observations became apparent. First, the bacteria which persisted in the prostate for years were not resistant organisms; on the contrary, they were highly sensitive, and thus we knew that bacterial resistance was not the cause of our failure to eradicate these bacteria from the prostate. Second, we made major efforts to achieve serum concentrations of antimicrobial agents that exceeded by severalfold the MIC of the bacteria persisting in the prostate. For example, the *E. coli* of J.H. (Table 7.14) was even treated with intravenous polymyxin-B sulfate in doses as high as 225 mg/day, a dose that was high enough to produce nephrotoxicity, and yet highly sensitive *E. coli* (<0.5 μg/ml polymyxin-B) could still be cultured from the EPS on the 8th day of the 10-day course of polymyxin therapy. In patient L.P. (Table 7.9), treatment for 4 months with nalidixic acid, at a dosage level which would have produced at least 20 μg of nalidixic acid/ml of plasma[45] against an *E. coli* sensitive to 2 μg/ml, never produced a sterile prostatic fluid. Long-term therapy fared no better than short-term: in Table 7.12, 35 days of ampicillin (14 of them at 500 mg every 6 hours) was no better than 10 days of oral penicillin-G; in fact, recovery of sensitive *E. coli* from the prostate at 35 days of ampicillin therapy appeared similar to cultures obtained 7 days after ampicillin was discontinued.

These clinical observations suggested very clearly that the antimicrobial agents simply had not been reaching the site of bacterial persistence in the prostate. We did not know then (or now) whether the bacteria are in the interstitial tissue of the prostate, but we did know from our method of culture that some bacteria had to be in the prostatic fluid. Since prostatic fluid is a secretion and is separated from the interstitial tissue and stroma of the prostate by epithelial cells that form the tubuloalveolar glands, we turned to the canine model used by Dr. C. Huggins in his classic studies of prostatic secretion.[46]

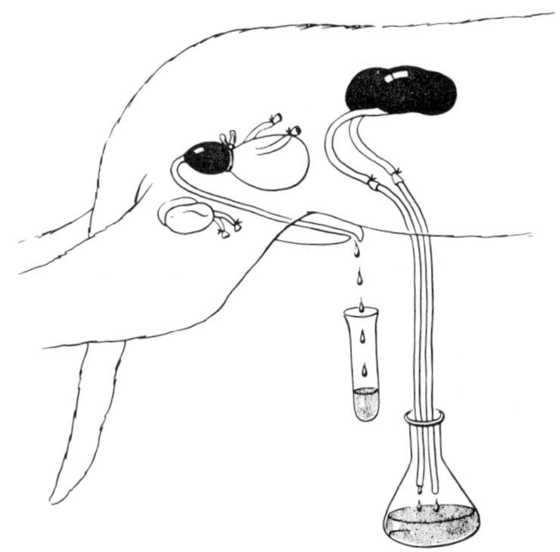

Figure 7.10 Experimental model used to study diffusion of antimicrobial drugs from plasma into prostatic fluid. A ligature is placed around the bladder just proximal to prostate, the ureters are ligated and cannulated above the bladder, the vasa deferentia are ligated, and the foreskin is incised and sutured to the abdominal wall to expose the glans. With pilocarpine stimulation, prostatic fluid is collected directly into a flask placed under the glans penis.

Experimental Observations

Dr. Donald Winningham and I studied a large number of antimicrobial drugs in terms of their diffusion kinetics from plasma to prostatic fluid.[47, 48] Male mongrel dogs of 25–40 kg were anesthetized with pentobarbital, 25 mg/kg body weight, followed by maintenance doses as needed. Urinary diversion was accomplished by placing a double ligature around the bladder neck proximal to the prostate and introducing polyethylene catheters through bilateral ureterotomies. The bladder was emptied by needle aspiration. Since seminal vesicles and bulbourethral glands are absent in the dog, ligation of the vasa deferentia permitted the collection of essentially pure prostatic secretion. The abdominal incision was closed, the penis was circumcised, and the dog was placed on his ventral surface for direct collection of prostatic fluid (Figure 7.10). Normal saline was infused at 10–20 ml/minute to initiate a brisk urine flow rate; 100–200 ml of blood were removed slowly through a femoral artery cannula, and the control plasma was saved for subsequent preparation of antibacterial standards as well as dilutions of plasma unknowns. Control urine was collected for subsequent dilution of urine unknowns. An intravenous loading dose of the antibacterial agent was followed by a maintenance infusion at a rate estimated to equal the expected excretion of the antibiotic; 5 minutes later a plasma sample was taken from the femoral cannula to estimate the peak plasma level. After approximately 30–60 minutes of equilibration time, two successive 15-minute clearance periods were obtained with appropriate urine and plasma samples. After completion of the clearances, 25 mg of intravenous pilocarpine were given to stimulate prostatic secretion; simultaneous plasma, urine, and prostatic fluid samples were collected. Prostatic fluid (PF) was collected in consecutive 2- to 5-ml aliquots. A typical protocol is shown in Table 7.18.

The samples were assayed in a deep well, agar diffusion system employing a large plate.[49] Two milliliters of the assay organism, prepared in the log phase of growth, were added to agar cooled to 45°C which was then mixed, poured into 15 × 24 inch autoclaved plates, and allowed to gel on a leveling table. After a short refrigeration period to harden the agar, circular wells 8 mm in diameter were cut in the agar with

Table 7.18
Failure of Cephalothin to Diffuse from Plasma to Prostatic Fluid Despite High Plasma Concentrations

Time	Procedure	Results	
		Antibiotic concentration	Antibiotic and creatinine clearance
min		*μg/ml*	*ml/min*
−130	Intravenous pentobarbital; begin surgical procedure		
−60	Completion of surgery; begin normal saline infusion at 20 ml/min		
−20	End of saline infusion; begin collection of control urine		
−10	Begin collection of control plasma		
−5	End collection of control plasma and urine		
0	Intravenous cephalothin load; begin cephalothin maintenance infusion		
5	Collect plasma for peak level of antibiotic (P_0).[a]	$P_0 = 65$	
25	Plasma sample P_1	$P_1 = 65$	
	Start collection of U_1	$U_1 = 940$	Antibiotic 67
40	End collection of U_1		Creatinine 106
	Plasma sample P_2	$P_2 = 67$	
	Start collection of U_2	$U_2 = 1083$	Antibiotic 67
55	End collection of U_2		Creatinine 109
	Plasma sample P_3	$P_3 = 62$	
	Intravenous pilocarpine, 25 mg		
56–59	Prostatic fluid sample PF_1	$PF_1 < 0.4$	
59–63	Prostatic fluid sample PF_2	$PF_2 < 0.4$	
63–67	Prostatic fluid sample PF_3	$PF_3 < 0.4$	
67–70	Prostatic fluid sample PF_4	$PF_4 < 0.4$	
70	Plasma sample P_4	$P_4 = 65$	
71	End of cephalothin maintenance infusion		

[a] P = plasma; U = urine; PF = prostatic fluid.

a cork borer and the agar was removed. Volumes of 0.15 ml were pipetted into each hole. Each sample was pipetted twice; the duplicate was placed in a well on the diagonally opposite side of the plate. After appropriate incubation, zone diameters of antibiotic inhibition were measured to the nearest 0.1 mm, using fine callipers. Standard curves in duplicate were constructed for each drug in the same assay plate with the unknowns. Saline standards were used to measure the levels in urine and PF, and plasma standards were used to measure the plasma concentration. Plasma and urine unknowns were determined at two different concentrations by diluting the unknown sample with control plasma or urine. The pH, incubation temperature, assay organism, the need for prediffusion, and the agar concentration for each of the antibacterial assays, together with the data on sensitivity and linearity of the assay, have been published in the original paper.[47] Control PF, placed on the agar wells, produced no zone. There was no inhibition of antimicrobial activity when the antibiotic was added to normal PF and placed in the agar wells. Nitrofurantoin and the sulfonamides were determined biochemically by methods published in the original papers.[48, 50]

The results of these studies are presented in Table 7.19. Except for the basic macrolides, erythromycin, and oleandomycin, none of the antimicrobial drugs could be detected in prostatic fluid, even when the plasma concentrations were extremely high. At the time of pilocarpine stimulation, the basic macrolides not only were detectable, but actually attained concentrations in prostatic fluid which were several times greater than the simultaneous plasma level. These observations seemed to explain why

Table 7.19
Diffusion of Nine Antimicrobial Agents from Plasma to Prostatic Fluid in the Dog[a]

Only erythromycin and oleandomycin were detectable in prostatic fluid. Note that prostatic fluid concentrations of these two antibiotics exceeded the plasma levels by 2 to 3 times.

Drug	Plasma	Prostatic Fluid
	μg/ml	*μg/ml*
Ampicillin	54	<0.2
Penicillin-G	62	<0.2
Cephalothin	63	<0.4
Kanamycin	41	<2.0
Oxytetracycline	10	<2.0
Polymyxin B	14	<0.5
Nalidixic acid	53	<5.0
Erythromycin	16	38.0
Oleandomycin	12	39.0

[a] Reproduced by permission from T. A. Stamey *et al.*, J. Urol. **103:** 187, 1970.[18]

sensitive bacteria were persisting in the prostatic fluid of our patients—those antibiotics useful against Gram-negative enteric pathogens cannot cross the prostatic epithelium into prostatic fluid. However, the interesting observation was the diffusion and concentration of the basic macrolides in prostatic fluid, interesting because elucidation of this mechanism might offer some leverage in searching for antimicrobial drugs that can diffuse and concentrate in prostatic fluid. Erythromycin and oleandomycin have no antimicrobial activity against the usual Gram-negative bacteria which cause urinary infections, except at an alkaline pH and in high concentrations.

Theoretical Considerations. The explanation for these seemingly contradictory observations lies in the principles governing the passage of drugs across biologic membranes and, in particular, the role of nonionic diffusion of weak acids and bases between membranes with different hydrogen ion concentrations. Almost all antimicrobial drugs are either weak acids or bases, and noninflammed prostatic fluid is distinctly acid, about pH 6.4,[51] compared to the pH of plasma, 7.4. These principles have been studied extensively in the absorption of drugs from the gastrointestinal lumen,[52–54] but they are rarely considered in the infectious disease literature in relation to antimicrobial therapy. Although the principles of drug diffusion are probably the same for all epithelial membranes, the prostate gland is perhaps the only organ where pathogenic bacteria residing in secretory fluid directly infects other major organs—the bladder and kidneys. To appreciate the therapeutic challenge of chronic bacterial prostatitis, one must consider the physiology of drug diffusion across prostatic epithelium.

The factors determining diffusion and concentration, in the absence of specific secretory or active transport mechanisms, are listed in Figure 7.11. If an antimicrobial drug is lipid-insoluble (a low lipid/water partition coefficient at pH 7.4), its distribution is limited to extracellular fluids because it cannot cross epithelial membranes.* Most of the clinically useful antimicrobials are completely lipid-insoluble (Table 7.20)

Even when a drug is lipid-soluble, only the uncharged fraction can cross lipid membranes; *i.e.*, the charged or ionized fraction is lipid-insoluble. Thus, if there is no pH gradient across the biologic membrane and the drug is lipid-soluble, the degree of ionization in the plasma (determined by the pKa of the drug) directly determines the uncharged fraction available for diffusion. Protein binding in the plasma can impose a further limitation on the fraction available for diffusion. Antibiotics like ampicillin, penicillin-G, and cephalothin not only are lipid-insoluble but also are acids with pKa values of 2.7, 2.5, and 2.5, respectively. At a plasma pH of 7.4, they are 99.99% in the charged form, which assures their exclusion from prostatic fluid (even if they were lipid-soluble). In Table 7.20, I have summarized these physical characteristics that determine diffusion as well as the concentration gradients between plasma and prostatic fluid found in our canine studies.

In addition to these factors determining simple diffusion, the presence of a pH gra-

* Some small molecules, if they are water soluble and of the correct shape, can cross biologic membranes as a part of the free diffusion of water.

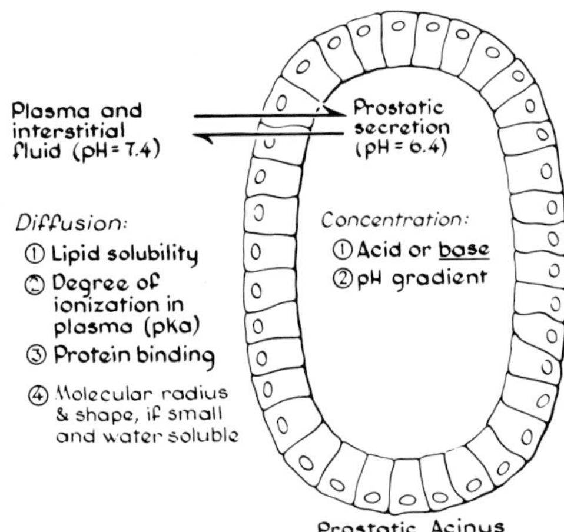

Figure 7.11 Factors determining diffusion and concentration of antimicrobial drugs across epithelium of prostatic acinus.

dient of considerable magnitude across prostatic epithelium (a 10-fold difference in hydrogen ion concentration) introduces the phenomenon of ion trapping. It is this phenomenon that accounts for the concentration of the basic macrolides in prostatic fluid (Table 7.19). In a stable system, the uncharged fraction of a lipid-soluble drug will eventually equilibrate on both sides of the membrane. However, the charged fraction will be greater on one side or the other depending on the pH. Thus, at equilibrium, there will be more total drug (charged plus uncharged) on the side of the greatest ionization. Figure 7.12*A* depicts these events for an acid of pKa 5.4 and Figure 7.12*B* illustrates a base of pKa 8.4. An antimicrobial substance in the plasma which dissociates as an acid will have 10 times more molecules in the charged form than can exist in prostatic fluid at pH 6.4 (Figure 7.12*A*). The ionized molecules are thereby trapped on the plasma side. Since the uncharged form is equal on both sides, there will be almost 10 times more total drug in the plasma than in prostatic fluid. With acids of higher pKa values, less of the drug is charged, more is in the uncharged form, and eventually the concentration in prostatic fluid of lipid-soluble acids with pKa values of 8.4 or greater can approach the plasma level (Figure 7.13). Note, however, that acid antimicrobial drugs, even with favorable pKa values of 8.4 or more, can never exceed the plasma concentration. A rearrangement of the Henderson-Hasselbalch equation, derived by Jacobs in 1940,[55] is useful for calculating the total concentration of any drug across a biologic membrane at equilibrium. This equation, which appears at the bottom of Figure 7.12, was used to calculate the limiting curves in Figure 7.13.

With antibacterial bases, the ion trapping occurs in the prostatic fluid. Figure 7.12*B* shows the theoretical concentration gradient, 101/11, that would be expected in prostatic fluid for a lipid-soluble, antimicrobial base of pKa 8.4 (erythromycin has a pKa of 8.8) at a prostatic fluid pH of 6.4. From Figure 7.13 (which was calculated using a prostatic fluid pH of 6.6 rather than 6.4), the maximal ion trapping in prostatic fluid occurs with bases of pKa values of 9.0 and above.

Returning to Table 7.20, one notes that nalidixic acid is lipid-soluble. However, it is an acid and 95% bound to plasma proteins.[45] Therefore, its diffusion into prostatic fluid is limited. Nitrofurantoin is also an acid. It has a favorable dissociation constant (40% is uncharged in plasma), and it is minimally lipid-soluble.[56] The major difficulty is that the plasma concentrations of nitrofurantoin are so low that, even if diffusion occurs, the concentrations are insignificant. Despite attaining pathological plasma concentrations of nitrofurantoin in the dog during intravenous infusion of the drug, we detected only minimal diffusion into prostatic fluid.[50]

Sulfonamides. The foregoing studies suggested that lipid solubility, pKa, protein binding, and nonionic diffusion were important in determining diffusion of antimicrobial drugs from plasma into prostatic fluid. Sulfonamides, as a general class of drugs, are many times more lipid-soluble than the antibiotics in Table 7.19, with the exception of the basic macrolides. On the other hand, their dissociation constants (pKa) vary over a wide range. Dr. Winningham and I[48] measured the diffusion of 17 different sulfonamides from plasma to prostatic fluid in 22 dogs.

Table 7.20
Diffusion Gradients Between Plasma and Prostatic Fluid in the Dog and the Physico-Chemical Characteristics that Determine Diffusion

Antimicrobial Drug	Plasma μg/ml	Prostatic Fluid μg/ml	Acid or Base	Lipid Soluble at pH 7.4	pKa	Percent Uncharged in Plasma
Penicillin-G	62	<0.2[a]	Acid	No	2.7	0.001
Ampicillin	54	<0.2	Acid	No	2.5	0.001
Cephalothin	63	<0.4	Acid	No	2.5	0.001
Nitrofurantoin	15	3.2	Acid	Slightly	7.2	39.0
Nalidixic acid	53	<5.0	Acid	Yes	6.0	4.0
Sulfisoxazole	15	0.3	Acid	Yes	5.0	0.4
Sulfamethoxazole	12.6	1.3	Acid	Yes	6.0	4.0
Sulfadimidine	8.5	4.6	Acid	Yes	7.7	67.0
Oxytetracycline	10	<2.0	Amphoteric	No	3.5, 7.6, 9.2	
Tetracycline	19	4.0	Amphoteric	Partial	3.3, 7.7, 9.7	
Polymyxin B	14	<0.5	Base	No	8–9	8.0
Kanamycin	41	<2.0	Base	No	7.2	39.0
Erythromycin	16	38.0	Base	Yes	8.8	4.0
Oleandomycin	12	39.0	Base	Yes	8.5	8.0
Trimethoprim	4	7.0	Base	Yes	7.3	56.0

[a] Indicates the lower limits of sensitivity of the bioassay.

Our general data are presented in Table 7.21. The different sulfonamides are arranged in descending order of their approximate molecular complexity. In general the plasma concentration at the time of pilocarpine stimulation had been established for at least 60 minutes, since prostatic fluid stimulation occurred after estimating the plasma clearance of the sulfonamide. The prostatic fluid concentrations vary from complete equilibration with plasma (P) (PF/P ratio of 0.98) in the case of sulfanilamide to virtual exclusion of sulfisoxazole and sulfamethizole from prostatic fluid (PF/P ratios of 0.02 and 0.03).

In Table 7.22, the PF/P ratios correspond closely to the dissociation constants (pKa) for each drug. This linear relationship is more readily seen in Figure 7.14.

The relative lipid solubilities of the sulfonamides in a 1:1 chloroform to sodium phosphate buffer at pH 7.4 (Table 7.22) are taken from the data of Rieder.[57]

These studies (Table 7.22 and Figure 7.14) establish that the diffusion of sulfonamides from plasma to prostatic fluid is determined by the pKa of the particular sulfonamide. Killman and Thaysen[58] also showed that the pKa determined the salivary fluid/plasma ratio in patients receiving sulfonamides of different dissociation constants. When we began these studies, we were not aware that all sulfonamides dissociate as acids; that is, they donate a proton in solution (Figure 7.15). Strong acid sulfonamides like sulfamethizole (pKa 5.4) will have about 100 charged ions in plasma of pH 7.4 for every uncharged one, while weak acids like sulfanilamide (pKa 10.4) will have only 1 charged ion for every 1000 uncharged. Since only the uncharged ion can cross the lipid layer of cells, sulfanilamide in prostatic fluid approaches the plasma concentration; sulfamethizole, with only a fraction of the drug in plasma in the freely diffusible uncharged form, can barely be detected in prostatic fluid. Because none of these sulfonamides dissociate as bases at the pH of plasma (Figure 7.15), they cannot be concentrated in more acidic prostatic fluid.

The relative lipid solubilities of the sulfonamides in Table 7.22 do not seem to play a major role in determining diffusion into prostatic fluid. For example, sulfanilamide with a PF/P ratio of 0.98 has about 1/30 the relative lipid solubility of sulfadimethoxine, which has a PF/P ratio of only 0.07. It is

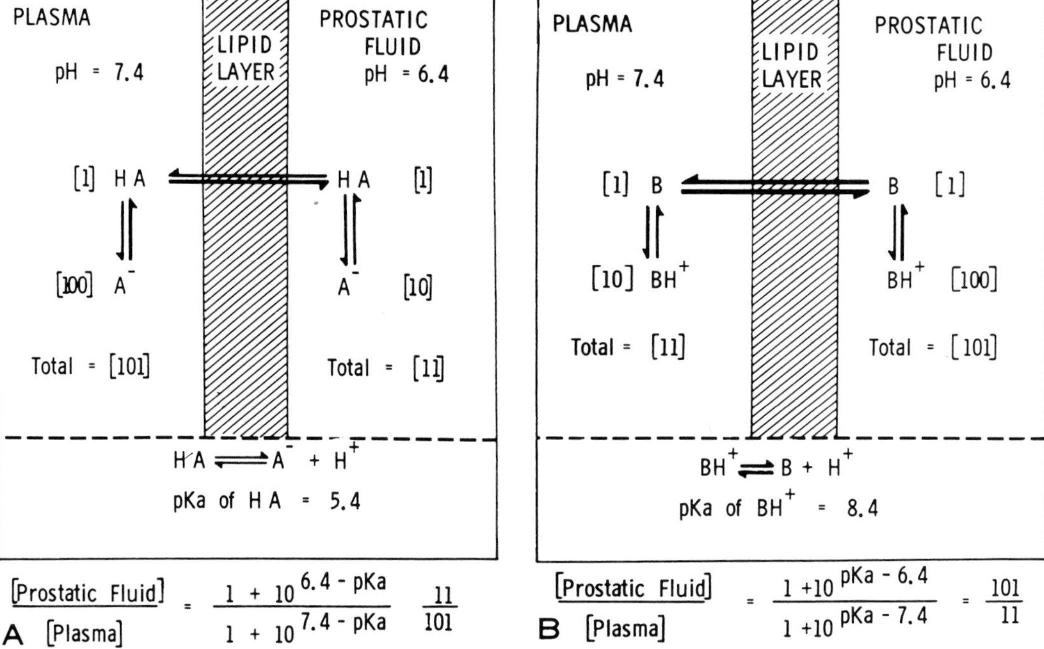

Figure 7.12 *A*, Nonionic diffusion of an antibacterial acid at equilibrium. Diagrammatic partition of an antibacterial acid of pKa 5.4 at theoretical equilibrium between plasma and prostatic fluid. A useful rearrangement of the Henderson-Hasselbalch equation that describes concentration ratios of total drug on both sides of membrane, as determined by ion trapping, is presented at bottom of figure. *B*, Diagrammatic partition of an antibacterial base of pKa 8.4 at theoretical equilibrium between plasma and prostatic fluid. Rearrangement of Henderson-Hasselbalch equation for concentration ratios of antimicrobial base due to ion trapping is presented at bottom.

probably that once a general level of lipid solubility is obtained, relative differences in lipid solubility are not important in determining diffusion across epithelial membranes. For the sulfonamides, these studies establish that the pKa, not the lipid solubility, determines the diffusion into prostatic fluid.

It should be emphasized that these data only establish which sulfonamides can diffuse into prostatic fluid. The degree of diffusion (PF/P ratio) is determined and, therefore, can be predicted by the pKa of the drug. Antibacterial activity of the drug, once the sulfonamide is present in prostatic fluid, is a separate question which we have not studied. For example, prostatic fluid is acidic to plasma by at least 1 pH unit. Many of our dogs consistently excreted prostatic fluid with a pH of 6.0. With sulfanilamide, all of the drug in prostatic fluid will be in the uncharged fraction. Studies of sulfonamide bacteriostasis *in vitro* at pH 7.0 have shown that the most effective antibacterial activity occurs when dissociation is about 50%, that is half in the charged form and half uncharged.[59] Thus, the possibility exists that a sulfonamide like sulfadiazine (pKa 6.5), with a PF/P ratio of 0.20, might be more antibacterial in prostatic fluid than sulfanilamide, with a PF/P ratio of 0.98.

Finally, we have had no clinical experience with any of these sulfonamides except sulfisoxazole and sulfamethizole. These drugs have not been helpful in patients with chronic bacterial prostatitis, and the studies reported here show the reason. However, it is noteworthy that sulfamethazine (sulfadimidine) with a PF/P ratio of 0.57 is the most commonly used sulfonamide for both urinary infection and meningitis in Britain.[60] In terms of diffusion across nonin-

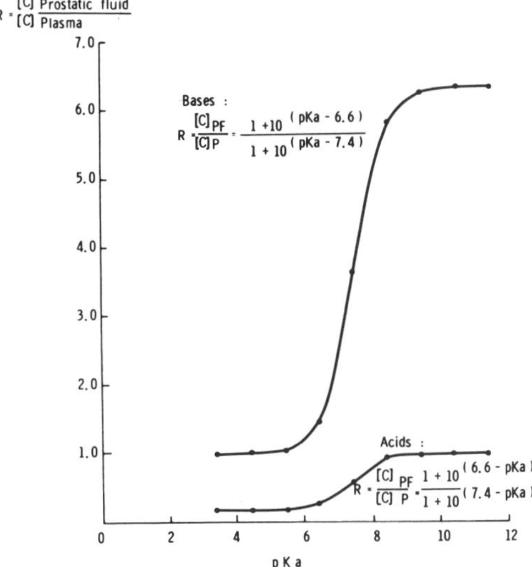

Figure 7.13 Theoretical partition ratios of antibiotics between prostatic fluid and plasma. From the Henderson-Hasselbalch derivations at bottom of Figure 7.12, theoretical limits for concentration ratios are presented for acids and bases of different pKa values. *R*, ratio of total drug in prostatic fluid to plasma; *C*, total concentration of each drug, charged and uncharged; *PF*, prostatic fluid; *P*, plasma; pKa, negative logarithm of acid or base dissociation constant; 6.6 and 7.4, negative logarithms of hydrogen ion concentration in prostatic fluid and plasma. Note that *R* can only approach ratio of 1.0 for antimicrobial acid, but can exceed 6.0 for antimicrobial base.

flammed membranes, it clearly has theoretical advantages over sulfisoxazole and sulfamethizole. It is strange that it is not available in this country. Lastly, if other sulfonamides are used clinically in an attempt to take advantage of diffusion into prostatic fluid, the clinician must be cautious for side effects such as precipitation of sulfonamide crystals in the renal tubules.

Tetracyclines. Dr. John Hessl and I published some studies on four tetracycline analogues.[61] We measured the diffusion gradients from plasma to prostatic fluid in four different tetracyclines of widely varying lipid solubility and serum protein binding (Table 7.23). Because the acidic dissociation constants are virtually the same for these tetracycline derivatives (Table 7.23), the relative number of charged and uncharged molecules in the plasma will be similar for each derivative. Under these circumstances, only the relative lipophilicity and protein binding should determine the degree of diffusion. Both canine and human protein binding of the tetracyclines are well documented.[62] The percentage of each drug bound to canine serum is presented in Table 7.23, along with the theoretical concentration ratio expected in prostatic fluid if it is assumed that only the nonprotein-bound fraction of each derivative is free to diffuse into prostatic fluid. As can be seen, the theoretical diffusion ratio, based on the plasma fraction of drug free for diffusion, agrees remarkably well with the experimental ratios found for tetracycline, α-6-deoxyoxytetracycline, and 6-demethyl-6-deoxytetracycline. Oxytetracycline, however, with 73% of the drug free in plasma, could not be detected in prostatic fluid, perhaps because it is virtually lipid-insoluble. These data suggest that once a certain degree of lipid solubility is present (*i.e.*, that of tetracycline), protein binding is more important in determining diffusion across prostatic epithelium than is a marked increase in lipophilicity.

These data explain the failure of tetracyclines to eradicate the sensitive bacteria from the prostatic fluid. With such limited diffusion into prostatic fluid, none of the oral tetracyclines could possibly come close to the mininal inhibitory concentration of even sensitive Gram-negative bacteria. Tetracycline hydrochloride (56% bound to plasma proteins in man) given intravenously at a dose of 500 mg every 6 hours[63] might be useful, but the danger of hepatic necrosis is a serious limitation.

Unique Position of Trimethoprim. The studies reviewed above suggest that if an antimicrobial drug is lipid-insoluble, whether it be acid like the penicillins and cephalosporins or a base like the polymyxins, it cannot cross the normal prostatic epithelium into prostatic fluid. Once a certain level of lipophilicity is present, however, the pKa of the antibiotic is important because the dissociation constant determines the percentage of uncharged mole-

Table 7.21
General Data

The diffusion of 17 different sulfonamides from plasma into prostatic fluid. I.V. = intravenous; peak [P] = plasma level of sulfonamide 5 minutes after intravenous injection; [PF] = prostatic fluid concentration of sulfonamide in mg%; [P] = plasma concentration of sulfonamide in mg%; [PF]/[P] = ratio of prostatic fluid concentration to that in the plasma; [U] = concentration in urine in mg%; UV/P = plasma clearance before pilocarpine stimulation. The plasma clearances of the sulfonamides represent only approximations because no attempt was made to obtain a steady state or to insure reproducibility of consecutive clearance periods. Nevertheless, they serve as gross estimates; the long acting sulfonamides like sulfamethoxypyridazine had low clearances, while the short acting drugs had high clearances (sulfadiazine).

Sulfonamide	$H-N(H)-C_6H_4-S(O_2)-N(H)-R$ R =	Dog no. and Wt.	I.V. Dose	Peak [P]	Simultaneous Concentrations [PF]	[P]	[PF]/[P]	Clearance data[a] Sulfonamide [U]	UV/P	Creatinine [U]	UV/P
		(lb)	*(g)*	*(mg%)*	*(mg%)*	*(mg%)*		*(mg%)*	*(ml/min)*	*(mg%)*	*(ml/min)*
Sulfanilamide	–H	1—55	2.0	11.1	6.20	6.31	0.98	49	55		
Sulfacetamide	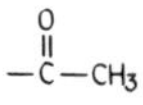 $-C(=O)-CH_3$	2—60	2.0	14.4	0.24	3.20	0.08	80	115		
Sulfapyridine	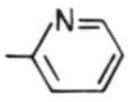 N	3—51	2.0	10.2	4.70	6.45	0.73	19.5	41	2.9	84
Sulfadiazine[b]	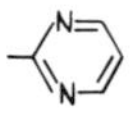 N, N	4—49	2.0	19.8	1.68	10.10	0.17	47	100	2.9	122
		5—44	2.0	13.3	1.89	8.06	0.23	38.5	61	3.9	99
Sulfamerazine[b]	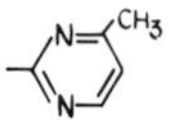 N, N, CH_3	6—46	2.0	14.5	2.70	10.30	0.26	34.5		5.4	
		7—44	2.0	10.3	2.10	5.70	0.37	31.1	91	3.4	127
Sulfamethazine[b] (sulfadimidine)	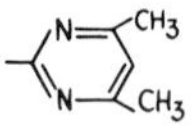 N, N, CH_3, CH_3	8—57	2.0	21.3	4.57	8.46	0.54	31.1	30	4.9	72
		9—60	2.0	19.9	4.37	7.25	0.60				
Sulfameter (Sulla)	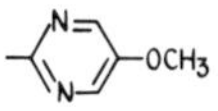 N, N, OCH_3	10—54	2.0	13.8	1.50	10.70	0.14	70.5	9.6		
Sulfamethoxy-pyridazine (Kynex)	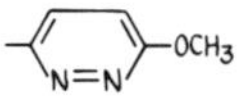 N=N, OCH_3	11—55	2.0	36.1	7.68	21.20	0.36	81	4.7		
Sulfisomidine (Elkosin)	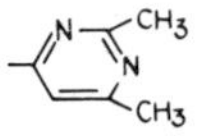 N, N, CH_3, CH_3	12—51	2.0	22.5	3.72	12.60	0.30	69	55	5.1	59
Sulfadimethoxine (Madribon)	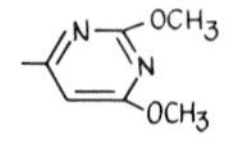 N, N, OCH_3, OCH_3	13—45	2.0	17.9	0.89	9.45	0.09	12.3	11.2	4.4	63
		14—65	2.0	16.1	0.56	12.00	0.05	6.7	10.5	3.9	62
Sulformethoxine	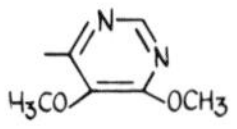 N, N, H_3CO, OCH_3	15—57	1.0	11.4	0.49	7.00	0.07	30.7	29.5		
		16—60	2.0	18.9	0.90	11.60	0.08	71	31.6		
Sulfathiazole	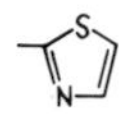 S, N	17—42	2.0	20.3	0.85	8.33	0.10	43	60	2.9	57
Sulfamethizole (Thiosulfil)	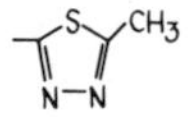 S, N–N, CH_3	18—52	4.0	75.0	0.94	32.50	0.03				
Sulfaethidole (Sul-Spantao)	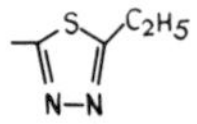 S, N–N, C_2H_5	19—69	2.0	18.7	0.25	15.30	0.02	92.5	123	5.9	106
Sulfisoxazole (Gantrisin)	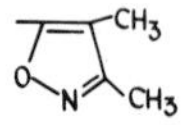 O, N, CH_3, CH_3	20—58	2.5	22.5	0.28	15.10	0.02				
	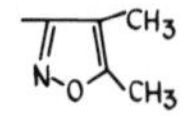 N–O, CH_3, CH_3	21—48	2.0	22.8	1.28	12.60	0.10	30.8	13.2	6.4	60
Sulfaphenazole (Sulfabid)	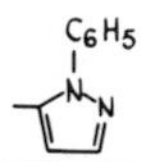 C_6H_5, N, N	22—48	2.0	34.8	1.20	22.50	0.05	22.3	9.5		

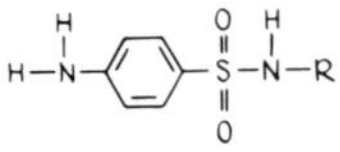

[a] Clearance data uncorrected.

[b] Usual mixture of triple sulfa combinations.

Table 7.22
Relationship of pKa, PF/P Concentration Ratio, and Lipid Solubility for Acid Sulfonamides[a, b]

Sulfonamide	pKa	Experimental PF/P	Lipid Solubility[c]
Sulfanilamide	10.43	0.98	2.6
Sulfapyridine	8.43	0.73	
Sulfamethazine	7.70	0.57	75.8
Sulfamethoxypyridazine	7.20	0.36	68.6
Sulfamerazine	6.98	0.32	48.6
Sulfisomidine	7.57	0.30	17.8
Sulfadiazine	6.52	0.20	11.9
Sulfameter	7.02	0.14	51.1
Sulfathiazole	7.25	0.10	6.8
Sulfamethoxazole	6.05	0.10	9.6
Sulfacetamide	5.78	0.08	0.7
Sulformethoxine	6.10	0.07	
Sulfadimethoxine	6.32	0.07	74.1
Sulfaphenazole	6.09	0.05	53.6
Sulfamethizole	5.45	0.03	
Sulfisoxazole	5.00	0.02	3.8
Sulfaethidole	5.65	0.02	3.6

[a] Reproduced by permission from D. G. Winningham and T. A. Stamey, J. Urol. **104:** 559, 1970.[48]

[b] PF = prostatic fluid; P = plasma.

[c] Percentage distribution of drug in lipid layer of a mixture of chloroform and sodium phosphate buffer in a 1 to 1 ratio.

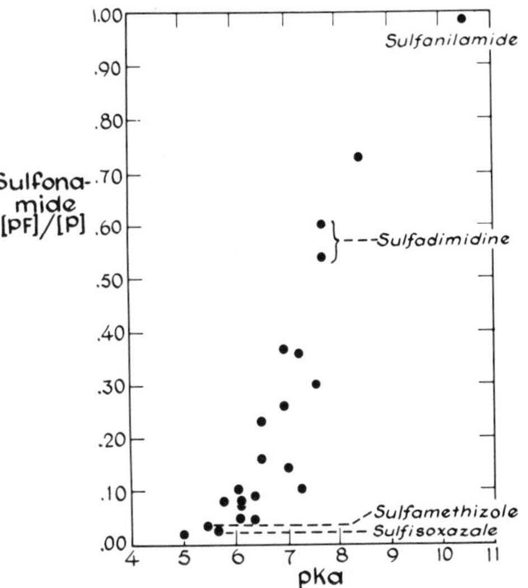

Figure 7.14 Relationship between pKa and prostatic fluid/plasma (PF/P) ratio of 17 different sulfonamides in 22 dogs.

cules in the plasma available for diffusion. Protein binding, as in the case of nalidixic acid and the more lipid-soluble tetracyclines, can exert a profound limitation on diffusion.

What is clearly needed, however, is a base that is lipid-soluble and has antimicrobial activity against Gram-negative bacteria at pH 6.0–6.5 (the pH of prostatic fluid). While a pKa of 8.6 or more would take optimal advantage of the ion-trapping potential in prostatic fluid (Figure 7.13), it must be remembered that the stronger the base (the higher the pKa) the smaller the percentage of the molecules that will be in the uncharged form in plasma. The mathematical derivations in Figure 7.13 assume complete equilibrium on both sides of the prostatic epithelium. A base, however, with a pKa of 10.4 will have only one uncharged molecule available for diffusion in the presence of a 1000 charged ions; understandably, the process of ion trapping will take longer than with a base of pKa 7.4 where half the molecules in plasma are immediately available for diffusion. This is undoubtedly the main reason that our original studies with the basic macrolides showed ion trapping with prostatic fluid concentrations exceeding the plasma levels for only a limited period following pilocarpine stimulation (Figure 7.16*A*). During the 60 minutes in Figure 7.16*A* before the prostate was stimulated, there was enough time for the 8% uncharged molecules to diffuse and become ion-trapped by more dissociation in the more acidic prostatic fluid. Once this fluid was emptied by pilocarpine stimulation, however, continuous secretion by the prostatic glands was too rapid for further ion trapping in the presence of only 4% of the plasma molecules available for diffusion. The diffusion of oleandomycin in Figure 7.16*A* is in sharp contrast to trimethoprim in 7.16*B* because 56% of trimethoprim molecules are available for diffusion.

When TMP (a compound of the 2,4-diaminopyrimidine series[64]) became available in England in the late 1960s and early 1970s, Reeves and Ghilchick[65] recognized that it met all of the requirements discussed above for diffusion into prostatic fluid. TMP is

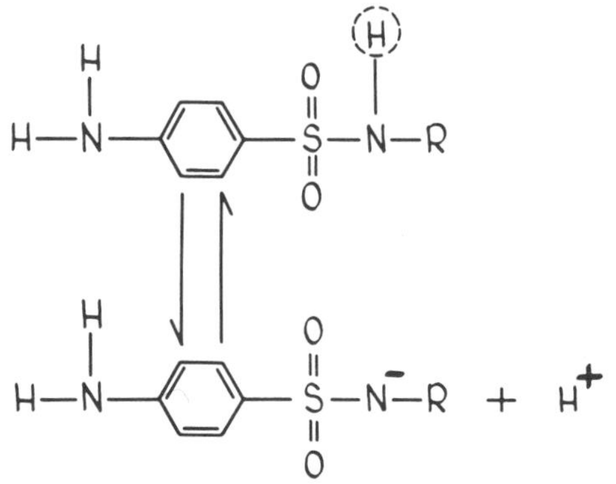

Figure 7.15 Ionizations of a sulfonamide. All the sulfonamides in Table 7.21 ionize as acids, as illustrated in this figure. The P-amino nitrogen group (to the left of the benzene ring), with a pKa between 2 and 3 (sulfanilamide), accepts a proton (acts as a base) only in highly acid solutions. Its ionization as a base, therefore, can be ignored in physiologic solutions.

lipid-soluble, it is a base, and with its pKa of 7.3, over 50% of the molecules in plasma are available for diffusion in the uncharged form. In canine studies similar to our model, Reeves and Ghilchick[65] reported that concentrations of TMP in PF exceeded those in serum (S) by 2.6 times. Because Robb *et al.*[66] found PF/S ratios as high as 16, and our group at Stanford found ratios in 13 dogs that varied between 2 and 10,[67] we wondered whether there was an active transport mechanism for TMP in prostatic epithelium because such large gradients exceeded the theoretical ratios (PF/S of 3.4 at a PF pH of 6.6 and a plasma pH of 7.4) expected from diffusion alone. In order to test for the presence of an active secretory site, we attempted to saturate the system by increasing the intravenous dosage every 30 minutes. In addition, prostatic fluid and arterial blood pH had to be monitored closely if the theoretical diffusion gradients were to be accurately calculated. All of the bioassays were performed at the Wellcome Research Laboratories by Drs. S. R. M. Bushby and Carl Sigel; the results were interesting.[68] As seen in Table 7.24 and illustrated in Figure 7.17, despite serum concentrations of TMP that increased 300 times (from 0.63 to 185 μg/ml) over 4 ½ hours of infusion, TMP in PF continued to rise in substantial increments. More importantly, when the theoretical diffusion ratios of PF/S were calculated during the periods when arterial pH was accurately measured, the actual PF/S ratios found in the experiments never exceeded the theoretical ratios expected from simple, nonionic diffusion alone (Table 7.24). Madsen *et al.*,[69] however, believe active transport is present because of studies in one 26-year-old man with urinary diversion; their PF/S ratios were 19 to 44 in the presence of a prostatic fluid pH of 6.9, which does exceed by severalfold the theoretical diffusion gradient.

In addition to excluding an active transport mechanism, these experiments established the extraordinary rapidity with which TMP concentrates in PF by nonionic diffusion and subsequent iontrapping. For example, compare the data in Figure 7.17 and Figure 7.16*B* with the diffusion characteristics of oleandomycin in Figure 7.16*A*. Although oleandomycin could be concentrated in PF, the PF/S ratio never exceeded 2.3 and required long periods of equilibration from plasma to PF before initiating PF secretion; more revealing is the observation that the PF/S ratio of >1.0 was short-lived and limited to the first few milliliters of PF obtained from the prostate. By contrast, and despite the fact that PF secretion was started simultaneously with the first intravenous dose of TMP (pilocarpine and TMP were injected intravenously in the same syringe), the very first PF to appear (moments after the intravenous injection of TMP and pilocarpine) already exceeded the plasma concentration of TMP by several times (Figures 7.16*B* and 7.17). When oleandomycin is given in the same syringe with pilocarpine and accompanied by the PF flow rates we obtained, then the concentration of oleandomycin never exceeds the plasma level. These differences in rapidity of diffusion and ion trapping are undoubtedly related to the difference in pKa between oleandomycin (8.5) and TMP (7.3); the former allows 8% of the molecules to exist in plasma in the uncharged form while TMP has 56% uncharged molecules available for diffusion. Finally, since salivary

Table 7.23
Lipid Solubility, Protein Binding, and Diffusion into Canine Prostatic Fluid of Four Tetracyclines

Tetracycline	Lipid Solubility $K\left[\frac{CHCl_3}{H_2O}\right] \times 10^3$	Acidic Dissociation Constants	Protein Binding in Canine Serum	Theoretical Concentration Ratio[a] PF/P[c]	Experimental Concentration Ratio[b] PF/P[c]
			%		
6-Demethyl-6-deoxytetracycline	6250	3.14, 7.93, 9.32	92	0.08	0.11
α-6-Deoxyoxytetracycline	475		83	0.17	0.16
Tetracycline	95	3.30, 7.68, 9.69	80	0.20	0.22
Oxytetracycline	7.2	3.27, 7.32, 9.11	27	0.73	0.00

[a] Assumes complete diffusion of the unbound fraction of the tetracycline derivative from plasma to prostatic fluid.
[b] Each ratio represents the average of at least two dogs.
[c] PF = Prostatic fluid; P = plasma.

fluid is alkaline to plasma (Table 7.24), these experiments show that ion trapping of a base must occur on the plasma side (the more acidic side) of the epithelial membrane; for this reason, the salivary fluid/serum ratio is less than 1.0.

The best experimental study based on direct assay of human prostatic tissue obtained surgically at the time of prostatectomy is by Dabhoiwala, Bye, and Claridge[70] in 1976 who found a prostatic tissue: plasma ratio for TMP of 2.03 in patients treated preoperatively for 1 week with 320 mg/1600 mg of TMP/SMX/day. It should be noted, however, that depending on the volume of EPS in prostatic tissue, a 2.0 ratio is compatible with a much higher ratio of TMP in PF compared to P.

Rosamicin. Rosamicin, a new macrolide antimicrobial agent that resembles erythromycin, was found by Baumueller *et al.*[71] to diffuse and concentrate in canine and human prostatic fluid at levels far exceeding those of erythromycin. Because rosamicin is more effective against Enterobacteriaceae and P. *aeruginosa in vitro* than erythromycin, clinical trials of this drug in patients with bacterial prostatitis may prove interesting.

Clinical Observations

Trimethoprim - sulfamethoxazole. TMP is a sulfonamide potentiator[72] and for this reason was combined with SMX, a sulfonamide with a reasonably similar blood half-life (about 9 hours for SMX, 10 hours for TMP). SMX blocks the bacterial production of folinic acid at the link between *p*-aminobenzoic acid and dihydrofolic acid; TMP blocks the bacterial production of folinic acid at the link between dihydrofolic acid and tetrahydrofolic acid; therefore, both TMP and SMX break the bacterial metabolic chain of purine synthesis that leads to the production of nucleic acids (Figure 7.18). Thus, sulfonamides and TMP are antifolate drugs but they show selective toxicity for bacteria. Because humans derive their dihydrofolic acid from dietary exogenous sources, sulfonamides do not affect the production of folates in man. TMP has a 100,000 times greater affinity (binding power) for the target enzyme (dihydrofolate reductase) of bacteria than it has for the same enzyme in humans.[73] Indeed, the biochemical evolution of TMP by George Hitchings[73] at Burroughs Wellcome from 2,4-diamino-5-benzylpyrimidine with a succession of molecular modifications to achieve greater binding to bacterial dihydrofolate reductase without significant increase in binding to mammalian reductase, makes TMP, and its discoverer, unique in the history of chemotherapy.

After preliminary clinical reports from England in 1969,[74–76] there have been numerous reports in this country and abroad on the clinical efficacy of TMP-SMX. Sev-

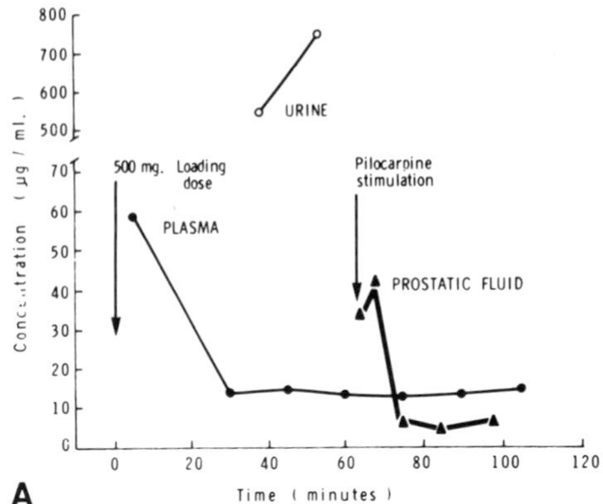

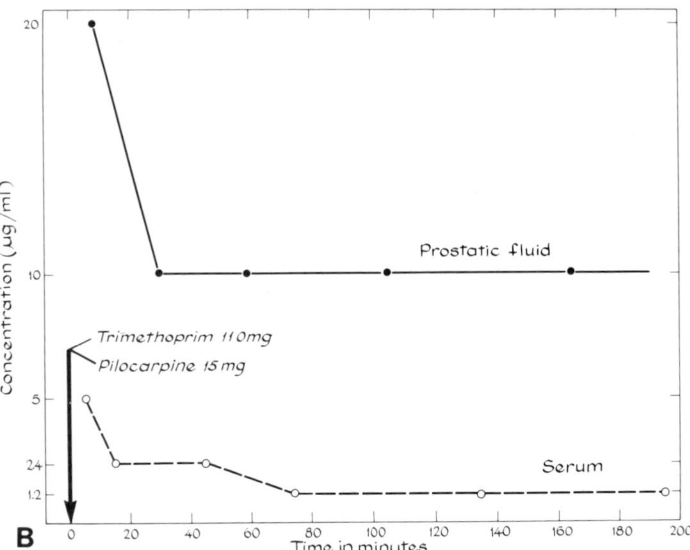

Figure 7.16 *A*. The diffusion of a basic macrolide (oleandomycin, dog 698) from plasma to prostatic fluid in the dog. Observe that pilocarpine stimulation occurred 60 minutes after high levels of antibiotic were established in the plasma. Only the first two collections of prostatic fluid showed antibiotic levels that exceeded the plasma. As noted in the text, this is related both to the pK_a of the antimicrobial base and to the rapid prostatic fluid flow rate. (Reproduced by permission from D. G. Winningham *et al.* Nature **219:** 139, 1968.[47]) *B*, Simultaneous administration of trimethoprim (TMP) and pilocarpine in a 22-kg dog. TMP and pilocarpine are given simultaneously in the same syringe. Observe that not only does the concentration of TMP exceed the serum level by several times, but as prostatic fluid secretion continues, levels of TMP in prostatic fluid continue to exceed the serum concentration by about 10 times. The differences in diffusion characteristics between *Part A* (oleandomycin) and *B* (TMP) are related to the number of uncharged molecules available for diffusion, 8% (pKa = 8.5) for oleandomycin and 56% (pKa = 7.3) for TMP.

eral excellent reviews and symposiums have been published; the best one on the combination of TMP-SMX is in the November 1973, supplement to the *Journal of Infectious Diseases* (volume 128, S425–S816) and the best review of TMP alone is published in the *Annals of Clinical Research* (Volume 10, Supplement 22, 1978) from Torku, Finland. Although the unique use of TMP-SMX in my view is in the prophylactic prevention of recurrent urinary infections in females (and is treated fully in Chapter 4), the clinical question in this Chapter relates to TMP-SMX efficacy in chronic bacterial prostatitis.

The best data, because of the 6-month follow-up and the care with which monthly prostatic localizations were performed, are from Stanford as reported by Meares.[77, 78] In this 1973 report, 13 patients were treated for 14 days with TMP-SMX at full dosage of 160/800 mg twice daily[77]; there were 2 cures and 11 failures, although 9 of the failures were considered improved because the responsible pathogenic bacterium could not be cultured from the EPS or VB_3 during

Table 7.24
Concentrations of Trimethoprim in Canine Serum, Prostatic, and Salivary Fluid During Successive Intravenous Dosing[a]

Collection period[b]	Dosage IV at 30-min intervals (mg/kg)	Serum[b]		Prostatic Fluid			Salivary Fluid			Diffusion Ratio PF/S	
		pH	TMP[c] (μg/ml)	Volume (ml)	pH	TMP (μg/ml)	Volume (ml)	pH	TMP (μg/ml)	Actual	Theoretical
1	1.5	7.33	0.63	8.5	6.3	2.41	56.0	7.8	0.57	3.83	5.60
2	2.5		1.88	11.0	6.0	16.55	31.0	8.1	1.41	8.80	
3	5.0	7.30	4.23	18.0	5.9	27.25	28.0	8.4	3.98	6.44	13.06
4	10.0		10.98	7.0	5.8	91.75	18.0	8.1	8.05	8.36	
5	20.0	7.24	25.63	7.0	5.7	234.5	15.0	7.8	17.00	9.14	18.98
6	40.0		61.63	4.5	5.8	342.5	8.5	8.0	25.55	5.56	
7	60.0		98.44	4.5	5.2	630.0	3.5	8.0	46.46	6.40	
8	60.0		152.50	3.5	5.2	885.0	1.0	8.3	60.50	5.60	
9	60.0		185.00	3.5	5.1	1555.0	0.5	8.4	68.37	8.41	

[a] Reproduced by permission from T. A. Stamey *et al.*, from J. of Infect. Disease **128 (Suppl.):** S686, 1973.[68]
[b] Blood for serum assays was drawn at the midpoint of each collection period.
[c] TMP = trimethoprim; PF = prostatic fluid; S = serum.

therapy. Since these patients are asymptomatic on any drug to which their prostatic bacteria are sensitive, it is important to note that the categories of cure, improved, and failure are bacteriologic definitions and not clinical ones. Failure meant that the responsible bacterium could be recovered from the EPS and/or VB_3 in the presence of TMP-SMX therapy. Because only 15% of patients were cured on 2 weeks of TMP-SMX therapy, 23 patients were treated for 3 months on full dosage therapy. Nineteen of these 23 patients were reported by Meares[78] in 1975. The results of the 23 patients were: 7/23 cured (30.5%), 10/23 improved (43.5%), and 6/23 failed (26%). Because 8/23 of these patients had previously been treated with the earlier 14-day course of therapy and therefore could have been preselected for failure, I have removed them for analysis of the 2 week versus the 12 week treatment results (Figure 7.19). Both series are too small for statistically significant analysis, but there were 3 times (six patients) as many cures in the 12-week treatment group as in the 2-week group which is suggestive of some increased benefit from prolonged, full-dosage therapy (even though the figures are statistically insignificant). In a randomized study of 30 patients, Smith and his colleagues[128] treated antibody-coated, bacteriuric infections—half of whom were proven to have prostatic infections—with either a 10-day or 12-week course of TMP-SMX; 9 of the 15 patients (60%) were cured by the 12-week course while only 3 of 15 were cured by 10 days of therapy (P = 0.06).

Whatever the cause of the failures, it is indisputable that TMP-SMX can cure chronic bacterial prostatitis, even with a short 14-day course of therapy. In Table 7.25, previously reported by Meares,[77] the bacteriologic course of G.C.B., a 39-year-old white male, is documented. His recurrent urinary infections with *E. coli* began in 1963 at the age of 31 and he had multiple recurrences each time antimicrobial therapy was stopped. In 1970 and early 1971, four different efforts to cure his recurrent infections failed; each time he recurred with *E. coli* bacteriuria. When referred to Stanford in June 1971, on nitrofurantoin 100 mg twice daily, the first two sets of cultures did not show *E. coli* because EPS was not obtained. However, the cultures on 7/21/71 and 9/1/71 proved the presence of *E. coli* in his prostate. An intravenous urogram was normal; there was no residual urine. An ejaculate culture on 8/29/71 showed large numbers of *E. coli* at a time when the bladder was sterile on suprapubic needle aspiration. In follow-up cultures for 9 months, off all antimicrobial therapy, there

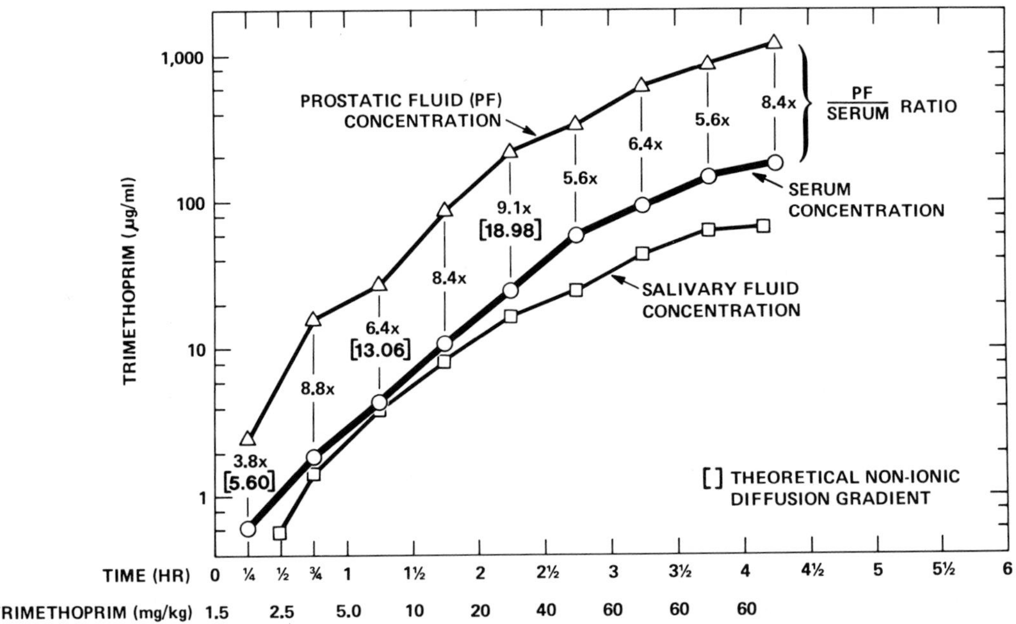

Figure 7.17 Diffusion of trimethoprim from plasma into prostatic and salivary fluid in the dog (plotted from data in Table 7.24). (Reproduced by permission from T. A. Stamey *et al.* J. Infect. Dis. **128 (Suppl):** S686, 1973.[68])

has been no recurrence of bacteriuria, no *E. coli* in the VB_3 or EPS, and his serum bacterial agglutination titers fell four tubes to normal level. The usefulness of an ejaculate culture, as advocated by Mobley,[79] is also apparent in Table 7.25. As Mobley[79] has pointed out, the VB_1 and VB_2 voided urine culture, obtained just prior to ejaculation, should be free of Gram-negative bacteria; 45% of ejaculate cultures will contain normal urethral bacteria like *S. epidermidis*, α-streptococci, and diptheroids,[79] and the number of these bacteria per milliliter of ejaculate will exceed the number in the VB_1.[80]

A search for the cause of the 40–60% failure rate in those patients treated for 12 weeks with TMP-SMX seems important. Dr. S. R. M. Bushby at Burroughs Wellcome determined the minimal inhibitory concentrations for each of the 18 strains causing chronic bacterial prostatitis in the 15 patients receiving TMP-SMX for 12 weeks (Figure 7.19). These data, previously published by Meares,[81] are reproduced in Table 7.26 because they indicate that neither the bacteriologic failures nor the improved group can be explained by *in vitro* sensitivities. For example, except for the one naturally resistant *P. aeruginosa*, all of the infecting strains were sensitive to 0.5 µg/ml or less of TMP regardless of the bacteriologic result; SMX resistance occurred in three of the six cures and in none of the four failures. Moreover, there was no significant change in the sensitivity of the strains during or after therapy with TMP-SMX.

These data seem important because bacteriologic persistence in the prostate as a cause of failure seems unrelated to the presence or development of bacterial resistance. The patients who were cured as well as those who were improved bacteriologically (no positive cultures from the EPS or VB_3 during therapy) certainly fit the experimental data that TMP gets into the prostate. It is true that the pH gradient for ion trapping of TMP may not exist in the inflamed human prostate.[82, 83] Nevertheless, TMP in prostatic fluid should approach the serum concentration which still should exceed the

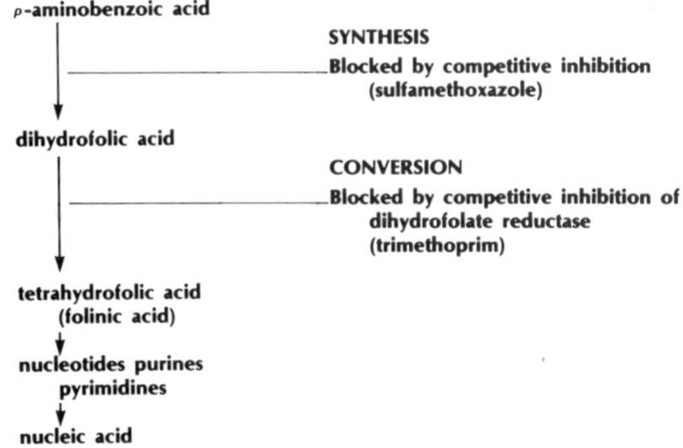

Figure 7.18 The antifolate blockade by sulfonamides and trimethoprim.

MIC of most infecting strains of Enterobacteriaceae. It is interesting that Baumueller and Madsen,[84] using an excellent model of experimental bacterial prostatitis in the dog, showed no change in the pH of prostatic secretion in either the acute or chronic phase of inflammation. In addition, and in the same experimental model, nonionic diffusion and concentration of TMP and erythromcycin in prostatic fluid were unimpeded in the presence of bacterial prostatitis.[85] Nevertheless, the recent data by Fair *et al.*[86] on 41 samples of EPS from 14 patients with chronic bacterial prostatitis (pH of EPS = 8.32 ± 0.07) is impressive.

I am impressed with the similarity of the improved group (sterile EPS and VB_3 cultures on therapy and sometimes for considerable periods after stopping therapy) with the behavior of renal infection stones during therapy. I expect the major cause of bacteriologic failure is bacterial persistence of the infecting organism in prostatic ductal concentrations wherein the TMP cannot penetrate the mucoprotein matrix of corpora amylacea.[29] We certainly have proven bacterial persistence in prostatic calculi and there is no reason to believe that the more common corpora amylacea may not serve as a nidus for bacterial persistence, thereby explaining the absence of radiologically detectable calcifications in the prostate.

Kanamycin. One of our early patients in 1966 was cured of his chronic bacterial prostatitis by 5 days of kanamycin therapy (Table 7.12). Pfau and Sacks[87] reported on

	14 DAYS	12 WEEKS
CURED	2 (15%)	6 (40%)
IMPROVED	9 (70%)	5 (33%)
FAILURE	2 (15%)	4 (27%)
	13 PATIENTS	15 PATIENTS

Figure 7.19 Results of trimethoprim-sulfamethoxazole therapy in patients with chronic bacterial prostatitis.

6 well-documented patients with chronic bacterial prostatitis all of whom recurred after short periods (10–30 days) of treatment with TMP-SMX. All six were then treated with 4 months of TMP-SMX, and three were cured. Two of the remaining three received kanamycin for 10–14 days and one received streptomycin for 12 days; all three were cured with minimal follow-up of 19 months. Apparently, all 6 patients were free of prostatic calculi on x-ray examination.

Therapeutic Recommendations. Given a patient with documented chronic bacterial prostatitis and recurrent bacteriuria due to Enterobaceriaceae sensitive to TMP-SMX, I would first treat him with 160 mg of TMP and 800 mg of SMX every 12 hours for 3–4 months. I would obtain localization cultures with VB_1, VB_2, EPS, and VB_3 specimens every 2 weeks after the start of therapy for the 1st month; if the pathogenic organism can be isolated from the EPS or VB_3, treatment should be discontinued because the patient will certainly be a bacteriologic failure. I would then try 10–14 days of kanamycin, probably using the Pfau and Sacks[87] regimen of 1000 mg intramuscularly twice daily for 3 days and then 500 mg twice daily for the rest of the period.

If long-term, full dosage TMP-SMX therapy and kanamycin both failed, I would offer the patient the alternative of chronic prophylaxis (½ tablet TMP-SMX, 40/200 mg nightly) on which regimen he will be totally asymptomatic, or offer him the possibility of a bacteriologic cure by "radical" transurethral prostatectomy. He will then ask how good is the possibility of a surgical

Table 7.25
Bacteriologic History of G.C.B., a 39-Year-Old White Man with an 8-Year History of Recurrent Urinary Tract Infections[a]

Date	Drug, days on (+) or off (−)	VB_1[b]	VB_2	EPS	VB_3	Organism	Antibody Titer
			Colonies/ml				
6-17-71	Nitrofur (+14)	0	0		0		
6-24-71	Nitrofur (+21)	0	0		0		
7-1-71	Nitrofur (−8)	20	0		0	*Klebsiella pneumoniae*	
7-11-71	Nitrofur (−19)	100,000	100,000			*Escherichia coli*	
7-12-71	Nitrofur (+1)	0	0		500	*E. coli*	
7-15-71	Nitrofur (+4)	0	0		0		
8-29-71	Nitrofur (+45)	Ejaculate = 100,000				*E. coli* 06	
8-30-71	Nitrofur (−1)	SPA = 0					
9-1-71	Nitrofur (−3)	0	0	3,000	30	*E. coli* 06	
9-9-71	Nitrofur (−11)	20	0	40	20	*E. coli* 06	1:320
9-30-71	TMP-SMX (+7)	0	0	0	0		1:320
10-7-71	TMP-SMX (+14)	0	0	0	0		1:320
10-21-71	TMP-SMX (−14)	0	0	0	0		1:160
11-18-71	TMP-SMX (−42)	0	0	0	0		1:160
12-16-71	TMP-SMX (−70)	0	0	0	0		1:160
12-21-71	TMP-SMX (−75)	Ejaculate = 0					
2-3-72	TMP-SMX (−120)	0	0	0	0		1:160
5-4-72	TMP-SMX (−213)	0	0	0	0		
6-29-72	TMP-SMX (−270)	0	0	0	0		1:80

[a] Reproduced by permission from E. M. Meares, Jr., J. Infect. Dis. **128:(Suppl):** S679, 1973.[77]

[b] VB_1 = first voided 10 ml of urine (urethral culture); VB_2 = midstream urine aliquot (bladder culture); EPS = expressed prostatic secretions (prostatic culture); VB_3 = first voided 10 ml of urine immediately after prostatic massage (prostatic culture); SPA = suprapubic needle aspiration of bladder (bladder culture); TMP-SMX = trimethoprim-sulfamethoxazole; Nitrofur = nitrofurantoin. Solid transverse line divides longitudinal cultures into major periods of significance.

cure? I expect it is about 33%, and I cannot believe it is 100% as reported by Silber.[24]

In terms of bladder prophylaxis, it should be remembered that almost any antimicrobial agent to which the prostatic organism is sensitive will suffice in small doses; tetracycline should be used for *Pseudomomas* prostatitis.

URETHRAL OR PREPUTIAL COLONIZATION WITH ENTEROBACTERIACEAE AS A CAUSE OF RECURRENT URINARY INFECTIONS

Most of this chapter on *Urinary Infections in Males* has dealt with the diagnosis and treatment of chronic bacterial prostatitis because it is the major cause of recurrent bacteriuria in males. There are, however, a few rare individuals in whom the site of bacterial persistence in between episodes of bacteriuria is not the prostate but the urethra and the prepuce. They can be recognized because localization cultures in between episodes of bacteriuria show the urethra (VB_1) and not the prostate (EPS, VB_3) as the site of bacterial persistence.

One example is that of J.K., a 15-year-old Caucasian man, who was first seen on 11/6/62 after his third attack of urinary urgency, frequency, terminal dysuria, and suprapubic pain; there was no known history of fever or chills. These episodes began suddenly, and the midstream urine contained large numbers of leukocytes and Gram-negative bacilli. The three infections occurred in 2 years; each one was treated

Table 7.26
Minimal Inhibitory Concentrations of Trimethoprim and Sulfamethoxazole to 18 Strains Causing Chronic Bacterial Prostatitis in 5 Patients[a]

Patient	Organism and Serogroup	MIC[a] (μg/ml)		Bacteriologic Result
		TMP	SMX	
M.E.O.	*Escherichia coli* 04	0.15	7.35	Cured
E.P.W.	*E. coli* 011	0.15	245	Cured
P.F.D.	*Proteus mirabilis*	0.5	7.35	Cured
F.G.S.	*E. coli* NT	0.15	245	Cured
R.H.	*E. coli* NT	0.5	9.5	Cured
D.E.G.	*E. coli* NT	0.15	>950	Cured
E.D.S.	*Mima*	0.5	>950	Cured
E.D.S.	*E. coli* 07	0.15	9.5	Improved
J.A.B.	*Klebsiella pneumoniae*	0.5	24.5	Cured
J.A.B.	*E. coli* 022	0.5	24.5	Improved
W.J.H.	*E. coli* 06	0.15	245	Improved
W.H.W.	*E. coli* 06	0.5	245	Improved
A.P.	*E. coli* 022	0.15	9.5	Improved
A.P.	*Pseudomonas aeruginosa*	15.0	95	Failure
J.S.A.	*E. coli* 06	0.15	7.35	Failure
R.E.V.	*E. coli* 06	0.5	7.35	Failure
H.E.W.	*E. coli* NT	0.15	7.35	Failure
A.J.	*Enterobacter aerogenes*	0.15	2.45	Failure

[a] MIC = minimal inhibitory concentration; TMP = trimethoprim; SMX = sulfamethoxazole; NT = nontypable.

with a sulfonamide, 1.0 g four times a day, and symptoms disappeared 48–72 hours after starting therapy. When first seen, he had just completed 10 days of sulfonamide therapy. An intravenous urogram was normal; there was no postvoiding residual urine. The segmented cultures obtained on 11/6/62, and all subsequent cultures, are presented in Table 7.27. Physical examination revealed a healthy boy; the penis was uncircumcised, the glans was clean, and the prostate was not remarkable. The cultures on 11/6/62 showed 40 colonies of *Klebsiella*/ml and a sterile midstream urine. The cultures from 11/6/62 through 9/3/63 established the presence of a chronic, asymptomatic *Klebsiella* infection of the urethra. Although a subsequent attack of cystitis did not occur during this period, the presence of these pathogenic bacteria in large numbers left little doubt as to the etiology of his acute infections. Accordingly, he was admitted on 9/3/63. A urethrogram and cystoscopy were both normal. Urethroscopy revealed flocculent material in the lumen of the urethra which readily washed from the dull, pale appearing urethral mucosa—an appearance, in our experience, frequently associated with urethral infection. Tube dilution sensitivities of the *Klebsiella* indicated that penicillin-G was bacteriostatic at 100 μg/ml. He was started on 400,000 units of oral penicillin-G every 6 hours (Table 7.27). He remained asymptomatic; several cultures during the next 12 months showed no Gram-negative bacteria. He was well until November 1965, when he experienced, while in the U.S. Air Force, the first of five urinary infections. Each episode was characterized by dysuria, frequency, chills, fever (101–102°C), cloudy urine, and fatigue. Midstream urine cultures, obtained by Air Force physicians, were said to confirm the presence of bacteriuria. Each infection responded immediately to oral penicillin-G, tetracycline, or sulfonamides. His last infection occurred in March 1970. When again examined at Stanford University Hospital in June 1971, his intravenous urogram was normal; urine cultures showed 10 colonies of *Achromobacter* species in the VB_1 specimen. Moreover, EPS contained neither leukocytes nor oval brown macrophages, thereby excluding the

Table 7.27
Urethral Persistence of Enteric Pathogenic Bacteria as a Cause of Recurrent Bacteriuria in J.K., a 15-Year-Old, Caucasian Man

Date	Days on (+) or off (−) Drug	Drug	Dose	VB$_1$[a]	VB$_2$	VB$_3$	Organism	
							Type	Sensitivity
				bacterial/ml[b]				
11/6/62	−1	Sulf	1.0 g q 6 h	40	0		*Klebsiella*	Pen-G
12/5/62	−1 mo			1,714	36		*Klebsiella*	(250 μg/ml)[c]
2/20/63	−4 mo			100,000	26	300	*Klebsiella*	
5/7/63	−7 mo			3,600	120	19	*Klebsiella*	
8/12/63	−10 mo			66,000	208	1020	*Klebsiella*	
9/3/63	−11 mo			150,000	70[d]	900	*Klebsiella*	Pen-G (250 μg/ml)[c]
9/5/63	Rx Pen-G, 250 mg q 8 h by mouth (for 7 days), then 250 mg q 6 h (for 12 days)							
9/10/63	+5	Pen-G.	250 mg q 8 h	0	0			
9/24/63	−2	Pen-G.	250 mg q 6 h	0	0			
10/8/63	−16	Pen-G.		0	0			
11/12/63	−6 wk			0	0			
12/25/64	−5 mo			0	0			
9/1/64	−12 mo			0	0			
6/28/71	−8 yr *(See text)*			10	0	0[e]	*Achromobacter species*	

[a] VB$_1$ = first voided 5–10 ml of urine from urethral meatus; VB$_2$ = midstream aliquot of urine; VB$_3$ = first voided 5–10 ml of urine from urethral meatus after prostatic massage; sulf = sulfisoxazole (Gantrisin); Pen-G = penicillin-G.
[b] Small counts of Gram-positive organisms are not included in the table.
[c] Pen-G was bacteriostatic at a concentration of 100 μg/ml and bactericidal at 250 μg/ml.
[d] Suprapubic bladder aspiration revealed 0 colonies/ml on 9/3/63.
[e] EPS also sterile.

prostate as the cause of his previous infections. It is likely that sexual intercourse, which began some months after the sterile cultures in late 1964, established new pathogens on the urethra which reached the bladder and upper tracts. With 16 years of retrospection, J.K. should have been circumcised in 1962, as the followoing case history illustrates.

J.H. was a 47-year-old white male electrician who had been in good health all his life until 1 year before he was seen at Stanford when he developed dysuria, urgency, suprapubic discomfort, and hematuria. He was treated with a sulfonamide but his symptoms soon recurred; an intravenous urogram and cystoscopy were normal. He was then maintained on sulfisoxazole until 10 days before his appointment at Stanford. When first seen on 10/12/72 he was bacteriuric with an *E. coli* and was placed on nitrofurantoin macrocrystals (Table 7.28); after 3 weeks of therapy, however, the localization study on 11/2/72 was inconclusive because of too many *E. coli* in the VB$_1$. On that date, however, his bacilluria and pyuria had cleared, but his EPS contained 15–20 WBC/hpf and 4–5 oval fat macrophages/low power field. A repeat intravenous urogram was normal. Next, on the 14th day of cephalexin therapy, there were no bacteria in any of the segmented cultures. Further attempts with nitrofurantoin and penicillin-G to prove the prostate as the site of bacterial persistence was unsuccessful. EPS was obtained on 1/11/73; it showed 5–10 RBC/hpf, but no WBC or oval fat macrophages. The *E. coli* causing his bacteriuria on 4/12, 5/22, and at the time of cystoscopy on 6/11/73, was a nontypable *E. coli* (highly resistant to penicillin-G: >1170 μg/ml), and his serum antibody titer on 4/12/73 to this *E. coli* was <1:5. At cystoscopy, ureteral catheterization studies

Date	Days on (+) or off (−) Drug	VB_1[a]	VB_2	EPS	VB_3	Organism	Comments
10/12/72	−10 Sulf	>100,000	>100,000	>100,000	>100,000	*Escherichia coli*	
11/2/72	+20 Nitrofur (100 mg q.i.d.)	7,000 400	1,000 1,000	10,000 500	10,000 1,000	*E. coli* Enterococci	
11/17/72	+14 Cephalexin (250 mg q.i.d.)	0	0	0	0		
11/22/72	+4 Nitrofur (50 mg b.i.d.)	10 110 10	0 20 0			*E. coli* *Proteus mirabilis* Enterococci	
12/9/72	+21 Nitrofur	10,000 5,000	10,000 500	10,000 5,000	10,000 400	*P. mirabilis* Enterococci	
12/21/72	+9 Pen-G (500 mg q.i.d.)	0	0				SPA 0
1/11/73	+20 Pen-G	580	0	1,040	80	*E. coli*	
4/12/73	+111 Pen-G (500 mg b.i.d.)	100,000	100,000		100,000	*E. coli* NT (Serum titer = <1:5)	Foreskin *E. coli* 330 *Klebsiella* 10
5/22/73	+151 Pen-G	100,000	100,000			E. coli NT	
6/10/73	−19 Pen-G	100,000	100,000			E. coli	
6/11/73	Cystoscopy, upper tract localization, bladder biopsy, circumcision		CB 12,000	WB 1,500		E. coli NT	LK_1 0 RK_1 0 LK_2 0 RK_2 0 LK_3 0 RK_3 0 LK_4 0 RK_4 0
6/12/73	+1 gentamicin (80 mg × 5 doses)	0	0				
6/26/73	+14 Nitrofur (100 mg q.i.d.)	0	0				
7/10/73	−14 Nitrofur	0	0	0	0		
8/21/73	−56 Nitrofur	0	0				
11/20/73	−147 Nitrofur	0	0	Semen 0	0		
5/21/74	−329 Nitrofur	0	0		0		
12/10/74	−1 yr, 5-1/2 mos. Nitrofur	0	0				
12/29/78	−5-1/2 yr Nitrofur	0	0	0	0		

[a] VB_1 = first voided 5–10 ml of urine from urethral meatus; VB_2 = midstream aliquot of urine; VB_3 = first voided 5–10 ml of urine from urethral meatus after prostatic massage; Pen-G = penicillin-G; Nitrofur = nitrofurantoin (Furadantin); Sulf = sulfisoxazole; SPA = suprapubic needle aspiration of the bladder; EPS = expressed prostatic secretion; NT = nontypable; CB = catheterized bladder urine; WB = washed bladder; LK_1 to LK_4, serial catheterized left kidney urines, and RK_1 to RK_4, serial catheterized right kidney urines, each had 0 colonies/ml. Solid transverse line divides longitudinal cultures into major periods of significance.

showed both renal urines were sterile; the vesical neck appeared contracted and there was 3+ trabeculation of the bladder wall. More importantly, the prostatic mucosa in the area of the verumontanum appeared rough and irregular; a biopsy of this area showed urethral epithelium, ejaculatory ducts, and a "prominent number of plasma cells and lymphocytes in the underlying connective tissue." He was then circumcised; the foreskin showed no significant abnormality. Immediately following the cystoscopic procedures, he was given 120 mg of gentamicin intavenously before leavingf the cystoscopy room, and he received 5 additional doses of 80 mg at 8-hour intervals before being discharged on nitrofurantoin macrocrystals, which were stopped 2 weeks later. All cultures over the next 18 months showed no further Enterobacteriaceae, including one ejaculate culture. He has remained well since 1974, except for some mild obstructive symptoms (nocturia × 2 and occasional posturinary dribbling). When last seen on 12/29/78, his midstream urine (VB_2) contained no sediment on examination and his EPS had 3–5 WBC/hpf and 4–6 RBC/hpf. His segmented cultures (Table 7.28) showed no Gram-negative bacteria in any of the specimens; his VB_1 contained 200 *S. epidermidis*, 10^5 diphtheroids, and 2000 γ-streptococci/ml of urine. The VB_2, EPS, and VB_3 contained the same urethral bacteria but not enough to suggest the prostate as the source of the organisms.

I am aware that the bacteriologic localization data in Table 7.28 are less than satisfactory because he was bacteriuric in 5 of the 10 precystoscopic localizations, segmented cultures were sterile in 1 of the 5 nonbacteriuric collections (while on cephalexin), and in 2 of the remaining 4 collections EPS and VB_3 cultures were not obtained. This leaves only 2 localizations (unfortunately!) that really count: 11/2/72 and 1/11/73, and neither localizes the infection to the prostate because the *E. coli* in the EPS and VB_3 can be accounted for by the addition of urethral *E. coli*. I believe the urethra and preputium were the site of bacterial persistence because (1) there were no serum agglutinating antibodies to the *E. coli* causing his infection, (2) the two segmented cultures on 11/2/72 and 1/11/73 failed to prove a focus in the prostate, and (3) the cultures show that the *Proteus mirabilis* on the urethra on 11/22/72 caused a bacteriuria on 12/9/72 while he was on nitrofurantoin macrocrystals; this was the only time in 2 years the *P. mirabilis* was ever seen in the 18 times he was cultured. It is also of some interest that I resisted the urge to do a transurethral resection of his prostate (TURP) despite the findings of a contracted vesical neck and 3+ bladder trabeculation at cystoscopy; otherwise, the cure of his recurrent infection might be attributed to resection of a prostatic focus. The cystoscopic and biopsy findings in the prostatic urethra are best assigned to a secondary posterior urethritis; he had been bacteriuric for at least 2 months prior to the cystoscopy.

Origin of Enterobacteriaceae on the Male Urethra

Since the urethral meatus of the male is not in juxtaposition to the rectum, how do enterobacteria from the fecal flora reach the urethra or prostate? One mechanism might be by direct lymphatic connections between the mucosal surface of the lower bowel and the prostate; while this mechanism cannot be excluded as a possibility, I know of no evidence to support such bacterial freeways between these two organ systems.

A more likely explanation is that enterobacteria on the male urethra (and beneath the prepuce of the uncircumcised male) are acquired during sexual intercourse from those women whose introitus is colonized with enterobacteria. In the first eight women with recurrent bacteriuria in whom we monitored their vaginal flora with *E. coli* serotyping, we were surprised to find that four out of the seven male consorts whom we cultured had the same *E. coli* serogroup on their urethral mucosa as was present in the vaginal introitus of their sexual partners.[88] Since only a few random cultures were made in these males, we thought this observation was meaningful. To further document this finding, we chose a 25-year-old married woman with several episodes of bacteriuria and whose vaginal introitus was usually colonized with *E. coli.* Her 25-year-old husband was completely healthy, circumcised, and absolutely free of any genitourinary symptoms. For 2 years (Figure 7.20 *A* and *B*), every time she came to clinic for cultures, she also brought his first voided VB_1 urine of that day. Note that in 1971 when she was colonized vaginally with an *E. coli* 054 that he had three consecutive cultures, 2 weeks apart, in which he carried the same 054 on his urethra; later in the year, the same relationship occurred with her nontypable (NT) *E. coli.* In 1972, she was mainly colonized with an *E. coli* 06 and on many occasions he had the same 06 on his urethra. The *E. coli* 0X3, a very rare serotype, detected just prior to her bacteriuria in late 1972, is particularly interesting and emphasizes the direct relationship between her introital colonization and his urethral cultures. It needs to be emphasized that he was, and still is in 1978, completely free of any genitourinary symptoms or signs of disease. In fact, in July 1971 when I performed a vasectomy on him at the time his wife stopped her birth control pills (Figure 7.20*A*), I cultured his VB_1 followed by a culture of his fresh ejaculate. The VB_1 showed 350 *E. coli,* 1500 *S. epidermidis,* 3000 diphtheroids, and 60 enterococci/ml of urine. The ejaculate showed 160 *E. coli* and 560 *S. epidermidis*/ml, bacteria that are clearly accounted for by urethral contamination of a sterile seminal plasma. It should be emphasized that at no time did he receive antimicrobial therapy for any purpose; his wife was treated for 10 days with cephalexin at her single episode of bacteriuria in 1971 and 1972.

Normal Urethral Flora of the Adult Male

In the mid-1960s we obtained urethral, midstream, and postprostatic massage cultures (VB_3 only) on 37 "normal" volunteers at a Veterans Administration Hospital. None of these men was hospitalized on the urologic service, none had urologic complaints or was receiving antibiotics at the time of the culture, and all denied a past history of urologic symptoms and instrumentation. Within the validity of this denial, and remembering that they were ambulatory, hospitalized patients, the results of their cultures are presented in Table 7.29.

Gram-negative, enteric pathogens are obviously rare. Diphtheroids, (*S. epidermidis*), and streptococci (including enterococci) comprised the bulk of their urethral flora. These data are similar to the urethral swab and urine cultures reported by Philpot[89] on 50 normal made volunteers.

At the time of this study, we were not aware that the same Gram-negative bacteria found on the introitus of women with recurrent bacteriuria could be present on the urethral mucosa of their male consorts. This observation means that the incidence of pathogenic, Gram-negative bacteria on the urethral mucosa of normal men depends in part on the infection history of their wives at the time of the culture.

Despite these obvious concerns, I regard the presence of enteric, Gram-negative bacteria in the VB_1 culture of the adult male as a potential source of harm. The presence of these bacteria at the time of bladder catheterization clearly relates to catheter-induced infections, most certainly to acute bacteremia and septicemia in those instances of difficult instrumentation and to unexplained post-TURP fever and bacteriuria in patients whose midstream urine was sterile prior to resection. In addition, the persistence of these bacteria, in men with reduced host defense mechanisms is probably the etiologic cause of acute and chronic bacterial prostatitis.

If the simple presence of Enterobacteriaceae on the male urethra was all that was required to get a urinary infection, we would expect the incidence of urinary infections in the male to more closely approach the incidence in women, which is clearly not the case. Therefore, for men to develop bacterial prostatitis, either acute or chronic, there must be some defect in their host defense mechanism that allows potentially pathogenic bacteria on the urethral mucosa to ascend the urethra to the prostatic ducts and acini. The most logical defect would be in the prostatic antibacterial factor since

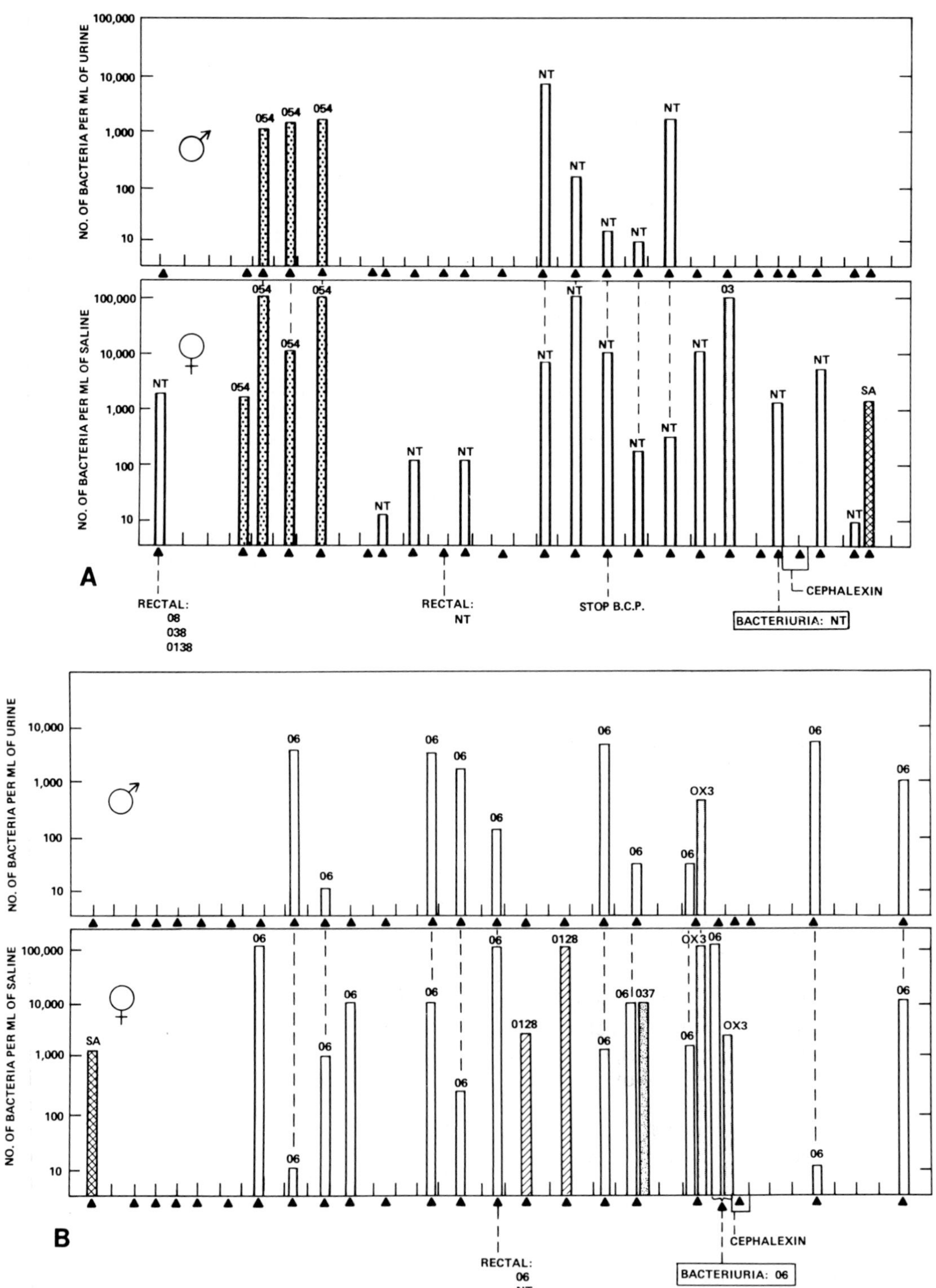

Figure 7.20 *Escherichia coli* in simultaneous collections at 2-week intervals from the ♂ urethra and the ♀ introitus. *A*, Vaginal introital cultures at biweekly intervals from a 25-year-old married patient obtained during 1971 (*lower columns*) compared to simultaneous first morning VB_1 (urethral) urine cultures from her husband (*upper columns*). The absence of columns over the black wedge markers (▲) indicates there were no detectable Gram-negative bacilli on culture.

prostatic immunoglobulins are actually increased in chronic bacterial prostatitis.[36] What is the prostatic antibacterial factor and is there evidence for a defect in its secretion in patients with chronic bacterial prostatitis?

Antibacterial Nature of Prostatic Fluid

One of the factors that determines bacterial persistence on the urethra of the male may be the natural antibacterial activity of prostatic fluid. We first observed this activity quite by accident.[90] During our experiments in dogs on diffusion of antimicrobial agents from plasma into prostatic fluid, we collected normal prostatic fluid in order to exclude antibiotic inactivation and to serve as a diluent in the bioassay. We observed that prostatic fluid rarely became contaminated, suggesting that it was inhibitory for bacteria. We then added a number of Gram-negative, enteric pathogens to natural prostatic fluid and incubated it; appropriate subcultures during incubation showed that natural prostatic fluid was remarkably bactericidal. The reproducibility of this phenomenon was shown by adding an *E. coli* 06 test strain, isolated from a patient with urinary infection, to the prostatic fluid of 20 different dogs (Table 7.30). When a number of different urinary tract pathogens were added to pooled canine prostatic fluid (Table 7.31), the same bactericidal activity was observed to occur with many different infecting strains. Most of the bacteria were killed by 4 hours of incubation; only 3 of 29 strains were viable after 6 hours of incubation.

Because of these observations in the dog, prostatic secretion from normal human volunteers was examined for antibacterial activity. Midstream (VB_2) and VB_3 urines were obtained; the midstream urine supported bacterial growth, while the same bladder urine following prostatic massage (VB_3) was bactericidal (Figure 7.21).

With this evidence that the antimicrobial factor was not an isolated observation limited to the dog, we proceeded to define further the nature of this antibacterial factor.[90]

The survival of *E. coli* in saline is compared to the death rate in prostatic fluid in Figure 7.22. In saline, two-thirds of the original inoculum were viable at 24 hours, whereas all *E. coli* in prostatic fluid were killed in 4 hours. Moreover, when prostatic fluid was boiled for 5 minutes, the antibacterial activity was lost and bacterial growth was comparable to that in trypticase soy broth (Figure 7.22). Ater boiling, a large protein precipitate was formed with a clear supernatant. When the coagulated protein was removed, even the supernatant contained enough nutrients to permit luxurious bacterial growth. Thus, the decrease in the number of viable bacteria in prostatic fluid is not due to a nonnutritious environment.

An 06 strain of *E. coli* was added to fresh normal blood serum and prostatic fluid from the same dog; the serum supported bcterial growth, while the prostatic fluid was bactericidal (Figure 7.23), an observation that was easily reproducible in different dogs (Table 7.32). The pH of canine prostatic fluid varied from 6.1 to 7.0; the pH of the pooled samples from 12 dogs was 6.5. Thus, pH alone was not a factor in the inhibition of bacterial growth.

Stability. Bacterial assays showed no loss of antibacterial activity after prostatic fluid had been frozen for 4 months; samples thawed and refrozen did not lose their activity. Antibacterial activity was not changed when prostatic fluid was stored at room temperature for 3 weeks.

Bacteriuria occurred only once near the end of 1971. Rectal cultures, in addition to routine introital cultures, were obtained as indicated. Observe the concurrence of the *E. coli* 054 on the male urethra at the time she was colonized vaginally with the same *E. coli*, as well as the same phenomenon later in the year with an *E. coli* NT. NT = nontypable; B.C.P. = birth control pills. *B*, A continuation of the biweekly cultures through 1972. Observe the concurrence of the *E. coli* 06 in both sexual partners and especially the recovery of the *E. coli* 0X3 (a very rare serotype) from his urethral urine at the same time his wife was colonized with the *E. coli* 0X3.

Table 7.29
Segmented Urine Cultures in 37 Hospitalized Normal Men

VB_1 (urethral), VB_2 (midstream), and VB_3 (first voided 10 ml after prostatic massage) specimens were cultured by surface streaking 0.1 ml of urine on appropriate agar plates and by placing 1.0 ml of urine into 9.0 ml of thioglycollate broth.

Patient	Age	VB_1	Organism	VB_2	Organism	VB_3	Organism
	yr	*bacteria/ml*		*bacteria/ml*		*bacteria/ml*	
J.E.	47	3,000	*Staphylococcus epidermidis*; γ-streptococcus	148	67% γ-*Streptococcus*; 33% *S. epidermidis*	260	80% γ-*Streptococcus*; 20% *S. epidermidis*
C.H.	56	1,560	*S. epidermidis*; *Streptococcus*[b]	3	*S. epidermidis*	76	*S. epidermidis*[a]; diphtheroids and *Streptococcus*[b]
H.D.	85	1,320	*S. epidermidis*[a]; *Streptococcus*[b]	22	*S. epidermidis*	236	*S. epidermidis*[a]; *Streptococcus*[b]
J.P.	66	1,140	*S. epidermidis*[a]; diphtheroids	140	*S. epidermidis*[a]; diphtheroids[b]	0	
J.L.	83	1,080	*S. epidermidis*[a]; diphtheroids	88	*S. epidermidis*	90	*S. epidermidis*; diphtheroids
H.F.	42	1,080	Diphtheroids[a]; *S. epidermidis*	45	Diphtheroids[a]; *S. epidermidis*	5	Diphtheroids[a]; *S. epidermidis*
B.B.	24	1,020	*Streptococcus faecalis*; *S. epidermidis*	1	*Klebsiella* and Gram-positive cocci[b]	30	*S. faecalis*
F.T.	48	900	67% *S. epidermidis*; 33% γ-streptococcus	29	*S. epidermidis*	100	*S. epidermidis*
R.T.	66	840	83% *S. epidermidis*; 17% *S. faecalis*	11	67% *S. epidermidis*; 33% *S. faecalis*	78	60% *S. faecalis*; 40% *S. epidermidis*
N.A.	33	780	*S. epidermidis*	12	*S. epidermidis*	500	*S. epidermidis*
J.C.	24	780	β-Enterococcus and γ-streptococcus[a]; *S. epidermidis*	1	β-Enterococcus; γ-streptococcus	25	β-Enterococcus; γ-*Streptococcus*
H.S.	63	660	96% *S. faecalis* and β-enterococcus; 4% *S. epidermidis*	4	*S. faecalis*; β-enterococcus	34	*S. faecalis*; β-enterococcus
F.D.	52	528	80% diphtheroids; 10% *S. epidermidis*; 10% group A *Streptococcus*	2	Diphtheroids	25	Diphtheroids[a]; *S. epidermidis* and *Streptococcus*[b]
S.C.	41	470	*S. epidermidis*	1	*S. epidermidis*	212	*S. epidermidis*
N.D.	43	396	*S. epidermidis*; *S. faecalis*	108	*S. epidermidis*; γ-*Streptococcus*	96	*S. epidermidis*; γ-*Streptococcus*; diphtheroids
E.C.	47	376	67% group A *Streptococcus*; 33% *S. epidermidis*	148	57% group A *Streptococcus*; 43% *S. epidermidis*	602	70% *S. epidermidis*; 30% group A *Streptococcus*
D.H.	30	280	*S. epidermidis*	1	*S. epidermidis*	51	*S. epidermidis*

E.B.	47	278	*S. epidermidis*	0	*S. epidermidis*[b]	3	*S. epidermidis*
L.M.	40	250	70% diphtheroids; 30% *S. epidermidis*	4	Diphtheroids	34	70% *S. epidermidis*; 30% diphtheroids
R.S.	42	240	*S. epidermidis*; *Streptococcus*	16	*S. epidermidis*; *Streptococcus*	56	*S. epidermidis*; *Streptococcus*
W.W.	69	212	55% diphtheroids; 30% *Streptococcus*; 15% *S. epidermidis*	2	*S. epidermidis*; *Streptococcus*	0	Diphtheroids*; *S. epidermidis*[b]
G.P.	36	208	*S. epidermidis*; *Streptococcus*	0	*S. epidermidis* and *Streptococcus*[b]	0	*S. epidermidis* and *Streptococcus*[b]
C.M.	40	172	*S. faecalis*	5	*S. faecalis*	5	*S. faecalis*
N.S.	41	158	*S. epidermidis*	39	*S. epidermidis*; diphtheroids	480	*S. epidermidis*
A.D.	42	96	60% *S. faecalis*; 40% *S. epidermidis*	0	Diphtheroids[b]	1	*S. faecalis*[a]; *S. epidermidis*
H.B.	55	60	*S. epidermidis*	2	*S. epidermidis*	27	*S. epidermidis*
W.S.	34	60	*Escherichia coli*	15	*E. coli*	50	*E. coli*
W.S.[c]	34	1	*S. epidermidis*	0		2	*S. epidermidis*
L.C.	38	53	*S. epidermidis*	0	*S. epidermidis*[b]	6	*S. epidermidis*[b]
R.P.	38	46	*S. epidermidis*; γ-*Streptococcus*	0		0	*S. epidermidis*, *Streptococcus* and diphteroids[b]
M.V.	47	40	*S. epidermidis*	0		0	*S. epidermidis*[b]
G.W.	53	40	*S. epidermidis*; *E. coli* intermediate[b]	3	*S. epidermidis*	2	*S. epidermidis*
R.W.	36	27	*Streptococcus*	2	*Streptococcus*; diphtheroids; *S. epidermidis*	1	*Streptococcus*
W.A.	47	16	β-Enterococcus	2	β-Enterococcus; *S. epidermidis*	5	*S. epidermidis*
A.C.	71	2	*S. epidermidis*	0		0	
L.C.	38	1	Gram-negative rods[b]	0		0	
L.D.	52	0		0		0	
M.C.	20	0		0		0	

[a] Predominant organism.

[b] Bacteria found only in thioglycollate broth and not on the agar plates, indicating an exceedingly low colony count (such as 1 bacteria/ml of urine) of that particular organism.

[c] Repeat culture.

Table 7.30
Bactericidal Effect of Prostatic Fluid against an *E. Coli* 06[a]

The *E. coli* 06 were grown in trypticase soy broth, diluted 10^5 with saline, and 0.1 ml added to 1.9 ml of prostatic fluid. Subcultures were performed at 0, 1, 2, 4, 6, and 24 hours of incubation at 37°C.

Dog Number	Bacteria after Incubation for:					
	0 hr	1 hr	2 hr	4 hr	6 hr	24 hr
	bacteria/ml					
1	770	600	120	0	0	0
2	310	240	50	10	0	0
3	450	70	0	0	0	0
4	1800	200	0	0	0	0
5	450	70	0	0	0	0
6	770	600	740	135	0	0
7	310	0	0	0	0	0
8	430	330	350	270	210	30
9	510	10	20	0	0	0
10	310	0	0	0	0	0
11	385	165	70	0	0	0
12	335	0	0	0	0	0
13	530	380	370	350	270	0
14	1600	70	10	0	0	0
15	260	120	0	0	0	0
16	1090	1400	1120	700	460	0
17	800	100	30	0	0	0
18	260	280	210	200	145	0
19	1200	720	220	0	0	0
20	1380	540	100	60	0	0

[a] Reproduced by permission from T. A. Stamey *et al.*, Nature **218:** 444, 1968.[90]

Filtration. Filtration through a 0.22-μ Millipore filter attached to the end of a sterile glass syringe produced a clearer and less viscous prostatic fluid but did not change its antibacterial acitivity.

Effect of Temperature. Samples of canine prostatic fluid were inoculated with bacteria, and separate aliquots were placed in a refrigerator (6°C), left at room temperature (24°C), and incubated at 37°C (Figure 7.24). Complete sterility was obtained in all tubes maintained at 24 or 37°C, although 24 hours was required at 24°C. Prostatic fluid at 6°C showed no decrease in the number of bacteria/ml after 24 hours in the refrigerator.

Heating. Prostatic fluid was heated to 56°C for 30 minutes to inactivate complement, to 56°C for 120 minutes, and to boiling for 5–15 minutes. There was progressive loss of activity with increased exposure to temperature (Figure 7.25).

Acid Phosphatase Content in Relation to Antibacterial Activity. Many enzymes are present in prostatic fluid, but the availability of valid measurements for acid phosphatase led us to compare the concentration of acid phosphatase with the antibacterial activity of serial aliquots collected under pilocarpine stimulation (Figure 7.26). Acid phosphatase activity was determined in successive 10-ml collections by a modification of the method described by Bessey *et al.*[91] As expected, only the first few 10-ml samples of prostatic secretion contained large amounts of acid phosphatase; by contrast, the bactericidal activity of consecutive aliquots was not diminished. In fact, the first few aliquots were sometimes less bactericidal than the later ones. Repeated efforts to find a decrease in antibacterial activity in samples collected near the end of pilocarpine stimulation were unsuccessful; this is surprising since 100–200 ml of prostatic secretion were sometimes collected before completion of the experiment.

Lysozyme. The standard photometric determination of lysozyme activity was used by plotting the increase in transmittance of a solution that contained a known weight of *Micrococcus lysodeikticus* cells lyophilized in saline buffered with phosphate. The decrease in optical density was determined at 420 nm in a spectrophotometer using the interval between 30 seconds and 3 minutes to express lysozymal activity.[92] There was no change in optical density when the suspension of *M. lysodeikticus* was treated with prostatic fluid, whereas the lysozyme standard produced marked changes at a concentration of 10 μg/ml (Figure 7.27).

Considerable effort was required to separate the antibacterial fraction present in prostatic fluid. Because the final measurement of activity was based on a bacteriologic assay, isolation was complicated by the need to maintain the chromatography system sterile as the fluid passed through the column, the spectrophotometer, and into the fraction collector. The cation exchange resin, carboxymethylcellulose, used in previous studies to isolate prostatic fluid

Table 7.31
Antibacterial Spectrum of Pooled Canine Prostatic Fluid[a]

Different strains are identified by the patients' initials. Each pathogen was grown in trypticase soy broth diluted 10^5 with saline, and 0.1 ml was added to 1.9 ml of pooled prostatic fluid. Subcultures were performed at 0, 1, 2, 4, 6, and 24 hours of incubation at 37°C.

Organism (Patient)	Bacteria after Incubation for:					
	0 hr	1 hr	2 hr	4 hr	6 hr	24 hr
			bacteria/ml			
Klebsiella (B.W.)	920	380	70	10	0	0
Klebsiella (T.I.)	2400	20	0	0	0	0
Klebsiella (J.S.)	1000	1000	500	110	0	0
Klebsiella (H.S.)	1500	1100	800	0	0	0
Escherichia coli (L.L.)	600	180	110	0	0	0
E. coli (J.R.)	1040	310	90	10	0	0
E. coli (M.M.)	800	380	560	140	0	0
E. coli (M.F.)	1500	160	240	0	0	0
E. coli (A.M.)	1200	370	360	30	0	0
E. coli (B.M.)	1600	180	80	0	0	0
E. coli (B.B.)	1600	140	150	0	0	0
E. coli (N.L.)	1500	1400	1100	170	0	0
E. coli (J.N.)	2250	1120	800	20	0	0
E. coli (S.M.)	3500	2200	1100	0	0	0
E. coli (M.R.)	1800	1700	420	0	0	0
E. coli (F.P.)	1300	800	410	50	0	0
E. coli (W.W.)	1600	840	340	0	0	0
Proteus mirabilis (L.J.)	1200	1000	1600	2200	1200	1800
P. mirabilis (C.W.)	1520	1500	600	20	0	0
P. mirabilis (T.S.)	2100	2400	1200	40	0	0
P. mirabilis (R.W.)	10^4	10^4	10^4	10^4	10^5	10^5
Proteus vulgaris (L.M.)	3000	1800	2200	180	0	0
Pseudomonas (C.C.)	3600	3000	1680	0	0	0
Pseudomonas (J.K.)	960	250	70	10	0	0
Paracolon (C.S.)	1200	900	680	10	10	0
Paracolon (M.R.)	2100	1200	660	50	0	0
Streptococcus faecalis (J.A.)	3000	2200	2500	2800	2200	10^5
Staphylococcus aureus (J.L.)	3000	1500	1000	340	0	0
Staphylococcus epidermides (H.J.)	1400	60	30	0	0	0

[a] Reproduced by permission from T. A. Stamey *et al.*, Nature **218:** 444, 1968.[90]

components,[93] was not helpful; the higher concentrations of phosphate buffer needed to elute the 2-carboxymethylcellulose prevented bacterial growth. With sterile technique, the molecular sieve Sephadex G-10, a nonionic polymeric carbohydrate with an exclusion limit of approximately 700 molecular weight (for polysaccharides), produced a remarkably constant peak for antibacterial activity (Figure 7.28). Because only pure prostatic fluid and distilled water were placed on the Sephadex column, no interfering components were present.

A large protein peak was found consistently within the void volume, representing the large molecular weight proteins in prostatic fluid. The next peak contained all the antibacterial activity (Figure 7.28); we have called this peak the prostatic antibacterial fraction (PAF) in contrast to the activity in natural prostatic fluid. Serial aliquots from both peaks were lyophilized separately and

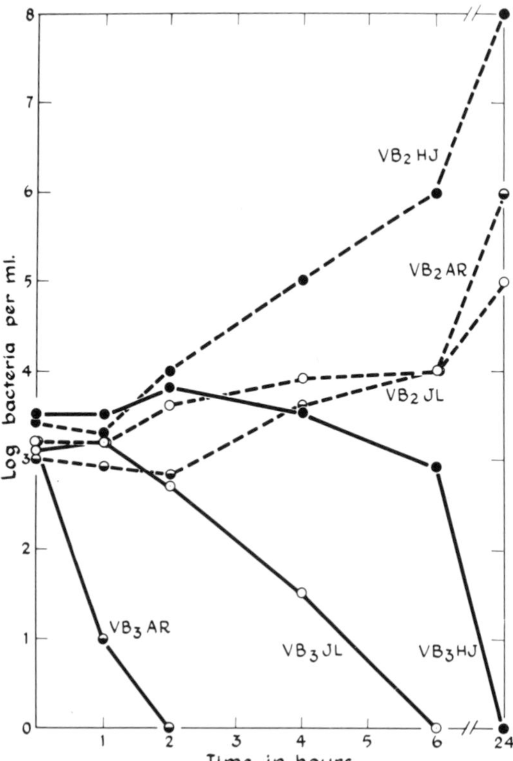

Figure 7.21 The bactericidal effect of human prostatic fluid (VB_3) assayed against *Escherichia coli* 06. Midstream (VB_2) and postprostatic (VB_3) urine aliquots from normal volunteers were Millipore-filtered, inoculated with between 1000 and 5000 *E. coli* 06/ml of urine, and incubated at 37°C. Subcultures showed the expected lag phase in the midstream urine followed by rapid growth. The VB_3 urine was bactericidal.

later reconstituted with saline to a final volume of 2.0 ml. To each tube was added 0.1 ml of a 10^4 dilution of an *E. coli* 06. All of the tubes within the *A peak* supported bacterial growth. The antibacterial activity of intact, untreated prostatic fluid is compared in Table 7.33 with a representative tube from the *A peak* and a tube from the second or *PAF peak*; a saline control is also included.

The antimicrobial characteristics of the prostatic antibacterial fraction isolated from the Sephadex column were similar to those of intact prostatic fluid. The antibacterial spectrum was identical to that in Table 7.31; the rate of bactericidal activity was usually enhanced (Table 7.33). As expected from the small molecular weight, there was no lysozymal activity. PAF, like intact prostatic fluid, was inactivated by either blood serum or trypticase soy broth.

The chief difference between PAF and intact prostatic fluid was the complete heat stability of the former. PAF could be boiled for 30 minutes and retain all of its antibacterial activity. The loss of antimicrobial activity when intact PF is heated (Figure 7.22) may be due to binding by the denatured proteins.

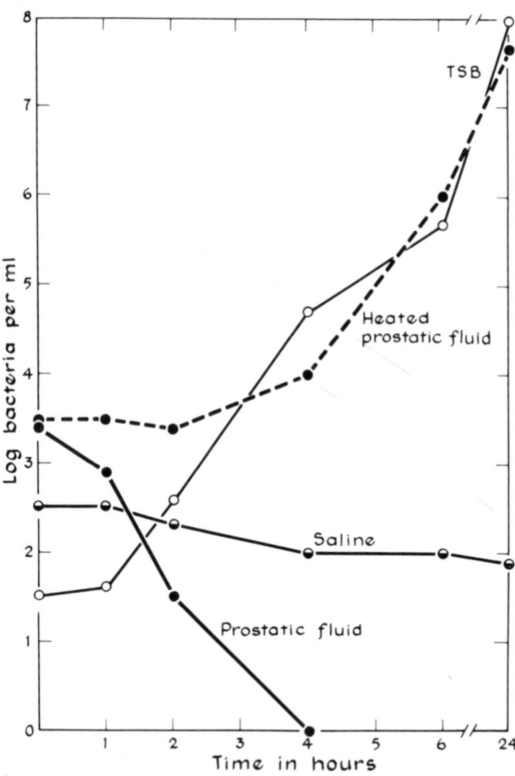

Figure 7.22 Comparative growth curves of *Escherichia coli* in prostatic fluid, heated prostatic fluid, trypticase soy broth (TSB) and normal saline. *E. coli* grown in TSB and diluted in saline were incubated at 37°C in 2-ml volumes of normal prostatic fluid, prostatic fluid heated to 100°C for 5 minutes, saline, and TSB. Subcultures were quantitated after 0, 1, 2, 4, 6, and 24 hours of incubation. (Reproduced by permission from T. A. Stamey *et al*, Nature **218:** 444, 1968.[90])

E. coli and *P. mirabilis*, exposed to PAF at 37°C, were viewed under the phase microscope and compared with the same strains similarly exposed to bactericidal concentrations of penicillin-G, nalidixic acid, and polymyxin-B sulfate. Bacteria exposed to PAF showed none of the features characteristic of cell death caused by penicillin-G (L-forms from cell wall inhibition) or nalidixic acid (elongated forms from DNA inhibition[94]). Death induced by PAF seemed similar to cells exposed to polymyxin-B sulfate, a surface-active bactericide[95]; the exposed bacilli developed punctate areas and gradually faded without aberrant changes in gross morphology.

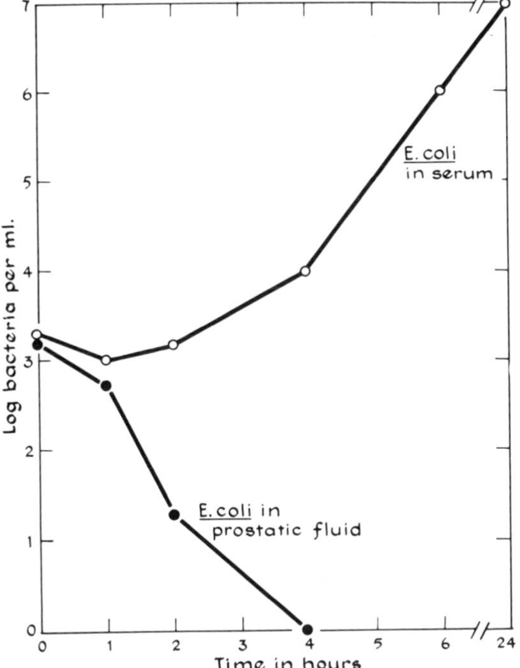

Figure 7.23 The effect of canine prostatic fluid and serum against an *Escherichia coli* 06 test organism.

Spermine, a basic polyamine, has been reported as possessing a definite antibacterial action against Gram-positive organisms.[96] It is this substance that is responsible, at least in part, for the antibacterial effect of human semen, described by Rozansky and associates.[97] The antibacterial spectrum of spermine and spermidine is almost entirely confined to Gram-positive organisms, whereas our data showed that Gram-negative pathogens were exquisitely sensitive to PAF. More importantly, Dr. William Fair and Miss Nancy Wehner in our unit have reported their studies on the antibacterial action of spermine.[98] They concluded that spermine plays little, if any, role in natural resistance to urinary tract infections. In another publication, Fair and Wehner[99] showed that the antibacterial factor in prostatic fluid cannot be spermine for the simple reason that canine prostatic fluid, unlike human prostatic fluid, contains no spermine!

When we began this work in 1965, we were not aware of the original description by Youmans, Liebling, and lyman[100] entitled *The Bactericidal Action of Prostatic Fluid in Dogs*, and did not reference his work in our report in Nature.[90] I apologised

Table 7.32[a]
Bacterial Assays for Pooled Prostatic Fluid[a] **and Individual Dog Serum**

Time	*E. coli* (J.N.)[b]		*E. coli* (N.L.)[b]		*E. coli* (M.R.)[b]		*Klebsiella* (T.I.)[b]	
	Prostatic fluid	Serum dog 113	Prostatic fluid	Serum dog 34	Prostatic fluid	Serum dog 429	Prostatic fluid	Serum dog 56
hr	*bacteria/ml*							
0	7750	6840	6840	8550	9700	11900	6700	11400
1	2240	10^4	3100	10^4	6000	3400	2400	10^4
2	410	10^4	510	10^4	1210	9100	20	10^5
4	0	10^4	490	10^5	0	4560	0	10^5
6	0	10^5	250	10^5	0	3500	0	10^5
24	0	10^5	0	10^5	0	2040	0	10^5

[a] Pooled prostatic fluid from 12 dogs.
[b] Patient isolate. *E. coli* = *Escherichia coli.*

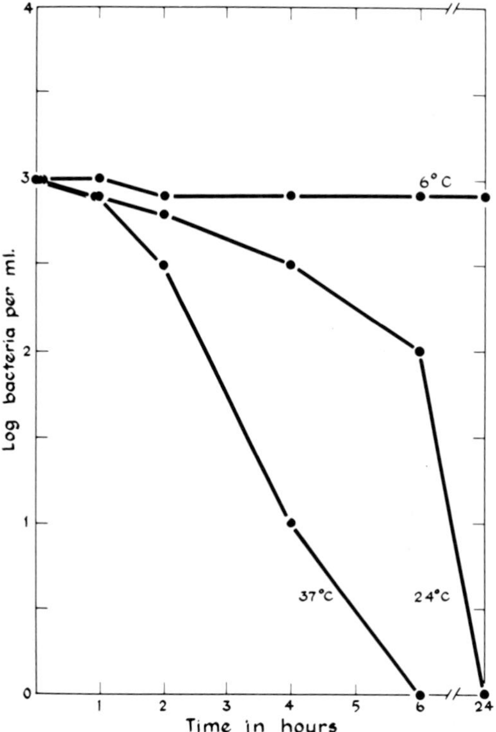

Figure 7.24 The effect of temperature on bactericidal activity of prostatic fluid.

to Dr. Youmans by letter, which he graciously accepted. It is interesting that Youmans in 1938 was also investigating the possibility of an antimicrobial agent being excreted in prostatic fluid at the time he observed the natural fluid to be bactericidal. Gip and Molin[101] have recently demonstrated activity of human prostatic fluid against *C. albicans.*

Fair, Wehner, and Couch, in their clinical and laboratory investigations at Stanford between 1969 and 1975, were able to purify and finally isolate the prostatic antibacterial factor. They showed in 1973 that the antibacterial activity in canine prostatic fluid and human seminal plasma was not spermine[102] and, after a 5000-fold purification, they knew it was a low molecular weight cationic substance.[103] In 1976, they conclusively showed that the antibacterial factor was a zinc salt, and that prostatic fluid zinc levels were substantially lower in men with chronic bacterial prostatitis than in normal men resistant to urinary infections.[104] Serum zinc levels, however, were not decreased in men with chronic bacterial prostatitis, nor could the depressed zinc levels in their prostatic fluid be raised by administration of exogenous zinc.[104] The isolation and identification of this antimicrobial substance in prostatic fluid is a great credit to Fair and his associates because there is no other naturally liberated secretory fluid known to possess antimicrobial activity against Gram-negative enteric bacteria.[105,106]

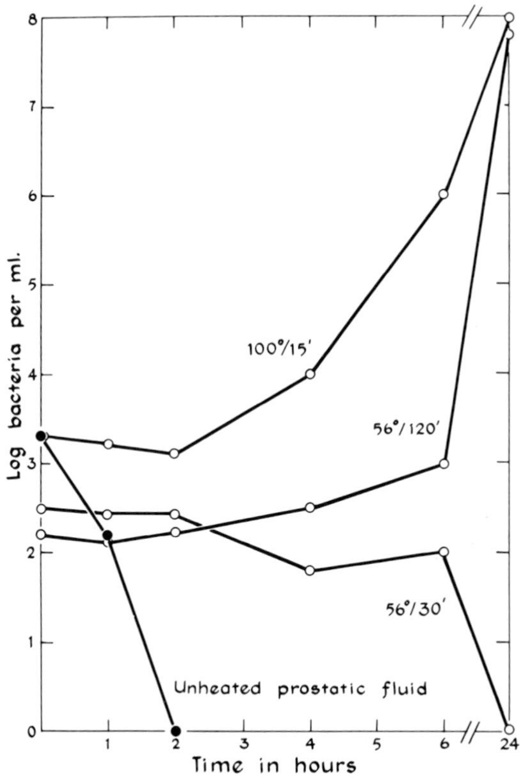

Figure 7.25 The effect of heating prostatic fluid (assay organism: *Escherichia coli* 06). Canine prostatic fluid was heated for 30 minutes at 56°C, heated for 120 minutes at 56°C, and boiled for 15 minutes at 100°C. Control prostatic fluid was bactericidal at 2 hours. Heating produced a progressive loss of activity.

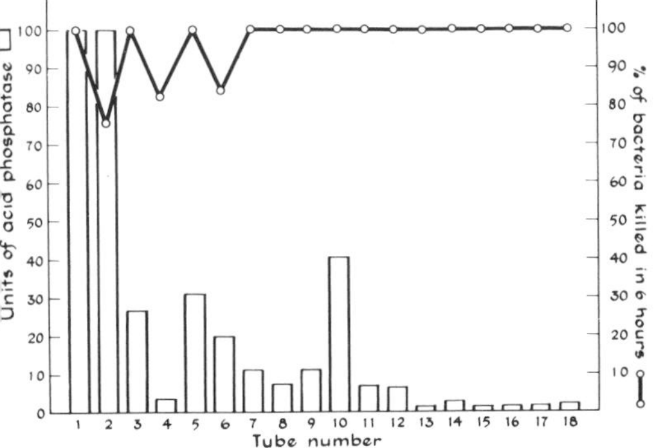

Figure 7.26 Comparison of acid phosphatase content and bactericidal activity in consecutive 10-ml collections of canine prostatic fluid (dog 13). Successive 10-ml aliquots of prostatic fluid were collected in consecutive tubes. Acid phosphatase activity rapidly fell with progressive secretion, but within the error of our biological test system we could detect no diminution in antimicrobial activity.

SEMINAL VESICULITIS: THE QUESTION OF GENITAL INFECTION IN INFERTILE MALES

It is virtually impossible to make the diagnosis of seminal vesiculitis unless the seminal vesicle is palpable as a hard swollen mass in the presence of urinary infection or sepsis. Since this rarely occurs, even in the presence of acute bacterial prostatitis, it is unlikely the seminal vesicles are involved in most acute bacterial infections that otherwise cause acute inflammation in the prostate, bladder, and kidney.

The question of asymptomatic seminal vesiculitis is even more difficult because there is no way to culture the fluid in the seminal vesicles and exclude bacteria from the prostate and urethra. We have attempted on a few occasions to cannulate the scrotal vas prior to a vaso-seminal vesiculogram (for example, R.F. in Table 7.13 and Figure 7.8) but have been unable to obtain seminal fluid for culture. Some investigators have tried to prove infection of the seminal vesicles by culturing the split ejaculate in which the prostate fraction occurs early and the seminal vesicular portion occurs late in the stream of ejaculate; this method is so bacteriologically ridiculous that it hardly deserves comment. That patients with gross bacterial infection of the "posterior urethra and upper urinary tract" ("selected from hundreds of necropsies") may have secondary involvement of the seminal vesicles was shown by Hyams, Kramer, and McCarthy in a postmortem study in 1931.[107] Sixty-six of 84 autopsied cases showed evidence of prostatitis; of these 66, 16 cases showed substantial seminal vesiculitis.

The basic question of seminal vesiculitis does not relate to patients with chronic bacterial prostatitis and recurrent bacteriuria, even though it would be interesting to know whether or not these patients have an associated seminal vesiculitis. The real question is whether asymptomatic infertile males have a genital infection (vas, epididymis, prostate, seminal vesicles) to account for their infertility. Since these patients almost never have recurrent bacteriuria, what is the objective evidence that they have any infection to warrant the widespread practice of treating them with antimicrobial therapy? There is almost no objective evidence based on adequate culture techniques to support this practice, a practice which is especially widespread in Europe. I was recently invited to Paris to speak before their national infertility soci-

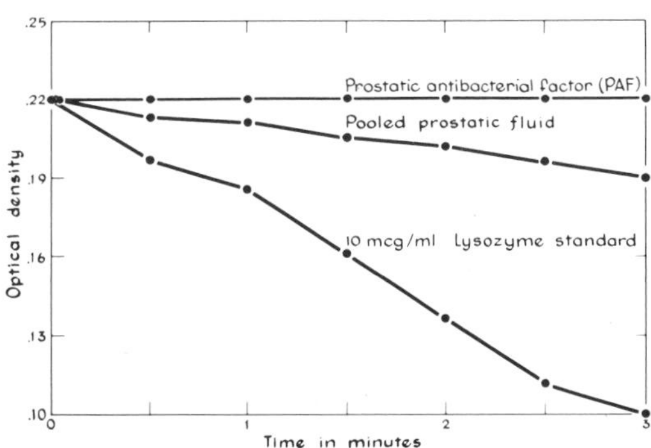

Figure 7.27 Lysozyme assay of prostatic fluid (lysis of *Micrococcus lysodeikticus*).

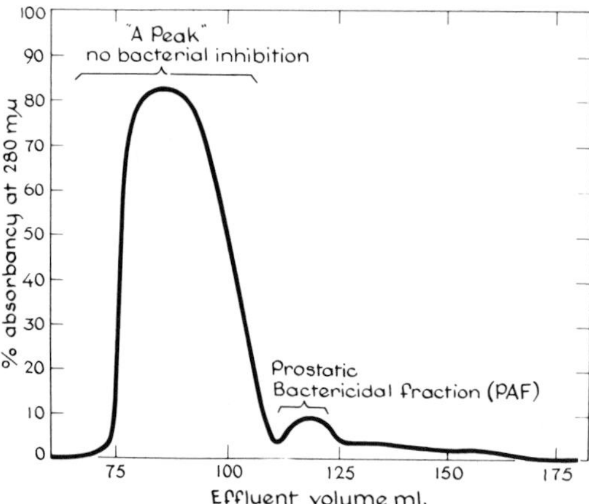

Figure 7.28 The separation of the prostatic antibacterial fraction (PAF) using Sephadex G-10. Ten milliliters of canine prostatic fluid were placed on a 45- × 2.5-cm column of Sephadex G-10 (Pharmacia), followed by a continuous flow of sterile, distilled water. A flow-through cell in an A-O Spectronic 600 spectrophotometer was used with a direct recording of transmittance at 280 nm. The void volume of the column was approximately 75 ml. (Reproduced by permission from T. A. Stamey *et al.*, Nature **218:** 444, 1968.[90])

ety on the role of prostatic infections and male infertility; I had to decline the invitation because, as I told them, I know of no relationship between bacterial prostatitis and infertility. Let us briefly review some of the evidence.

Because patients with proven chronic bacterial prostatitis have indisputable evidence of secretory dysfunction (the concentration of zinc, spermine, and cholesterol are reduced compared to normal controls),[83] and because 25% of infertile males have evidence of secretory dysfunction in their seminal plasma[108] which could theoretically affect adversely sperm viability and fertility, it is appealing to andrologists to believe that a subclinical infection often exists in the accessory genital glands. So appealing is this concept that a recent review of infertility and genitourinary infections by Caldamone and Cockett[109] begins with the statement "genitourinary infection is now recognized as a major factor in the etiology of infertility." I would suggest that the clinical and bacteriologic methodology is so controversial in this field that the issue is far from certain. For example, Caldamone and Cockett[109] in their review report that Dahlberg[110] found positive prostatic fluid cultures in 180 of 190 infertile male partners. Dahlberg,[110] in his paper entitled *Asymptomatic Bacteriospermia*, did not even culture the prostatic fluid; he cultured the ejaculate only, and "to avoid contamination from the skin or urethra," the infertile males had the "top of the penis washed" and they urinated before ejaculation. I hope it is clear to even the most casual reader that Dahlberg's[110] 180/190 positive cultures were nothing more than indigenous urethral bacteria (the species cultured was not even reported). If VB_3 urine and EPS cultures are commonly contaminated by urethral bacteria after a VB_2 culture has been obtained (which washes the urethra), can you imagine how many urethral bacteria reaccumulate during masturbation to contaminate the ejaculate? Moreover, Dahlberg's[110] report of finding *Trichomonas vaginalis* in 89% of the 190 ejaculates is as-

Table 7.33
Antibacterial Effect of Respresentative Aliquots from the Sephadex Column (Figure 7.28) Compared with Intact Prostatic Fluid and Normal Saline[a]

After passing through the spectrophotometer, 5-ml aliquots from the fraction collector were lyophilized and later reconstituted to 2.0 ml with saline. After 0.1 ml was removed for culture, 0.1 ml of a 10^4 dilution of *Escherichia coli* was added to each tube, as well as to 2 ml of saline and to a sample of the original intact prostatic fluid. Subcultures were made at 0, 1, 2, 4, 6, and 24 hours.

Time	"A" Peak	PAF Peak	Intact Prostatic Fluid	Saline Control
hr		*bacteria/ml*		
0	1980	1880	2000	1930
1	2180	1620	2200	1800
2	3500	200	1400	1640
4	10^4	0	900	1440
6	10^5	0	610	1440
24	10^6	0	0	1200

[a] Reproduced by permission from T. A. Stamey *et al.*, Nature **218:** 444, 1968.[90]

tonishing; it is not clear how he identified *T. vaginalis* under the microscope. Perhaps he used a dry smear where many different cells can be confused with *Trichomonas*.

The absolute necessity for controlled clinical trials is emphasized by the reported results of Derrick and Dahlberg[111] who achieved a 30% pregnancy rate by treating 100 infertile men who had prostatitis (>20 WBC/hpf of prostatic fluid) with methenamine hippurate. Since absolutely no formaldehyde could have been released from the methenamine in either the prostatic fluid (pH > 7.5) or interstitial fluid (pH 7.4), the 30% pregnancy rate could not have been due to the methenamine hippurate. A controlled clinical trial has been done by Harrison *et al.*[112] on the controversy over whether *U. urealyticum* causes infertility. These investigators randomly divided infertile couples into untreated, placebo treated, and doxcycline treated and found no difference in the conception rate between the three groups; they had previously shown a 52.6% isolation rate of *U. urealyticum* among fertile couples compared to a 57.2% isolation rate among infertile couples.[113]

Except for the studies of Ulstein *et al.*,[80] it is difficult to find an investigation that combined acceptable bacteriologic culture techniques with quantitation of leukocyte counts in the ejaculate together with a semen analysis in asymptomatic fertile and infertile men. These investigators showed that mycoplasmas, chlamydiae, and viruses were unrelated to male infertility, but three patients were thought to have aerobic bacterial infection (*P. mirabilis*, *E. coli*, and *S. epidermidis*) of their prostate gland; in two of these, the infection apparently caused diminished sperm viability and was corrected by antibacterial therapy.[80] The most critical review of this controversy is by Meares[114] who correctly emphasizes the importance of methodology and who nicely demonstrates the conflicting evidence.

When the question has been reversed, how many men with prostatic inflammatory disease have evidence of an abnormal sperm analysis, there is no evidence of an effect on seminal quality.[38,115] Since the prostatic inflammation (largely nonbacterial prostatitis in Colleen and Mardh's[38] patients) was also associated with subnormal levels of zinc and magnesium in their seminal plasma, the absence of semen abnormalities places the burden of proof on those who believe that a relationship actually exists between prostatic infection and infertility.

The interested clinician who looks for inflammatory cells in the ejaculate must also remember that the distinction between polymorphonuclear leukocytes and nonseparated spermatids, as well as between early spermatids and lymphocytes, is not simple and requires special stains.[116] Perhaps the simplest differential stain is the peroxidase stain for polymorphonuclear leukocytes.[117]

I hope it is clear that most of the difficulty with the infertility literature, as was equally true of the early prostatitis literature, is the failure of the investigators in this field to recognize urethral contamination of the ejaculate and the prostatic fluid. One cannot swab-culture the prostatic fluid, even after careful retraction of the prepuce and thorough washing and drying of the glans, and even have the patient urinate first, and expect the EPS or seminal fluid to be free of urethral organisms. This is the difficulty with the bacteriological analysis of accessory gland fluids proposed by Eliasson.[118]

URETHRITIS

The two major forms of symptomatic urethritis in males are gonococcal and nongonococcal (NGU); NGU accounts for over half of all cases of urethritis in sexually active males attending veneral disease clinics.[119,120] The distinction between the two is easy: in gonococcal urethritis, the discharge is usually purulent, of short duration, and the Gram stain is almost always unequivocally positive; when the Gram stain shows typical intracellular gram-negative diplococci, culture for gonococci is positive in 98% of cases.[119] In NGU, the discharge is more mucoid, not so heavy, the symptoms are usually of longer duration, and the Gram stain is negative. Twenty percent of equivocal Gram stains (atypical Gram-negative diplococci) will be culture positive for gonococci.[119] Dr. J. D. Oriel at University College Hospital in London contrasts the differences between gonorrhea and NGU in a very interesting way (Table 7.34).

The etiology of nongonococcal urethritis is *Chlamydia trachomatis* in about 40% of cases.[121] *U. urealyticum* unquestionably causes urethritis[122] but the proportion of patients with NGU caused by this mycoplasma remains controversial; it probably represents another 40% of patients with NGU, leaving 20% due to unknown causes. Since both *C. trachomatis* and *U. urealyticum* are sensitive to tetracyclines, the differential diagnosis between the two is probably not clinically significant. Because some 70% of sexual consorts of men with chlamydial urethritis have chlamydial infection of the cervix,[120] Schachter[123] makes the sensible plea that the sexual partner be treated in parallel with the patient. Moreover, the physician should remember that several investigators agree that *Chlamydia* is responsible for about 70% of postgonococcal urethritis.[124] The increasing importance of *Chlamydia* as the cause of genital infections in the female is emphasized in the recent review by Schachter.[123] Evidence that *C. trachomatis* is the major cause of acute "idiopathic" epididymitis has just been reported by the Seattle group.[125]

Table 7.34
Differences Between Gonorrhoea and Nongonococcal Urethritis (NGU)[a]

	Gonorrhoea	NGU
Infecting agent	Single	Multiple
Ethnic group affected	Mostly Black	Mostly White
Socioeconomic group affected	Lower	Higher
Prevalence in homosexual men	High	Low
Partner change admitted	85%	70%
Diagnosis of infected women	Easy	Difficult
Host factors	Not Important	May be Important
Antimicrobial therapy	Simple	May Be Complex

[a] Courtesy of Dr. J. D. Oriel, University College Hospital, London.

Swartz and his colleagues[126] at the Center for Disease Control in Atlanta, GA have contributed substantially to the diagnosis of NGU by defining urethral inflammation on the basis of polymorphonuclear cells (PMN) per hpf seen in Gram-stained smears of urethral secretions. A calcium alginate swab is passed into the urethra and then rolled once over a 2 × 1 cm area of a glass slide. Sixty of 61 patients with gonococcal urethritis had >50 PMN/hpf, while 25 monogamous control men had 0 to 2.2 PMN/hpf (mean 0.8 ± 0.07). An analysis of urethral smears in patients with NGU led the authors to define NGU as any patient with a urethral discharge and/or a count of more than four PMN/hpf in their urethral smear accompanied by a negative culture for *N. gonorrhoeae*.

Since urethritis is an inflammatory disease, this definition allows the inclusion of asymptomatic NGU which is clearly important.Since the final story as to the etiology of NGU is far from over, the direct assessment of urethral inflammation as proposed by Swartz *et al.*[126] should allow a tighter definition of nongonococcal urethritis.

Urethritis secondary to enterobacteria (*E. coli*, etc.), in the absence of cystitis, must be extremely rare and I am not sure I have ever documented a case. Colonization of the urethral mucosa, however, by Enterobacteriaceae from the introital mucosa of the female sexual partner is not uncommon (as I have shown earlier in this chapter).

J.B., a 26-year-old, part-time college student, is an instructive patient with nongonococcal urethritis. I saw him in July 1971, at which time he was complaining of a urethral discharge and dysuria of 6 days duration. Three-and-a-half years before he had developed a thin, white, urethral discharge and terminal dysuria that failed to respond to sulfonamide but cleared with tetracycline therapy (*U. urealyticum* is resistant to sulfonamides while *C. trachomatis* is sensitive). One year ago a similar discharge and dysuria responded again to tetracycline. On 7/2/71, 10 days after sexual intercourse with a new consort for the first time, he developed a moderately thin, white, profuse urethral discharge accompanied by terminal dysuria. Examination of the urethral meatus showed a thin, whitish discharge. A bacteriologic wire loop was inserted 2 cm down the urethra for cultures and for Gram stain; the latter showed many polymorphonuclear leukocytes per hpf but no intracellular diplococci. Wire loop cultures were streaked on chocolate blood agar and Thayer-Martin agar in the examining room; no gonococci were isolated from either plate. A VB_1, VB_2, and VB_3 urine showed only 80 diphtheroids and 10 *S. epidermidis*/ml in the VB_1, but *U. urealyticum* grew at 22,900 colony-forming units/ml in the VB_1, 2900/ml in the VB_2, and 4300/ml in the VB_3. The VB_2 urine sediment, centrifuged, contained only a rare

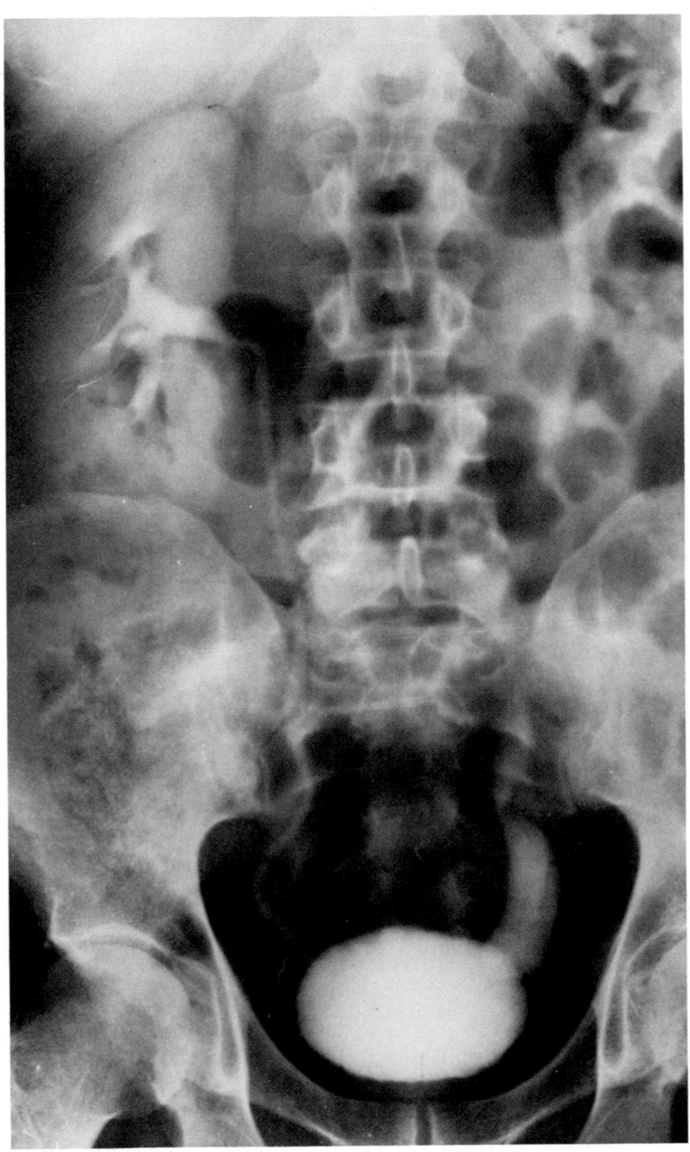

Figure 7.29 An intravenous urogram on a 56-year-old, white man. The right kidney is hypertrophied (14.7 × 8 cm) without evidence of obstruction or disease. The left kidney is small (9.4 × 6.3 cm), the calyces distorted, and the left ureter is dilated, especially in the lower one-third.

WBC per hpf. Because the patient had had five sexual partners in the past 3 years, and it would have been difficult to treat them, I elected not to treat him despite his urethritis. He returned in October of 1971 to report that his discharge and dysuria subsided and finally disappeared spontaneously, despite continued intercourse with the same consort responsible for the last episode of urethritis. He had no further episodes until August 1977, when he was seen again with a "yellow-green" discharge and dysuria; Gram stain and gonococcal cultures were negative (but loaded with polymorphonuclear leukocytes), but this time mycoplasma could not be isolated from the VB_1 urine. He was treated with 5 days of tetracycline and has remained asymptomatic since. Presumably, the latest episode was due to *C. trachomatis*. A follow-up telephone call in February 1979, indicated that he has remained free of any urethral discharge since the August 1977 episode.

CYSTITIS AND PYELONEPHRITIS

Urinary infection of the bladder and the kidneys in the male with a nonobstructed urinary tract, and in the absence of renal calculi, is almost always secondary to bacterial persistence in the prostate; the diagnosis of pyelonephritis should rarely be made as a primary disease. Even in the presence of "infection stones" in the kidney, the prostate must be excluded as the real cause of the original *Proteus* urinary infection; otherwise, as in W.D., Table 7.11, the infected renal stone will be removed but the same infection recurs because of bacterial persistence in the prostate.

When Alphonse Pfau, Professor of Surgery at the Hadassah Medical Organization in Jerusalem, Israel, was spending some sabbatical time with us at Stanford in 1977, he showed me a fascinating patient that makes this point very well indeed. With his permission, the case is reproduced here.

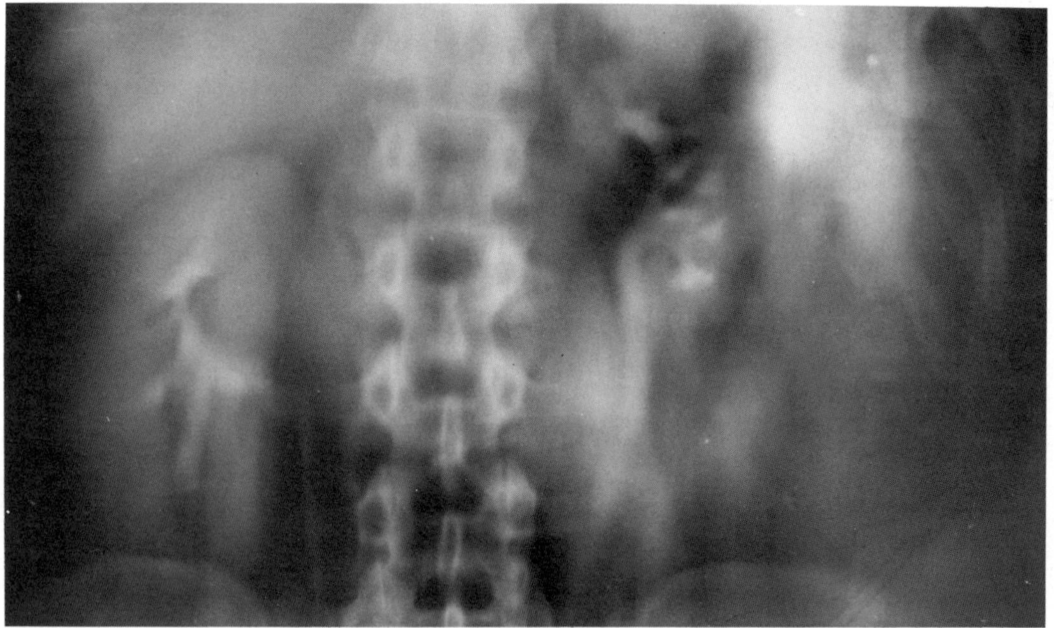

Figure 7.30 A nephrotomogram made during the intravenous urogram illustrated in Figure 7.29. The calyceal distortion and narrow cortex is compatible with atrophic pyelonephritis.

A 56-year-old man was first seen by Dr. Pfau on 1/15/75 because of recurrent urinary tract infections for the last 30 years. At the age of 12 years, the patient had experienced left flank pain accompanied by high fever. A left ureterocele was diagnosed and a transurethral ureteral meatotomy was done in 1936 at the age of 17 years. Following this intervention, the patient felt well for a number of years but after the Second World War he started to experience recurrent urinary tract infections, accompanied by frequency, urgency, and dysuria and sometimes by fever, chills and left flank pain. Antibacterial therapy was usually effective and the symptoms disappeared within a number of days each time he was treated. In 1973, the episodes of urinary tract infection became more frequent (4–5 times a year) and the urine cultures always grew *E. coli*. An intravenous urogram done in 1974 revealed prompt secretion from a hypertrophied right kidney (14.7 × 8 cm) which had a normal pyelo-calyceal system (Figure 7.29); the small left kidney (9.4 × 6.3 cm), however, showed irregular borders, deformed calyces, and delayed secretion of the contrast medium (Figure 7.30). The left ureter was substantially dilated in its lower third (Figure 7.29). The bladder was normal and emptied without residual urine. A cystogram revealed reflux into the lower one-third of the ureter (Figure 7.31). The previous *E. coli* urinary infection had occurred at the beginning of January 1975 and antibacterial therapy, completed on 1/10/75, had sterilized the urine. Several urologists consulted by the patient had advised him to have the left kidney and ureter removed because they believed the contracted left kidney was the source of the recurrent urinary infections.

Physical examination revealed a patient in good general condition with a slightly enlarged, smooth and nontender prostate. Blood pressure was 145/90 mm Hg. Sequential urine and EPS cultures on 1/27/75 grew 100,000 colonies/ml of *E. coli* in all specimens, clearly indicating that he was bacteriuric (Table 7.34). The patient received 500 mg of ampicillin four times a day for the next 2 weeks. Repeated localization studies in February 1975 showed on three occasions that the prostate was the source of the recurrent *E. coli* infections (Table 7.35). Two weeks after the ampicillin treatment, he was again bacteriuric with the *E. coli* (2/26/75). Endoscopy revealed diffuse inflammatory changes in the bladder, a normal right ureteral orifice, and a gaping left ureteral orifice, but no specific changes in the prostatic urethra. Differential ureteral catheterization studies showed the right kidney was sterile, the left kidney infected

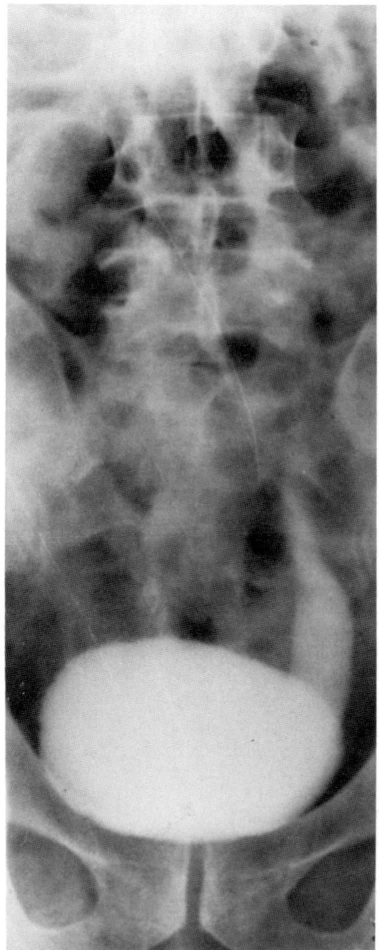

Figure 7.31 A cystogram, demonstrating left ureteral reflux, in the same patient as illustrated in Figures 7.29 and 7.30.

Table 7.35
Bacteriologic History of a 56-year-old Man with an Atrophic Left Kidney, Left Ureteral Reflux, and Recurrent Bacteriuria

Date	Days On (+) or Off (−) Drug	Drug	VB_1[a]	VB_2	EPS	Organism	pH of EPS
				Colonies/ml			
1/27/75			100,000	100,000	100,000	*Escherichia coli*	
2/7/75	+10	Amp	0	0	200	*E. coli*	
2/10/75	+13	Amp	0	0	1,900	*E. coli*	
2/14/75	−2	Amp	0	0	0		
2/20/75	−8	Amp	0	0	30,000	*E. coli*	
2/26/75	−14	Amp	100,000	100,000	100,000	*E. coli*	
2/28/75	Cystoscopy + localization						
			CB	100,000		*E. coli*	
			WB	1,200		*E. coli*	
			RK_1 0	LK_1 100,000		*E. coli*	
			RK_2 0	LK_2 50,000		*E. coli*	
			RK_3 0	LK_3 50,000		*E. coli*	
3/2/75	+6	Amp	0	0	0		
3/17/75	−11	Amp	100,000	100,000	100,000	*E. coli*	
3/24/75	+3	Kana	0	0	0		
4/4/75	−1	Kana	0	0	0		
4/11/75	−8	Kana	0	0	0		
4/18/75	−15	Kana	0	0	0		
5/2/75	−29	Kana	0	0	0		
5/23/75	−50	Kana	0	0	1,000	*E. coli*	8.0
5/30/75	−57	Kana	100	0	200	*E. coli*	
6/75	+8	TMP-SMX	0	0	0		
6/27/75	+28	TMP-SMX	0	0	0		8.3
7/25/75	+56	TMP-SMX	0	0	0		
8/29/75	+91	TMP-SMX	0	0	0		7.4
10/17/75	+140	TMP-SMX	0	0	0		
10/24/75	−7	TMP-SMX	0	0	0		
11/7/75	−21	TMP-SMX	0	0	0		
12/5/75	−50	TMP-SMX	0	0	0		7.9

1/9/76	−84	TMP-SMX	0	0	0	8.0
3/13/76	−147	TMP-SMX	0	0	0	
6/11/76	−237	TMP-SMX	0	0	0	
8/13/76	−300	TMP-SMX	0	0	0	
9/20/76	−338	TMP-SMX	0	0	0	
12/24/76	−433	TMP-SMX	0	0	0	
4/15/77	−544	TMP-SMX	0	0	0	
8/13/77	−665	TMP-SMX	0	0	0	
12/9/77	−754	TMP-SMX	0	0	0	7.9

[a] VB_1 = first voided 5–10 ml of urine from urethral meatus; VB_2 = midstream aliquot of urine; VB_3 = first voided 5–10 ml of urine from urethral meatus after prostatic massage; EPS = expressed prostatic secretion; TMP-SMX = trimethoprim-sulfamethoxazole; Amp = ampicillin; Kana = kanamycin; CB = catheterized bladder urine; WB = washed bladder (after 3000-ml sterile water irrigation); LK_1 to LK_4, serial catheterized left kidney urines, and RK_1 to RK_4, serial catheterized right kidney urines, each had 0 colonies/ml. Solid transverse line divides longitudinal authors into major periods of significance.

with *E. coli*. A 10-day course of ampicillin (2 g/day) again sterilized the urine, but 11 days after completion of therapy the urine was infected with *E. coli* (3/17/75).

He was treated with kanamycin for 13 days, 1 g intramuscularly twice a day for the first 3 days and then 500 mg twice daily for the next 10 days. Fifty days after completion of therapy (5/23/75), *E. coli* were recovered again from the prostate. TMP-SMX (160–800 mg) twice daily was then given for 140 days. The prostatic fluid became sterile and remained so on repeated cultures for over 2 years, which represented the first time in 30 years he had been free of recurrent, symptomatic pyelonephritis (Table 7.35). In mid-1978, an asymptomatic *S. epidermidis* and enterococcal bacteriuria was detected, two organisms that he commonly carried on his urethra. He was treated for 10 days with ampicillin and kanamycin; his urines have remained sterile since, the last culture recorded was in January 1979.

This patient clearly documents that the cause of a 30-year history of recurrent symptomatic pyelonephritis in an atrophic, refluxing kidney, is not to be found in the kidney *per se*; in the absence of renal calculi and in the presence of reasonable renal function, the kidney is almost never the cause of recurrent pyelonephritis. In the male, the physician must exclude the prostate as the cause of recurrent pyelonephritis.

REFERENCES

1. Freedman, L. R., Phair, J. P., Seki, M., Hamilton, H. B., Nefzger, M. D., and Hirata, M.: The epidemiology of urinary tract infections in Hiroshima. Yale J. Biol. Med. **37:** 262, 1965.
2. Miall, W. E., Kass, E. H., Ling, J., and Stuart, K. L.: Factors influencing arterial pressure in the general population in Jamaica. Br. Med. J. **2:** 497, 1962.
3. Kunin, C. M., Zacha, E., and Paquin, A. J.: Urinary tract infections in school children. I. Prevalance of bacteriuria and associated urologic findings. N. Engl. J. Med. **266:** 1287, 1962.
4. O'Shaughnessy, E. J., Perrino, P. S., and White, J. D.: Chronic prostatitis—Fact or fiction? J. Am. Med. Assoc. **160:** 540, 1956.

5. Gonder, M. J.: Prostatitis, Surg. Clin. N. Am. **45:** 1449, 1965.
6. Drach, G. W., Meares, E. M., Fair, W. R., and Stamey, T. A.: Classification of benign diseases associated with prostatic pain: prostatitis or prostatodynia? J. Urol. **120:** 266, 1978.
7. Blacklock, N. J.: Some observations on prostatitis. In D. C. Williams, M. H. Briggs, and M. Staniford (Eds.), Advances in the Study of the Prostate. London, William Heinemann Medical Books, 1969, p. 37.
8. Pfau, A., Perlberg, S., and Shapira, A.: The pH of the prostatic fluid in health and disease: implications of treatment in chronic bacterial prostatitis. J. Urol. **119:** 384, 1978.
9. Jameson, R. M.: Sexual activity and the variations of the white cell content of the prostatic secretion. Invest. Urol. **5:** 297, 1967.
10. Pai, M. G., and Bhat, H. S.: Prostatic abscess. J. Urol. **108:** 599, 1972.
11. Dajani, M. D., and O'Flynn, J. D.: Prostatic abscess. Br. J. Urol. **40:** 736, 1968.
12. Kelalis, P. P., Greene, L. F., and Harrison, E. G., Jr.: Granulomatous prostatitis. J. Am. Med. Assoc. **191:** 287, 1965.
13. Bowers, J. E., and Thomas, G. B.: The clinical significance of abnormal prostatic secretion. J. Urol **79:** 976, 1958.
14. Bourne, C. W., and Frishette, W. A.: Prostatic fluid analysis and prostatitis. J. Urol. **97:** 140, 1967.
15. Schmidt, J. D., and Patterson, M. D.: Needle biopsy study of chronic prostatitis. J. Urol. **96:** 519, 1966.
16. Stamey, T. A., Govan, D. E., and Palmer, J. M.: The localization and treatment of urinary tract infections; the role of bactericidal urine levels as opposed to serum levels. Medicine **44:** 1, 1965.
17. Drach, G. W.: Problems in diagnosis of bacterial prostatitis: Gram-negative, Gram-positive and mixed infections. J. Urol. **111:** 630, 1974.
18. Stamey, T. A., Meares, E. M., and Winningham, D. G.: Chronic bacterial prostatitis and the diffusion of drugs into prostatic fluid. J. Urol. **103:** 187, 1970.
19. Meares, E. M., and Stamey, T. A.: Bacteriologic localization patterns in bacterial prostatitis and urethritis. Invest. Urol. **5:** 492, 1968.
20. Huggins, C., and Bear, R. S.: The course of the prostatic ducts and the anatomy, chemical and x-ray diffraction analysis of prostatic calculi. J. Urol. **51:** 37, 1944.
21. Friedlander, A. M., and Braude, A. I.: Experimental prostatitis: relationship to pyelonephritis. J. Infect. Dis. **126:** 645, 1972.
22. McNeal, J. E.: Regional morphology and pathology of the prostate. Am. J. Clin. Pathol. **49:** 347, 1968.
23. Smart, C. J., and Jenkins, J. D.: The role of transurethral prostatectomy in chronic prostatitis. Br. J. Urol. **45:** 654, 1973.
24. Silber, S. J.: Transurethral Resection. New York, Appleton-Century-Crofts, 1977.
25. Smart, C. J., Jenkins, J, and Lloyd, R. S.: The painful prostate. Br. J. Urol. **47:** 861, 1976.
26. Fox, M.: The natural history and significance of stone formation in the prostate gland. J. Urol. **89:** 716, 1963.
27. Meares, E. M., Jr.: Infection stones of prostate gland. Laboratory diagnosis and clinical management. Urology **4:** 560, 1974.
28. Eykyn, S., Bultitude, M. I., and Lloyd-Davies, R. W.: Prostatic calculi as a source of recurrent bacteriuria in the male. Br. J. Urol. **46:** 527, 1974.
29. Smith, M. J. V.: Prostatic corpora amylacea. Monographs in the Surgical Sciences **3:** 209, 1966.
30. Percival, A., Brumfitt, W., and de Louvois, J.: Serum-antibody levels as an indication of clinically inapparent pyelonephritis. Lancet **2:** 1027, 1964.
31. Meares, E. M., Jr.: Serum antibody titers in urethritis and chronic bacterial prostatitis. Urology **10:** 305, 1977.
32. Meares, E. M., Jr.: Serum antibody titers in treatment with trimethoprim-sulfamethoxazole for chronic prostatitis. Urology **11:** 142, 1978.
33. Zollinger, W. D., Dalrymple, J. M., and Artenstein, M. S.: Analysis of parameters affecting the solid phase radioimmunoassay quantitation of antibody to meningococcal antigens. J. Immunol. **117:** 1788, 1976.
34. Chodirker, W. B., and Tomasi, T. B.: Gamma globulins: quantitative relationships in human serum and nonvascular fluids. Science **142:** 1080, 1963.
35. Ablin, R. J., Gonder, M. J., and Soanes, W. A.: Localization of immunoglobulins in human prostatic tissue. J. Immunol. **107:** 603, 1971.
36. Gray, S. P., Billings, J., and Blacklock, N. J.: Distribution of the immunoglobulins G. A, and M in the prostatic fluid of patients with prostatitis. Clin. Chim. Acta **57:** 163, 1974.
37. Riedasch, G., Ritz, E., Möhring, K., and Ikinger, U.: Antibody-coated bacteria in the ejaculate: a possible test for prostatitis. J. Urol. **118:** 787, 1977.
38. Colleen, S., and Mårdh, P.-A.: Studies on non-acute prostatitis. Clinical and laboratory findings in patients with symptoms of non-acute prostatitis. In D. Danielsson, L. Juhlin, and P.-A. Mårdh (Eds.), Genital Infections and Their Complications. Stockholm, Almqvist & Wiksell International, 1975, p. 121.
39. Mårdh, P.-A., and Colleen, S.: Search for urogenital tract infections in patients with symptoms of prostatitis. Studies on aerobic and strictly an-

aerobic bacteria, mycoplasmas, fungi, trichomonads and viruses. Scand. J. Urol. Nephrol. **9:** 8, 1975.

40. Nilsson, I.-K., Colleen, S., and Mårdh, P.-A.: Relationship between psychological and laboratory findings in patients with symptoms of non-acute prostatitis. In D. Danielsson, L. Juhlin, and P.-A. Mårdh (Eds.), Genital Infections and their Complications. Stockholm, Almqvist & Wiksell International, 1975, p. 133.
41. Nielsen, M. L., and Justesen, T.: Studies on the pathology of prostatitis. A search for prostatic infections with obligate anaerobes in patients with chronic prostatitis and chronic urethritis. Scand. J. Urol. Nephrol. **8:** 1, 1974.
42. Gordon, H. L., Miller, D. H., and Rawls, W. E.: Viral studies in patients with non-specific prostato-urethritis. J. Urol. **108:** 299, 1972.
43. Mårdh, P.-A., Ripa, K. T., Colleen, S., Treharne, J. D., and Darougar, S. Role of *Chlamydia trachomatis* in non-acute prostatitis. Br. J. Vener. Dis., **54:** 330, 1978.
44. Messing, E. M., and Stamey, T. A.: Interstitial cystitis. Early diagnosis, pathology, and treatment. Urology **12:** 381, 1978.
45. Stamey, T. A., Nemoy, N. J., and Higgins, M.: The clinical use of nalidixic acid; a review and some observations. Invest. Urol. **6:** 582, 1969.
46. Huggins, C.: The prostatic secretion. Harvey Lect. **52:** 148, 1946–47.
47. Winningham, D. G., Nemoy, N. J., and Stamey, T. A.: Diffusion of antibiotics from plasma into prostatic fluid. Nature **219:** 139, 1968.
48. Winningham, D. G., and Stamey, T. A.: Diffusion of sulfonamides from plasma into prostatic fluid. J. Urol. **104:** 559, 1970.
49. Kavanagh, F.: Analytical Microbiology. New York, Academic Press, 1963.
50. Dunn, B. L., and Stamey, T. A.: Antibacterial concentrations in prostatic fluid. I. Nitrofurantoin. J. Urol. **97:** 505, 1967.
51. Mann, T.: Biochemistry of Semen and of the Male Reproductive Tract. London, Methuen and Co., 1964.
52. Brodi, B. B., and Hogben, A. M.: Some physicochemical factors in drug action. J. Pharm. Pharmacol. **9:** 345, 1957.
53. Schanker, L. S., Shore, P. A., Brodi, B. B., and Hogben, C. A. M.: Absorption of drugs from the stomach. I. The rat. J. Pharmacol. Exp. Ther. **120:** 528, 1957.
54. Shore, P. A., Brodi, B. B., and Hogben, C. A. M.: The gastric secretion of drugs: A pH partition hypothesis. J. Pharmacol. Exp. Ther. **119:** 361, 1957.
55. Jacobs, M. H. Some aspects of cell permeability to weak electrolytes. Cold Spring Harbor Symp. Quant. Biol. **8:** 30, 1940.
56. Conklin, J. D., and Hollifield, R. D.: Studies on the movement of nitrofurantoin across the dog urinary bladder. Invest. Urol. **5:** 244, 1967.
57. Rieder, J.: Physicochemical and biological studies on sulfonamides. I. Pharmacologically interesting physicochemical characteristics of 21 sulfonamides and 6 sulfonamide metabolites. Arzneim. Forsch. **13:** 81, 1963.
58. Killman, S. A., and Thaysen, J. H.: Permeability of human parotid gland to series of sulfonamide compounds, paraaminohippurate and inulin. Scand. J. Clin. Lab. Invest. **7:** 86, 1955.
59. Bell, P. H., and Roblin, R. O., Jr.: Studies in chemotherapy; theory of relation of structure to activity of sulfanilamide type compounds. J. Am. Chem. Soc. **64:** 2905, 1942.
60. Garrod, L. P., and O'Grady, F.: Antibiotics and Chemotherapy. London, E. & L. Livingstone, 1968, p. 12.
61. Hessl, J. M., and Stamey, T. A.: The passage of tetracyclines across epithelial membranes with special reference to prostatic epithelium. J. Urol. **106:** 253, 1971.
62. Schach von Wittenau, M., and Yeary, R.: The excretion and distribution in body fluids of tetracyclines after intravenous administration in dogs. J. Pharmacol. Exp. Ther. **140:** 258, 1963.
63. Wood, W. S., Kipais, G. P., Spies, H. W., Dowling, H. F., Lepper, M. H., and Jackson, G. G.: Tetracycline therapy. Arch. Intern. Med. **94:** 351, 1954.
64. Roth, B., Falco, E. A., Hitchings, G. H., and Bushby, S. R. M.: 5-Benzyl-2, 4-diaminopyrimidines as antibacterial agents. 1. Synthesis and antibacterial activity *in vitro*. J. Med. Pharm. Chem. **5:** 1103, 1962.
65. Reeves, D. S., and Ghilchick, M. B.: Secretion of the antibacterial substance trimethoprim in the prostatic fluid of dogs. Br. J. Urol. **42:** 66, 1970.
66. Robb, C. A., Carroll, P. T., Tippett, L. O., and Langston, J. B.: The diffusion of selected sulfonamides, trimethoprim, and diaveridine into prostatic fluid of dogs. Invest. Urol. **8:** 679, 1971.
67. Granato, J. J., Jr., Gross, D. M., and Stamey, T. A.: Trimethoprim diffusion into prostatic and salivary secretions of the dog. Invest. Urol. **11:** 205, 1973.
68. Stamey, T. A., Bushby, S. R. M., and Bragonje, J.: The concentration of trimethoprim in prostatic fluid: nonionic diffusion or active transport? J. Infect. Dis. **128(Suppl.):** S686, 1973.
69. Madsen, P. O., Kjaer, T. B., and Baumueller, A.: Prostatic tissue and fluid concentrations of trimethoprim and sulfamethoxazole. Experimental and clinical studies. Urology **8:** 129, 1976.
70. Dabhoiwala, N. F., Bye, A., and Claridge, M.: A study of trimethoprim-sulfamethoxazole in the human prostate gland. Br. J. Urol. **48:** 77, 1976.
71. Baumueller, A., Hoyme, U., and Madsen, P. O.:

Rosamicin—a new drug for the treatment of bacterial prostatitis. Antimicrob. Agents Chemother. **12:** 240, 1977.
72. Bushby, S. R. M., and Hitchings, G. H.: Trimethoprim, a sulphonamide potentiator. Br. J. Pharmocol. Chemother. **33:** 72, 1968.
73. Burchall, J. J., and Hitchings, G. H.: Inhibitor binding analysis of dihydrofolate-reductases from various species. Mol. Pharmocol. **1:** 126, 1965.
74. Brumfitt, W., Pursell, R. E., Faiers, M. C., Reeves, D. S., and Turnbull, A. R.: Bacteriological, pharmacological, and clinical studies with trimethoprim-sulfonamide combination. Postgrad. Med. J., Suppl. **45:** 56, 1969.
75. Reeves, D. S., Faiers, M. C., Pursell, R. E., and Brumfitt, W.: Trimethoprim-sulphamethoxazole: comparative study in urinary infection in hospital. Br. Med. J. **1:** 541, 1969.
76. Pines, A., Greenfield, J. S. B., Raafat, H., Rahman, M., and Siddiqui, A. M.: Preliminary experience with trimethoprim and sulfamethoxazole in the treatment of purulent chronic bronchitis. Postgrad. Med. J., Suppl. **45:** 89, 1969.
77. Meares, E. M., Jr.: Observations on activity of trimethoprim-sulfamethoxazole in the prostate. J. Infect. Dis. **128(Suppl.):** S679, 1973.
78. Meares, E. M., Jr.: Long-term therapy of chronic bacterial prostatitis with trimethoprim-sulfamethoxazole. Can. Med. Assoc. J. **112:** 22S, 1975.
79. Mobley, D. F.: Semen cultures in the diagnosis of bacterial prostatitis. J. Urol **114:** 83, 1975.
80. Ulstein, M., Copell, P., Holmes, K. K., and Paulsen, C. A.: Nonsymptomatic genital tract infection and male infertility. In E. S. E. Hafez (Ed.) Human Semen and Fertility Regulation in Men. St. Louis, Mosby, 1976, p. 355.
81. Meares, E. M., Jr.: Urinary tract infections in men. In J. H. Harrison *et al.* (Eds.), Campbell's Urology, 4, Ed., Vol. 1. Chap. 13, Philadelphia, W. B. Saunders, 1978, p. 527.
82. Blacklock, N. J., and Beavis, J. P.: The response of prostatic fluid pH in inflammation. Br. J. Urol. **46:** 537, 1974.
83. Anderson, R. U., and Fair, W. R.: Physical and chemical determinations of prostatic secretion in benign hyperplasia, prostatitis, and adenocarcinoma. Invest. Urol. **14:** 137, 1976.
84. Baumueller, A., and Madsen, P. O.: Experimental bacterial prostatitis in dogs. Urol. Res. **5:** 211, 1977.
85. Baumeller, A., and Madsen, P. O.: Secretion of various antimicrobial substances in dogs with experimental bacterial prostatitis. Urol. Res. **5:** 215, 1977.
86. Fair, W. R., Crane, D. B., Schiller, N., Heston, W. D. W.: A re-appraisal of treatment in chronic bacterial prostatitis J. Urol. **121:** 437, 1979.
87. Pfau, A., and Sacks, T.: Chronic bacterial prostatitis: new therapeutic aspects. Br. J. Urol. **48:** 245, 1976.
88. Stamey, T. A., Timothy, M., Millar, M., and Mihara, G.: Recurrent urinary infections in adult women. The role of introital enterobacteria. Calif. Med. **115:** 1, 1971.
89. Philpot, V. B. Jr. The bacterial flora of urine speciments from normal adults. J. Urol. **75:** 562, 1956.
90. Stamey, T. A., Fair, W. R., Timothy, M. M., and Chung, H. D.: Antibacterial nature of prostatic fluid. Nature **218:** 444, 1968.
91. Bessey, O. A., Lowry, P., and Brock, M. J.: A method for the rapid determination of alkaline phosphatase with five cubic millimeters of serum. J. Biol. Chem. **164:** 321, 1946.
92. Litwack, G.: Photometric determination of lysozyme activity. Proc. Soc. Exp. Biol. Med. **89:** 401, 1955.
93. Rosenkrantz, H., and Kirdani, E. S.: The proteolytic enzymes of canine prostatic fluids. Cancer Chemother. Rep. **15:** 9, 1961.
94. Goss, W. A., Deitz, W. H., and Cook, T. M.: Mechanism of action of nalidixic acid on *Escherichia coli.* J. Bacteriol. **88:** 1112, 1964.
95. Newton, B. A.: The properties and mode of action of the polymyxons. Bacteriol. Rev. **20:** 14, 1956.
96. Rozansky, R., Bachrach, U., and Grossowicz, N.: Studies on the antibacterial action of spermine. J. Gen. Microbiol. **10:** 11, 1954.
97. Rozansky, R., Gurevitch, J., Brezezinsky, A., and Ekerling, B.: Inhibition of the growth of *Staphylococcus aureus* by human semen. J. Lab. Clin Med. **34:** 1526, 1949.
98. Fair, W. R., and Wehner, N.: Antibacterial action of spermine; effect on urinary tract pathogens. Appl. Microbiol. **21:** 6, 1971.
99. Fair, W. R., and Wehner, N.: Further observations on the antibacterial nature of prostatic fluid. Infection and Immunity **3:** 494, 1971.
100. Youmans, G. P., Leibling, J., and Lyman, R. Y.: The bactericidal action of prostatic fluid in dogs. J. Infec. Dis. **63:** 117, 1938.
101. Gip, L., and Molin, L.: On the inhibitory activity of human prostatic fluid on *Candida albicans.* Mykosen **13:** 61, 1970.
102. Fair, W. R., and Wehner, N.: The antibacterial action of canine prostatic fluid and human seminal plasma in an agar diffusion assay system. Invest. Urol. **10:** 262, 1973.
103. Fair, W. R., Couch, J., and Wehner, N.: The purification and assay of the prostatic antibacterial factor (PAF). Biochem. Med. **8:** 329, 1973.
104. Fair, W. R., Couch, J., and Wehner, N.: Prostatic antibacterial factor: identity and significance. Urology **7:** 169, 1976.

105. Skarnes, R. C., and Watson, D. W.: Antimicrobial factors of normal tissues and fluids. Bacteriol. Rev. **21:** 273, 1957.
106. Hirsch, J. G.: Antimicrobial factors in tissue and phagocytic cells. Bacteriol. Rev. **24:** 133, 1960.
107. Hyams, J. A., Kramer, S. E., and McCarthy, J. F.: The seminal vesicles and the ejaculatory ducts: histopathologic study. J. Am. Med. Assoc. **98:** 691, 1932.
108. Eliasson, R.: Correlation between the sperm density, morphology and motility and the secretory function of the accessory genital glands. Andrologia **2:** 165, 1970.
109. Caldamone, A. A., and Cockett, A. T. K.: Infertility and genitourinary infection. Urology **12:** 304, 1978.
110. Dahlberg, B.: Asymptomatic bacteriospermia: cause of infertility in men. Urology **8:** 563, 1976.
111. Derrick, F. C., Jr., and Dahlberg, B.: Male genital tract infections and sperm viability. In E. S. E. Hafez (Ed.), Human Semen and Fertility Regulation in Men. St. Louis, Mosby, 1976, p. 389.
112. Harrison, R. F., de Louvois, J., Blades, M., and Hurley, R.: Doxycycline treatment and human infertility. Lancet **1:** 605, 1975.
113. de Louvois, J., Blades, M., Harrison, R. F., Hurley, R., and Stanley, V.: Frequency of mycoplasma in fertile and infertile couples. Lancet, **1:** 1073, 1974.
114. Meares, E. M., Jr.: Influence of infections of the male accessory glands on secretory function, sperm viability and fertility. In E. S. E. Hafez and E. Spring-Mills (Eds.), Accessory Glands of the Male Reproductive Tract. Ann Arbor, Ann Arbor Science Publishers, 1979.
115. Boström, K.: Chronic inflammation of human male accessory sex glands and its effect on the morphology of the spermatozoa. Scand. J. Urol. Nephrol. **5:** 133, 1971.
116. Couture, M., Ulstein, M., Leonard, J., and Paulsen, C. A.: Improved staining method for differentiating immature germ cells from white blood cells in human seminal fluid. Andrologia **8:** 61, 1976.
117. Prescott, L. F. and Brodie, D. E. A simple differential stain for urinary sediment. Lancet **2:** 940, 1964.
118. Eliasson, R.: Clinical examination of infertile men. In E. S. E. Hafez (Ed.), Human Semen and Fertility Regulation in Men. St. Louis, Mosby, 1976, p. 321.
119. Jacobs, N. F., and Kraus, S. J.: Gonococcal and nongonococcal urethritis in men. Clinical and laboratory differentiation. Ann. Intern. Med. **82:** 7, 1975.
120. Holmes, K. K., Handsfield, H. H., Wang, S. P., Wentworth, B. B., Turck, M., Anderson, J. B., and Alexander, E. R.: Etiology of nongonococcal urethritis. N. Engl. J. Med. **292:** 1199, 1975.
121. Dunlop, E. M. C., Jones, B. R., and Darougar, S.: *Chlamydia* and non-specific urethritis. Br. Med. J. **2:** 575, 1972.
122. Taylor-Robinson, D., Csonka, W., and Prentice, M. J.: Human intraurethral inoculation of ureaplasmas. Q. J. Med., New Series, **46:** 309, 1977.
123. Schachter, J.: Medical progress. Chlamydial infections (second of three parts). N. Engl. J. Med. **298:** 490, 1978.
124. Schachter, J.: Medical progress. Chlamydial infections (first of three parts). N. Engl. J. Med. **298:** 428, 1978.
125. Berger, R. E., Alexander, E. R., Monda, G. D., Ansell, J., McCormick, G., and Holmes, K. K.: *Chlamydia trachomatis* as a cause of acute "idiopathic" epididymitis. N. Engl. J. Med. **298:** 301, 1978.
126. Swartz, S. L., Kraus, S. J., Herrmann, K. L., Stargel, M. D., Brown, W. J., and Allen, S. D.: Diagnosis and etiology of nongonococcal urethritis. J. Infect. Dis. **138:** 445, 1978.
127. Anderson, R. U., and Weller, C.: Prostatic secretion leukocyte studies in nonbacterial prostatitis (prostatosis). J. Urol. **121:** 292, 1979.
128. Smith, J. W., Jones, S. R., Reed, W. P., Tice, A. D., Deupree, R. H. and Kaijser, B.: Recurrent UTI in men. Characteristics and response to therapy. Ann. Intern. Med. **91:** 544, 1979.

CHAPTER 8

Infection Stones*

THE relationship between urea-splitting organisms in the urine, mainly *Proteus mirabilis*, and stones composed of struvite (magnesium ammonium phosphate) and apatite (calcium phosphate) is well known.[2–4] It was probably first suggested by Marcet in 1817.[5] Surgical treatment, although affording immediate relief from the morbidity of pyelonephritis and obstruction, is usually followed by persistence of the infection and recurrence of the stone; in several reports published before and after the introduction of antibiotics, the recurrence rate has been as high as 50 to 70%.[6,7]

Using a method of stone culture that distinguishes surface contamination from infection within the stone (see Chapter 1), we have demonstrated urea-splitting organisms to be deeply imbedded in the stone, protected from the action of antibacterial agents. Thus, even minute particles left at surgery represent foci of persistent infection which may result in recurrent stone formation. Although a variety of surgical techniques have been advocated,[8–10] none insures total removal of macroscopic fragments.

To reduce the recurrence rate of such "infection stones," surgery was supplemented by chemical dissolution of residual fragments in the presence of a bacteriologically sterile urine. I show first our initial experience with 14 consecutive patients, seen over a period of 7 years (1962 to 1969), in whom neither stones nor infections have recurred, in order to present several observations and principles of management.

SURGICAL, BACTERIOLOGICAL, AND BIOCHEMICAL MANAGEMENT

Fourteen patients with infection stones—struvite calculi due to urea-splitting bacteria—in the kidney were seen between 1962 and 1969 (Table 8.1). Each had recurrent urinary tract infections on admission: eight had lower tract symptoms (dysuria, frequency, urgency), three had upper tract symptoms (intermittent fever, flank pain), and three asymptomatic bacteriuria. In three patients, formation of stones had recurred after surgical removal elsewhere.

In addition to special bacteriologic and roentgenographic studies, the following laboratory determinations were made in each patient: a complete blood cell count (CBC), blood urea nitrogen (BUN), creatinine, serum electrolytes, calcium, uric acid, total

* Part of the material presented in this chapter was originally published in J. Am. Med. Assoc. **215:** 1470, 1971.[1]

Table 8.1
Clinical Summary[a]

Patient	Sex	Age	Location of Stone	Size	Infecting Organism	Surgical Procedure	Stone[b] Analysis	Size of Postoperative Residual Fragments[c]	Duration of Renacidin Irrigation
		yr		*mm*				*mm*	*days*
1	F	39	Right middle infundibulum and calyx	20 × 15	*Proteus mirabilis*	Pyelolithotomy	Struvite, apatite	None	None
2	F	16	Right lower pole	12 × 2	*P. mirabilis*	Pyelolithotomy	Struvite, apatite	None	None
3	F	37	Right upper pole	15 × 10	*P. mirabilis*	Pyelolithotomy	Struvite, apatite	None	None
4	M	66	Left upper pole	25 × 15	*P. mirabilis*	Pyelolithotomy	Struvite, apatite	4	3
5	F	30	Right renal pelvis	16 × 12	*P. mirabilis*	Pyelolithotomy	Struvite, apatite	None	None
6	F	34	Right upper pole	35 × 12	*P. mirabilis*	Pyelolithotomy	Struvite, apatite	None	None
7	F	31	Left renal pelvis	20 × 15	*Klebsiella*	Pyelolithotomy	Struvite, apatite	None	None
8	F	37	Right renal pelvis, infundibula and calyces	55 × 22	*P. mirabilis*	Pyelolithotomy	Struvite, apatite	None	3
			Left renal pelvis	22 × 17	*P. mirabilis*	Pyelolithotomy	Struvite, apatite	None	2
9	F	37	Left lower pole	17 × 4	*P. mirabilis*	Partial nephrectomy	Struvite, apatite	5	14
10	F	51	Left upper pole	38 × 15	*P. mirabilis*	Pyelolithotomy	Struvite, apatite	>1	1
11	F	46	Right lower pole	30 × 10	*P. mirabilis*	Pyelolithotomy	Lost	8	10
12	M	26	Left renal pelvis, infundibula and calyces	40 × 20	*P. mirabilis*	Cystoscopy, placement of ureteral catheters		None	30
13	F	42	Left upper pole	30 × 25	*P. mirabilis*	Cystoscopy, placement of ureteral catheters		None	14
14	F	50	Left renal pelvis	6 × 4	*Klebsiella*	Cystoscopy, placement of ureteral catheters		None	12

[a] Reproduced by permission from N. J. Nemoy and T. A. Stamey, J. Am. Med. Assoc. **215:** 1470, 1971.[1]
[b] Struvite signifies magnesium ammonium phosphate ($MgNH_4PO_4 \cdot 6H_20$); apatite signifies calcium phosphate ($Ca_{10}(PO_4)_6(OH)_2$).
[c] As shown on plain film tomograms.

protein, serum albumin, alkaline phosphatase, and serum glutamic oxaloacetic transaminase (SGOT).

Roentgenography

In addition to the routine scout x-ray film and intravenous urogram (IVU), plain film tomograms were taken at 0.5-cm cuts. With this technique, calculi that were relatively nonopaque and too soft to be seen on routine x-ray films were easily visualized, and small fragments left at surgery were more likely to be detected.

Bacteriology

Urine specimens for culture were obtained by either a physician or a trained urologic nurse (Chapter 1). Localization of the urinary tract infection was performed with ureteral catheters as previously described in Chapter 1.

Bacterial identification and quantitative counts were done as in earlier studies; antibacterial agents were chosen on the basis of their bactericidal activity at urinary concentrations (Chapter 2).

At surgery, before the renal pelvis was opened, urine was obtained for culture by needle aspiration (Figure 8.1). The stone was removed, immediately placed in a sterile tube containing 5 ml of saline solution, and cultured by a technique described in Chapter 1, and illustrated in Figure 8.1.

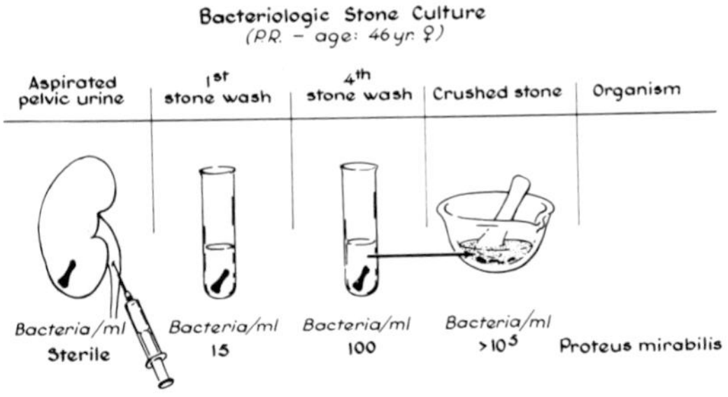

Figure 8.1 Illustrative method of stone culture (patient 11). This technique is presented in detail in Chapter 1 (Reproduced by permission from N. J. Nemoy and T. A. Stamey, J. Am. Med. Assoc. **215:** 1470, 1971.)[1]

Surgical Techniques

Antibacterial therapy was begun at least 1 week prior to surgery; a sterile urine culture was mandatory prior to operative intervention, and the intramuscular form of the orally effective antibiotic was given with the preoperative medication. An intrarenal sinus pyelolithotomy[8] was performed in five patients, a standard pyelolithotomy in five patients, and a partial nephrectomy in one patient. In an attempt to remove all stone fragments at surgery, the renal pelvis and collecting system were irrigated copiously with sterile saline solution by means of a malleable nozzle attached to a high pressure syringe. In five patients (six kidneys) a small nephrostomy tube was inserted to allow for postoperative irrigation (Figure 8.2). A polyethylene tube with multiple holes, such as occurs in the Hemovac drainage set, is ideal.

Three patients who were considered poor surgical candidates had dissolution of their calculi by means of irrigation through ureteral catheters which were passed into the renal pelvis. The irrigating solution was instilled through a 5 Fr polyethylene catheter and drained through a 7 Fr polyethylene catheter (Stamey Ureteral Catheters, American Latex Corp., Sullivan, Ind.)

Biochemical Dissolution of Struvite and Apatite Fragments

Following surgery, the nephrostomy tube was connected to dependent drainage to expedite healing of the pyelotomy incision. Appropriate antibacterial treatment (usually penicillin-G potassium or ampicillin for Proteus-containing stones) was continued, usually by intramuscular injection, in order to maintain a sterile urine.

Daily samples of urine were obtained from the nephrostomy tube for culture. *Sterile urine was a mandatory prerequisite to irrigation of the renal pelvis.*

Irrigation of the renal pelvis with saline solution was begun on the 4th or 5th postoperative day at a rate of 120 ml/hour for 24–48 hours. The height of the irrigating bottle was maintained at the lowest level above the kidney commensurate with a flow rate of 120 ml/hour. Leakage around the

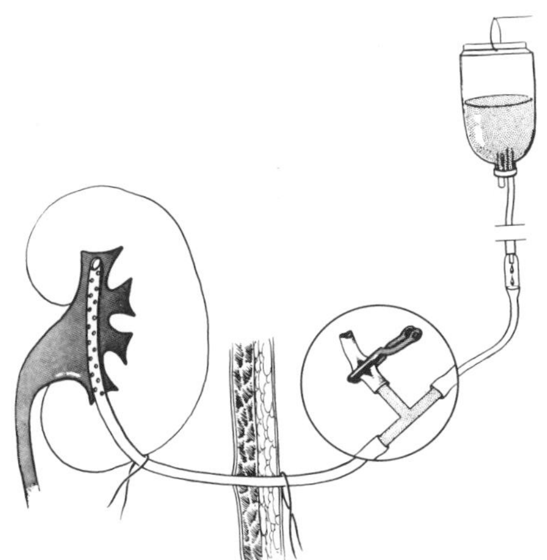

Figure 8.2 Precautions for renal irrigation with Renacidin. All the holes in the polyethylene tubing must be placed within the collecting system. The tube is fixed by suture ligature to both the capsule of the kidney and the skin or muscle of the abdominal wall. A pinch-clamp on a Y-tube intersection is located well within reach of the patient. The height of the bottle should be no higher than is necessary to deliver the desired flow rate (about 120 ml/hour).

surgical drain indicated incomplete healing of the pyelotomy incision, and further irrigation was temporarily discontinued.

If no leakage, fever, or flank discomfort occurred, a multivalent, buffered organic acid solution (10% hemiacidrin [Renacidin]) was then started at 120 ml/hour through the nephrostomy tube.

The patients were carefully instructed how to release the pinch-clamp themselves at the first sign of flank discomfort, even before notifying the nurse. This important precaution allows immediate reduction of intrarenal pressure in the presence of temporary outflow obstruction. The pinch-clamp arrangement in Figure 8.2 is convenient.

Plain film tomograms of the kidney were obtained to detect macroscopic residual fragments. It is best to remove all wound drains except the nephrostomy tube before obtaining the plain film tomograms because their radiologic visibility interferes with detection of residual struvite fragments. In the absence of visible particles, Renacidin irrigation was discontinued after 24–48 hours. In the presence of fragments, the irrigation was continued until subsequent tomograms indicated complete dissolution. Occasionally, a patient may require a bladder catheter to prevent vesical irritation from the Renacidin; in these patients, the rate of irrigation may be reduced to 50 ml/hour, or saline solution (1000 ml) may be alternated with each liter of Renacidin. In the presence of irritation, the concentration of Renacidin may be reduced from 10 to 5%, thereby decreasing the irritation in some patients.

We have observed in some patients, especially in those who develop symptoms of cystitis, that the ureteral and renal pelvic mucosa show radiologic signs of ureteritis cystica or mucosal spiculation, as we have called it.[11] This edematous appearance to the uroepithelium can interfere with free irrigation, but it completely disappears within 1–4 days of stopping the Renacidin. The potentially obstructive nature of this mucosal edema serves as a further reason for never irrigating in the presence of urinary infection.

Absolute contraindications to continued irrigation are infected urine, fever, persistent flank discomfort, or an obstructed outflow system.

The clinical data on all 14 patients are summarized in Table 8.1. Nine of the 14 were under 40 years of age; 12 were women. One patient had bilateral renal calculi. The infecting organism was *P. mirabilis* in 12 patients, and *Klebsiella* in 2 patients. The stones were located in the upper pole of five kidneys; the lower pole of three kidneys; within the renal pelvis of four kidneys; in the renal pelves, infundibula, and calyces of two kidneys; and in the middle infundibulum and calyx of one kidney.

Ten patients had 11 pyelolithotomies (patient 8 had bilateral stones); one patient had a partial nephrectomy. Among the three patients who were considered poor surgical risks and had dissolution of their calculi by irrigation through ureteral catheters was patient 14, who had a solitary kidney and a creatinine level of 3.5 mg/100 ml.

Analysis of 10 stones showed each to be composed of struvite and apatite, with struvite the predominant component.

Residual fragments, shown by plain film tomography, were left in four patients; their size varied from a tiny fleck in patient 10 to an 8 × 4 mm fragment in patient 11. The efficacy of dissolution with Renacidin irrigation was demonstrated in these four patients and in the additional three patients judged to be poor surgical risks.

Renacidin irrigation (10%) was used in nine kidneys (eight patients). The duration of irrigation varied from 1 to 30 days, depending upon the persistence of residual fragments. In no patient did Renacidin have to be discontinued because of complications. Each patient was given an appropriate antibacterial agent during the entire period of Renacidin therapy; daily cultures or urine from the involved kidney remained sterile in every instance. Determinations of creatinine, BUN, serum electrolyte, calcium, SGOT, and alkaline phosphatase levels were made on alternate days, and no changes were noted during or after Renacidin therapy.

Urine and Stone Cultures

Since the publication of these original eight patients, Nemoy and I[12] reported the successful management of 35 patients in 1976, including the details of two with solitary kidneys. We continue to use Renacidin irrigation as a routine in all postoperative patients with struvite infection stones.

Preoperatively, the infection was always localized to the kidney with the calculus (Table 8.2). Patient 11 had bilateral renal

Table 8.2
Preoperative Bacteriologic Localization Studies[a]

Patient	Organism	CB[b]	WB	RK_1	RK_2	RK_3	RK_4	LK_1	LK_2	LK_3	LK_4	Location of Stone
					bacteria/ml							
1	*Proteus mirabilis*	$>10^5$	1000	$>10^4$	8,600	6500	7000	0	0	0	0	Right middle infundibulum and calyx
2	*P. mirabilis*	$>10^4$	74	9,000	1,260	798	342	0	0	0	0	Right lower pole
3	*P. mirabilis*	$>10^5$	lost	32,000	13,000			270	0			Right upper pole
4	*P. mirabilis*	$>10^5$	110	0	0	0		$>10^4$	$>10^4$	$>10^4$		Left upper pole
5	*P. mirabilis*	$>10^5$	240	900	550	380		0	0	0		Right renal pelvis
6	*P. mirabilis*	$>10^5$	1000	$>10^5$	$>10^5$	$>10^5$		$>10^3$	50	0		Right upper pole
7	*Klebsiella*	100	0	Not catheterized				570	270			Left renal pelvis
8	No localization study											
9	*P. mirabilis*	4000	600	0	0	0	0	4000	3700	3700	3500	Left lower pole
10	*P. mirabilis*	$>10^5$	800	20	0	0	0	$>10^4$	$>10^4$	$>10^4$	$>10^4$	Left upper pole
11	*P. mirabilis*	$>10^5$	3000	4000	2200	1400	920	0	0	0	0	Right lower pole Left lower pole

[a] Reproduced by permission from N. J. Nemoy and T. A. Stamey, J. Am. Med. Assoc. **215:** 1470, 1971.[1]

[b] CB = culture of bladder urine obtained through cystoscope. WB = culture of bladder-irrigating fluid (after washing bladder with 2 liters of sterile water) immediately prior to passing ureteral catheters up ureters. RK_1, LK_1, RK_2, LK_2, RK_3, etc. = paired, simultaneous cultures obtained from right (R) and left (L) kidneys through ureteral catheters during water diuresis.

calculi (Figure 8.3), but her infection was present in only the right kidney (the central density in the left renal stone suggested a calcium oxalate nucleus, rather than an infection stone).

Bacteriologic cultures of the stones are summarized in Table 8.3. All patients were receiving antibacterial therapy at the time of surgery; cultures of urine aspirated from the renal pelvis were sterile in all cases.

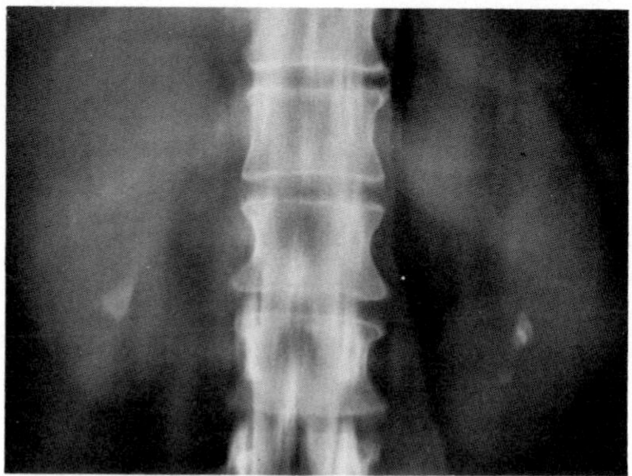

Figure 8.3 Preoperative plain film tomograms of kidneys (patient 11). Infection localized to stone in the right kidney only; urine from left kidney was sterile (Table 8.2). (Reproduced by permission from N. J. Nemoy and T. A. Stamey, J. Am. Med. Assoc. **215:** 1470, 1971.)[1]

Cultures of the first and fourth saline washes often yielded low counts of bacteria and probably represented surface growth (perhaps from manipulation of soft stones at surgery). Patients 5 and 9, however, had sterile stones prior to crushing; the stones from patients 4, 8, and 11 had insignificant wash counts compared with the crush counts. The high counts of bacteria observed in the crushed stone cultures of patients 4, 5, 8, 9, and 11, compared to the negligible bacterial counts obtained from washing the surface of the stone, confirm the presence of bacteria within the inner portion of the stones. The organism recovered from within the calculus was always the same as that originally cultured from the pretreatment urine.

That this is not always true, however, is shown by the analysis Thompson and I[13] did on the results of stone cultures in 49 patients with struvite stones. As can be seen in Table 8.4, only two of the struvite stones were sterile, and both were obtained from patients with documented recurrent *P. mirabilis* infections. Thirty-four of the patients were women and 15 were men. In this group there were 44 renal stones and 5 bladder stones. If one excludes the 5 bladder stones (primarily from paraplegic patients) and the renal stones in those pa-

Table 8.3
Stone Cultures[a]
See Chapter 1 for details and Figure 8.1 for illustration.

Patient	Aspirated Pelvic Urine	1st Stone Wash	4th Stone Wash	Crushed Stone	Organism
			bacteria/ml		
1	Sterile	15	100	$>10^5$	*Proteus mirabilis*
2	Not obtained				
3	Not obtained				
4	Sterile	10	0	1600	*P. mirabilis*
5	Sterile	0	0	2500	*P mirabilis*
6	Sterile	450	20	7000	*P. mirabilis*
7	Sterile	1300	170	$>10^5$	*Klebsiella*
8 (Stone in right kidney)	Sterile	10	10	$>10^5$	*P. mirabilis*
9	Sterile	0	0	$>10^3$	*P. mirabilis*
10	Sterile	1000	1000	$>10^5$	*P. mirabilis*
11	Sterile	20	20	3000	*P. mirabilis*

[a] Reproduced by permission from N. J. Nemoy and T. A. Stamey, J. Am. Med. Assoc. **215:** 1470, 1971.[1]

Table 8.4
Results of Stone Cultures in 49 Patients with Struvite Stones[a]

Organism	Number of Stones Infected	Total
Single		28
Proteus mirabilis[b]	21	
Klebsiella	2	
Staphylococcus aureus[c]	2	
Pseudomonas[c]	1	
Escherichia coli[b]	1	
Yeast[b]	1	
Multiple		19
P. mirabilis with *Klebsiella*;[b] *E. coli*; *Pseudomonas*; *Streptococcus*; *Providencia*; *Proteus rettgeri*; *Proteus morganii*; *Proteus vulgaris*; *Enterobacter cloacae*;[b] *Staphylococcus*; *Enterobacter aerogenes*[b]	17	
P. rettgeri with yeast[c]	1	
Streptococcus with *E. coli*[c]	1	
Sterile		2

[a] Reproduced by permission from R. B. Thompson and T. A. Stamey, Urology **2:** 627, 1973.[13]

[b] Indicates stones containing calcium oxalate (4 patients) or protein (2 patients).

[c] Indicates patients who also had previous *P. mirabilis* urinary infections.

tients with chronic urinary infection secondary to an indwelling bladder catheter or ileal loop, the marked preponderance of women with infected renal calculi is even more striking. The ratio is then 28 women to 7 men. That is, the majority of infected struvite stones in men were associated with a source of chronic urinary infection, such as an indwelling catheter. Only 4 women with infected struvite stones were paraplegic and had indwelling catheters.

The bacteria cultured from the struvite stones are shown in Table 8.4. Of the 47 patients with infected struvite stones, 28 were infected with a single organism in pure culture, and 19 contained more than one organism. *P. mirabilis*, however, was the predominant organism in both groups.

The organism most frequently found in struvite stones infected with only one organism was *P. mirabilis.* Twenty-one of 28 struvite stones infected with only one organism contained *P. mirabilis* (Table 8.4). Two patients had recurrent *Klebsiella* infections, and only *Klebsiella* (urease-positive) was cultured from the stone. Two patients had only *Staphylococcus aureus* (urease-positive) present in their stones; one of these also had recurrent infections with *Proteus* organisms, the other patient possibly acquired his staphylococcal infection following surgery elsewhere for a previous renal stone. In one paraplegic patient only *Pseudomonas* (urease activity unknown) was cultured from her renal stone, but she also had documented recurrent infections with *P. mirabilis.* In fact, both *P. mirabilis* and *Pseudomonas* had been localized preoperatively to the kidney containing the stone. Only two patients in this group had a urease-negative organism (*Escherichia coli*, yeast) cultured from their stones, and neither had a history to suggest previous infection with a urease-positive organism. However, these two stones were not typical of the other struvite stones in this series, since other elements were present and struvite constituted a smaller portion of the stone in both. The yeast-infected stone was approximately one-third whewellite, struvite, and hydroxyl apatite; the stone containing *E. coli* was composed of whewellite, struvite, and carbonate apatite. The presence of Ca oxalate suggests that the original stone was sterile and became secondarily infected.

More than one organism was present inside the stones obtained from 19 of the 47 patients with infected struvite calculi (Table 8.4). The number of different organisms within a stone varied from two, in 11 patients, up to seven contained in the bladder stone of a paraplegic man. However, only 7 of these 19 patients were paraplegic or had a chronic indwelling catheter to account for infection with multiple organisms. The large number of stones containing *P. mirabilis* is again evident. Only 2 of the 19 stones did not contain *P. mirabilis*, and both of these patients had had urinary tract infections with *P. mirabilis*. The bacteria associated with *P. mirabilis* are listed in

Table 8.4 in order of decreasing frequency of occurrence. No one organism was predominantly associated with *P. mirabilis.* The most frequently associated bacteria were *E. coli* and *Klebsiella*, and each was cultured from 6 stones. Eleven stones contained only two different organisms, and *P. mirabilis* and *E. coli*, occurring in five cases, was the most frequent pattern. It should be noted that many of the associated organisms may also split urea.

Incorporation of *E. coli* into a *P. mirabilis Infection Stone*

Since most P. mirabilis urinary tract infection (UTI) occur in women susceptible to recurrent urinary infections, it should not be surprising that some struvite infection stones formed by *P. mirabilis* then incorporate strains of subsequent UTI. Longitudinal studies on patients with struvite infection stones are required to show that this occurs.

Incorporation of a second organism (*E. coli*) into a pure *P. mirabilis* struvite stone is illustrated by the longitudinal studies on a 24-year-old white woman. She was first seen at Stanford in the prenatal clinic during her first pregnancy in November 1970. Although asymptomatic, she had experienced intermittent episodes of cystitis since the age of 18 years. Urinalysis showed 10–15 white blood cells/high-power field; urine culture was not obtained. Three symptomatic episodes of dysuria and frequency between February and early May 1971 were treated with short courses of ampicillin and later nalidixic acid; cultures were positive for *P. mirabilis* on all three occasions. On the 5th day of treatment with nalidixic acid, she was admitted to the hospital with a temperature of 104°F, right flank pain, a white blood count of 18,600, and a serum creatinine of 1.4 mg/100 ml. She was treated with intravenous cephalothin and intramuscular kanamycin for 3 days, and then placed on oral penicillin-G, a regimen that kept her urine free of *P. mirabilis.* A soft, staghorn calculus filling the left kidney was visible on a single plain film radiograph. Serum creatinine fell to 1.1 mg/100 ml 4 days after admission. One month later she delivered a normal, full term infant. While waiting 3 months for the normal hydroureteronephrosis of pregnancy to subside, an acute *E. coli* urinary infection developed (resistant to penicillin-G) that was treated with tetracycline. On tetracycline, the *P. mirabilis* again grew in the urine because it was resistant to tetracycline. She was admitted to the hospital on September 9, 1971. Tetracycline was stopped, but by mistake she received two doses of oral penicillin-G before cystoscopy the following day. Cystoscopic localization studies showed the right renal urine to be sterile and the left infected with both *E. coli* and *P. mirabilis.* She was placed on gentamicin, and the left staghorn calculus was removed 3 days later. Cultures of the stone showed both *E. coli* and *P. mirabilis* in the stone at a time when the urine was sterile. After 3 days of postoperative Renacidin irrigations, she was discharged on nalidixic acid which was discontinued 14 days later. She remained without UTI until 1973 when she again developed recurrent infections due to *E. coli.* In late 1975, she was placed on 6 months of trimethoprim-sulfamethoxazole (TMP-SMX) prophylaxis, which she completed in 1976. She has remained asymptomatic without UTI since that time.

Nonstruvite Infection Stones

We have several clinical examples where it is clear that sterile calcium oxalate stones have become secondarily infected, usually by instrumentation of the urinary tract, but occasionally by natural history. When this occurs, they behave bacteriologically exactly like struvite infection stones (see Figure 8.4). In the analysis of stone cultures, Thompson and I[13] did, only five nonstruvite stones were found to be infected. All five patients, three female and two male, had documented recurrent urinary tract infections, only one of which was with a urea-splitting organism. Bacteria cultured from the infected nonstruvite stones, together with the composition and site of origin, are listed in Table 8.5. Four of the five infected stones were removed from the kidney and were basically calcium oxalate stones. Recurrent *E. coli* infections were present in

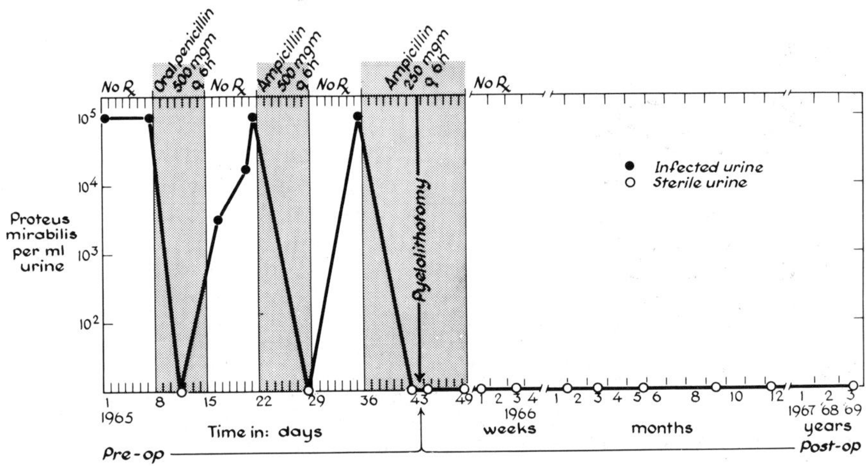

Figure 8.4 Preoperative and postoperative bacteriologic course of patient 1. Note recurrence of *P. mirabilis* infection each time antibiotic therapy was stopped. Eradication of infection was achieved only after removal of stone from right kidney. (Reproduced by permission from N. J. Nemoy and T. A. Stamey, J. Am. Med. Assoc. **215:** 1470, 1971.)[1]

Table 8.5
Results of Stone Cultures in Five Patients with Infected Nonstruvite Stones[a]

Origin	Composition	Bacteria	Urease
Renal	Calcium oxalate uric acid	*Escherichia coli*	–
Renal	Calcium oxalate	*E. coli*	–
Renal	Calcium oxalate	*Proteus mirabilis*	+
Renal	Calcium oxalate	*Herbicola-Lathyri*	–
Bladder	Brushite	*Pseudomonas*	+, –

[a] Reproduced by permission from R. B. Thompson and T. A. Stamey, Urology **2:** 627, 1973.[13]

the first two patients, and *E. coli*, urease-negative, was cultured from their stones. The third patient, the only one with *P. mirabilis* in this group, had a history of four episodes of cystitis during the preceding 2 years. Four months preoperatively she had a single episode of colic suggesting a renal calculus. Three months preoperatively *P. mirabilis* cystitis developed which differed from previous episodes of cystitis in that prompt recurrence was noted whenever antibiotics were stopped. When the small renal stone which was believed to be the source of the recurrent bacteriuria was removed, it did contain *P. mirabilis*; but on analysis it proved to be an oxalate stone without any struvite elements. The last renal stone was removed from a woman with a 5-year history of passing small ureteral calculi without urinary infections. Preoperatively, she suffered with fever, chills, and flank pain. Urine culture elsewhere showed 100,000 Gram-negative bacteria, apparently *E. coli.* An intravenous urogram revealed a partially obstructing stone at the left ureteropelvic junction and a small, nonobstructing stone in the right kidney. The stone at the left ureteropelvic junction was removed and contained low numbers of an uncommon organism, *Herbicola-Lathyri*, which was urease-negative. Stone analysis revealed a pure oxalate stone.

The only bladder stone in this group was removed from a man who had a catheter for approximately 1 month following the onset of traumatic paraplegia but who was without a catheter when transferred for rehabilitation. Midstream urine culture showed *Pseudomonas*, *Serratia*, and enterococcus. Several small calculi of the bladder were seen on an otherwise normal urogram. Stone cultures showed two different *Pseudomonas*, one urease-positive and one urease-negative. The stone was brushite which is formed at a lower pH than struvite.

Incorporation of bacteria *in vivo* into a previously sterile stone has been documented in patient 11 (Figure 8.3). She was first seen in 1968 with a history of bilateral renal calculi and recurrent *P. mirabilis* urinary infections. A soft calculus was present in the right kidney; a stone of greater density was present in the left kidney. Localization studies showed that the kidney containing the stone on the left side was completely sterile whereas *P. mirabilis* was cultured from the kidney containing the stone on the right side (Table 8.2). The right renal stone was removed in January 1969, and shown to contain *P. mirabilis.* In the subsequent years the patient was asymptomatic and maintained a sterile urine without the use of antibiotics as shown on culture. The left renal stone did not change in size. In April 1971, more than 2 years after the removal of the infected stone, she was hospitalized elsewhere for bilateral oophorectomy. Postoperatively, she had a pulmonary embolus and had a bladder catheter indwelling for 5 days. Immediately following discharge she became symptomatic of upper and lower urinary tract infection. Antibiotic treatment eliminated her symptoms, but cultures were positive each time antibiotics were stopped. She was again seen at Stanford in July 1971, and localization studies were performed. These studies demonstrated that the originally infected right kidney was completely sterile. The originally sterile left kidney containing a previously sterile stone was now infected with *Klebsiella* and *Streptococcus faecalis.*

Thus, this patient had bilateral renal stones, one infected and one sterile. Surgical removal of the infected stone followed by Renacidin irrigation cured the patient of recurrent bacteriuria for over 2 years. Subsequently she again became infected, presumably following catheterization; the bacteria then became incorporated into the originally sterile stone, and produced the classic picture of recurrent urinary infection each time antibiotics were stopped.

Long Term Follow-Ups

The follow-up data are summarized in Table 8.4. The duration of follow-up for the 14 patients was 4–89 months (mean, 34 months). The urine cultures obtained at the last follow-up visit were sterile in 13 patients; 1 patient, a paraplegic with an indwelling catheter, had infected urine. Antibacterial therapy was stopped 2–4 weeks following surgery in each case (patient 14, with azotemia, solitary kidney, and medullary sponge kidney, received a maintenance dose of sulfisoxasole). Roentgenographic studies, also obtained at the last follow-up visit, showed each patient to be free of recurrent stone formation. As this chapter is revised in 1979, I am disappointed that I am unable to add longer term follow-ups to the 14 patients in Table 8.1. The original identifying numbers have been lost and, despite an extensive search, we are unable to locate the names of these early patients.

Persistence of Bacteria within Struvite Stones

Surgery by itself, as evidenced by the high recurrence rate, [6, 7] is usually an inadequate treatment for infection stones. Failure is probably due to residual fragments left behind at surgery which harbor urea-splitting organisms. We have demonstrated that, whereas the urine and stone surface are readily sterilized in the presence of appropriate antibacterial treatment (Table 8.3), the original infecting organism continues to exist below the surface of the stone. Thus, discontinuation of drug therapy, in the presence of either the original stone or its residual fragments, results in recurrence of the infection. The inability of antimicrobial agents to kill the bacteria within the stone necessitates complete removal of the stone in order to eradicate the infection. This phenomenon is well illustrated by the preoperative and postoperative course of patient 1 (Figure 8.4). A *P. mirabilis* infection was localized to the right kidney, which contained a 20- × 15- mm stone (Tables 8.1 and 8.2). Although the urine was sterilized repeatedly with antibiotics, the infection recurred each time therapy was stopped. Ampicillin was no more effective than orally administered penicillin-G. Cure of the infection was achieved only by removing its source—the calculus in the right kidney. Longer term therapy (8–12 weeks) in other patients has been equally unsuccessful; recurrence with the original infecting organism has occurred within 48–72 hours of discontinuation of antibacterial therapy.

These bacteriologic studies do not represent the first time that bacteria have been noted within the depths of infection stones. Hellström[2] was able to stain tissue sections of infection stones with Gram stain; the urea-splitting *Staphylococcus epidermidis* was demonstrated to be deeply layered within the interstices of the stone. The implication of our studies, that a major reason for failure to cure recurrent pyelonephritis may be bacteria embedded in macroscopic interstitial calcifications rather than bacteria embedded in renal tissue, has not escaped us.

Rocha and Santos[14] placed bladder stones from patients with urinary infections in iodine and alcohol for 6 hours; despite sterilization of the external surface of the stone, viable bacteria were recovered from the interior of the calculi.

Precautions with Renacidin Irrigation

When an infection stone is small and lying free within the renal pelvis, its total removal is easily accomplished, and a good prognosis is insured. Difficulty, however, is encountered with those stones that have extensions into the infundibula and calyces. As a rule they are soft and friable; small particles, despite copious irrigation at the time of surgery, are often left behind. Barney[15] reported leaving residual fragments in 45% of his patients; both Comarr *et al.*[16] and Oppenheimer[17] left fragments in 33% of their patients with infection stones. With the use of plain film tomograms to detect small particles, 36% of our patients were found to have residual fragments. Almost certainly, the frequency of particles left behind which are too small to be seen roentgenographically is higher. These fragments, because of their imbedded bacteria, must be eliminated to prevent urea-splitting alkalinization of the urine with its concomitant precipitation of struvite crystals.[18]

Although no complications developed in the three poor risk patients who could not be operated upon, constant attention was necessary to overcome mechanical problems during irrigation. The ureteral catheters frequently became obstructed by debris and required irrigation with saline solution; repositioning of the catheter was often necessary. The patient is bedridden during the period of irrigation (with nephrostomy irrigation, the patient is usually ambulatory), and the length of time required to dissolve the stone is long. Because of these factors, irrigation through ureteral catheters should probably be limited to patients who are poor surgical risks. The hazards are increased in paraplegic patients because of their inability to appreciate flank discomfort, and irrigation in such patients should be approached with caution.

Because struvite and apatite calcifications are so readily dissolved, surgical removal should be followed by Renacidin irrigation. Renacidin (10%) contains, besides several multivalent organic acids buffered to pH of 3.7, 639 ± 42 mEq/liter of magnesium (mean and SD of six different batches); its action is probably due to an ion exchange in which the calcium of the stone is replaced with magnesium to form the equivalent magnesium salt which is soluble in the gluconocitrate solution, as noted by A. M. Globus (written communciation, April 1969).

The compound was introduced in 1959, and Mulvaney and others[16, 19, 20] reported encouraging results with dissolution of renal calculi. However, because of several unfavorable reports,[21–23] the drug was withdrawn for use in the renal pelvis by the Federal Drug Administration. Four deaths were reported[21]; two patients were paraplegic, one had poliomyelitis, and one had multiple sclerosis. All four were febrile for 24–48 hours before death; blood cultures were not obtained, and findings of urine cultures were not reported. Findings at autopsy showed multiple renal abscesses with areas of necrosis and pulmonary edema. The clinical course and postmortem findings in these patients were most consistent with septicemia as the cause of death. It is possible that even saline irrigation of the renal pelvis of these patients, under gravity pressure and in the presence of infected urine, would have produced the same result. A further report noted, at autopsy, the presence of widespread necrotic abscesses filled with numerous neutrophils together with a "striking abundant growth of bacterial colonies."[22] The third, and remaining, unfavorable report[23] described a patient who, in the presence of an untreated urinary tract infection, had irrigation of the renal pelvis through ureteral catheters. It is abundantly clear from these reports that if the physician is unwilling to assume responsibility for a sterile renal urine prior to and during irrigation of the renal pelvis with saline solution and Renacidin, he should not attempt dissolution of infection stones. Daily urine cultures from the nephrostomy tube or ureteral catheters, prior to and during irrigation, must be sterile. To prevent pyelovenous backflow, the patient is instructed to disconnect the inflow at the first sign of flank discomfort before calling the nurse. This precaution allows immediate reduction of intrapelvic pressure in the presence of temporary outflow obstruction. Paraplegic patients, unable to appreciate flank discomfort, may be more prone to complications resulting from high intrarenal pressure. Fever is obviously a contraindication to renal irrigation.

With use of Renacidin in our first eight patients (nine kidneys), we encountered no difficulty; five of the patients (six kidneys) had nephrostomy tubes. One patient required a Foley catheter to relieve bladder spasms caused by the irrigation. Frequent determinations of serum creatinine, BUN, serum calcium, serum alkaline phosphatase, and SGOT levels during treatment showed no changes. Serum citric acid levels were measured in two patients who were receiving such irrigations and were normal in both. We have infused Renacidin intravenously in dogs to determine what biochemical changes might be monitored by the clinician as a measure of gross Renacidin absorption.[24] Ten dogs, infused intravenously for 8 hours with 10% Renacidin at a rate equivalent to total absorption intravenously of 120 ml/hour/70 kg in a human, showed a rise in serum magnesium proportional to the rate of infusion, an early leukocytosis, and a 24-hour delayed elevation in the SGOT and serum creatinine (Figures 8.5 and 8.6). All of the chemical pathology could be reproduced by a simple solution containing only $MgCl_2$ in the same concentration. By 96 hours, all parameters returned to control values. From these studies, intravenous absorption of Renacidin during dissolution of renal stone fragments can be monitored in patients by following the serum magnesium. A white blood cell count and determinations of SGOT and serum creatinine levels may be of value, *but the presence of a sterile urine during irrigation must remain the primary concern of the physician.*

Importance of Postoperative Cultures and Follow-up

Because reinfection with urea-splitting organisms can lead to new stone formation, all patients given this treatment deserve close attention following surgery. Urine cultures should be obtained every 1–2 months during the 1st year, and at regular intervals thereafter. In fact, we tell every patient with infection stones that surgical removal

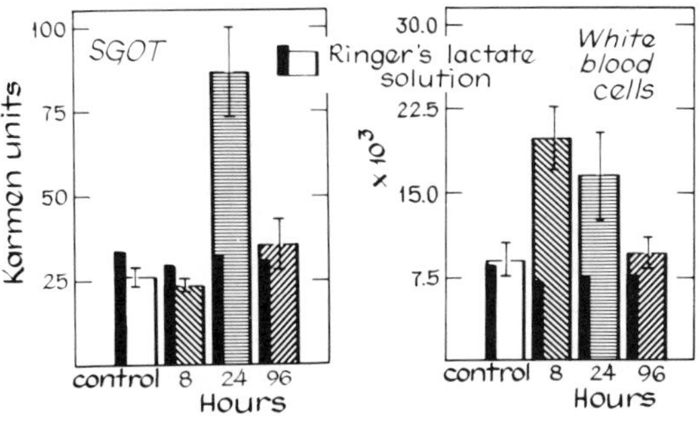

Figure 8.5 The mean values of serum glutamic oxaloacetic transaminase (SGOT) and the white blood cell count are shown at 8, 24, and 96 hours after the start of the infusion of 10% Renacidin in six surviving dogs and in two dogs receiving $MgCl_2$; the means of the control values prior to infusion are represented by the *open bar*. The values for the two control dogs given Ringer's lactate are indicated by the *solid bars*.

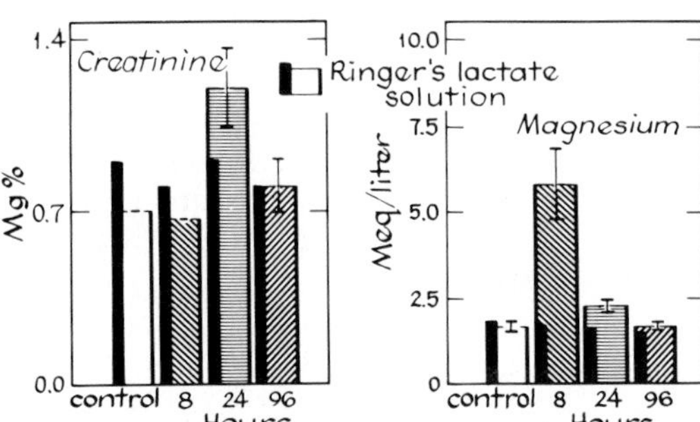

Figure 8.6 The mean values of serum creatinine and serum Mg^{++} are shown at 8, 24, and 96 hours after the start of the infusion of 10% Renacidin in six surviving dogs and in two dogs receiving $MgCl_2$; the means of the control values prior to infusion are represented by the *open bar*. The values for the two control dogs given Ringer's lactate are indicated by the *solid bars*.

solves only half the problem. Equally important is close follow-up to prevent reinfection. After all, *P. mirabilis* is not an uncommon urinary infection. I emphasized in Chapter 1 that half of all bacteriurias in adult women involve one or both upper tracts,[25] an observation confirmed by others [26, 27]; thus, bacteriuria caused by urea-splitting organisms will ascend to the renal pelvis in about 50% of the patients. As also pointed out in Chapter 1, *P. mirabilis* is present in the fecal flora of at least one out of every four normal individuals. Indeed, I believe an argument can be made that as long as reinfections in women are caused by *E. coli*, *Klebsiella*, and sometimes even *Pseudomonas*, there is little danger to the patient *in the absence of pregnancy* or other obstructive disease. But the presence of *P. mirabilis* should make the careful clinician extra cautious. To be sure, *P. mirabilis* often occurs in bacteriuria and can be readily cleared without posing any special threat. On the other hand, chronic, long-standing bacteriuria with *P. mirabilis* is not so benign. Most of our patients with *P. mirabilis* and struvite stones have had their infection for at least 6 months or longer.

I believe the clinical data presented here on infection stones are best interpreted by considering the infection as the primary event in the initiation and propagation of struvite stones. If a metabolic abnormality is at fault the stones should reform in the absence of infection. This is not the case (Table 8.6). Moreover, Elliot [28] could show

Table 8.6
Postoperative Results[a]

Patient	Duration of Follow-Up	Urine Culture	Roentgenographic Evidence of Recurrent Stone
	mo[b]	*mo off therapy*	*mo after surgery*
1	41	Sterile (40)	None (41)
2	46	Sterile (45)	None (46)
3	89	Sterile (88)	None (89)
4	25	Sterile (24)	None (24)
5	29	Sterile (28)	None (29)
6	26	Sterile (25)	None (26)
7	30	Sterile (29)	None (29)
8	16	Sterile (15)	None (16)
9	34	Sterile (33)	None (34)
10	4	Sterile (3)	None (4)
11	5	Sterile (4)	None (5)
12 (Paraplegic, indwelling Foley catheter)	60	$>10^5$ pseudomonas organisms $>10^5$ proteus organisms	None (60)
13	65	Sterile (64)	None (65)
14	5	Sterile[c]	None (4)

[a] Reproduced by permission from N. J. Nemoy and T. A. Stamey, J. Am. Med. Assoc. **215:** 1470, 1971.[1]
[b] *mo* = months.
[c] Patient receiving long term sulfisoxasole therapy because of medullary sponge kidney.

no difference in calcium, magnesium, or phosphorus excretion in patients forming struvite or apatite (basic calcium phosphate) stones compared to normal individuals, whereas oxalate stone patients tend to excrete more calcium and oxalic acid.

The importance of these observations is clear. Reinfection with urea-splitting bacteria must be prevented, or detected early and cleared, in the infection stone former. For this reason, surgical removal is only half the obligation of the clinician.

Nonsurgical Management of Infection Stones

Elliot's publications[28, 30–36] on the physicochemical factors involved in struvite and apatite stone formation ("phosphate" stones) are important contibutions. Before his work, few investigators distinguished between phosphate and oxalate stones. Since infection stones are invariably struvite with some apatite (Table 8.1), the factors that determine crystallization—and especially dissolution—are critically important in management. Elliot, after reviewing the literature on spontaneous dissolution of renal calculi (mostly stones of recumbency) and adding several cases of his own,[29] commented that "this phenomenon can be explained only on the basis of a change in chemical equilibrium in the urine favoring solubility of the salts composing the calculus." In a remarkable succession of papers on phosphate stones,[28, 30–36] he showed that (1) normal urines are undersaturated with tricalcium phosphate and not supersaturated, as commonly believed, in the presence of protective colloids[30]; (2) struvite occurs as a crystalline phase, in urines saturated with calcium phosphate, only above a pH of 7.2[31] (apatite above a pH of 6.6); (3) the mean urinary pH of normal individuals (5.85)[33] is less than that required for the crystallization of apatite and well below that required for struvite; (4) the major conditions required for struvite precipitation in urine are a pH of 7.1 or greater and a calcium to magnesium ratio that is lower than the normal mean[34]; and, finally, (5) the solubility of calcium phosphate and hence the formation and growth of the apatite calculus are influenced principally by pH of the urine.[35]

From these studies, it is not unreasonable that sterile apatite stones formed during recumbency, or in the alkaline urine characteristic of quadriplegia,[36] renal tubular acidosis, or antacid therapy for duodenal ulcer,[28] are capable of dissolution in the presence of a normally acid urine. But is dissolution of struvite stones, complicated by the presence of urea-splitting organisms, also a medical possibility? Because we prefer to remove surgically the bulk of struvite-apatite calcifications, followed by Renacidin irrigations, we have not treated large infection stones by sterilization of the urine and concomitant acidification to attempt dissolution. This is clearly a distinct possibility, however, as shown by the course of the following patient.

L.V., a 42-year-old Caucasian mother of two children, was referred to us in 1967 with a 7-year history of recurrent urinary infections associated with chills, fever, and flank pain. Without a preceding history of urinary infections in childhood or during her two normal pregnancies, she had two infections per year between 1960 and 1966. Intravenous urography showed bilateral medullary sponge kidneys. In 1966, six infections occurred and in 1967 she had one each month until her referral in late April 1967. *P. mirabilis* was known to be responsible for most (if not all) of her infections. Hospitalization was required in February and March of 1967; she was treated with chloramphenicol on both occasions and discharged on methenamine mandelate, 1.0 g every 6 hours. Her family history revealed no instances of renal disease or calculi.

Upon admission to the hospital, her urine was pH 7.5 and infected with *P. mirabilis* (Table 8.7). Serum chemistries were within normal limits, including a creatinine of 0.9 mg%. Intravenous urography confirmed the diagnosis of medullary sponge kidneys (Figure 8.7), but plain film tomograms showed multiple opaque calculi in both kidneys. A 5- × 6-mm stone was present in the middle calyx of the left kidney with multiple smaller stones in the lower calyces. In the

Table 8.7
L.V., a 42-year-old, Caucasian Mother with Struvite Infection Stones and Medullary Sponge Kidney: Effect of Conservative Treatment[a, b]

Date	Days On (+) or Off (−) Therapy		Vaginal Vestibule		Urethral		Midstream	
			bacteria/ml		*bacteria/ml*		*bacteria/ml*	
4/25/67	+14	methenamine mandelate 1.0 g q. 6 hr					SPA[a]	100,000
							Proteus mirabilis	
5/1/67	−6	methenamine mandelate 1.0 g q. 6 hr					*Localization*	
							CB = *P. mirabilis*	100,000
							WB = *P. mirabilis*	2,000
							RK (1–4) *P. mirabilis*	10,000
							LK (1–4) *P. mirabilis*	10,000
5/4/67	+4	tetracycline 500 mg q. 6 hr	*Staphylococcus epidermidis*	40	*P. mirabilis*	10^4	*P. mirabilis*	10^4
					Escherichia coli	10	*E. coli*	80
5/9/67	+5	streptomycin 500 mg q. 6 hr (I.M.)	*S. epidermidis*	70	*P. mirabilis*	90	*P. mirabilis*	90
			γ-streptococcus	30	*S. epidermidis*	2,000	*S. epidermidis*	2,500
					γ-streptococcus	1,000	γ-streptococcus	1,000
					E. coli	140	*E. coli*	70
5/23/67	+14	sulfamethazole 500 mg q. 6 hr	γ-streptococcus	10			SPA	
							P. mirabilis	10^5
6/6/67	−7	kanamycin					SPA	0
	+10	methenamine mandelate						
6/20/67	+24	methenamine mandelate					SPA	0
7/18/67	+52	methenamine mandelate	*S. epidermidis*	150			*S. epidermidis*	5,000
							E. coli	20
7/25/67	+60	methenamine mandelate	Yeast	10			CB	0
8/22/67	+90	methenamine mandelate					*S. epidermidis*	3,000
							Diphtheroids	Few
11/20/67	+180	methenamine mandelate	*S. epidermidis*	430	*S. epidermidis*	770	*S. epidermidis*	260
			Diphtheroids	570			γ-streptococcus	100
1/29/68	+250	methenamine mandelate			Yeast	1,290	Yeast	350
					γ-streptococcus	20		
3/25/68	+340	methenamine mandelate			*S. epidermidis*	440	*S. epidermidis*	700
					Pseudomonas	60	*Pseudomonas*	20
					γ-streptococcus	10	γ-streptococcus	210

Table 8.7—*Continued*

Date	Days On (+) or Off (−) Therapy		Vaginal Vestibule		Urethral		Midstream	
			bacteria/ml		*bacteria/ml*		*bacteria/ml*	
4/8/68	+360	methenamine mandelate	*S. epidermidis*	20	*S. epidermidis*	$>10^4$	*S. epidermidis*	$>10^4$
					P. miribalis	100	*P. mirabilis*	40
6/10/68	+410	methenamine mandelate			*S. epidermidis*	5,000	*S. epidermidis*	650
6/24/68	+425	methenamine mandelate	*S. epidermidis*	10		0		0
7/8/68	+440	methenamine mandelate			Yeast	360	Yeast	>40
7/30/68	+460	methenamine mandelate			*S. epidermidis*	960	*S. epidermidis*	600
					E. coli	610	*E. coli*	70
8/5/68	+466	methenamine mandelate					SPA	0
9/16/68	+500	methenamine mandelate			*S. epidermidis*	400	*S. epidermidis*	190
11/12/68	+560	methenamine mandelate		0			SPA	0
12/9/68	+587	methenamine mandelate					SPA	0
3/10/69	+678	methenamine mandelate					SPA	0
6/2/69	+762	methenamine mandelate					SPA	0
10/16/69	+898	methenamine mandelate					SPA	0
2/12/70	+1017	methenamine mandelate					SPA	0
6/9/70	+1134	methenamine mandelate					SPA	0

[a] SPA = suprapubic aspiration of bladder; CB = catheterized bladder urine; WB = washed bladder; RK = right kidney; LK = left kidney.
[b] Solid transverse line divides longitudinal cultures into major periods of significance.

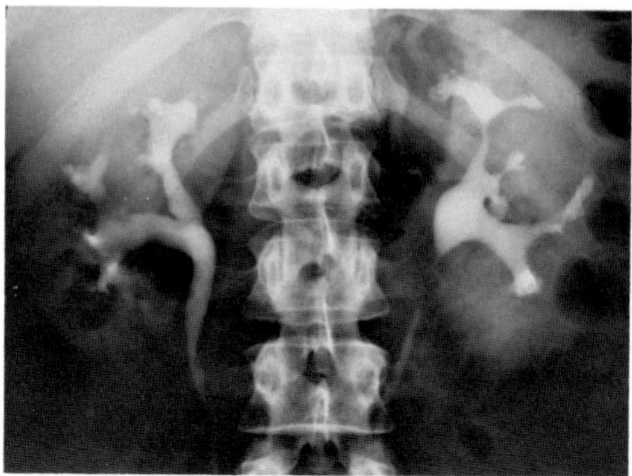

Figure 8.7 Intravenous urogram on L.V., a 42-year-old white woman with *Proteus mirabilis* urinary infection and multiple, small struvite-apatite calcifications seen on plain film tomography in both kidneys.

right kidney, a 5-mm stone was present in the lower calyx with multiple smaller ones. Serial urines examined for pH were all 7.5 or greater. On April 30, 1967 she spontaneously passed a 3-mm stone which consisted of 92% struvite and 8% apatite.

Cystoscopy and ureteral catheterization studies on May 1, 1967 showed *P. mirabilis* in high counts in four consecutive serial cultures from each kidney (Table 8.7). Because of a marked sensitivity to penicillin, she was started on tetracycline 500 mg every 6 hours despite *in vitro* evidence of resistance. As seen in Table 8.7, tetracycline was ineffective, and she was switched to streptomycin to which the *P. mirabilis* was sensitive. On the 5th day of apparent success (unless the 90 *P. mirabilis*/ml represent suppression) with streptomycin, sulfamethazole 500 mg was started as a possible oral suppressive agent. Fourteen days later, we knew that this sulfamethazole regimen was also a failure. Kanamycin, 500 mg intramuscularly every 6 hours, was promptly started for 7 days. Methenamine mandelate and ascorbic acid, 1.0 g of each four times a day, were added a few days after starting kanamycin. As can be seen in Table 8.7, the methenamine and ascorbic acid were continued indefinitely. All urines during the period of her 3-year follow-up remained sterile. Her serum creatinine in March 1969, was 0.9 mg%. Plain film tomograms, repeated in June 1968, and February 1970, showed complete disappearance of all calcifications.

The course of this patient suggests that if the urine can be kept sterile in the presence of struvite stones and urea-splitting bacteria, acidification of the urine may result in dissolution of the calculi. I know now that ascorbic acid in doses under 12 g/day probably does not acidify the urine, which I did not know in 1970. Indeed, except for NH_4Cl, we lack an effective urinary acidifier. Fortunately, a nondiuretic, normal urine is quite acid.

Of equal importance is the possibility that if surgery and Renacidin irrigations fail to leave the urinary tract free of infection calculi, acidification of the urine may dissolve the remaining stones. For most patients with *P. mirabilis* struvite stones, sterilization with penicillin-G and acidification with NH_4Cl would offer an ideal regimen.

Griffith *et al.*[37] have published their clinical results in controlling infection-induced staghorn calculi by using acetohydroxamic acid (AHA). They reported 16 patients with 21 stone-containing kidneys who took AHA—a specific inhibitor of bacterial urease—for 6–30 months. After 1–4 months of AHA alone, however, most patients were given "culture-specific antibiotics." Since the latter drugs alone can be effective in dissolving struvite infection stones, we really do not know how effective AHA is in dissolving renal calculi. Even with the combination, if I understand their data correctly, of their 16 patients, 7 had surgical removal of their stones, 4 patients showed "evidence of stone dissolution," and in 7 patients there was slight growth (I am aware this adds up to 18 patients; perhaps residual calculi in some of their surgical patients are included in their observations). Apparently no patient treated with AHA, with or without antibiotics, had complete dissolution of their stones with sterile urine after treatment, which is the usual outcome we observe with surgery and Renacidin irrigation. At best, then, and including antibiotic therapy, 4 of 16 or 4 of 18 showed some reduction in size of the calculi—all of which could have been from the antibiotic effect on the bacteria.

I personally interpret these data[37] as a disappointing response to AHA, and it is clearly incomparable to what can be accomplished with surgical removal, Renacidin irrigation, and careful attention to bacteriologic reinfection. On the other hand, there is no doubt that keeping the urine sterile on continuous antimicrobial therapy prevents bacterial growth in the urine and all the consequences of bacterial urease and alkalinization of the urine with subsequent struvite precipitation; under these circumstances there is a chance for struvite dissolution, as we pointed out in 1972.[38] In the report by Griffith *et al.*[37] five of nine patients had significant stone dissolution by just keeping the urine sterile with antimicrobial agents alone, but we are not told the amount of dissolution that occurred and apparently none was complete. To conclude, my own opinion is that AHA remains unproven as to its efficacy in stone dissolution, and the results by the Baylor group[37] are disappointing. Moreover, even when antimicrobial therapy alone keeps the urine sterile for months and years, I am afraid that patients like L.V. in Table 8.7 are extremely rare, and dissolution of struvite in the presence of a sterile urine is a tedious and unrewarding exercise for most patients. Its greatest benefit is to keep those patients who are poor operative risks asymptomatic in terms of urinary tract morbidity regardless of what happens to their calculi.

SOME SELECTED EXPERIMENTAL STUDIES

While calcium oxalate stones commonly show evidence of calyceal origin by the presence of a papillary depression at the base of a calyceal-shaped stone,[39] it is equally clear from Table 8.1 that most infection stones begin in the calyces as well. Only 2 of the 14 patients had their infection stones limited to the renal pelvis. Interestingly, these were the only two patients in whom the urea-splitting bacteria were not *P. mirabilis.*

Braude's[40] method of producing pyelonephritis in rats, using *Proteus morganii* as the infecting organism, was accompanied by a 20% incidence of struvite stone formation in the kidneys. These stones formed in direct continuity with the calyx, often showing papillary indentations. Thus, Braude's data and ours (Table 8.1) suggest that urea-splitting organisms begin struvite crystallization at the papillary tip; some experimental studies of the papillus in the earliest phase of struvite stone formation would be interesting to confirm these gross impressions.

Vermeulens[41–43] systematic and scientifically appealing series of papers on experimental urolithiasis contains several excellent publications on struvite stones. His work in 1951[41] demonstrated that not only did an acid urine prevent struvite stone formation in his model, but, when acidification was begun after stones had already been formed, complete dissolution of the calculi occurred in 14 of 20 animals.

In 1954, Vermeulen and Goetz[43] studied the effects of six different organisms on the rate of stone growth. While the urea-splitting organisms produced a striking increase in stone formation, nonurea-splitting bacteria augmented stone growth of the "calcium" type (nonstruvite or apatite stones). This observation is of interest to us because we have several instances in which *E. coli* have been recovered from within the depths of nonstruvite stones.

Vermeulen's[42] accidental but characteristically careful observation that at least one species of bacteria, *Salmonella enteritidis,* prevents and even dissolves struvite stones—in the absence of a change in pH—is interesting. Further experiments to understand the nature of this unexpected inhibition could be most rewarding.

The importance of infection and pH in struvite and apatite stone formation has also been demonstrated by experiments in mink.[44, 45] Urinary calculi in mink are composed chiefly of struvite; large scale feeding of NH_4Cl on mink ranches is known to reduce the incidence of struvite stones.[44] Nielsen,[45] however, in a most elegant paper, elucidated the pathogenesis of these calculi;

there are striking similarities to struvite stone formation in man. A urea-splitting *S. epidermidis* was present in most mink that formed calculi while normal mink had sterile urine. *P. mirabilis* and *Proteus* species were not uncommon. Reminiscent of Hellström's[2] studies in man, Gram-positive cocci were found deep in the stones within concentric layers of the matrix. Nielsen[45] also carefully investigated the question of renal plaque formation at the papillary tip, which he found to be common in both normal and calculus-forming mink. He concluded that infection of the urinary tract, chiefly with urea-splitting, hemolytic strains of *S. epidermidis,* is the basic etiology of struvite stone formation in ranch mink.

More recently, Griffith and Musher[46–48] at Baylor University have been active in experimental studies on bacterial urease—the enzyme with which *Proteus* and other bacteria split urea and thereby alkalinize the urine—and urease inhibitors; these studies have been an exciting part of their efforts to inhibit bacterial urease by AHA.

THREE INSTRUCTIVE PATIENTS WITH LONG TERM FOLLOW-UPS

Bilateral, Recurrent, Staghorn Infection Calculi in an Azotemic Patient

A.N., a 36-year-old Oriental, was first seen at Stanford by the Renal-Transplant group in 1967. Around 1956, at 25 years of age, she first experienced bilateral flank pain with recurrent low grade fevers. Bilateral staghorn calculi were found, and these

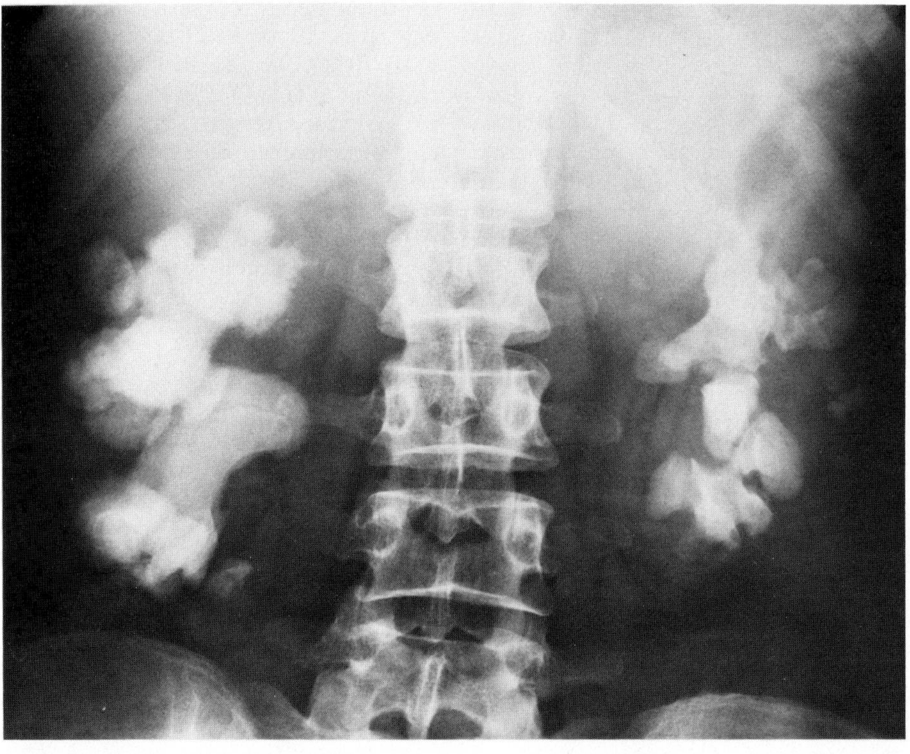

Figure 8.8 Plain film x-ray (August 1971) of A.N., a 40-year-old woman with a 15-year history of bilateral staghorn calculi, chronic *Proteus mirabilis* and *Escherichia coli* urinary tract infection and an unsuccessful attempt at bilateral nephrolithotomies in 1955 and 1956. Serum creatinine 1.5–2.5 mg%.

were partially removed in 1956 and 1957, but they soon recurred to full staghorn stones. Between 1957 and 1967, she was intermittently symptomatic with a mixed growth of *P. mirabilis* and *E. coli*; in May 1967, she was hospitalized for symptoms of an acute UTI, during which time her serum creatinine reached a peak of 2.7 mg%, but returned to 1.5 mg% by discharge. Several creatinines between 1967 and 1971, when I first saw her, were in the 1.5 mg% range, her blood pressure was always normal, and she was always infected with a hemolytic *E. coli* and a *P. mirabilis* regardless of antimicrobial therapy. Urinalysis invariably showed heavy pyuria, bacilli, and 10–50 mg% of protein. Her major symptoms were fatigue, backache, episodic dysuria, and some urinary frequency (two times nocturia). The *E. coli* and *P. mirabilis* had mutually exclusive sensitivities: the former was sensitive to tetracycline (1–2 μg/ml) and the latter to penicillin-G (2 μg/ml), ampicillin (1 μg/ml) and cephaloridine (1.5 μg/ml). She was tried on various antimicrobial agents when symptomatic between 1967 and 1971; not one culture out of many was ever free of the hemolytic *E. coli* or the *P. mirabilis.* The sensitivities to antimicrobial agents never changed: the *P. mirabilis* was always exquisitely sensitive to penicillin-G and its analogues (to which the *E. coli* was resistant) and the E. coli was always sensitive to tetracycline (to which the *P. mirabilis* was resistant).

I first saw her in August 1971. Her creatinine clearance was 28 ml/minute (uncorrected) and her serum creatinine 1.4 mg% (she weighed 53 kilograms). Her blood pressure was 110/80 mm Hg. A plain film of the abdomen showed massive staghorn calculi in both kidneys (Figure 8.8) which does not look much different from the 15-minute IVU (Figure 8.9). Because of the nonfunc-

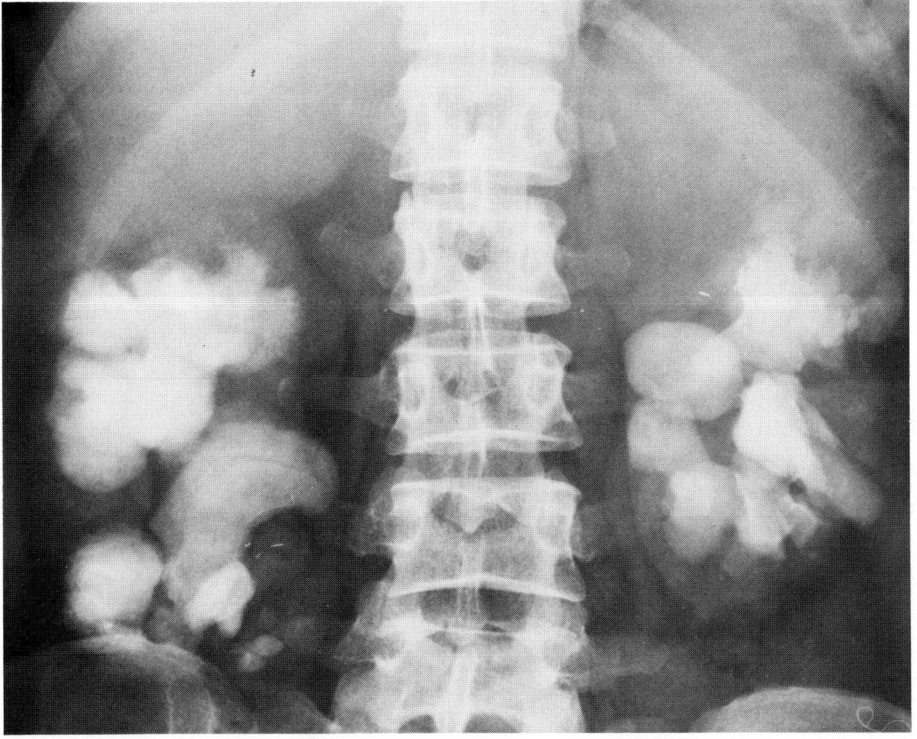

Figure 8.9 A 15-minute intravenous urogram (August 1971). Some contrast excretion can be seen when compared to Figure 8.8.

tioning upper half of the left kidney, a percutaneous needle aspiration showed a purulent, cyst-like cavity that grew hemolytic *E. coli* and *P. mirabilis* (Figure 8.10). A serum creatinine on admission to the hospital was 2.8 mg%, which was surprising; her CO_2 was 20 mEq/liter and her BUN was 30 mg%. A voiding cystourethrogram showed no reflux to either kidney.

The left kidney was operated upon in late August 1971; preoperative and intraoperative gentamicin was given, to which both bacteria were sensitive. The left renal "cyst" proved to be a dilated upper calyx with renal calculus extending through the infundibulum; three other cystic calyces were also unroofed in the lower two-thirds of the kidney, each filled with purulent urine, and each requiring closure of the exposed infundibulum after the protruding calculi were removed. An intraoperative x-ray film appeared to be free of residual calculi (Figure 8.11), but the irregularity of the kidney cortex from her previous surgery, calyceal obstruction, and infection was substantial, and clearly not ideal for radiographic visualization of soft struvite fragments. As is our routine, a multi-holed, polyethylene catheter was left in the kidney for postoperative irrigation. Plain film tomograms on the fourth postoperative day showed a single residual calculus in the upper pole of the left kidney (Figure 8.12); a nephrostomy injection with saline and contrast agent showed no extravasation and good filling of the renal calyces (Figure 8.13). After 24 hours of saline irrigation at 120 ml/hour without difficulty, she was started on Renacidin irrigation on the 5th postoperative day. Because of bladder

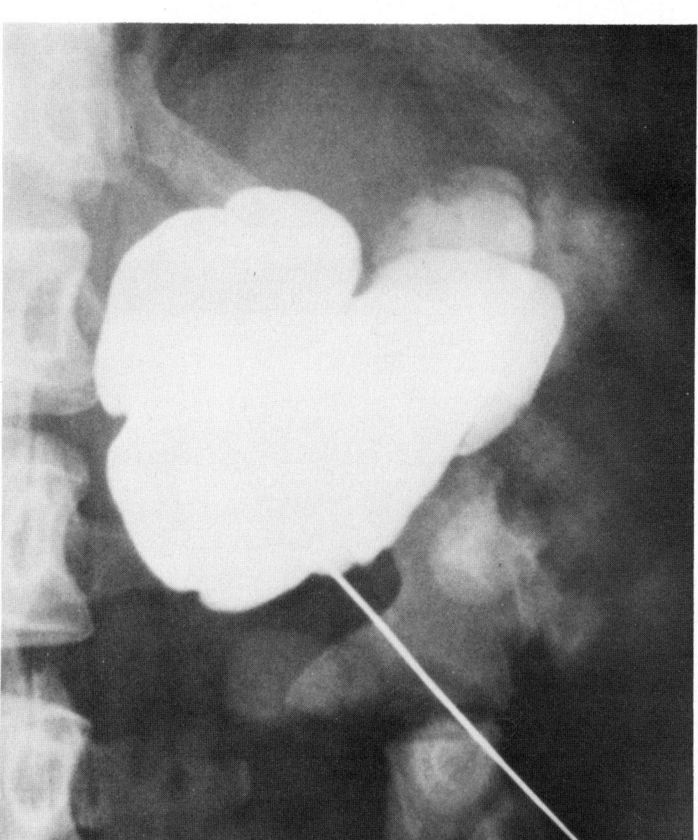

Figure 8.10 Infected calyceal, cystic dilatation in left renal upper pole of A.N. See text.

spasms 48 hours later, a ureteral catheter was passed to the left renal pelvis and used as the inflow tube for irrigation. Between cephalothin and tetracycline, the urine from the nephrostomy tube was kept sterile, but irrigation was stopped for 3 days in order to regain sterile control of the nephrostomy drainage. By the 5th day of Renacidin irrigation, only a faint trace remained of the upper calyceal stone; by the 7th day of irrigation no stones were visible on tomograms. She was discharged on the 17th postoperative day and readmitted for surgery on the right staghorn calculus 3 days later. Her serum creatinine was 1.7 mg% on discharge.

The right kidney was operated upon in mid-September 1971; the findings were about the same as with the left kidney. Much of the stone was removed utilizing the surgical approach of Boyce and Smith.[10] The calculi (from both kidneys) were "88% struvite and 12% carbonate apatite." As would be expected, the pathologist found evidence of extensive pyelonephritis and squamous metaplasia of the calyceal epithelium in both kidneys. Again, the intraoperative film appeared free of residual cal-

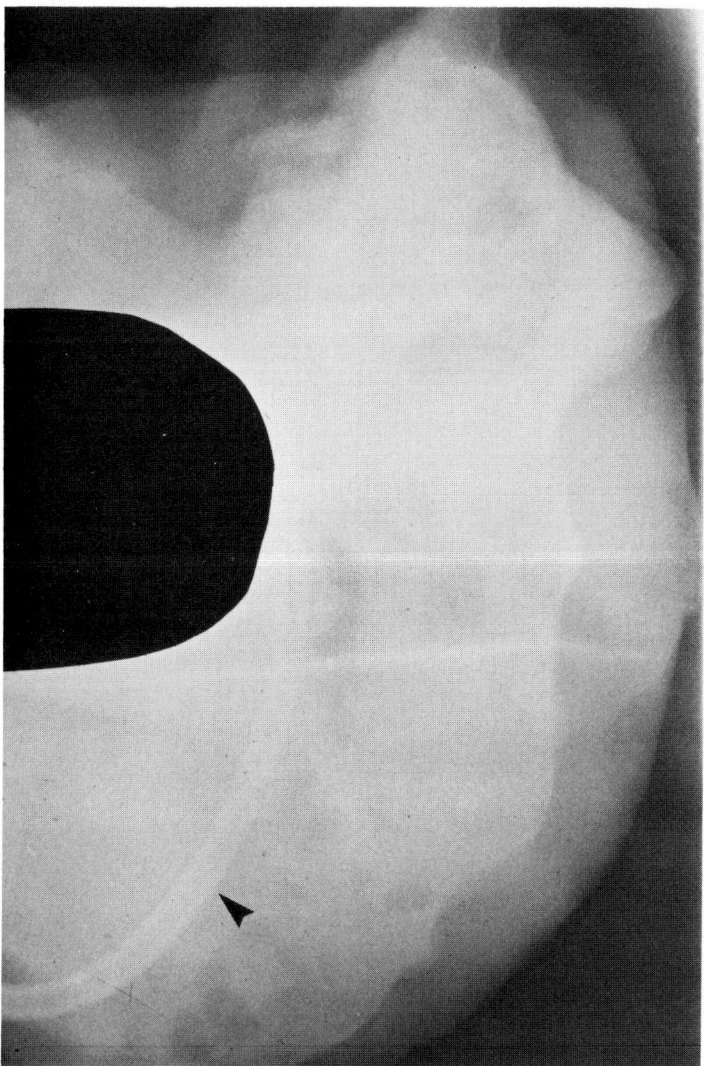

Figure 8.11 Intraoperative x-ray film of the left kidney after removing the staghorn calculus in A.N. in August 1971. *Arrow* marks the multiholed polyethelene catheter left for nephrostomy drainage and later irrigation with Renacidin.

culi (Figure 8.14) but, as can be seen, the renal cortex was very bumpy and irregular. Postoperative tomograms on the 4th day showed one fragment of calculus almost resting at the tip of the multi-holed polyethylene catheter (Figure 8.15). After 24 hours of saline irrigation through a ureteral catheter (placed at the time of surgery) and out the nephrostomy tube, without any morbidity, 10% Renacidin was begun. By the 8th day of irrigation, the stone was dissolved (Figure 8.16) and the Renacidin irrigation discontinued 24 hours later. The polyethylene nephrostomy tube can be seen in Figure 8.16, as well as the fact that no residual stone fragments are seen in either kidney. She was discharged on the 15th postoperative day on cephalexin, but the appearance of her old hemolytic *E. coli* at the first outpatient visit required the addition of tetracycline. Her serum creatinine was 2.3 mg% on discharge.

On this regimen of tetracycline and cephalexin therapy, her midstream urine remained free of any colonies of Enterobacteriaceae although she grew *Candida albicans* in her urine almost from the first postoperative culture. She was maintained

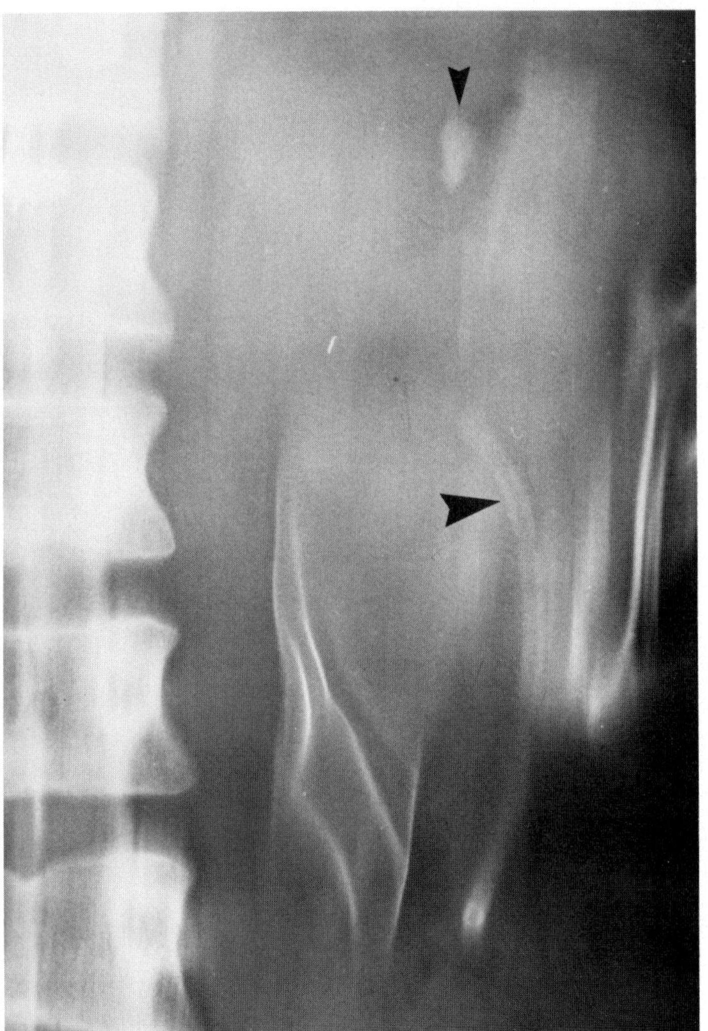

Figure 8.12 Tomogram on 4th postoperative day of A.N. showing residual stone fragment in left upper pole (*small arrow*), polyethelene nephrostomy tube (*large arrow*), and the Penrose drain, which should be removed before taking tomographic x-rays.

on 250 mg of tetracycline and cephalexin twice daily from November 1971 until July 1973; 10 urine cultures during this interval showed only *C. albicans* in the urine. She felt great, was asymptomatic, and had the most energy she had felt in over a decade. Her serum creatinine varied between 1.5 mg% and 1.7 mg%.

In August 1973, 2 years after removing all her calculi, all antibiotics were stopped. A bladder aspiration 30 days later showed 500 *C. albicans*/ml of urine but nothing else. Because cultures at 2 weeks and 4 weeks after stopping her antibiotics had shown *P. mirabilis*, *E. coli*, and *Klebsiella* on the vaginal introitus, I started her on one-half tablet of TMP-SMX each night rather than risk a recurrence of her urinary infection, especially the *P. mirabilis*. She has remained on TMP-SMX prophylaxis for all of these 6 years. Several cultures per year have never shown a single colony of Enterobacteriaceae on the introitus or in the urine. She is continually infected with *C. albicans* without any apparent harm. I did sterilize her urine in August 1973, with 10 days of 5-fluoro-cytosine, 500 mg every 6 hours, but the *C. albicans* returned immediately after stopping it. All her urines continually show 30–60 glitter cells/high power field in the spun sediment, but she has no protein (3% sulfasalicylic acid method), and her serum creatinines have remained unchanged in the range of 1.5 mg%–2.0 mg%. Her last creatinine on June 1, 1979 was 1.8 mg%, her BUN was 31 mg%, and her CO_2 was 25 mEq/liter.

Plain film tomograms and intravenous urograms have been repeated every 1–2 years. Representative films, including the

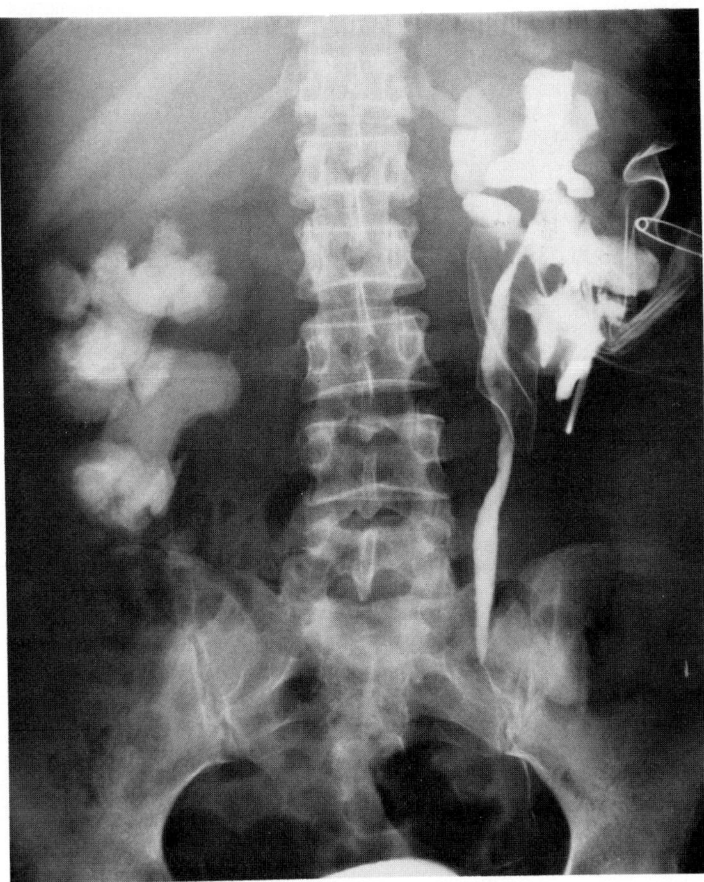

Figure 8.13 Nephrostomy injection by gravity in A.N. on the 4th postoperative day showing no extravasation and good filling of the kidney in the area of the residual stone (Figure 8.12).

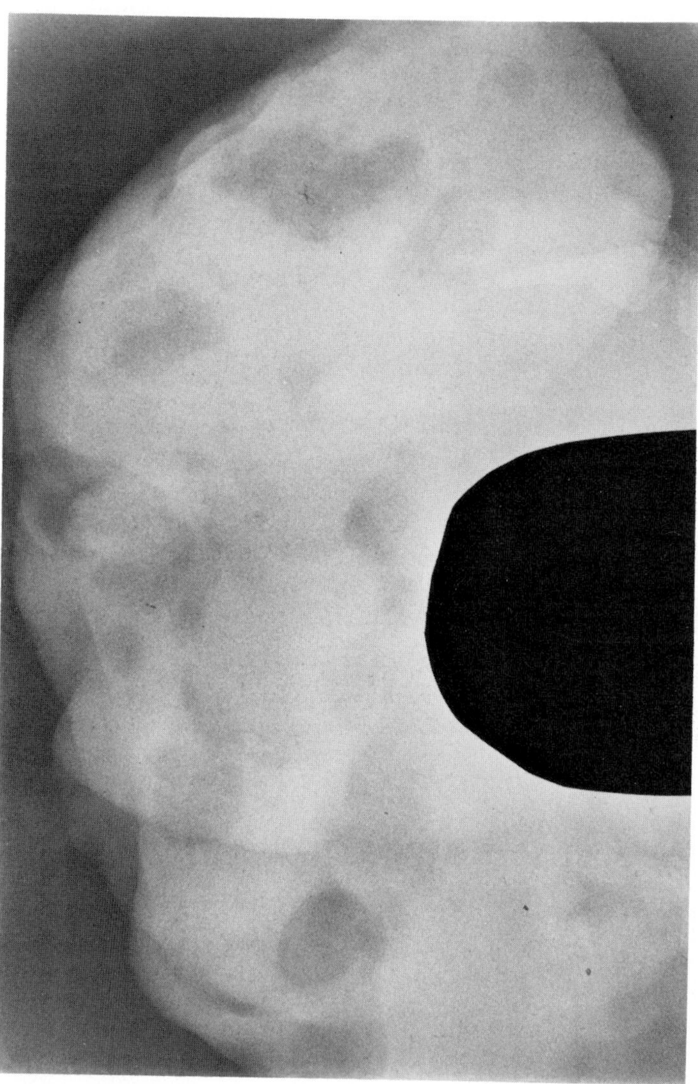

Figure 8.14 Intraoperative x-ray film of right kidney in A.N. following removal of the staghorn calculus. Note the irregularity of the renal cortex from previous surgery, obstruction, and infection.

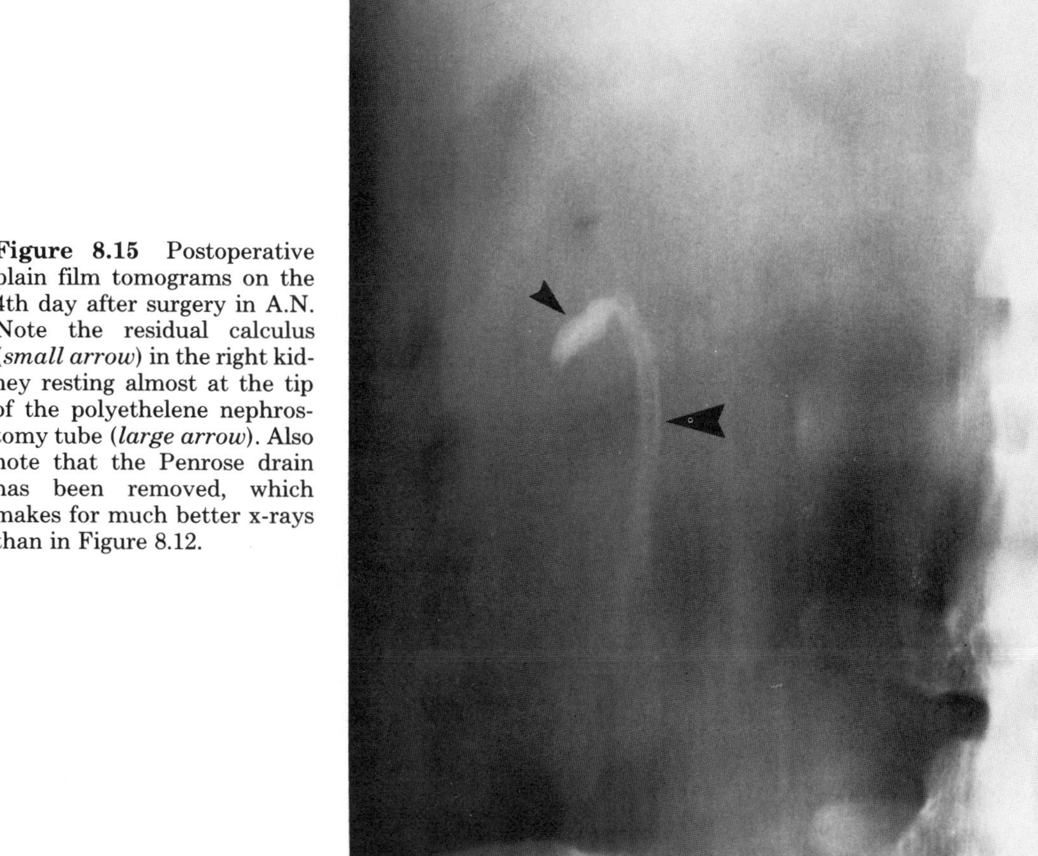

Figure 8.15 Postoperative plain film tomograms on the 4th day after surgery in A.N. Note the residual calculus (*small arrow*) in the right kidney resting almost at the tip of the polyethelene nephrostomy tube (*large arrow*). Also note that the Penrose drain has been removed, which makes for much better x-rays than in Figure 8.12.

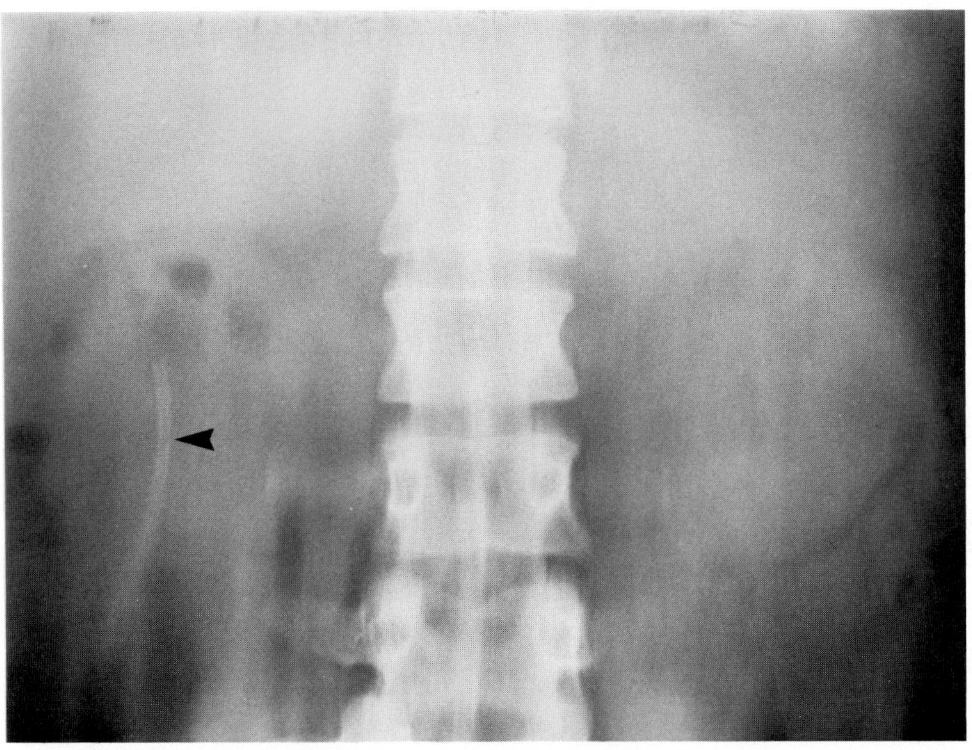

Figure 8.16 Final plain film tomogram in A.N. after 8 days of irrigating the right kidney with 10% Renacidin. The stone is dissolved; the polyetheline catheter for nephrostomy irrigation is easily seen (*arrow*). Compare to Figure 8.15.

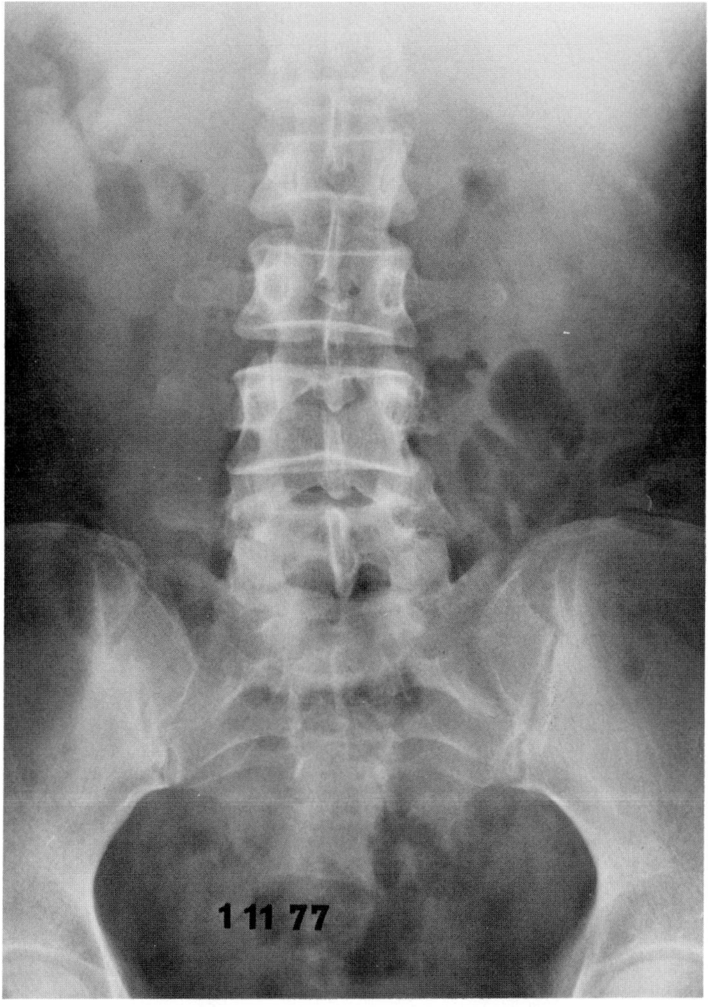

Figure 8.17 Plain film x-ray of an intravenous urogram on A.N. made 5½ years after surgical removal and Renacidin dissolution of bilateral staghorn calculi. There are no residual calculi.

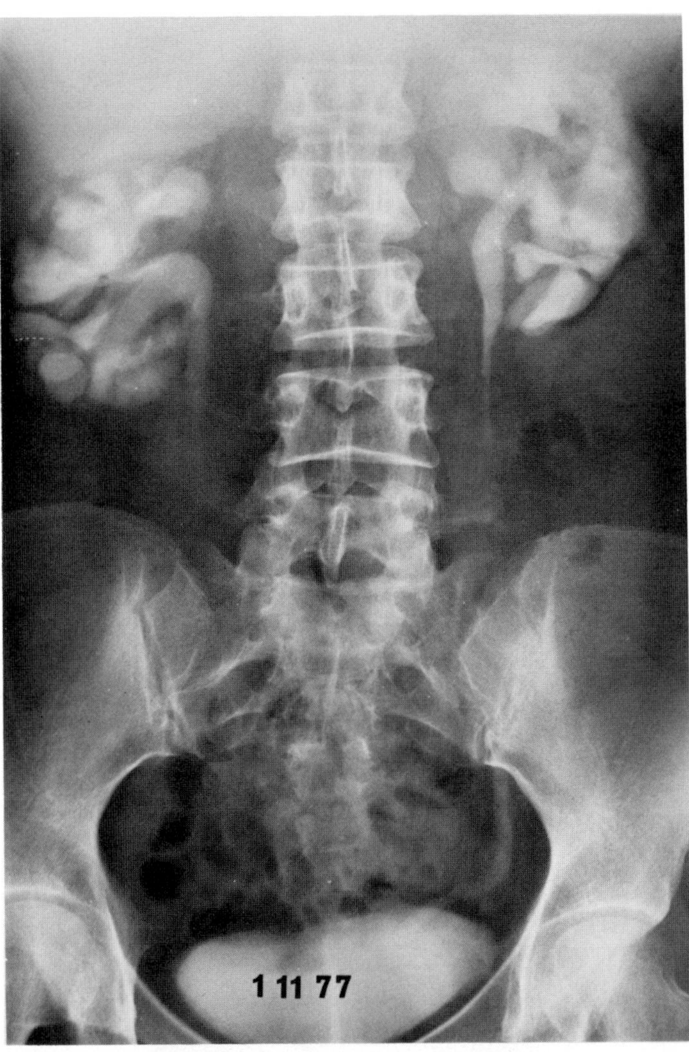

Figure 8.18 A 30-minute intravenous urogram 5½ years after surgical removal of staghorn calculi in A.N. Serum creatinine 1.7 mg%.

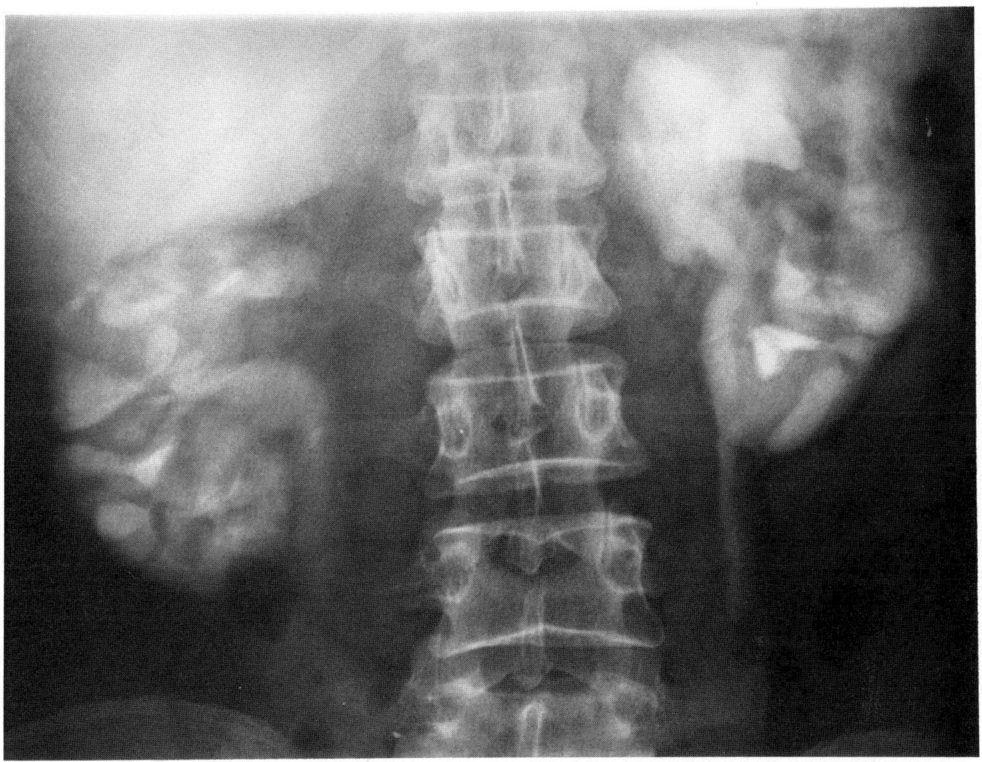

Figure 8.19 A 10-minute intravenous urogram on June 12, 1979, 8 years after bilateral staghorn surgery on A.N. The right kidney measures 10.0 cm and the left 11.3 cm. This film was made immediately after release of ureteral compression. It should be compared to Figures 8.8 and 8.9.

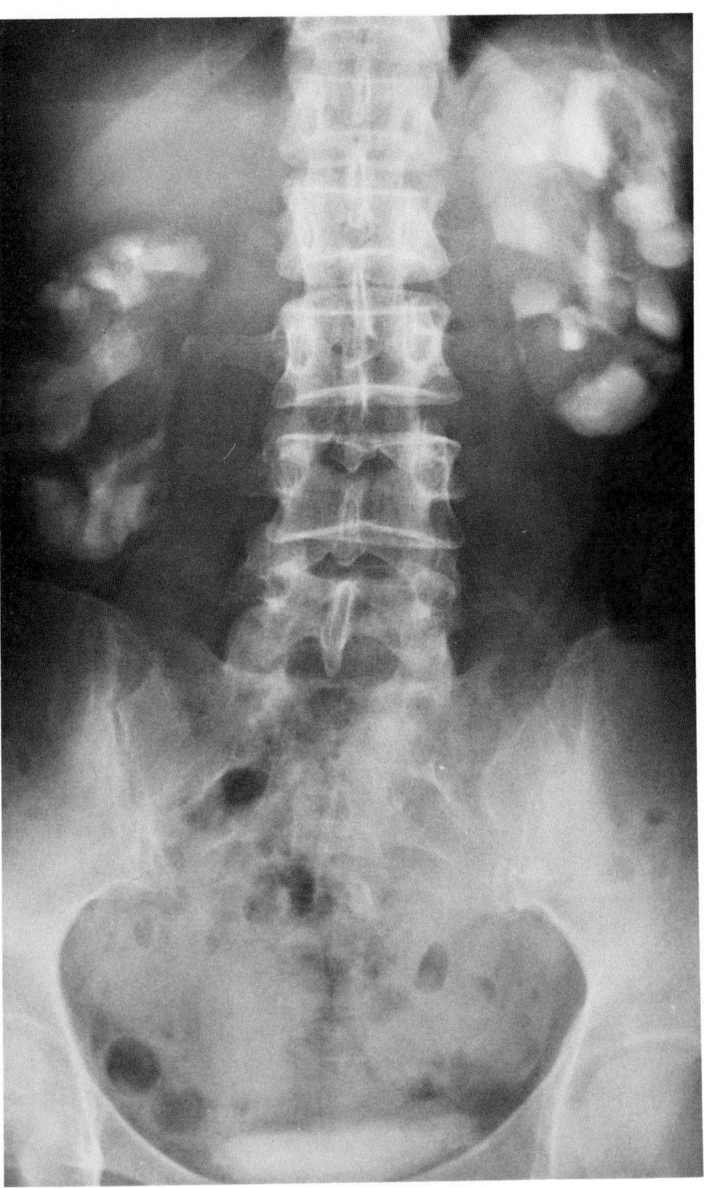

Figure 8.20 A postvoid, upright film from the intravenous urogram on A.N. from June 12, 1979. Her serum creatinine was 1.8 mg%, her blood pressure was 110/70 mm Hg (on propranolol and hydrochlorothiazide), and she is much healthier than in 1971 (Figures 8.8 and 8.9) when she had bilateral staghorn calculi with hydronephrosis and infection.

most recent IVU, are presented in Figures 8.17–8.20.

In November 1973, 2 years after removing the staghorn calculi, she was found to be hypertensive, in fact, 175/105 mm Hg. She was immediately treated with propranolol and hydrochlorothiazide and remains on these drugs to this day, but her blood pressure is normal (110/70 mm Hg in June 1979). I attribute her steady renal function as much to controlling her hypertension as to the prophylactic prevention of further infections due to *P. mirabilis* and a recurrence of her staghorn calculi.

Lastly, I should add that liberal renal biopsies at the time of both of my surgeries showed extensive squamous metaplasia of the renal pelvic and calyceal epithelium. Because of this, I have obtained cytologies of her bladder urine twice a year, but all her squamous cells have remained benign.

I believe this patient is a classic example of what can be accomplished in severe staghorn calculi if Renacidin irrigation is used postoperatively to dissolve any residual fragments and if a careful bacteriologic vigil is maintained to prevent reinfection with *P. mirabilis.* To be sure, careful control of the blood pressure is equally important in any patient with renal disease.

The Subtlety of Early Infection Stones and the Importance of Plain Film Tomograms

S.S., a 25-year old white gravida 3, para 3 patient was admitted to Stanford for the first time on August 22, 1971 with an 8-year history of recurrent UTI, which apparently began with her early pregnancies. Some of her infections were considered to be kidney infections, and she had considerable flank discomfort with two of her pregnancies. An IVU obtained in August 1969 (Figures 8.21

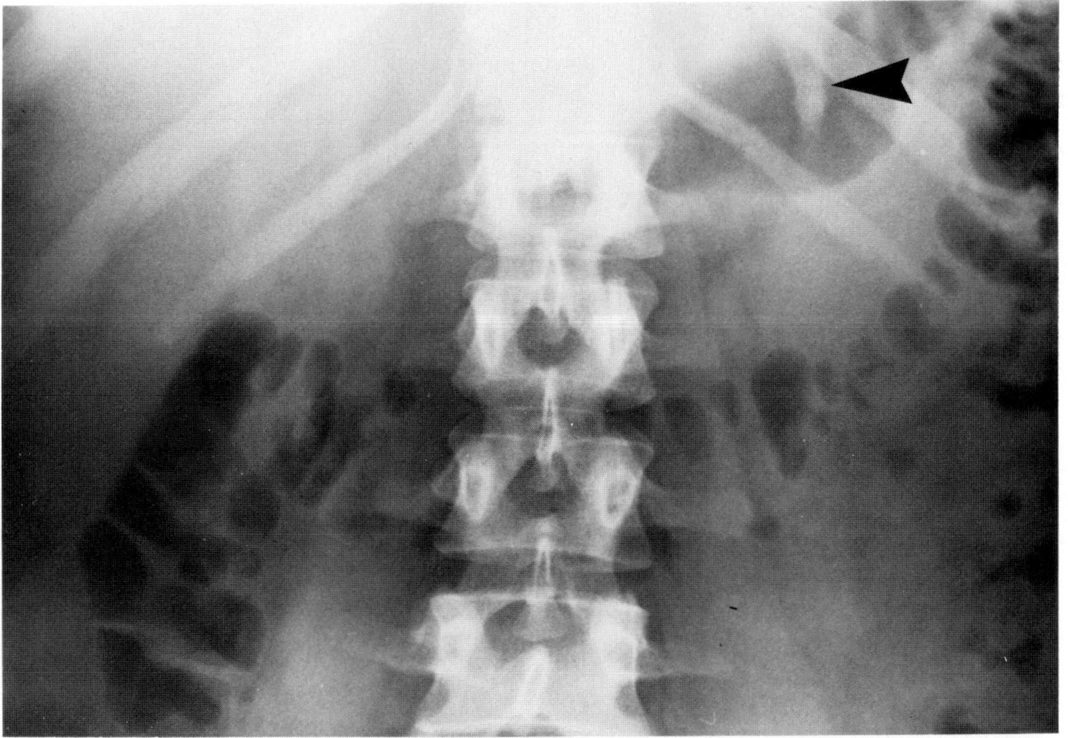

Figure 8.21 A plain film x-ray on S.S., a 25-year-old white woman with an 8-year history of recurrent urinary tract infection. This film, made when she was 23 years old, was considered normal; the *arrow* indicates what must have been thought to be normal gastric shadows, but what was, in fact, a struvite calculus.

-8.23) showed substantial right ureterectasis and pyelectasis but the calyces were delicate and drained well (Figure 8.23); a right nephropexy was done following exploration of the right ureter. Her recurrent infections were not improved. In January 1971, she was seen by another urologist who recognized a staghorn calculus in the left kidney (Figure 8.24); at fluoroscopy, he noted the right ureter was dilated and atonic with poor peristalsis, and both ureteral urines apparently cultured *P. mirabilis*. There was no reflux on an excellent voiding cystourethrogram. He placed her on penicillin-G and ascorbic acid and referred her to me at Stanford.

We obtained plain film tomograms (Figures 8.25 and 8.26) which should be compared to Figures 8.21 and 8.24; the value of tomographic cuts when there is overlying bowel gas or feces is clearly apparent. We stopped her penicillin-G and cystoscoped her the following day. The catheterized bladder urine contained 30 *P. mirabilis*/ml, and the washed bladder culture obtained immediately before passing the ureteral catheters to the kidneys (see Chapter 1) was sterile. Four consecutive cultures from

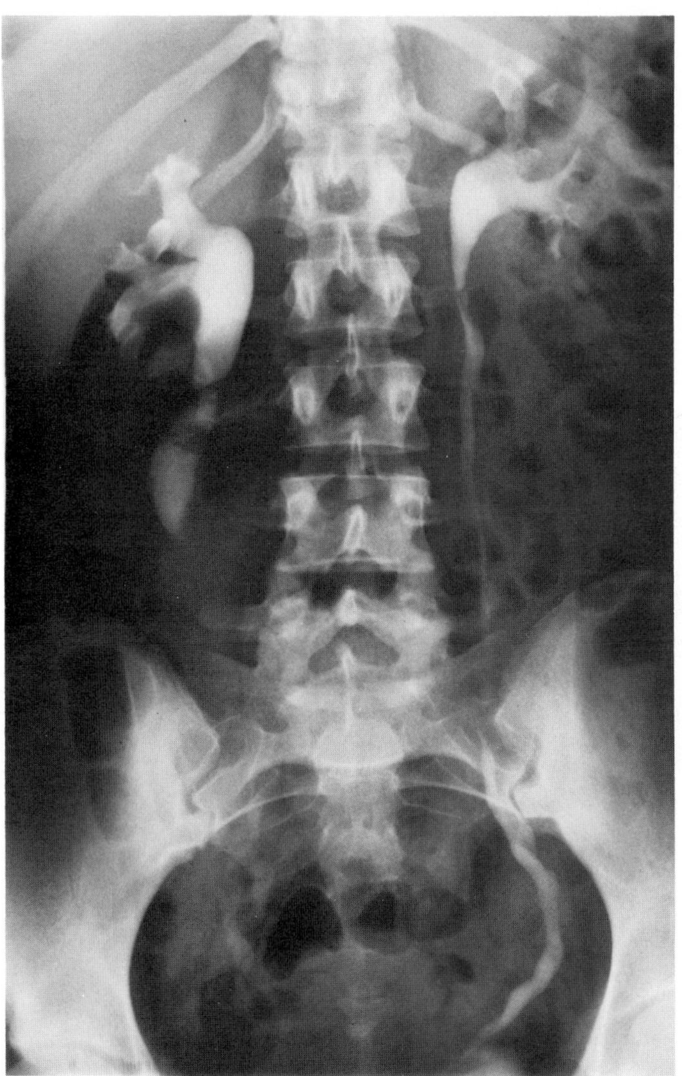

Figure 8.22 An intravenous urogram made immediately after the plain film shown in Figure 8.21. Note the delicate left renal structures and the obvious right renal ureterectasis and pyelectasis. In retrospect, the filling defect in the left upper infundibulum and calyx are easily seen; the overlying gas from the stomach probably made this difficult to detect.

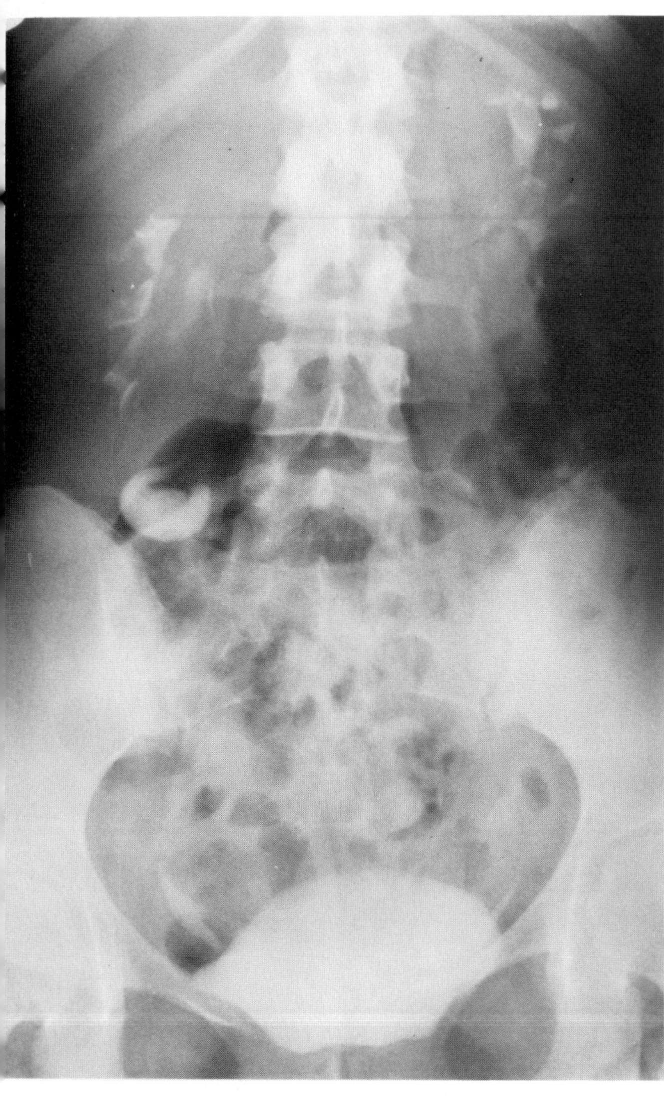

Figure 8.23 A delayed, upright film from the intravenous urogram in Figures 8.21 and 8.22. Note the midureteral dilatation, the poor drainage from the left upper calyces, and the absence of obstruction in the lower ureters.

the right kidney were sterile, but the four from the left kidney showed *P. mirabilis* (Table 8.8).

At the time of ureteral catheteriztion, three consecutive collection periods for renal function studies were obtained without bladder leakage around the polyethylene Stamey catheters. These three clearances are averaged and presented in Table 8.9. They show the hallmarks of renal function when an infected kidney is compared to a contralateral sterile one (see Chapter 3): although the left kidney has substantially less renal function than the right kidney in terms of the creatinine clearance, the left kidney excretes much more water and sodium than the contralateral kidney. Gentamicin was started immediately after removing the ureteral catheters.

She was explored the next day, on August 25, 1971, through a flank incision using the Boyce technique.[10] The calculi were extracted and an intra-operative x-ray showed all the stone was apparently removed (Figure 8.27). I show this film so the reader can contrast it with Figures 8.11 or 8.14; intra-operative radiographs are infinitely more reliable in the absence of renal scarring.

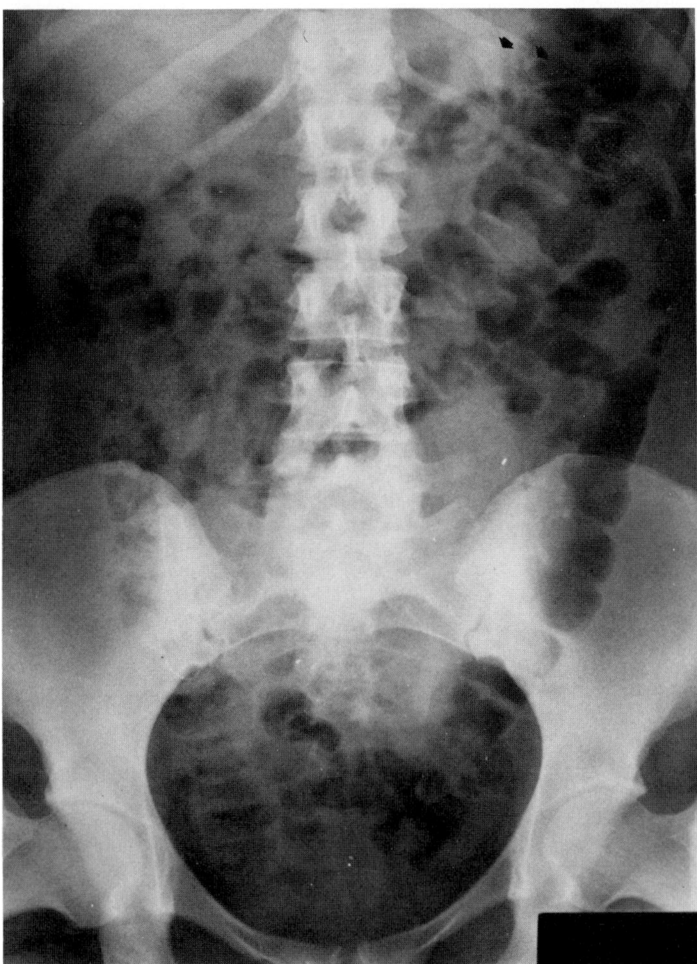

Figure 8.24 Plain film from an intravenous urogram on S.S. made in January 1971 from which the upper pole left renal calcifications were first identified (indicated by the *two arrows*).

Despite this film showing no possibility of residual calculi, we left the small, multi-holed polyethylene tube in the kidney for nephrostomy drainage and irrigation with Renacidin. On the 4th postoperative day, plain film tomograms confirmed the absence of radiologically visible calculi, a nephrostogram showed no extravasation (Figure 8.28), and after 24 hours of saline irrigation, 10% Renacidin was run through the kidney at 120 ml/hour for 24 hours. Her urine remained sterile on gentamicin throughout her hospitalization, and she was discharged on the 12th postoperative day.

The stone culture showed 10 *P. mirabilis*/ml in the first wash (see Figure 8.1), none in the fourth wash, and 450 *P. mirabilis*/ml in the crushed stone culture. The stone analysis showed "82% struvite, 18% carbonate-apatite."

She has been followed by her referring urologist since discharge because she lives out of state. IVUs on July 26, 1972, October 2, 1974, and July 1976 showed no calculi in either kidney and the right kidney has not changed its ureterectasis. At least one *E. coli* infection was documented with lower tract symptoms in 1974 for which she was placed on TMP-SMX prophylaxis. Cultures since then have been sterile (as expected) and she has remained asymptomatic.

This young woman illustrates how subtle a beginning staghorn calculus can be (Fig-

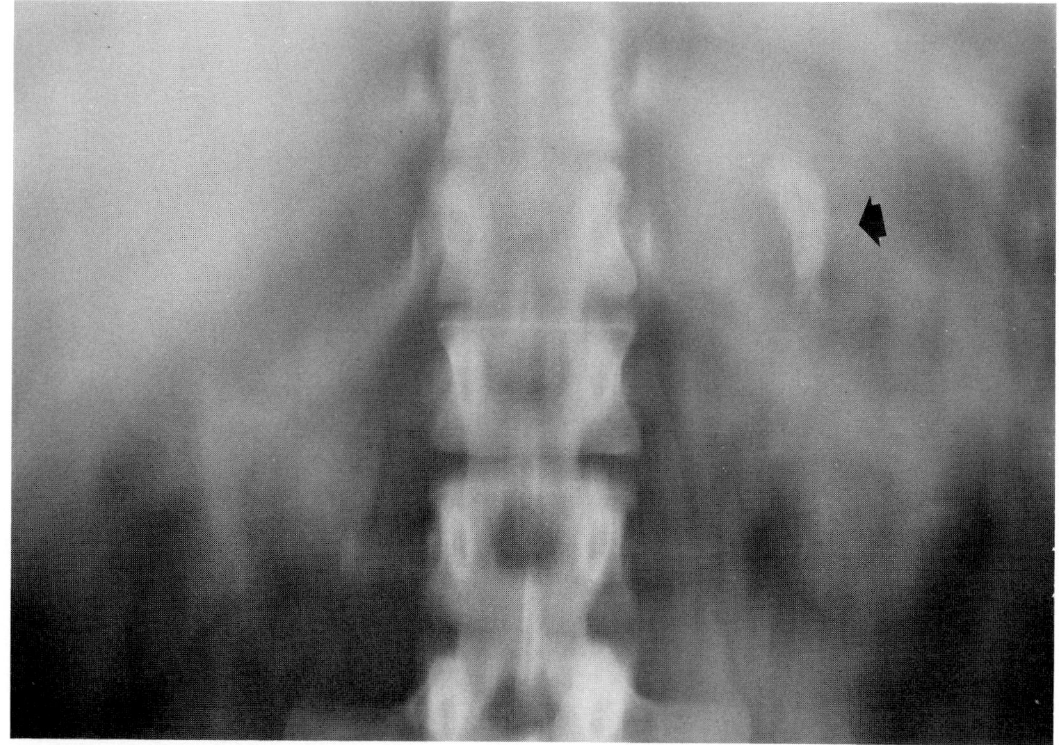

Figure 8.25 Plain film tomograms made at Stanford in August 1971. Note how dramatically plain film tomography allows soft, struvite renal stones (*arrow*) to be seen. Compare this figure to Figures 8.21 and 8.24.

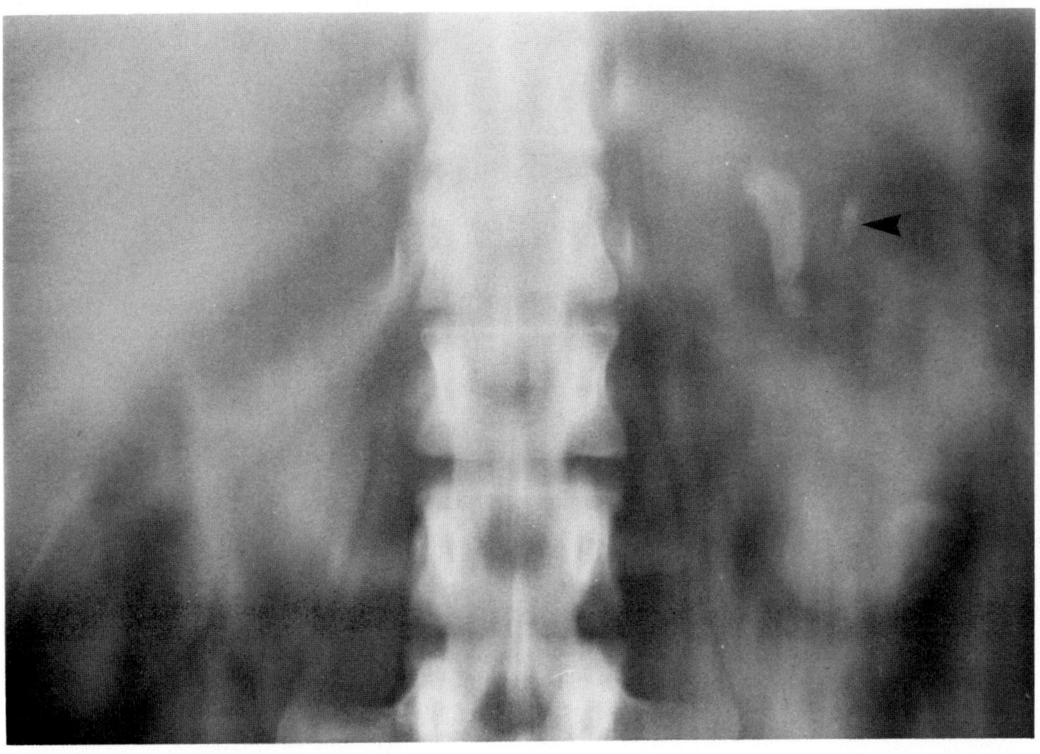

Figure 8.26 A plain film tomogram from the same series as Figure 8.25, but 0.5 cm different in depth. The small calyceal stone is indicated by the *arrow*.

ure 8.21) and how easily missed on a plain film x-ray that has overlying gas or feces; and yet, how obvious it can be with plain film tomography. Without question, the easiest way to make the diagnosis is to recognize that repeated cultures which show *P. mirabilis* must be associated with an infection stone. But in the absence of culture data like those in Figure 8.4, the physician should obtain plain film tomograms in his search for the cause of recurrent bacteriuria if the regular plain film of the IVU has overlying gas or feces.

The second reason for presenting this patient is how well she illustrates the fruits of our urologic teachings that residual urine predisposes the patient to urinary infection. Without question the right ureter was atonic and there was residual urine on that side compared to the delicate, nonobstructed left kidney. And yet, the *P. mirabilis* did not infect the atonic right renal system but rather the nonobstructed, delicate left kidney. It is perhaps understandable why the right kidney was explored in an effort to stop her recurrent infections, but much of the fault lies with us because we have taught that residual urine predisposes the patient to UTI. I do not believe that it does.

Table 8.8
Bacteriologic Localization Studies on Patient S.S., a 25-Year-Old Female

Source	Culture
	Proteus mirabilis/ml
CB[a]	30
WB	0
RK1	0
RK2	0
RK3	0
RK4	0
LK1	340
LK2	960
LK3	100
LK4	320

[a] CB = catheterized bladder; WB = washed bladder; K1–K4 = Serial cultures from the left (L) and right (R) kidney.

Reinfection with *P. Mirabilis* in a 4 Year-Old Girl after Complete Removal of a Staghorn Infection Calculus

T.K., a 4 year-old white girl, was admitted to Stanford in June, 1977. In 1973, at the age of 8 months, she had a febrile illness that resolved with antibiotics. During 1976 her mother noticed several episodes of foul-smelling urine. In January 1977, she had an episode of hematuria which was treated with antibiotics without a culture. Her first documented UTI was early April 1977 when she had a fever to 102°F.; *P. mirabilis* was cultured from the urine and her infection resolved on ampicillin therapy. An IVU (Figures 8.29 and 8.30) on April 13, 1977 showed a complete staghorn calculus filling every calyx; a voiding cystourethrogram (VCU) showed no reflux (Figure 8.31). She was cystoscoped and the *P. mirabilis* localized to the right kidney (Table 8.10); the bladder and ureteral orifices were normal. She was treated with TMP-SMX for 2 weeks after the cystoscopy; when it was stopped, her fever and *P. mirabilis* returned and she again responded to TMP-SMX. Her urinalysis was always loaded with glitter cells (polymorphonuclear leukocytes) and 10–50 red blood cells/high power field.

On admission to Stanford on June 6, 1977 she was started on gentamicin, 20 mg every 8 hours. A complete blood count was nor-

Table 8.9
Differential Renal Function Studies on Patient S.S.

	Urine Flow Rate	L/R	Sodium Concentration	L/R	Creatinine Concentration	L/R	Creatinine Clearance	L/R
	ml/min		*mEq/L*		*mg %*		*ml/min/1.73*	
Left kidney	1.89	2.3	48.6	2.0	15.5	0.22	32	0.57
Right kidney	0.82		24.0		69.6		56	

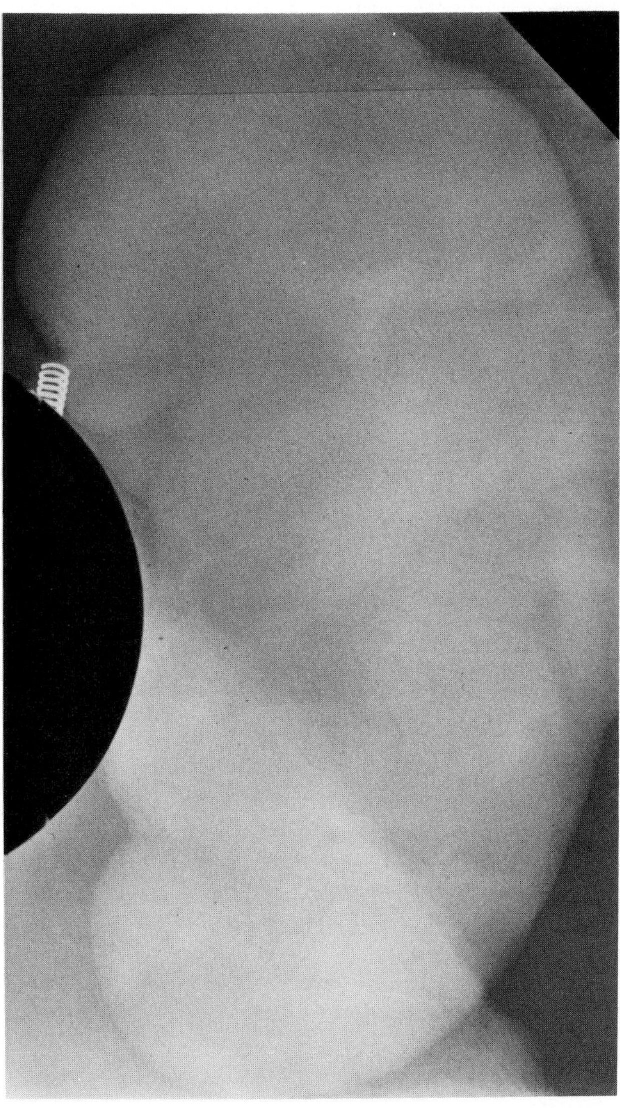

Figure 8.27 Intraoperative plain film of the kidney after removing all the calculi from the left upper pole of the kidney. This smooth detailed x-ray should be compared with Figures 8.11 and 8.14. Films such as this one are much more reliable in excluding residual fragments than those in scarred, irregular kidneys.

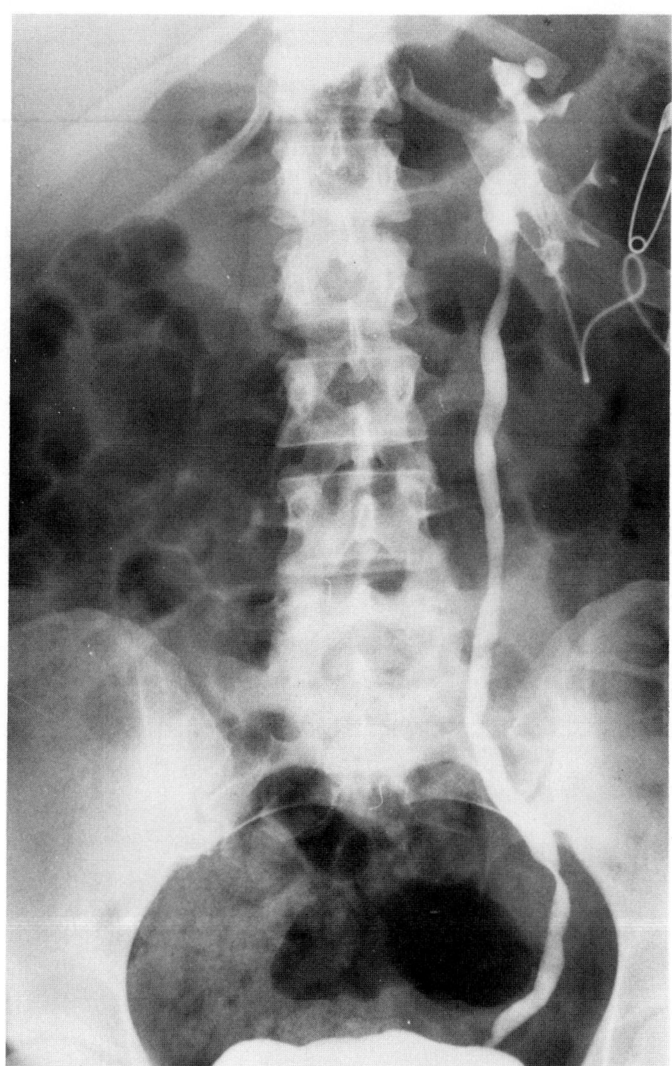

Figure 8.28 Gravity nephrostogram in patient S.S. on the 4th postoperative day. There was no extravasation of contrast agent. The Penrose drain, which should have been removed, overlies the medial portion of the kidney. Note the minimal distortion of the operated calyces.

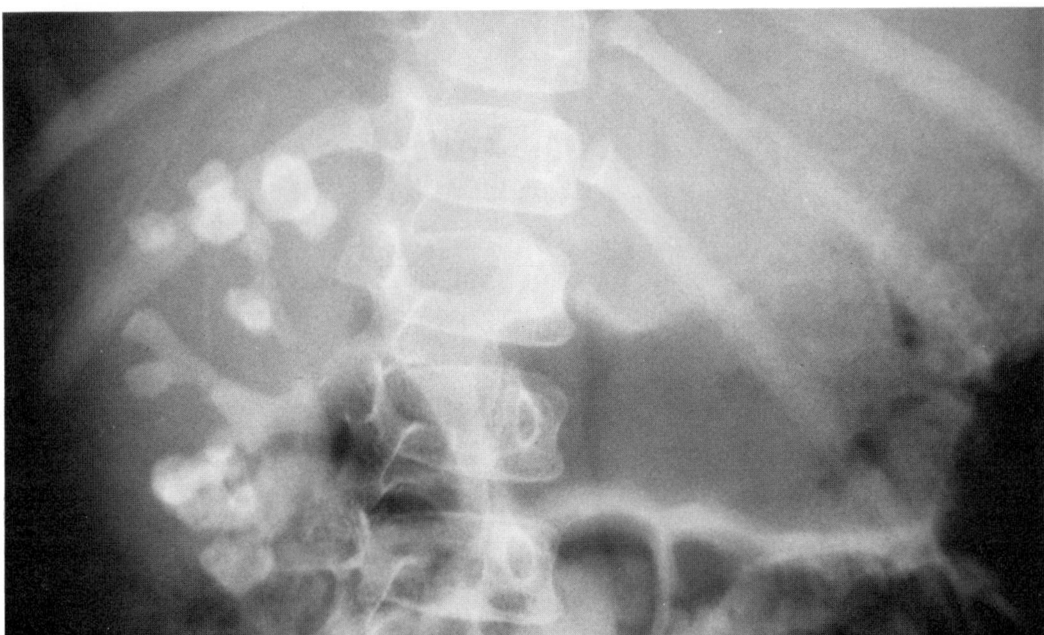

Figure 8.29 Plain film x-ray from intravenous urogram of April 13, 1977 on T.K., a 4-year-old white girl with recurrent *P. mirabilis* urinary tract infection.

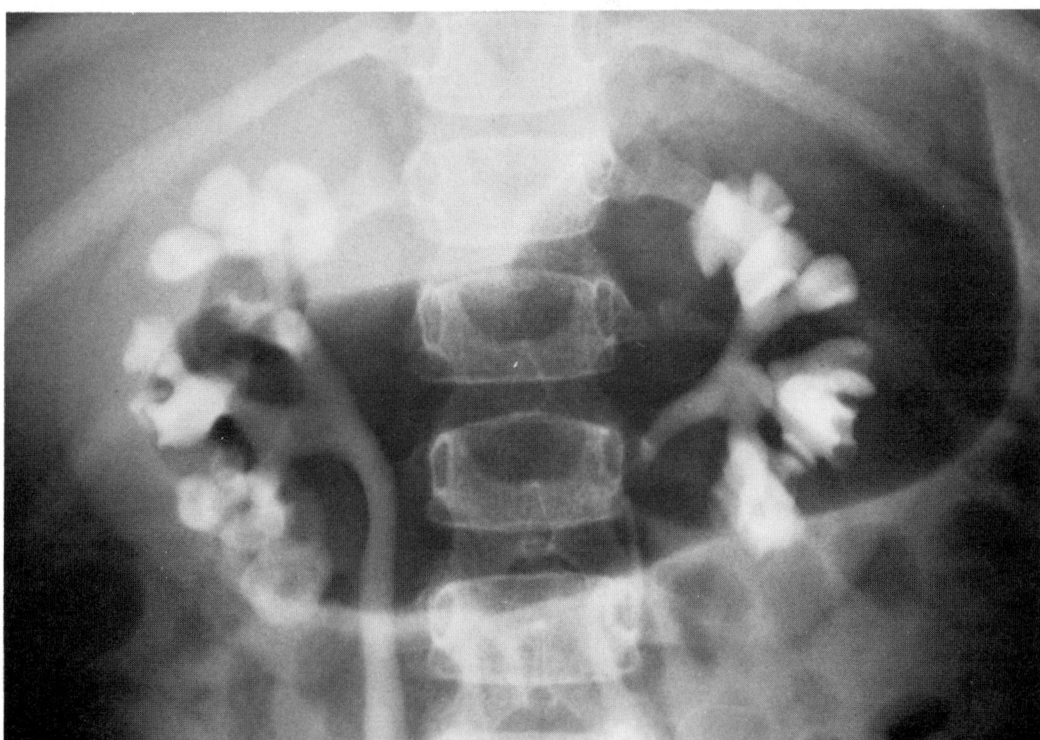

Figure 8.30 A 15-minute intravenous urogram from examination of April 13, 1977 on T.K. Note the smooth renal cortex in the right kidney despite the staghorn calculus (Figure 8.29).

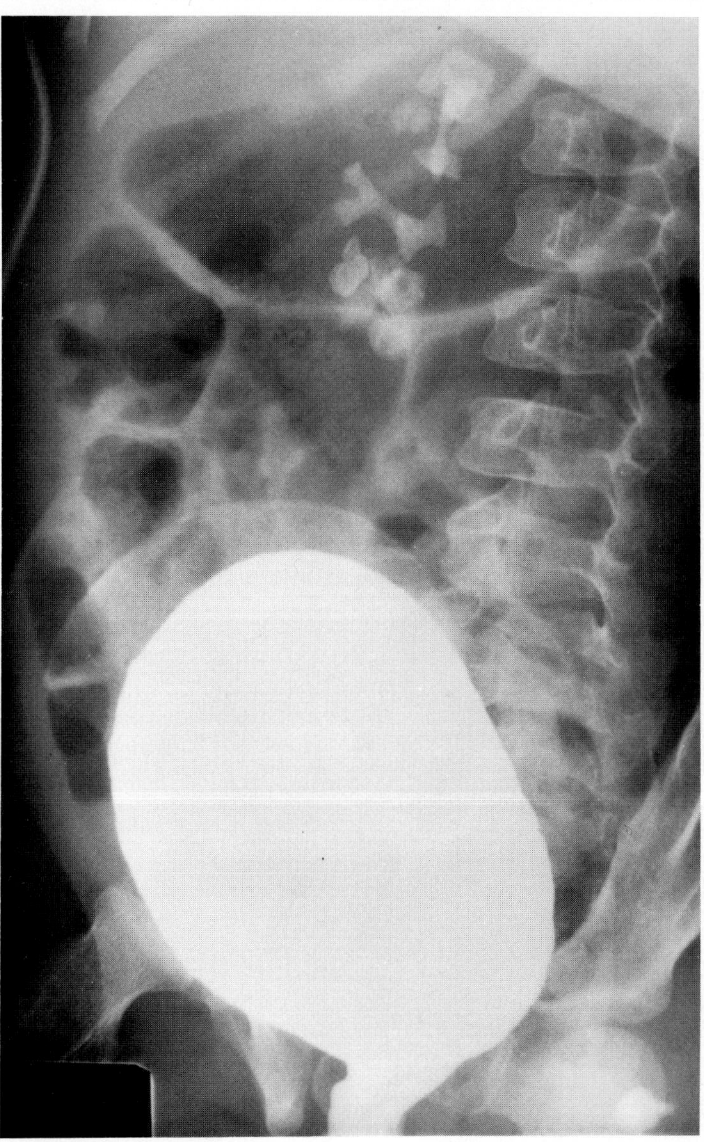

Figure 8.31 Voiding cystourethrogram on T.K. There is no reflux. The right staghorn calculus is seen nicely on this oblique view.

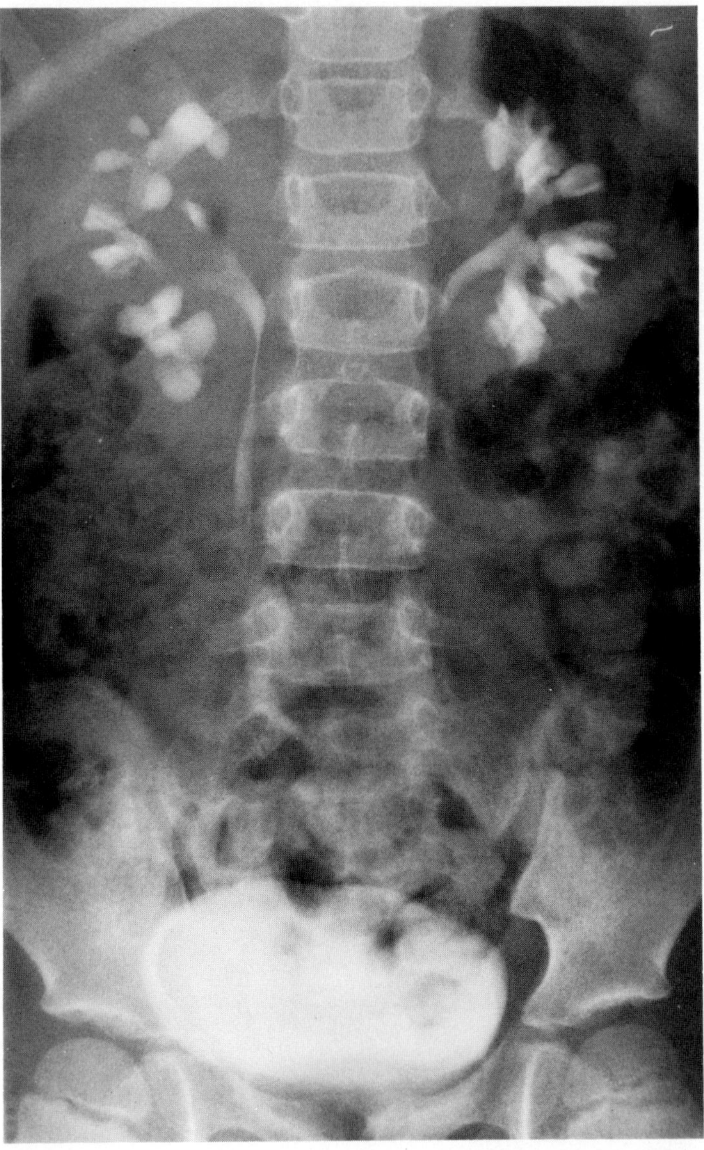

Figure 8.32 An intravenous urogram on T.K. made 10 weeks after removal of the staghorn calculus. The plain film x-ray showed no residual calculi.

mal, her serum calcium was 9.9 mg%, uric acid 2.2 mg%, and a serum creatinine was 0.5 mg%. Her blood pressure was normal as was her height and weight for her age. A urine culture on June 7 was sterile and she was operated on June 8, 1977. All of the calculi were removed, and a multi-holed polyethylene catheter left in place as a nephrostomy tube. Four days after surgery, plain film tomograms showed no residual calculi, a nephrostogram was done on the 6th day without extravasation, saline irrigation was begun on the 7th day, and 10% Renacidin was run through the kidney for 32 hours on the 8th and 9th postoperative days. Her nephrostomy tube was removed and she was discharged on the 10th postoperative day. Her nephrostomy cultures were all sterile throughout the postoperative period but she was maintained on penicillin-G, upon which she was also discharged. Her oral penicillin-G was stopped on June 30, 1977, 3 weeks after surgery. Urine cultures were sterile on July 8, 22, and August 24, 1977. An IVU on August 23, 1977 showed no residual stones on the plain film and no obstruction with good excretion on the 15-minute film (Figure 8.32).

Interestingly, and the main reason for presenting her, is that she developed a symptomatic *P. mirabilis* UTI on September 23, 1977—14 weeks after removing the staghorn calculus. She was treated for 2 weeks with TMP-SMX which was then stopped. Many cultures (more than 12) since that time have been sterile, but she continues to be followed closely.

The staghorn calculus was composed of the usual "80% struvite and 20% apatite"—actually monotonous reports, if true. The stone culture showed 70 *P. mirabilis*/ml in the first wash, 10 *P. mirabilis* in the fourth wash, and 5000/ml in the crushed stone. This 4-year-old girl probably formed this stone in infancy which was the cause of her unexplained fever at age 8 months. Our youngest patient was a 3-month-old girl with a full staghorn calculus also due to *P. mirabilis.*

It is clear that with such susceptibility to UTI, and especially to *P. mirabilis*, these children and women must be watched closely for reinfections. If not, the price paid must be similar to A.N. whose tragic story is shown in Figures 8.8 to 8.20.

Table 8.10
Bacteriologic Localization Studies on Patient T.K., a 4-Year-Old Girl

Source	Culture
	Proteus mirabilis/ml
CB[a]	5000
WB	10
LK1	60
LK2	0
LK3	0
LK4	0
RK1	3000
RK2	5000
RK3	5000
RK4	5000

[a] CB = catheterized bladder; WB = washed bladder; K1–K4 = serial cultures from the left (L) and right (R) kidneys.

REFERENCES

1. Nemoy, N. J., and Stamey, T. A.: Surgical bacteriological, and biochemical management of "infection stones." J. Am. Med. Assoc. **215:** 1470, 1971.
2. Hellström, J.: The significance of staphylococci in the development and treatment of renal and ureteral stones. Br. J. Urol. **10:** 348, 1938.
3. Higgins, C. C.: Factors in recurrence of renal calculi. J. Am. Med. Assoc. **113:** 1460, 1939.
4. Chute, R., and Suby, H. I.: Prevalence and importance of urea-splitting bacterial infections of the urinary tract in the formation of calculi. J. Urol. **44:** 590, 1940.
5. Butt, A. J.: Etiologic Factors in Renal Lithiasis. Springfield, Il, Charles C Thomas, 1956.
6. Rovsing, C. M.: On infection as a cause of recurrence following operations for kidney stone. Acta Chir. Scand. **57:** 387, 1924.
7. Sutherland, J. W.: Recurrence following operations for upper urinary tract stone. Br. J. Urol. **26:** 22, 1954.
8. Gil-Vernet, J.: New surgical concepts in removing renal calculi, Urol. Int. **20:** 255, 1965.
9. Hanley, H. G., Joekes, A. M., and Wickham, J. E. A.: Renal hypothermia in complicated nephrolithotomy. J. Urol. **99:** 517, 1968.
10. Smith, M. J. V., and Boyce, W. H.: Anatrophic nephrotomy and plastic calyrhaphy. J. Urol. **99:** 521, 1968.
11. Cunningham, J. J., Friedland, G. W., and Stamey, T. A.: Radiologic changes in the urothelium during Renacidin irrigations. J. Urol. **109:** 556, 1973.

12. Nemoy, N. J., and Stamey, T. A.: Use of hemiacidrin in management of infection stones. J. Urol. **116:** 693, 1976.
13. Thompson, R. B., and Stamey, T. A.: Bacteriology of infected stones. Urology, **2(6):** 627, 1973.
14. Rocha, H., and Santos, C. S.: Relapse of urinary tract infection in the presence of urinary tract calculi: The role of bacteria within the calculi. J. Med. Microbiol. **2:** 372, 1969.
15. Barney, J. D.: The question of recurrent renal calculi. Surg. Gynecol. Obstet. **35:** 743, 1922.
16. Comarr, A. E., Kawaichi, G. K., and Bors, E.: Renal calculosis of patients with traumatic cord lesions. J. Urol. **87:** 647, 1962.
17. Oppenheimer, G. D.: Nephrectomy versus conservative operation in unilateral calculous disease of the upper urinary tract. Surg. Gynecol. Obstet. **65:** 829, 1937.
18. Elliot, J. S., Sharp, R. F., and Lewis, L.: The solubility of struvite in urine. J. Urol. **81:** 366, 1959.
19. Mulvaney, W. P.: The clinical use of Renacidin in urinary calcifications. J. Urol. **84:** 206, 1960.
20. Ries, S. W., and Malament, M.: Renacidin: A urinary calculi solvent. J. Urol. **87:** 657, 1962.
21. Fostvedt, G. A., and Barnes, R. W.: Complications during lavage therapy for renal calculi. J. Urol. **89:** 329, 1963.
22. Kohler, F. P.: Renacidin and tissue reaction. J. Urol. **87:** 102, 1962.
23. Auerbach, S., Mainwaring, R., and Schwarz, F.: Renal and ureteral damage following clinical use of renacidin. J. Am. Med. Assoc. **183:** 61, 1963.
24. Rosen, D. I., Nemoy, N. J., Wolf, P. L., and Stamey, T. A.: Intravenous infusion of Renacidin in dogs. Invest. Urol. **9:** 31, 1971.
25. Stamey, T. A., Govan, D. E., and Palmer, J. M.: The localization and treatment of urinary tract infections: The role of bactericidal urine levels as opposed to serum levels. Medicine **44:** 1, 1965.
26. Fairley, K. F., Bond, A. G., and Adey, F. D.: The site of infection in pregnancy bacteriuria. Lancet **1:** 939, 1966.
27. Reeves, D. S., and Brumfitt, W.: Localization of urinary tract infection. A comparative study of methods. In F. O'Grady and W. Brumfitt (Eds.), Urinary Tract Infection. London, Oxford University Press, 1968, p. 53.
28. Elliot, J. S.: Calcium stones: The difference between oxalate and phosphate types. J. Urol. **100:** 687, 1968.
29. Elliot, J. S.: Spontaneous dissolution of renal calculi. J. Urol. **72:** 331, 1954.
30. Elliot, J. S.: Calcium phosphate solubility in urine. J. Urol. **77:** 269, 1957.
31. Elliot, J. S., Quaide, W. L., Sharp, R. F., and Lewis, L.: Mineralogic studies of urine: The relationship of apatite, brushite and struvite to urinary pH. J. Urol. **80:**269, 1958.
32. Elliot, J. S., Adamson, J. P., and Lewis, L.: The dissolution of renal phosphatic calculi by retrograde irrigation. J. Urol. **81:** 56, 1959.
33. Elliot, J. S., Sharp, R. F., and Lewis, L.: Urinary pH. J. Urol. **81:** 339, 1959.
34. Elliot, J. S., Sharp, R. F., and Lewis, L.: The solubility of struvite in urine. J. Urol. **81:** 366, 1959.
35. Elliot, J. S., Todd, H. E., and Lewis, L.: Some aspects of calcium phosphate solubility. J. Urol. **85:** 428, 1961.
36. Elliot, J. S., and Todd, H. E.: Calculous disease in patients with poliomyelitis. J. Urol. **86:** 484, 1961.
37. Griffith, D. P., Moskowitz, P. A., and Carlton, E. C., Jr.: Adjunctive chemotherapy of infection-induced staghorn calculi. J. Urol. **121:** 711, 1979.
38. Stamey, T. A. Urinary Infections. Baltimore, Williams & Wilkins, 1972.
39. Prien, E. L.: Studies in urolithiasis. II. Relationships between pathogenesis, structure and composition of calculi. J. Urol. **61:** 821, 1949.
40. Shapiro, A. P., Braude, A. I., and Siemienski, J.: Hematogenous pyelonephritis in rats. IV. Relationship of bacterial species to the pathogenesis and sequelae of chronic pyelonephritis. J. Clin. Invest. **38:** 1228, 1959.
41. Vermeulen, C. W., Ragins, H. D., Grove, W. J., and Goetz, R.: Experimental urolithiasis. III. Prevention and dissolution of calculi by alteration of urinary pH. J. Urol. **66:** 1, 1951.
42. Vermeulen, C. W., Helsby, C. R., and Goetz, R.: Experimental urolithiasis. V. Prevention and dissolution of foreign body calculi by infection with *Salmonella enteritidis.* J. Urol **68:** 790, 1952.
43. Vermeulen, C. W., and Goetz, R.: Experimental urolithiasis. IX. Influence of infection on stone growth in rats. J. Urol. **72:** 761, 1954.
44. Leoschke, W. L., and Elvehjem, C. A.: Prevention of urinary calculi formation in mink by alteration of urinary pH. Proc. Soc. Exp. Biol. Med. **85:** 42, 1954.
45. Nielsen, I. M.: Urolithiasis in mink: Pathology, bacteriology and experimental production. J. Urol. **75:** 602, 1956.
46. Griffith, D. P., Musher, D. M., and Itin, C.: Urease: the primary cause of infection-induced urinary stones. Invest. Urol. **13:** 346, 1976.
47. Griffith, D. P.: Struvite stones. Kidney Int. **13:** 372, 1978.
48. Musher, D. M., Griffith, D. P., Yawn, D., and Rosen, R. D.: Role of urease in pyelonephritis resulting from urinary tract infection with *Proteus.* J. Infect. Dis. **131:** 177, 1975.

CHAPTER 9

Urologic Abnormalities as a Cause of Bacterial Persistence in Urinary Tract Infections

THERE are two questions that deserve serious and detailed consideration: (1) Does the presence of residual urine predispose to urinary infections? (2) When infection is present, what is the importance of urologic abnormalities?

QUESTION OF RESIDUAL URINE

Although there is widespread belief, especially among urologists, that residual urine predisposes to urinary infection, there is little evidence to support it. The view that patients with residual urine are more likely to become infected than those without is easy to understand: most patients with residual urine are eventually examined by a method involving insertion of an instrument and hence are often secondarily infected; moreover, once the infection is present, eradication can be difficult, although it is by no means impossible. But these are circumstantial points; they have little to do with the basic question of whether the presence of residual urine *per se* makes a person more likely to become infected in the absence of instrumentation.

Both the clinical and experimental data suggest that residual urine does not predispose to urinary infection. Guze and Beeson showed that the affected kidneys in rabbits and rats with chronic, unilateral hydronephrosis were barely more susceptible to hematogenous pyelonephritis than were the contralateral, nonobstructed kidneys,[1] whereas total ureteral occlusion always caused severe pyelonephritis.[2] Vivaldi *et al.*,[3] in 1959, found in experiments with rats that if they ligated one ureter before inducing a bladder infection, the obstructed kidney remained sterile while pyelonephritis developed in the contralateral, unobstructed kidney. Although the rat refluxes, and infection in the nonobstructed kidney would be expected, it is interesting that the obstructed kidney remained sterile in the presence of so much urinary infection.

Because much of the clinical impression of the relationship between infection and residual urine is derived from experience with patients who have prostatic obstruction, the studies of Hasner[4] are interesting.

In 221 patients with prostatic obstruction who needed prostatectomy and who had 50 ml or more of residual urine, he found a spontaneous infection rate (in the absence of instrumentation) of only 8.6%. Of the 19 patients who presented with obstruction and infection, 7 were 60–69 years old and 12 were 71–85 years old. Nine of the 19 patients had the severest form of obstruction in his classification—azotemia with pronounced electrolyte and water disorders—and all 19 had had prolonged illness (average, 3.1 years) before seeking consultation. These data are suggestive that most, although not all, of the infection in patients with prostatic obstruction is iatrogenic. Clearly then, the practice of determining residual urine—as an indication for prostatectomy—is not only hard to justify, but potentially hazardous and unnecessary in patients who have sterile urine and no ureteral abnormality on intravenous urography (IVU). In the 24 years that I have been practicing urology, I have never been disappointed by encouraging the patient to tell *me* when his symptoms are severe enough to warrant prostatectomy. As long as his IVU shows only minimal dilatation of the lower ureters, and a yearly serum creatinine remains normal, the size of his prostate or the amount of sterile residual urine should not influence the decision for prostatectomy. A postvoiding residual urine determined by IVU is adequate enough to exclude those rare individuals who have massive residual urine and who, perhaps, are in danger of developing a "decompensated" bladder from obstruction. Indeed, there is no evidence that these rare cases of large bladders which fail to regain adequate emptying capacity after prostatectomy are due to the obstruction, or that their malfunction could have been altered by an earlier prostatectomy. For example, they are just as likely to be caused by superimposed autonomic damage to the detrusor. Except for these rare, debatable exceptions of massive residual urine, readily determined by IVU, or better still by abdominal palpation of the bladder, there is no excuse for catheterizing a patient with obstructive urologic symptoms; the amount of residual urine is not a justifiable indication for prostatectomy. With the advent of ultrasound to determine hydronephrosis, even the IVU can be dispensed with in the clinical evaluation.

The question can be reversed by asking how many patients with bacteriuria have residual urine. Williams *et al.*[5] determined the residual urine in 100 women, 4–6 months after delivery, who had been treated for asymptomatic bacteriuria during pregnancy. When the 32 patients in whom bacteriuria persisted were compared with the 64 who had sterile urine, residual urine was the same in both groups.

Ureteral reflux is a form of residual urine. We reviewed in Chapter 6 the evidence that the correction of reflux does not change the incidence of urinary infections.[6]

In Winberg, Larson, and Bergström's[7] comparison of the natural history of urinary tract infection (UTI) in 21 children who refluxed with 34 who did not reflux, the two groups could not be distinguished in terms of (1) the number of febrile recurrences; (2) the number of symptomatic, afebrile recurrences; or (3) the number of asymptomatic recurrences. In fact, the nonrefluxing group had more of all three types of recurrences than the refluxing group. Mean follow-up time for the nonrefluxers was 4.4 years and for the refluxers was 5.7 years. If residual urine is a determinant of susceptibility to recurrent infections, there should be an increased susceptibility in those children who reflux compared to those who do not; in fact, they cannot be distinguished by clinical history.

There are two investigations, one in children[8] and one in adults[9] using ^{131}I-Hippuran that show residual urine is more common in bacteriuric than in nonbacteriuric female subjects. Most of these residual urine samples were not large (less than 50 ml in most bacteriuric subjects). It is possible that bacteriuria of a prolonged duration does cause some functional failure to completely empty the bladder; the study in children was done on asymptomatic subjects whose bacteriuria was detected during screening surveys[8] and hence was probably of a long duration. The presence of residual urine in the isotope study in adults also correlated with increasing age; the mean age of the roup with the most significant residual ırine was 47 years. Since Williams *et al.*[5] lid not find any difference in residual urine n their study of infected and noninfected ostnatal patients, the fact that these pa-ients were younger and probably had their acteriuria for a shorter period of time may ccount for the absence of significant resid-ıal urine in this study.

And finally, although firm statistics are ıot available, in the vast majority of pa-ients with ureteropelvic junction obstruc-ion, the urine is sterile and there is no istory of urinary infections. A particularly nstructive patient is N.B. (Tables 9.4 and).5), presented in the following section.

IMPORTANCE OF UROLOGIC ABNORMALITIES

When the large group of cases of reinfec-tion in children (Chapter 6) and premeno-pausal adult women (Chapter 4) are ex-cluded, we are surprised at how often a recurrent urinary infection, caused by bac-terial persistence within the urinary tract, is due to a specific urologic abnormality; if the abnormality is recognized and cor-rected, the patient is usually cured of the infection. The 14 urologic abnormalities that have caused bacterial persistence in our patients at Stanford University Hospi-tal are listed in Table 9.1. Because these patients can be cured, and because the un-derlying abnormality is rarely obvious, Ta-ble 9.1 should serve as a deliberate check list in the investigation of any patient with recurrent bacteriuria due to bacterial per-sistence; the reader should briefly review the classification of UTI presented in Chap-ter 1.

Infection stones (predominantly in women), chronic bacterial prostatitis, and infected unilateral atrophic kidneys (also mainly in women) are by far the most common; infected pericalyceal diverticula (sometimes nonfunctioning), infected ure-teral stumps, vesical fistulas, and infected urachal cysts are much less frequent. All of the abnormalities in Table 9.1 have one thing in common—the persistence of bac-teria in a site that communicates directly or indirectly (urethral diverticulum and perilabial persistence) with the urinary tract.

Infection Stones

I have shown in the preceding chapter several clinical examples of bacterial per-sistence inside struvite infection stones. The characteristic bacteriologic history is illustrated in Figure 8.4 where the urine is easily sterilized with antibacterial therapy but the infection recurs because of bacterial persistence inside the stone. While many cases diagnosed late in the course of their disease are obvious (Figures 8.29–8.32), other patients with early struvite crystali-zation are not so obvious (Figures 8.21–8.28).

Although the documentation of this most important of all causes of bacterial persist-ence is extensive in Chapter 8, as well as the demonstration that other bacteria than *Proteus mirabilis* can persist in calculi, I would like to present an additional patient who illustrates the important point that the presence of contralateral bacteriuria to an ipsilateral source of infection is not a deter-rent to cure with ipsilateral nephrectomy.

M.P., a 51-year-old white female patient, was first seen at Stanford on 6/13/76, with a life-time history of intermittent cystitis which had caused her little symptomatic difficulty. The reason for her referral was a 2-year documentation of continuous pyuria with *Klebsiella* bacteriuria, and three epi-sodes of chills and fever with right flank pain, two of them in the past year. She had been told she had "kidney stones" but did not know when this information was given to her; she had never had renal colic or passed any stones.

Upon admission, her serum creatinine was 1.1 mg/100 ml, her BUN 8 mg/100 ml, and her electrolytes and SMA-12 chemis-tries were all normal; her serum calcium was 9.3 mg/100 ml and her serum phospho-rus 2.7 mg/100 ml. Her hematocrit was 45%, hemoglobin 14 g/100 ml, but her white blood cell count was 14,600 with 73% poly-morphonuclear leukocytes. A ^{131}I-Hippuran renogram showed a renal plasma flow of 373 ml/minute to the right kidney but

Table 9.1
Correctable Urologic Abnormalities that Cause Bacterial Persistence and Recurrent Urinary Tract Infection

1. Infection stones	8. Unilateral medullary sponge kidneys
2. Chronic bacterial prostatitis	9. Nonrefluxing, normal appearing, infected ureteral stumps following nephrectomy
3. Unilateral infected atrophic kidneys	10. Infected urachal cysts
4. Vesicovaginal and vesicointestinal fistulas	11. Infected communicating cysts of the renal calyces
5. Ureteral duplication and ectopic ureters	12. Papillary necrosis in a single calyx
6. Foreign bodies	13. Paravesical abscess with fistula to bladder
7. Urethral diverticula and infected paraurethral glands	14. Labial persistence in Bartholin's ducts(?)

only 37 ml/minute to the left kidney (which approximates tissue background). Her urine culture on admission showed 10,000 *Klebsiella* and 2,000 *Escherichia coli*/ml of voided urine. The *E. coli* was pansensitive to all antimicrobial agents, while the

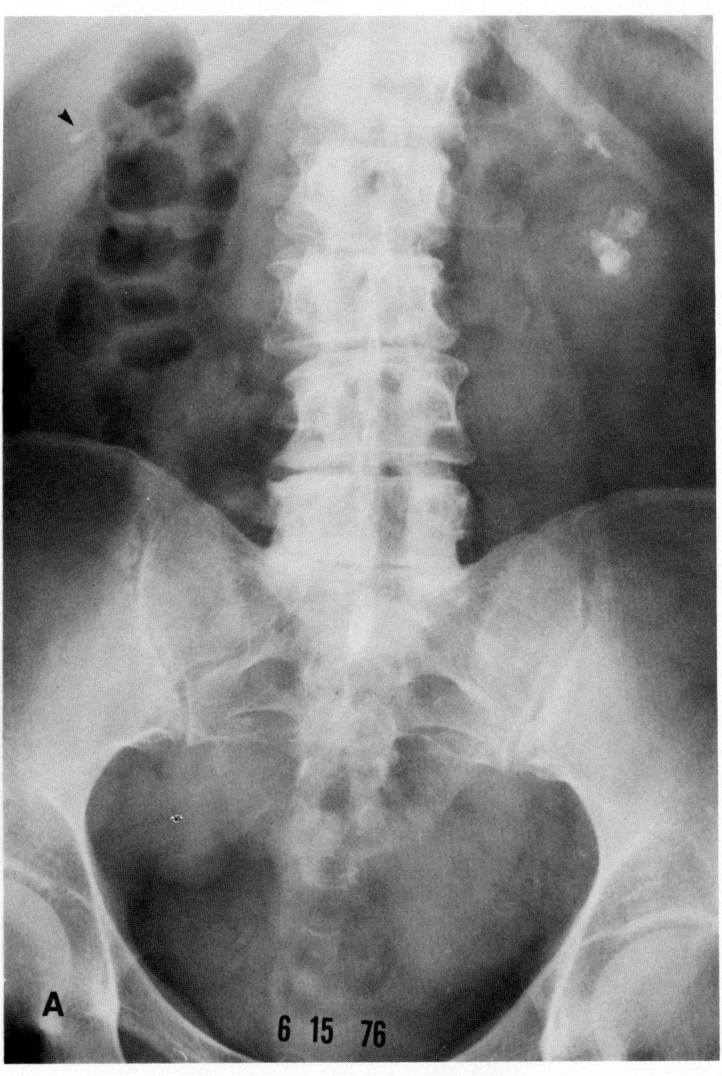

Figure 9.1 (*A*) Plain film of the abdomen on M.P. prior to the tomographic films and the intravenous urogram. Neither renal shadow is well seen, but the calcifications in the left kidney are apparent and a single teardrop-shaped calculus is probably in the right kidney. (*B*) (facing page) A 9-cm tomographic cut showing the right renal stone (*arrow*) to be within the depth of the kidney in M.P.

Klebsiella was resistant to tetracycline, nitrofurantoin, and sulfonamide. Urinalysis showed 30–40 white blood cells/high power field (WBC/hpf), a pH of 6.0, and no protein or casts.

An IVU was obtained on 6/15/76, with plain film tomographic cuts of the upper abdomen from 7 cm through 13 cm (Figures 9.1–9.4). The left kidney was nonfunctioning, atrophic without obstruction (Figure 9.5), and probably represented atrophic pyelonephritis. The soft-appearing, amorphous calcifications within the collecting system (Figures 9.1–9.5) are probably secondary to earlier urea-splitting bacteria; one culture from her referring physician's office reported *Klebsiella* and *Proteus* species in March 1974. The 1-minute nephrogram phase of the IVP (Figure 9.2) is the best film to study the renal contour for scarring; none are seen in the right kidney. No nephrogram is seen in the left kidney. The excretory films seen in Figures 9.3 and 9.4 also failed to show pyelonephritic scarring in the right kidney although the infundibulae appear somewhat atonic, perhaps reflecting the *Klebsiella* infection in this kidney (Table 9.2).

On 6/16/76, she was cystoscoped. The bladder mucosa showed many lymphoid nodules, especially on the posterior bladder wall and near the internal vesical neck on all sides. Both ureteral orifices were normal. The bacteriologic localization studies are shown in Table 9.2. After washing the bladder thoroughly with several liters of sterile water, number 7 Fr Stamey ureteral catheters were passed to the midureters of each kidney. Five milliliters of the right renal urine was centrifuged; the sediment showed 2–4 WBC/hpf, 3–6 RBC/hpf, and many ureteral and pelvic epithelial cells without tubular casts or bacilli. The left kidney, which made no urine, was irrigated with 2- to 5-ml aliquots of sterile saline; an unspun drop showed 0–4 WBC/hpf, 6–8 RBC/hpf, occasional bacterial rods, and some renal pelvic epithelial cells. Several consecutive, timed collections of urine from the right ureteral catheter at a urine flow rate of 7–8 ml/minute showed a creatinine clearance of 85 ml/minute, uncorrected for her 94-kg

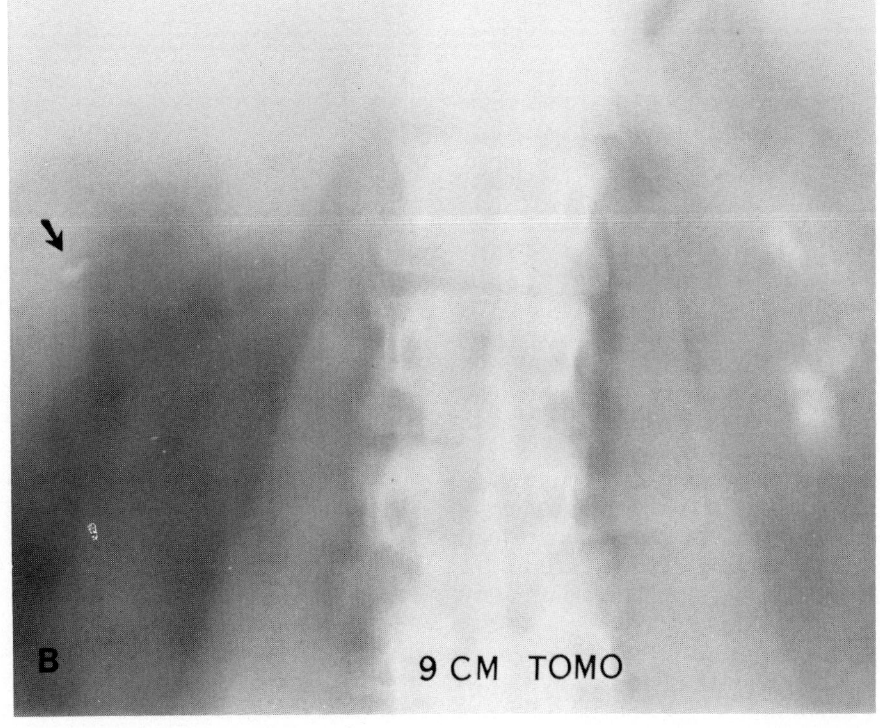

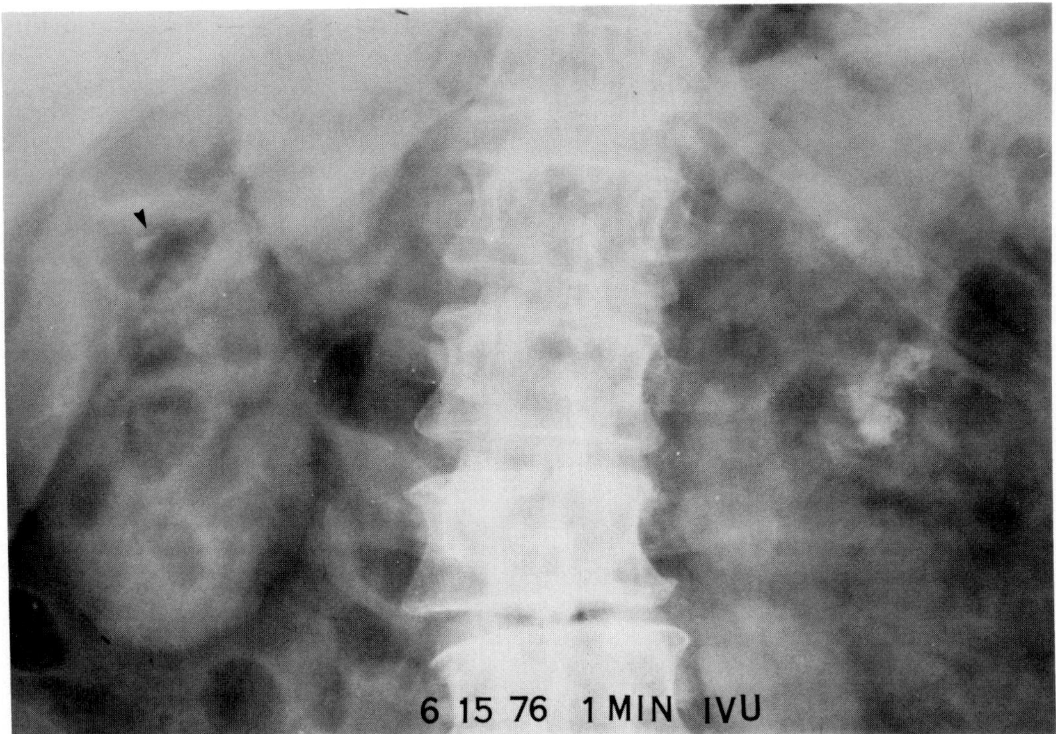

Figure 9.2 A 1-minute nephrogram phase of the intravenous urogram on M.P. The right renal border appears reasonably smooth; the right kidney measures 17.3 cm. No definite nephrogram can be detected in the left kidney.

body weight and 5-½ foot height. A retrograde urogram was obtained of the left ureter and kidney at the end of the study (Figure 9.5).

She was given 80 mg of gentamicin before leaving the cystoscopy room and every 8 hours thereafter. The right ureteral catheter was removed the following day and the left kidney was excised the next day through a flank incision. The distal end of the left ureter at surgery was cannulated with a ureteral catheter which was brought out through the wound and infused with gentamicin for 48 hours before removing it. This precaution kills the residual bacteria on the ureteral mucosa in a nonrefluxing ureter, and prevents the normal ureter from serving as another site of bacterial persistence.

The kidney measured 7 × 5 × 2.5 cm (Figure 9.6*A*). The bivalved kidney showed markedly atrophic cortex and medulla measuring 0.7 cm in average thickness (Figure 9.6*B*). The stones were brown to black in color (Figure 9.6*A*), but porous and soft. Identification of the crystals under polarized light showed the calculi were almost pure apatite with microscopic amounts of whewellite (calcium oxalate monohydrate). Representative thin slices of the cortex and medulla were removed at surgery for tissue culture. The results of these tissue cultures and stone cultures in Table 9.3 suggest that the bacteria are more in the stone than in the tissue.

It is interesting that although this atrophic, infected kidney made no detectable urine, the bacteria obtained by washing the renal pelvis preoperatively were antibody-coated by fluorescent antibody studies (Table 9.2); the reader may wish to review this technique in Chapter 1. As seen in Figure 9.6 *C* and *D*, the lining of the pelvis and dilated calyces contained many

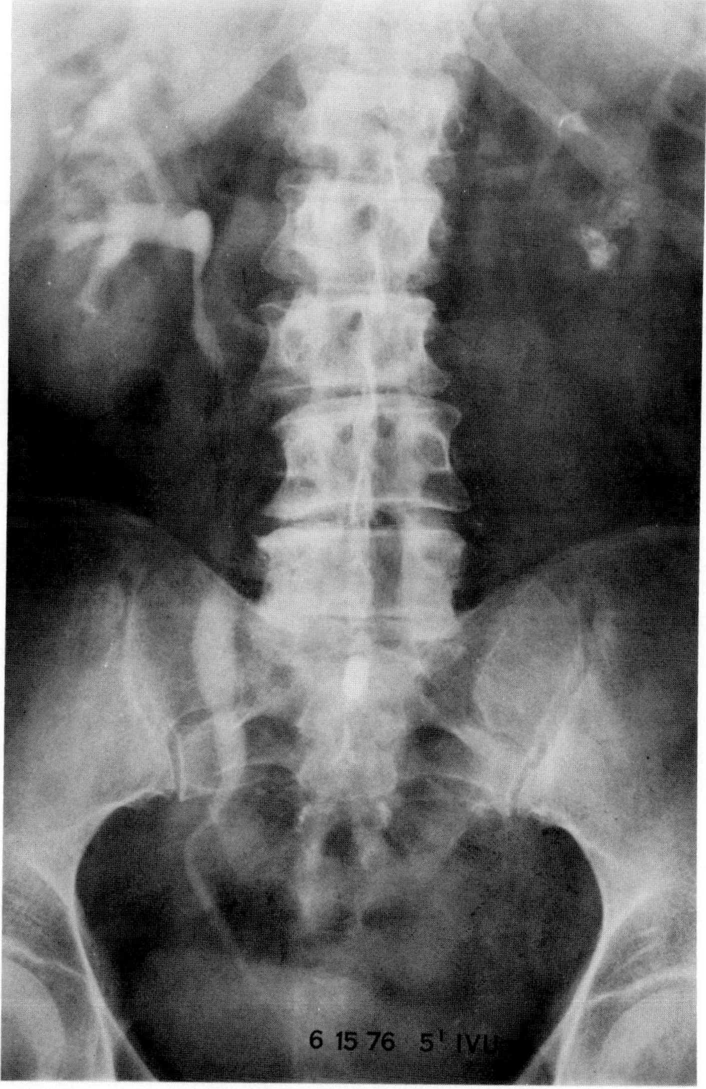

Figure 9.3 A 5-minute excretory film from the intravenous urogram on M.P. There is mild dilatation of the midportion of the right ureter at the level of the pelvic brim. No excretion is detected in the left kidney.

lymphoid nodules with germinal centers undoubtedly producing the antibody that coated the bacteria. The uroepithelium showed extensive lymphocytic and plasmacytic infiltrates everywhere (Figure 9.6*E*), consistent with pyelonephritic atrophy. While a rare glomerulus and its nephron seemed spared (Figure 9.6*F*), virtually all of the glomeruli were hyalinized (Figure 9.6*G*) and the tubules showed extensive atrophy and thyroidization (Figure 9.6*B*). An occasional glomerulus showed the typical periglomerular fibrosis of pyelonephritis (Figure 9.6*H*).

Following her nephrectomy on 6/18/76, she received gentamicin for 5 days and was discharged on cephalexin 250 mg every 6 hours on the 7th postoperative day. Urine cultures 3 days and 7 days after nephrectomy were sterile and she had no Gram-negative bacteria on the introitus. The cephalexin was stopped on 8/15/76. Multiple cultures were obtained over the next 6 months, all of them off antimicrobial ther-

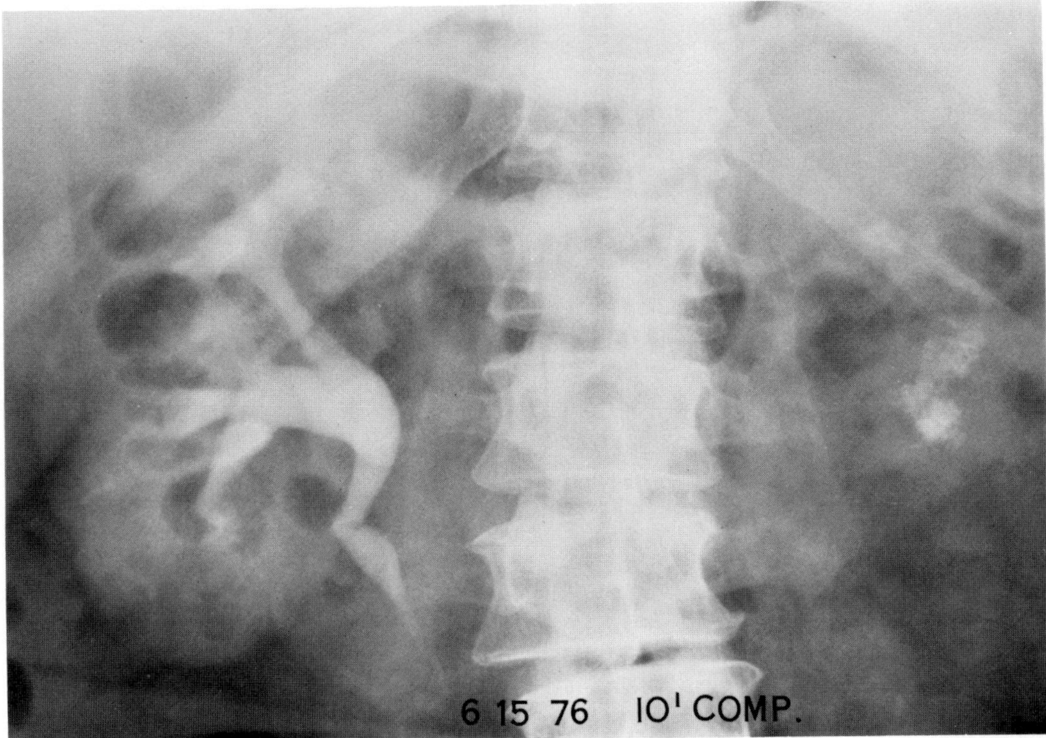

Figure 9.4 A 10-minute compression film from the intravenous urogram on M.P. The right renal calculus lies in an upper, middle lobe calyx. The left kidney does not excrete the contrast medium.

apy, and all of them were sterile without a single colony of Enterobacteriaceae on the introitus.

Because stress urinary incontinence was a complaint of 10 years in duration when I first saw her, I performed our operation of endoscopic suspension of the vesical neck for stress urinary incontinence[10] in early December 1976, 6 months after her nephrectomy. Although her bladder looked normal and the lymphoid nodules in the submucosa seen 6 months earlier were gone, I took a 2-cm long transurethral biopsy in the floor behind the trigone; it was interesting that the submucosa showed edema with acute and chronic inflammatory cells with even a lymphoid nodule on one edge. The mucosa and muscle were unremarkable. I learned from this patient that 6 months of a sterile urine was not long enough for the submucosal inflammatory response to a long-standing bacteriuria to disappear. It should also be noted that her bladder capacity under a general anesthesia at 72 cm of water pressure was 1750 ml! Finally, she had a large ventral urethral diverticulum in the floor of the urethra 1.5 cm from the vesical neck, which clearly was unrelated to her recurrent bacteriuria.

The important lessons from this patient are:

1. The *Klebsiella* infection in the right kidney contralateral to the nonfunctioning left kidney did not prevent cure of her bacteriuria by a left nephrectomy—even though the *Klebsiella* in the right renal urine were fluorescent antibody positive (FA+), indicating an immunologic response in the right kidney and more than just superficial colonization of the uroepithelium on the right side. This is not the first time we have observed contralateral clearing of bacteriuria when the ipsilateral focus of infection is cured, but it is the heaviest infection

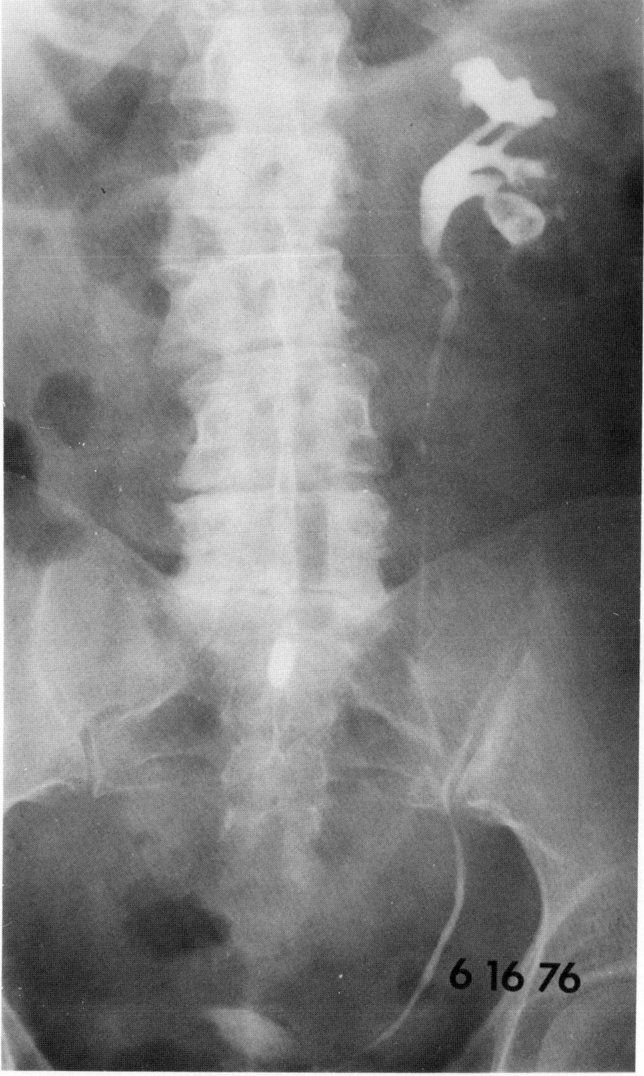

Figure 9.5 A left retrograde urogram made the day following the intravenous urogram on M.P. The ureter is nonobstructed. Filling defects from the calculus material are seen in the lower and middle calyces.

(>10^5 *Klebsiella*/ml in all serial right renal urines) we have ever observed and the demonstration of FA+ bacteriuria seems unique.

Of greater concern to me was the possibility that the small teardrop-shaped stone in the right upper middle calyx (Figure 9.1, *A* and *B*) might be an infection stone. Indeed, with the heavy *Klebsiella* infection in the right renal urine I gave some thought to removing this stone at the time of the left nephrectomy. Her clinical course has shown the wisdom of not doing so and that somehow the *Klebsiella* had not become trapped in the interstices of the stone, as so often happens in other cases.

2. The nonfunctioning, atrophic left kidney—clearly due to pyelonephritis (Figure 9.6, *A–H*)—with porous apatite stones is also of interest from the bacteriologic view. For one thing, the bacteria irrigated from the renal pelvis were also antibody-coated (FA+) in the absence of detectable urine flow from the kidney. The lymphoid nodules with active germinal centers (Fig-

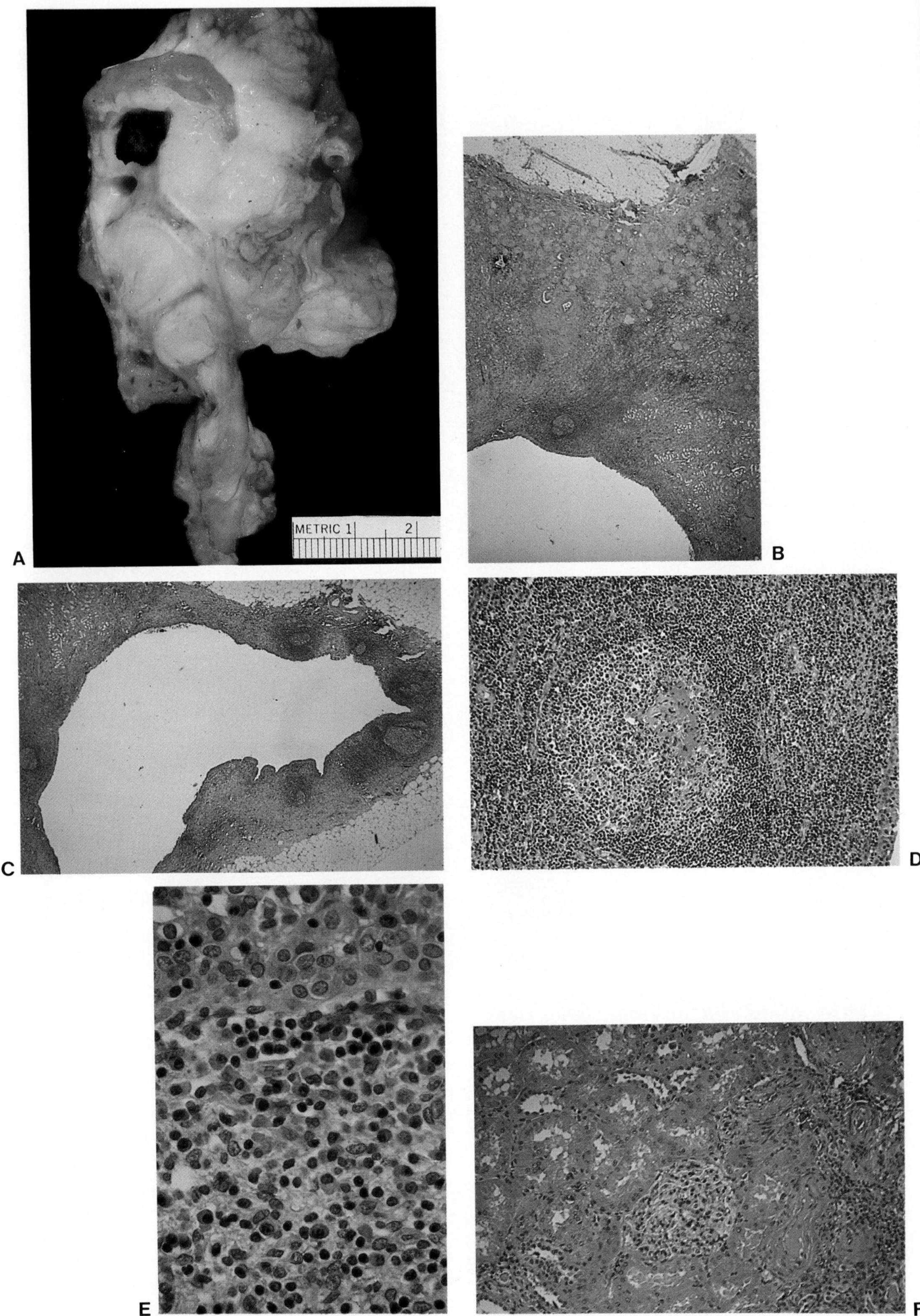
METRIC 1
2

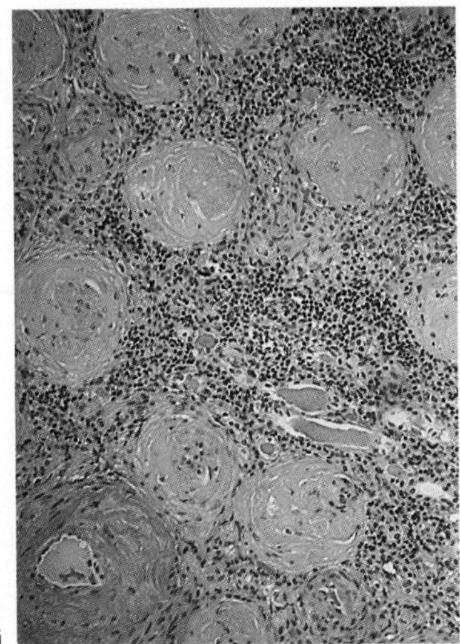

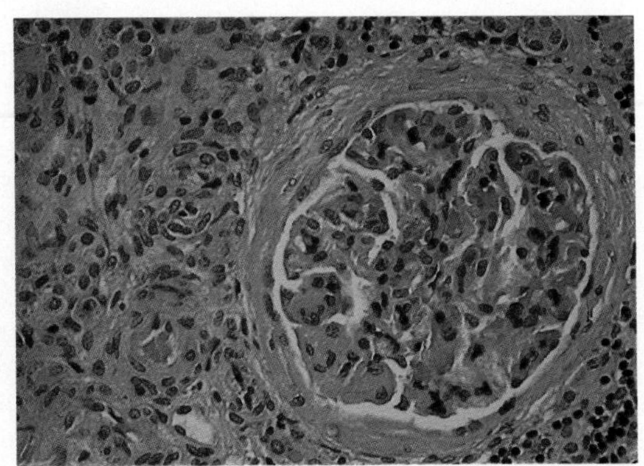

Figure 9.6 Gross and microscopic features of the atrophic pyelonephritic kidney of M.P. which emphasize the source of renal antibody that coated the *Escherichia coli* and *Klebsiella* recovered from this kidney preoperatively, even though the kidney made no urine. (*A*) A 7 × 5 × 2.5 cm kidney showing the brown to black apatite stones in one calyx; (*B*) macroscopic view showing the full thickness (0.7 cm) of the cortex and medulla, as well as the extensive hyalinization of the glomeruli and thyroidization of the tubules; (*C*) macroscopic view of a dilated calyx with many active lymphoid follicles with (*D*) germinal centers; (*E*) although the interstitium showed a heavy chronic inflammatory infiltrate, as seen in *B*, it was most marked around the calyces and pelvis beneath the uroepithelium as shown in this figure with the urothelium at the top; (*F*) normal glomeruli and tubules were rare; (*G*) Extensive hyalinization of the glomeruli were present with (*H*) some periglomerular fibrosis typical of pyelonephritis.

Table 9.2
Bacteriologic Localization Studies on M.P.[a]

Source[a]	*Klebsiella*	*Escherichia coli*	Fluorescent Antibody-Coated Bacteria
	bacteria/ml	*bacteria/ml*	
CB	10,000	2000	4+
WB	2,000	30	
RK_{1-6}	>100,000	0	4+
LK_1	5,000	200	
LK_2	170	1000	
LK_{3-6}	5,000	2000	4+

[a] CB = catheterized bladder count, WB = washed bladder count before urethral catheterization, RK_{1-6} = six consecutive serial urine samples from the right kidney, LK_{1-6} = six consecutive cultures from the nonfunctioning left kidney obtained by irrigating with 2–5 ml of sterile saline for each culture.

ure 9.6, *C* and *D*) undoubtedly account for the immunologic response; the only detectable abnormality in her blood was a WBC of 14,600 and 15,100 on admission which 6 months later was 9,900.

3. It is interesting that both the *Klebsiella* and the *E. coli* appear to be more in the apatite stone than in the renal tissue (Table 9.3). Indeed, the *E. coli* counts in the ground tissue are almost within the range of surface contamination; moreover, since the *E. coli* were several logs more numerous in the stone than the *Klebsiella*, the slices of renal cortex and medulla were more apt to be contaminated by *E. coli* than *Klebsiella*. If this observation is true, as it appears to be, it is one more piece of evidence that it is renal calcifications that cause bacteria to persist in human kidneys rather than invasion of the renal tissue *per se*.

In closing this section, I would mention one additional experience with infection stones which may be more common than

Table 9.3
Bacteriologic Cultures of the Kidney and the Apatite Stone[a]

Source	*Klebsiella*	*Escherichia coli*
	bacteria/ml	*bacteria/ml*
Stone:		
Wash 1	30	10,000
Wash 4	10	5,000
Crushed stone	500	>100,000
Renal cortex:		
Wash 1	0	110
Wash 4	0	10
Ground tissue	0	100
Renal medulla:		
Wash 1	0	130
Wash 2	0	50
Ground tissue	0	440

[a] Wash 1 = initial wash of stone or tissue in 5 ml sterile saline, wash 4 = fourth wash of stone or tissue in 5 ml sterile saline, crushed stone = bacterial count after crushing stone in fourth wash, ground tissue = bacterial count after grinding tissue in fourth wash. See Chapter 1 for greater details.

we think, although I have proven only one such case. In 1969 I saw a 51-year-old white woman with a lifetime history of recurrent UTI at 6-month to 2-year intervals. Three months before I saw her, she began having recurrent episodes of chills, fever, and right flank pain with passage of small renal calculi; she had never passed stones before but passed a "pillbox" full during that 3-month interval before referral. All urine cultures reportedly grew *Proteus*. She was admitted to the hospital on several occasions, either with pain or fever or both. Bilateral ureteral catheterization by her referring urologist had shown $>10^5$ *P. mirabilis*/ml from both kidneys. Stone analysis had shown struvite and apatite. She was transferred directly from a local hospital to our service; she was not on antimicrobial therapy. During the transfer, or shortly before, she passed a small 3-mm yellow stone which was washed and crushed for culture in our laboratory: wash 1, wash 4, and the crushed stone all grew $>10^5$ *P. mirabilis*/ml. Our dilemma, however, was that all her urine cultures were sterile! In fact, except for our second culture showing a few colonies of *Pseudomonas aeruginosa* and *P. mirabilis* on the introitus, there were no Gram-negative bacteria anywhere in her urine specimens or on the introitus. Her admission urine contained 20–30 WBC/hpf (spun), but she soon lost her pyuria. An IVU and plain film tomograms showed evidence of bilateral pyelonephritis (without stones) and her serum creatinine was 1.4 mg/100 ml. I followed her closely for 5 years without antimicrobial therapy but did give her 2.0 g/day ascorbic acid; her urine pH values were 4.5–6.0 whether she took the ascorbic acid or not. She never had another UTI in the 5 years I followed her. She had clearly cured herself of *P. mirabilis* struvite infection stones by passing the last one in the 48 hours before transfer to Stanford in 1969.

Chronic Bacterial Prostatitis

Several clinical examples of bacterial persistence in prostatic fluid were presented in Chapter 7. The urologic abnormality that favors the establishment of these pathogenic bacteria in prostatic fluid is probably a biologic defect; it certainly is not a mechanical one such as obstruction or residual urine. Whatever the basic cause—perhaps the absence of the prostatic antibacterial factor in a man whose urethra contacts the pathogenic introital bacteria of a female who has recurrent urinary infections (Chapter 7)—chronic bacterial prostatitis is the most common cause of recurrent bacteriuria in men. The problems relating to the therapeutic control, and occasionally cure, of this recurrent infection, where the bacteria persist in the prostatic fluid between episodes of bacteriuria, were presented in Chapter 7.

Unilateral Infected Atrophic Kidneys

Several of our most gratifying cures have occurred in patients with unilateral, atrophic kidneys in whom the contralateral kidney has remained sterile despite years of continuous bladder infection. When antimicrobial therapy, especially serum level bactericidal therapy, has failed to cure these patients, nephrectomy can offer them a lifetime free of chronic infection, chills,

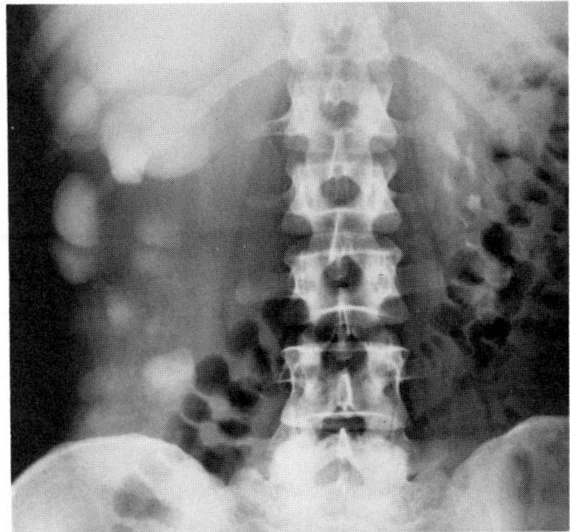

A

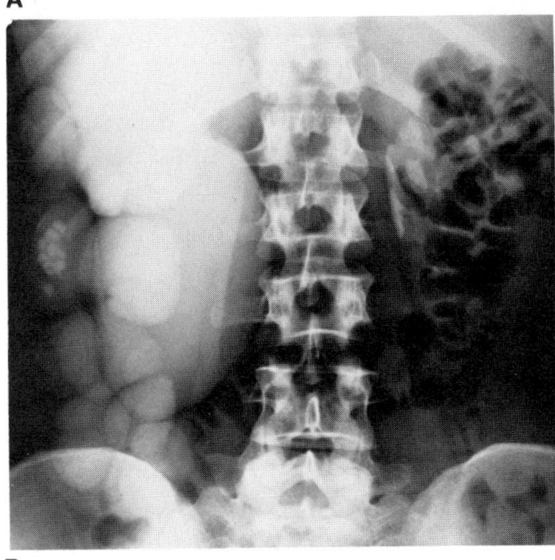

B

Figure 9.7 (*A*) N.B., a 27-year-old, Caucasian woman with unilateral, atrophic infected kidney on the left and a sterile, ureteropelvic junction obstruction on the right. This x-ray film was made 5 minutes after a second injection of intravenous contrast solution. Date of examination: 9/19/68. (*B*) X-ray film from same intravenous urogram in part *A* but taken 95 minutes after injection. Note the giant hydronephrosis and hydropelvis of the right kidney, the multiple small stones in the middle calyx of the right kidney, and the small left kidney.

and fever. A detailed report on one such patient with Pseudomonas pyelonephritis (and small pericalyceal calcifications) was presented in Chapter 3. The patient shown in Figures 9.1–9.6 is another example of atrophic pyelonephritis, albeit with renal calcification in addition.

An equally instructive case is that of N.B., a 27-year-old, Caucasian woman who had been married for 10 years at the time of her initial visit to Stanford University Hospital in October 1968. She experienced multiple episodes of left flank and lower abdominal pain during childhood days but, because of her religion, did not seek medical advice. After her marriage in June 1958, two severe urinary infections occurred in September and December accompanied by sharp right flank pain and fever which responded to antibacterial drugs. Severe fevers, pains, and even pleural effusion complicated her only pregnancy in 1961, forcing an abortion at 7 months. From 1961, however, to 1968, she was asymptomatic except for a single, transient episode of right flank pain in 1967. Because of a "brownish urine," her family physician obtained an IVU (Fig. 9.7) and referred her to Stanford.

Upon admission on 10/2/68, her blood pressure was 138/90 mm Hg, the fundi were normal, but a mass was easily palpable in the right flank. Her urine was infected with *E. coli* (Table 9.4); numerous white and red blood cells and bacterial rods were visible in the sediment. The serum creatinine was 0.9 mg/100 ml. Except for a serum chloride of 110 mEq/liter and a CO_2 of 22 mEq/liter, all other electrolytes and blood studies were normal. Serum calcium was 9.5 mg/100 ml. A voiding cystourethrogram on 10/3/68 showed no reflux on filling, at the point of urgency, or during micturition. There was no residual urine on the postvoiding film or at the time of catheterization for the cystourethrogram (20 ml). Cystoscopy, ureteral catheterization studies to localize the *E. coli* bacteriuria (Table 9.4), differential renal function studies, and bilateral retrogrades were performed the following day under local anesthesia. Both ureteral orifices and their submucosal tunnels were normal. A No. 7 Fr polyethylene Stamey catheter was first passed to the left renal pelvis and a Foley catheter placed in the bladder to collect the right renal urine. Two consecutive 30-minute periods were col-

Table 9.4
Bacteriologic Course of N.B., a 27-year-old White Woman[a]

Date	Days On (+) or Off (−) Therapy	Vaginal Vestibule		Urethral (VB_1)		Midstream (VB_2)	
		bacteria/ml		*bacteria/ml*		*bacteria/ml*	
10/2/68	−several years					*Escherichia coli*	10,000
10/3/68	−several years					CB:	
						E. coli	>100,000
10/4/68	−several years					CB = *E. coli*	> 100,000
						WB = *E. coli*	> 10,000
						RK_{1-3} = sterile	
						LK_1 = *E. coli*	> 100,000
						LK_2 = *E. coli*	> 100,000
						LK_3 = *E. coli*	> 100,000
10/7/68	+3 ampicillin 500 mg q 6 hr	Left nephroureterectomy, right pyeloplasty an extraction of 13 calcium oxalate stones		Stone wash 1 0		Irrigation of left renal pelvis	0
				Stone wash 4 0			
				Ground stone 0		Aspiration of right renal pelvis	0
10/10/68	+6 ampicilln 500 mg q 6 hr					Nephrostomy tube	0
10/12/68	+8 ampicillin 500 mg q 6 hr					Nephrostomy tube	0
10/15/68	−1 ampicillin 500 mg q 6 hr					Nephrostomy tube	0
10/17/68	+1methenamine 500 mg q 6 hr					Nephrostomy tube	0
10/22/68	+5 methenamine 500 mg q 6 hr					Nephrostomy tube	0
10/25/68	+8 methenamine 500 mg q 6 hr					Nephrostomy tube	0
						Staphylococcus epidermidis	850
10/29/68	+12 methenamine 500 mg q 6 hr			*S. epidermidis*	740	*S. epidermidis*	40
				γ-Streptococcus	40	γ-Streptococcus	10
11/12/68	+26 methenamine	*S. epidermidis*	400		0		0

Date	Days On (+) or Off (−) Therapy	Vaginal Vestibule		Urethral (VB_1)		Midstream (VB_2)	
			bacteria/ml		*bacteria/ml*		*bacteria/ml*
	500 mg q 6 hr	γ-Streptococcus	700				
		Diphtheroids	1,500				
11/22/68	−5 methenamine	*Bacillus subtilis*	150	*B. subtilis*	20		0
	500 mg q 6 hr	*S. epidermidis*	750	γ-Streptococcus	10		
				Diphtheroids	3,000		
12/3/68	−16 methenamine	γ-Streptococcus	100		0		0
	500 mg q 6 hr	*S. epidermidis*	110				
1/7/69	−51 methenamine	γ-Streptococcus	<100		0	*S. epidermidis*	10
	500 mg q 6 hr	*S. epidermidis*	<1,000				
		Diphtheroids	10,000				
7/1/69	−8 mo	Enterococci	500	Enterococci	120		0
		S. epidermidis	20	*S. epidermidis*	110		
		Diphtheroids	100,000	Diphtheroids	>100,000		
7/29/69	+9 nitrofurantoin	*S. epidermidis*	1,000	*S. epidermidis*	60		0
		Diphtheroids	10,000	Diphtheroids	10,000		
8/5/69	−1 nitrofurantoin	*E. coli*	130	*E. coli*	50		0
		Enterococci	>1,000	Enterococci	10,000		
		S. epidermidis	1,000	*S. epidermidis*	500		
		Diphtheroids	100,000				
8/19/69	−15 nitrofurantoin	*Achromobacter lwoffii*	80	*Achromobacter lwoffii*	90		0
		S. epidermidis	750	*S. epidermidis*	60		
		Diphtheroids	10,000	Diphtheroids	100		
10/9/69	−66 nitrofurantoin	Enterococci	70	Enterococci	10		0
		Diphtheroids	1,000	*S. epidermidis*	30		
				Diphtheroids	50		
10/23/69	−80 nitrofurantoin	*E. coli*	40	Enterococci	40	Enterococci	10
		Enterococci	240	*S. epidermidis*	10		
		S. epidermidis	200				
		Lactobacilli	10,000				
12/18/69	−137 nitrofurantoin			*S. epidermidis*	10		
		Diphtheroids	1,000	Diphtheroids	1,000		
		Lactobacilli	100,000	Lactobacilli	30	Lactobacilli	3,000
3/10/70	−217 nitrofurantoin	*S. epidermidis*	2,000	*S. epidermidis*	2,000		0
4/16/70	−263 nitrofurantoin	*E. coli*	60	*E. coli*	100		0

Table 9.4, *Continued*

Date	Days On (+) or Off (−) Therapy	Vaginal Vestibule		Urethral (VB_1)		Midstream (VB_2)	
			bacteria/ml		*bacteria/ml*		*bacteria/ml*
		γ-Streptococcus	20				
		S. epidermidis	500	*S. epidermidis*	1,000		
8/20/70	−1 yr	Diphtheroids	1,000	Diphtheroids	1,000		0
1/14/71	−1 yr, 5 mo	*E. coli*	1,000	*E. coli*	40		
		Enterococci	6,000	Enterococci	390	Enterococci	20
		S. epidermidis	3,000	*S. epidermidis*	190		
		γ-Streptococcus	100,000	γ-Streptococcus	5,000		
				α-Streptococcus	1,000		
3/4/71	−1 yr, 7 mo	*S. epidermidis*	80	*S. epidermidis*	20		0
		Diphtheroids	500	Diphtheroids	200		
		Lactobacilli	10,000	Lactobacilli	10,000		
9/9/71	−2 yr, 1 mo	*S. epidermidis*	450	*S. epidermidis*	1,000		0
		Diphtheroids	120	Diphtheroids	500		
		Lactobacilli	100,000	Lactobacilli	1,000		

[a] CB = catheterized bladder urine, or in the presence of a Foley catheter CB represents urine aspirated from the Foley. WB = culture of residual irrigation fluid after washing bladder with several liters of sterile irrigating fluid. RK = right kidney; RK_1, RK_2, etc. = serial cultures from RK. LK = left kidney; LK_1, LK_2, etc. = serial cultures from LK. SPA = suprapubic needle aspiration of bladder. Solid transverse line divides longitudinal cultures into major periods of significance.

Table 9.5
Differential Renal Function Studies on N.B., a 27-year-old White Woman[a]

Sample	Flow Rate		Sodium		Potassium		Creatinine Concentration		Creatinine Clearance	
	ml/min	*ratio L/R*	*mEq/liter*	*ratio L/R*	*mEq/liter*	*ratio L/R*	*mg/100 ml*	*ratio L/R*	*ml/min*	*ratio L/R*
Serum			139.0		4.0		0.9			
LK_1	0.19	0.04	34.5	1.08	7.0	0.54	11.7	0.39	2.5	0.01
RK_1	5.47		32.0		13.0		30.1		185.1	
LK_2	0.11	0.05	34.5	1.33	6.0	0.55	7.3	0.32	0.9	0.005
RK_2	6.73		26.0		11.0		23.2		175.5	

[a] LK = left kidney; RK = right kidney. Both collections were 30-minute periods using an oral water diuresis.

ected during an oral water diuresis (Table 9.5); as can be seen, the excretion from the small left kidney was negligible. Three consecutive cultures over a 90-minute period from the left kidney all showed >10^5 *E. coli*/ml (Table 9.4). The Foley catheter was then removed, the cystoscope was reintroduced, and a No. 5 Fr Stamey ureteral catheter was passed to the middle of the right ureter; urine from the right kidney was sterile. Bilateral retrograde urograms were performed with neomycin in the contrast medium (Fig. 9.8). No contrast would pass from the right ureter into the right renal pelvis, but the ureterogram showed a widely patent upper ureter. The left retrograde ureterogram showed malrotation of the left kidney with the ureteropelvic junction displaced laterally; the pelvis and calyces appeared minimally dilated. At the conclusion of the cystoscopic study, she was started on ampicillin 500 mg every 6 hours; the *E. coli* were sensitive to all antimicrobial drugs tested.

Three days later she was explored through a midline incision. A left nephroureterectomy was performed first. The left kidney weighed 65 g, measured 11 × 3 × 1.5 cm, and microscopically showed extensive periglomerular fibrosis, chronic interstitial inflammation, and dilatation of tubules with hyaline casts. Irrigation of the renal pelvis and ureter with saline at the time of surgery surprisingly produced a sterile fluid (Table 9.4), but she had received 500 mg of ampicillin every 6 hours for 3 days and the last dose was given intramuscularly on the morning of surgery. After the left kidney and ureter were removed, the right renal pelvis was inspected; intrapelvic pressure was less than 3 or 4 cm of water, and the urine was sterile. The renal pelvis was resected together with the intrinsic ureteral stricture, 13 small stones were removed from the calyces, the calyces were copiously irrigated, and an Anderson-Hines pyeloplasty was performed. Because of the enormous dilatation of the calyces, we decided to insert a nephrostomy tube at the time of surgery. A biopsy of the right renal cortex showed only an occasional focal area of inflammatory cells. Cultures of the stones were sterile (Table 9.4); crystallographic analysis showed them to be composed of 90% calcium oxalate monohydrate with 10% hydroxyl apatite (minute superficial patches). Her postoperative course was uneventful. The chemical evidence of hyperchloremic acidosis disappeared by the 5th postoperative day. She was discharged on the 11th postoperative day on methenamine 500 mg 4 times a day, and the nephrostomy tube was removed 1 week later on 10/25/68. She continued the methenamine for 3 additional weeks, discontinuing all therapy on 11/17/68, 5 weeks after surgery.

Cultures for the first 3 years after her nephroureterectomy are presented in Table 9.4. She may have had a single infection while on vacation in late July 1969, but there was no fever, cultures were not obtained, and she returned from holiday on nitrofurantoin. In the 11 years since her left nephrectomy, she has had one documented *E. coli* UTI on 5/27/77 for which she was treated with trimethoprim-sulfamethoxazole (TMP-SMX) for 5 days. All subse-

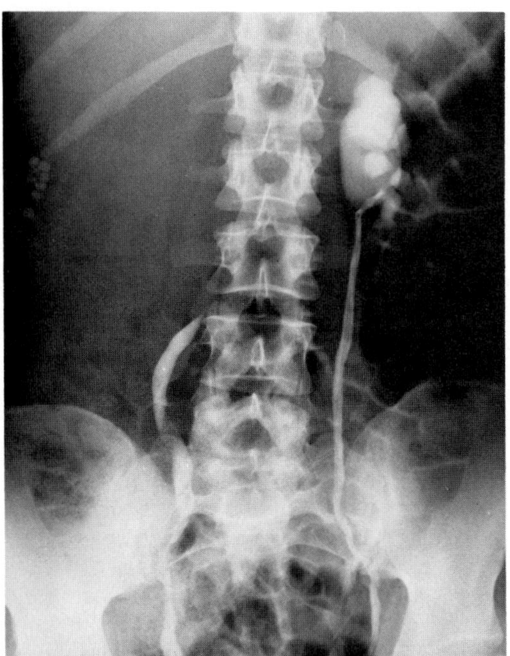

Figure 9.8 Preoperative retrograde urogram performed at the end of the differential function studies in Table 9.5.

quent cultures since 1977, including the last one on 3/23/79, have been sterile. Except for her one bacteriuric episode, 15 cultures since the last one shown in Table 9.4 have failed to grow a single colony of Enterobacteriaceae on the introitus. Multiple urinalyses have shown no protein, acid urines (pH 5.5–6.0), and no inflammatory cells. Her serum creatinine was 1.1 mg/100 ml on 3/4/71. Representative films from an IVU, performed 28 months after surgery, are reproduced in Figure 9.9. Her blood pressure is normal. Table 9.4 is particularly interesting because it shows that her introital bacteriology is comparable to that of our normal controls (Chapter 5); that is, *E. coli* appear on the introitus only transiently (4 of 17 cultures) and in small numbers.

With removal of the chronically infected, atrophic left kidney, she has had only 2 episodes of bacteriuria in 11 years. Her blood pressure remains 125/85, her serum creatinine was 1.0 mg/100 ml on 3/23/79, and her urinalyses never show protein or significant sediment. With a normal introital flora, she is not susceptible to recurrent infections. It is also of interest that, although her history of infection clearly dates back to childhood, reflux was not present and the left ureteral orifice was normal. Residual urine was never present in the bladder. Of even more importance is the observation that, despite a long standing bacteriuria, the right renal urine was sterile and the calcifications were oxalate—not phosphate—stones, suggesting that the enormously hydronephrotic right kidney (Fig. 9.7) was never infected. In view of the sterile hydronephrosis in the right kidney in the presence of a long standing bacteriuria from the left kidney, how can one posssibly defend the urologic thesis that the presence of residual urine *predisposes* the urinary tract to infection?

Vesicovaginal and Vesicointestinal Fistulas

Vesicovaginal Fistula with Urinary Tract Infection but No Leakage of Urine

N.K., a 35-year-old, married mother of 2 children, ages 8 and 15, was first seen at Stanford University Hospital on 7/17/69. In April 1969, after 1–2 months of feeling tired and fatigued, she developed a fever of 102°F and occasional nocturia. Her gynecologist, who had performed a hysterectomy for endometriosis in 1966, found a urinary infection and referred her to a urologist. Intravenous urography and cystoscopy were said to be normal. Several antibiotics failed to clear her bacteriuria. Except for malaise and some mild lower abdominal discomfort, she had no other symptoms from her chronic bacteriuria.

She was seen numerous times as an outpatient between 7/17/69 and 11/13/69 before being admitted to the hospital for bacteriologic localization studies and intramuscular cephaloridine therapy. The first six cultures in Table 9.6 established (1) the unusual chronicity of her bacteriuria despite the selection of antimicrobial agents on the basis of *in vitro* sensitivities; (2) that at least two (*E. coli* and *Enterobacter*) and probably four (*Klebsiella* and enterococci) different bacteria had caused her bladder

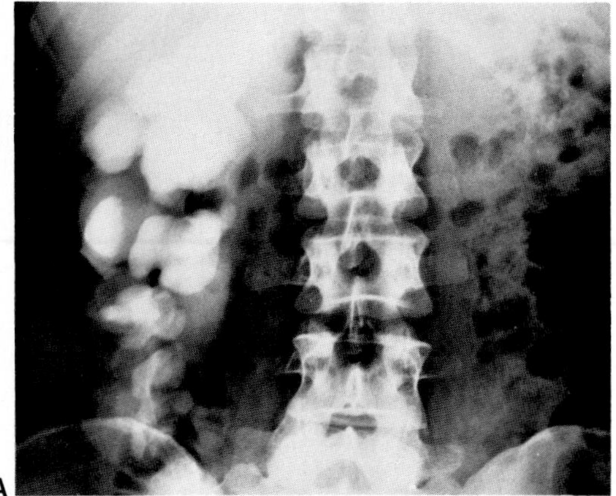

A

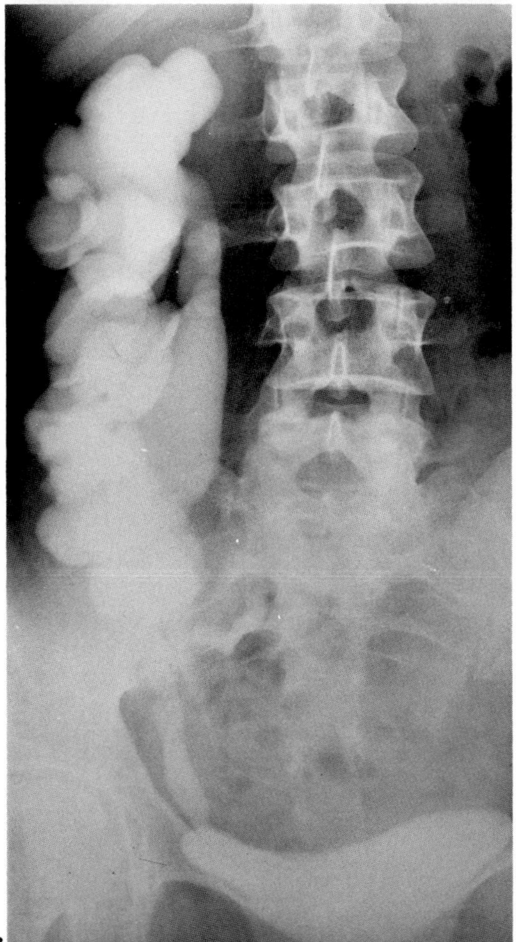

B

Figure 9.9 (*A*) A 10-minute intravenous urogram from a February, 1971, study of N.B. Note the prompt appearance of the contrast agent, the smaller calyces, and the absence of a dilated pelvis. There were no calculi on the preinjection plain film x-ray. (*B*) A delayed upright x-ray film from the same study as part *A*.

infections; (3) several of the midstream cultures suggested more than one bacterial species in the bladder since the colony count was the same in the midstream as in the urethral specimens; and (4) the vaginal cultures seemed unusually heavy in terms of pathogenic bacteria. These observations on the equivalence of VB_1 and VB_2 bacterial counts representing bladder infection were possible because all specimens were collected on the cystoscopy table under direct control of a nurse, as described in Chapter 1, Figures 1.25 and 1.26. Her outside IVU was reviewed and found to be normal; a voiding cystourethrogram on 8/13/69 showed a bladder capacity of 600 ml, no reflux despite the presence of bacteriuria, and no residual urine.

Upon admission to the hospital in November 1969, her serum creatinine was 0.7 mg/100 ml, the white blood cell count was 5500 with 57% segmented neutrophils, and the remainder of her blood and serum studies were normal. An IVU showed minimal dilatation of the right upper ureter and pelvis without caliectasis; there were no calcifications. Cystoscopy was normal. Ureteral catheters were passed to each kidney for bacteriologic localization studies (Table 9.6, 11/14/69). The bacteriuria clearly involved the right renal urine and probably the left. Cephaloridine 1.0 g every 8 hours was given intramuscularly for 10 days. The urine became sterile, and the cephaloridine was changed to oral cephalexin. On the 18th day of oral cephalexin, her urine was infected with *Enterobacter,* which had been present in the vagina on the 10th day of cephaloridine therapy (11/24/69). The *Enterobacter,* resistant to cephaloridine (minimal inhibitory concentration, MIC, >1500 μg/ml) was sensitive to nalidixic acid (MIC, 5 μg/ml). Despite therapy with nalidixic acid, the *Enterobacter* developed immediate resistance. In the first 4 months of 1970, she was treated in succession with oxytetracycline, nitrofurantoin, penicillin-G, nalidixic acid, and again with nitrofurantoin—

Table 9.6
N..K., a 35-year-old White Woman with a Vesicovaginal Fistula[a]

Date	Days On (+) or Off (−) Therapy	Vaginal Vestibule		Urethral (VB_1)		Midstream (VB_2)		Procedures and Comment
		bacteria/ml		*bacteria/ml*		*bacteria/ml*		
7/17/69	1st visit							
7/24/69	+7 sulfamethizole 500 mg q 6 hr	*Escherichia coli* Enterococci	>100,000 <10,000	*E. coli* Enterococci	>100,000 <10,000	*E. coli* Enterococci	>100,000 <10,000	Equal counts of Enterococci in the VB_1 and VB_2 suggest enterococci in the bladder as well as the *E. coli*
8/7/69	−11 sulfamethizole 500 mg q 6 hr	*E. coli* *Klebsiella*	>100,000 <10,000	*E. coli* *Klebsiella*	>100,000 <10,000	*E. coli* *Klebsiella*	>100,000 <10,000	*Klebsiella*, as well as *E. coli*, in the bladder
8/13/69	Cystourethrogram							First voiding cystourethrogram
9/16/69	+32 nalidixic acid 500 mg q 6 hr	*E. coli* *Klebsiella* Enterococci	>100,000 4,000 100	*E. coli* *Klebisella* Enterococci	>100,000 4,000 100	*E. coli* *Klebsiella* Enterococci	>100,000 4,000 100	All three species may be in the bladder
10/7/69	+19 nitrofurantoin 100 mg q 6 hr	*E. coli* Enterococci *Staphylococcus epidermidis*	100,000 5,000 5,000	*E. coli* Enterococci *S. epidermidis*	100,000 5,000 5,000	*E. coli* Enterococci *S. epidermidis*	6,000 3,000 2,000	Bladder urine probably sterile
10/28/69	+18 penicillin-G 500 mg q 6 hr	*E. coli* *Enterobacter*	1,000 10,000	*E. coli* *Enterobacter*	1,000 100,000	*E. coli* *Enterobacter*	1,000 100,000	Both species in the bladder
11/11/69	+10 sulfamethizole 500 mg q 6 hr	*E. coli*	>100,000	*E. coli*	>100,000	*E. coli*	>100,000	
11/14/69	−2 sulfamethizole 500 mg q 6 hr	*E. coli* Lactobacilli	1,000 10,000	CB *E. coli* 100,000 WB *E. coli* 4,000 LK_1 *E. coli* 540 LK_2 *E. coli* 520 LK_3 *E. coli* 550 LK_4 *E. coli* 230		RK_1 *E. coli* 10,000 RK_2 *E. coli* 5,000 RK_3 *E. coli* 5,000 RK_4 *E. coli* 5,000		Cystoscopy normal Both kidneys are infected
11/17/69	+3 cephaloridine 1.0 g q 8 hr				0	*Enterobacter*	10	
11/24/69	+10 cephaloridine 1.0 g q 8 hr	*Enterobacter*	4,000				0	
12/12/69	+18 cephalexin 250 mg q 6 hr	*Enterobacter*	>100,000	*Enterobacter*	>100,000	*Enterobacter*	>100,000	
12/30/69	+12 nalidixic acid 500 mg q 6 hr	*Enterobacter* γ-Streptococcus	>10,000 1,000	*Enterobacter*	>100,000	*Enterobacter*	>100,000	
4/2/70	Vesicovaginal fistula identified (Figure 9.10)							
4/19/70	−35 nitrofurantoin	*Enterobacter* Enterococci Gram-negative cocci	1,000 10,000 >100,000	*Enterobacter* Gram-negative cocci	190 >100,000	*Enterobacter* Gram-negative cocci	90 >100,000	Second voiding cystourethrogram
4/22/70	Vesicovaginal fistula fulgerated							

	100 mg q 6 hr							
5/17/70	+10 nalidixic acid 500 mg q 6 hr			*Enterobacter*	>100,000	*Enterobacter*	>100,000	
5/18/70	Suprapubic excision of vesicovaginal fistula							
5/18/70	+1 gentamicin 30 mg q 8 hr	*Enterobacter*	110		0		0	
		Proteus mirabilis	5,000					
5/22/70	+5 gentamicin					CB	0	
5/27/70	+3 nitrofurantoin 100 mg q 6 hr	*Enterobacter*	5,000			CB *Enterobacter*	130	Foley catheter removed
		P. mirabilis	10,000			*P. mirabilis*	120	
		Deep vaginal:						
		Enterobacter	5,000					
		P. mirabilis	10,000					
6/11/70	+17 nitrofurantoin 100 mg q 6 hr	*P. mirabilis*	>100,000	*P. mirabilis*	>100,000	*P. mirabilis*	>100,000	This *P. mirabilis* was overlooked in the Foley catheter at the time of its removal on 5/27/70
		Deep vaginal:						
		P. mirabilis	>100,000					
6/25/70	+10 nalidixic acid 500 mg q 6 hr	*P. mirabilis*	10,000	*P. mirabilis*	350	*P. mirabilis*	100	
		Enterococci	10,000	Enterococci	500	Enterococci	220	
		Midvaginal:						
		P. mirabilis	10,000					
		Enterococci	10,000					
7/9/70	−6 nalidixic acid	*P. mirabilis*	100,000	*P. mirabilis*	8,000	*P. mirabilis*	4,000	
		Enterobacter	520	*Enterobacter*	10			
		Enterococci	1,000	Enterococci	310	Enterococci	1,000	
		Midvaginal:						
		P. mirabillis	100,000					
		Enterobacter	30					
		Enterococci	750					
8/4/70	−32 nalidixic acid	*P. mirabilis*	300	*P. mirabilis*	310	*P. mirabilis*	240	
		Enterobacter	30			*Enterobacter*	20	
		Enterococci	750	Enterococci	20	Enterococci	320	
9/19/70	−78	*P. mirabilis*	100	*P. mirabilis*	20	*P. mirabilis*	20	
		Enterobacter	10,000	*Enterobacter*	4,000	*Enterobacter*	2,500	
				Enterococci	240	Enterococci	70	
1/29/71	−209	*S. epidermidis*	220					
		Lactobacilli	100,000	Lactobacilli	3,000	Lactobacilli	200	
6/10/71	−340	*P. mirabilis*	10	*P. mirabilis*	20		0	
		Enterobacter	20					
		Enterococci	130	Enterococci	20			
		S. epidermidis	1,000	*S. epidermidis*	150			
		Diphtheroids	1,000					
		Lactobacilli	10,000					

[a] Abbreviations as in Table 9.4. Solid transverse line divides longitudinal cultures into major periods of significance.

all with similar results (these nine cultures are not shown in Table 9.6 because the pattern is almost the same as in the earlier studies). The bladder urine was sterilized in March with nitrofurantoin, and, in the absence of sexual intercourse, a Gram-negative coccus caused the next bacteriuria; the same, unidentifiable organism was present (4/19/70) in large numbers in the vagina (Table 9.6).

During these early months of 1970, several deep vaginal cultures were obtained with a vaginal speculum; they were always similar to cultures of the vaginal vestibule and were characterized by thousands of Gram-negative bacteria and enterococci. Not once was free fluid found in the vaginal vault, nor had the patient ever noticed fluid coming from the vagina. Further discussion with the patient, however, did reveal that some leakage of urine per vagina had occurred for a few days following her hysterectomy for endometriosis in 1966; she had seen a urologist for a single silver nitrate cauterization and the leakage had ceased.

Because of her bacteriologic course and this additional history, the bladder was filled to capacity with indigo carmine in saline and the vaginal vault was carefully inspected. There was no staining; except for a slight cufflike indentation in one corner of the posterior vaginal fornix, which had been inspected on several occasions before, there were no visible abnormalities. Nevertheless, three cotton balls were packed into the vagina before the speculum was removed. She was asked to walk around for 10 minutes and then empty her bladder. The cotton balls were carefully removed; the deepest one was dark blue in the area of the cufflike indentation in the lateral fornix (Fig. 9.10).

She was admitted to Stanford University Hospital on 4/19/70. Because the previous voiding cystourethrogram had shown no fistula, the studies were repeated. The bladder was filled to 700 ml with 50% Hypaque; numerous lateral views during voiding showed no evidence of a fistula. A 3-hour postvoiding film did not demonstrate contrast in the vagina. A repeat IVU was normal.

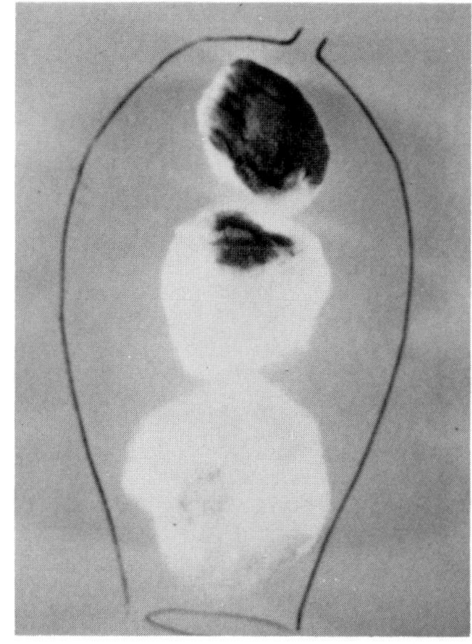

Figure 9.10 A photograph of the three cotton balls removed from the vagina of N.K. (see text). A vaginal outline is drawn around the cotton balls. The introitus is at the bottom of the picture, the cufflike indentation of the posterior vaginal fornix at the top.

At cystoscopy, using general anesthesia and fiberoptic illumination, three different observers, including the author, could not detect a fistulous opening. A 75-ml Foley bag catheter was then placed in the vagina and inflated to 150 ml, and the posterior vagina was filled under pressure with saline containing indigo carmine. Repeat cystoscopy now showed a column of blue dye jetting out of a 2-mm, noninflamed lip of mucosa on the back wall of the bladder above the trigone. The fistula site in the bladder was catheterized with a Bugby electrode which surprisingly passed easily into the vagina. The entire fistulous tract was fulgurated, a Foley catheter was left in the bladder for 2 weeks, and the urine was sterilized with 5 days of gentamicin followed by nitrofurantoin (Table 9.6). By the 14th day of Foley catheter drainage, however, she was leaking profuse amounts of urine into the vagina. The catheter was removed, the leakage continued, and she was readmitted for suprapubic excision of the fistula, which was performed on 5/18/

70. Gentamicin, started the day before surgery, again sterilized the urine. After 5 days, the gentamicin was changed to nitrofurantoin. The Foley catheter was removed on 5/27 and she was discharged on nitrofurantoin. Although her first follow-up visit on 6/11/70 showed a *P. mirabilis* bacteriuria (Table 9.6), it is clear that this organism was in the urine aspirated from the Foley catheter at the time of removal (Table 9.6, 5/27/70). Nalidixic acid, to which the *P. mirabilis* was sensitive (MIC, 4 μg/ml), cleared the bacteriuria. There have been no further infections in the 9 years since clearing this catheter-induced *P. mirabilis* bacteriuria.

This patient is presented in detail to emphasize how subtle bacteriologic fistulas can be between the urinary tract and adjacent structures. Two voiding cystourethrograms failed to demonstrate a fistula, and the second one was performed knowing it was there. The patient, a fastidious, attractive woman, had never observed leakage of fluid from the vagina. Several cystoscopists had seen nothing abnormal in the bladder; indeed, three of us, knowing the fistula was there and using optimal instruments and general anesthesia, could not detect the slightest evidence for a fistulous opening until blue dye was made to efflux from the vagina into the bladder.

The rather boring and repetitive bacteriology shown in Table 9.6 is presented because the interested observer will quickly recognize that the vaginal bacteriology in this patient is substantially different from that in any patient presented in Chapter 4. While the introitus of women with recurrent urinary infection may occasionally show pathogenic bacterial growth to this magnitude, few have been as persistent in carrying such enormous numbers. Moreover, when antimicrobial therapy is administered on the basis of *in vitro* sensitivities, it is virtually impossible to have such poor results as occurred in this patient without the urinary tract having immediate access to a reservoir of new pathogens. I am inclined to believe that only 2 or 3 ml of urine per day, leaking into the vagina of this patient, destroyed the bactericidal nature of the normal vagina and thereby allowed the free proliferation of enteric pathogens to the numbers observed in Table 9.6.

There are other vesical fistulas that cause persistent urinary infections, but these are obvious for the most part, and detailed examples will not be presented. We have all seen vesicoileal fistulas from regional enteritis and vesicocolic fistulas from diverticulitis of the colon. Rarely, though, do these patients present as seemingly uncomplicated urinary infections as in the case of N.K. (Table 9.6). Postoperative or cancer fistulas, as a complication of operative technique or radiation, are clearly obvious. In the male child, rectourethral and the even rarer rectovesical fistulas, persisting after repair of imperforate rectums, must always be considered. Fortunately, those fistulas in the female associated with an imperforate anus at birth are embryologically converted to rectovestibular fistulas rather than urethral or vesical ones.[11]

Vesicoileal and Vesicoappendiceal Fistulas

Most vesicointestinal fistulas are reasonably obvious if the patient has gastrointestinal symptoms, a UTI, and is passing gas per urethra. We see, however, one or two patients each year who deny intestinal symptomatology, who have localized regional ileitis, and who clearly have had their vesicointestinal fistula longer than necessary. One of these patients was a 50-year-old white man who 5 years before seeing us developed dysuria, frequency, pyuria, and cloudy odorous urine. He was cystoscoped three times and each time was diagnosed as having prostatitis. Multiple courses of antimicrobial therapy were given, but each time the infection recurred after stopping treatment. Two years before seeing us in 1973 he began having suprapubic discomfort immediately before voiding and observed gas in his urine. A right inguinal hernia was repaired in 1972 as a possible cause of his suprapubic discomfort. When seen at Stanford in April 1973, he was on ampicillin, his urine was sterile and contained no WBCs or RBCs. Cystoscopy showed a small, noninflamed fistulous opening on the right posterior lateral wall of the bladder above the

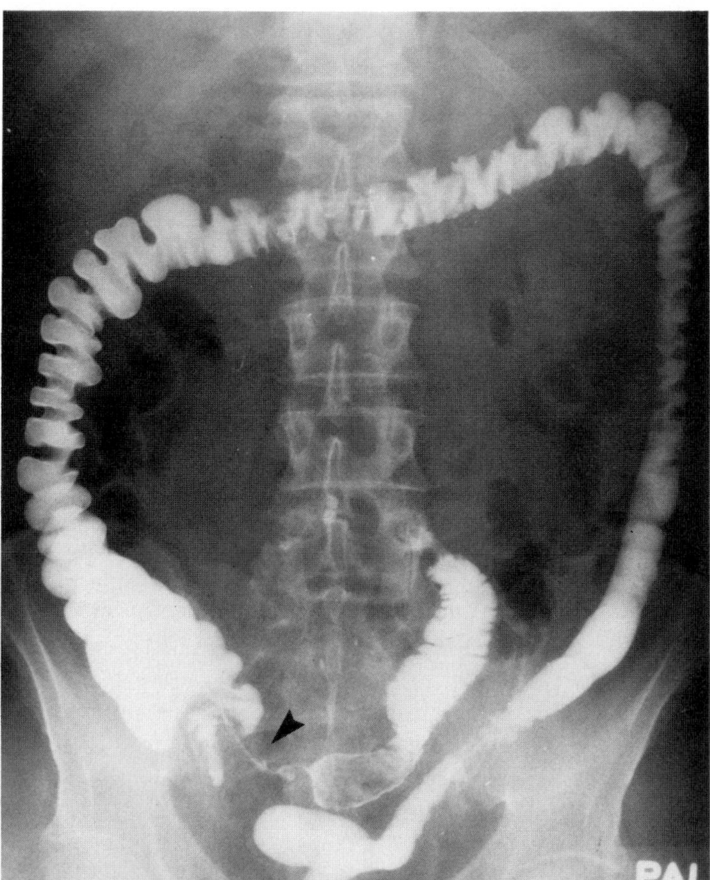

Figure 9.11 Barium enema showing that the rectum, sigmoid colon, and flexures are normal. The cecum appears unremarkable with an appendiceal stump. The terminal ileum is straight and narrow (*arrow*), consistent with regional enteritis.

ureteral orifice; the absence of mucosal edema was remarkable. A barium enema (Figure 9.11) and an upper gastrointestinal (GI) series (Figure 9.12) both showed an abnormal terminal ileum with straightening and stricture formation consistent with regional enteritis. A cystogram performed the following day by suprapubic puncture showed no fistula on the filling films, but contrast medium passed from the right posterior lateral aspect of the bladder toward the terminal ileum during voiding (see arrow in Figure 9.13). The following day, 16 cm of terminal ileum and 6.0 cm of cecum were resected along with part of the bladder wall containing the fistulous tract between the ileum and the bladder. The patient was discharged on the 9th postoperative day. He has had no further UTI in the past 6 years; multiple cultures off antibiotics during the first postoperative year were sterile. The VB_1 contained only a few colonies of *Staphylococcus epidermidis*.

Even more subtle than the previous patient is a 25-year-old white man from Michigan whom I saw for the first time in September 1978. He had experienced continuous urinary infections for 2½ years; the initial infection was caused by *P. mirabilis*, but *E. coli* had been grown on numerous occasions. Antimicrobial therapy included ampicillin, nitrofurantoin, and TMP-SMX; discontinuation of therapy was always followed promptly by severe symptoms of bladder irritation and infection. He was cystoscoped twice, the last time 7/11/77, and spotty inflammation of the bladder wall was observed with edema along the right lateral wall; cup biopsies showed cystitis cystica. Bilateral retrograde urograms were normal. *E. coli* was cultured at the time of cystoscopy. Cultures for tuberculosis were negative but, because of a positive tuberculin skin test, he was treated with isoniazid and vitamin B_6 for 1 year. Because of a past history of intermittent diarrhea, especially an episode in 1972 of 3 weeks of severe abdominal cramps and diarrhea, he had had several upper and lower bowel x-ray contrast studies, all of which were repeated in July 1977 as well as a sigmoidoscopy. The upper GI series was compatible with regional ileitis. Because he was mostly asymptomatic from the intestinal standpoint, it was decided that neither medical nor surgical treatment of his ileum was indicated.

When I saw him in September 1978, he had been on ampicillin continuously for 6 months; despite this therapy, he observed that the urine was often cloudy and that he had noticed terminal pneumaturia on three occasions which had been explained to him as "gas-producing bacteria." I had asked him to stop his ampicillin 5 days before seeing me. Upon examination, his urine was loaded with leukocytes and *P. mirabilis* $> 10^5$ bacteria/ml. His expressed prostatic secretion was also loaded with clumps of leukocytes and oval fat macrophages, compatible with bacterial prostatitis (see Figure 7.1). The *P. mirabilis* were strongly coated with fluorescent antibody, and showed the usual sensitivities to antimicrobial agents, that is, sensitive to all agents at urinary levels except the polymyxins, tetracyclines,

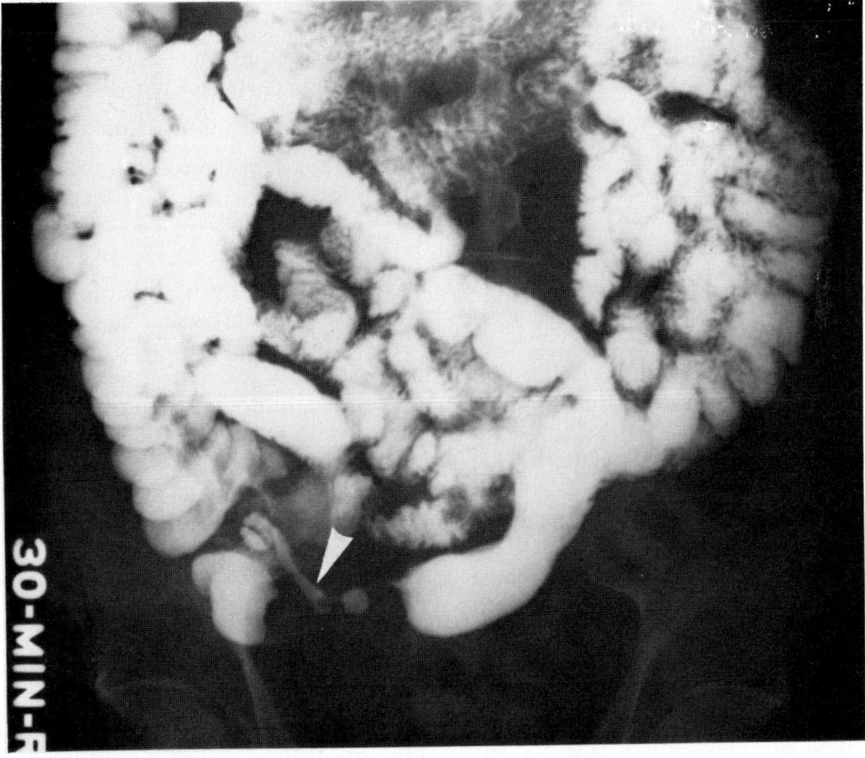

Figure 9.12 Small bowel series from an upper gastrointestinal study. The small bowel appears normal except for the terminal strictured area of the ileum (*arrow*); some of the ileum is dilated just before the stricture. Special radiographic techniques are required if the terminal ileum is to be well seen in small bowel series. If the patient does not have an incompetent ileocecal valve (Figure 9.11), the terminal few centimeters of ileum may not be visualized unless special care is taken with the small bowel series.

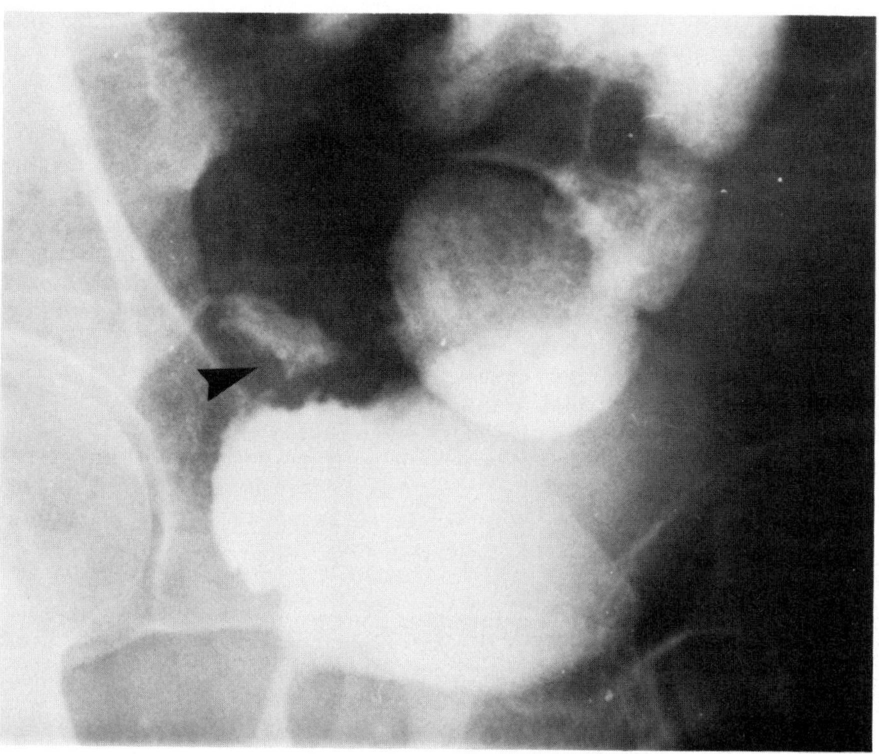

Figure 9.13 Cystogram via suprapubic puncture. No fistula was observed during the filling phase. With voiding, contrast is seen to pass through a fistula toward the region of the terminal ileum (*arrow*). Residual contrast medium from the upper gastrointestinal series is seen also.

and nitrofurantoins. *P. mirabilis* and *E. coli* were the predominant aerobic Enterobacteriaceae on rectal culture.

He was started on gentamicin 80 mg every 8 hours and 24 hours later, prior to cystoscopy under a saddle anesthesia, had a lower tract bacterial localization: VB_1 = 80 β-streptococci/ml, VB_2 = 10 β-streptococci/ml, expressed prostatic secretion (EPS) = 20 *P. mirabilis*/ml and 80 β-streptococci/ml, and VB_3 = 60 β-streptococci/ml, apparently indicating a *P. mirabilis* bacterial prostatitis (see Chapter 7). His EPS was again observed to be purulent with oval fat macrophages.

Cystoscopy confirmed some edema on the back wall of the bladder. By pressing the abdomen, purulent material exuded from one area and I was able to pass a No. 5 Stamey ureteral polyethylene catheter into the hole for about 3 cm. Injection with contrast medium (Figure 9.14, *A–C*) showed progressive filling of the rectosigmoid and ultimately the descending colon. The following day, an upper GI, a small bowel, and colon follow-through series showed the cecum, sigmoid, and distal ileum matted together in the pelvis; an enterocolic fistula was demonstrated by the appearance of contrast agent in the cecum and sigmoid at the same time before filling of the transverse and descending colon. The vesicointestinal fistula was not identified by the intestinal x-rays. Only the proximal part of the appendix was filled. Our radiologist did not feel that Crohn's disease was a likely diagnosis because of the limited segment of ileum that would have to be involved; they favored either a periappendiceal abscess with fistula formation between the ileum and sigmoid and a vesicocolic fistula, or a foreign body abscess with subsequent fistula formation.

On the third day of hospitalization, I

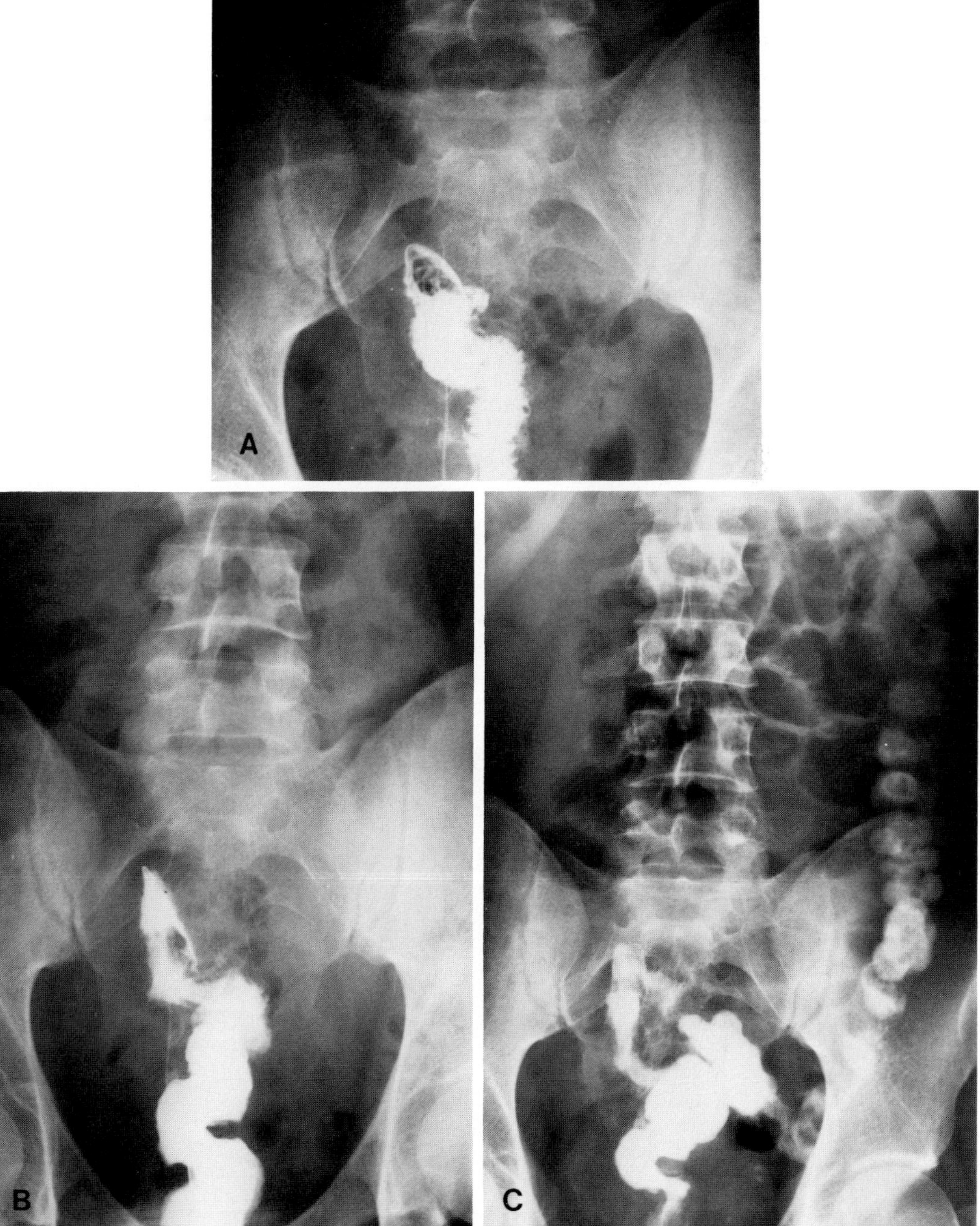

Figure 9.14 Fistulogram made by injecting the 5 Fr polyethelene Stamey ureteral catheter passed at cystoscopy: (*A*) 5 ml of contrast medium, (*B*) an additional 10 ml, and (*C*) an additional 20 ml. Figures show a progressive filling of the sigmoid colon with ultimate filling of the descending colon.

resected a 30-cm segment of terminal ileum with 10 cm of cecum all of which was matted together in the pelvis. The vesicocolic fistula was identified and the back wall of the bladder resected with the fistula. The enterocolic fistula was also identified and the sigmoid colon closed in layers at the fistula site. After resection of the specimen, the appendix was difficult to find; the wall was thickened and there was fibrous obliteration of much of the appendix. Except for granulation tissue in the fistula sites, there was no evidence of inflammatory bowel disease and our pathologist found no evidence of Crohn's disease. We believe the patient probably had a ruptured appendix during his 3-week illness in 1972 and fistula formation a few years later.

A Foley catheter was left in the bladder for 7 days; his gentamicin was stopped 48 hours after surgery. On the 6th postoperative day, 4 days after stopping the gentamicin and 1 day before removing the Foley catheter, the urine was again infected with *P. mirabilis* which was again fluorescent antibody-positive. He was started on cephalexin 250 mg every 6 hours after the Foley catheter was removed. Prostatic localization cultures 24 hours after starting cephalexin showed VB_1 = 0 bacteria/ml, VB_2 =

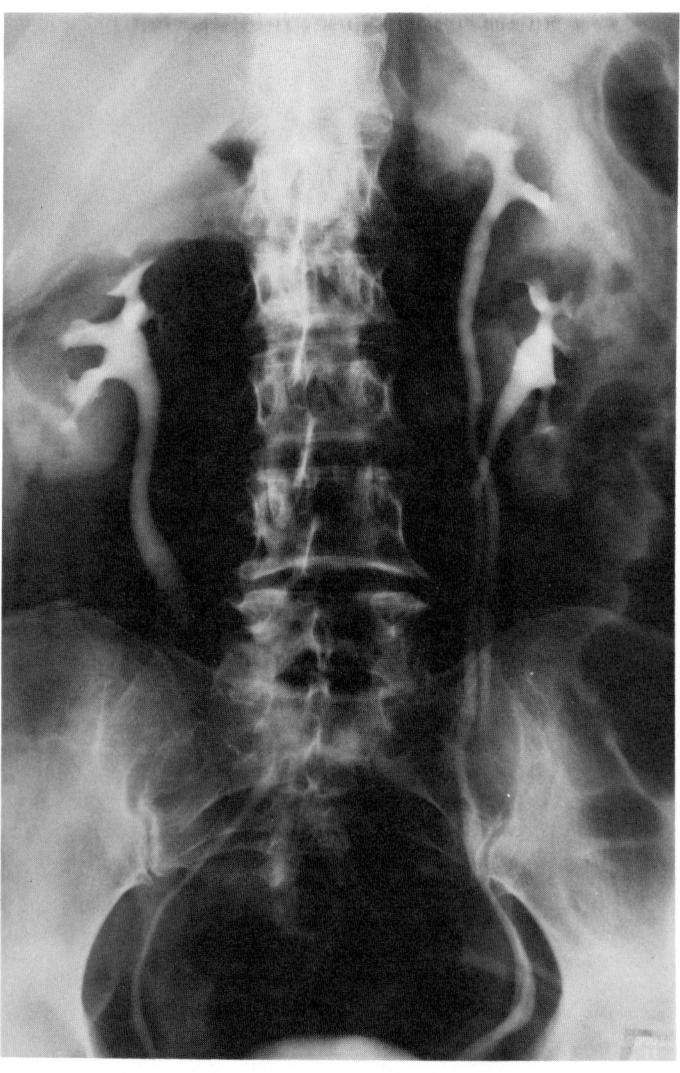

Figure 9.15 Intravenous urogram on a 52-year-old, white woman with a 12-year history of recurrent Pseudomonas urinary tract infection. The right and left renal outlines are well seen with a single ureter on the right and a double ureter on the left. Observe how normal the right kidney appears to be.

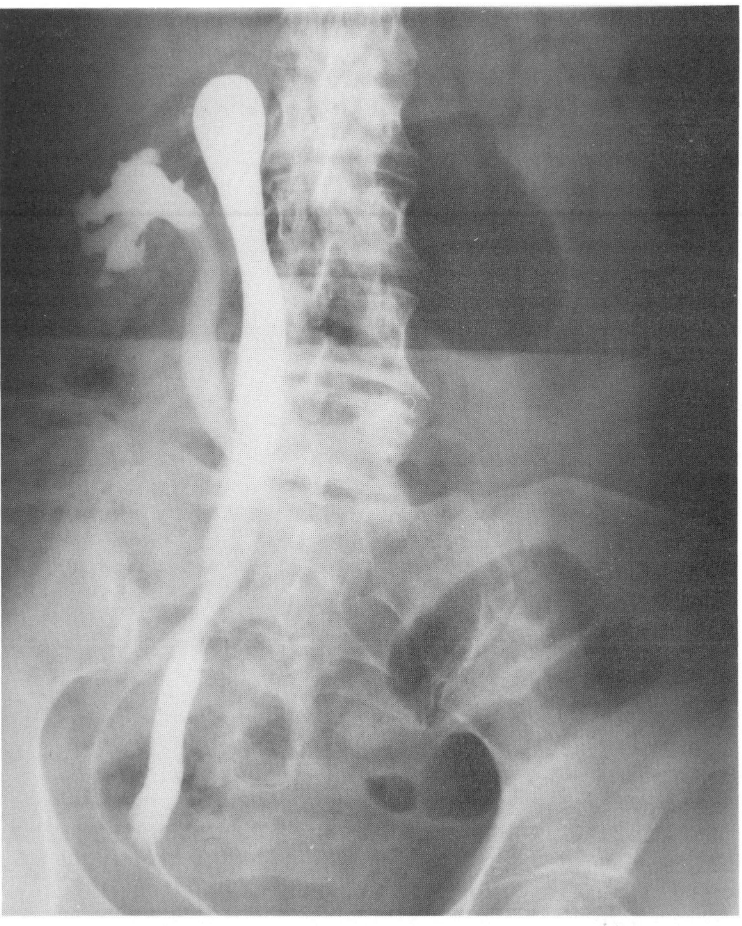

'igure 9.16 Retrograde urogram of the upper pole ectopic ureter filled with *Pseudomonas aeruginosa*; the lower pole ureter has also been catheterized. Resection of the duplicated, ectopic ureter resulted in cure of her recurrent Pseudomonas infections and pyuria, but did not prevent further *Escherichia coli* urinary tract infection. Same patient as in Figure 9.15.

0 bacteria/ml, EPS = 620 *P. mirabilis*/ml, and VB_3 = 10 *P. mirabilis*/ml. He returned to Michigan on the 10th postoperative day, stopped the cephalexin after several weeks, and has had no further UTI. My last follow-up was January 1980. The prostate was probably infected with *P. mirabilis* secondary to the UTI from the intestinal fistula; whatever the cause, the *P. mirabilis* prostatitis appears to be cleared from the cephalexin therapy.

In closing this section, I am aware that vesicointestinal fistulas theoretically belong to reinfections of the urinary tract, as I have outlined in my classification in Chapter 1, rather than as a cause of bacterial persistence. I have included them here, however, because most patients do recur with the same organism which represents the predominant bacteria present in the intestinal tract.

Ureteral Duplication and Ectopic Ureters

Ureteral duplication, especially when associated with ectopic ureters emptying into the urethra, are often infected and may give rise to recurrent bacteriuria with the organism which persists in the ectopic, duplicated segment. At least 80% of ectopic ureters in females are duplicated ureters[12] which means that the nonectopic ureter of the duplication may appear as a completely normal kidney thereby confusing the physician. For example, look at the normal-appearing kidneys in Figure 9.15. Who would have suspected that the right kidney in this 52-year-old woman with a 12-year history of recurrent *P. aeruginosa* infections had an ectopic ureter filled with *P. aeroginosa* emptying into her urethra, as shown in Figure 9.16? Her symptoms had always been dysuria and urgency incontinence; when I first saw her with a bacteriuria due to *P. aeruginosa*, cystoscopy and urethroscopy were normal and ureteral catheterization studies showed all three ureters in Figure 9.15 were uninfected. Even when I found the ectopic opening, I thought it was an accessory urethra because injection with contrast medium filled only the urethral portion of the tube; only after I had resected the "accessory urethra," and her recurrent bacteriuria with *P. aeruginosa* continued, did I suspect that I was dealing with a duplication. The lesson is that duplications with ectopic ureters can be extremely subtle. Since one-third will empty into the urethra,[13] and many of these will have hypoplasia or dysplasia of the upper pole segment, this congenital anomaly is a perfect setup for infection which will then persist and cause recurrent bacteriuria with the same organism. In retrospect, the right ureter in Figure 9.15 is deviated medially by the grossly dilated ectopic ureter (Figure 9.16). More importantly, any female patient with recurrent bacteriuria caused by bacterial persistence of the same organism, who has a complete duplication of the ureter on one side and not on the other, is a prime suspect for an infected ectopic ureter emptying into the urethra.

Since resection of the duplicated ureter on 9/10/73, she has had multiple cultures and urinalyses. The pyuria disappeared and *P. aeruginosa* has not been seen since surgery, not even on the introital cultures. Her urine was sterile for the first year after resection of the duplication, but she had an asymptomatic bacteriuria without pyuria in August 1974 (an *Enterobacter*), an *E. coli* in December 1974, an enterococcus in Jan-

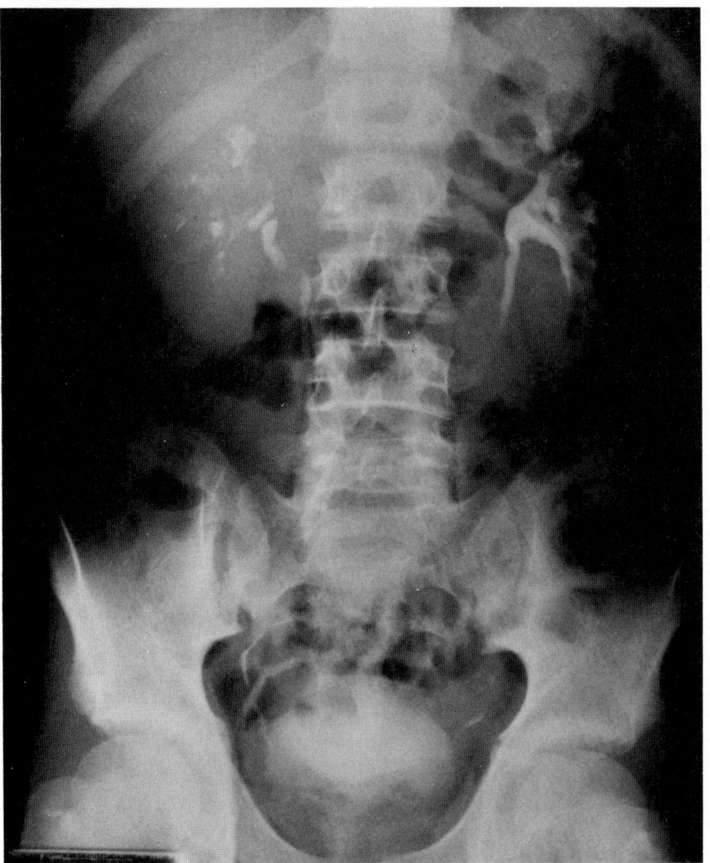

Figure 9.17 Intravenous urogram on a 15-year-old boy with pyuria and *Pseudomonas aeruginosa* infection. The film appears normal except for some atonicity to the right collecting system.

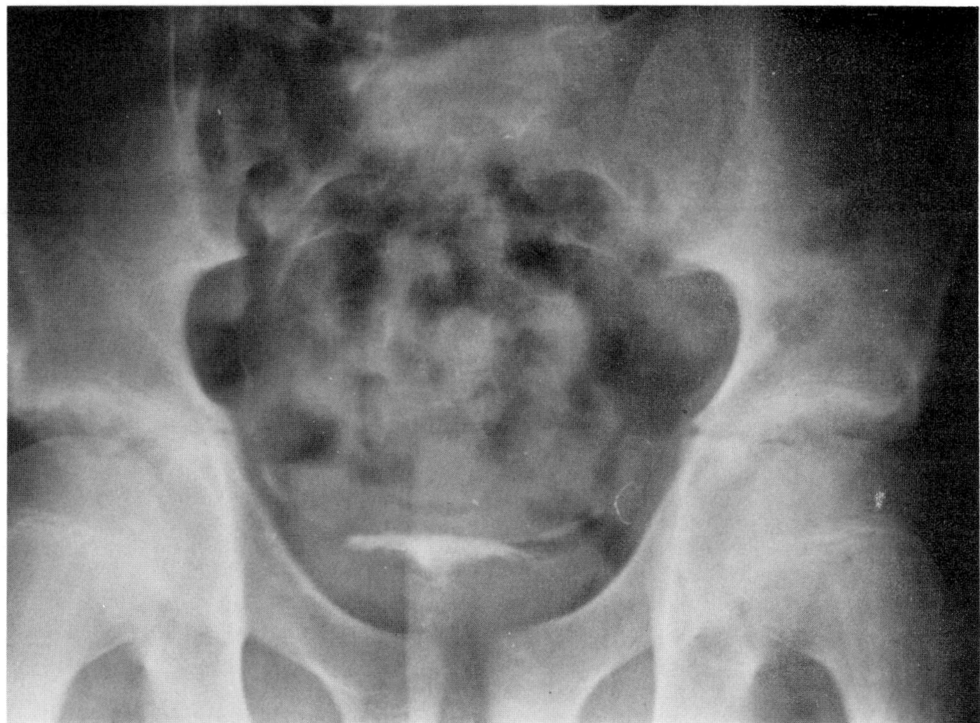

Figure 9.18 Postvoiding intravenous urogram from the same series as Figure 9.17 on the 15-year-old boy with Pseudomonas urinary tract infection. Note that the nylon fishing-line cannot be seen in the bladder even on the emptying film. Removal of the coil of nylon from the bladder cured the infection.

uary 1975, another *E. coli* in March 1975, and still another *E. coli* in February 1976. It is interesting that every one of these infections were symptomless, accompanied by less than 3 WBC/hpf in the spun urine, and easily cleared with a few days of antimicrobial therapy.

These recurrent infections show that resecting an infected congenital abnormality that had caused recurrent infections due to bacterial persistence of *P. aeruginosa* did not prevent her susceptibility to further reinfections. It is likely that it was this basic susceptibility to infections that caused the anomaly to become infected in the first place. The lesson should be clear to every urologist: do not promise a female patient that surgical excision of an abnormality that has caused UTI to recur with the same infecting strain will necessarily cure her of recurrent infections. It certainly will cure her of the persisting strain causing the recurrent bacteriuria, and she may feel much better as did this patient, but the basic cause of reinfections is a biologic one, not a surgical one.

Foreign Body

A 15-year-old boy was seen in consultation for an asymptomatic *P. aeruginosa* UTI with pyuria discovered during a routine physical examination. His VB_1 and VB_2 grew *P. aeruginosa* $> 10^5$ bacteria/ml. A 15-minute x-ray film from his IVU is shown in Figure 9.17 and a postvoiding film from the same study in Figure 9.18; both films are considered normal, although the calyces in the right kidney appear somewhat atonic and may represent the consequences of ascending infection on that side.

On 3/11/77, he was cystoscoped to obtain more bacteriologic information. Within the bladder, and with one end protruding to the external sphincter, was a coiled string of nylon fishing line which was grasped and removed. At no time prior to cystoscopy did he admit to inserting foreign objects into his urethra. He was treated with gentamicin for 3 doses and discharged on 10 days of sulfisoxazole, to which his *P. aeruginosa* was also sensitive *in vitro* (I will comment more on this not uncommon finding in the following chapter). All follow-up cultures off therapy have been sterile and his pyuria disappeared.

A much more subtle foreign body as a cause of bacterial persistence—iatrogenic rather than self-inflicted—is detailed in the following case study of a 58-year-old white woman who was first seen in 1965 with renal colic, small bilateral renal stones, and an appearance on IVU that suggested bilateral medullary sponge kidneys, but neither the calcifications nor the disease appeared severe.

She passed a small, calcium oxalate stone and her colic disappeared. Her urine was uninfected and a metabolic stone workup unrevealing. In 1967 she had a total vaginal hysterectomy with an anterior urethroplasty for stress urinary incontinence. In 1968 she was seen for recurrent urinary frequency, urgency, and *E. coli* urinary infections; cystoscopy showed a normal urethra and bladder. Ureteral catheterization studies in the presence of *E. coli* bacteriuria indicated the right kidney was infected, the left sterile (Table 9.7). Between 1968 and 1972 she had multiple infections with *S. epidermidis, Klebsiella,* and *E. coli,* but from 1972 until 1978 all her infections were due to *P. aeruginosa.* When she was symptomatic, tetracycline (MIC = 30 μg/ml) usually alleviated her symptoms. Because all of her voided urine specimens were obtained on the cystoscopy table, rather than self-caught specimens, her bacterial cultures are extremely interesting and I have reproduced all of her cultures from the first time we documented *P. aeruginosa* on 8/16/72 (Table 9.8). These cultures clearly suggest a urethral rather than a vaginal source of her *P. aeruginosa.* Because of this, she was again cystoscoped on 3/13/78. In the middle of the urethra, just beneath

Table 9.7
Bacteriologic Localization Studies in August 1968[a]

Source	*Escherichia coli*
	bacteria/ml
CB	10^4
WB	1140
LK_1	0
LK_2	0
LK_3	0
LK_4	0
RK_1	5000
RK_2	1400
RK_3	1000
RK_4	2000

[a] *CB* = catheterized bladder count, *WB* = washed bladder count before ureteral catheterization, K_1–K_4 = serial kidney urines from each side.

a mucosal fold, one could see the top of a yellow stone deeply buried in the mucosa. Further inspection failed to show a diverticulum, just a deep-lying linear, yellow calcification extending across the urethra but deeply buried in the mucosa. The calcification could not be palpated vaginally. Bilateral ureteral catheterization studies showed both kidneys were uninfected (Table 9.9), unlike the localization 10 years earlier when *E. coli* were present in the right ureteral urine (Table 9.7). A plain film x-ray of the pelvic area showed the transverse-lying stone (Figure 9.19). The stone (10.6 × 7.3 × 5.7 mm) was removed with an anterior vaginal incision; to our surprise a calcified fibrous suture protruded from both ends of the transverse stone extending for 2 cm at one end, obviously representing a suture placed through the urethra at the time of the vaginal hysterectomy 11 years earlier. The stone analysis showed predominantly apatite surrounding the catgut suture, but there was some whewellite (calcium oxalate monohydrate), obviously adventitial from her propensity to form calcium oxalate stones (which have not recurred since 1965). The stone culture results are shown in Table 9.9. She received tobramycin on call to the operating room and for 5 days thereafter (80 mg every 12 hours) and was discharged on one-half tablet TMP-SMX for 1 month. As seen in Table 9.8, her introital, urethral (VB_1) and

Table 9.8
Bacteriologic Course of a 58-year-old Woman with an 11-year history of a Urethral Foreign Body[a]

Date	Days On (+) or Off (−) Drug	Drug	Introitus		VB_1[b]		VB_2[b]	
			bacteria/ml		*bacteria/ml*		*bacteria/ml*	
8/16/72	− 7	Nitrofurantoin	*Escherichia coli*	20	*Pseudomonas aeruginosa*	5,000	*P. aeruginosa*	2,000
8/22/72	+ 6	Nalidixic acid	*P. aeruginosa*	40	*P. aeruginosa*	6,000	*P. aeruginosa*	820
8/28/72	+ 3	Tetracycline		0	*P. aeruginosa*	40	*P. aeruginosa*	40
9/11/72	− 7	Tetracycline		0	*P. aeruginosa*	6,000	*P. aeruginosa*	2,000
9/21/72	−17	Tetracycline		0	*P. aeruginosa*	5,000	*P. aeruginosa*	2,000
6/29/76	Postcoital	Penicillin-G	*P. aeruginosa*	4,000	*P. aeruginosa*	10,000	*P. aeruginosa*	2,000
1/10/78	+10	Sulfisoxazole	*P. aeruginosa*	1,000	*P. aeruginosa*	3,000	*P. aeruginosa*	2,000
1/17/78	− 7	Sulfisoxazole		0	*P. aeruginosa*	7,500	*P. aeruginosa*	5,000
1/24/78	−14	Sulfisoxazole	*P. aeruginosa*	280	*P. aeruginosa*	10,000	*P. aeruginosa*	3,000
2/7/78	− 5	Tetracycline		0	*P. aeruginosa*	10,000	*P. aeruginosa*	2,500
2/14/78	−12	Tetracycline	*P. aeruginosa*	250	*P. aeruginosa*	2,500	*P. aeruginosa*	2,000
3/13/78	−42	Tetracycline	Cystoscopy and bacteriologic localization; see Table 9.9				*P. aeruginosa (CB)*	10,000
4/5/78		Day of surgical excision; See Table 9.9 for stone culture results.						
4/6/78	+ 2	Tobramycin					(CB)	0
4/14/78	+ 4	TMP-SMX (½ tab q h.s.)		0		0		0
5/16/78	+36	TMP-SMX (½ tab q h.s.)		0		0		0
6/20/78	−35	TMP-SMX		0		0		0
8/28/79	−1 yr 3 mo	TMP-SMX		0		0		0

[a] CB = catheterized bladder, TMP-SMX = trimethoprim-sulfamethoxazole. Solid transverse line divides longitudinal cultures into major periods of significance.

[b] All cultures were obtained from the cystoscopy table by the nurse; see Chapter 1, Figures 1.25 and 1.26.

Table 9.9
Bacteriologic Localization Studies in March 1978 and Stone Culture Results in April 1978[a]

Source	Pseudomonas
A. Cystoscopy Results	
	bacteria/ml
CB	10^4
WB	10^3
LK_1	40
LK_2	0
LK_3	0
LK_4	0
RK_1	10
RK_2	0
RK_3	0
RK_4	0
B. Stone Culture Results	
W1	60
W4	1,140
Crushed stone	10,000

[a] CB = catheterized bladder count, WB = washed bladder count before ureteral catheterization, K_1–K_4 = serial kidney urines from each side, W1 = initial stone wash of 5 ml, W4 = fourth stone wash of 5 ml, crushed stone = bacterial count after crushing stone in fourth wash. Pseudomonas was a *P. aeruginosa*.

midstream (VB_2) cultures have not shown a single colony of a Gram-negative bacillus since removal of the infected urethral stone.

It is interesting that a urethral suture, present for 11 years, could cause such substantial susceptibility to UTI. It is easy to understand how once the bacteria, especially the *P. aeruginosa*, were imbedded in the apatite deposits around the suture, that all bacterial recurrences were caused by persistence of the *P. aeruginosa* on the urethra. It is also interesting how the cultures in Table 9.8 clearly suggest that the site of bacterial persistence was the urethra. This is one of the advantages, among others, of collecting the voided urine on the cystoscopy table with a nurse in attendance, and is why we continue this practice over 15 years after we started it.

Urethral Diverticula and Paraurethral Glands

Urethral diverticula in the female are common (Huffman[14] would probably say they are normal from his study of paraurethral glands), but infected diverticula as a cause of recurrent UTI or the urethral syndrome are exceedingly rare. Andersen[15] reported the incidence of urethral diverticula to be about 3% in 300 women with carcinoma of the cervix. If the physician uses the double-balloon pressure system described by Davis and TeLinde,[16] urethral diverticula can be found in a large series of symptomatic women very quickly. It cannot be emphasized too strongly, however, that 99% or more of these diverticula have no relationship to recurrent UTI. I am unaware of a single report that has shown the course of UTIs in women with diverticula to be changed by resection of the diverticulum. The reason to excise urethral diverticula is because of pressure symptoms and discomfort from the mass *per se*, usually occurring with sexual intercourse; urethral diverticula should not be excised because of a false hope to change the biologic susceptibility to recurrent urinary infections in the female. The following patient surely illustrates, in a rather dramatic way, that even a large urethral diverticulum—residual urine and all—does not predispose the patient to UTI; indeed, she developed her first UTI *after* the resection of the diverticulum, not before.

S.H., a 34-year old, Caucasian woman, was first seen in December 1969. Her referring internist had found pyuria, sterile urethral and midstream cultures for Gram-negative bacteria, and a palpable urethral diverticulum. An intelligent woman, she denied any history even slightly suggestive of urinary infections. She had been married for several years but was unable to become pregnant. Her only symptoms were some stress incontinence, and she had observed on occasions an egg-sized vaginal lump. On examination, her urethral urine contained many "glitter cells" which were rare in the midstream specimen. An egg-sized, urethral diverticulum was readily palpable vaginally and easily emptied with massage. An IVU was normal, a cystogram showed no reflux, and her residual urine was nil after voiding 180 ml before inserting the Foley catheter for the cystogram.

Because she was not bothered by this

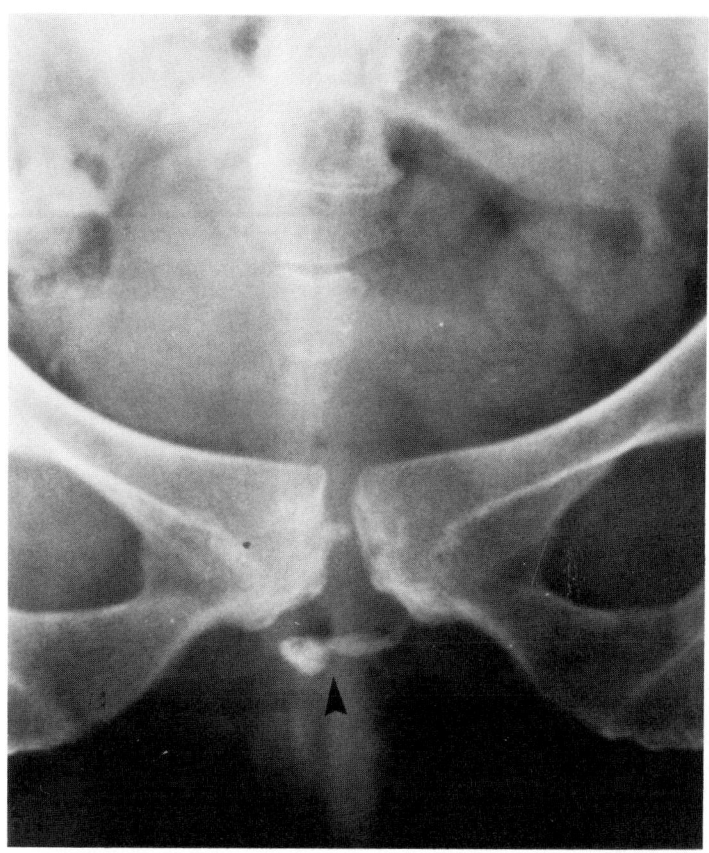

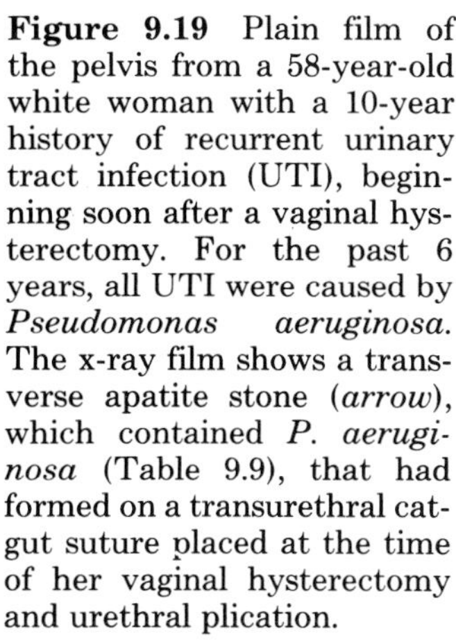

Figure 9.19 Plain film of the pelvis from a 58-year-old white woman with a 10-year history of recurrent urinary tract infection (UTI), beginning soon after a vaginal hysterectomy. For the past 6 years, all UTI were caused by *Pseudomonas aeruginosa.* The x-ray film shows a transverse apatite stone (*arrow*), which contained *P. aeruginosa* (Table 9.9), that had formed on a transurethral catgut suture placed at the time of her vaginal hysterectomy and urethral plication.

urethral diverticulum, she was followed with only occasional cultures (Table 9.10). Observe that not only was she never infected, but there were no *E. coli* bacteria on the introitus or urethra from which she could become infected. Repeated cultures of the fluid within the diverticulum, obtained after the VB_1 by urethral massage, showed only normal introital bacteria and never in numbers greater than present in the VB_1 (Table 9.10). The diverticulum was excised vaginally on 5/11/70; the opening into the floor of the urethra, easily visible at cystoscopy, was in the midline in the proximal half of the urethra. Examination by surgical pathology revealed the diverticulum to be a Gartner's duct cyst with evidence of chronic inflammation in the wall. An indwelling Foley catheter was left in the bladder, and daily aspirations were sterile; she was never given antimicrobial agents of any kind. An introital culture on 5/15/70, the day before removing her catheter, showed 2000 *E. coli*/ml of transport broth. These introital *E. coli* persisted for 1 week (5/21/70) and then disappeared. Sexual intercourse was not resumed until after her visit on 6/18/70. On 9/3/70, the urethral urine showed no further evidence of inflammatory cells.

On 1/21/71, she suddenly developed urinary frequency every half-hour, dysuria, and tenesmus. Cultures the next day confirmed an *E. coli* bacteriuria. She was not treated and her symptoms gradually subsided. One week later, while still mildly symptomatic, her cultures had reverted to normal and have remained so. Careful questioning confirmed that she had received no medication of any kind.

The bacteriologic data in this 34-year old patient with an egg-sized Gartner's duct cyst in the floor of the urethra illustrate that (1) the presence of this congenital di-

Table 9.10
S.H., a 34-year-old, Caucasian Woman with a Large Urethral Diverticulum[a]

Date	Days On (+) or Off (−) Therapy	Introital Cultures		Urethral (VB_1)		Midstream (VB_2)	
		bacteria/ml		*bacteria/ml*		*bacterial/ml*	
12/11/69	None	*Staphylococcus epidermidis*	300	γ-Streptococcus	10^3	*S. epidermidis*	40
		γ-Streptococcus	150				
				Diphtheroids	10^4	Diphtheroids	60
				Urethral massage:			
				Diphtheroids	30		
12/16/60	None	Catheterization for cystogram				CB	0
4/3/70	None	*S. epidermidis*	40	*S. epidermidis*	250		0
				Diphtheroids	16		
				Urethral massage:			
				S. epidermidis	10		
4/8/70	None	Enterococci	20	Enterococci	160	Enterococci	60
		S. epidermidis	300	*S. epidermidis*	10^3	*S. epidermidis*	310
				Urethral massage:			
				Enterococci	160		
				S. epidermidis	2,000		
4/23/70	None	Enterococci	20	Enterococci	560	Enterococci	210
				Citrobacter	110	Citrobacter	10
				Urethral massage:			
				Citrobacter	10		
				Enterococci	10		
5/10/70	None			Enterococci	30	Enterococci	10
				S. epidermidis	4,000	Enterococci	70
5/11/70	None	Excision of urethral diverticulum and plication of urethra					
5/12/70	None	Indwelling Foley catheter				CB*	0
5/13/70	None	Indwelling Foley catheter				CB*	0
5/14/70	None	Indwelling Foley catheter				CB*	
						Escherichia coli	10
5/15/70	None	Indwelling Foley catheter				CB*	0
							0
5/15/70	None	*E. coli*	2,000	Indwelling Foley catheter		CB*	0
		Enterococci	10^3				
		Diphtheroids	230				
5/16/70	None					*E. coli*	30
5/21/70	None	*E. coli*	1,000	*E. coli*	1,500	*E. coli*	100
				Enterococci	30		
				S. epidermidis	170	*S. epidermidis*	90
6/18/70	None		0	Diphtheroids	60	Diphtheroids	50
						S. epidermidis	20
9/3/70	None	γ-Streptococcus	390	γ-Streptococcus	260	γ-Streptococus	90
		Lactobacillus sp.	10^4	*S. epidermidis*	100	*S. epidermidis*	10
1/22/71	None	*E. coli*	70	*E. coli*	>100,000	E. coli	>100,000
		Enterococci	30				
		Diphtheroids	70	Diphtheroids	160	Diphtheroids	60
1/28/71	None	Enterococci	140	Enterococci	300		0
		S. epidermidis	600	*S. epidermidis*	10^3		
		Diphtheroids	400	Diphtheroids	2,000		
		Lactobacillus sp.	10^4				
5/20/71	None	Enterococci	10	Enterococci	20		0
		S. epidermidis	20	*S. epidermidis*	130		

[a] CB = catheterized bladder urine. CB* = urine aspirated from indwelling Foley catheter. Solid transverse line divides longitudinal cultures into major periods of signficance.

verticulum with substantial residual urine never predisposed this patient to urinary infections, despite the probability of its presence all her life; (2) a constant residual urine in a vulnerable position also did not predispose her to UTI; and (3) her resistance to UTI, even during 5 days of hospitalization with an indwelling Foley catheter while on no antibiotics, was related to her vaginal biology that prevented colonization of the introitus with Enterobacteriaceae (Table 9.10). It is somewhat of an anachronism that her first and only UTI occurred 7 months after the resection of her urethral diverticulum.

Saga of an *Escherichia coli* 023

Except for iatrogenic foreign bodies, the female urethra is virtually never the cause of bacterial persistence in recurrent bacteriuria. I have seen one exception in nearly 20 years of looking at this problem. She is interesting enough, however, to justify presention in some detail. In 1974, while Schaeffer and I were observing that hysterectomy prolonged introital carriage of *E. coli* on the vaginal vestibule of the rabbit[17] (see Chapter 5 for details), we wondered if the prevalence of bacteriuria was higher in hysterectomized women than in women who had not had a hysterectomy (a question that still remains unanswered). In the course of screening some hysterectomized women, we cultured R.S., a 48-year-old white woman, who had a total abdominal hysterectomy and a Marshall-Marchetti operation for stress urinary incontinence 4 years before, in 1970. She had experienced intermittent episodes of cystitis beginning with her first pregnancy. Following her hysterectomy, she experienced multiple episodes of *E. coli* UTI, always with lower tract symptoms of cystitis. She had been through many courses of antimicrobial therapy, but her infections always recurred within a few weeks of completing therapy. An IVU was normal except for a calyceal diverticulum in the upper pole calyx of the right kidney.

As seen in Table 9.11, she was infected with an *E. coli* 023 when we first cultured her. Introital, urethral, midstream, and anal cultures were obtained as described in Chapter 1, but she was unable to void from the cystoscopy table and accordingly collected the first voided and midstream urine samples herself. I have divided these interesting longitudinal studies into seven time periods, separated by appropriate spacing to make the lessons we learned from each period and the data easier to follow.

During the first 4 months that we followed her, she was treated four different times for recurrent bacteriuria with 4 g a day of nalidixic acid for 10 days. The data in Table 9.11 show that the first recurrence was an *E. coli* 06 bacteriuria (3/25/75), but the second (4/25/75) and third (5/19/75) were caused by the same *E. coli* 023 with which she was originally infected; these recurrences were detected, 37, 21, and 14 days, respectively, after stopping nalidixic acid. She had mild suprapubic discomfort at each occurrence. From the data in the first period of our study, it is also interesting that the *E. coli* 023 was detected on three occasions among the fecal bacteria obtained from the anal canal; the *E. coli* 023, however, was never the predominant anal strain and it was only present at the time of her bacteriuric episodes. One might argue from these data that the anal canal can be colonized transiently by the organism causing the bacteriuria (see Chapter 4 on the rectal reservoir).

With her third bacteriuric recurrence (5/19/75), 10 days of nalidixic acid was followed by prophylaxis with 100 mg of nitrofurantoin macrocrystals each night. In this second period of study (Table 9.11), we learned that her midstream voided urine often contained small numbers of *E. coli* 023 in the absence of significant introital colonization. After 136 days of effective prophylaxis (in terms of preventing bacteriuria) with nightly doses of nitrofurantoin, she was again bacteriuric and symptomatic with an *E. coli* 023 27 days after stopping prophylaxis. Ten days of nalidixic acid was again effective, but 9 days after stopping it she was infected for the fifth time (11/25/75) in 9½ months.

Study period three begins in Table 9.11 with TMP-SMX prophylaxis which began

Table 9.11
Clinical Course of R.S., a 48-year-old White Woman with Recurrent Urinary Tract Infection due to the Same *Escherichia coli*—or the "Saga of the 023 *Escherichia coli* 023"[a]

Date	Days On (+) or Off (−) Therapy	Vaginal Introitus		Urethral		Midstream		Anal Canal[b]	
			bacteria/ml		*bacteria/ml*		*bacteria/ml*		*bacteria/ml*
2/6/75		*E. coli* 023	20	*E. coli* 023	$>10^5$	*E. coli* 023	$>10^5$	*E. coli* 06	10^4
				(CB)		(CB)		*E. coli* 051	10^4
2/12/75	+ 6 Nalidixic acid		0				0	*E. coli* 06	40
								E. coli 051	110
2/21/75	− 5 Nalidixic acid		0				0		0
3/6/75	− 18 Nalidixic acid	*E. coli* 023	10			E. coli 023	10	*E. coli* 051	5000
3/25/75	− 37 Nalidixic acid	*E. coli* 06	600			E. coli 06	$>10^5$	*E. coli* 06	600
		E. coli 023	50					*E. coli* 023	500
								E. coli 051	10^4
3/31/75	+ 6 Nalidixic acid		0				0	*E. coli* 051	10
4/11/75	− 7 Nalidixic acid		0				0	*E. coli* 051	10
4/25/75	− 21 Nalidixic acid	*E. coli* 023	10	*E. coli* 023	10^4	*E. coli* 023	10^4	*E. coli* 023	20
								E. coli	200
5/2/75	+ 7 Nalidixic acid		0	*E. coli*	30	*E. coli* 023	20	*E. coli* 051	10
5/9/75	− 4 Nalidixic acid		0				0		0
5/19/75	− 14 Nalidixic acid	*E. coli* 023	10			*E. coli* 023	$>10^5$	*E. coli* 023	40
								E. coli 051	800
5/27/75	+ 8 Nalidixic acid	*E. coli*	10			*E. coli*	10	*E. coli*	$>10^4$
END OF FIRST PERIOD OF STUDY									
7/7/75	+ 41 Nitrofurantoin[c]		0				0	*E. coli*	10^4
8/4/75	+ 69 Nitrofurantoin	*E. coli*	220			*E. coli* 023	10^3	*E. coli*	10^5
9/2/75	+ 98 Nitrofurantoin		0			*E. coli* 023	1000	*E. coli*	10^5
10/10/75	+136 Nitrofurantoin		0			*E. coli* 023	70	*E. coli*	10^4
								E. coli	$<10^4$
								Klebsiella	20
11/6/75	− 27 Nitrofurantoin		0			*E. coli* 023	$>10^5$[d]	*E. coli*	10^4
11/12/75	+ 6 Nalidixic acid		0				0	*E. coli* NT	10^3
								E. coli 051	30
								E. coli NT	10
11/25/75	− 9 Nalidixic acid	*E. coli* 023	190			*E. coli* 023	10^5	*E. coli* NT	$>10^4$
								E. coli NT	$>10^4$

END OF SECOND PERIOD OF STUDY								
12/2/75	+ 7	Nalidixic acid		0		0		0
1/14/76	+ 43	TMP-SMX[e]		0		0		0
2/3/76	+ 63	TMP-SMX		0		0		0
3/2/76	+ 91	TMP-SMX		0		0		0
4/6/76	+126	TMP-SMX		0		0		0
5/11/76	+161	TMP-SMX		0	*E. coli* 023	30		0
6/15/76	+196	TMP-SMX		0	*E. coli* 023	60		0
7/13/76	− 28	TMP-SMX	*E. coli*	10	*E. coli* SA	$>10^{5}$[d]	*E. coli*	10^{5}
END OF THIRD PERIOD OF STUDY								
7/20/76	+ 7	Sulfamethizole		0	*E. coli* 023	50	*Klebsiella*	10^{4}
7/28/76	− 5	Sulfamethizole		0	*E. coli* 023	$<10^{5}$[d]	*Klebsiella*	4000
8/3/76	− 1	Nitrofurantoin		0	*E. coli* 023	200	*Klebsiella*	20
8/10/76	+ 7	Nitrofurantoin		0	*E. coli* 023	300	*E. coli* 023	3000
9/7/76	+ 35	Nitrofurantoin		0	*E. coli* 023	30	*E. coli* 023	700
							E. coli NT	3000
10/5/76	+ 63	Nitrofurantoin		0	*E. coli* 023	30	*E. coli* 023	3000
							SA *E. coli*	10^{5}
11/2/76	+ 91	Nitrofurantoin		0	*E. coli* 023	10	*E. coli* 023	10^{5}
END OF FOURTH PERIOD OF STUDY								
11/9/76	+ 7	TMP-SMX (160 mg TMP/ 800 mg SMX, q 12 hr)		0		0	*E. coli* 023	40
11/16/76	− 4	TMP-SMX		0		0		0
12/14/76	− 32	TMP-SMX	NT *E. coli*	40	NT *E. coli*	$>10^{5}$[d]	*E. coli* 023	4000
1/4/77	− 11	TMP-SMX		0	*E. coli* 023	250	*E. coli* 0125	500
END OF FIFTH PERIOD OF STUDY								
3/1/77	+ 56	TMP-SMX		0	*E. coli* 023	20		0
3/22/77	+ 78	TMP-SMX		0	*E. coli* 023	30		0
4/27/77	+114	TMP-SMX		0	*E. coli* 023	50		0
5/25/77	+142	TMP-SMX		0	*E. coli* 023	10		0

Table 9.11, *Continued*

Date	Days On (+) or Off (−) Therapy	Vaginal Introitus	Urethral		Midstream		Anal Canal[b]	
		bacteria/ml		*bacteria/ml*		*bacteria/ml*		*bacteria/ml*
6/22/77	+170 TMP-SMX	0				0		0
7/26/77	+204 TMP-SMX	0	*E. coli* 023	20[f]		0[f]		0
8/23/77	+232 TMP-SMX	0	*E. coli* 023	300[f]		0[f]		0
8/30/77	+239 TMP-SMX	0	*E. coli* 023	80[f]		0[f]		0
		0	*E. coli* 023	800[f]		0[f]		0
9/13/77	+253 TMP-SMX Cystoscopy	0	*E. coli* 023 (Ureteral catheter-tip culture)	10[4]				
9/27/77	+267 TMP-SMX	0				0		
10/19/77	+289 TMP-SMX	0	*E. coli* 023	750[f]	*E. coli*	20[f]		
10/24/77	Rupture and fulgeration of submucosal urethral gland		*E. coli* 023	3000				
		END OF SIXTH PERIOD OF STUDY						
10/27/77	+297 TMP-SMX	0		0		0		0
11/7/77	+308 TMP-SMX	0		0		0		0
11/22/77	+323 TMP-SMX	0		0		0		0
12/7/77	− 15 TMP-SMX	0				0		0
12/14/77	− 22 TMP-SMX	0		0	*Klebsiella*	10	*P. mirabilis*	10
							Enterobacter	10[5]
							Klebsiella	10[5]
1/4/78	− 43 TMP-SMX	0				0	NT *E. coli*	10[4]
							Enterobacter	100
2/1/78	− 71 TMP-SMX	0			*Klebsiella*	10	SA *E. coli*	10[4]
							Klebsiella	10[4]
							Enterobacter	1000
							Enterobacter	20
3/22/78	−120 TMP-SMX	0				0	*E. coli* 075	10[4]
4/23/78	Urethral pain and hematuria				*E. coli* 075	600		
4/24/78	+ 1 TMP-SMX	0				0	NT *E. coli*	<10[5]
							NT *E. coli*	5000

5/1/78	− 2 TMP-SMX	0		0	*E. coli* 075	50
6/21/78	− 53TMP-SMX	0	*Klebsiella*	20	*Klebsiella*	10^4
10/23/78	−177 TMP-SMX	0		0	NT *E. coli*	10^5
					NT *E. coli*	3000
					Klebsiella	3000
5/1/79	−366 TMP-SMX	0		0		
END OF SEVENTH PERIOD OF STUDY						

[a] CB = catheterized bladder urine, SA = self-agglutinating, NT = nontypable, TMP-SMX = trimethoprim-sulfamethoxazole. Solid transverse line divides longitudinal cultures into major periods of significance.

[b] When more than one *E. coli* is listed in the anal cultures, the morphology of the strains appeared to be different and hence were isolated as separate strains.

[c] Nitrofurantoin in the form of macrocrystals (Macrodantin®), 100 mg nightly.

[d] No antibody-coated bacteria on fluorescent antibody studies.

[e] TMP-SMX in the form of Septra®, ½ tablet nightly (40 mg trimethoprim, 200 mg sulfamethoxazole).

[f] Cultures obtained from the cystoscopy table under control of the nurse. All others are self-caught by patient.

immediately after obtaining sterile urine for the sixth time with nalidixic acid. As we have reported previously,[18] one-half tablet of TMP-SMX nightly (40 mg TMP and 200 mg SMX) cleared all introital, urinary, and rectal Enterobacteriaceae so that not a single colony remained. On the 161st and 196th day of TMP-SMX prophylaxis, however, an important observation was made: with no *E. coli* on the introitus or in the rectum, small numbers of *E. coli* 023 were being picked up from somewhere in the lower urinary tract by the voided urine! On the 28th day after stopping TMP-SMX prophylaxis, she had her sixth recurrence of bacteriuria, this one due to a self-agglutinating (SA) *E. coli* that prevented O-serogrouping. It could have been an altered strain of the *E. coli* 023.

The fourth period of study begins on the 7th day of therapy of sulfamethizole for the SA *E. coli*, which cleared the infection, but the *E. coli* 023 recurred 5 days after stopping the sulfonamide (the 7th recurrence). It should be noted in this fourth period that the 023 was detected 3 times in the urine from 7/20/76 to 8/3/76 when no *E. coli* were detectable in the rectal flora (presumably from the sulfamethizole therapy). This observation, like the one from the third period, suggested a source other than the usual rectal reservoir. After the *E. coli* 023 infection on 7/28/76, she was treated for 5 days with nitrofurantoin 400 mg a day before resuming prophylaxis with 100 mg each night. These cultures on nitrofurantoin prophylaxis are similar to the ones during study period two except complete O-grouping of the rectal *E. coli* during this period shows that the *E. coli* 023 was present at every culture in the rectum and was the predominant and only *E. coli* present on the 91st day of nitrofurantoin prophylaxis.

The fifth study period begins with full dosage TMP-SMX (160 mg TMP and 800 mg SMX) twice daily; this was tried because the one-half tablet prophylactic data in period three was the first time we had seen complete disappearance of the *E. coli* 023 without any colonies detectable in the voided urine. We thought full dosage therapy with TMP-SMX might permanently cure the infections with the *E. coli* 023. As can be seen in this fifth period of study, 4 days after completing 10 days of full dosage TMP-SMX (11/16/76), it appeared as if we had succeeded. Thirty-two days later, however, she was infected with a nontypable *E. coli*, and was again treated with TMP-SMX at full dosage for 10 days; to our surprise the *E. coli* 023 was present once more in the voided urine 11 days after stopping TMP-SMX (1/4/77).

The sixth period of study begins on 3/1/77, on continuous one-half tablet TMP-SMX and extends to the time of her surgery which cured her in late October 1977, a period of almost 8 months. She was seen monthly during this interval and never had a single *E. coli* or any other Gram-negative aerobic rod on the introital mucosa or in the rectal flora. During this time, the *E. coli* 023 was present in almost every voided urine, but in small numbers. On four different visits, we carefully cultured the labia majora, the labia minora, and especially the area of Bartholin's glands (both before and after massage) with moistened cotton swabs without detecting a single colony of *E. coli* anywhere on the labial hair or perineal area. These culture studies excluded the area below the urethra as a source for the *E. coli* 023 which were clearly being added to the voided stream from somewhere.

We next persuaded the patient to void from the cystoscopy table (as 80–90% of our patients do) despite her reluctance and failure to do so early in our studies. As can be seen in study period six on 7/26/77, 8/23/77, and 8/30/77, she was finally able to do so—and the diagnosis was made! The *E. coli* 023 appeared only in the first voided urethral urine and not in the later midstream aliquot. Two separate collections were made on 8/30/77, both confirmatory.

She was cystoscoped on 9/13/77, still on TMP-SMX, with a saddle anesthesia. In the middle one-third of the floor of the urethra was a small opening through which a yellow toothpaste-like material could be seen coming from the urethra. The orifice was probed submucosally for only 1 cm with a 5 Fr polyethylene Stamey ureteral catheter. The distal 1 cm of the catheter, however, filled with this yellow material through the three holes in the catheter. The catheter was removed and the distal 1 cm cut off into 5 ml of transport broth. As seen on 9/13/77, this catheter tip culture grew 10^4 *E. coli* 023/ml.

We had to delay surgical excision of the urethral site of her bacterial infections for 5 weeks. Another nurse-collected urethral and midstream urine was obtained on 10/19/77 which showed that probing the submucosal gland had not cleared the infection.

On 10/24/79, the urethra was dilated to a 40 Fr sound and the area inspected with a nasal speculum. The yellow material was seen to cover the floor of the urethra. A swab culture of this material in 5 ml transport broth grew 3000 *E. coli* 023/ml. The submucosal gland was again observed to probe only 1 cm and to remain just beneath the mucosa. In the process of probing it with a Kelly clamp, the submucosal tunnel ruptured and became part of the urethra. The area was fulgurated lightly with the resectoscope and I injected the floor of the urethra with 80 mg of gentamicin in 5 ml of saline; no further surgery was performed. A Foley catheter was left in place for 24 hours and the patient discharged the following day on the same one-half tablet TMP-SMX prophylaxis.

The seventh and last study period begins after hospital discharge where three consecutive cultures contained no Gram-negative aerobic bacteria in the vagina, urine, or rectum. The TMP-SMX was stopped on 11/22/77. We have never seen the *E. coli* 023 again—not in the voided urine, on the introitus, or among the rectal flora. Thus ends the saga of the *E. coli* 023.

As noted in Table 9.11, she had one episode of urethral discomfort with hematuria in April 1978, but a home-caught culture before she started TMP-SMX for 5 days showed only 600 colonies of an *E. coli* 075. No further episodes of symptoms or bacteriuria have occurred in the 16 months since that time.

What did we learn from this extensively documented longitudinal study? Several observations interest me:

1. I am surprised that an infected, para-

urethral submucosal gland, or possibly a minute diverticulum lying in the middle of the urethra, could cause such unrelenting recurrent bacteriuria. Eight infections occurred within a period of 24 months and for 17 of those months she was on antimicrobial therapy, which always prevented her bacteriuric episodes. We are fortunate that bacterial persistence in infected urethral ducts or glands occurs only rarely.

2. How do we explain the *E. coli* 023 in the rectum during the fourth study period when she was on nitrofurantoin prophylaxis (8/10/76 to 11/2/76)? I can perhaps understand the *E. coli* 023 in the anal canal during the first period at a time when she was bacteriuric if voided urine somehow runs across the anus, but in the fourth period, the numbers of *E. coli* 023 added to the urine from the urethra were small; moreover, the 023 became the predominant and only rectal *E. coli.*

   If this paraurethral gland or duct became infected during the postoperative period of her hysterectomy in 1970 (and her infections certainly accelerated after that period), why should the *E. coli* 023 also be present in the rectal flora many years later?
3. The diagnostic usefulness of TMP-SMX was crucial in wiping out all vaginal and rectal carriage of Enterobacteriaceae in our search for a persistent site of bacterial infection on the perineum of this patient; these studies could not have been accomplished without such a drug.
4. The diagnostic usefulness of our technique of nurse-collected urethral and midstream urine samples from the cystoscopy table is apparent from the cultures on 7/26/77, 8/23/77, and 8/30/77. When specimens are collected in this manner, the investigator does not have to be concerned with sites of bacterial persistence below the urethra on the labia minora or perineum. The critical usefulness of this technique was also shown in the patient illustrated in Table 9.8 who had the urethral stone infected with *Pseudomonas.*
5. The extraordinary usefulness of nitrofurantoin macrocrystals and TMP-SMX in the prophylactic prevention of recurrent bacteriuria is again demonstrated (see Chapter 4).
6. Two of the eight bacteriuric episodes that occurred were not caused by the *E. coli* 023: the *E. coli* 06 on 3/25/75 and the NT *E. coli* on 12/14/76. How did the presence of a paraurethral gland infected with an *E. coli* 023 predispose to infections with these other *E. coli* from the rectal reservoir? Since she had been susceptible to UTI all her married life, it is possible that the 06 and nontypable (NT) *E. coli* from the rectal reservoir acquired dominance through the usual colonization route. I am inclined to believe that the 06 and NT *E. coli* infections were related to the infected paraurethral gland, but I do not understand how she acquired these two *E. coli* rather than the ever-present 023.

Unilateral Medullary Sponge Kidneys*

Medullary sponge kidney was first described by Lenarduzzi[20] in 1939 and occurs in about 0.005 per cent of the population.[21, 22] While most patients are asymptomatic, gross and microscopic hematuria, recurrent stone formation, and urinary infection occur in some. Complicated medullary sponge kidney is one cause of renal failure.[23, 24]

A 51-year-old white woman was first seen on my service in January 1971 with persistent bacteriuria. Her past history included surgical repair of a left ureteropelvic junction obstruction in 1955 at the age of 32 after an episode of hematuria in the last trimester of pregnancy. No early records were available, but in 1965 she had one episode of right flank pain and fever; an IVU showed a medullary sponge kidney with calcifications in the right kidney and

* This patient was first presented in *Urology* **8:** 373, 1976.[19] It is reproduced here with the publisher's permission.

hydronephrosis in the left kidney. Slight enlargement of the stones in the right kidney was thought to have occurred between 1966 and 1969. Except for the ease with which fatigue developed, few specific symptoms were present during these years. One episode of chills, fever, gross hematuria, dysuria, and frequency occurred in the fall of 1970.

At admission to Stanford University Medical Center in January 1971 the patient's urine was found to be infected with *E. coli*, and ureteral catheterization studies showed both kidneys to be severely infected (Table 9.12). The bladder capacity was 500 ml, the ureteral orifices were edematous and erythematous bilaterally, and transurethral biopsy of yellow patches near the trigone confirmed cystitis glandularis. Radiologic studies showed no reflux, a medullary sponge kidney on the right side, and internal hydronephrosis in the larger left kidney (Figure 9.20). Calculi were visible in the medullary cyst of the right kidney (Figure 9.21) which filled well with IVU and poorly on retrograde studies (Figure 9.22). The internal hydronephrosis without pelvic outlet obstruction was presumably secondary to the previously operated ureteropelvic obstruction but, without the original films, congenital calycosis cannot be excluded. Her serum creatinine was 1 mg/100 ml; blood and electrolytes were normal. Blood pressure was 150/90 mm Hg.

The patient's mother died of "nephritis" while giving birth to the patient, but three brothers and one sister were presumed healthy. Three sibling daughters were healthy also, although none had radiologic studies.

The *E. coli* bacteriuria, when treated with nitrofurantoin, was immediately replaced with *P. aeruginosa*. Because of what appeared to be bilateral renal disease of different etiologies, and certainly bilateral renal infection, she was treated from January 1971 to July 1974 with a variety of antimicrobial agents, but either *E. coli* or *P. aeruginosa* was present in all 21 cultures. Antimicrobial therapy included, besides nitrofurantoin, gentamicin, oxytetracycline, tetracycline, methenamine, ascorbic acid, ampicillin, carbenicillin, and chloramphenicol; none was effective in even sterilizing the urine, let alone curing the infection. Despite this failure, the serum creatinine remained constantly between 0.9 and 1.2 mg/100 ml. The urine never contained more than a trace of protein (<30 mg/100 ml), but never less than 10–20 fresh leukocytes per high power field (spun).

In early March 1973, chills, fever, right flank pain, and foul-smelling urine developed. Repeat IVU showed no change in the

Table 9.12
Bacteriologic Localization Studies[a]

Source	Bacteria/ml	Organism
January 6, 1971		
CB	10^5	*Escherichia coli*
WB	10^5	*E. coli*
LK_1	10^5	*E. coli*
LK_2	10^5	*E. coli*
LK_3	10^5	*E. coli*
LK_4	10^5	*E. coli*
RK_1	10^5	*E. coli*
RK_2	10^5	*E. coli*
RK_3	10^5	*E. coli*
RK_4	10^5	*E. coli*
March 28, 1974		
CB	10^5	*E. coli*
WB	10^4	*E. coli*
LK_1	10^4	*E. coli*
LK_2	10^4	*E. coli*
LK_3	10^4	*E. coli*
LK_4	10^4	*E. coli*
RK_1	10^4	*E. coli*
RK_2	10^4	*E. coli*
RK_3	10^4	*E. coli*
RK_4	10^4	*E. coli*
July 16, 1974		
CB	5,000	*Pseudomonas aeruginosa*
WB	360	*P. aeruginosa*
LK_1	60	*P. aeruginosa*
LK_2	90	*P. aeruginosa*
LK_3	80	*P. aeruginosa*
LK_4	70	*P. aeruginosa*
RK_1	2,000	*P. aeruginosa*
RK_2	10,000	*P. aeruginosa*
RK_3	5,000	*P. aeruginosa*
RK_4	5,000	*P. aeruginosa*

[a] CB = catheterized bladder urine, WB = washed bladder specimen (after 2–3 L of sterile water irrigation), LK_1 to LK_4 = serial left renal urines, RK_1 to RK_4 = serial right renal urines.

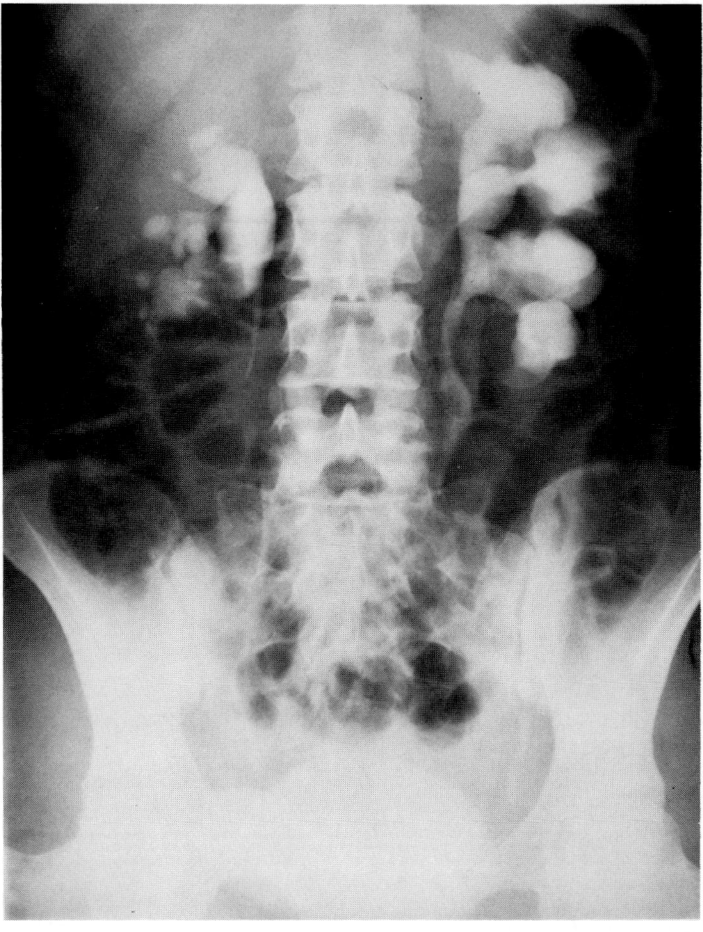

Figure 9.20 Twenty-minute intravenous urogram showing medullary cysts in right kidney communicating with calyces. Left kidney shows internal hydronephrosis without obstruction at ureteropelvic junction. (Reproduced by permission from H. Huland *et al.*, *Urology* **8:** 373, 1976.[19])

size or position of the stones, but the right kidney appeared 0.6 cm smaller than in 1971. Intravenous furosemide demonstrated excellent washout of the contrast medium in the pelvis of the right kidney.

Ureteral catheterization studies were repeated on 3/28/74, when she had been off all medication for 7 days and again on 7/16/74, when she was receiving nitrofurantoin. As seen in Table 9.12, *E. coli* in March involved both kidneys (as in January 1971), and *P. aeruoginosa* in July was present in higher counts in the right kidney.

Differential renal function studies performed immediately after the localization study on 7/16/74, showed a 3:1 difference in urine flow and renal plasma flow with equivalent concentrations of PAH (*p*-aminohippuric acid) (Table 9.13). With this evidence that the right medullary sponge kidney was contributing only one-third of the total renal function and that all of the stones were limited to the right kidney, and despite the finding of bilateral renal infection on three separate localization studies, a simple right nephrectomy was performed on 7/21/74. Because we wished to avoid a nonrefluxing ureteral stump as a cause of persistent bacteriuria, a ureteral catheter was left in the proximal end of the right ureter and irrigated with polymyxin B sulfate for 3 days after nephrectomy. The patient received 60 mg of gentamicin every 8 hours for 6 days prior to surgery and, because of viable *P. aeruginosa* in the renal pelvic urine at the time of nephrectomy, was changed to 75 mg of polymyxin E every 8 hours after surgery for 6 days. The serum

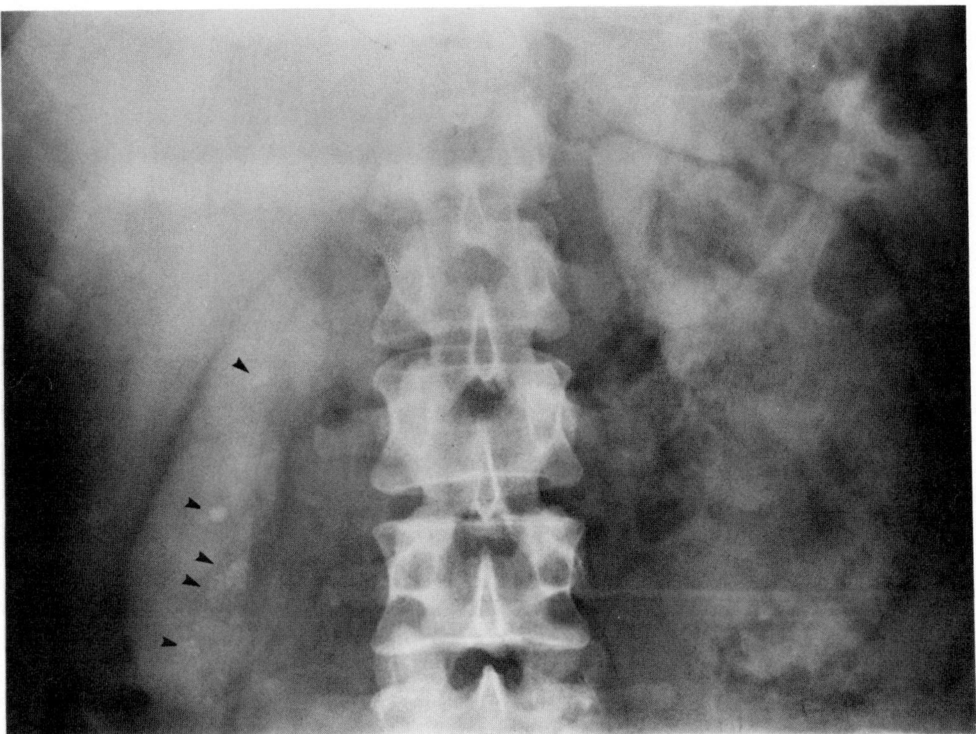

Figure 9.21 One-minute intravenous urogram showing cortical outlines of both kidneys and presence of medullary calculi in right kidney (*arrows*). Plain film tomograms showed no stones in left kidney. (Reproduced by permission from H. Huland *et al.*, *Urology* **8:** 373, 1976.[19])

creatinine did not change after nephrectomy. Three weeks after surgery (2 weeks off all antimicrobial agents) the urine was clear and sterile for the first time in the 4 years since her first visit to Stanford in 1971. In the 5 years since nephrectomy, she has had two *E. coli* reinfections with lower tract symptoms, both responding to short courses of nitrofurantoin.

She was last seen in June 1978. There had been no further infections. Her blood pressure was 130/80 mm Hg and her urine was sterile. The introital cutlure showed 10 *Klebsiella* with 10^5 lactobacilli, 10^4 corynebacteria, and 500 *S. epidermidis*/ml of transport broth.

The right kidney, measuring 11 × 5 × 2 cm and weighing 70 g, was opened on the operating table and none of the calculi was present in the calyces. On sectioning the kidney, nine stones, composed of pure calcium apatite, were removed from medullary cysts. Cultures of both stones and medullary renal tissue surprisingly failed to grow either *E. coli* or *P. aeruginosa*, although the latter was cultured from the pelvic urine (20 colonies/ml). The capsule stripped with difficulty revealing a focally scarred renal cortex. In the medulla a number of renal papillae contained several small circumscribed cysts measuring from 2 to 3 mm in diameter and filled with straw-colored murky fluid (Figure 9.23*A*). The papillary cysts did not appear to communicate with the calyces, and many contained small spherical black calculi (apatite).

Microscopically, the kidney showed the features of medullary sponge kidney (Figure 9.23, *B* and *C*). The medullary cysts were filled with proteinaceous fluid and lined by low cuboidal or transitional epithelium, some appeared to communicate with the renal pelvis. Most of the collecting ducts proximal to the cyst appeared normal al-

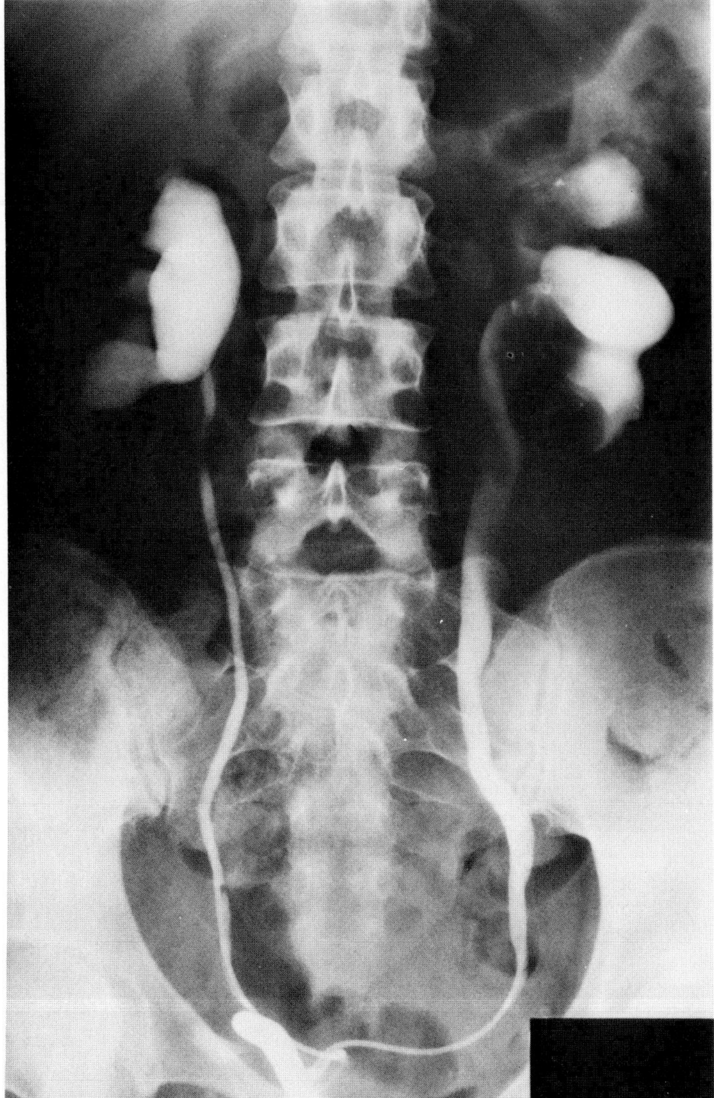

Figure 9.22 Retrograde urogram. Note that medullary cysts fail to fill by retrograde injection (compare with Figure 9.20). There is pyelectasis and a narrow ureteropelvic junction in right kidney. (Reproduced by permission from H. Huland *et al.*, *Urology* **8:** 373, 1976.[19])

Table 9.13
Differential Renal Function Study[a]

Source	Urine Flow	Ratio R/L	PAH Concentration	Ratio R/L	Renal Plasma Flow	Ratio R/L
	ml/min		*mg/100 ml*		*ml/min*	
RK_1	2.37	0.33	73.0	0.95	108.1	0.31
LK_1	7.20		76.7		344.9	
RK_2	2.30	0.29	65.7	0.95	94.4	0.28
LK_2	7.90		69.4		342.2	
RK_3	2.75	0.47	65.7	1.00	112.9	0.47
LK_3	5.85		65.7		240.2	
Mean $RK_{1\text{-}3}$	2.47	0.35	68.1	0.96	105.1	0.34
$LK_{1\text{-}3}$	6.98		70.6		309.1	

[a] LK_1 to LK_3 = serial left renal urines; RK_1 to RK_3 = serial right renal urines; PAH = *p*-aminohippuric acid.

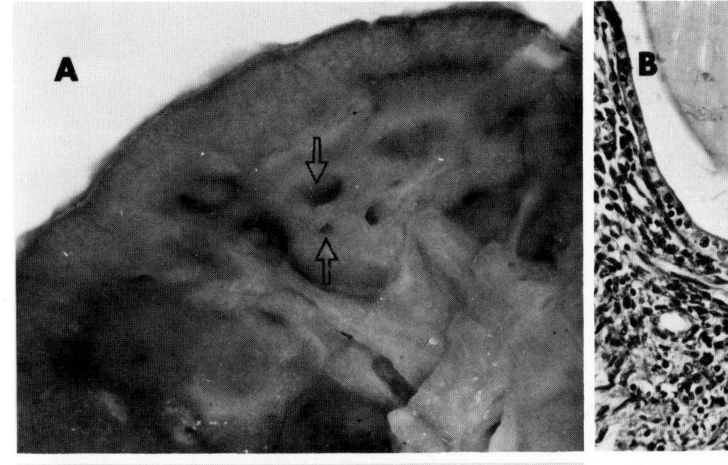

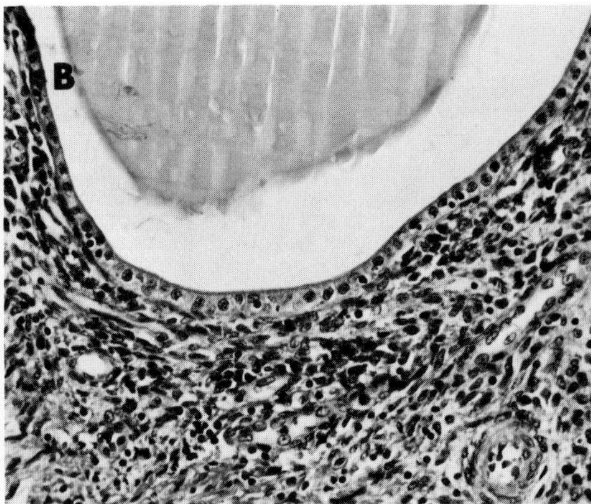

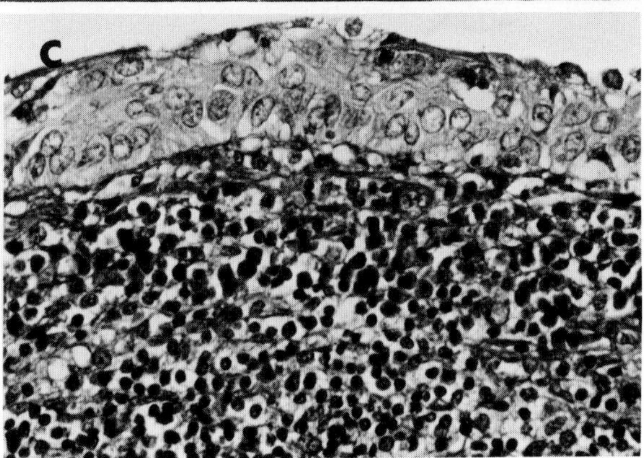

Figure 9.23 Medullary sponge kidney. (*A*) Gross picture of part of hemisected kidney, showing three medullary cysts (*arrows*). Note also focal cortical thinning. (*B*) Photomicrograph of medulla showing a colloid filled cyst lined by low cuboidal epithelium and surrounded by dense chronic inflammatory infiltrate (hematoxylin and eosin stain, ×250). (*C*) Photomicrograph of portion of medullary cyst showing transitional epithelial lining and surrounding dense chronic inflammatory infiltrate (hematoxylin and eosin stain, ×400). (Reproduced by permission from H. Huland *et al.*, *Urology* **8:** 373, 1976.[19])

though a few were dilated. A number of cysts were filled with cellular debris and numerous polymorphonuclear leukocytes, and there was a dense acute and chronic inflammation of the medulla around the cysts. The kidney also showed changes of chronic pyelonephritis with focal interstitial chronic inflammation and fibrosis extending from the cortex to the renal pelvis, tubular atrophy, thyroidization, glomerulosclerosis, and periglomerular fibrosis. This involved about 20% of the kidney.

Our differential renal function studies in Table 9.13 show no differences in total water reabsorbtion between the two kidneys (urinary PAH concentrations), but the contralateral kidney was not a normal control. Studies have been reported, however, where unilateral disease was compared to a contralateral normal kidney[25]; the concentration of urine creatinine, osmolality, urea, and sodium were all substantially reduced in the medullary sponge kidney compared to the contralateral kidney, but because urine flow was so increased from the diseased kidney, osmolar clearance was actually increased in comparison to the normal kidney.

In terms of persistent bacteriuria, the infection was probably present for more than 20 years. In the 4 years we followed the patient, specific antibiotic therapy—usually based on *in vitro* sensitivities—was never capable of even sterilizing the urine. Since the urine in other patients with infection stones in the calyces can be sterilized, we suspect the presence of infection in the medullary cyst prevented sterilization. Our hesitancy in removing the right kidney was based on finding the bacteria in the contralateral hydronephrotic kidney and our overestimation of the total function in the right kidney as judged by the intravenous urogram. We should have performed differential function studies sooner, because this is not the first patient in whom contralateral bacteriuria has been present without preventing cure of persistent bacteriuria from an ipsilateral cause (Figures 9.1–9.6, Table 9.2).

A review of the English literature shows that of 156 cases of complicated medullary sponge kidney, 24 have been operated on for infection by either nephrectomy or partial nephrectomy in unilateral instances of complicated medullary sponge kidney (Table 9.14). Although postoperative bacteriologic results have rarely been documented, there were apparently 23 patients in whom the bacteriuria was alleviated. Ekstroëm *et al.*,[23] in their excellent follow-up of 44 patients with complicated medullary sponge kidney, observed that the only patients cured of their infection were those in whom the stones and medullary cysts were excised by either nephrectomy (3 cases) or partial nephrectomy (5 cases). Ram and Chisholm[32] have also presented an interesting case of unilateral disease that required nephrectomy for hemorrhage and infection; they properly point out that the cysts are confined to the renal pyramids in medullary sponge kidneys and have suggested the name cystic disease of the renal pyramids for this condition. Our patient's life has been dramatically changed by nephrectomy; she has gained weight and energy and is free from recurrent chills and fever as well as costly, ineffective antimicrobial agents. It is also clear why less conservative surgery than partial or complete nephrectomy will not remove the focus of infection; the stones are not amenable to calyceal extraction.

Nonrefluxing, Normal Appearing, Infected Ureteral Stumps Following Nephrectomy

Y.L., a 26-year-old, married woman, was first seen in 1959 for dysuria and suprapubic aching. Her symptoms were minimal, but she was greatly concerned because 2 years before she had undergone an emergency right nephrectomy elsewhere for *P. mirabilis* calculous pyonephrosis and septicemia. In 1959, we were not aware of the importance of introital cultures, but many suprapubic needle aspirations of the bladder were being performed. Repeated needle aspirations of her bladder, in the absence of antimicrobial therapy, always showed *P. mirabilis* in numbers less than 5000 bacteria/ml. An IVU was normal except for the absence of the right kidney. She had no residual urine, and a cystogram showed no reflux. At cystoscopy, both ureteral orifices appeared normal; bacteriologic localization studies indicated a sterile left renal urine but suggested an infected ureteral stump (Table 9.15). A right ureterogram demonstrated the ureter to be of normal caliber and configuration; it terminated at L3. Despite several courses of various antimicro-

Table 9.14
Infection Results from Surgical Excision in Unilateral, Medullary Sponge Kidney[a]

References	Cases Reported		Type of Surgery	Infection Result
	Total No.	Unilateral		
Ekstroëm *et al.*[23]	44	3 Unilateral	Nephrectomy	3 Cured
		5 Localized	Partial nephrectomy	5 Cured
Abeshouse and Abeshouse[24]	5	2 Unilateral	Nephrectomy	—
Mulvaney and Collins[26]	1	1 Unilateral	Nephrectomy	1 Cured
Lindvall[27]	35	9 Unilateral	Resected or nephrectomy	9 Cured
Morris *et al.*[28]	20	1 Unilateral	Heminephrectomy	1 Cured
Powell[29]	1	1 Unilateral	Nephrectomy	1 Cured
Harrison and Williams[30]	10	1 Unilateral	Nephrectomy	1 Cured
Lalli[31]	40	1 Unilateral	Partial nephrectomy	1 Cured
Totals	156	24		23

[a] Postoperative bacteriology was not reported.

Table 9.15
Y.L., a 26-year-old, White Woman with Bacterial Persistence in a Normal Ureteral Stump: Bacteriologic Localization Studies[a]

Source	*Proteus mirabilis*
	bacteria/ml
CB	2100
WB	15
LK_1	0
LK_2	0
LK_3	0
LK_4	0
RUS 1	600
RUS 2	500

[a] CB = bladder urine obtained through cystoscope. WB = After irrigating the bladder with 2000 ml of distilled water, about 100 ml are left in the bladder to facilitate catheterization of the ureters. WB represents the bacterial count in this 100 ml of irrigating fluid. LK = left kidneys. RUS = right ureteral stump irrigated with 2 ml of sterile saline after ureteral catheterization.

bial agents, the *P. mirabilis* always returned after discontinuing each antibiotic. At exploration through a midline incision, the ureter appeared normal and excellent peristalsis was observed with forceps stimulation. The entire ureter, including a cuff of bladder, was excised; after placing a ligature around the lower end of the ureter, 2–3 ml of sterile saline were flushed in and out of the ureter using a needle and syringe. Two different irrigations each cultured 2500 *P. mirabilis*/ml of saline. Histologic sections of the ureter were all normal. She had an uneventful recovery from surgery and penicillin-G was discontinued 10 days later. All subsequent suprapubic aspirations during the next 2 years of follow-up were sterile.

That an entirely normal ureter can persist with viable, pathogenic bacteria on its mucosal surface, seeding the bladder and potentially endangering the remaining contralateral kidney, is of some concern. It is clear that a nonrefluxing ureter with bacteria "trapped" on its mucosal surface presents the same pharmacologic problem in drug diffusion across a normal epithelial surface as does the prostatic epithelium (Chapter 7). Indeed, if the urine is not sterile at the time an infected kidney is removed, it is better to leave a refluxing ureteral stump (where antibacterial drugs in the urine can reach the mucosal surface of the ureter) than a nonrefluxing stump.

Infected Urachal Cysts

I have had two patients in 24 years, both young adult males, with recurrent bladder infections and epididymitis in whom the site of the infection was a small urachal cyst in the dome of the bladder. In both instances, the opening of the cyst was behind the air bubble and was missed on outpatient cystoscopy under local anesthesia. Neither cyst was larger than 3 cm, and the opening into the bladder appeared as a small fistula behind the air bubble. Infected urachal cysts represent the rarest of all causes of bacterial persistence in the urinary tract.

Infected Communicating Cysts of the Renal Calyces

J.L., a 20-year-old, married Caucasian woman was referred to Stanford in October 1968 because of persistent pyuria in the presence of sterile urine. In brief, she had experienced frequent episodes, "all her life" of urinary frequency, urgency, and terminal dysuria lasting 5–10 days and usually responding to antibiotics. They were sometimes accompanied by fever and left flank pain. Three to four episodes occurred each year during childhood. She reportedly had meningitis at the age of 18 months, leaving her with minimal residual weakness in the left arm and leg. Her infections, at least by history, ceased at the age of 16 years. She married at age 17 and became pregnant the following year, and her symptoms recurred during the first trimester accompanied by left flank pain. After a normal delivery of a healthy infant, she remained essentially asymptomatic but continued to run a pyuria without positive urine cultures. Intravenous urograms, cystoscopy, and ureteral urine samples collected for cultures in November 1967 were interpreted as normal except for a "single calcified structure in the left renal parenchyma," thought not to communicate with the collecting system and to "probably represent an old calcified abscess or cyst." Between November 1967 and the time of her referral to Stanford University Hospital in October 1968, she continued to show pyuria—even on catheterized bladder urine samples—but urine cultures, including examinations for tuberculosis, were sterile. In the words of her referring family doctor, after describing a recent course of kanamycin therapy, "she has had every other antibiotic in good concentrations over long periods of time—sometimes it (the pyuria) has improved but not completely."

When she was first seen on 10/29/68 at Stanford (Table 9.16), 14 days after completion of kanamycin therapy, it was easy to confirm by suprapubic needle aspiration of the bladder that the urine was sterile, but contained 20–30 polymorphonuclear leukocytes (many of them "glitter cells") per high power field accompanied by both fine and coarse granular casts. When admitted to the hospital on 12/9/68, voided urine cultures confirmed the absence of bacteriuria, but some *P. mirabilis* were present on the introitus. Plain film tomograms at 0.5-cm intervals showed a 15 × 10 mm calcification in the upper pole of the left kidney posteriorly (Figure 9.24), best seen on the 6-cm film. The calcification showed an outer rim of dense calcium and an inner lucent area. The right kidney measured 12.5 cm and the left 13.6 cm. No other calcifications were seen on tomography. Following injection of 60 ml of Hypaque, prompt excretion was observed bilaterally, and the left pyelocalyceal system appeared separate from the calcification (Figure 9.25). On the right posterior oblique view, a slight bulging of the renal outline adjacent to the calcification was observed (Figure 9.26). The Stanford radiologists considered vascular malformations or tumor as possibilities. Dr. C. J. Hodson, who was visiting professor in the Division of Urology on the day these radiologic studies were done, considered tuberculosis and pointed out that the middle calyces just below the calcification seemed attenuated (Figures 9.25 and 9.26).

Cystoscopy on 12/10/68 showed a normal bladder and intravesical ureters. The 10 *P. mirabilis*/ml in the catheterized urine, when the vaginal vestibule contained 920/ml of transport broth, probably reflected carriage of introital organisms into the bladder from the urethra. After the bladder was washed with 200 ml of normal saline, the WB culture was sterile (Table 9.16). In an attempt to localize the pyuria to the left kidney, bilateral ureteral catheterization showed no white blood cells from either ureter, but her urine was too dilute from overhydration; one granular cast was seen in the unspun aliquot from the left renal urine. Acid-fast stains and urine cultures were negative for tuberculosis; her skin test was tuberculin-negative. The blood pressure was normal. White blood counts were 7,700 and 6,900, both with about 50% lymphocytes.

Because aspirated urine from the bladder showed evidence of inflammatory disease, and because the parenchymal calcification was in the left kidney, an exploratory biopsy of the left kidney was performed on 12/11/68. A slight cortical bulge was easily found on the posterolateral surface of the upper pole. An incision for a wedge biopsy was made over the soft bulge; a gelatinous, leather-like, white material exuded from the incision. With removal of the wedge, a cavity was clearly present, and the stone was located in the cavity within the gelatinous mass. The stone and the leather-like gelatinous mass are shown in Figure 9.27. The latter was cut with scissors and cultured for aerobes, fungi, anaerobes, and tuberculosis. As seen in Table 9.16 (12/11/68), both the stone and the gelatinous debris were loaded with *P. mirabilis despite the presence of a sterile urine 43 days after completion of kanamycin therapy.* Frozen sections disclosed pyelonephritis in the tissue adjacent to the cavity, but a biopsy at the lower pole of the kidney was normal. Crystallographic analysis of the stone showed 70% hydroxyl apatite and 30% protein matrix; no struvite.

At surgery, the roof of the cavity was widely resected, a drain was left in place, and the incision was closed. Two days after surgery, although urethral catheterization

Table 9.16
Bacteriologic Course of J.L., 20-year-old White Woman[a]

Date	Days On (+) or Off (−) Therapy	Vaginal Vestibule		Urethral (VB_1)		Midstream (VB_2)	
			bacteria/ml		*bacteria/ml*		*bacteria/ml*
10/29/68	−14 (kanamycin 300 mg/ 24 hr × 7 days)	*Staphylococcus epidermidis*	10		0	SPA	0
12/9/68	−41	*Proteus mirabilis*	20	*P. mirabilis*	20	*P. mirabilis*	20
		S. epidermidis	400	*S. epidermidis*	20	*S. epidermidis*	10
12/10/68	−42	*P. mirabilis*	920			CB *P. mirabilis*	10
		S. epidermidis	1,200			WB	0
12/11/68	−43 left renal exploration			Stone wash 1 = *P. mirabilis*	10,000		
				Stone wash 4 = *P. mirabilis*	10,000		
				Ground stone = *P. mirabilis*	10,000		
				Tissue wash 1 = *P. mirabilis*	100,000		
				Tissue wash 4 = *P. mirabilis*	>100,000		
				Ground tissue = *P. mirabilis*	>100,000		
12/13/68	−45	*P. mirabilis*	100,000	*P. mirabilis*	>100,000	*P. mirabilis*	>100,000
		Escherichia coli	1,000				
12/15/68	+1 Nalidixic acid 500 mg q 6 hr					Diphtheroids	190
						S. epidermidis	30
12/17/68	+3 Nalidixic acid 500 mg q 6 hr	Diphtheroids	10	*S. epidermidis*	20		0
		S. epidermidis	160				
12/29/68	−12 Nalidixic acid 500 mg q 6 hr		0	*P. mirabilis*	100,000	*P. mirabilis*	100,000
12/31/68	+2 Nalidixic acid 500 mg q 6 hr	*S. epidermidis*	90	*P. mirabilis*	340	*P. mirabilis*	390
1/14/69	−7 Nalidixic acid 500 mg q 6 hr	*P. mirabilis*	30	*P. mirabilis*	100,000	*P. mirabilis*	100,000
		E. coli	160				
		S. epidermidis	180				
1/16/69	−9 Nalidixic acid 500 mg q 6 hr	*P. mirabilis*	60	CB *P. mirabilis* 4,000			
		Diphtheroids	600	WB *P. mirabilis* 970			
		S. epidermidis	800	LK_1 70		RK_1 40	
				LK_2 120		RK_2 20	
				LK_3 160		RK_3 30	
				LK_4 50		RK_4 80	
				LK_5 20		RK_5 20	
1/21/69	+5 Nalidixic acid 500 mg q 6 hr	*S. epidermidis*	20	*P. mirabilis*	310	*P. mirabilis*	290

	500 mg q 6 hr					*P. mirabilis*	210
2/4/69	+7 Sulfamethizole	*E. coli*	260		0	SPA	0
	500 mg q 6 hr	*S. epidermidis*	180				
2/11/69	−4 Sulfamethizole	*S. epidermidis*	80	*P. mirabilis*	200	*P. mirabilis*	200
	500 mg q 6 hr	γ-Streptococcus	10	γ-Streptococcus	30	*S. epidermidis*	10
2/27/69	−20 Sulfamethizole	*P. mirabilis*	1,000	*P. mirabilis*	100	*P. mirabilis*	200
	500 mg q 6 hr	γ-Streptococcus	700	γ-Streptococcus	20	SPA	
		Diphtheroids	120			*P. mirabilis*	1,320
3/3/69	−24 Sulfamethizole	*P. mirabilis*	680	*P. mirabilis*	10,000	*P. mirabilis*	10,000
	500 mg q 6 hr	*S. epidermidis*	200			CB:	
		Diphtheroids	280			*P. mirabilis*	10,000
3/4/69	+1 Cephaloridine	γ-Streptococcus	330	*P. mirabilis*	60	*P. mirabilis*	60
	1.0 g q 8 hr i.m.						
3/6/69	+3 Cephaloridine		0		0		0
	1.0 g q 8 hr i.m.						
3/8/69	+5 Cephaloridine	*Proteus vulgaris*	20		0		0
	1.0 g q 8 hr i.m.	*S. epidermidis*	10				
3/10/69	+7 Cephaloridine	*P. vulgaris*	540	*P. vulgaris*	10		0
	1.0 g q 8 hr i.m.	*S. epidermidis*	200				
		γ-Streptococcus	150			CB	0
3/12/69	+9 Cephaloridine	*P. vulgaris*	90		0		0
	1.0 g q 8 hr i.m.	γ-Streptococcus	70				
		S. epidermidis	30				
3/18/69	−5 Cephaloridine	*P. mirabilis*	40	*P. mirabilis*	>10,000	*P. mirabilis*	10,000
	1.0 g q 8 hr i.m.	*E. coli*	40				
		Enterococci	3,000				
4/1/69	+14 Nalidixic acid	*E. coli*	200				
	500 mg q 6 hr	Enterococci	3,000				
	but intermittently	Diphtheroids					
		S. epidermidis	1,000		0	*P. mirabilis*	40
4/27/69	−4 Nalidixic acid	*P. mirabilis*	50	*P. mirabilis*	3,000	*P. mirabilis*	3,000
	500 mg q 6 hr	γ-Streptococcus	110				
	but intermittently						
4/28/69	−5 Nalidixic acid			CB *P. mirabilis* 60			
	500 mg 6 hr			WB *P. mirabilis* 20			
	but intermittently						
				LK_1 70		RK_1 0	
				LK_2 60		RK_2 20	
				LK_3 20		RK_3 10	
				LK_4 690		RK_4 20	
				LK_5 90		RK_5 20	

Table 9.16, *Continued*

Date	Days On (+) or Off (−) Therapy	Vaginal Vestibule		Urethral (VB_1)		Midstream (VB_2)	
4/29/69	+1 Cephaloridine	*P. mirabilis*	10,000	*P. mirabilis*	50		0
	1.0 g q 8 hr i.m.	γ-Streptococcus	<100				
4/30/69	+2 Cephaloridine	Surgical excision		Stone wash 1 = *P. mirabilis*			10,000
	1.0 g q 8 hr i.m.	of communicating		Stone wash 4 = *P. mirabilis*			600
		cyst, left kidney		Stone (crushed) = *P. mirabilis*			100,000
5/3/69	+4 Cephaloridine	*P. mirabilis*	10				
	1.0 g q 8 hr i.m.	*P. aeruginosa*	10,000	*P. aeruginosa*	550	*P. aeruginosa*	1,520
		S. epidermidis	160				
		γ-Streptococcus	100				
5/6/69	+7 Cephaloridine	*P. aeruginosa*	90		0		0
	1.0 g q 8 hr i.m.	*S. epidermidis*	80				
		Enterococci	10				
5/7/69	−1 Cephaloridine	*S. epidermidis*	100		0		0
	1.0 g q 8 hr i.m.	γ-Streptococcus	20				
5/8/69	−2 Cephaloridine	*P. aeruginosa*	140				
	1.0 g q 8 hr i.m.	*Klebsiella*	90				
		Enterococci	300				
		S. epidermidis	160				
5/20/69	−14 Cephaloridine	*S. epidermidis*	60				
	1.0 g q 8 hr i.m.	γ-Streptococcus	390	*E. coli*	10		
		Diphtheroids	10,000	Diphtheroids	160	Diphtheroids	40
6/3/69	−28 Cephaloridine	Enterococci	2,000	Enterococci	50		0
	1.0 g q 8 hr i.m.	*S. epidermidis*	30	*S. epidermidis*	220		
		Diphtheroids	>10,000	Diphtheroids	1,000		
7/1/69	−56 Cephaloridine	*E. coli*	30	*E. coli*	140		0
	1.0 g q 8 hr i.m.	*S. epidermidis*	60	*S. epidermidis*	120		
		γ-Streptococcus	80	γ-Streptococcus	20		
		Diphtheroids	440	Diphtheroids	340		
10/23/69	−170 Cephaloridine	*E. coli*	20	*E. coli*	10		0
	1.0 g q 8 hr i.m.	*S. epidermidis*	1,000				
		Enterococci	5,000	Enterococci	170		
		Lactobacilli	10,000	Lactobacilli	10,000		

[a] Abbreviations as in Table 9.4. Solid transverse longitudinal line divides cultures into periods of significance.

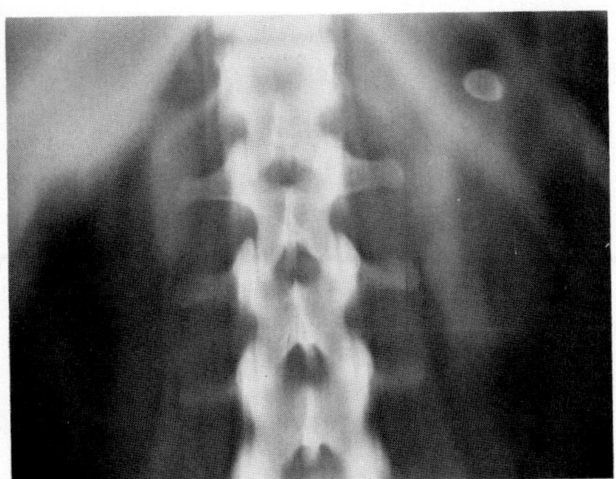

Figure 9.24 Plain film tomographic cut at 6 cm in J.L., a 20-year-old woman with pyuria, sterile bladder urine, and a history of urinary infections since childhood. The 15 × 10 mm calcification is present in the upper pole of the left kidney.

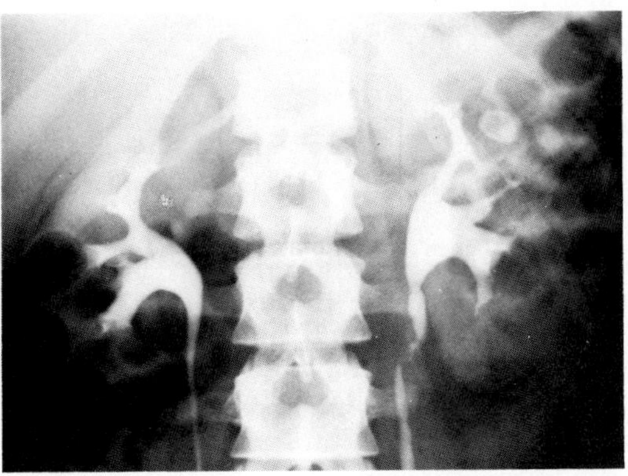

Figure 9.25 A compression x-ray film made 10 minutes after injecting 60 ml of Hypaque intravenously in J.L. The calcification appears separate from the collecting system; the calyces are delicate.

had not occurred, the midstream urine was heavily infected with *P. mirabilis*. Nalidixic acid, 500 mg every 6 hours, sterilized the urine within 24 hours (Table 9.16, 12/15/68), and she was discharged on the 7th postoperative day with instructions to stop the nalidixic acid 6 days after returning home. She was seen in our out-patient facility on 12/29/68 complaining of dysuria and frequency, she was 12 days off therapy, and she was again infected with *P. mirabilis*. Realizing that *P. mirabilis* was on the vaginal vestibule when she was originally seen with a sterile urine, the possibility existed that her recurrence was from the introitus and not the left kidney. Accordingly, nalidixic acid was restarted on 12/29/68 for 10 days with instructions to abstain from sexual intercourse until she returned on 1/14/69. Despite abstinence, and al-

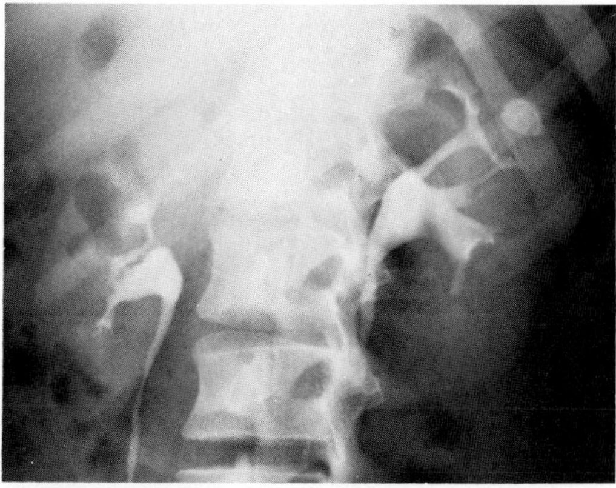

Figure 9.26 A right posterior oblique view (from the same urogram series as Figure 9.25) showing a slight bulge in the renal outline adjacent to the calcification.

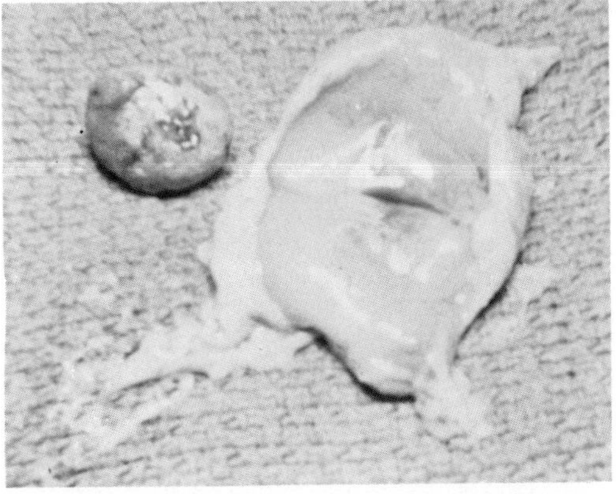

Figure 9.27 A black and white reproduction from a Kodachrome film made at the time of surgery on J.L. The stone is shown beside the leather-like, gelatinous mass that had to be divided with scissors to separate segments for culture. Both the stone and the gelatinous mass contained *Proteus mirabilis* despite the presence of a sterile urine (Table 9.16).

though asymptomatic, she was again infected with *P. mirabilis* (Table 9.16).

A ureteral catheter localization study was not convincing on 1/16/69 that the left kidney was the site of her infection (Table 9.16). Suprapubic bladder aspiration, performed after restarting nalidixic acid for 12 days on 1/28/69, showed only suppression and not sterilization of the *P. mirabilis*, a fact strongly suggested by the voided cultures on 1/21/69 and 12/31/68.

Sulfamethizole, to which the *P. mirabilis* was also sensitive, sterilized the urine, but she was infected by the 4th day of discontinuing therapy—at first in small numbers, but gradually increasing to higher counts (Table 9.16).

She was readmitted to the hospital on 3/3/69 and started on intramuscular cephaloridine 1.0 g every 8 hours. The urine promptly became sterile, but 5 days after completing the 10-day course of therapy the *P. mirabilis* had recurred. Plain film and infusion nephrotomograms made on the 10th day of cephaloridine therapy clearly confirmed the reason for bacterial persistence: the cavity was not an isolated renal cyst, but a communicating calyceal cyst connected with the renal collecting system (Figure 9.28); moreover, a new stone had formed within the cavity (Figures 9.28 and 9.29). With the recurrence following cephaloridine therapy, she was placed again on nalidixic acid, which she took intermittently because she felt well.

Her last admission to the hospital occurred on 4/27/69. A ureteral catheterization localization was again suggestive of infection in both sides, but certainly heavier on the left (Table 9.16). Cephaloridine 1.0 g every 8 hours was started preparatory to reexploration of the left kidney and excision of the communicating cyst. The surgery was surprisingly easy with simple wedge resection. A stone 0.6 × 0.3 cm had reformed in the cyst (the lucent defect in

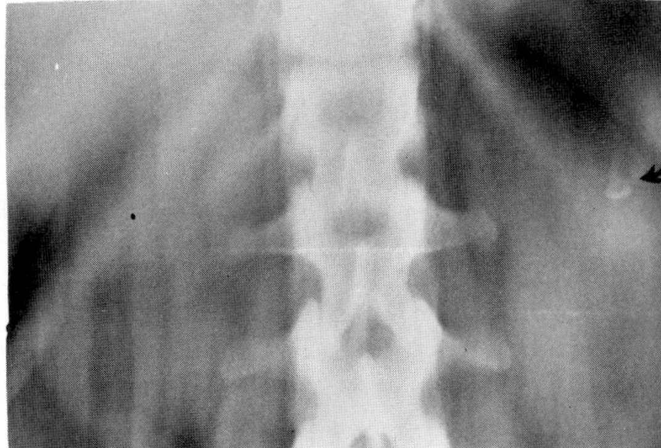

Figure 9.29 A 6-cm plain film tomograph made just before the infusion nephrotomogram in the preceding figure. The new calcification in the old cavity measured 7 × 7 mm (*arrow*); crystallographic analysis showed it to be 80% struvite and 20% apatite. The original stone (Figure 9.24 and Figure 9.27), however, present in a closed cavity without apparent contact with urine salts, was 70% apatite and 30% protein matrix.

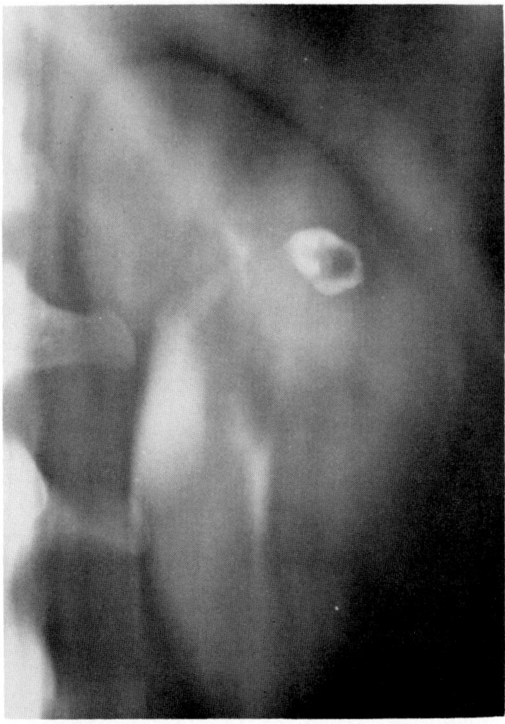

Figure 9.28 Infusion nephrotomogram (J.L., 3/13/69). This 6-cm cut of the left kidney shows that the intravenous Hypaque now fills the cavity previously identified at surgery, confirming a calyceal or infundibular connection with the renal collecting system. The radiolucent defect is a new struvite stone (Figure 9.29) formed in the 3-month interval since surgery (12/11/68).

Figure 9.28); *P. mirabilis* was again cultured from the stone, but crystallographic analysis this time showed 80% struvite and 20% carbonate apatite. At the time of surgical excision, urine could be seen entering the cyst through a small connection with the infundibulum. Histology showed the cavity to be lined with transitional epithelium, surrounded by severe chronic inflammation bordered by normal renal cortical tissue.

Her postoperative course was uneventful. Cephaloridine was continued only for 7 days. Six consecutive cultures during the next 170 days failed to show a single colony of *P. mirabilis* in any specimen (Table 9.16). When last seen on 10/23/69, she had returned to work, was totally asymptomatic, and a centrifuged urine specimen showed only a rare squamous epithelial cell. A follow-up telephone conversation on 7/8/71 revealed that she had been totally free of all urinary symptoms since her last visit on 10/23/69. In fact, she became pregnant with her second child in March of 1970, delivering a full term, healthy baby in January 1971. Throughout her pregnancy, monthly cultures by her obstetrician never showed any evidence of urinary infection. Delivery was uncomplicated and the postpartum period equally free of infection.

Seven of the nine women with communicating cysts reported by Williams *et al.*[33] had urinary infection and renal pain, although bacteriologic details are not given. None of the communicating cysts in this report involved the lower calyces; seven originated from the upper calyces, nine from the middle calyces. In my patient, the origin was from either the upper calyx or the upper middle infundibulum (Figures 9.25 and 9.26).

The reason bacteria persist in these communicating cysts once they become infected is probably because the neck of the cyst where it drains into the calyx is narrow and functions poorly; this undoubtedly accounts for the poor drainage of these cysts often seen on intravenous urography. The fact that some are barely or not at all seen on IVU compared to their easy demonstration with retrograde urography emphasizes that antimicrobial agents may not back diffuse through the neck into the cyst, thereby making sterilization of the urine difficult.

What makes J.L. unusual is that the communicating duct between the cyst and the calyceal system had closed off; the *P. mirabilis* could not get out of the cyst into the urine (perhaps sealed by the gelatinous debris shown in Figure 9.27), nor could contrast outline the cyst by back diffusion from below. Not until the stone and gelatinous debris were removed was free communication again established between the cyst and the calyces. Even so, there was rapid formation of a struvite stone from the *P. mirabilis* and the urine within 3 months (Figure 9.29).

The important point is that communicating cysts of the kidney represent a perfect situation for bacterial persistence once they become infected. Since they may be poorly seen on the IVU, or not seen at all if the communication is blocked, the wary physician should keep communicating cyst of the kidney in mind when seeking a cause for bacterial persistence in his patient.

Papillary Necrosis in a Single Calyx

A 41-year-old white woman consulted me in October 1977 with a 4-year history of constant right flank discomfort, occasional chills and fever, and recurrent bacteriuria.

Her urinary infections began at the age of 18 years with her first pregnancy. The next four pregnancies were all characterized by recurrent bacteriuria; the fifth and last one at age 24 required almost continuous antimicrobial therapy. Except for passing two kidney stones at age 22 and 27, she was well after her last pregnancy until she had a total abdominal hysterectomy and bilateral öophorectomy in 1973 at the age of 37 years. From then until October 1977, when I first saw her, she had almost continuous infections, apparently all due to *E. coli*, but accompanied by constant right flank aching with occasional chills and fever. Cystoscopy, voiding cystourethrogram, and IVU had been done twice and were said to be normal except for a small stone in the lower pole of the right kidney.

Her urine showed numerous fresh WBCs and she was infected with a SA *E. coli*, which was sensitive only to carbenicillin, kanamycin, gentamicin, and colistin. A plain film tomogram and a 15-minute IVU with compression is shown in Figures 9.30–9.32. These x-ray films suggested a filling defect with papillary necrosis in the right lower medial calyx. On the 3-minute film, contrast was observed to rim the intracavitary filling defect, but it is not reproduced here because of its faintness. The tubular ectasia, especially in the middle calyx of the right kidney (Figures 9.31 and 9.32), was also compatible with mild medullary sponge disease. Three first AM urine samples were negative for tuberculosis on stain or culture.

She was treated with carbenicillin for 5 days which sterilized the urine, but the SA *E. coli* recurred by the 8th day after stopping therapy (Table 9.17). She was cystoscoped and her infection localized 12 days after stopping carbenicillin (Table 9.18). These data show that the SA *E. coli* and the pyuria were localized to the right kidney. The bacteria were FA+. A retrograde urogram was performed on the right side

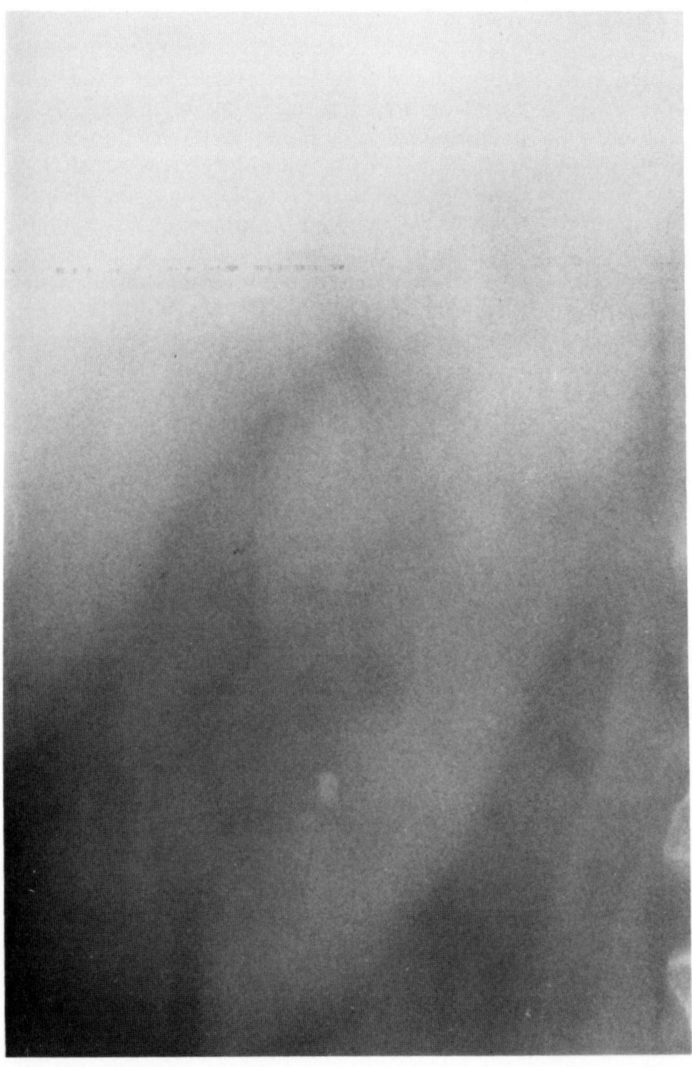

Figure 9.30 Plain film tomogram, showing a small calculus in the lower pole of the right kidney.

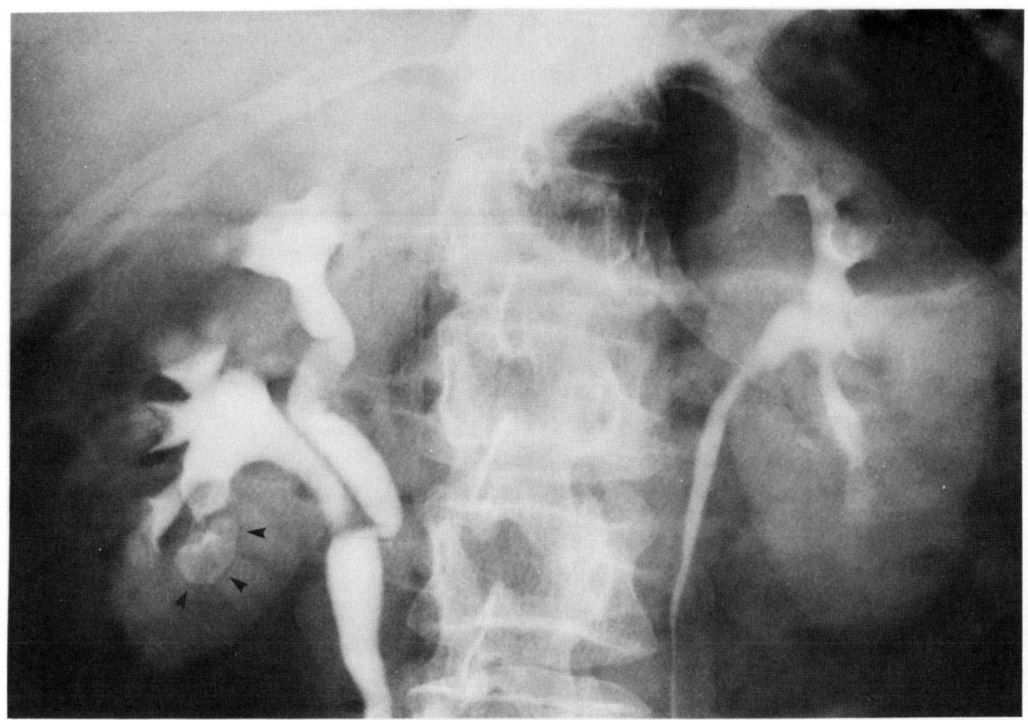

Figure 9.31 A 15-minute compression film from an intravenous urogram. The right kidney shows a filling defect in the right lower medial calyx with a narrowed infundibulum (*arrows*). The middle calyces show some ectasia suggestive of medullary sponge kidney. The left kidney is normal.

before removing the catheter (Figure 9.33). The filling defect in the diseased lower calyx is again seen and it appears to extend into the lower infundibulum. At the end of the out-patient study, she was given 80 mg of gentamicin and a 2-day supply of carbenicillin before returning home.

As seen in Table 9.17, subsequent cultures were all positive for the same SA *E. coli.* As would be expected, fluorescent antibody studies for antibody-coated bacteria were strongly positive in both the right renal and bladder urine samples. (Table 9.18).

A lower pole nephrectomy was performed on 12/5/77 and the SA *E. coli* has not been seen since. Her pyuria disappeared. She has had two reinfections with an *E. coli* 016, two with an enterococcus, and one with a nontypable *E. coli* in the 19 months since her partial nephrectomy. All her reinfections have been easy to clear with short term antimicrobial therapy with nitrofurantoin or cephalexin. None of these reinfections have shown antibody-coating of the bacteria. She was placed on 50 mg of trimethoprim nightly as prophylaxis for 6 months beginning 9/21/78 (after the second *E. coli* 016 recurrence); she has had no bacteriuric episodes during those 6 months or 4 months after stopping prophylaxis on 4/26/79. The catheterizations since 5/7/79 have been to instill dimethyl sulfoxide for interstitial cystitis.

Pathologic examination of the lower pole of the kidney showed a small oval calculus, 5 × 3 × 3 mm, that proved to be apatite with some calcium oxalate monohydrate, lying within a black, necrotic papillus; reticulum stains showed an architecture highly suggestive of a sloughed papillus. Lymphocytes and plasma cells surrounded the transitional cell-lined calyceal cavity, but the renal parenchyma of the entire lower pole was histologically normal without any evidence of interstitial inflammation.

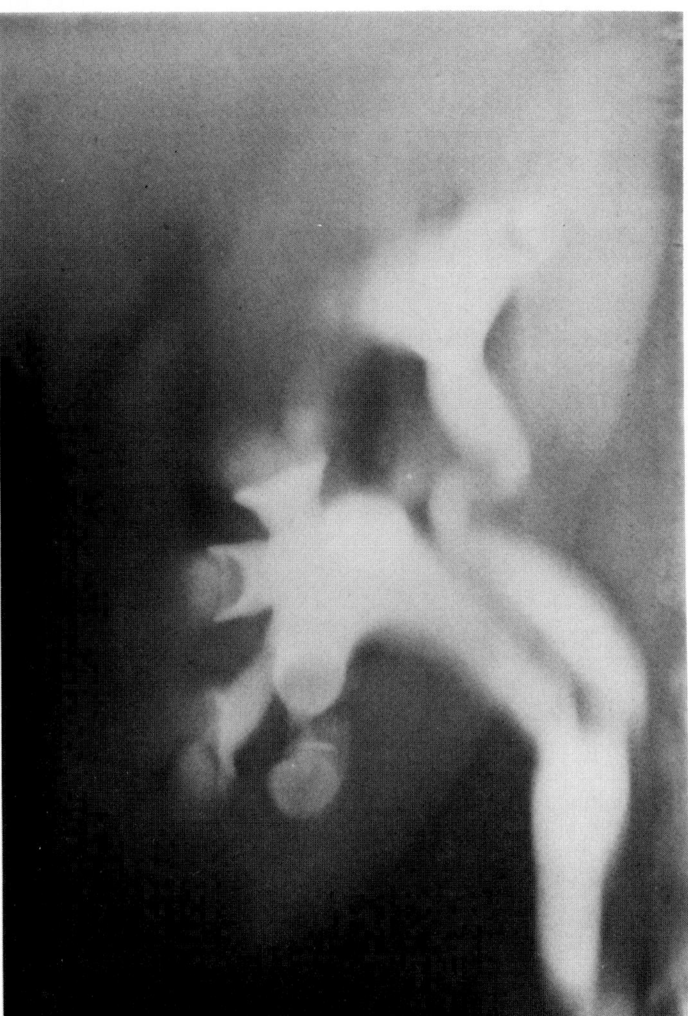

Figure 9.32 Tomographic cut from same intravenous urogram as shown in Figure 9.31 with slight rotation.

Table 9.17
Bacteriologic Course of a 41-year-old Woman with Papillary Necrosis of Right Lower Pole Calyx[a]

Date	Source	WBC in Urine	Antibody-Coated Bacteria	Midstream VB_2	Days On (+) or Off (−) Drug
				bacteria/ml	
10/6/77	VB_2	9.0×10^3/ml	ND	SA *Escherichia coli* (>10^5)	−17 Nf
10/11/77	VB_2	2.3×10^4/ml	—	*Klebsiella* (300)	+4 Carbenicillin
10/20/77	VB_2	1.2×10^4/ml	Pos	SA *E. coli* (10^4)	−8 Carbenicillin
10/24/77	CB	3.4×10^4/ml	Pos (see Table 9.18)	SA *E. coli* (10^5)	−12 Carbenicillin
11/7/77	VB_2	8.4×10^4/ml	ND	SA *E. coli* (10^4)	+7 Tetracycline
11/15/77	VB_2	1.6×10^6/ml	Pos	SA *E. coli* (> 10^5)	−5 Tetracycline
11/22/77	VB_2	1.2×10^4/ml	Pos	SA *E. coli* (10^4)	−12 Tetracycline
11/29/77	VB_2	1.0×10^5/ml	ND	SA *E. coli* (10^5)	−19 Tetracycline
12/5/77	Right lower pole nephrectomy				

Table 9.16, *Continued*

Date	Source	WBC in Urine	Antibody-Coated Bacteria	Midstream VB_2	Days On (+) or Off (−) Drug
12/13/77	VB_2	ND	—	Sterile	−1 Tobramycin
12/20/77	VB_2	1–2 WBC/hpf	—	Sterile	−8 Tobramycin
1/3/78	VB_2	6×10^4/ml	—	Sterile	−24 Tobramycin
1/18/78	VB_2	0–1 WBC/hpf	—	Sterile	−39 Tobramycin
2/10/78	VB_2	7–8 WBC/hpf	Neg	*E. coli* 016 (10^5)	−62 Tobramycin
2/15/78	VB_2	6–7 WBC/hpf	ND	*E. coli* 016 (10^4)	−67 Tobramycin
2/22/78	VB_2	1–2 WBC/hpf	—	Sterile	−1 Nf
3/7/78	VB_2	0–1 WBC/hpf	—	Sterile	−14 Nf
3/28/78	VB_2	3×10^3/ml	Neg	Enterococci (10^4)	−35 Nf
4/3/78	VB_2	0–2 WBC/hpf	—	Sterile	−1 Nf
5/10/78	VB_2	1–2 WBC/hpf	—	Sterile	−38 Nf
5/18/78	VB_2	2–3 WBC/hpf	ND	Enterococci (2000)	−46 Nf
5/23/78	VB_2	0/ml	Neg	Enterococci (10^5)	−51 Nf
5/24/78	VB_2	0–1 WBC/hpf	—	Sterile	+1 Nf
6/27/78	VB_2	1–2 WBC/hpf	—	Sterile	−30 Nf
7/18/78	VB_2	5.5×10^3/ml	—	Sterile	−51 Nf
8/1/78	VB_2	10–12 WBC/hpf	Neg	NT *E. coli* (> 10^5)	−65 Nf
9/7/78	VB_2	5×10^4/ml	Neg	*E. coli* 016 (> 10^5)	−32 Cephalexin
9/8/78	VB_2	9×10^3/ml	—	Sterile	+1 Cephalexin
9/21/78	VB_2	0/ml	—	Sterile	−8 Cephalexin
9/28/78	VB_2	2×10^3/ml	—	Sterile	+7 TMP prophylaxis
11/10/78	VB_2	0/ml	—	Sterile	+50 TMP prophylaxis
1/10/79	VB_2	6×10^2/ml	—	Sterile	+111 TMP prophylaxis
3/7/79	VB_2	6×10^2/ml	—	Sterile	+167 TMP prophylaxis
4/11/79	VB_2	1.2×10^3/ml	—	Sterile	+202 TMP prophylaxis
4/26/79	VB_2	0/ml	—	Sterile	+217 TMP prophylaxis
5/3/79	VB_2	1.0×10^3/ml	—	Sterile	−7 TMP prophylaxis
5/7/79	CB	0/hpf	—	Sterile	−11 TMP prophylaxis
5/14/79	CB	0/hpf	—	Sterile	−18 TMP prophylaxis
5/23/79	CB	0 WBC/hpf	—	Sterile	−27 TMP prophylaxis
5/30/79	CB	0 WBC/hpf	—	Sterile	−34 TMP prophylaxis
6/6/79	CB	1.2×10^3/hpf	—	Sterile	−41 TMP prophylaxis
6/18/79	CB	0 WBC/hpf	—	Sterile	−53 TMP prophylaxis
8/17/79	VB_2	6×10^2/ml	—	Sterile	−113 TMP prophylaxis

[a] White blood cells in urine = either quantitated per ml unspun or reported as WBC/high power field (hpf) in the spun sediment, CB = catheterized bladder, VB_2 = self-caught, midstream urine, ND = not done, SA = self-agglutinating *E. coli*, Nf = nitrofurantoin, TMP = trimethoprim. Antibody-coated bacteria: Pos = 25% or more show fluorescence, Neg = no fluorescence or <25% of bacteria show fluorescence. Solid transverse line divides longitudinal cultures into major periods of significance.

This patient has had no further right flank discomfort and has returned to her pattern of reinfection. As to why she should slough a single papillus in the absence of diabetes or analgesic abuse remains a mystery. It is quite feasible that the calyceal stone obstructed the infundibulum producing a pressure necrosis in the presence of her *E. coli* infection. The self-agglutinating nature of the *E. coli* suggests that it had been present for a considerable time period in order to lose its outer cell wall O-group specificity (see Chapter 5).

Table 9.18
Bacteriologic Localization Data in a 41-year-old Woman with Papillary Necrosis in a Lower Pole Calyx of the Right Kidney[a]

Source	SA *Escherichia coli*	Pyuria
	bacteria/ml	
CB	$>10^5$[b]	3+
WB	600	
LK_1–LK_5	0	0
RK_1–RK_5	5000[b]	2+

[a] SA = self-agglutinating *E. coli*. Other abbreviations as in Table 9.12.

[b] 4+ antibody-coated bacteria.

Whatever the cause, bacteria can persist in a necrotic calyx and cause recurrent infection with the same organism. When the necrotic calyx is localized to one pole of the kidney, the patient can be cured of her bacterial persistence by partial nephrectomy.

Paravesical Abscess with Fistula to Bladder

Most pelvic infections with sinus tracts to the bladder are clinically obvious, but not always.

R.B. was a 46-year-old white man referred to me in July 1972 for persistent *E. coli* bacteriuria of several month's duration. The initial development of his symptoms

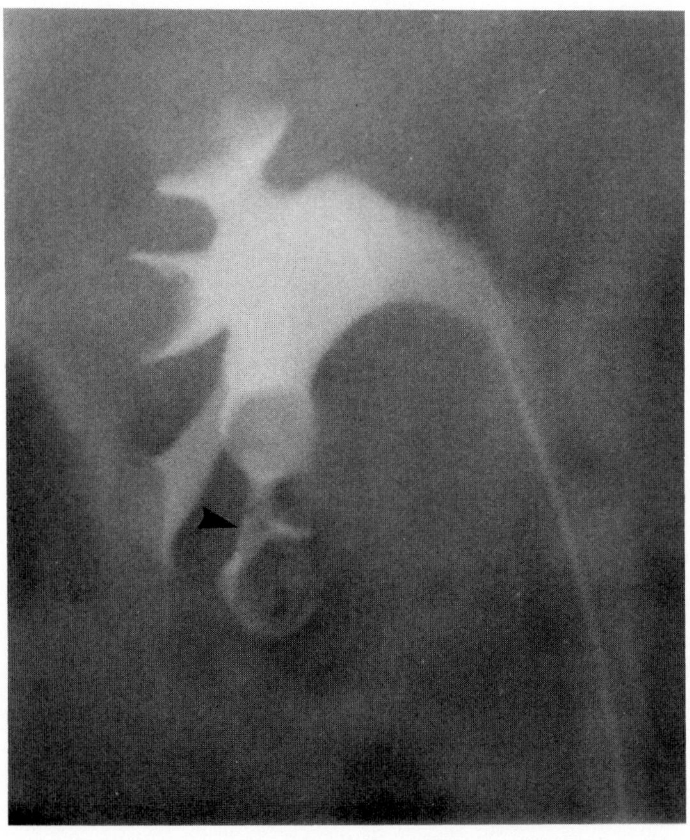

Figure 9.33 Retrograde urogram confirming filling defect in right lower calyx but showing extension into the infundibulum (*arrow*) probably accounting for its strictured appearance on the intravenous urogram (Figures 9.31 and 9.32).

was interesting. In December 1971, he first noticed a sensation of penile itching and discomfort. The urine was uninfected when examined in January by an excellent urologist in Sacramento who also felt the prostate was normal. To his surprise, 3 weeks later the patient returned with full-blown cystitis with severe dysuria and fever; the urine cultured *E. coli*, which cleared on tetracycline, but the pyuria persisted. An IVU was normal. Cephalexin and nitrofurantoin failed to clear the pyuria. Cystoscopy was normal. Nalidixic acid, followed by several weeks of penicillin-G, was also ineffective in influencing the pyuria. He was admitted to his local hospital where cystoscopy was again normal, bilateral ureteral catheterization studies showed both kidneys were infected with $>10^5$ *E. coli*/ml, and a perineal needle biopsy of the prostate was also culture negative but showed some mild periglandular chronic inflammation. At every culture, the *E. coli* was pansensitive to all antimicrobial agents. Several urines for acid-fast bacilli were negative by stain and culture.

His past history included an episode of dysuria in 1962 which was diagnosed as prostatitis and treated with sulfonamides. Following some rectal bleeding, he had a transrectal colon biopsy in 1969 for a benign tumor; the biopsy apparently perforated the colon and required an open surgical repair through a left paramedian incision. He had an indwelling Foley catheter for 3 days, and then developed a urinary and wound infection which required opening and packing the wound. He recovered without further complications and was discharged from the Air Force in June of 1970 in apparently good health.

When I first saw him on 7/13/72, 2 days off antimicrobial therapy, his urine contained 50–75 WBC/hpf (spun) with clumps of glitter cells, no protein, and the pH was 6.5. As seen in Table 9.19, his VB_1 grew 140 *E. coli*/ml, his VB_2 80 *E. coli*/ml, and his EPS was sterile. The *E. coli* was exquisitely sensitive to all antimicrobial agents at urinary levels. His EPS contained 6 WBC/hpf but his VB_1 urine was observed to be more cloudy than his VB_2. Through a misunderstanding, he restarted his combination tablets of methenamine mandelate and sodium acid phosphate; after only three tablets, repeat cultures the next day were surprisingly sterile. He again stopped this therapy, and the bladder was aspirated 48 hours later (7/17/72); the aspirate was loaded with WBCs but grew only 40 *E. coli*/ml. After the aspiration, prostatic localization cultures failed a second time to show the prostate as the site of the persisting *E. coli* (Table 9.19).

A retrograde urethrogram, sigmoidoscopy, barium enema, and upper GI series were all normal and showed no evidence of intestinal disease to suggest a vesicointestinal fistula.

By July 20 (Table 9.19), 6 days off antimicrobial therapy, his bladder aspirate was loaded with *E. coli* and WBCs. Interestingly, an EPS obtained that day showed many WBCs and 10–30 fat macrophages/lpf of prostatic fluid (see Figure 7.1), strongly suggesting prostatic inflammation. He was started on low doses of nitrofurantoin, 25 mg 4 times a day, on July 21.

Three days later he was cystoscoped as an out-patient under a saddle anesthesia. Suprapubic aspiration before cystoscopy showed only 10 *E. coli*/ml and prostatic localization studies for the third time failed to implicate the prostate; a drop of EPS, however, again confirmed the presence of oval fat macrophages, suggesting prostatic inflammation. Before I cystoscoped him, I was ready to accept the diagnosis that he probably had *E. coli* bacterial prostatitis and that I simply could not prove the *E. coli* in his prostate despite three attempts to do so. I was perplexed, however, by the persistent pyuria.

At cystoscopy, the urethra and prostate were normal. Number 5 Fr Stamey ureteral catheters were passed to each kidney, 4 ml of urine collected, spun, and examined under the microscope: not a single WBC was present in either renal urine. After removing the ureteral catheters, the bladder was inspected a second time. In the dome of the bladder there was a small tented area which appeared to trap the normal air bubble. On closer inspection, behind the air bubble was

Table 9.19
Bacteriologic Course of a 46-year-old White Man with a Subrectus Abscess (*Escherichia coli* 06) Presenting Three Years Later as a Urinary Tract Infection[a]

Date	Days On (+) or Off (−) Drug	Drug	Dose	VB_1	VB_2	EPS	VB_3	Organism	Serum Agglutination Titer	Comment
				bacteria/ml						
7/13/72	− 2	Methenamine and NaH_2PO_3	1 gm q 12 hr	140	80	0		*E. coli* 06		Pyuria
7/14/72	+ 1	Methenamine and NaH_2PO_3	500 mg q 8 hr	0	0	0	0			Pyuria
7/17/72	− 3			30	10		20	*E. coli* 06		SPA = 40 *E. coli* 06/ml; loaded with WBC
7/18/72	− 4			20	0					
7/20/72	− 6			10^4	10^4	100	10^4	*E. coli* 06	1:640	EPS = many WBC; 10–30 oval fat macrophages/1pf; pyuria
7/24/72	+ 3	Nitrofurantoin	25 mg q 6 hr	0	10	0	0	*E. coli* 06	1:1280	SPA = 10 *E. coli* 06/ml; loaded with WBC; cystoscopy shows sinus tract
9/10/72	+ 55	Nitrofurantoin	50 mg q 6 hr	0	0	0	0			Pyuria
9/13/72	+ 3 hr	Gentamicin	80 mg	Surgical excision of abdominal abscess and partial cystectomy						Bladder urine = sterile; sinus tract = 2000 *E. coli* 06/ml transport broth
10/12/72	+ 21	Nitrofurantoin	100 mg q.i.d.	0	0	0	0		1:640	5–10 WBC/hpf in urine
11/16/72	− 2			0	0	0	0			No pyuria
12/14/72	− 28			0	0					No pyuria
3/15/73	− 91			0	0				1:160	No pyuria
3/29/73	− 105			0	0	0	0		1:160	No pyuria; EPS = 1–3 WBC/hpf, 0 oval fat macrophages
8/20/79	− 7 yr; telephone call, well and healthy									

[a] SPA = suprapubic aspiration of bladder urine. See Table 7.2 for other abbreviations. Only Gram-negative bacteria shown in table. Small numbers of urethral *Staphylococcus epidermidis*, none of which localized to the prostate, are excluded. Solid transverse line divides longitudinal cultures into major periods of significance.

a small, pinpoint red hole which I thought at first was the puncture site of the needle aspiration. On further inspection, however, and with suprapubic pressure, I was able to express both pus and blood from this tiny hole that had no epithelial edema surrounding it. I was unable to introduce a catheter into the opening.

I felt the patient had a urachal cyst in the dome of the bladder which had become secondarily infected; he was scheduled for surgical excision, at his convenience, after summer vacation.

He was admitted to the hospital on 9/10/72. He had been on nitrofurantoin 50 mg 4 times a day during the summer. His admission urine showed a pH of 5.5, 0–3 WBC in his VB_1 and 10–12 WBC with clumps of glitter cells in the VB_2 urine. His EPS had 3–4 WBC/hpf and only 0–1 oval fat macrophage. Segmental urine cultures showed only normal urethral flora in all specimens. A complete blood count was normal; the WBC was 5500 with 54% segmented neutrophils, 30% lymphocytes, 9% monocytes, but interestingly 7% eosinophils. An IVU and voiding cystourethrogram were obtained; the kidneys were normal, the ureters undeviated, and the apex of the bladder showed some elongation or peaking toward the anterior abdominal wall.

At surgical exploration, the peritoneal cavity was benign. No bowel was stuck to the bladder. A mass measuring 5 × 5 × 2 cm extended from the superior aspect of the bladder under the left rectus muscle into the medial border of the right rectus muscle. The mass was resected with a portion of the bladder wall to include the sinus tract (Figure 9.34). A swab culture of the

A

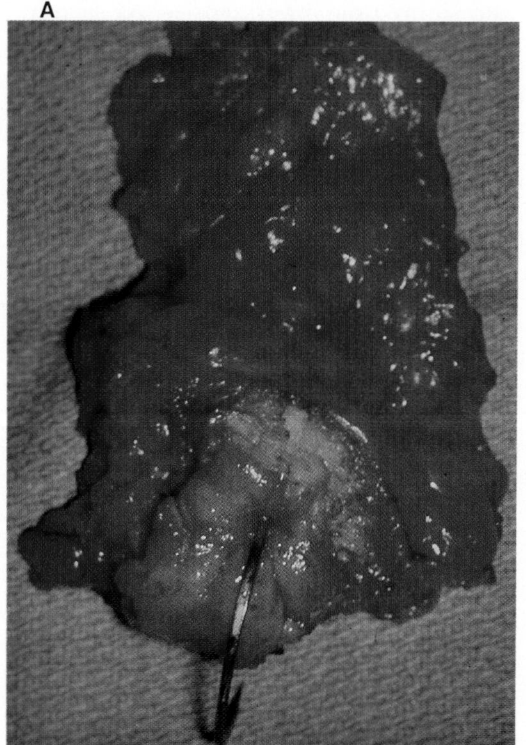

B

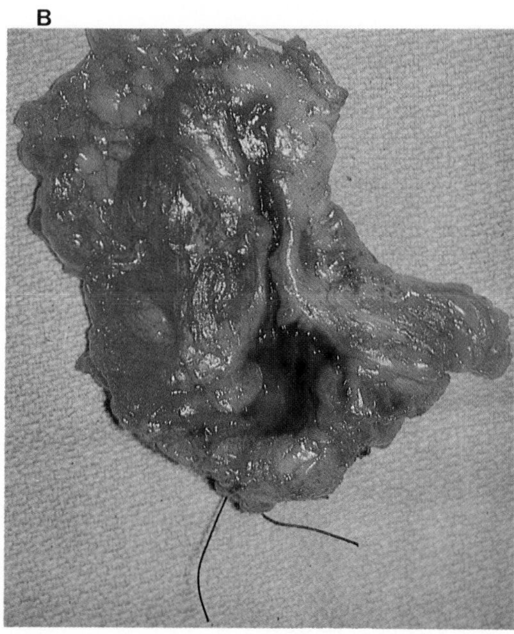

Figure 9.34 Surgical specimen from R.B., a 46-year-old man with a subrectus abscess (*Escherichia coli* 06) presenting 3 years later as a urinary tract infection. (*A*) The bladder mucosa with the blunt end of a curved needle in the sinus opening is seen at the bottom of the 5 × 5 × 2 cm mass. (*B*) The back side of the extravesical mass with the sinus tract opened showing the extensive fibrosis; the bladder mucosa is on the other side, marked by the suture at the bottom of the photograph.

sinus tract showed 2000 *E. coli*/ml of transport broth at a time when the bladder urine was sterile (80 mg of gentamicin was given on call to surgery). Histologically, the sinus tract extended for 6 cm and was lined with transitional epithelium; it ended extravesically in intense fibrosis, with acute and chronic inflammation of the tissues. There was no abscess cavity *per se*. The bladder wall showed acute and chronic transmural inflammation. He was discharged on the 9th postoperative day on nitrofurantoin 100 mg 4 times a day, which was discontinued on 11/14/72. As can be seen in Table 9.19, all subsequent cultures have contained only normal urethral flora—no *E. coli*. His EPS has been normal. His pyuria was gone by 11/16/72 and he has remained asymptomatic and well. A telephone conversation in August 1979 indicated he had been in good health without urinary symptoms.

All of his *E. coli* were serogroup 06. Bacterial agglutination titers in his serum were 1:640 to 1:1280 preoperatively; eight months later they were normal, 1:160 (Table 9.19).

It is surprising that a paravesical wound abscess due to *E. coli* could lie so dormant from 1969 to early 1972 when it is documented that he had his first UTI. It is even more surprising that the inflammatory reaction would break into the bladder and present as a UTI. These are the facts, however, and the data support them.

The distinguishing diagnostic features of this case are that despite leukocytes and oval fat macrophages in the prostatic fluid, chronic bacterial prostatitis does not leave residual bladder pyuria once the cystitis has cleared after a few days of antimicrobial therapy. When ureteral catheterization excluded the presence of leukocytes in his renal urine, there had to be a fistula or sinus tract emptying into his bladder.

Labial Persistence in Bartholin's Ducts (?)

The greater vestibular glands of Bartholin have long ducts which open at the sides of the vaginal orifice. Unfortunately, the vaginal opening of these ducts is impossible to see or find except occasionally in the presence of an abscess of Bartholin's gland. Nevertheless, if the urethra can be excluded as the site of bacterial persistence by nurse-collected, table-voided specimens by the technique successfully used as described in Tables 9.8 and 9.11, and if the rectum can be cleared of all *E. coli* by TMP-SMX therapy (as shown in Table 9.11), persistence of *E. coli* in the labial area is probably from Bartholin's ducts because there are no other ductal structures in the region.

F.P. was a 52-year-old, white, married woman when I first saw her in 1970. Her first UTI occurred 2 months after her marriage, but she had only three infections in the next 25 years. A partial hysterectomy in 1966, however, was followed by multiple urinary infections. Several IVUs were normal and at least one voiding cystourethrogram showed no abnormalities. As seen in Figure 9.35, which extends from 9/18/70 to 3/5/71, her introitus was colonized with an 023 *E. coli* at every visit, and a symptomatic bacteriuria due to *E. coli* 023 occurred at the end of the period shown in Figure 9.35. The first culture shown in Figure 9.36 is identical to the last culture in Figure 9.35; thus, the figures are consecutive. Notice in Figure 9.36 that another *E. coli* 023 infection occurred in May 1971 but her next infection was due to an *E. coli* 06 (July, 1971) despite the 023 also being on the introitus as well as in the urethra at the time of her bacteriuria; she was away the month of June 1971, and the 06 colonization of the introitus may have occurred at that time. It is interesting that the 023 and 06 persisted together on the introital and urethral mucosa during July, but by August the 06 had acquired dominance and was present in pure culture.

She always took small daily doses of oral conjugated estrogens. The pH of her introital mucosa was consistently 4.0–4.5 and most readings with a direct surface electrode were 4.0–4.3 pH.

She was placed on a vaginal jelly called "Aci-Jel" which contains acetic acid, oxyquinoline sulfate, ricinoleic acid, and boric acid to mention a few of its components that might exert some local biological

Figure 9.35 Enterobacterial relationship of the vaginal vestibule, urethral, and mid-stream cultures in a 52-year-old, white, married woman (F.P.). The only Gram-negative enterobacterial cultures were *Escherichia coli*; the culture symbol (▲), without overlying vertical bars, indicates the complete absence of Gram-negative enterobacterial. The serogroup of *E. coli* appears at the top of each solid bar; NT is a nontypable *E. coli*. Her first urinary infection occurred 2 months after marriage, followed by only three infections in the next 25 years. A partial hysterectomy in 1966 was followed by multiple urinary infections. The *E. coli* 023 bladder infection illustrated in this figure was preceded by the constant presence of *E. coli* 023 on the introitus in pure culture, despite the fecal *E. coli* consisting of 91% *E. coli* 013, 5% *E. coli* NT, and only 4% *E. coli* 023. The last culture in this figure was obtained on 3/5/71. Figures 9.36 and 9.37 follow consecutively in time.

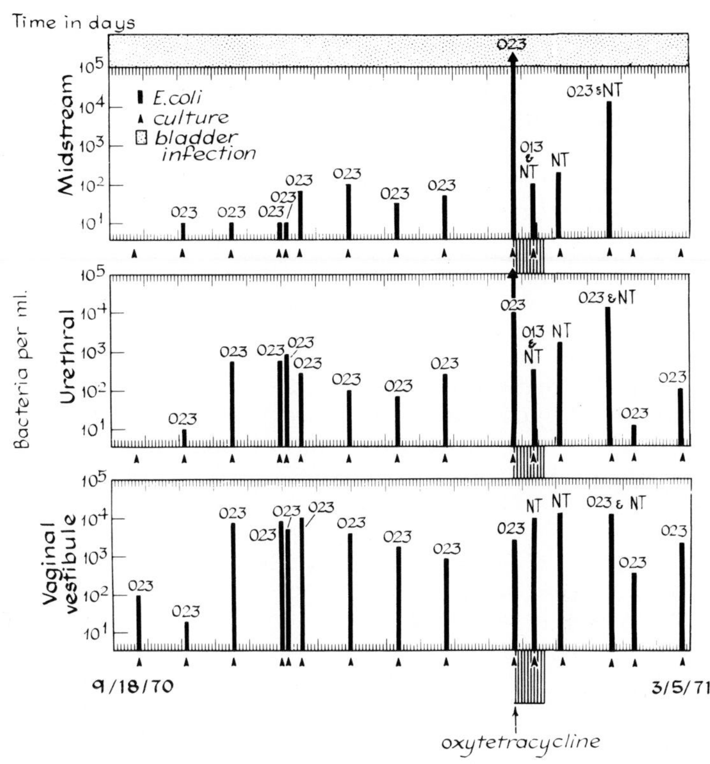

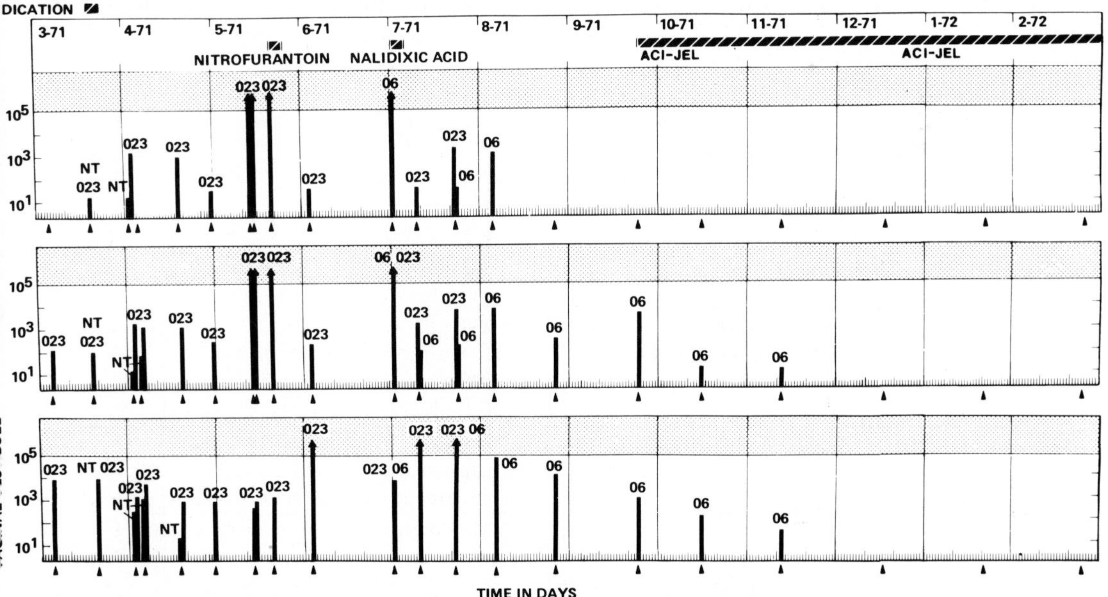

Figure 9.36 The first culture in this figure is a repeat of the last culture (3/5/71) in Figure 9.35. Observe the appearance of the *Escherichia coli* 06 for the first time at the bacteriuric episode early in 7/71, and its ultimate dominance of the vaginal flora in pure culture by 8/71. Vaginal application of Aci-jel reduced the colonization to below detectable levels, but discontinuation was followed by reappearance of the *E. coli* 06 (Figure 9.37).

effect. To our surprise the introital carriage of the *E. coli* 06 completely disappeared as seen in Figure 9.36 which continues chronologically into Figure 9.37. Within 1 month of stopping the Aci-Jel (Figure 9.37), however, she was again growing the *E. coli* 06 on the introitus and had an *E. coli* 06 UTI. The apparent effect of Aci-Jel vaginal application was not due to pH; in fact, her introital pH *rose* from the 4.0–4.5 range before Aci-Jel to the 5.0–6.0 range during application. Because of stress urinary incontinence which had been present for years, I corrected her incontinence with an endoscopic suspension of her vesical neck for which she received a few doses of gentamicin for tissue prophylaxis and was discharged on nitrofurantoin prophylaxis for a few days. As can be seen in Figure 9.37, from August 1972 through February 1973 she had five bacteriuric episodes with this *E. coli* 06 which was constantly on the introitus at every culture between her infections. All her bacteriuric episodes, most of which were symptomatic, always responded promptly to nitrofurantoin which she usually took for 10 days.

The remainder of her interesting bacteriologic history is presented in Tables 9.20–9.22 because it can be divided into three convenient periods of observation. The interested reader should concentrate on the general pattern of each table rather than attempt an individual study of each set of cultures. During the 8 months that elapsed between the last cultures in Figure 9.37 (February 1973) and the first culture in Table 9.20 (December 1973), we repeated the Aci-Jel vaginal application for 6 months without any change in her vaginal carriage of *E. coli* 06. Her introital pH again rose from 4.0–4.5 to 5.0–6.0, but the *E. coli* 06 was present at every culture. I can only surmise that the 06 became resistant to one of the organic acids in the Aci-Jel mixture which contained so many different substances. One other experiment was done during these 8 months. Our pharmacy made up 10% lactic acid (pH 2.0!) in a methylcellulose base which was placed in the vagina each morning and evening with a syringe. The acidity of her mucosal pH again rose from her normal pH of 4.0–4.5 to 5.0–6.0, and the *E. coli* 06 continued happily on the introitus.

The information given in Table 9.20 was

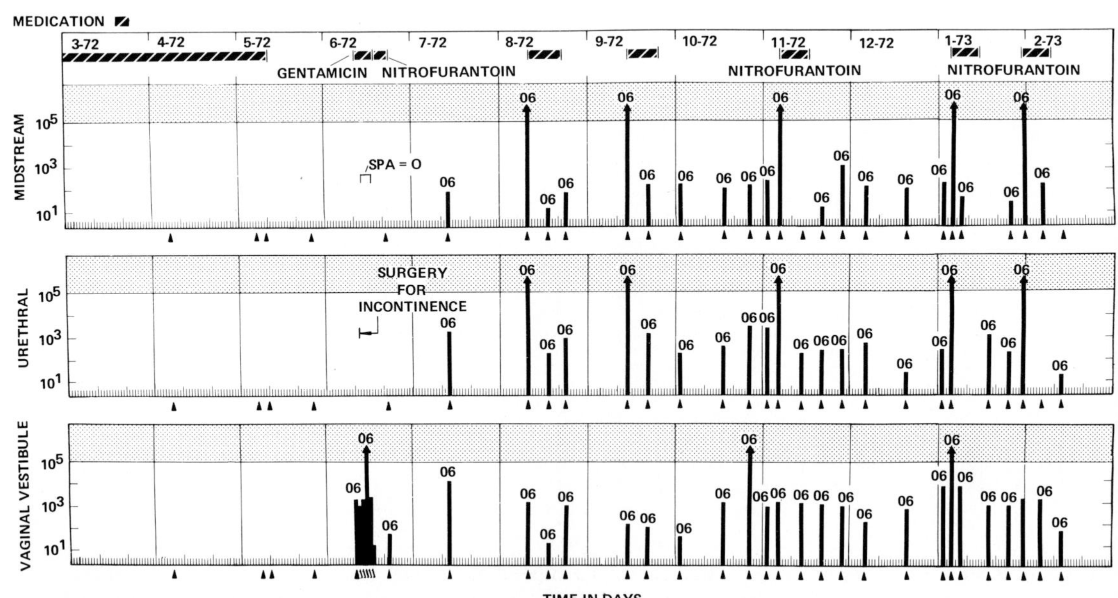

Figure 9.37 See legend to Figures 9.35 and 9.36. Discontinuation of Aci-Jel in May 1972 was followed by reappearance of the *Escherichia coli* 06 and multiple bacteriuric episodes from it.

Table 9.20
Bacteriologic History of F.P. during TMP-SMX Prophylaxis with ½ Tablet Each Night[a]

Date	Days On (+) or Off (−) Therapy	Vaginal Introitus		Urethra		Midstream		Anal Canal	
			bacteria/ml		*bacteria/ml*		*bacteria/ml*		*bacteria/ml*
12/10/73	+11 Nitrofurantoin	*Escherichia coli* 06	4100	*E. coli* 06	850[b]	*E. coli* 06	70[b]	SA *E. coli* 015	10^5
12/17/73	+7 TMP-SMX (40 mg TMP, 200 mg SMX nightly)		0		0[b]		0[b]	*Pseudomonas*	5000
1/7/74	+27 TMP-SMX		0		0[b]		0[b]	*E. coli* 02	500
								Proteus mirabilis	10
								Klebsiella	500
								Pseudomonas	50
1/14/74	+34 TMP-SMX	*E. coli* 06	30		0[b]		0[b]	*Klebsiella*	10
								Pseudomonas	650
1/21/74	+41 TMP-SMX	*E. coli* 06	10		0[b]		0[b]	*Pseudomonas*	60
2/4/74	+55 TMP-SMX		0		0[b]		0[b]	*Pseudomonas*	4000
2/19/74	+70 TMP-SMX	*E. coli* 06	10		0[b]		0[b]	*Pseudomonas*	300
3/4/74	+83 TMP-SMX		0	Urethral swab	0		0	*Pseudomonas*	10^4
4/1/74	+110 TMP-SMX	*E. coli* 06	10	Urethral swab	0		0	*Pseudomonas*	3000
4/29/74	+138 TMP-SMX	*E. coli* 06	210	Urethral swab	0		0	*Pseudomonas*	120
5/13/74	+152 TMP-SMX	*E. coli* 06	20	Urethral swab	0		0	NT *E. coli*	400
								Pseudomonas	10^4
6/25/74	+195 TMP-SMX		0	Urethral swab	0		0	*Pseudomonas*	10^3
7/23/74	+223 TMP-SMX		0	Urethral swab	0		0	*Pseudomonas*	900
9/3/74	+265 TMP-SMX	*E. coli* 06	10	Urethral swab	0		0	*Pseudomonas*	1500
10/28/74	+320 TMP-SMX	*E. coli* 06	10				0	*Pseudomonas*	750
12/2/74	+355 TMP-SMX	*E. coli* 06	10				0	NT *E. coli*	200
								Pseudomonas	3000
12/16/74	+369 TMP-SMX	*E. coli* 06	10				0	*Pseudomonas*	5000

[a] TMP-SMX = trimethoprim-sulfamethoxazole, SA = self-agglutinating, NT = nontypable.
[b] Nurse-collected, table caught urine samples; all other urine samples self-caught.

Table 9.21
Bacteriologic History of F.P. during Nitrofurantoin Macrocrystals Prophylaxis with 100 mg Each Night[a]

Date	Days on (+) or off (−) Therapy	Vaginal Introitus		Urethra		Midstream		Anal Canal	
			bacterial/ml		*bacteria/ml*		*bacteria/ml*		*bacteria/ml*
1/2/75	− 16 TMP-SMX					*Escherichia coli* 06	$>10^5$		
1/3/75	− 17 TMP-SMX	*E. coli* 06	5000			*E. coli* 06		*E. coli* 06, 0113 *Pseudomonas*	$>10^4$
1/10/75	+ 7 Nitrofurantoin (400 mg/day)	*E. coli* 06	2000			*E. coli* 06	2000	*E. coli* 06, 0113 *Pseudomonas*	1600 500
1/17/75	+ 17 Nitrofurantoin (100 mg nightly)	*E. coli* 06	800	*E. coli* 06	1250[b]	*E. coli* 06	160[b]	*E. coli* 0113 *Klebsiella* *Pseudomonas*	300 310 20
2/20/75	+ 51 Nitrofurantoin	*E. coli* 06	10^3			*E. coli* 06	750	NT *E. coli* *Pseudomonas*	10^4 300
3/21/75	+ 80 Nitrofurantoin	*E. coli* 06	5000			*E. coli* 06	410	*E. coli* 06, 036 *Pseudomonas*	$>10^3$ 110
4/17/75	+107 Nitrofurantoin	*E. coli* 06	750			*E. coli* 06	200	SA *E. coli* 06 *Pseudomonas*	2200 1500
5/22/75	+151 Nitrofurantoin	*E. coli* 06	3000			*E. coli* 06	450	*E. coli* 06 *Pseudomonas*	190 2000
7/7/75	+197 Nitrofurantoin		0				0	NT *E. coli* *Pseudomonas*	10^3 2000
9/2/75	+253 Nitrofurantoin	*E. coli* 06	3000			*E. coli* 06	220	*E. coli* 075 *Enterobacter* *Pseudomonas*	3000 250 3000
10/6/75	+287 Nitrofurantoin	*E. coli* 06	10^3			*E. coli* 06	90	NT *E. coli*, *Pseudomonas*	$<10^4$ 3000
11/3/75	+315 Nitrofurantoin	*E. coli* 06	50			*E. coli* 06	10	*E. coli* 075 *Pseudomonas*	10^5 10^4
11/18/75	− 4 Nalidixic acid[c] (1000 mg/day)	*E. coli* 06	500			*E. coli* 06	100	*Pseudomonas*	700
12/8/75	+ 20 Nitrofurantoin (100 mg nightly)	*E. coli* 06	1250			*E. coli* 06	240	NT *E. coli* *Klebsiella* *Proteus morganii* *Pseudomonas*	$>10^5$ 200 2000 1000

[a] TMP-SMX = trimethoprim-sulfamethoxazole, SA = self-agglutinating, NT = nontypable.
[b] Nurse-collected, table-caught urine samples; all other samples self-caught.

important in detecting the site of her bacterial persistence, but we were unaware of it at the time. All of the urine specimens were self-caught by the patient except those indicated as being table-caught specimens. Observe that the *E. coli* 06 was detected on the introitus on 1/14/74, 1/21/74, and 2/19/74 when there was not a single colony of 06 in the rectum, the urethra, or the bladder. Moreover, urethral swab cultures were also sterile on 4/1/74, 4/29/74, and 5/13/74 at a time when the introital cultures were also positive. These six positive introital cultures at a time when the urethra was also cultured and found to be without *E. coli* strongly suggest the introital area as the site of *E. coli* persistence. This table should be contrasted with Table 9.11 where cultures collected in the same way showed the introitus and the rectum contained no *E. coli* but the 023 was clearly coming from the urethra.

Additional evidence was obtained on 9/3/74 and 9/4/74 that we were dealing with introital persistence inside the labia minora. On each of these days, we carefully obtained moistened swab cultures of the left and right labia majora, the left and right labia minora before massage of Bartholin's glands, and the labia minora after massage. On 9/3/74, both cultures of the labia majora were sterile, the right labia minora was sterile, the left labia minora showed 30 *E. coli* 06/ml premassage but 70 *E. coli*/ml postmassage. On 9/4/74, the only *E. coli* detected in the whole series was 20 *E. coli* 06 from the postmassage left labia minora.

These data clearly suggested that the site of 06 persistence was probably the duct or gland of Bartholin on the left side, but I could see and feel nothing abnormal. Attempts to determine exactly where the duct from Bartholin's gland might be, even with gynecologic consultation, were futile.

Not knowing what else to do, we returned to nitrofurantoin prophylaxis, as shown in Table 9.21. The major observation from this table is the almost immediate increase in introital density of the *E. coli* 06 and, of course, the return of *E. coli* to the rectal flora.

Table 9.22 tells the whole story. We realized that we had used only prophylactic doses of TMP-SMX, which had drastically reduced the colonization density without completely clearing the *E. coli* 06 from the vaginal introitus. We wondered if full dosage TMP-SMX might obliterate the site of 06 persistence since prophylactic dosage had almost done so. Accordingly, we began TMP-SMX at full dosage (160 mg TMP and 800 mg SMX twice daily) for 10 days on 1/14/76, followed by one-half tablet prophylaxis each night afterward for 5 months, after which all antimicrobial therapy was stopped. As can be seen in Table 9.21, the full dosage TMP-SMX apparently cured her. For the first and only time after a therapeutic effort, there were no further *E. coli* 06 or any other Enterobacteriaceae on the introitus. The introitus has been colonized only twice since that time and with *E. coli* 04 rather than *E. coli* 06. She had one documented infection on 6/18/78 which she cultured at home with a Uricult dip slide and self-treated herself with TMP-SMX. The *E. coli* was a nontypable organism. She further treated herself, without cultures, in February and June of 1979 for what she thought to be symptoms of bacteriuria.

These data strongly suggest that the *E. coli* 06 were persisting at some site communicating with the introitus since the 06 could be cultured there and nowhere else—neither the rectum nor the urethra or the bladder—while on TMP-SMX prophylaxis. The only logical site anatomically is one of the long ducts from the greater vestibular glands of Bartholin.

URINARY INFECTIONS IN PATIENTS WITH NEUROLOGIC DISEASE

Of all patients who have urinary infections, no group compares in severity and morbidity to those with spinal cord injury. Nearly all require catheterization because of spasticity, or flaccidity of the bladder, and in a significant proportion ureterectasis, hydronephrosis, reflux, or renal calculi develop.

Table 9.22
Bacteriologic History of F.P. During and Following Full Dosage TMP-SMX Therapy for Bacterial Persistence of *Escherichia Coli* 06 on Introitus[a]

Date	Days On (+) or Off (−) Therapy	Vaginal Introitus		Urethra	Midstream		Anal Canal	
		bacterial/ml		*bacteria/ml*	*bacteria/ml*		*bacteria/ml*	
1/13/76	+ 56 Nitrofurantoin (100 mg nightly)				*E. coli* 06	$>10^5$		
1/14/76	+ 1 Nitrofurantoin (400 mg daily)	*E. coli* 06	1500		*E. coli* 06	40	*E. coli* 011	1500
							Klebsiella	500
							Pseudomonas	2500
1/24/76	+ 10 TMP-SMX (160 mg TMP-800 mg SMX g 12 hr)		0			0	NT *E. coli*	250
							Pseudomonas	1040
2/13/76	+ 30 TMP-SMX (40 mg TMP, 200 mg SMX nightly)		0			0		0
3/24/76	+ 60 TMP-SMX		0			0	*Pseudomonas*	10^3
5/5/76	+102 TMP-SMX		0			0	*Pseudomonas*	1000
6/23/76	+151 TMP-SMX		0			0	*Pseudomonas*	200
10/6/76	−105 TMP-SMX		0			0	*E. coli* 018	5000
							Pseudomonas	1000
11/3/76	−133 TMP-SMX		0			0	*E. coli* 04, 018	6000
							Proteus mirabilis	500
							Pseudomonas	40
12/13/76	−173 TMP-SMX		0			0	*E. coli* 018, NT *E. coli*	4000
							P. Mirabilis	200
							Pseudomonas	2000
1/12/77	−202 TMP-SMX		0			0	*E. coli* 018	4000
							Pseudomonas	1000
3/16/77	−265 TMP-SMX	*E. coli* 04	10			0	*E. coli* 04, 01	7000
							Pseudomonas	500
6/17/77	−358 TMP-SMX	*E. coli* 04	80		*E. coli* 04	10	*E. coli* 018, 01	$>10^4$
							Pseudomonas	120
2/27/78	−1 yr, 8 mo TMP-SMX		0			0	NT *E. coli*, 016	$>10^4$
							E. coli 08	
							Pseudomonas	1000

5/30/78	−1 yr, 11 mo TMP-SMX	0		0	*E. coli* 04, NT *E. coli*	5000
					E. coli 01	
					Pseudomonas	2000
6/18/78	−1 yr, 11.5 mo TMP-SMX		NT *E. coli* (Uricult)	$>10^5$		
10/25/78	−4 mo TMP-SMX	0		0	NT *E. coli*,	$>10^5$
					E. coli 04	
2/16/79	+3 TMP-SMX[b] (160 mg TMP/800 mg SMX g 8 hr)	0		0	SA *E. coli*, *E. coli* 064	8000
					Pseudomonas	2500
6/20/79	− 14 TMP-SMX[c]	0		0		

[a] TMP-SMX = trimethoprim-sulfamethoxazole, NT = nontypable, SA = self-agglutination.
[b] Self-treated for symptoms, no culture on 2/13/79.
[c] Self-treated for symptoms 6/1 to 6/6, no culture on 6/1.

Table 9.23
Comparison of Bacterial Species Isolated from Paraplegic Patients with Those from Bacteriuric Schoolgirls and Adult Females

	Paraplegics[33]	Schoolgirls[34]	Adult Females[35]
Total isolates	724	122	107
Escherichia coli	67	102	90
Proteus mirabilis	126	1	9
Klebsiella-Aerobacter	126	12	2
Pseudomonas	222	1	0
Others	183	6	6

Severe pathologic changes in the bladder and pelvic musculature require frequent instrumentation of the urinary tract; the bacterial species cultured from the urine of paraplegic patients reflects the consequences of the need for repeated catheterization. In Table 9.23, the organisms found on bladder puncture by Govan *et al.*[34] in 724 positive cultures from patients with neurogenic bladder dysfunction are compared to the species distribution reported by Kunin *et al.*[35] and Sussman *et al.*[36] in nonhospitalized general populations. In paraplegic patients, *Pseudomonas*, *Klebsiella*, and *P. mirabilis* replace *E. coli* as the most common strains.

Bacteriuria occurs in at least 80% of patients with spinal cord injury,[37] renal calculi in 12% within the first 3 years of injury (almost all due to *Proteus*),[37] and reflux in about 18% in long term followups.[38] Stovall *et al.*[39] studied the incidence of renal bacteriuria in paraplegic patients who had had indwelling catheters for 3 months to 15 years; they reported that 83% of the ureteral urine specimens were sterile, but their bacteriologic technique could not have detected small numbers of bacteria (for example, all of their bladder cultures after washing with 2000 ml of sterile water were sterile). Nevertheless, Govan *et al.*[34] reported a similar figure—sterile ureteral urine in 42 of 55 patients with "neurogenic bladder dysfunction" (76%). These studies suggest that the kidneys are relatively well protected in many paraplegic patients with chronic bacteriuria, but these differences may be due to a greater resistance of the male to upper tract bacteriuria, an observation suggested in our early localization studies in 1965.[40] Future studies of patients with spinal cord injuries would be more useful if females were distinguished from males and the spinal cord level of paralysis and the duration of the disease were noted. For example, Jacobson and Bors[37] noted more hydronephrosis associated with lower motor neuron than with upper motor lesions, but reflux is more common with upper motor neuron lesions.[38]

The major advance in the bacteriuria of spinal cord injuries is undoubtedly Guttmann's[41] introduction of intermittent catheterization in 1954. Catheterization, done only by technicians using a "nontouch" technique, was performed two or three times every 24 hours until spontaneous bladder function returned. Antibiotics were used if cultures became positive. Guttmann and Frankel[42] reported their 10-year experience on 476 patients in 1966, a paper that must have startled rehabilitation centers around the world. Of the 476 patients admitted within 14 days of injury (most within 48 hours), 77% had sterile urine on admission and 62% on discharge; only a further 7% drop occurred in sterility during subsequent follow-up. Most importantly, hydronephrosis was reduced to 7.4%, ureteral reflux to 4.4%, and renal calculi to 1.7%. Moreover, there were no urethral fistulas or diverticula from periurethral abscesses, whereas this difficult complication develops in 25–30% of paraplegics with indwelling catheters.[43] If these data are confirmed, as Bors's[43] initial study indicates, public health money in this country might be better spent by adopting Gutmann's technique of managing spinal cord injuries than by screening our asymptomatic bacteriuric populations. Even more convincing than Guttmann's data, J. W. Pearman (an internist with the Royal Perth Rehabilitation Hospital in Perth, Australia) has presented some remarkable data on intermittent catheterization in patients with spinal cord injury.[44] In this report, patients were catheterized every 6 hours following acute traumatic spinal cord injury until bladder function returned. At each catheterization the urine was cultured, and 150 mg of kanamycin and 30 mg of colistin sulfate in 25 ml of sterile water were left in the bladder. Of 3036 catheterizations performed in 27 male patients, 16 episodes of bacteriuria occurred (an incidence of 1 per 190 catheterizations or 0.5%). Of 1547 catheterizations performed in 9 female patients, 9 instances of bacteriuria occurred (an incidence of 1 per 172 catheterizations or 0.6%). Almost all the resistant organisms were enterococci and *S. epidermidis*. For the 18 patients of the 36 who acquired bacteriuria (50%), the rate of occurrence was 15.7 infections per 1000 patient days of intermittent catheterization. Rhame and Perkash[45] have reported similar data without a catheter team and even with the patients themselves doing their own catheterization; about 50 ml of a neomycin-polymyxin irrigant was left in the bladder and urethra after each catheterization. Nevertheless, Pearman[46] makes a strong argument for a catheter team, and has recently updated his statistics and described his team approach; with nearly 15,000 catheterizations in men and 5,500 in women, the incidence of significant bacteriuria (>1,000 bacteria/ml in three consecutive catheterizations) was still 0.56% in men and 0.97% in women. In a more recent study,[47] where half the patients on intermittent catheterization had 50 mg of kanamycin and 10 mg of colistin base in 25 ml of water left in their bladder at each catheterization, while the other half served as controls and had nothing left in their bladder, the incidence of significant bacteriuria was cut in half by the instillation. The interested reader should note that the Perth group has cut their concentrations of kanamycin and colistin base to 1/3 of their original recommendation apparently without changing their results.

Perhaps more important than the incidence of infection is the reduction in urinary tract complications achieved by intermittent catheterization regimens. In addition to Guttmann and Frankel's[42] report in 1966, we now have Pearman's[48] report of 99 patients followed for an average of 36 months after discharge from the hospital. Forty-six percent of the men and 59% of the women did not have a single infection after discharge. Among the males, there were no instances of epididymitis, urethral stricture, or bladder calculi; one male had a urethral diverticulm (for a 1.3% incidence) and one developed renal calculi (1.3%). Seventy of the 75 male patients had a normal IVU either at discharge or at later follow-ups; most of the IVUs, however, were apparently made at discharge and we lack long term follow-ups on the status of the kidneys in this series. Price *et al.*[49] reported on the 8th year of a 10-year study on renal function evaluation in 228 patients with quadriplegia and paraplegia. Seventy-eight percent had good function, 13% showed mild deterioration, 4% moderate deterioration, and 5% severe deterioration. It is interesting that there were no substantial differences in renal clearances and tubular function among patients with sterile urine, intermittent bacteriuria, or constant bacteriuria; 75% of their patients were constantly infected.

Nevertheless, the results of intermittent catheterization appear to have substantially changed urinary tract morbidity from spinal cord injury. Marosszeky *et al.*,[50] however, have reported almost as good results by using an indwelling catheter during the

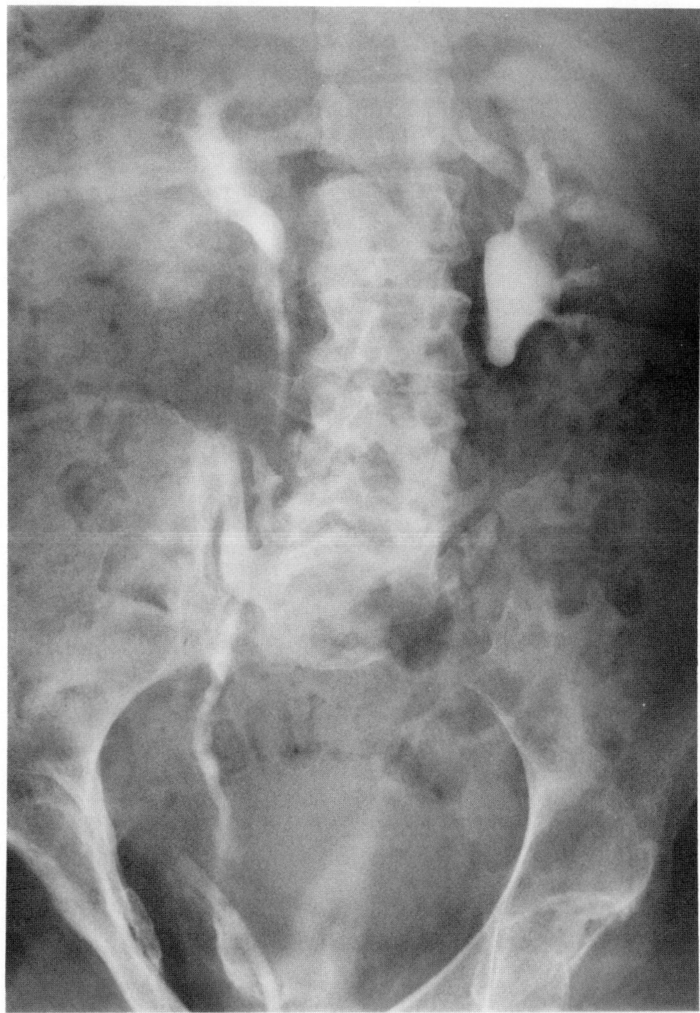

Figure 9.38 An intravenous urogram from May 15, 1975, on a T4 paraplegic woman, managed with an indwelling Foley catheter since her gunshot wound in 1954.

initial period of acute spinal cord trauma in 77 patients, suggesting that how the patient is managed in the initial period is perhaps not so important as long as the catheter is removed as soon as possible. I am reminded of the story that whereas most of us think streptomycin marked the end of the era of pulmonary tuberculosis, that in fact, if you plot the declining incidence of tuberculosis against time in years, you cannot tell when streptomycin was introduced into our culture. Perhaps more than just intermittent catheterization is responsible for the dramatic change in urinary tract morbidity from spinal cord injury, but whatever it is, it is a most welcome change.

Before concluding this section on urinary infection in patients with neurologic disease, I should point out that although Lapides and Costello[51] believe that the uninhibited neurogenic bladder is a common cause of recurrent urinary infection in normal women, I know of no evidence to support this suggestion. In fact, Walter *et al.*[52] tested this hypothesis by looking at the incidence of urinary infection in 579 pa-

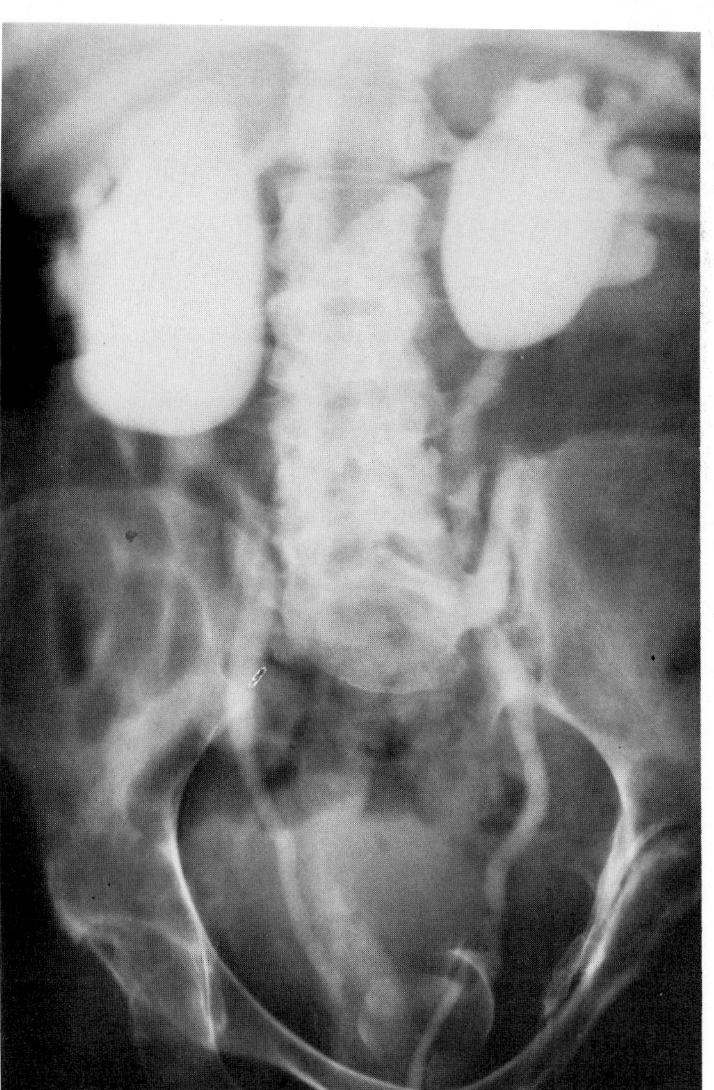

Figure 9.39 An intravenous urogram from November 10, 1977, on the same paraplegic patient described in Figure 9.38. She had experienced 8 months of lowback pain and low grade fever without seeking medical advice. The Foley catheter was open and draining throughout this examination.

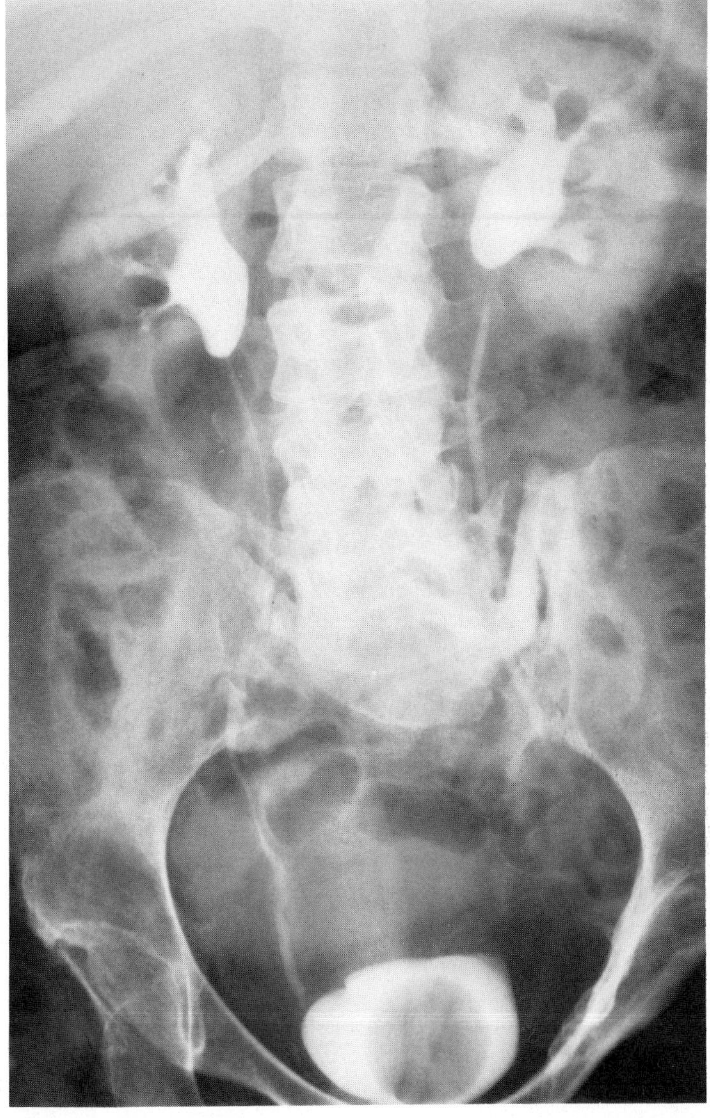

Figure 9.40 A repeat intravenous urogram on February 23, 1978, after 3½ months of ampicillin therapy. Her urine was sterile despite the Foley catheter. Compare to Figures 9.39 and 9.38.

tients with detrusor hyperreflexia; they found no correlation between the cystometric finding and the presence of bacteriuria.

On the other hand, there can be no doubt that infection adversely affects the smooth muscle of the urinary tract. David Cumes, Assistant Professor of Urology at Stanford, recently managed a remarkable case that emphasizes this point very strongly. A 43-year-old women was referred in February 1978 for urinary diversion because of severe bilateral hydronephrosis. She was a T_4 paraplegic from a gunshot wound in 1954 and was always managed with an indwelling Foley catheter. Spontaneous detrusor contractions with leakage around the catheter began in 1965, but IVUs were normal in 1972 and 1975 (Figure 9.38). Grade 1, left-sided reflux was known to be present. Throughout 1977, she experienced low grade fever and backaches for which she did not seek medical attention until November 1977; an IVU showed extensive bilateral hydronephrosis (Figure 9.39) and a cystogram Grade 1, left-sided reflux. Her urine was infected with *P. mirabilis.* She had been treated with ampicillin in the interim before referral by her family physician and on admission her urine culture was sterile. A repeat IVU showed complete disappearance of the hydronephrosis (Figure 9.40); the collecting system was now comparable to the IVU in 1975 (Figure 9.38). It is unusual in these days for a patient to go so many months with low grade fever and backache without receiving antimicrobial agents, but in preantibiotic days it is clear that such changes were not so uncommon.[53] This paraplegic patient, then, is an excellent example of hydroureteronephrosis from untreated, symptomatic UTI. We should not forget that this can occur, even in these days of better medicine.

CONCLUDING COMMENTS

Many observers have commented upon the high failure rate of antibacterial therapy in the presence of urologic abnormalities.[54, 55] But these general statistics are not really helpful because either the diagnosis of the presence of infection was inadequate (before 1956),[54] or the specific urinary tract abnormalities were not indicated in the analysis of failures.[55] A few patients with infection stones and a few others with chronic bacterial prostatitis can make any series of chemotherapeutic attempts look dismal. And yet, these patients can be sorted out satisfactorily. Table 9.1 is presented because these abnormalities *cause* infections to persist and become chronic; with careful bacteriologic techniques, the site of these abnormalities can be accurately localized and the patients then cured of their infections by the appropriate surgical procedure.

I hope these clinical examples show, however, that the cause of bacterial persistence is often subtle. Without plain film tomograms, for example, the soft putty-like foci of struvite stones in *P. mirabilis* urinary infections will frequently be missed. The diagnosis of unilaterally infected, atrophic kidneys requires both time and knowledge of cystoscopic localization techniques, as well as careful bacteriology; in N.B., Figure 9.7, a casual or hurried observer might turn immediately to the gigantic hydronephrosis in the right kidney (which also contained sterile calculi) without taking the required diagnostic time to prove that the cause of the infection was the atrophic left kidney. In the male, the persistence of pathogenic bacteria in prostatic fluid requires even more careful clinical technique and equally knowledgeable bacteriologic methodology based on the ability to culture small numbers of bacteria. Thus, although considerable effort and care are required to prove the site of bacterial persistence in patients with recurrent urinary infections, the rewards can be measured only in terms of a lifetime free of both infection and the danger of progressive renal failure.

A final word of precaution: when acute urinary obstruction, usually from an infection stone or sometimes ureteral instrumentation, occurs in the presence of a urinary infection, the obstruction must be relieved immediately. Failure to act decisively usually leads to renal abscesses, wedge-shaped areas of tubular destruction, and, ultimately, renal atrophy. With good radiology now available to all physicians, every adult patient (with the possible exception of pregnant women) who presents with high fever, chills, and flank pain should have an emergency IVU to exclude acute renal obstruction. The price of procrastination, so often observed on even good medical services, is one of our modern medical tragedies.

REFERENCES

1. Guze, L. B., and Beeson, P. B.: Experimental pyelonephritis; II. Effect of partial ureteral obstruction on the course of bacterial infection in the kidney of the rat and the rabbit. Yale J. Biol. Med. **30:** 315, 1958.
2. Guze, L. B., and Beeson, P. B.: Experimental pyelonephritis; I. Effect of ureteral ligation on the course of bacterial infection in the kidney of the rat. J. Exp. Med. **104:** 803, 1956.
3. Vivaldi, E., Cotran, R., Zangwill, D. P., and Kass, E. H.: Ascending infection as a mechanism in pathogenesis of experimental nonobstructive pyelonephritis. Proc. Soc. Exp. Biol. Med. **102:** 242, 1959.
4. Hasner, E.: Prostatic urinary infection. Acta Chir. Scand. Suppl. **285:** 1, 1962.
5. Williams, G. L., Davies, D. K. L., Evans, K. T., and

Williams, J. E.: Vesicoureteric reflux in patients with bacteriuria in pregnancy. Lancet **2:** 1202, 1968.

6. Govan, D. E., and Palmer, J. M.: Urinary tract infection in children—the influence of successful antireflux operations in morbidity from infection. Pediatrics **44:** 677, 1969.
7. Winberg, J., Larson, H., and Bergström, T.: Comparison of the natural history of urinary infection in children with and without vesico-ureteric reflux. In P. Kincaid-Smith and K. F. Fairley (Eds.), Renal Infection and Renal Scarring, Mercedes Publishing Services, 1970, p. 293.
8. Lindberg, U., Bjure, J., Haugstvedt, S., and Jodal, U.: Asymptomatic bacteriuria in schoolgirls; III. Relation between residual urine volume and recurrence. Acta Paediatr. Scand. **64:** 437, 1975.
9. Shand, D. G., Nimmon, C. C., O'Grady, F., and Cattell, W. R.: Relation between residual urine volume and response to treatment of urinary infection. Lancet **1:** 1305, 1970.
10. Stamey, T. A.: Endoscopic suspension of the vesical neck for urinary incontinence. Surg. Gynecol. Obstet. **136:** 547, 1973.
11. Stephens, F. D.: Congential Malformations of the Rectum, Anus and Genitourinary Tracts. Edinburgh, E. & S. Liningstone, 1963, pp. 145, 224.
12. Schulman, C. C.: The single ectopic ureter. Eur. Urol. **2:** 64, 1976.
13. Ellerker, A. G.: The extravesical ectopic ureter. Br. J. Surg. **45:** 344, 1958.
14. Huffman, J. W.: The detailed anatomy of the paraurethral ducts in the adult human female. Am. J. Obstet. Gynecol. **55:** 86, 1948.
15. Andersen, M. J. F.: The incidence of diverticula in the female urethra. J. Urol. **98:** 96, 1967.
16. Davis, H. J., and TeLinde, R. W.: Urethral diverticulum: an assay of 121 cases. J. Urol. **80:** 34, 1958.
17. Schaeffer, A. J., and Stamey, T. A.: The effect of hysterectomy on colonization of the vaginal vestibule with Escherichia coli. Invest. Urol. **14:** 10, 1976.
18. Stamey, T. A., Condy, M., and Mihara, G.: Prophylactic efficacy of nitrofurantoin macrocrystals and trimethoprim-sulfamethoxazole in urinary infections. N. Engl. J. Med. **296:** 780, 1977.
19. Huland, H., Lewin, K., and Stamey, T. A.: Unilateral sponge kidney. Urology **8:** 373, 1976.
20. Lenarduzzi, G.: Reperto pielografico poco commune: dilatazione delle vie urinarie intrarenali. Radiol. Med. **26:** 346, 1939.
21. Mayall, G. F.: The incidence of medullary sponge kidney. Clin. Radiol. **21:** 171, 1970.
22. Palubinskas, A. J.: Medullary sponge kidney, Radiology **76:** 911, 1961.
23. Ekstroëm, T., Engfeldt, B., Lagergren, C., and Lindvall, N.: Medullary Sponge Kidney, Stockholm, Almquist and Wiksell, 1959.
24. Abeshouse, B. J., and Abeshouse, G. A.: Sponge kidney: A Review of the literature and a report of five cases. J. Urol. **84:** 252, 1960.
25. Igawa, K.-I., and Miyagishi, T.: Unilateral medullary sponge kidney: report of a case with some observations on urine osmotic pressure. J. Urol. **112:** 556, 1974.
26. Mulvaney, W. P., and Collins, W. T.: Cystic disease of the renal pyramids, J. Urol. **75:** 776, 1956.
27. Lindvall, N.: Roentgenologic diagnosis of medullary sponge kidney, Acta Radiol. **51:** 193, 1959.
28. Morris, R. C., Yamauchi, H., Palubinskas, A. J., and Howenstine, J.: Medullary sponge kidney, Am. J. Med. **38:** 883, 1965.
29. Powell, R. E.: An unusual congenital deformity of the kidney, Can. Med. Assoc. J. **60:** 48, 1949.
30. Harrison, A. R., and Williams, J. P.: Medullary sponge kidney and congenital hemihypertrophy, Br. J. Urol. **43:** 552, 1971.
31. Lalli, A. F.: Medullary sponge kidney disease, Radiology **92:** 92, 1969.
32. Ram, M. D., and Chisholm, G. D.: Cystic disease of renal pyramids (medullary sponge kidney). Br. J. Urol. **41:** 280, 1969.
33. Williams, G., Blandy, J. P., and Tresidder, G. C.: Communicating cysts and diverticula of the renal pelvis. Br. J. Urol. **41:** 163, 1969.
34. Govan, D. E., Butler, E. D., and Engelsgjerd, G. L.: Pathogenesis of urinary tract infections in patients with neurogenic bladder dysfunction. Urol. Digest **7:** 16, 1968.
35. Kunin, C. M., Deutscher, R., and Paquin, A. J.: Urinary tract infection in school children: An epidemiologic, clinical and laboratory study. Medicine **43:** 91, 1964.
36. Sussman, M., Asscher, A. W., Waters, W. E., Evans, J. A. S., Campbill, H., Evans, K. T., and Williams, J. E.: Asymptomatic significant bacteriuria in the nonpregnant woman; I. Description of a population. Br. Med. J. **1:** 799, 1969.
37. Jacobson, S. A., and Bors, E.: Spinal cord injury in Vietnamese combat. Paraplegia **7:** 263, 1970.
38. Mihaldzic, N., Leal, J. F., and Brewer, R. D., Jr.: Incidence of vesicoureteral reflux in paraplegia as related to the level of injury and the type of urinary drainage. Proc. Ann. Clin. Spinal Cord Inj. Conf. **15:** 136, 1966.
39. Stovall, C. W., Mihaldzic, N., and Lloyd, F. A.: Incidence of renal bacteriuria in the presence of long standing bladder infections. Proc. Ann. Clin. Spinal Cord Inj. Conf. **16:** 172, 1967.
40. Stamey, T. A., Govan, D. E., and Palmer, J. M.: The localization and treatment of urinary tract infections: The role of bactericidal urine levels as opposed to serum levels. Medicine **44:** 1, 1965.

41. Guttmann, L.: Statistical survey on one thousand paraplegics and initial treatment of traumatic paraplegia. Proc. Roy. Soc. Med. **47:** 1099, 1954.
42. Guttmann, L., and Frankel, H.: The value of intermittent catheterization in the early management of traumatic paraplegia and tetraplegia. Paraplegia **4:** 63, 1966.
43. Bors, E.: Intermittent catheterization in paraplegic patients. Proc. Ann. Clin. Spinal Cord Inj. Conf. **15:** 127, 1966.
44. Pearman, J. W.: Prevention of urinary tract infection following spinal cord injury. Paraplegia **9:** 95, 1971.
45. Rhame, F. S., and Perkash, I.: Urinary tract infections occurring in recent spinal cord injury patients on intermittent catheterization. J. Urol. **122:** 669, 1979.
46. Pearman, J. W.: The catheter team: an essential service for rehabilitating neurogenic bladders. Aust. N. Z. J. Surg. **47:** 339, 1977.
47. Pearman, J. W.: The value of kanamycin-colistin bladder instillations in reducing bacteriuria during intermittent catheterization of patients with acute spinal cord injury. Br. J. Urol., **51:** 367, 1979.
48. Pearman, J. W.: Urological follow-up of 99 spinal cord injured patients initially managed by intermittent catheterization. Br. J. Urol. **48:** 297, 1976.
49. Price, M., Kottke, F. J., and Olson, M. E.: Renal function in patients with spinal cord injury; the eighth year of a ten-year continuing study. Arch. Phys. Med. Rehabil. **56:** 76, 1975.
50. Marosszeky, J. E., Farnsworth, R. H., and Jones, R. F.: The indwelling urethral catheter in patients with acute spinal cord trauma. Med. J. Aust. **2:** 62, 1973.
51. Lapides, J. and Costello, R. T., Jr.: Uninhibited neurogenic bladder: a common cause for recurrent urinary infection in normal women. J. Urol. **101:** 539, 1969.
52. Walter, S., Andersen, J. T., Hebjørn, S., and Vejlsgaard, R.: Detrusor hyperreflexia and bacteriuria. Urol. Int. **32:** 117, 1977.
53. Cumming, R. E., and Jarre, H. A.: Roentgen symptomatology of infected urinary passages in combination with a classification of urinary tract infections. J. Urol. **28:** 455, 1932.
54. Rhoads, P. S., and Billings, C. E.: Antibacterial management of urinary tract infections. J. Am. Med. Assoc. **148:** 165, 1952.
55. Garrod, L. P., Shooter, R. A., and Curwen, M. P.: The results of chemotherapy in urinary infections. Br. Med. J. **2:** 1003, 1954.

CHAPTER 10

General and Specific Principles of Therapy

I presented in Chapter 1 our classification of urinary tract infections which has substantial therapeutic implications, and which the reader may wish to review. Of the four categories—first infections, unresolved bacteriuria, bacterial persistence, and bacterial reinfections—I pointed out that understanding the causes of unresolved bacteriuria may be the most important aspect of the classification. Unless the bacteriuria is resolved, there can be no cure of the urinary infection.

IMPORTANCE OF INITIAL STERILIZATION OF URINE

Successful antimicrobial cure of a urinary tract infection is always accompanied by sterilization of the urine within a few hours of beginning therapy.[1] For example, in Figure 10.1 we plotted the bacterial counts in successive urine cultures from two patients following the start of oral nalidixic acid therapy. Usually within 6–9 hours, and nearly always by 24 hours, the urine is sterile if treatment is going to be successful. This principle has at least two practical implications. First, if the physician performs his own urine cultures in the office in an inexpensive way (Chapter 1),[2] better medicine is practiced, at less expense to the patient, if a culture is repeated 48–72 hours after starting therapy than if a useless antimicrobial agent is continued for 10 days in the face of ineffective therapy. Unfortunately, the patient's symptomatic response is a poor criterion of successful therapy; alleviation of symptoms commonly occurs with minimal suppression of bacteriuria. Second, rapid sterilization of the urine following oral antimicrobial therapy explains the occasional dilemma of the physician who admits a patient to the hospital with an overt urinary infection only to find the urine culture sterile. The mistake of ordering both a urine culture and antimicrobial therapy simultaneously in the nurse's order book is apparent: the patient receives the

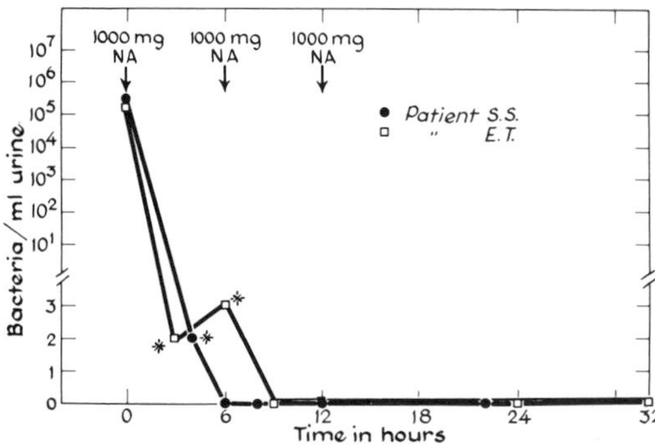

Figure 10.1 Urine cultures, performed at about 3, 6, 9, 12, 24, and 32 hours after beginning nalidixic acid (NA), 1000 mg every 6 hours, in two patients with *Escherichia coli* urinary infections. The cultures at 3, 4, and 6 hours (*) were actually sterile by the standard method of streaking 0.1 ml of urine on appropriate agar. When 5 ml of urine were Millipore-filtered and washed with 20 ml of saline solution and the filter disc was cultured, 2–3 *E. coli*/ml of urine were recovered in these three specimens. All later cultures were sterile by both methods. The minimal inhibitory concentration of NA for these *E. coli* was 25 μg/ml, as determined by both tube dilution and quantitative disc (Chapter 2) studies.

medication, cannot void, and the urine culture is obtained 3 or 4 hours after the start of therapy.

Urine cultures obtained during therapy must not contain any—not even one organism—of the original bacterial strain; that is, treatment is inadequate, and the bacteriuria will recur, if the colony count is reduced from 10^8 bacteria/ml to 10^2/ml. If any number of the original infecting bacteria are present in the midstream voided urine during therapy, there is no way to be certain that initial sterilization of the urine has occurred. Even when our technique of culturing the introital bacteria demonstrates a bacterial count several logs higher than in the midstream specimen, it is impossible to be absolutely certain that a sterile bladder urine has been obtained during therapy. We have repeatedly demonstrated suppression of a pretreatment bacteriuria of 10^8 bacteria/ml to less than 10^3 organisms/ml on suprapubic needle aspiration of the bladder at the height of antimicrobial therapy only to have immediate regrowth of the infecting strain to 10^8 bacteria/ml upon discontinuing therapy. For this reason, and despite the possibility of introital persistence and contamination of the midstream urine specimen, a careful clinician will demand that none of the original infecting organisms be present in the midstream urine during therapy. Alternatively, a sterile bladder urine, in the presence of introital persistence, can be confirmed by suprapubic needle aspiration. This principle is the cardinal basis for successful antimicrobial therapy because without initial sterilization of the urine there can be no successful therapy and therefore no further consideration as to whether the basic problem is one of bacterial persistence or reinfection at the next recurrence.

A high correlation exists between immediate urinary sterilization and *in vitro* antibiotic sensitivities.[1] The reason infections with bacteria which are resistant *in vitro* are often cured with an antimicrobial agent thought to be ineffective from sensitivity studies is due to the low antibiotic content of some discs. Many discs, like penicillin-G and tetracycline, reflect the concentrations of drug that can be obtained in the serum, not in the urine. A real need exists for a second set of antibiotic discs, for urinary infections only, that will represent more closely the minimal urinary concentration.[1, 3]

The reason that 80–88% of uncomplicated infections,[4] including bacteriuria of pregnancy,[5] respond to almost any form of antimicrobial therapy—sulfonamides, nitrofurantoins, antibiotics—is precisely because the infecting bacteria are sensitive at urinary concentrations to the drug on *in vitro* studies. We have commented previously on the almost uniform correlation between *in vitro* tube dilution sensitivity studies and *in vivo* results.[1, 3]

When bacteria are added *in vitro* to soy broth (or urine) containing antimicrobial agents, placed in the incubator at 37°C and subcultured, they are rapidly killed, depending upon the organism, the antimicrobial agent, and the concentration of the antimicrobial drug. For example, with

Escherichia coli and polymyxin-B sulfate, the rate of cell death is extremely rapid (Figure 10.2). Using an inoculum of 10^6 bacteria/ml, all of the organisms were killed within 5 minutes at concentrations of polymyxin-B sulfate between 50 and 500 μg/ml; at 10 μg/ml a period of 30 minutes to 2 hours was required to kill the *E. coli*. Hence, both *in vivo* (Figure 10.1) and *in vitro* (Figure 10.2) rates of cell death are rapid, especially at concentrations achieved in the urine.

Despite these correlations between what happens in the test tube and what occurs in the urinary tract, the clinician must remember this cardinal principle of therapy: *without initial sterilization of the urine, there can be no successful therapy*. Because introital persistence of the organism responsible for the bacteriuria can confuse the interpretation of the midstream urine culture obtained during antimicrobial therapy, suprapubic needle aspiration (SPA) of the urine (described in detail in Chapter 1) is sometimes necessary to decide if a sterile urine has been achieved. The disadvantage of catheterizing the bladder to determine the presence of a sterile urine during therapy is obvious: not only are introital bacteria likely to be introduced, but, as shown in Chapter 4, they may be resistant to the antimicrobial agent in the urine.

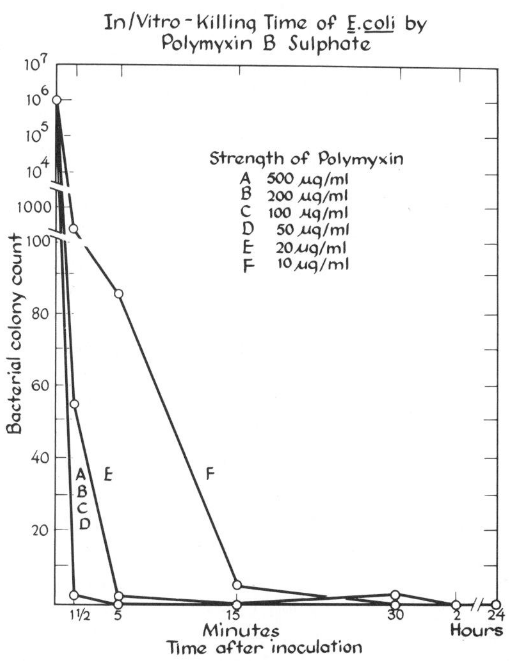

Figure 10.2 In vitro-killing time of *Escherichia coli* by polymyxin B sulfate. *E. coli*, 10^6/ml, were added to decreasing concentrations of polymyxin-B sulfate in soy broth, incubated at 37°C, and subcultured on surface agar at frequent intervals. Cell death was extremely rapid.

DURATION OF THERAPY

Once initial sterilization of the urine is achieved, we treat all patients when first seen—virtually regardless of how many recurrences they have had—for 5–10 days and no longer. There are at least three reasons for this. First, it is a rare referral when the consulting physician can be absolutely certain that a sterile urine was achieved at the time of previous antimicrobial efforts. Failure to culture the urine during therapy, or within a few days of completing therapy, does not allow assessment of the first basic question: Has the urine ever been sterilized? The second reason for limiting initial therapy to 5–10 days is the natural tendency of urinary infections, once a sterile urine is obtained, to undergo long term remissions. This tendency in adults is well documented in Chapter 4 (Figure 4.2) in women,[6] and in Kunin's[7] (Figure 6.13) and Govan's[8] (Figure 6.18) data which suggest a 20% long-term remission with each 10-day course of therapy in children, almost regardless of the number of previous recurrences. Third, there are few data to indicate that full dosage therapy for longer than 5–10 days is any better than short-term therapy. For example, Kincaid-Smith and Fairley[9] found no difference between 2 weeks and 6 weeks of therapy and Kincaid-Smith, Friedman, and Nanra[10] showed no difference between 1 and 2 weeks of treatment; both studies involved substantial numbers of patients and their infections were proven by catheterization and many were localized by Fairley's bladder-washout technique. In symptomatic children, with and without reflux, there was no difference in cure rates between 10 days and 60 days of sulfonamide therapy.[11] Thus, antimicrobial therapy for longer than 5–10 days for the purpose of curing a specific infection seems unjustified. But what about periods of therapy shorter than 5 days?

SINGLE DOSE THERAPY

Although my preference continues to be 5–10 days of antimicrobial therapy for the type of infection I see in my practice, if the patient presents with acute lower tract symptoms, it appears that single-dose therapy is highly effective in curing urinary infections. In 1967, Grüneberg and Brumfitt[12] treated 22 of 25 symptomatic patients successfully with "long-acting" sulfonamide and Williams and Smith[13] in 1970 treated 55 of 95 pregnant patients successfully with a single 2-g dose of a "long-acting" sulfonamide. Both of these efforts were based on the prolonged duration (serum half-life of 150 hours) of these sulfonamides in the serum and urine of the patient. Brumfitt *et al.*[14] cured only 44% of ambulatory bacteriuric women with a single 2-g dose of cephaloridine.

The recent era of single-dose, short-acting antimicrobial therapy for urinary infections was ushered in by Ronald and his associates[15] at Winnipeg, Canada when they treated 100 bacteriuric women with a single 500-mg dose of kanamycin intramuscularly. All patients had a Fairley bladder-washout localization of their bacteriuria (see Chapter 1) before treatment. Thirty-six of 39 infections confined to the bladder were cured (92%) compared to only 18 of the 65 patients with upper tract localization (28%). Since the patients were not cultured until 7 days after the single dose of kanamycin, we do not know whether the 28% of renal infections in patients who were cured were the only ones who achieved a sterile urine following therapy, similar to that observed in Figure 10.1. This paper clearly established that single-dose, short-acting therapy was adequate for infections limited to the bladder, that 28% of renal infections could be cured by a single dose, and that those whose bacteriuria was still present at 1 week (perhaps unresolved from the start) had a high probability of representing upper tract infections.

Fang, Tolkoff-Rubin, and Rubin[16] divided 61 bacteriuric women into those with and without antibody-coated bacteria (FA+ or FA−). Of 43 patients with FA− bacteria, 22 were cured with a single 3-g dose of amoxicillin and 21 were cured by 10 days of amoxicillin, 250 mg four times a day. Of 18 patients with FA+ bacteria, 9 recurred within 1 week of completing 10 days of amoxicillin therapy. Six of these 9 patients were then cured by 14–21 days of either ampicillin or sulfisoxazole; the three who recurred again within 1 week of completing therapy surprisingly had normal intravenous urograms. As in Ronald's study,[15] we do not know whether the urine was sterilized during therapy in these subjects who had bacterial persistence during treatment; thus, it is possible they represent instances of unresolved bacteriuria rather than "relapse."

Bailey and Abbott have reported 75–80% cures with single doses of amoxicillin (3 g)[17] and trimethoprim-sulfamethoxazole TMP-SMX (480 mg of TMP and 2400 mg of SMX)[18]; conventional dosage therapy with both drugs was no better than single dosage.

Ludwig *et al.*[19] have presented a prospective study on 83 unselected consecutive women with acute lower urinary tract symptoms who were randomized to four different single-dose regimens. All regimens were effective and there was no statistical difference between sulfisoxazole in 1- or 2-g doses or TMP-SMX in a dose of 160/800 mg or 320/1600 mg of TMP and SMX, respectively. The 160/800-mg dose of TMP-SMX (the "double-strength" tablet) is one-third the dose used by Bailey.[18] Not only does this study suggest that mega-doses appear unnecessary in single dosage therapy, but of 10 patients in their series who were FA+ on antibody-coated studies, only 2 recurred after single-dose treatment. They concluded that single-dose therapy with a number of regimens was effective in adult women with cystitis regardless of the antibody-coated bacterial status of their infection.

The therapeutic implications of these single-dose studies are obvious, and we all should treat for shorter periods of time, but what do they mean in terms of pathogenesis of urinary infections? First, it must be remembered that these studies are in women with acute urinary tract infections and for the most part limited to the lower urinary tract. We must not forget Mabeck's[20] studies which showed that 80% of such women achieve sterile urine with placebo therapy within 5 months, and that 71% are sterile within 1 month; it is not known how many are sterile within 1 week, but it is surely substantial. In this setting, it is not surprising that the addition of a single dosage of antimicrobial therapy cures 80% of the patients. Moreover, the clinician should not underestimate the considerable duration of antimicrobial inhibitory levels in the urine that follows single-dosage therapy, especially when that dosage is in grams rather than in milligrams or if the drug has a long half-life in the serum such as TMP-SMX. Without doubt, many of these urines, if not most, will be inhibitory on the 3rd day after single-dose therapy.

Second, these surprising results of therapeutic efficacy—in both upper and lower tract infections—with single-dosage therapy should just about bury the concept once and for all that serum levels rather than urinary concentrations are important in the cure of most urinary tract infections. It should no longer be surprising that 10 days of oral penicillin-G therapy or nitrofurantoin cured upper tract infections in our 1965 report.[1]

Third, antimicrobial agents differ markedly in their pharmacologic and microbiologic activities even when chosen on the basis of sensitivity testing. If one selects an antimicrobial agent that is less potent in its rate of bactericidal activity (sulfonamides, for example) or its pharmacologic penetration (ampicillin, for example), then it is absolutely certain that those patients who also have bacteria in their upper tracts will not be cured at the same rate as those whose bacteriuria is confined to the bladder. For one thing, among others, the transient time of the antimicrobial agent is many times shorter in the upper tract than in the bladder. If one wants to separate upper from lower tract infections on the basis of therapeutic efforts, methenamine should be the ideal drug because, as will be reviewed later in this chapter, it can only act in the bladder urine—and not in renal urine. Thus, there will be all gradations of effectiveness when therapy—either single dosage or conventional dosage—is prescribed with the knowledge of whether upper or lower tract infection is present at the institution of therapy. For example, would the nine patients in the excellent study by Fang *et al.*[16] who recurred with the same organism after 10 days of amoxicillin therapy or the the three who recurred after 2–3 weeks of sulfisoxazole or ampicillin therapy, have also recurred after 5–10 days of TMP-SMX therapy? I seriously doubt it in view of the patient's normal intravenous urograms, but if they would have recurred, the time had clearly come to look for the causes of bacterial persistence I discussed in Chapter 9.

The clinician should not lose sight of the need to persist with a more potent antimicrobial agent if the bacteria recur from the upper urinary tract following 5–10 days of therapy. I do not personally believe that longer-term therapy is the answer for bacterial persistence in the absence of the urologic abnormalities presented in Chapter 9. The answer is a different antimicrobial agent for a conventional, short period of therapy. Two examples are presented in the following section to document the importance of this practice.

Importance of Repeating Therapy With a Better Antimicrobial Agent in Women With Renal Infections Whose Infecting Organism Recurs Immediately After Successful Sterilization of Urine

Bacterial persistence in adult men, as demonstrated in Chapter 7, is not prevented by a progressive increase in the intensity of antimicrobial therapy because few of the clinically useful drugs diffuse into prostatic fluid. Nor can recurrences be prevented in women, regardless of the potency of the chemotherapeutic agent, when persistence is due to infection stones (Chapter 8) or the other 13 causes discussed in Chapter 9. But in the absence of these causes of bacterial persistence and renal failure, and despite the presence of major renal scars, we have cured a number of adult women with upper tract infections by following their recurrence with a similar short term course of a different antimicrobial agent. Without question, the only decision separating many of these women from a lifetime of chronic bacteriuria and one free of infection is a 5–10 day course of a single chemotherapeutic agent.

A particularly instructive patient with severe scarring from pyelonephritis is B.E., a 41-year-old, white mother of two children who was admitted to the Stanford University Hospital in June 1966, for a chronic *Enterobacter* infection. Fortunately, complete records from other hospitals were available from the beginning of her urologic history. A hysterectomy had been performed in 1950. She was first seen by a urologist in 1952, at the age of 27, for a recent history of urinary infections. After extracting cystoscopically a low lying, right ureteral calculus, he removed from the left renal pelvis a calcium phosphate stone that contained a "trace of carbonate and oxalate." Bilateral retrograde urograms were thought to be normal in December 1952, after the pyelolithotomy. *Enterobacter* was cultured postoperatively and failed to clear on oxytetracycline, methenamine mandelate, nitrofurantoin, and various sulfonamides.

Despite a chronic infection, her next acute symptomatic episode was not until 1961 and was due to a small, right ureteral calculus that was spontaneously passed. An intravenous urogram showed bilateral calyceal blunting diagnostic of bilateral pyelonephritis. There was no residual urine, and a cystogram showed no reflux. Because of persistent infection in the face of cycloserine, nitrofurantoin, demethylchlortetracycline, and chloramphenicol therapy, she was referred in December 1962, to the University of California—San Francisco Medical Center. Again, no residual urine or reflux was found. Bilateral ureteral catheterization recovered > 100,000 *Enterobacter* from both kidneys. Her serum creatinine was 1.4 mg/100 ml. She was thought to have incurable, bilateral pyelonephritis and was discharged on chronic sulfonamide therapy. Upon return to her referring urologist, he tried ampicillin and nalidixic acid without clearing the bacteriuria.

Upon admission to Stanford in June 1966, her serum creatinine was 1.5 mg/100 ml, and three consecutive 2-hour creatinine clearances were 78, 103, and 92 ml/minute. Urinalysis showed 1+ protein, several granular and cellular casts, bacteria, and numerous white blood cells (WBCs) with clumps. Urine culture from a suprapubic needle aspiration grew > 100,000 *Enterobacter* (Table 10.1). Tube dilution studies showed that nitrofurantoin was bactericidal in 24 hours at a concentration of 50 μg/ml, nalidixic acid at 50 μg/ml, and polymyxin-B sulfate at 0.5 μg/ml.

Plain film tomograms showed no calcifications, a voiding cystourethrogram demonstrated neither reflux nor residual urine, and an intravenous urogram (Figure 10.3) was characteristic of severe pyelonephritis. In fact, the calyceal distortion was so irregular that a mass lesion was suggested in the left kidney, and an arteriogram was performed to exclude a tumor (these studies are reproduced earlier in Chapter 1, Figure 1.22, *A* and *B*, as classic radiologic evidence of pyelonephritis).

Ureteral catheterization studies on 6/15/66 again proved bilateral involvement with *Enterobacter* (Table 10.1). Immediately after these studies, she was begun on nalidixic acid, which only suppressed the infection. Note, however, that the 650 *Enterobacter*/ml of voided urine indicates the bacteriuria was unresolved; I am concerned that therapeutic trials like those just reviewed[15, 16] where the first culture is 1 week after therapy would classify this therapeutic effort as a "relapse." Is is not because the urine was never sterilized, *i.e.*, the bacteriuria was never resolved. You cannot classify an infection as a relapse unless you know the urine was sterilized during therapy—which means there must be *no* bacteria present in the midstream urine. Coly-Mycin (colistin methane sulfonate) was then started with an initial dose of 150 mg followed by 75 mg every 12 hours for 10 days; the minimal inhibitory concentration was 1.0 μg/ml. Her serum creatinine remained 1.4 mg/100 ml; multiple blood pressures were in the range of 120/80 mm Hg, although her out-patient and admission pressures were 160/100. Although Coly-Mycin sterilized the urine, by the 9th day after therapy she had recurred with the *Enterobacter*. She was readmitted to the hospital and started on 50 mg of intravenous polymyxin-B sulfate every 8 hours, each 50 mg injected within a 1-hour period of infusion. Her urine, however, remained infected with *Enterobacter* on the 1st, 3rd, and 4th days of therapy; repeat tube dilutions showed resistance to polymyxin-B sulfate and Coly-Mycin (even at 20 μg/ml), suggesting that her unresolved bacteriuria was due to development of a resistant strain. Kanamycin tube dilution studies showed that 1.25 μg/ml was bacteriostatic and 2.5 μg/ml bactericidal. Accordingly, 1.0 g of kanamycin was given intramuscularly every 12 hours for two doses and then 0.5 g every 8 hours. Her urine was sterile within 24 hours and remained so on the 5th day of therapy. On 8/9/66, 17 days after completing a 10-day course of kanamycin therapy, and in the absence of sexual intercourse during the interim, voided urine cultures contained only a few colonies of introital *Staphylococcus epidermidis* and α-Streptococcus. Urinalysis indicated a pH of 5.5, no bacilli or WBCs in the sediment, but 50 mg% protein. During the 1 year of close follow-up, bacteriuria did not recur; indeed, even the introitus remained free of pathogenic bacteria (Table 10.1). It is clear that the 10-day course of kanamycin cleared her bacteriuria, which had been present for 14 years. Her blood pressure on 4/18/67 was 170/90 mm Hg, and proteinuria continued to be present at the level of 50–75 mg%. When seen in our outpatient unit on 7/18/67, her blood pressure was 150/90 mm Hg and only 5 mg% of protein was in the urine.

When examined 4 years later on 7/29/71, she had been in perfect health without the slightest urinary symptom in the intervening years. Sexual intercourse had occurred about twice a week. Although 46 years old, she had no menopausal symptoms. Her initial blood pressure was 180/95 mm Hg, falling to 160/90 mm Hg during the 30-minute interview. The serum creatinine was 1.2 mg/100 ml. Urinalysis showed a pH of 5.5, less than 20 mg% protein, and the centrifuged microscopic sediment contained only an occasional squamous epithelial cell. Her cultures showed that the bladder urine was sterile; there were no Gram-negative bacteria on the introitus. Since multiple serum creatinines in 1966 were always 1.4–1.5 mg/100 ml, it is reasonable to believe that progressive azotemia in this patient was reversed by cure of her chronic renal bacteriuria. It is equally important to realize that the severe scarring, irregular calyces, and cortical distortion seen in Figures 1.22 and 10.3 do *not* represent incurable, chronic pyelonephritis. It is unfortunate that I could not locate her for a further follow-up in 1979.

A second, equally instructive, case whose bacterial persistence in the renal urine occurred in the absence of calyceal or cortical scarring—and therefore is more comparable to the three cases of "relapse" reported by Fang *et al.*[16]—is that of C.B., a 39-year-old mother of three children who was first seen at Stanford University Hospital in April 1966. Except for some minor symptoms of vaginitis (pruritus) and a peculiar cerebral sensation of "trickling or wetness" on the right side of her head, she was asymptomatic and had never experienced any urinary symptoms whatsoever. A general examination in the Medical Clinic at Stanford uncovered a bacteriuria due to *Klebsiella* (Table 10.2). Tube dilution sensitivities showed bactericidal activity at urinary levels (Chapter 2) for virtually all antimicrobial agents except nitrofurantoin. Attention was devoted to clearing the *Klebsiella* bacteriuria. Accordingly, 30 days of oral penicillin-G at 500 mg every 6 hours, 11 days of nalidixic acid at 500 mg every 6 hours, and 5 days of ampicillin at 250 mg every 6 hours served only to suppress her

Table 10.1
B.E., a 41-year-old, White Woman with a 14-year History of Documented Bacteriuria due to Enterobacter

Date	Days on (+) or off (−) Therapy	Vaginal Vestibule		Urethral (VB$_1$)[a]		Midstream (VB$_2$)	
		bacteria/ml		*bacteria/ml*		*bacteria/ml*	
6/12/66	>30 off					SPA:	
						Enterobacter	>100,000
6/14/66	>32 off	Midvaginal					
		Enterobacter	<1,000	*Enterobacter*	>100,000	*Enterobacter*	>100,000
		α-Streptococcus	<100			CB:	
		Staphylococcus epidermidis	<100			*Enterobacter*	>100,000
		Diphtheroids	>100,000				
6/15/66	>33 off			CB = *Enterobacter*	>100,000		
				WB = *Enterobacter*	> 8,000		
				LK$_1$ *Enterobacter*	>100,000	RK$_1$ *Enterobacter*	>100,000
				LK$_2$ *Enterobacter*	>100,000	RK$_2$ *Enterobacter*	>100,000
				LK$_3$ *Enterobacter*	>100,000	RK$_3$ *Enterobacter*	>100,000
6/16/66	+1 nalidixic acid 500 mg q 6 hr					CB: *Enterobacter*	>10,000
6/17/66	+2 nalidixic acid 500 mg q 6 hr					CB: *Enterobacter*	650
6/20/66	+2 Coly-Mycin 75 mg q 12 hr	Enterococci	10,000	Enterococci	250		0
				S. epidermidis	50		
6/21/66	+3 Coly-Mycin 75 mg q 12 hr	Enterococci	<100				0
		α-Streptococcus	1,000	α-Streptococcus	1,000		
6/24/66	+6 Coly-Mycin 75 mg q 12 hr	Enterococci	<1,000				
		α-Streptococcus	10,000	α-Streptococcus	4,000	α-Streptococcus	180
		S. epidermidis	<1,000				
		Diphtheroids	<1,000				
6/27/66	+9 Coly-Mycin 75 mg q 12 hr					CB	0
6/28/66	+10 Coly-Mycin 75 mg q 12 hr	*S. epidermidis*, Diphtheroids }	>100,000	*S. epidermidis*, Diphtheroids }	9,000	*S. epidermidis*	10
7/7/66	−9 Coly Mycin 75 mg q 12 hr					SPA: *Enterobacter*	>100,000
7/10/66	+1 polymyxin 50 mg q 8 hr					SPA: *Enterobacter*	>100,000
7/12/66	+3 polymyxin 50 mg q 8 hr	*Enterobacter*	<1,000	*Enterobacter*	>100,000	*Enterobacter*	>100,000
		Enterococci	<1,000				
		S. epidermidis	10,000				

7/13/66	+4 polymyxin	*S. epidermidis*	9,000	*Enterobacter*	>100,000	*Enterobacter*	>100,000
	50 mg q 8 hr	Diphtheroids					
7/14/66	+1 kanamycin	Diphtheroids	10,000		0		0
	1.0 gm q 12 hr						
7/15/66	+2 kanamycin		0		0		0
	0.5 gm q 8 hr						
7/18/66	+5 kanamycin	Diphtheroids	>100,000		0		0
	0.5 gm q 8 hr						
8/9/66	−17 kanamycin	*S. epidermidis*	6,000	*S. epidermidis*	50	*S. epidermidis*	20
	0.5 gm q 8 hr	α-Streptococcus	3,000	α-Streptococcus	30		
8/30/66	−38 kanamycin	*E. coli*	40	*S. epidermidis*	600		0
		S. epidermidis	<1,000				
		α-Streptococcus	<1,000				
		Diphtheroids	10,000				
9/30/66	−68 kanamycin	*S. epidermidis*	10,000	*S. epidermidis*	9,000		
		Enterococci	<1,000	Enterococci	<1,000	Enterococci	90
11/1/66	−99 kanamycin	*S. epidermidis*	400	*S. epidermidis*	80		0
		Streptococcus	<100				
1/24/67	−183 kanamycin	*S. epidermidis*	2,000	*S. epidermidis*	600	*S. epidermidis*	420
4/18/67	−267 kanamycin	*S. epidermidis*	1,000	*S. epidermidis*	800	*S. epidermidis*	600
7/18/67	−358 kanamycin	Diphtheroids	10,000	*S. epidermidis*	310	*S. epidermidis*	50
		S. epidermidis	<1,000				
7/29/71	−5 years	Yeasts	10,000	β-Streptococci	10,000	β-Streptococci	80
		S. epidermidis	1,000	*S. epidermidis*	500		
		β-Streptococci	200	Yeasts	460		
		Enterococci	60				

[a] VB = voided bladder urine (VB_1 = urethral, VB_2 = midstream). CB = catheterized bladder urine, or in the presence of a Foley catheter CB represents urine aspirated from the Foley. WB = culture of residual irrigation fluid after washing bladder with several liters of sterile irrigating fluid. RK = right kidney. RK_1, RK_2, etc. = serial cultures from RK. LK = left kidney. LK_1, LK_2, etc. = serial cultures from LK. SPA = suprapubic needle aspiration of bladder. Solid transverse line divides longitudinal cultures into major periods of significance.

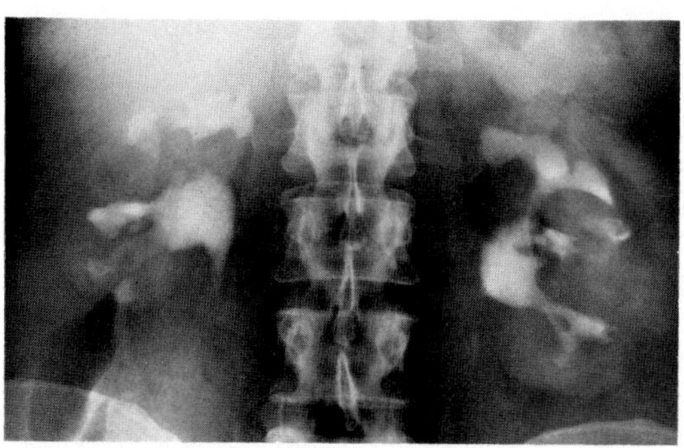

Figure 10.3 A 10-minute intravenous urogram (June 1966) from B.E., a 41-year-old Caucasian woman with a continuous history of *Enterobacter* bacteriuria since 1952. Further views of the left kidney are presented in Chapter 1 (Figure 1.22*A*) as well as a selective arteriogram in Figure 1.22*B*.

bacteriuria to about 1000 *Klebsiella*/ml (Table 10.2); after completing 11 days of nalidixic acid, she ran out of medicine and switched herself back to penicillin-G (5/6/66, Table 10.2). Note that the 900 colonies/ml of *Klebsiella* in the urethral and midstream specimens on 5/6/66, in the absence of introital *Klebsiella*, correctly indicated the presence of a low count bacteriuria, confirmed by SPA (1000 *Klebsiella*/ml). After each course of penicillin-G, nalidixic acid, and ampicillin, respectively, repeat tube dilution sensitivities showed the development of resistance to each one of these drugs in succession, thereby accounting for bacterial persistence in the presence of an originally sensitive organism.

A serum creatinine was 0.8 mg/100 ml. An intravenous urogram (Figure 10.4) on 6/1/66 showed delicate calyces, normal renal outlines, and no postvoiding residual urine. Cystoscopy on 6/21/66 was unremarkable except for a few inflammatory "polyps" in the proximal urethra at the vesical neck. Ureteral catheterization studies demonstrated that the *Klebsiella* was coming from the right kidney (6/21/66, Table 10.2). Polymyxin-B sulfate was bactericidal at 1.25 μg/ml, so she was given Coly-Mycin (polymyxin-E) 150 mg each day for 4 days as an out-patient. Four days after the last dose she was still infected with *Klebsiella*.

She was admitted to Stanford University Hospital on 10/2/66 and given 75 mg of Coly-Mycin every 12 hours for 9 days. Daily cultures showed sterilization by the 3rd day, but by the 9th day the *Klebsiella* was growing again in the urine (Table 10.2) and was resistant to 20 μg/ml of Coly-Mycin. Interestingly, cultures on the 3rd and 8th days of therapy suggested the urethra as the site of persistence. Realizing that the right kidney was infected, we performed plain film tomograms without finding any evidence of calcification. Even the intravenous urogram was repeated, paying close attention to the right kidney, but there was no evidence of calyceal distortion or scarring.

Kanamycin, in tube dilutions, was bacteriostatic at 5 μg/ml. Between 1/5/67 and 1/15/67, she received as an out-patient 0.5 g of kanamycin intramuscularly twice a day. All subsequent cultures have been sterile, including a follow-up of 7/22/71 (Table 10.2). She has remained well, and all introital cultures have been normal. Her serum creatinine on 7/22/71 was 0.7 mg/100 ml. These studies show that rapid resistance developed to penicillin-G, nalidixic acid, ampicillin, and Coly-Mycin, but not to kanamycin. The last antibiotic resulted in a permanent cure. Telephone conversation with her in August 1979, indicated that she had been well in the past 8 years without any urinary tract infections or symptoms.

The bacteriologic course of L.V. with *Proteus mirabilis* struvite stones and medullary sponge kidneys, presented in Table 8.7 (Chapter 8), also demonstrates the critical importance of repeating therapy with a different antibacterial drug in women with upper tract infection who recur immediately after therapy. Tetracycline for 4 days, streptomycin for 5 days, and sulfamethizole for 14 days all failed; 7 days of kanamycin resulted in a permanently sterile urine.

These three clinical examples should make it amply clear that in adult women with upper tract bacteriuria, who do not have the urologic abnormalities presented in Chapter 9 or azotemia, immediate recurrence of their bacteriuria means inadequate treatment and should always be followed by further therapeutic efforts.

Indications for Continuous Antimicrobial Therapy

There is no evidence, of which I am aware, that long-term antimicrobial therapy in the *continuing presence of bacteriuria*, so-called suppressive therapy, is beneficial either in terms of preventing further renal damage or even in preventing clinical episodes of pyelonephritis. Nor is it clear that continuous therapy in patients with indwelling catheters, for example, in paraplegic patients, is helpful. What is clear, however, is that continuous therapy in the presence of bacteriuria is accompanied by resistance of the bacteria to the antimicrobial agent; that these resistant bacteria are less virulent seems unlikely.

Long-term, or continuous antimicrobial therapy, then, is pointless in the presence of bacteriuria. The only justifiable use of continuous antimicrobial therapy is to maintain the presence of a sterile urine. Thus, even with prophylactic, long-term antimicrobial therapy, the importance of first obtaining a sterile urine cannot be overemphasized. Without a sterile urine, long-term therapy is doomed to failure before it starts. It should be emphasized, however, that the urine can be sterilized with TMP-SMX even in the presence of urinary tract obstruction and long-standing infection[21] or in the presence of chronic pyelonephritis, infection, and azotemia.[22]

There are, I believe, only two or possibly three indications for using continuous antimicrobial therapy after initially obtaining a sterile urine. They are (1) in patients with chronic bacterial prostatitis; (2) in females with frequent episodes of reinfection of the urinary tract; and, finally, (3) in patients with early infection stones in whom dissolution of the struvite stone may occur in the presence of a sterile, acid urine.

Chronic Bacterial Prostatitis

As discussed in Chapter 7, when TMP-SMX fails to cure chronic bacterial prostatitis—or possibly carbenicillin if the early data prove to be true—there is almost no alternative other than continuous, low dosage antimicrobial therapy. Such therapy is designed to maintain a bactericidal bladder urine in order to prevent symptomatic bladder and kidney infections from occurring when the prostatic bacteria inoculate the bladder urine. Continuous therapy is not designed to suppress bacterial growth in the prostate and thereby allow host defense mechanisms ultimately to kill the organisms, for this it apparently will not do. But by keeping the bladder urine bactericidal, the bacteria are limited to the prostatic fluid, where they do no apparent harm. Because these enteric bacteria virtually never change their antimicrobial sensitivity patterns, the choice of drug for long-term bladder prophylaxis is easy: the safest and least expensive drug that will maintain bactericidal urinary levels against the prostatic organism is a good choice. As seen in Chapter 7, nitrofurantoin and oral penicillin-G have been extremely useful for *E. coli*, and the tetracyclines are ideal for *Pseudomonas aeruginosa*. Any antibiotic that serves to sterilize the urine during a bladder or kidney infection will do admirably to maintain a bactericidal bladder urine; it usually can be administered at a substantially reduced dosage, such as one tablet in the morning and one in the evening. But since these bacteria are most often quite sensitive, the clinician should not prescribe an expensive drug for chronic therapy even if one was used during the acute urinary infection.

Since 1973, we have also used one-half tablet TMP-SMX (40 mg of TMP and 80 mg of SMX) successfully in these patients. Since the TMP does get into the prostate (see Chapter 7), there may be some merit to long-term suppression of prostatic bacteria as opposed to simply keeping the bladder urine bactericidal against the prostatic organism. Whether months or years of suppression with TMP-SMX will result in ultimate cure, remains to be seen.

Reinfections in Women

As emphasized in Chapter 4, the major problem in women and little girls is not recurrence from a persistent focus as occurs in infection stones (Chapter 8) or unilateral, atrophic pyelonephritis (Chapter 9), but rather reinfection of the bladder from En-

Table 10.2
C.B., a 39-year-old Caucasian Woman with Chronic *Klebsiella* Urinary Infection

Date	Days on (+) or off (−) Therapy	Vaginal Vestibule		Urethral (VB_1)[a]		Midstream (VB_2)	
		bacteria/ml		*bacteria/ml*		*bacteria/ml*	
4/1/66						*Klebsiella*	>100,000
4/12/66	+11 penicillin-G					*Klebsiella*	8,000
	500 mg q 6 hr						
4/15/66	+14 penicillin-G					*Klebsiella*	700
	500 mg q 6 hr						
4/19/66	+3 nalidixic acid						
	500 mg q 6 hr					*Klebsiella*	2,000
5/6/66	+5 penicillin-G	*Staphylococcus*	150	*Klebsiella*	900	*Klebsiella*	900
	500 mg q 6 hr	*epidermidis*					
		Streptococcus[b]	50			SPA:	
						Klebsiella	1,000
5/20/66	+5 ampicillin					SPA:	
	250 mg q 6 hr					*Klebsiella*	1,200
6/7/66	−7 ampicillin					SPA:	
						Klebsiella	>100,000
6/21/66	−211 ampicillin	Streptococcus	>100,000	CB = *Klebsiella* 2000			
				WB = *Klebsiella* 160			
				LK_1 = 0 RK_1 = *Klebsiella* 7000			
				LK_2 = 0 RK_2 = *Klebsiella* 6000			
				LK_3 = 0 RK_3 = *Klebsiella* 5000			
6/29/66	−4 Coly-Mycin	*Klebsiella*	<1,000	*Klebsiella*	>100,000	*Klebsiella*	>100,000
		Streptococcus	100,000				
7/5/66	−10 Coly-Mycin	*Klebsiella*	<1,000	*Klebsiella*	>100,000	*Klebsiella*	>100,000
		Enterococci	100,000				
9/27/66	−94 Coly-Mycin	*Klebsiella*	80	*Klebsiella*	>100,000	*Klebsiella*	>100,000
		Enterococci	2,000				
		S. epidermidis	500				
10/3/66	−100 Coly-Mycin						
						CB:	
						Klebsiella	>100,000
10/4/66	+1 Coly-Mycin			*Klebsiella*	170	*Klebsiella*	320
	75 mg q 12 hr	Enterococci	800	Enterococci	60		
10/5/66	+2 Coly-Mycin	Streptococcus	<100	Streptococcus	70	*Klebsiella*	30
	75 mg q 12 hr	*S. epidermidis*	2,000	*S. epidermidis*	130	*S. epidermidis*	130
10/6/66	+3 Coly-Mycin	Streptococcus }		*Klebsiella*	300	Streptococcus	50
	75 mg q 12 hr	*S. epidermidis* }	1,000			*S. epidermidis*	50
		Diphtheroids }					
10/7/66	+4 Coly-Mycin		0		0		0

	75 mg q 12 hr	*S. epidermidis*	650	*S. epidermidis*	60	*S. epidermidis*	10
10/11/66	+8 Coly-Mycin			*Klebsiella*	250	*Klebsiella*	80
	75 mg q 12 hr	*S. epidermidis*	10,000	*S. epidermidis*	750	*S. epidermidis*	250
10/12/66	+9 Coly-Mycin					CB:	
	75 mg q 12 hr					*Klebsiella*	1,000
10/14/66	−2 Coly-Mycin	*Klebsiella*	10	*Klebsiella*	>10,000	*Klebsiella*	>10,000
	75 mg q 12 hr	Streptococcus	70				
		S. epidermidis	100				
10/17/66	−5 Coly-Mycin	*Klebsiella*	<100	*Klebsiella*	8,000	*Klebsiella*	8,000
	75 mg q 12 hr	Streptococcus	10,000				
		S. epidermidis	100				
		Diphtheroids	10,000				
11/14/66	−33 Coly-Mycin	*Klebsiella*	20	*Klebsiella*	10,000	*Klebsiella*	10,000
		Streptococcus	10,000				
12/20/66	−69 Coly-Mycin	*Klebsiella*	10	*Klebsiella*	10,000	*Klebsiella*	10,000
		Streptococcus, Diphtheroids	10,000				
1/10/67	+5 kanamycin	Streptococcus	7,000	Streptococcus	130	Streptococcus	30
	500 mg q 12 hr						
1/23/67	−8 kanamycin	Streptococcus, *S. epidermidis*	200		0		0
	500 mg q 12 hr						
2/20/67	−35 kanamycin	Streptococcus, *S. epidermidis*, Diphtheroids	8,000	Streptococcus	10,000	Streptococcus	1,500
6/2/67	−6 months	Streptococcus, *S. epidermidis*, Diphtheroids	240	Streptococcus	100	Streptococcus	40
				S. epidermidis	300		
				Diphtheroids	100		
1/29/68	−1 year	*S. epidermidis*	800	*S. epidermidis*	10	*S. epidermidis*	80
		Diphtheroids	1,000				
7/22/71	−3½ years	Enterococci	90				
		S. epidermidis	300	*S. epidermidis*	10		0
		Diphtheroids	3,000	Diphtheroids	90		
		Lactobacillus sp.	>10,000				

[a] VB = voided bladder urine (VB_1 = urethral urine, VB_2 = midstream urine). CB = catheterized bladder urine, or in the presence of a Foley catheter CB represents urine aspirated from the Foley. WB = culture of residual irrigation fluid after washing bladder with several liters of sterile irrigating fluid. RK = right kidney. RK_1, RK_2, etc. = serial cultures from RK. LK = left kidney. LK_1, LK_2, etc. = serial cultures from LK. SPA = suprapubic needle aspiration of bladder. Solid transverse line divides longitudinal cultures into major periods of significance.

[b] Our records are not clear as to whether these and subsequent streptococci are α- or γ-streptococci; they are not enterococci.

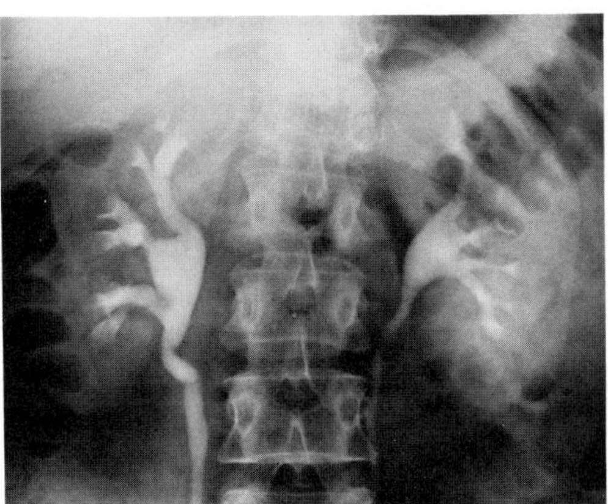

Figure 10.4 A 5-minute compression film from the intravenous urogram on C.B., a 39-year-old mother of three children. The right kidney, the site of the persistent *Klebsiella* urinary infection (Table 10.2), measures 13.8 cm in vertical length compared to 13.5 cm for the left kidney. All renal calyces are delicate. The slight dilatation and deviation of the right upper ureter is due to the compression balloon.

terobacteriaceae in the introital flora. As long as the frequency of these reinfections is limited to one, or sometimes two, infections per year, better medicine is probably practiced by treating each infection for a few days (or in some cases with single-dosage therapy) with the proper antibacterial agent; the physician should make sure that the bladder urine is sterile several weeks off therapy to avoid the consequences of an asymptomatic *Proteus* infection (see Chapter 8). When, however, the frequency of reinfections is several times a year, the clinician should begin prophylactic antimicrobial therapy[6] as I discussed in Chapter 4; the least expensive time in terms of cost and morbidity is when the second urinary tract infection (UTI) occurs within a 6-month period. Since most reinfections are caused by different bacteria at each recurrence, especially in prepubertal girls, the problem of keeping the bladder urine sterile is much more complicated than in men with chronic bacterial prostatitis where usually only one organism with a constant antimicrobial sensitivity pattern serves as the source of trouble.

I have reviewed in Chapter 4, in the section Prophylactic Prevention of Recurrent Bacteriuria, the antimicrobial effect on the bowel flora which is the major consideration in prophylactic therapy in the female. These data, which include the effect of prophylaxis on both the intestinal and vaginal flora, are important and represent the key to successful control of recurrent bacteriuria in the female.

Struvite Infection Stones

Although this subject, too, has been reviewed extensively in Chapter 8, a third reason for continuous antimicrobial therapy in the presence of a sterile urine is in patients with struvite infection stones. It is possible, as in the case of L.V., Table 8.7, Chapter 8, that if the urine can be kept sterile (and acid) in the presence of urea-splitting bacteria inside the stone, dissolution of the struvite stone may occur in the presence of an acid urine. Since most of these stones are caused by *P. mirabilis*, continuous penicillin-G, ampicillin, or TMP-SMX are the drugs of choice. If the infection stones are large and accompanied by substantial caliectasis, however, continuous antimicrobial therapy with oral antibacterial agents may not sterilize the urine even in the presence of *in vitro* sensitive bacteria. This rare example of lack of correlation between *in vitro* sensitivity and *in vivo* response is probably related to the "critical mass" of bacteria, a phenomena reviewed in Chapter 2.

We have a few patients with struvite infection stones who are poor operative risks, such as the elderly with severe cardiovascular disease or severely obese diabetic patients, in whom we keep their urines sterile on continuous antimicrobial thèrapy to prevent morbidity without any serious hope of dissolving their calculi. Without question, they feel better and are probably at less risk for septicemia or perirenal abscesses. In these efforts, we use the smallest dosage of antimicrobial agent that will maintain a sterile urine; TMP-SMX is by far the most successful in this context.

Prophylactic Antimicrobial Agents

Nitrofurantoin

In the case of nitrofurantoin, the urinary levels (see Chapter 2, Figures 2.3–2.7) are bactericidal for most *E. coli* and enterococci, but less effective against *Klebsiella* and *P. mirabilis*. The major advantage of nitrofurantoin for prophylaxis is that the intestinal flora is unaltered by continuous exposure to the drug and that resistance rarely develops. I have presented in Chapter 4 our own data on the prophylactic efficacy of nitrofurantoin macrocrystals as well as our studies on the fecal and vaginal flora during long-term administration of 100 mg each night.[23] An instructive patient is presented in Figures 4.16–4.22 to illustrate the efficacy and management of intractable urinary infections with nitrofurantoin prophylaxis. All things considered, this is an excellent long-term prophylactic antimicrobial agent for keeping the urine sterile in girls and women who have repeated reinfections of the urinary tract. As in the case of chronic bacterial prostatitis, a minimal dosage such as 50 mg once a night is adequate to maintain a sterile urine.

Trimethoprim-sulfamethoxazole

The physical and chemical determinants of trimethoprim (TMP) diffusion are presented in Chapter 7 in terms of penetration into prostatic fluid. In Chapter 4, the diffusion and ion trapping of TMP in vaginal fluid and its extraordinary efficacy in clearing all Enterobacteriaceae from the vaginal introitus at a dosage of only one-half tablet per day is presented in detail. The effect of TMP-SMX and TMP alone on the bowel flora is also considered at some length. Clinical examples, especially those shown in Figures 4.14 and 4.15, as well as the collective data in Tables 4.15 to 4.27, all serve to indicate that TMP-SMX is the most remarkable prophylactic agent for the prevention of urinary infections in the history of antimicrobial therapy.

Cephalexin

Besides nitrofurantoin, TMP-SMX, and methenamine, few antimicrobial agents have been well studied for prophylactic efficacy and almost no others have had a detailed analysis of their effects on the fecal and vaginal flora. The latter gap in our knowledge is particularly unfortunate because the effect of any antimicrobial agent on the bacteria at these two mucosal sites—intestinal and vaginal—determines their efficacy as a prophylactic agent for urinary tract infections.

Despite our lack of information on the effects of cephalexin at the vaginal and intestinal level, Fairley and his associates[24] at Melbourne studied the efficacy of 500 mg/day of cephalexin in preventing recurrent infections during a 6-month period. Seventeen of the 22 patients remained free of infection, 1 had a single infection, and 4 had two infections in the 6 months. Considering the information that three had renal calculi, four papillary necrosis, and three chronic pyelonephritis, efficacy in 17 of 22 patients may well mean that cephalexin is an important addition to our minimal armamentarium of good prophylactic drugs. The effect of cephalexin, however, on the intestinal and vaginal flora remains to be determined.

Methenamine

Methenamine (hexamethylenetetramine) is a colorless, odorless compound that is readily soluble in water, forming weakly basic solutions of pH 8.0–8.5. A tertiary amine, it has the properties of a monoacidic base in its salt formation and therefore can be combined with an unlimited number of organic and inorganic compounds. Various compounds and salts of methenamine are the active ingredients in over 200 pharmaceutical preparations.[25]

There is an extensive literature on methenamine. It was introduced by Nicolaier in 1894 for the treatment of urinary infections, and he was the first to show that formaldehyde was the active decomposition product of methenamine.[26] The classic paper by Hanzlik and Collins in 1913[27] established the widespread distribution of methenamine into every body fluid, including cerebrospinal, synovial, pericardial, and both the aqueous and vitreous humors of the eye. These investigators showed, however, that only methenamine, not formaldehyde, was present in these body fluids. With discriminating *in vitro* and *in vivo* experiments, they proved that: (1) methenamine, regardless of concentration, was not antibacterial in alkaline solutions; (2) formaldehyde could be liberated from methenamine only below a pH of 7.0; and (3) only two body fluids, gastric juice and urine, were capable of releasing formaldehyde (HCHO) from methenamine. These observations were confirmed and extended by Levy and Strauss[28] in a paper that contains the best review of the early literature prior to 1914, by Shohl and Deming,[29] and by De Eds.[30] Shohl and Deming made the interesting observation that, although methenamine was not antimicrobial in the presence of alkaline fluids, HCHO was equally bactericidal at acid and alkaline pH values.

Hanzlik and Collins[27] also observed HCHO in the freshly voided urine of the dog and "even in the urine from the pelvis of the kidney." Hinman,[31] however, on the basis of ureteral catheterization studies, concluded that methenamine was not active in renal urine and that antibacterial activity was present only in bladder urine, conclusions that were apparently confirmed by Levy and Strauss.[28]

The more recent studies on methenamine mandelate include those of Scudi and Reinhard,[32] Knight and associates,[33] and Gandelman.[34] Scudi and Reinhard, in clearance studies on dogs, showed that methenamine is distributed throughout total body water, and that the renal clearance is less than glomerular filtration rate.

Methenamine, through the liberation of free formaldehyde ($N_4(CH_2)6 + 6\ H_2O \leftrightarrows 4\ NH_3 + 6\ HCHO$), is theoretically an ideal drug. Significant resistance cannot be induced *in vitro*,[35] and almost all bacteria are susceptible to free formaldehyde at about the same concentration.[36] For example, the data in Table 10.3 were obtained by Millipore filtering a normal urine of pH 5.25, and adding to aliquots of it reagent grade HCHO from 10 μg/ml to 50 μg/ml. To each tube, including a control one that contained no HCHO, bacteria were added at a final concentration of 10,000/ml. Subcultures were performed at 6 and 24 hours after incubation at 37°C. Four strains each of *E. coli, Klebsiella, Pseudomonas*, and *P. mirabilis* were studied. As can be seen, HCHO at 20 μg/ml was bactericidal at 24 hours for 15 of 16 strains. The greater susceptibility of *Pseudomonas* and *P. mirabilis*, compared with *E. coli* and *Klebsiella*, is noteworthy and can be observed at the 6-hour subculture. Thus, between 15 and 25 μg of free HCHO must be made available through hydrolysis of methenamine if bactericidal activity is to occur in urine. Similar results have been reported by Musher and Griffith[37] but using a different technique.

What are the factors that determine the hydrolysis of methenamine to HCHO in urine? There are two: pH and time. Both have been recognized as being of major importance for over 50 years and were particularly well studied and emphasized by Heathcote in 1935.[38] Further studies, however, have been difficult because the early chemical methods for determining free HCHO are relatively insensitive; for example, the phenylhydrazine-nitroprusside and phloroglucin dilutional color reactions are accurate to about 10 μg/ml. Modern commercial methods sensitive to 1 μg/ml, such as Tanenbaum and Bricker's procedure,[39] cannot be used in the presence of methenamine because the acidity of the chemical reaction converts significant amounts of the methenamine to HCHO.*

Jane Jackson and I[40] have published a modification of the Riker method for determining free HCHO in the presence of methenamine. This method has allowed us to study the rate of hydrolysis of methenamine to free HCHO in natural urines of different pH. The critical importance of

* Our use of the Tanenbaum and Bricker[39] method proved to be a costly error for us and led to some false conclusions. In patients who had a ureteral catheter in one kidney and a Foley catheter in the bladder to collect urine from the contralateral kidney, we compared the free HCHO liberated in the renal pelvis to that formed by retention of urine in the bladder. We could show no difference between renal and bladder urine in free HCHO and reported this observation in the Urologists' Letter Club of 9/27/68. We discovered a few months later that the Tanenbaum and Bricker method was converting 15–25% of the total methenamine present in urine to free HCHO. Since in the bladder urine, even under conditions of maximal acidity and adequate time for hydrolysis, only about 2–10% of methenamine is normally converted to free HCHO, it is not surprising that we could detect no differences in free HCHO between renal and bladder urine in six patients.

Table 10.3
The Bactericidal Effect of Free HCHO In Urine on Gram-Negative Urinary Pathogens

A natural urine of pH 5.25 was filtered (Millipore) to remove contaminating bacteria and divided into multiple aliquots of 1.8 ml. Four different strains each of *Escherichia coli*, *Klebsiella*, *Pseudomonas*, and *Proteus mirabilis* were grown overnight in soy broth, diluted, and added in 0.1-ml volume to all tubes. The inoculum size was determined by culturing each tube at "zero" time; all tubes were incubated at 37°C and subcultured at 6 and 24 hours. All control tubes of urine (those without HCHO) supported bacterial growth. Reagent grade HCHO (0.1 ml) was added to all other tubes so that the final concentration varied between 10 and 50 μg/ml.

Organisms	Inoculum/ ml urine	Bacteria/ml after 6-hr Incubation of Urine Containing 10–50 μg/ml of HCHO									
		Control	10	15	20	25	30	35	40	45	50
E. coli	10^4	$>10^5$	$>10^5$	3×10^3	3×10^3	3×10^3	3×10^3	3×10^3	3×10^3	3×10^3	3×10^3
E. coli	10^4	$>10^5$	$>10^5$	$>10^4$	5×10^3	5×10^3	4×10^3	4×10^3	4×10^3	4×10^3	4×10^3
E. coli	10^4	$>10^5$	$>10^5$	3×10^3	3×10^3	680	850	870	640	240	380
E. coli	10^4	$>10^5$	$>10^5$	4×10^3	4×10^3	4×10^5	4×10^3	4×10^3	4×10^3	4×10^3	4×10^3
Klebsiella	3×10^3	$>10^5$	$>10^4$	$>10^4$	$>10^4$	$>10^4$	$>10^4$	$>10^4$	$>10^4$	$>10^4$	$>10^4$
Klebsiella	10^4	$>10^5$	$>10^4$	$>10^4$	$>10^4$	5×10^3	4×10^3	4×10^3	4×10^3	3×10^3	3×10^5
Klebsiella	10^4	$>10^5$	$>10^4$	5×10^3	5×10^3	5×10^3	5×10^3	5×10^3	5×10^3	4×10^3	510
Klebsiella	10^4	$>10^5$	$>10^4$	$>10^4$	$>10^4$	$>10^4$	$>10^4$	$>10^4$	$>10^4$	$>10^4$	$>10^4$
Pseudomonas	10^4	$>10^5$	3×10^3	0	0	0	0	0	0	0	0
Pseudomonas	10^4	$>10^5$	$>10^4$	0	0	0	0	0	0	0	0
Pseudomonas	10^4	$>10^5$	$>10^5$	$>10^4$	10	20	70	40	120	140	120
Pseudomonas	2×10^3	$>10^5$	1140	10	0	0	0	0	0	0	0
P. mirabilis	3×10^3	$>10^5$	$>10^4$	690	280	30	0	0	0	0	0
P. mirabilis	10^4	$>10^5$	$>10^5$	1110	600	270	50	10	0	0	0
P. mirabilis	2×10^3	$>10^4$	0	0	0	0	0	0	0	0	0
P. mirabilis	10^4	$>10^5$	4×10^3	4×10^3	4×10^3	4×10^3	3×10^3	3×10^3	820	600	290
		Bacteria/ml after 24-hr Incubation of Urine Containing 10–50 μg/ml of HCHO									
		Control	10	15	20	25	30	35	40	45	50
E. coli	10^4	$>10^5$	$>10^5$	0	0	0	0	0	0	0	0
E. coli	10^4	$>10^5$	$>10^5$	$>10^5$	0	0	0	0	0	0	0
E. coli	10^4	$>10^5$	$>10^5$	$>10^5$	0	0	0	0	0	0	0
E. coli	10^4	$>10^5$	$>10^5$	$>10^5$	0	0	0	0	0	0	0
Klebsiella	3×10^3	$>10^5$	$>10^5$	0	0	0	0	0	0	0	0
Klebsiella	10^4	$>10^5$	$>10^5$	0	0	0	0	0	0	0	0
Klebsiella	10^4	$>10^5$	$>10^4$	0	0	0	0	0	0	0	0
Klebsiella	10^4	$>10^5$	$>10^5$	0	0	0	0	0	0	0	0
Pseudomonas	10^4	$>10^5$	$>10^5$	0	0	0	0	0	0	0	0
Pseudomonas	10^4	$>10^5$	$>10^5$	0	0	0	0	0	0	0	0
Pseudomonas	10^4	$>10^5$	$>10^5$	$>10^5$	$>10^5$	0	$>10^5$	0	0	0	0
Pseudomonas	2×10^3	$>10^5$	$>10^5$	2×10^3	0	0	0	0	0	0	0
P. mirabilis	3×10^3	$>10^5$	$>10^5$	0	0	0	0	0	0	0	0
P. mirabilis	10^4	$>10^5$	$>10^5$	0	0	0	0	0	0	0	0
P. mirabilis	2×10^3	$>10^5$	0	0	0	0	0	0	0	0	0
P. mirabilis	10^4	$>10^5$	0	0	0	0	0	0	0	0	0

both pH and time in the hydrolysis of methenamine to free HCHO is shown in Figure 10.5. In these studies, methenamine was added to two separate aliquots of three Millipore-filtered natural urines of pH 5.38, 5.65, and 7.30 in concentrations of 0.15 mg/ml and 0.75 mg/ml. In normal subjects receiving methenamine, 0.75 mg/ml represents a reasonable concentration that should easily be achieved in the urine while 0.15 mg/ml is very minimal. HCHO, determined immediately and at frequent intervals during incubation at 37°C (Figure 10.5), showed that the liberation of HCHO, while highly pH-dependent, required 3 hours to reach 90% of the final equilibrium. After 5–6 hours, there is little or no further increase in HCHO. A negligible amount of HCHO was formed at pH 7.30.

These data on rates of hydrolysis should be interpreted clinically in relation to the studies in Table 10.3. That is, given an adequately acid urine, how much time is needed to reach or exceed the concentration of free HCHO needed to kill bacteria infecting the urinary tract? From Figure 10.5, at an average urinary methenamine concentration of 0.75 mg/ml, and at a quite acid pH, at least 1 hour is needed to exceed 25 μg/ml of free HCHO and probably 2 hours is safer; the zero time value in Figure 10.5, the amount of HCHO liberated by the chemical method per se,[40] must be subtracted from any value during hydrolysis. This rather prolonged time required to reach inhibitory concentrations virtually excludes any chance that methenamine is active during the short transit time down the renal tubules, calyces, and pelvis. Extreme dehydration with a highly acid urine, or some degree of obstructive renal residual urine, might provide rare exceptions. Musher *et al.*[41] used an *in vitro* model which simulated bladder filling and emptying; their hydrolysis curves are very similar to Figure 10.5.

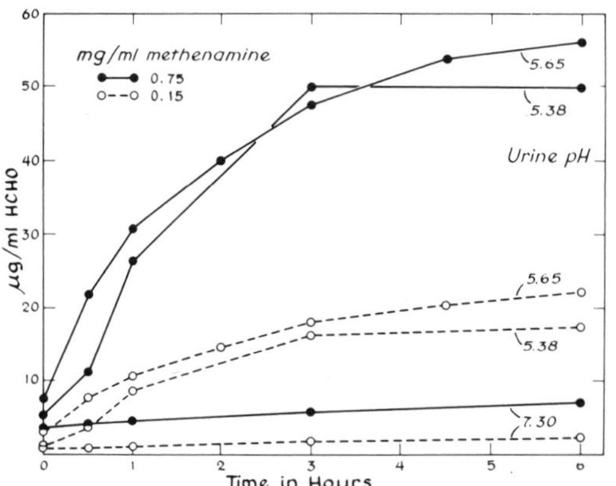

Figure 10.5 The hydrolysis of methenamine (at concentrations of 0.15 and 0.75 mg/ml) to HCHO in three urine samples of different pH values when incubated at 37°C. The final concentration of HCHO depends on pH, amount of methenamine available for hydrolysis, and the time allowed for hydrolysis. Ninety % of the final equilibrium is reached in 3 hours, with little change after 6 hours. (Reproduced by permission from J. Jackson and T. A. Stamey, Invest. Urol. **9:** 124, 1971.[40])

Miller and Phillips[42] have published an excellent paper on correlating antibacterial activity in urine with pH and the concentration of free HCHO and methenamine. No urine with a pH >6.4 was bacteriostatic. All urines were inhibitory that contained 18 μg/ml or more of free HCHO, and a direct relationship was observed between urine pH, free HCHO, and bacteriostasis. They also observed an increased sensitivity of *Pseudomonas* and *P. mirabilis* to free HCHO excreted in the urine of their volunteers. An equally informative paper on male paraplegic urine is that of Pearman, *et al.*[43] They make a good case for using NH_4Cl to acidify the urine if effective concentrations of HCHO are going to occur in human urine.

Thus, the factors determining successful use of methenamine in preventing reinfection of the bladder are: (1) the bacteria must not be in the kidney, or failure will certainly occur; (2) the urine must be acid, preferably below pH 6.0; (3) there must be time for hydrolysis of methenamine to occur: 3 hours is required to reach 90% of the final equilibrium, but with a pH of 5.4–5.6 (Figure 10.5) and 0.75 mg/ml of methenamine in the urine, 2 hours of hydrolysis will produce bactericidal levels of free HCHO; (4) there must be adequate concentrations of methenamine in the urine (0.15 mg/ml of methenamine is clearly inadequate as shown in Figure 10.5); and (5) it is probably best not to force fluids for two reasons. First, a diuretic urine is always more alkaline. Second, diuresis can easily reduce the concentration of free HCHO to a noninhibitory level; about 20 μg/ml of free HCHO is required to kill bacteria, but even under optimal conditions the limiting equilibrium from hydrolysis of methenamine is about 40–60 μg/ml.

Even with all these precautions, I am the first to admit that methenamine can be a frustrating drug when bacteriuria occurs in a child whose mother assures the clinician that not a single dosage was missed. Even in the highly successful study of Holland and West,[44] the prevention of recurrences in female children was by no means complete. Similar observations on its prophylactic efficacy in recurrent UTI in women have been made by Harding and Ronald[45] and Kincaid-Smith *et al.*[10]; in the latter study, however, efficacy was confined to bladder infections. In patients with indwelling catheters and others on intermittent catheterization, Vainrub and Musher[46] reported that 4 g/day each of methenamine mandelate and ascorbic acid was ineffective in either preventing or suppressing bacteriuria.

I suspect, without being able to prove it, that the major difficulty with keeping the bladder urine bactericidal is that every time the patient voids, the urine is no longer bactericidal until hydrolysis of new methenamine in the bladder occurs with time (at least 1–2 hours). That this hydrolysis is also dependent on the pH of urine formed in the distal tubules of the kidney is no help. Moreover, the subcultures in Table 10.3 for *E. coli* and *Klebsiella* in urine containing high concentrations of free HCHO show a disappointing rate of bactericidal activity after 6 hours of incubation. Other antimicrobial agents, for example, those in Figures 10.1 and 10.2, kill bacteria with greater rapidity. This observation suggests another reason besides hydrolysis considerations as to why frequent voidings are detrimental to the successful use of methenamine.

Despite these difficulties, methenamine can be a useful drug in preventing reinfections of a sterile bladder urine, especially if there is residual urine and if NH_4Cl is added. A few comments on dosage, the different methenamine salts that are available, and the usage of urinary-acidifying drugs in conjunction with methenamine are appropriate.

Since methenamine is distributed through total body water,* including that of red blood cells, and since clearance from the blood is considerably less than glomerular filtration rate,[32] its half-life in blood is quite long. Moreover, in the presence of an optimally acid urine, only 2–10% of the methenamine present is converted to free HCHO, and it is, therefore, not surprising that a dosage schedule of every 12 hours is perfectly adequate for antibacterial activity.

As mentioned in the first paragraph of this section, some 200 different pharmaceutical preparations contain methenamine as the active antibacterial agent. There is no evidence, of which I am aware, that the particular acid form of the salt contributes in any way to the antibacterial activity of methenamine. For example, mandelic acid was apparently used to form the salt with methenamine because of Rosenheim's observations in 1935[47] that of nine different keto- or hydroxy- acids, only mandelic acid was excreted in the urine unchanged and rendered it bactericidal. It is historically interesting that Rosenheim's studies were done because of Helmholz's observation[48]

* The pKa of methenamine is 4.8. Since it is a base (a proton acceptor), there is no dissociation in plasma of pH 7.4; all of the molecules are in the uncharged, freely diffusible form (see Chapter 7). We have performed experiments on methenamine diffusion from plasma to prostatic fluid using the canine model described in Chapter 7. Regardless of the rate or total volume of prostatic secretion, the concentration of methenamine in prostatic fluid was always the same as that in the plasma. Unfortunately, the pH of canine prostatic fluid (6.4) in these experiments was not acid enough to detect free HCHO, nor is the plasma concentration high enough from standard oral dosage to reach bactericidal levels of HCHO even if an acid pH promoted hydrolysis. Ion trapping of methenamine in prostatic fluid, as described in Chapter 7, is virtually impossible because of its low pKa.

that the urine of children treated for epilepsy with a diet designed to produce ketosis was bactericidal *in vitro*, and that this activity was not due to acidity *per se*. The important point about mandelic acid is that urine is not rendered inhibitory unless the acid is administered in doses of 12 g or more/24 hours. Since 1.0 g of methenamine mandelate contains 480 mg of methenamine and 520 mg of mandelic acid, 4 g of the salt supply only 2 g of mandelic acid, which could not possibly contribute to the antibacterial activity of the urine. The same is true for hippuric acid in the salt methenamine hippurate. Indeed, since it is known that these organic acids inhibit the metabolism of bacteria by virtue of their unionized molecules,[49] it is not surprising that mandelic and hippuric acid are equally effective, since they have essentially the same pKa (3.37 and 3.82, respectively). The important fact about the methenamine salts of organic acids, however, is that the dosage of the organic acid is a fraction of what is required in the urine to exert an antibacterial effect.

Since methenamine is a base, and since a highly acid urine (<6.0) is needed to release free HCHO effectively within a reasonable time of hydrolysis, the acid salts are widely thought to contribute to the lowering of the urinary pH. If true, this would be an advantage, but unfortunately there is no evidence that any of these acids—sodium or potassium acid phosphates, mandelic, hippuric, or sulfosalicylic acid—in the 2-g limitation/24 hours imposed by the combination with methenamine, influence in any way the pH of the urine. In fact, one of the unhappy chapters in renal physiology is the lack of a chronic acidifying agent for the urinary tract. Ammonium chloride in reasonable dosages will certainly acidify the urine for a short time, but a long term effect is debatable. Methionine, at one time recommended by Kass and his group as an effective antimicrobial agent[50] but later shown to be ineffective,[51] will acidify the urine in enormous doses (12–20 g a day). We have used ascorbic acid as a urinary acidifier in doses of 2.5 g/day following the report of McDonald and Murphy,[52] but we are aware of the suggestion that ascorbic acid, like methionine, must be given in prohibitively large doses in order to be effective.[53] Fortunately, normal urine, in the absence of a diuresis, is quite acid enough[54] to liberate some free HCHO from methenamine, probably accounting for the fact that therapeutic effectiveness does not depend on which salt of methenamine is prescribed. In fact, methenamine as the pure base is readily available in 500-mg tablets from Eli Lilly and Co. (methenamine tablets, N.F., No. 772); a prescription is not required, and patients in our area can buy 100 tablets for $2.50, making methenamine base the least expensive antimicrobial agent of our time. A more important advantage to prescribing the pure base form of methenamine is in patients with azotemia and slight acidosis. Since the acidifying ability of the renal tubules remains essentially intact in azotemia, these patients can convert the methenamine to free HCHO about as well as patients with normal renal function. The advantage to prescribing a pure base in the presence of acidosis is obvious: it avoids 1–2 g of extra acid that must be excreted. We have not observed any increased gastric distress by using the pure base form of methenamine, in either adults or children.

Comparative Clinical Trials

Several authors have compared the prophylactic efficacy of either nitrofurantoin and methenamine,[10] methenamine mandelate, SMX, and TMP-SMX,[45] or methenamine hippurate, nitrofurantoin, TMP, and TMP-SMX.[55] The first two studies included placebo-treated controls. It is clear that any regimen is better than placebo therapy, that nitrofurantoin is superior to methenamine, that methenamine is better than sulfonamides, and that TMP or TMP-SMX is superior to any other regimen. For example, in the controlled clinical trials of Harding and Ronald,[45] there were 3.6 infections/patient year in the placebo group, 2.5/patient year in the sulfamethoxazole group, 1.6/patient year in the methenamine mandelate (2 g) and ascorbic acid (2 g) group, and 0.1 infections/patient year in the TMP-SMX patients; it should be appreciated that the methenamine and ascorbic acid regimen was a substantial dose equal to half of the conventional full dosage regimen whereas the TMP-SMX dosage was only one-eighth of the conventional daily dose (40 mg of TMP/200 mg of SMX). In a later paper, the Winnipeg investigators[56] have shown that thrice-weekly dosage of 40 mg of TMP with 200 mg of SMX (one-half of the regular tablet) showed the same prophylactic efficacy as their earlier report,[45] an infection incidence of 0.1/patient year of therapy.

A Recommendation

In summary, if I had to design a therapeutic regimen for the treatment and prophylaxis of recurrent UTI in women with lower tract symptoms it would go like this:

1. For first infections, and for the occasional recurrent UTI (once or twice a year), I would treat the patient with a short-acting sulfonamide (0.5 g four times a day) or oral penicillin-G (250 mg four times a day) for 3 days. The reader will note that I am not psychologically prepared to recommend single-dosage therapy, but to go from 10 days therapy to 3 is quite a compromise! Dr. Wm. Fair at Washington University, St. Louis, has shown me his data where three days therapy is as good as 10 days; he studied TMP-SMX and penicillin-G.

2. For those who have more frequent infections, at the second occurrence within 6 months (see Chapter 4 on natural history), I would treat for 3 days with full-dosage TMP-SMX (160/800 mg twice daily for adults) and follow on the 4th day with 40/200 mg (one-half regular tablet) each night (Chapter 4, Tables 4.15–4.27) or even thrice-weekly as the Winnipeg group[56] suggest. In this instance, I have a valid reason for the 3 days of therapy because not only would the introitus be cleared of enterobacterial colonization by that time, but virtually all the Enterobacteriaceae would be cleared from the rectum and would then remain clear on the one-half tablet of daily prophylaxis.

My second choice would be nitrofurantoin, 50 mg four times a day, for 3 days (to be consistent) followed by 50 mg each night beginning on the fourth night.

It will be a rare individual who cannot tolerate one of these two regimens. If that occurs, my third choice—in the current absence of TMP alone—would be cephalexin or penicillin-G used in the same way. When TMP alone becomes available in this country, 100 mg twice a day for three days, followed by 50 mg each night (one-half a tablet) should represent effective treatment and prophylaxis; Kasanen's *et al.*[55] data indicate that trimethoprim alone is even better than TMP-SMX for prophylaxis.

For little girls, the same regimens apply but at reduced dosages.

3. I would like to emphasize that the above recommendation is for *symptomatic* female patients with lower tract complaints. For all others, I prefer 5–10 days of therapy with a culture during treatment so that I know the bacteriuria has been resolved.

Postintercourse Antimicrobial Therapy in Preventing Reinfections of the Bladder

We pointed out in 1965[1] that, in women in whom sexual intercourse is the initiating event in recurrent infections, a substantial reduction in recurrences can be achieved by a single tablet of an oral antimicrobial agent following sexual intercourse. These observations were made before we knew that pathogenic bacteria on the introitus determined bacteriuric recurrences (Chapter 4). It is now clear why this regimen was so effective: once pathogenic bacteria become established on the introitus, if sexual intercourse is the primary event causing inoculation of the bladder, bactericidal activity in the bladder urine can be produced by the drug before the second or third generation of the inoculated organisms. Since the number of bacteria inoculated into the bladder is likely to be small, the concentration of antimicrobial agent will be all the more effective (Chapter 2). Our routine is to ask the patient to empty her bladder after intercourse before taking the antimicrobial tablet, thereby preventing unnecessary dilution of the antibacterial agent when it reaches the bladder urine.

As emphasized throughout this final chapter, the clinician must know that he has cured the current bacteriuria before initiating this regimen. A useful routine is to treat the current infection for a few days with the appropriate drug and have the patient abstain from sexual intercourse for 10 days *after* completing therapy. If a culture at that time indicates a sterile bladder urine, we then begin the postintercourse regimen. Our favorite drug is oral penicillin-G in doses of either 250- or 500-mg tablets. Oral penicillin-G has three advantages: (1) it is a broad spectrum antibiotic at urinary concentrations (as will be reviewed in the next section of this chapter), (2) it is inexpensive, and (3) the serum levels, like those of nitrofurantoin, are so negligible in relation to Gram-negative pathogens that oral penicillin-G is most unlikely to alter the natural bacteria of the host. For example, Louria and Brayton[57] have shown that superinfection is related to the dose of penicillin-G; they found no instances of superinfection when pencillin-G was used in low doses.

Other antimicrobial agents like nitrofurantoin and ampicillin may be equally useful. The following patient with severe pyelonephritis and reflux is an excellent example of what can be accomplished with a postintercourse antimicrobial regimen.

D.O., a 27-year-old, white, married mother was first seen at Stanford University Hospital in January 1967, complaining of a dull backache, fatigue, and puffiness under the eyes. She recalled a childhood history of recurrent abdominal cramps which were never diagnosed. Her first overt urinary infection occurred as "honeymoon cystitis" followed shortly by an acute febrile illness with chills and back pain but no urinary symptoms; the infection responded well to sulfonamide therapy. Despite this history, her first pregnancy was uneventful, but during her second pregnancy sulfonamide therapy was required for 1–2 months. Urological evaluation in 1963, including cystoscopy and retrograde pyelograms, was said to be unremarkable. She continued to be asymptomatic until September 1966, when she consulted a local internist because of fatigue and eyelid edema. He found her blood pressure to be 120/80 mm Hg, but because the urine contained a trace of protein, white blood cells, and some red blood cells, she was treated with sulfasoxazole with complete clearing of her urine. In December 1966, he admitted her to the hospital because of fever and mild bilateral flank pain, more severe on the right, and a urine loaded with white blood cells. Within 48 hours of starting ampicillin, the fever and flank pain were gone. An intravenous urogram showed bilateral pyelonephritis, and she was referred to Stanford.

When first seen in January 1967, the most remarkable fact about her history was that she denied ever having dysuria, urinary frequency, or urgency. Her blood pressure was 160/100, and examination of the urine showed no protein, WBCs, or bacteria. Except for a blood urea nitrogen of 26 mg/100 ml and a serum creatinine of 1.5 mg/100 ml, all other chemistries and electrolytes were normal. When first seen on 1/12/67, she had been on ampicillin for 30 days; her urine culture showed *Klebsiella* on the vaginal introitus (Table 10.4). The ampicillin was stopped, and repeat cultures the next day showed the same *Klebsiella* on the introitus; an SPA was sterile. She was seen twice again in January and once each in February and March of 1967; all symptoms had disappeared, her blood pressure was normal, but the urine repeatedly contained 10–40 mg% protein. In late April 1967, she again experienced flank aching and was admitted to the hospital in May 1967, for complete evaluation. A catheterized urine specimen, obtained the day of admission (5/22/67) at the time a Foley catheter was placed in the bladder for a voiding cystourethrogram, grew >100,000 *E. coli*, sensitive to all antimicrobial agents. Residual urine was 10 ml at the time of catheterization. The cystogram demonstrated reflux into the distal left ureter when the bladder was filled to 300 ml, followed by marked reflux into the left caly-

D.O., a 27-year-old, Caucasian Woman with Grade III Reflux and Chronic Pyelonephritis Effectively Maintained on Postintercourse Ampicillin for 12 Years

Date	Days on (+) or off (−) Therapy	Vaginal Vestibule		Urethral (VB_1)[a]		Midstream (VB_2)	
		bacteria/ml		*bacteria/ml*		*bacteria/ml*	
1/2/67	+30 ampicillin	*Klebsiella*	500	*Klebsiella*	190	*Klebsiella*	70
		γ-Streptococcus	<100				
1/13/67	−1 ampicillin	*Klebsiella*	2,500	*Klebsiella*	700	*Klebsiella*	20
		γ-Streptococcus	<100			SPA = 0	
1/16/67	−4 ampicillin	*Escherichia coli*	300	*E. coli*	<100		
		Klebsiella	1,200	*Klebsiella*	600	*Klebsiella*	10
		γ-Streptococcus	100,000	γ-Streptococcus	>10,000	γ-Streptococcus	20
		S. epidermidis	<100	*S. epidermidis*	160	SPA = 0	
1/26/67	−14 ampicillin	*Klebsiella*	30	*Klebsiella*	10		
		S. epidermidis	70				
		Yeast	100,000	Yeast	1,500	Yeast	110
2/23/67	−42 ampicillin	γ-Streptococcus	100,000	γ-Streptococcus	10,000	γ-Streptococcus	7,000
		S. epidermidis	<100				
3/30/67	−77 ampicillin	γ-Streptococcus	<100	γ-Streptococcus	20		0
		S. epidermidis	<100	*S. epidermidis*	10		
		Diphtheroids	10,000				
5/22/67	−130 ampicillin					CB:	
						E. coli	>100,000
5/24/67	−132 ampicillin			CB = *E. coli* > 100,000			
				WB = *E. coli* > 100,000			
				LK_1 = >100,000		RK_1 = >100,000	
				LK_2 = >100,000		RK_2 = >100,000	
				LK_3 = >100,000		RK_3 = >10,000	
				LK_4 = >10,000			
5/25/67	+1 penicillin-G	*E. coli*	>10,000	*E. coli*	300	*E. coli*	700
	500 mg q 6 hr	*Klebsiella*		*Klebsiella*	60	*Klebsiella*	10
		γ-Streptococcus	<100				
6/8/67	−4 penicillin-G	*E. coli*	>100,000	*E. coli*	>100,000	*E. coli*	>100,000
6/22/67	+14 ampicillin	*Klebsiella*	10,000	*Klebsiella*	120	*Klebsiella*	10
	500 mg q 6 hr	γ-Streptococcus	<100				
7/6/67	−14 ampicillin	*E. coli*	10,000	*E. coli*	30		
	(no intercourse)	*S. epidermidis*	<100	γ-Streptococcus	1,000	γ-Streptococcus	50
		Diphtheroids	<100				
7/20/67	−28 ampicillin	*E. coli*	50	*E. coli*	20	*E. coli*	10
	(no intercourse)	γ-Streptococcus	>10,000	γ-Streptococcus	5,000	γ-Streptococcus	600

Table 10.4 *continued*

Date	Days on (+) or off (−) Therapy	Vaginal Vestibule		Urethral (VB_1)[a]		Midstream (VB_2)	
8/17/67	Postintercourse ampicillin: 1 mo	*E. coli*	<100			*E. coli*	30
		γ-Streptococcus	100,000	γ-Streptococcus	30	γ-Streptococcus	210
		S. epidermidis	<100			*S. epidermidis*	40
9/21/67	Postintercourse ampicillin: 2 mo	*E. coli*	>100,000	*E. coli*	80	*E. coli*	90
		Diphtheroids	10,000	Diphtheroids	3,000	Diphtheroids	3,000
						S. epidermidis	10
11/2/67	Postintercourse ampicillin: 3½ mo	*E. coli*	20				
		γ-Streptococcus	>100,000	γ-Streptococcus	>100,000	γ-Streptococcus	6,000
		S. epidermidis	<100	*S. epidermidis*	<100	*S. epidermidis*	<100
12/7/67	Postintercourse ampicillin: 4½ mo	γ-Streptococcus	>100,000	γ-Streptococcus	3,500	γ-Streptococcus	2,750
		S. epidermidis	30				
1/25/68	Postintercourse ampicillin: 6 mo	*E. coli*	220				
		γ-Streptococcus	>10,000	γ-Streptococcus	3,000	γ-Streptococcus	10
3/26/68	Postintercourse ampicillin: 8 mo	Diphtheroids	10,000	*Pseudomonas*	50	*Pseudomonas*	30
		S. epidermidis	<1,000	*S. epidermidis*	40	*S. epidermidis*	20
7/30/68	Postintercourse ampicillin: 12 mo	Diphtheroids	130				
		S. epidermidis	300	*S. epidermidis*	10		0
10/29/68	Postintercourse ampicillin: 15 mo	Diphtheroids	2,500	Diphtheroids	30	Diphtheroids	50
		S. epidermidis	30				
2/18/69	Postintercourse ampicillin: 19 mo	Diphtheroids	320	Diphtheroids	30		0
		S. epidermidis	40				
10/17/69	Postintercourse ampicillin: 27 mo	*E. coli*	2,000			*E. coli*	70
		Diphtheroids	4,000			Diphtheroids	4,000
2/25/70[b]	Postintercourse ampicillin: 31 mo	*E. coli*	>10,000			CB:	
						E. coli	10
8/11/70	Postintercourse ampicillin: 37 mo					CB	0
9/7/70	Postintercourse ampicillin: 38 mo	*S. epidermidis*	80	*S. epidermidis*	20		0
		Lactobacilli	100,000	Lactobacilli	10,000		

2/19/71	Postintercourse ampicillin: 43 mo	*S. epidermidis* Diphtheroids	30 10,000	*S. epidermidis* Diphtheroids	30 400	Diphtheroids	60
8/17/71	Postintercourse ampicillin: 49 mo					CB	0
2/11/72	Postintercourse ampicillin: 55 mo					CB	0
8/10/72	Postintercourse ampicillin 61 mo					CB	0
2/23/73	Postintercourse ampicillin: 67 mo					CB	0
4/17/74	Postintercourse ampicillin: 81 mo					CB	0
1/23/75	Postintercourse ampicillin: 90 mo					CB	0
7/10/75	Postintercourse ampicillin: 96 mo					CB	0
6/18/76	Postintercourse ampicillin: 107 mo					CB	0
7/20/77	Postintercourse ampicillin: 120 mo					CB	0
7/12/78	Postintercourse ampicillin: 132 mo					CB	0
8/23/79	Postintercourse ampicillin: 145 mo					CB	0

[a] VB = voided bladder urine (VB_1 = urethral urine, VB_2 = midstream urine). CB = catheterized bladder urine, or in the presence of a Foley catheter CB represents urine aspirated from the Foley. WB = culture of residual irrigation fluid after washing bladder with several liters of sterile irrigating fluid. RK = right kidney. RK_1, RK_2, etc. = serial cultures from RK. LK = left kidney. LK_1, LK_2, etc. = serial cultures from LK. SPA = suprapubic needle aspiration of bladder. Solid transverse line divides longitudinal cultures into major periods of significance.

[b] Following this catherization for creatinine clearances, she had an acute urinary infection characterized by chills, fever, and bilateral flank pain.

ceal system on voiding. No reflux at this time was demonstrated into the right ureter, despite the presence of bacteriuria. An intravenous urogram (Figure 10.6) showed diffuse bilateral blunting and distortion of the renal calyces typical of childhood pyelonephritis; the right kidney measured 9.6 cm and the left 12.3. Cystoscopy and ureteral catheterization studies (Table 10.4) confirmed that the *E. coli* were present in large numbers in both kidneys. Both ureteral orifices seemed somewhat relaxed, but there was very little submucosal tunnel on the left. After 10 days of oral penicillin-G (followed by recurrence 4 days later), ampicillin 500 mg every 6 hours was started and continued for 2 weeks. After stopping the ampicillin on 6/22/67, she abstained from intercourse for the next 4 weeks; cultures on 7/6/67 and 7/20/67 showed no infection despite the presence of *E. coli* on the introitus. Because of these *E. coli*, she was started on a regimen of 250 mg of ampicillin after each sexual intercourse, a regimen she has constantly maintained from 7/20/67 to the present examination,

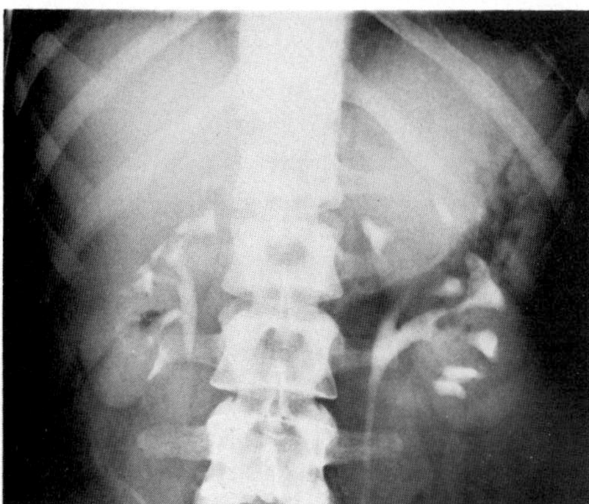

Figure 10.6 An intravenous urogram on D.O., a 27-year-old, white married woman with chronic pyelonephritis and bilateral ureteral reflux. The right kidney, measuring 9.6 cm, showed only a thin rim of cortex lateral to the middle and upper calyces, but a thick lower pole cortex. The left kidney (12.3 cm) was uniformly involved with calyceal distortion, characteristic of pyelonephritis.

Table 10.5
D.O., 27-year-old, Caucasian Woman with Grade III Reflux and Chronic Pyelonephritis: Serial Serum Creatinines and Creatinine Clearances during a 12-year Period While on an Ampicillin Postintercourse Regimen.

Date	Serum Creatinine	Creatinine Clearance
	mg%	*ml/min/1.73 M^2*
5/24/67	1.6	70
10/29/69	1.5	71
2/25/70	1.3	72
9/4/70	1.4	71
2/19/71	1.5	
8/17/71	1.5	65
2/11/72	1.7	68
8/10/72	1.6	63
2/23/73	1.4	71
4/17/74	1.5	64
1/23/75	1.7	57
7/10/75	1.5	52
6/18/76	1.7	66
7/20/77	1.7	52
7/12/78	1.8	66
8/23/79	1.6	65

August 23, 1979 (Table 10.4). All urinalyses have been acid (pH 5.0–6.5), protein has either been absent or about 10 mg%, and there have been no cells or casts in the urine. Creatinine clearances have been performed yearly without showing any deterioration in renal function (Table 10.5). She has gained 15 pounds in weight, her blood pressure is normal, and she has remained asymptomatic. Her intravenous urogram was repeated in October 1968 and on August 6, 1973; there was no change in comparison to Figure 10.6. A voiding cystourethrogram on 10/15/68 demonstrated bilateral, low pressure reflux with gravity filling (Figure 10.7). It is interesting that this cystogram showed bilateral reflux during filling at a time when her urine had been sterile for 16 months, whereas our original cystogram on 5/22/67 while she was bacteriuric showed reflux only into the left kidney, and then only during voiding. A repeat voiding cystourethrogram (VCU) on 8/6/73, 6 years later, was still identical to Figure 10.7. It is important to observe in Table 10.4 that the only urinary infection

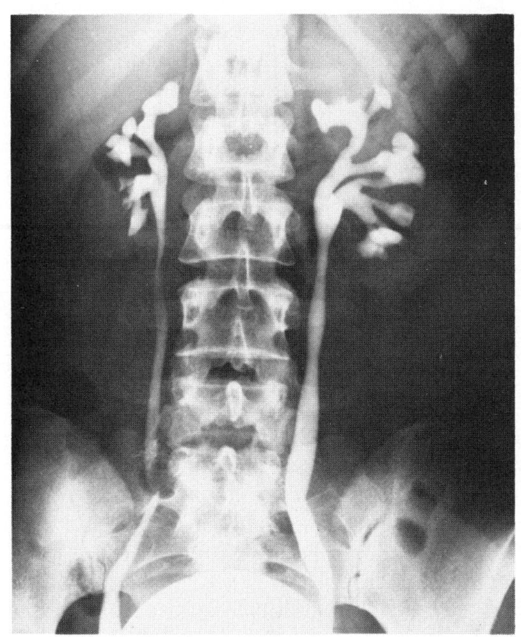

Figure 10.7 A cystourethrogram on D.O., 10/15/68, showing bilateral reflux during gravity filling of the bladder. Her urine had been sterile for 16 months. Despite this degree of reflux and pyelonephritis (Figure 10.6), a simple regimen of postintercourse ampicillin has kept her urine sterile (Table 10.4) and her renal function stable (Table 10.5) for over 12 years. A repeat voiding cystourethrogram (VCU) on 8/6/73 was identical to this figure (grade III reflux).

she experienced between June 1967 and August 1979 (the last date of follow-up) was immediately following the insertion of a Foley catheter for an out-patient creatinine clearance on 2/25/70. Of particular interest is that the introital culture just prior to the catheterization showed >10,000 *E. coli*/ml on the vaginal vestibule and even the catheterized bladder urine had 10 colonies of *E. coli*/ml on culture, leaving no doubt that introital *E. coli* were carried into the bladder with the catheter. Unfortunately, we neglected to give her ampicillin at the time of our catheterization! Her B.P. on 8/23/79 was 122/76 mm Hg on no medication. All the creatinine clearances in Table 10.5 have been three 1-hour clearances with an indwelling Foley catheter.

Although postintercourse antimicrobial therapy is sometimes a better alternative than continuous therapy in the sexually active woman, it is not always successful. If the Enterobacteriaceae become resistant to the oral antimicrobial agent, then reinfection will occur with the resistant bacteria. For example, the postintercourse regimen on K.S., presented in Figure 4.5 of Chapter 4, had been highly successful for 1 year (August 1969 to August 1970) with 250 mg of penicillin-G until she developed a nontypable *E. coli* bacteriuria which was resistant to penicillin-G (minimal inhibitory concentration (MIC) >1200 μg/ml) and tetracycline (see the first bacteriuria in Figure 4.5). Because of this kind of experience, I prefer continuous prophylaxis to postintercourse therapy. Moreover, drugs that have a powerful biological effect on the fecal flora like TMP-SMX are probably poor candidates for postintercourse therapy since an intermittent bactericidal effect on the *E. coli* of the bowel rationally should encourage resistance. If postintercourse therapy is to be used, nitrofurantoin would be the ideal drug since it does not influence the bowel flora.

Vosti[58] reported some interesting quantitative data on postintercourse regimens in 14 patients using 5 different antimicrobial agents. During 705 months without prophylaxis, there were 90 infections; during 761 months with postintercourse prophylaxis, there were only 19 infections. Of the 19 infections, the strains were usually resistant to the prophylactic agent the patients were receiving with the exception of nitrofurantoin. Penicillin-G, nitrofurantoin, cephalexin, and nalidixic acid were all successfull as prophylactic agents. Lastly, Vosti analyzed the occurrence of any Gram-negative bacteria found in the urine cultures while the patients were taking or not taking the prophylactic agents. While off prophylaxis, 394 of 571 cultures (69%) were positive for some Gram-negative bacteria, but only 181 of 384 (47%) were positive while on prophylactic therapy. These latter data implied that even intermittent therapy reduced the colonization incidence of Enterobacteriaceae on the vaginal introitus and urethra.

SOME PERSONAL OBSERVATIONS ON A FEW SELECTED DRUGS

Penicillin-G

We should not forget that the quantitative basis for diagnosing bacteriuria, and therefore the ability to assess results accurately in terms of cures and failures, was not firmly established until about 1956. By 1956, however, most infectious disease units had had 10 years' experience in the use of penicillin-G shortly followed by the so-called "broad spectrum" antibiotics; most of this experience, at least in terms of accurate assessment, was based on nonurinary tract tissue infections where serum concentrations are obviously important. It is not surprising, then that our report in January 1965,[1] that urinary—not serum—concentrations determined cure of renal infections was met with considerable opposition.[59] These observations were made possible because most of our patients between 1960 and 1965 with urinary infections were being localized at cystoscopy with ureteral catheterization studies (Chapter 1) and then treated on the basis of tube dilution determinations of bacterial sensitivity (Chapter 2). It was a simple matter to observe that patients with renal infections were cured by antimicrobial agents like oral penicillin-G and nitrofurantoin that produced bactericidal concentrations in urine when the serum levels had to be negligible. These observations served to convince us that the concentration in urine, and not serum, determined the course of the infection. But the most useful drug that proved this principle to us repeatedly was oral penicillin-G.

As observed in Chapter 2, 113 strains of *E. coli* (Figure 2.3) isolated from our patients in 1963 and 1964 and 144 strains (Figure 2.8) isolated after 1965 showed the same results when placed in tube dilutions with penicillin-G: about 80% were killed by 100 μg/ml but no organisms were inhibited at 5 μg/ml. These tube dilutions were done in soy broth without serum and therefore mean that 5 μg/ml of free, unbound penicillin-G will not inhibit *E. coli*. Even a cursory knowledge of penicillin-G pharmacology[60–62] leads to the conclusion that 500 mg (800,000 units) of penicillin-G taken every 6 hours by mouth will not produce an average serum concentration of 0.5 μg/ml of biologically active antibiotic. The concentration of active penicillin-G in the urine, however, will rarely fall below 100 μg/ml. Thus, urinary infections caused by *E. coli*, treated with oral penicillin-G, proved ideal to test the question of whether serum or urinary levels determined cure. As summarized in Figure 10.8, treatment of *E. coli* urinary infections with oral penicillin-G means that the maximal level obtained in the serum is about one-tenth of that needed to inhibit the most sensitive *E. coli*! In brief, we reported in 1965[1] that oral penicillin-G is a remarkably effective drug for urinary infections, an effectiveness that has to be based solely on its urinary concentrations. Palmer, Neal, and I[63] measured the concentrations of penicillin-G in midstream voided urines from nine volunteers during a 48-hour course of oral penicillin-G (Figure 10.9). The mean concentration exceeded 100 μg/ml in every individual. The median antibiotic concentration, a statistic of perhaps greater therapeutic significance, also exceeded 100 μg/ml except in volunteer J.T., who was receiving probenecid because

Dosage	Serum Conc.	Minimal Urine Conc.
800,000 units Q 6 H	<0.5 μg/ml	100 μg/ml

Penicillin-G Conc.	% *E. coli* killed
5 μg/ml	0
100 μg/ml	85

Figure 10.8 A composite summary of the average serum and urine concentrations of penicillin-G that can be expected in a 70-kg adult with normal renal function (and an average urine flow rate) compared to the percentage of *Escherichia coli* killed at 5 and 100 μg/ml of penicillin-G. Thus, even 5 μg/ml of penicillin-G, which exceeds by at least 10 times the average serum level produced by 800,000 units (500 mg) of oral dosage, would not be enough to inhibit the most sensitive *E. coli*. The urinary level, however, is bactericidal to about 85% of strains of *E. coli*.

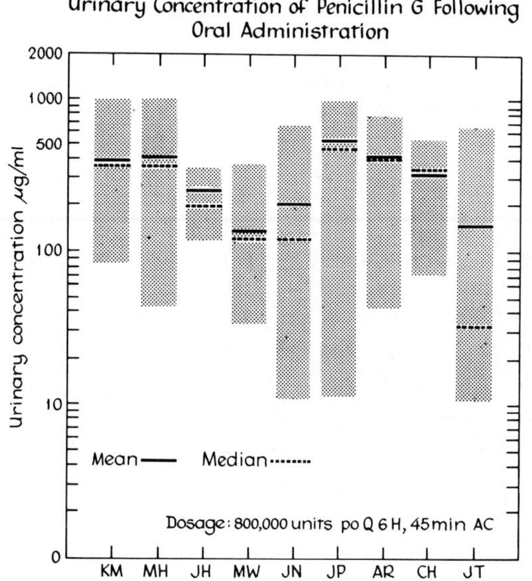

Figure 10.9 Urinary concentration of penicillin-G following oral administration. Bar graphs represent ranges in the concentration of penicillin-G obtained in midstream urines from nine volunteers who took 800,000 units of penicillin-G by mouth every 6 hours (45 minutes before ingestion of food). Mean and median levels are shown for each volunteer. J.T. was taking probenecid for gout. (Reproduced by permission from J. M. Palmer *et al.*, Progress in Antimicrobial and Anticancer Chemotherapy. Proceedings of the 6th International Congress of Chemotherapy, Vol. 1 Baltimore, University Park Press, 1970, p. 902.)

of gout. If penicillin-G sensitivities, then, are considered in terms of the urinary levels achieved during oral therapy, this drug becomes a "broad spectrum" antibiotic. Not only are 80% of *E. coli* killed by 100 µg/ml (Figures 2.3 and 2.8), but nearly 100% of *P. mirabilis* (Figures 2.5 and 2.10), all the enterococci, and about 25% of *Klebsiella* (Figures 2.4 and 2.9). These data, summarized graphically in Figure 10.10, are convincing that oral penicillin-G is a true "broad spectrum" antibiotic for infections of the urinary tract. The clinician, however, should realize that other penicillin derivatives (Figures 2.8 to 2.11), like penicillin-V and methicillin, are substantially inferior. Ampicillin, as seen in Figures 2.8–2.11, is more potent, but the difference at urinary

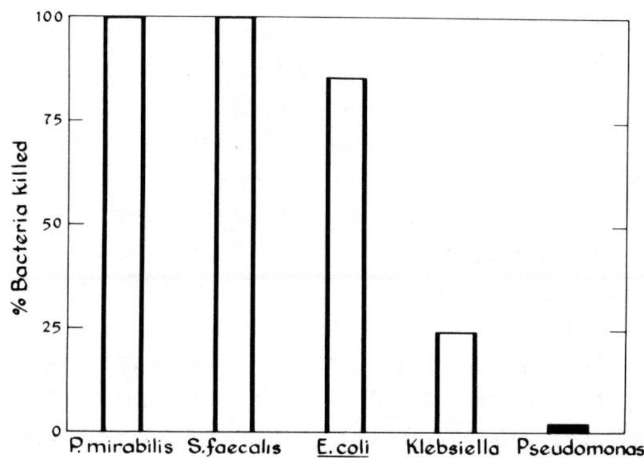

Figure 10.10 The percentage of *Proteus mirabilis*, enterococcus, *E. coli, Klebsiella*, and *Pseudomonas* killed in tube dilution studies (Figures 2.3–2.7, enterococci not shown) at the minimal urinary level of pencillin-G (100 µg/ml).

levels is small (Figure 2.8) and not worth the increased cost to the patient.

As apparent in Figure 10.8, the clinician cannot use penicillin-G for *E. coli* if he goes by the results of sensitivity testing; the Food and Drug Administration limits the content of penicillin-G discs to 10 µg, and therefore *E. coli* will always appear resistant. As seen in Chapter 2, Table 2.19, a disc content of at least 100 µg is required to detect the 80% of *E. coli* that are sensitive to the urinary concentrations of penicillin-G.

Tetracycline and *Pseudomonas*

The importance of urinary concentrations in determining cure of urinary infections is not limited to penicillin-G and nitrofurantoin. As I reviewed in Chapter 2 in discussing my concern with the Kirby-Bauer disc method of sensitivity testing, the choice of a 5 µg/ml level of tetracycline as a definition of sensitivity[59] can not be based on pharmacologic levels achieved in the serum during standard oral dosage regimens. If the true concentration of biologically active tetracycline actually achieved in the serum (<2.0 µg/ml) were honestly represented by *in vitro* sensitivity testing, almost none of the Gram-negative bacteria would ever be reported as sensitive. This would have excluded tetracycline from use in urinary infections, just as penicillin-G is excluded now because sensitivity discs reflect the serum levels. Figures 2.3–2.7 confirm that 1–2 μg/ml of either oxytetracycline or tetracycline are virtually never inhibitory for Gram-negative bacteria. Thus, the tetracyclines, like penicillin-G and nitrofurantoin, depend on urinary levels for their effectiveness in urinary infections. The average serum concentration in adult receiving oxytetracycline 250 mg orally every 6 hours[64] or tetracycline in the same dosage[65] is about 1.0 to 2.0 μg/ml, but the free unbound fraction is even less. The urinary concentrations average about 150 μg/ml and are slightly greater for oxytetracycline.[66]

Especially useful is the activity of tetracycline at urinary levels against *Pseudomonas*. In Figure 10.11, observe that strains of *Pseudomonas* are never inhibited by 5 μg of oxytetracycline and therefore will appear resistant to the standard disc used for sensitivity testing. But the 100 μg/ml urinary level of oxytetracycline (or tetracycline) is inhibitory for 80% of *Pseudomonas* strains (Figure 2.7). *Pseudomonas* urinary infections are not limited to those patients with complicated urinary tract disease, for we observe these infections in even outpatient girls and women. Indeed, we not infrequently find *Pseudomonas* transiently appearing on the vaginal introitus in patients susceptible to recurrent infections, indicating that the rectal flora is the reservoir. Whatever the cause, *Pseudomonas* urinary infections are not always complicated by stones or sites of persistence such as the prostate. Under these conditions, either tetracycline or oxytetracycline is ideal and is nearly always effective. Moreover, even low dosage tetracycline therapy can be extremely useful in keeping the bladder urine bactericidal and confining *Pseudomonas* to the prostatic fluid (Chapter 7). Indeed, one can make a good case for the following philosophy in treating *Pseudomonas* urinary infections: either the infection is uncomplicated and 5–10 days of tetracycline therapy will cure it, or the infection is caused by persistence of the *Pseudomonas* in stones or the prostate, in which event injectable drugs like tobramycin, the polymyxins, and gentamicin are most unlikely to cure the infection. The major use of these latter drugs in *Pseudomonas* infections of the urinary tract, then, is in the seriously ill patient who has bacteremia or septicemia, in which case they can be lifesaving; they are unlikely, however, to clear the infection permanently from its site of persistence in the urinary tract.

Dosage	Serum Conc.	Minimal Urine Conc.
250 mg Q 6 H	1-2 μg/ml	100 μg/ml

Oxytetracycline Conc.	% Pseudomonas killed
5 μg/ml	0
100 μg/ml	80

Figure 10.11 A composite summary of the average serum and urine concentrations of oxytetracycline that can be expected in a 70-kg adult with normal renal function (and an average urine flow rate) compared to the percentage of *E. coli* killed at 5 and 100 μg/ml of oxytetracycline. Although 5 μg/ml of oxytetracycline is not inhibitory to *Pseudomonas*, 100 μg/ml is bactericidal to 80% of the strains causing urinary infections.

Oral carbenicillin is of little use in *Pseudomonas* infections if the physician remembers that tetracycline is extraordinarily effective; indeed, the 20% of *Pseudomonas* that I see which are resistant to tetracycline have usually been resistant to carbenicillin as well.

For these reasons, it would be helpful if the clinician could know if *Pseudomonas* urinary infections are sensitive to the urinary level of the tetracyclines. From Table 2.19, however, this requires a tetracycline disc content of at least 100 μg. Until the Food and Drug Administration allows the manufacture of antimicrobial discs for urinary sensitivity testing, the practicing physician is excluded from an intelligent selection of these useful drugs for his patient. One of the advantages of a simple tube dilution system like that described in Figures 2.15 and 2.16 is that it allows the intelligent selection of drugs like penicillin-G for *E. coli* and tetracycline for *Pseudomonas*.

Sulfonamides

As every practicing clinician realizes, the sulfonamides are useful in the treatment of urinary infections. The two most commonly used ones in this country are sulfisoxazole and sulfamethizole. Both are "short-acting" in that they are rapidly excreted in the urine and they are primarily limited to the extracellular fluids in their distribution within the body. Sulfadimidine is the sulfonamide most used in England. As discussed in Chapter 7, diffusion into prostatic fluid (and across other epithelial membranes) is determined by the number of uncharged ions in the plasma (the pK_a of the sulfonamide). Because sulfisoxazole and sulfamethizole are relatively strong acids, their diffusion is limited to extracellular body fluids and they do not readily cross epithelial membranes. The pK_a of sulfadimidine, on the other hand, is near that of plasma and half its molecules are uncharged in plasma, accounting for its diffusion into prostatic fluid at a prostatic fluid to plasma ratio of 0.50. Sulfadimidine is not available in this country. It is interesting that in terms of sulfonamide diffusion, we are at a disadvantage in this country, in treating both bacterial prostatitis and meningococcal meningitis (the other major use of sulfonamide therapy where spinal fluid levels would clearly be helpful). Moreover, sulfadimidine does not accumulate in the plasma with renal failure,[67] undoubtedly due to the fact that so much of the drug is reabsorbed in the normal kidney that renal disease needs only to be associated with a decreased tubular reabsorption in order to maintain the plasma clearance.

Sulfonamides are usually inactivated by conjugation with acetate; the acetyl derivative is biologically inactive. This is important in terms of clinical usage because about 35% of sulfisoxazole is excreted in the urine as the acetyl derivative while less than 10% of sulfamethizole is inactivated.[68] On this basis alone, it is hard to justify the use of sulfisoxazole if sulfamethizole is available. It is historically interesting that sulfamethizole was first marketed as a 0.25-g tablet precisely because the activity in the urine was almost equivalent to 0.5 g sulfisoxazole. Apparently, however, the 0.25-g formulation was not acceptable to the prescribing profession. As soon as sulfamethizole was introduced as a 0.5-g tablet (the so-called "forte" preparation), sales increased substantially! While this story is hardly a credit to the rational use of antimicrobial drugs, it is worth noting that 0.5 g of sulfamethizole will produce nearly twice the urinary concentration of biologically active drug as 0.5 g of sulfisoxazole.

The activity of the clinically available sulfonamides, milligram for milligram of active drug in the urine, show few and insignificant variations.[69] There are substantial differences, however, in the susceptibility of the different species. *E. coli* is the most susceptible, followed by *Klebsiella*, *P. mirabilis*, and *Pseudomonas*; enterococci are resistant. Because virtually all nutrient broths contain *p*-aminobenzoic acid, which competitively blocks the action of sulfonamides on bacteria, susceptibility studies are best carried out by placing the sulfonamide in urine and adding the bacteria directly.[69]

In unpublished studies, we measured free, nonacetylated sulfamethizole in the 24-hour urine of 10 volunteers during the 4th day of therapy. Each volunteer received 250 mg of sulfamethizole four times a day, and the entire 24-hour urine output on the 4th day was collected and refrigerated. The mean concentration of active sulfonamide, using the Bratton and Marshall method,[70] was 688 μg/ml (range 355 to 1133 μg/ml). We then added sulfamethizole to normal. Millipore-filtered, pooled urine; the final concentrations, in two-fold dilution steps, varied between 1.56 and 800 μg/ml. To these urines, as well as a control aliquot containing no sulfonamide, we added 10 strains of *E. coli* sensitive to most antibiotics and 5 strains resistant to the urinary levels of most antibiotics, 10 unselected strains of *Klebsiella*, 10 strains of *Proteus* (5 indole-negative and 5 indole-positive), 5 strains of *P. aeruginosa*, and 5 strains each of *S. epidermidis* and enterococci. All bacterial strains were collected from patients with bacteriuria. The inoculum size varied between 1000 and 3000 bacteria/ml, and subcultures were performed at 0, 4, 8, 16, 24, 48, and 72 hours. All control urines had bacterial counts of >10^5/ml by the 8th hour and were turbid by 24 hours. The MIC was defined as the lowest concentration of sulfamethizole required to prevent bacterial growth to turbidity. The results are presented in Table 10.6. The 12 strains in the >800 μg/ml column showed turbid growth by 24 hours in all tubes, including the 800-μg tube, and undoubtedly represent a resistance to sulfonamides even at concentrations substantially greater than 800 μg/ml. Noteworthy are the total resistance of enterococci, the exquisite sensitivity of 4 out of 5 strains of *P. aeruginosa* (a fact which we have made good clinical use of in some patients), and the interesting observation that *E. coli* selected because of general resistance to antibiotics were more sensitive than *E. coli* exhibiting a high sensitivity to all antibiotics. These studies should be interpreted in terms of the mean sulfamethizole concentration (688 μg/ml) found in the urine of normal volunteers receiving 250 mg four times a day.

The sulfonamide disc technique, using Mueller-Hinton agar, as developed by Bauer and Sherris[71] is most useful for determining *in vitro* sensitivity, but Ericsson's quantitative disc technique described in Chapter 2 is equally applicable. We found that the distribution of sulfonamide sensitivities is so completely bimodal that we were unable to establish a regression curve; we read sulfonamide sensitivities on the Ericsson plate as either sensitive or resistant.

Sulfonamides differ from all other antimicrobial agents in the time required for their inhibitory action to stop bacterial growth. The growth curves of *E. coli* in soy broth, saline, and urine are shown in Figure 10.12 and compared to the growth curves in urine containing sulfamethizole at 50 and 400 μg/ml. In the first 3 hours of incubation with sulfamethizole, no effect on bacterial growth can be detected. Bacterial growth even continues during the 5th and 6th hours of incubation, albeit at a reduced rate compared to urine and soy broth containing no sulfonamide. Not until the 9th hour in the urine containing 400 μg/ml is there a definite decrease in bacterial numbers. This lack of inhibition during the first few hours is clearly different from other antimicrobial agents where, as in Figure 10.2, a decrease in viable bacteria can be detected after the first generation (within 1 hour). This characteristic of sulfonamides probably makes them unsuitable for use as a postintercourse antimicrobial agent.

Table 10.6
Minimal Inhibitory Concentration of Sulfamethizole for Urinary Pathogens

The minimal inhibitory concentration is defined as the first tube of urine that prevented bacterial growth to turbidity. The bacterial inoculum was between 1000 and 3000 bacteria/ml, and all control tubes (not shown in table) were turbid by 24 hours. The Millipore-filtered, pooled human urine to which the sulfamethizole was added had the following composition: osmolality 828 mOsm/liter, specific gravity 1.024, pH 6.4, creatinine concentration 256 mg/100 ml, Sodium 117 mEq/liter, and Potassium 123 mEq/liter.

Bacterial Strains Species and No. Tested	Concentration of Sulfamethizole in Urine, μg/ml										
	1.56	3.125	6.25	12.5	25	50	100	200	400	800	>800
10 "sensitive" *Escherichia coli*		1		3	1	3					2
5 "resistant" *E. coli*	3	2									
10 *Klebsiella*				1	2	2			1		4
10 *Proteus* species:											
5 *P. mirabilis*						2	1			2	
2 *P. vulgaris*					2						
3 *P. morganii*					2			1			
5 *Pseudomonas aeruginosa*	3	1									1
5 *Staphylococcus epidermidis*				3	1			1			
5 *Enterococcus*											5

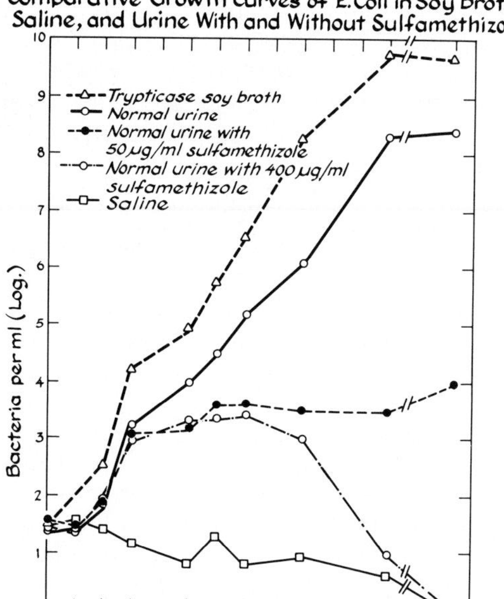

Figure 10.12 A strain of *Escherichia coli* was inoculated into trypticase soy broth, saline, and a Millipore-filtered aliquot of urine with and without sulfamethizole. During incubation at 37°C, subcultures were made every hour or two for 9 hours, at 12 hours, and at 24 hours. Bacterial growth in urine containing sulfamethizole paralleled the growth rate in control urine and soy broth for the first 3 hours, in sharp contrast to growth curves with other antimicrobial agents (Figure 10.2).

Sulfonamides are inexpensive, reasonably safe to use, and clearly useful in treating urinary infections. We have recently treated 50 consecutive bacteriuric outpatients with 250 mg of sulfamethizole four times a day without regard to the results of sensitivity testing. All patients had a culture on therapy and at least one culture 10 days after stopping therapy. The next 50 bacteriuric outpatients were all treated with 250 mg oxytetracycline four times a day and also without regard to the results of *in vitro* sensitivity testing. The results from both these studies are shown in Table 10.7, and the differences are not impressive. Other antimicrobial agents, such as penicillin-G or nitrofurantoin, may be better than oxytetracycline because only about 50% of *E. coli* are killed at the urinary levels of the tetracyclines (Figure 2.3). Since *E. coli* is the most common urinary pathogen, a rational use of antimicrobial agents would not include tetracycline as the first choice.

Nalidixic Acid

I have reviewed in both Chapters 2 and 4 some important aspects of our experience with nalidixic acid. The selection of resistant mutants seems to be, at least in part, a problem of under dosage (Figure 2.26)[72]; a good case can be made for forcing fluids to reduce the concentration of bacteria in the urine and then to give large doses of nalidixic acid (at least 4 g/day) for a few days depending upon the clinical setting of the bacteriuria. The effect on the vaginal and fecal flora is largely a beneficial one with clearance of Enterobacteriaceae from both reservoirs (Chapter 4). The place of nalidixic acid as a chemotherapeutic agent in the treatment of UTI probably rest with treatment of multiple-resistant Enterobacteriaceae since R factor plasmids do not carry resistance to nalidixic acid (Chapter 2).

The pharmacologic difficulty with nalidixic acid is that 95% of the urinary concentrations are inactive; the mean urinary level of 4 g/day is only about 75 µg/ml (Table 2.18). Cephalexin at this dosage, for example, would achieve several thousand micrograms/ml of urine. With nalidixic acid, then, large doses are needed if the MIC of infecting strains is to be exceeded by 10 to 20 times.

The medical profession will undoubtedly see a number of nalidixic acid-related antimicrobial agents introduced that have less inactivation in the urine and can be used in much smaller doses. One such drug is cinoxacin where 500-mg doses every 12 hours produces several hundred micrograms/ml of biologically active drug in the urine within the first four hours after dosing. Initial reports seem promising.

Cefoxitin

Because perirenal abscesses, intestinal fistulae, perineal abscesses, radiation abscesses, and other grossly complicated uri-

Table 10.7
Comparison of Sulfamethizole with Oxytetracycline in 100 Consecutive Bacteriuric Out-Patients

Drug and Dosage	No. of Patients Treated	No. Sterile on Therapy	No. Persisting on Therapy	No. Cured off Therapy[a]
Sulfamethizole				
250 mg q.i.d.	50	33/50	17/50	27/50
Oxytetracycline				
250 mg q.i.d.	50	29/48[b]	19/48[b]	31/50

[a] For purposes of this study, a cure was defined as a sterile urine 10 days or more after completing therapy.

[b] Two patients failed to obtain a culture during the 10 days of therapy but were cultured on later follow-up; both were sterile.

nary tracts are occasionally encountered with both anaerobic and aerobic bacterial infections, cefoxitin should be one drug in the antibiotic armamentarium of the hospital physician. It is a bactericidal antibiotic that inhibits Gram-positive cocci, Gram-negative bacilli, and most anaeorbic species. It must be used intravenously; most UTIs responded to 3 g of cefoxitin/day. Harold Neu[73] has an excellent review in 1979.

RENAL FAILURE AND ANTIMICROBIAL THERAPY

There are four aspects to renal failure in the treatment of urinary tract infections which every physician should remember.

The first is to make sure that treatment of the infection is really necessary. Unless there is symptomatic morbidity, the potential complications of therapy and the likelihood of therapeutic failure will often outweigh the potential benefit to the patient. I have already emphasized that the major causes of progressive renal deterioration are usually hypertension or analgesic abuse and not bacteriuria *per se*. The improvement in the serum creatinine in patient B.E. (Figure 10.3 and Table 10.1) is an exception to this general observation.

The second consideration is the therapeutic difficulties imposed by the renal failure in delivering enough antimicrobial agent into the urine to sterilize the infection. I have repeatedly emphasized throughout this book that the urine must be sterilized during therapy if the patient is to have a chance to bacteriologic cure: I know of no greater obstacle to achieving a sterile urine than the presence of renal failure with its accompanying diminutive urinary concentrations. Moreover, minimal urinary levels also encourage the emergence of resistant clones, which is not uncommon in the treatment of bacteriuria of renal failure.

The third important aspect, of course, is to adjust the dose of the antimicrobial agent and the interval between doses in such a way that adequate serum levels are obtained without producing cumulative systemic toxicity. These adjustments in dosage depend on the specific antimicrobial agent and the degree of renal failure. A number of antibiotics like doxycycline and chloramphenicol are hardly affected by renal failure whereas the aminoglycosides are greatly affected. Cephalexin is one of the few antimicrobial agents that can achieve reasonable urinary concentration without too much risk of systemic toxicity[74, 75]; intravenous penicillin-G in large doses is another excellent choice. McHenry and his associates[76] give excellent guidelines for using gentamicin in the presence of renal failure. Kunin[77] has an old, but excellent publication which I always find useful in selecting appropriate dosage schedules for several antimicrobial agents.

The fourth and last aspect every clinician must keep in mind when treating UTI in the presence of renal failure is the potential for antibiotic damage to already damaged kidneys. Many antimicrobial agents exhibit no nephrotoxicity for normal kidneys but can be devastating to already damaged nephrons. Since most of these patients can ill-afford further renal deterioration, the wise physician will be very careful. The aminoglycosides, cephaloridine, and cephalothin are all nephrotoxic. TMP-SMX may be nephrotoxic[78] in the presence of azotemia, but the issue is controversial[79]; it is also complicated by the possibility that

TMP may interfere with the tubular secretion of creatinine and thereby give a false indication of increasing azotemia.

FUNGURIA

Candida albicans, *Candida* species, and *Torulopsis glabrata* are pathogenic yeasts for man. While they do not occur in the normal urinary tract, they are present in the healthy oral cavity, the intestinal tract (including the stomach), and the vagina. For example, 10–20% of all our vaginal cultures from healthy, control women contain *Candida* species, usually *C. albicans*, and most of them deny any history of vaginitis.

Candida and *Torulopsis* invade the urinary tract of the female by the ascending route—rectum, vagina, urethra, bladder, kidney—in all probability, but the intestinal, lymphatic, thoracic duct, and blood stream cannot be excluded in some instances. For example, in the fascinating paper by Krause, Matheis, and Wulf,[80] a healthy volunteer ingested 80 g of *C. albicans*; blood cultures were positive at 3 and 6 hours while urine cultures were positive after 2-¾ and 3-¼ hours.

The 20–30% normal carriage of *Candida* in fecal cultures rises substantially in patients treated with antibiotics, especially the tetracyclines (see Chapter 4).

The predisposing factors to funguria have been known for years; they are antibiotic treatment, indwelling catheters, and probably duration of hospitalization.[81] In immunosuppressed patients, fungal infections are often disasterous; 10% of the 51% of renal transplants, who had fungi cultured from superficial sites, developed serious complications.[82] The susceptibility of these immunosuppressed patients, including other patients who have blood dyscrasias—especially leukopenia—from any cause, is easy to understand because the leukocyte is apparently the primary host defense mechanism against fungi.[83] In addition to cortisone and cytotoxic agents—including radiation therapy—it is well recognized that diabetics are especially prone to funguria. The most difficult patients we treat at Stanford with renal funguria are diabetic patients with papillary necrosis, sometimes complicated by analgesic abuse.

Except for these patients with papillary necrosis and renal funguria—and immunosuppressed patients of all kinds, of course—urinary tract funguria is a relatively benign suprainfection that disappears with discontinuation of antibiotics and indwelling catheters in most patients.

Candiduria can persist for years in the urinary tract, even with substantial pyuria, but apparently cause little damage, as clearly demonstrated by the clinical course of patient A.N. in Chapter 8, Figures 8.8–8.20; at every culture and urinalysis since removal of her bilateral staghorn calculi in September 1971, she has had about 5000 *C. albicans* in her urine accompanied by gross pyuria. She reminds me that the physician should not forget that funguria is rarely accompanied by 10^5 colony-forming-units/ml of urine, and hence bladder aspiration or catheterization is usually required to distinguish funguria from urinary contamination with vaginal *Candida*. Because candiduria can occur in small numbers and cause pyuria, funguria is one of the causes of "sterile" pyuria where the low numbers on culture are considered contaminants.

Some patients are symptomatic either from the aggregation of fungi to form large masses in the urinary tract—the so-called bezoars—or from the classic symptoms of cystitis, pyelonephritis, or even septicemia. Schönebeck[83] found that 14 of the 29 bezoars in his material occurred in diabetics; the rest were on antibiotics or were immunosuppressed.

Treatment is limited to systemic amphotericin-B (which is highly nephrotoxic) or 5-fluorocytosine which is virtually 100% excreted in the urine and relatively nontoxic. The disadvantage of the latter is the substantial resistance which can occur during therapy. Nevertheless, 5-fluorocytosine is the first line of therapy; where possible all antibiotics should be stopped and certainly indwelling catheters removed before 5-fluorocytosine therapy is begun. The recommended dose is 50 mg/kg body weight every 6 hours[83]; with renal failure, the dose must be reduced proportionally.

We have had little experience with systemic amphotericin-B therapy because the patients in whom we have needed it already have damaged kidneys. On the other hand, we have had substantial success in using amphotericin-B as a local irrigant in both upper and lower tract candidiasis. The infections are first localized as with *E. coli* (Chapter 1). If the kidneys are infected, we place two Stamey polyethylene ureteral catheters—one small and one large—for continuous irrigation as described for disolving struvite infection stones in Chapter 8. I realize that the experimental data and common sense would indicate that the *Candida* must be in the distal tubules and that this therapy should be doomed to failure. This has not been the case and it can be recommended in certain clinical situations.

In concluding this section, I wish to point out that almost everything the physician needs to know about funguria is contained in the 1972 monograph by Jan Schönebeck[83]; it is carefully written, informative, and I consult it frequently.

ANTIBACTERIAL MANAGEMENT OF PROSTATECTOMY

There is no excuse for patients to have a prostatectomy in the presence of an infected urine. There are several antimicrobial drugs available—gentamicin, tobramycin, cephalothin, cefoxitin, TMP-SMX, cephalexin—to name only a few, that are capable of sterilizing the urine if therapy is begun 24 hours prior to prostatectomy. The rewards are obvious: less fever, bacteremia, and no septicemia.

One cause of bacteremia and postoperative fever in the presence of a sterile midstream urine needs to be discussed. About 5% of men carry Enterobacteriaceae on their urethra even though the midstream urine is sterile (Chapter 7). Although many of these men could be detected by recovering small numbers of Enterobacteriaceae in their midstream urine, the widespread bacteriologic practice of culturing urine with a calibrated wire loop of 0.01 or 0.001 ml volume will prevent detection of this pathogenic colonization. Urethral colonization with Enterobacteriaceae or enterococci is the major cause of fever, bacteremia, and UTI in the immediate postoperative period following transurethral prostatectomy.

My own practice is to always culture the first voided bladder (VB_1) urines as well as midstream (VB_2) urines in the preoperative evaluation for a prostatectomy. If the VB_1 urine is positive for Enterobacteriaceae or enterococcus, the patients receive 80 mg of gentamicin (or tobramycin) the evening before surgery and on call to the operating room the next morning. If enterococci are present, I use ampicillin or a cephalosporin in the same regimen. I also give one or two, but no more, 80-mg doses postoperatively at 8-hour intervals.

If the VB_1 and VB_2 urines preoperatively contain only normal indigenous bacteria from the urethra, I do not give preoperative or intraoperative antimicrobial therapy unless there is a danger of causing bacterial endocarditis on a diseased or prosthetic heart valve.

As will be seen in the next and last section of this book, the clinical rule should be never to treat a patient with antimicrobial therapy while an indwelling catheter is present in the bladder unless the patient has systemic signs of toxicity from his infection. In the presence of a foreign body, antibiotics can only select resistant strains. One of the difficult questions, however, is whether a patient who has had a prostatectomy should be given prophylactic antimicrobial therapy when the bladder catheter is removed. Theoretically, if the VB_1 and VB_2 urines were sterile before prostatectomy, and if a catheter-aspirated urine is sterile at the time the urethral catheter is removed, there should be no reason to prophylactically treat the male patient. Unfortunately, I have had the rare patient who—with all those sterile urine cultures—develops fever to 104°F, epididymitis, and UTI with *E. coli* within 48 hours of removing the Foley catheter. It is obvious that a sterile urine aspirated from a Foley prior to removal does not assure the surgeon there are no *E. coli* or other pathogens along the outside of the catheter on the urethra. Indeed, the study by Hills *et al.*[84] shows that full dosage antimicrobial therapy with even as powerful a drug as TMP-SMX will not change the pathogens in the periurethral catheter area. The rather dramatic interruption of an otherwise benign postprostatectomy course by chills and epididymitis, which surely can be prevented by oral antimicrobial agents started at the time of removing the Foley catheter, only has to happen to you once or twice before you become an advocate of short-term antimicrobial prophylaxis at the time the catheter is removed. For this reason, I start my patients on TMP-SMX or nitrofurantoin simultaneously with removal of the indwelling catheter.

There are some well-documented, highly effective regimens in the literature of the last 15 years, especially in the prophylactic management of patients undergoing prostatectomy who have a sterile urine prior to surgery. Before reviewing these regimens, however, I would like to outline my own management because it is somewhat more inclusive than some reports. I can assure the practicing physician that if he follows the regimen outlined below, bacteremia and septicemia will be almost nonexistent and very few of his prostatectomy patients who were sterile before surgery will be infected afterwards.

I. For patients whose prostatism occurs in the absence of bacteriuria, make sure the VB_1 urine contains only normal urethral bacteria before admission to the hospital. If this is impractical, or made impossible by the calibrated-loop methodology of the bacteriologic laboratory, assume the urethra is colonized with Enterobacteriaceae and follow this regimen:

(1) Give 80 mg of gentamicin or tobramycin the night before surgery and on call to the operating room the next morning.

(2) Postoperatively, give two additional 80-mg doses at 8-hour intervals from the time of the "on call" dose.

(3) When the Foley catheter is removed, and not before, start TMP-SMX at full dosage, 160 mg of TMP and 800 mg of SMX, every 12 hours for 5 days followed by 1 tablet (80/400 mg) each day for an additional 5 days. Since most patients will be discharged 24 hours after removing the Foley catheter, this regimen should mean that TMP-SMX is administered in the hospital for not more than 24 hours before discharge. The 4 doses of gentamicin will not cause fecal resistance because it is not an oral drug and cannot influence the rectal bacteria. Widespread use of TMP-SMX in the hospital could cause resistance and should be avoided; for this reason, the urologist should try to limit therapy with TMP-SMX to the 24 hour period before discharge.

II. For patients whose prostatism is accompanied by bacteriuria without an indwelling catheter, and whose kidneys are free of calculi or other causes of persistent bacteriuria (see Chapter 9), the regimen should be as follows:

(1) Give 80 mg of gentamicin or tobramycin the evening before and on call to the operating room providing the infecting organism is sensitive to aminoglycosides; if it is resistant, use the safest injectable antimicrobial agent suggested by the sensitivities. One milligram per killogram per 8 hours of gentamicin is adequate dosage for UTI.

(2) Continue the same injectable antimicrobial agent throughout the hospitalization with due regard for renal function and potential systemic toxicity in the presence of azotemia.

(3) At discharge, start the patient on TMP-SMX, as above, at full dosage for 5 days followed by 5 additional days of one tablet each day; if the preoperative infection was caused by *Pseudomonas*, the discharge antimicrobial agent should be tetracycline rather than TMP-SMX.

III. If the catheter cannot be removed the day before surgery (starting gentamicin the moment it is removed), the regimen outlined in II is probably adequate. The disadvantage of leaving the catheter indwelling is that systemic antimicrobial therapy will not be as effective in sterilizing the pathogenic flora between the catheter and the urethral mucosa; for this reason, epididymitis and bacteremic fevers may not be wholly prevented.

The incidence of bacteriuria following prostatectomy in untreated patients whose urine was sterile preoperatively is reported to be 26–70%.[85–90] Gonzalez *et al.*,[89] using parenteral cephalothin preoperatively and for a short period postoperatively followed by cephalexin for 10 days, and Morris *et al.*,[88] using preoperative kanamycin followed by 3 weeks of TMP-SMX, simultaneously reported that the postoperative incidence of bacteriuria could be reduced to about 5%. The secret to these results, as opposed to other postoperative prophylactic studies,[86, 87] undoubtedly lies with the institution of antibiotic therapy *before* surgery (in keeping with basic prophylactic principles) as well as the continuation of therapy for a brief period after removal of the catheter. Plorde *et al.*[85] reported only a 7.7% incidence of bacteriuria in patients receiving kanamycin, 0.5 g preoperatively and every 8 hours until removal of the catheter; the numbers, however, were small (1 out of 12 patients).

Matthew and his associates,[90] following up on their cephalosporin studies,[89] reported on 87 patients undergoing transurethral prostatectomy. Of the 40 who received no prophylaxis, 13 developed bacteriuria by the fourth postoperative week (33%); of the 47 patients who received 100 mg of nitrofurantoin macrocrystals 6 hours before surgery and three times daily until the tenth postoperative day, *none* of the 42 patients for whom cultures were available developed bacteriuria! How do you beat that?

The key, then, is probably a combination of preoperative dosage to clear the urethra *prior* to transurethral resection and to continue the prophylaxis at least 10 days into the postoperative period.

Hills *et al.*[84] conducted the only double-blind trial of prophylaxis of which I am aware. Nineteen of 36 patients (53%) who received placebo developed bacteriuria, while only 2 of 38 (5%) who were treated with full dosage TMP-SMX from the morning of surgery until discharge from the hospital became bacteriuric. Each patient received their first treatment prior to, but on the morning of surgery; all were cultured every other day for 10 days. It is clear from this careful study that postprostatectomy infections can be virtually eliminated in the immediate postoperative period. I am concerned, however, as were the authors, that this practice on a urologic ward would soon negate the usefulness of TMP-SMX because of bacterial resistance. I prefer, as outlined above, to use an injectable drug which cannot cause intestinal resistance in the hospital and follow it with TMP-SMX on discharge or 24 hours before in those cases who were sterile prior to surgery.

To be sure, it can be argued that each infection could be treated as it develops, but this is an older population of patients and should be spared the morbidity of symptomatic infections as well as the occasional death from septicemia.

MANAGEMENT OF INDWELLING URINARY CATHETER

Bacteriuria occurs soon after placement of an indwelling catheter in most patients; it occurs sooner in females than males if the catheter is placed through the urethra. Bacteriuria can be greatly delayed if the catheter is passed percutaneously through the suprapubic area—far removed from the contaminated perineum—into the bladder. For this reason, acute urinary retention should be relieved by a percutaneous suprapubic tube when possible rather than by a urethral catheter. In the male, passage of the percutaneous tube with local anesthesia is less painful than passage of a urethral catheter and, more importantly, avoids potential trauma to the urethra and prostate; without trauma, the patient is more likely to urinate later if edema of the urethra and prostate have been avoided. Lastly, placement of a percutaneous suprapubic tube allows the patient to be tested for voiding capability without recatheterization; the suprapubic tube is simply clamped until the bladder is full and, if the patient is unable to void, the tube is unclamped. Removal and reinsertion of Foley catheters in those who cannot void can be difficult for the patient and potentially dangerous in terms of bacteremia. For these reasons, we have designed a Malecot-like, winged catheter that can be placed directly through the suprapubic skin into the full bladder with 5–10 ml of local anesthesia. A hollow needle obturator allows the physician to know when he is within the bladder before removing the obturator and allowing the Malecot wings to re-expand (Figure 10.13). The 14 Fr size has a urine flow rate capacity of 400 ml/minute and is no more difficult to introduce than the 10 Fr size. This percutaneous suprapubic catheter can be obtained from Vance Products, Inc., 165 South Main Street, Spencer, IN 47460.

When a conventional catheter must be passed through the urethra, it should be connected to a closed drainage system. How do bacteria reach the bladder if the closed system is intact, besides the obvious route of direct inoculation of urethral bacteria at the time of catheterization? There are two obvious routes: one is directly up the inside of the catheter from the bag reservoir once the reservoir becomes infected, and the other is periurethral colonization at the urethral meatus and ascent up the outside of the catheter. Almost all investigators have observed a relationship between the duration of catheter drainage and the development of bacteriuria. In the 1977 study of males by Islam and Chapman,[91] for example, there was a 9% infection rate when the catheter was *in situ* for no longer than 3 days but a 50% rate when maintained for longer than 6 days.

Bultitude and Eykyn[92] investigated the ascent of bacteria outside the urethral catheter in males undergoing prostatectomy. Periurethral swabs were compared bacteriologically to the results of catheter aspi-

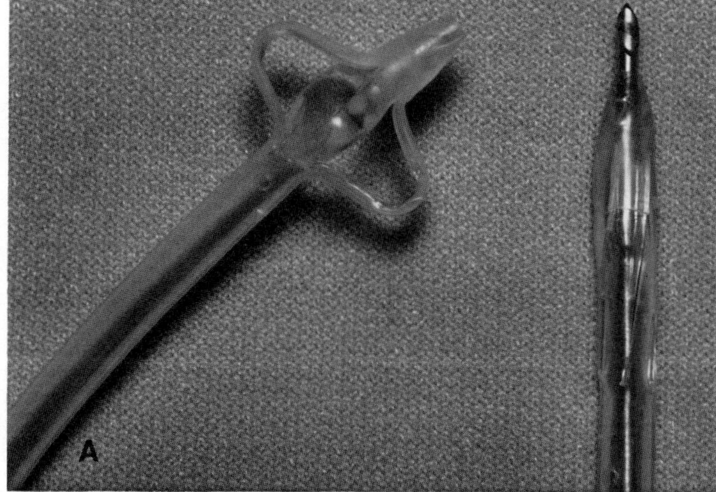

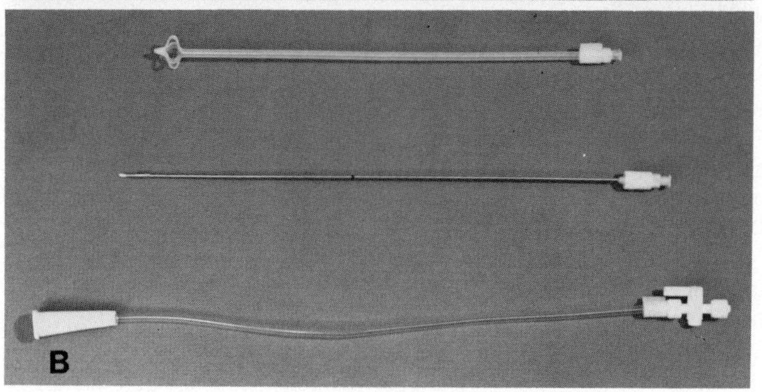

Figure 10.13 The Stamey percutaneous suprapubic catheter. *A*, The four open wings of the Malecot-like polyethelene catheter are shown on the *left*. On the *right*, the needle obturator has been introduced down the inside of the catheter prior to suprapubic puncture. Upon withdrawal of the hollow, needle obturator, the catheter assumes the position seen on the left. *B*, The catheter set is comprised of the catheter (*top*), the needle obturator which Leur-locks into the catheter upon insertion and straightening of the open Malecot wings (*middle*), and the connecting tubing with the Teflon valve on one end to Leur-lock to the catheter, and a polyvinyl connector which fits any form of drainage tubing on the other end (*bottom*).

ration. Twenty-five of the 56 patients developed bacteriuria; in 17 of the 25, the bacteria infecting the bladder were the same ones previously cultured from the urethra. In most instances, the periurethral organism reached the bladder in 1–3 days.

Maizels and Schaeffer[93] have recently studied 31 consecutive acute spinal cord injury patients from the time of admission with sterile urine to the time of bacteriuria from their indwelling catheter. By sampling daily the periurethral bacteria at the meatus, the urine in the catheter, and the urine in the bag, they determined that the closed system drainage bag was the reservoir for ascending infection in 32% of bacteriuric episodes and that this route of bladder infection could be completely prevented by periodically placing 30 ml of 3% hydrogen peroxide into the drainage bag. This interesting and potentially useful investigation deserves careful study.

Continuous irrigation of three-way Foley catheters with a neomycin-polymyxin solution was no better than nonirrigated catheters in preventing acquired bacteriuria.[94]

Except for the studies by Bultitude and Eykyn[92] and Maizels and Schaeffer[93] I am unaware of any work since 1972 which has served to elucidate further the pathogenesis or the prevention of catheter-induced infections. Schaeffer's investigations at Northwestern make me believe that the opportunities for tracing the bacteria from the time of catheterization to the occurrence of bacteriuria have not been as exploited as they should have been. With better understanding of the pathogenesis of catheter-induced bacteriuria will come better preventive medicine, as Schaeffer has already suggested with hydrogen peroxide.

Because there is little else that is new in the care of the indwelling catheter, I would like to repeat what Dr. E. M. Meares, Jr., now Professor and Chairman of Urology at Tufts University in Boston, wrote in 1971 when he was an Assistant Professor of Urology here at Stanford serving on the Infection Control Board of the Stanford University Hospital. He was responsible for instituting a "closed" system of urinary catheter drainage throughout the hospital at that time. His practical and scholarly essay was distributed to all physicians and nurses. The 15 references for general reading that accompanied Dr. Meares's remarks appear in the bibliography at the end of this chapter as reference numbers 95–109. The following is his report, reproduced verbatim.

The indwelling urethral catheter continues to play an indispensable role in medical care. In 1958 Beeson pointed out that the urethral catheter was a serious cause of morbidity and mortality. Although his article initially resulted in unfounded fears of the catheter by many internists (many would withhold urethral catheterization at all costs) and cries of heresy from surgeons and urologists, its overall effect was to stimulate a decade of renewed interest in the indications for and management of the indwelling urethral catheter. Despite continuing controversy regarding urethral catheterization, two undeniable facts remain: (1) urethral catheters are sources of patient morbidity and mortality, and (2) urethral catheterization is mandatory for the management of a variety of medical conditions; indeed, morbidity and mortality may result from the injudicious avoidance of urethral catheterization.

The logical answers to this controversy are (1) the indications for urethral catheterization must be sound, (2) strict principles of asepsis and atraumatic catheterization must be employed, (3) every effort must be made throughout the period of catheter drainage to prevent catheter-induced infections, and (4) the physician must ensure that the patient is left with a sterile urinary tract after the catheter is removed.

Kass and many others have clearly shown that 95–100% of patients develop significant bacteriuria within 96 hours of "open" urinary catheter drainage. Although intermittent catheter irrigation by the "open technique" (the catheter is disconnected from the drainage tubing and is irrigated via a syringe) is occasionally necessary to unplug the catheter and assure proper drainage, experience has shown that intermittent irrigation with saline, acid solutions, or various antibiotic solutions is generally ineffective in preventing or clearing bacteriuria. This technique, indeed, often *induces* bacteriuria.

Several investigators have shown that the morbidity associated with temporary indwelling catheterization is significantly reduced by the use of either a strictly closed system of urinary drainage or a three-way Foley catheter with *continuous* bladder irrigation with an antibiotic solution (such as 40 mg of neomycin and 20 mg of polymyxin in 1000 ml of isotonic saline). So effective was the latter that Martin reported a 24% reduction in annual Gram-negative bacteremias, a 48% reduction in Gram-negative bacteremias secondary to acute pyelonephritis, and a 46% reduction in annual deaths from Gram-negative bacteremia at the Jersey City Medical Center. Kunin has reported similarly impressive results in his study of the closed urinary drainage system at the University of Virginia. Several investigators have found that cultures taken from the drainage bag are often positive from 1–6 days before cultures taken by catheter aspiration become positive, indicating that infection of the bag urine actually precedes infection of the bladder urine. Roberts has shown that, in addition to closed drainage, the addition of a small quantity of 10% formalin to the drainage receptacle is highly effective in preventing catheter-induced bladder infections. Webb and Blandy have found that, in addition to closed drainage, the addition of 10 ml of 5% chlorhexidine (Hibitane) to disposable plastic bags with one-way valves at the junction of the drainage tubing with the drainage bag likewise significantly reduces the incidence of catheter-induced bacteriuria.

The establishment of a closed system on a hospital-wide basis does require the active cooperation of everyone—physicians, nurses, orderlies, technicians, aides, students, and the patients themselves. Although such a system probably has merit for all patients who have indwelling catheters, the main objective is to assure maximum protection for those patients who require only temporary catheter drainage (1–30 days). While the principles of closed drainage are simple, they require strict adherence.

Catheterization Technique: (1) Catheterization of male patients should be done only by a physician or a person who is thoroughly familiar with aseptic, atraumatic catheterization techniques. (2) The genitalia should be thoroughly cleansed with pHisoHex or other suitable antibacterial agents. (3) Fresh draping is then applied and the physician changes to fresh sterile gloves. (4) To protect against inducing urethral pathogens into the bladder, it is recommended that a tube (5 g) of Lubasporin ointment should be instilled into the urethra. (5) Some two to three minutes after Lubasporin has been instilled into the urethra, a well lubricated #16 or #18 French Foley catheter, which is already attached to the drainage tubing and drainage bag, is gently passed through the urethra into the bladder. If the catheter does not pass easily, force should not be used; instead, a sterile water soluble lubricant (such as Lubafax or K-Y Jelly) is gently injected through the urethra via a sterile asepto syringe. Inability to pass the catheter after this maneuver probably means that a urethral stricture or other forms of urethral pathology exist. At this point, the physician may want to seek urological consultation. Every effort should be made to minimize urethral trauma. (6) The Foley balloon should not be inflated until the physician is sure that the catheter is draining properly and that it is actually within the bladder. Inflation of the balloon within the urethra is painful to the patient and causes urethral trauma. (7) If the patient is uncircumcised, the foreskin should be properly replaced over the glans penis. Paraphymosis may develop if the foreskin is allowed to remain retracted. (8) The catheter should be taped to the patient's abdomen and the bag should be attached to the patient's bed to assure good dependent urinary drainage. Taping the catheter to the patient's leg causes a pressure point on the urethra at the penoscrotal angle and can eventually lead to formation of a urethrocutaneous fistula.

Closed Urinary Drainage: (1) The catheter should already be attached to the drainage apparatus at the time of catheterization. (2) Strictly aseptic technique must be used for catheterization. (3) To prevent residual urine within the bladder and to minimize the time required for urine to traverse the drainage apparatus and enter the drainage bag, free flow through the system must be assured. (4) If the catheter is plugged and not draining, the system should be checked for kinks or other mechanical causes of obstruction. Gentle milking of the drainage tubing will often unplug the catheter and make irrigation unnecessary. Should this fail, however, strictly aseptic technique must be used to disconnect the catheter from the drainage tubing and to gently irrigate the catheter with sterile saline via a syringe. If this is successful in unplugging the catheter, the end of the catheter and the end of the drainage tube should be rinsed with alcohol prior to reunion. If irrigation of the catheter fails to reestablish satisfactory drainage, the entire system probably needs to be replaced. (5) Since the urine within the drainage bag is considered contaminated, at no time should the bag be raised above the level of the patient's bladder; reflux of contaminated urine into the bladder from the bag will otherwise occur. (6) The air chamber that connects the distal drainage tubing to the drainage bag must be in the vertical, upright position at all times.

(7) The drainage bag must be emptied from the *bottom* often enough to assure that urine cannot back up in the system above the level of the air chamber. Since the better drainage bags hold 2000 ml of urine, the bags rarely require emptying oftener than once every eight hours (or once per nursing shift). (8) The system ordinarily should not require replacement oftener than every 10–14 days; however, urethral catheters should usually be changed after 14 days of closed drainage. Some physicians may prefer to change the catheter after 7–10 days. (9) Although the urometer drainage apparatus facilitates the monitoring of hourly urinary outputs, everyone must realize that this apparatus is not a closed system of urinary drainage. Patients who have compromised renal function are often the very patients who will benefit the most from a strictly closed system of urinary drainage. Each physician must, therefore, carefully weigh the slight convenience of urometer drainage against the extra protection afforded by closed urinary drainage. (10) Ascending infection along the urethra can be minimized by good perineal care, frequent cleansing of the mucous secretions from the urinary meatus, and application of Lubasporin ointment about the meatus every eight hours. (11) Since disconnecting the catheter from the drainage tubing opens the system, the preferred way to obtain urine cultures from the bladder of a patient who is under closed urinary drainage is needle aspiration of the catheter itself. The technique suggested consists of cross-clamping the drainage tubing near the junction with the catheter, swabbing the hub of the catheter with an alcohol sponge, and aspirating a small volume of urine by using a 25-gauge needle attached to a sterile 2-ml syringe. One should not aspirate the shaft of the catheter, lest the Foley bag be accidentally deflated. (12) The routine use of oral or parenteral antibiotics *during the time* of closed urinary drainage is controversial and must be left to the individual physician's discretion. It is the responsibility of each physician, however, to assure that the patient is left with a sterile urinary tract following the discontinuation of urinary catheter drainage.

Continuous Catheter Irrigation: Continuous bladder irrigation via a closed three-way catheter system may have special merit for specific patients. Because of the expense of three-way catheters, the expense of the irrigant, and the extra attention required of the nursing staff to maintain such a system, this system should probably be reserved for selected patients. The use of this system is an accepted form of closed urinary drainage, however, and can be used if the physician desires.

Summary: Experience has shown that the morbidity and mortality associated with indwelling urethral catheters can be minimized by use of closed urinary drainage. Important features of aseptic, atraumatic urethral catheterization and closed urinary drainage have been outlined and rationale for closed urinary drainage has been discussed. The need for total cooperation of all hospital personnel in making the system work has been stressed.

REFERENCES

1. Stamey, T. A., Govan, D. E., and Palmer, J. M.: The localization and treatment of urinary tract infections: The role of bactericidal urine levels as opposed to serum levels. Medicine **44:** 1, 1965.
2. Stamey, T. A.: Office bacteriology. J. Urol. **97:** 926, 1967.
3. Stamey, T. A., Fair, W. R., Timothy, M. M., Millar, M. A., Mihara, G., and Lowery, Y. C.: Serum versus urinary antimicrobial concentrations in cure of urinary-tract infections. N. Engl. J. Med. **291:** 1159, 1974.
4. Garrod, L. P., Shooter, R. A., and Curwen, M. P.: The results of chemotherapy in urinary infections. Br. Med. J. **2:** 1003, 1954.
5. Williams, J. D., Reeves, D. S., Condie, A. P., Franklin, I. S. N., Leigh, D. A., and Brumfitt, W.: The treatment of bacteriuria in pregnancy. In F. O'Grady and W. Brumfitt (Eds.), Urinary Tract Infection. London, Oxford University Press, 1968, p. 160.
6. Kraft, J. K., and Stamey, T. A.: The natural history of symptomatic recurrent bacteriuria in women. Medicine **56:** 55, 1977.
7. Kunin, C. M.: The natural history of recurrent bacteriuria in schoolgirls. N. Engl. J. Med. **282:** 1443, 1970.
8. Govan, D. E., Fair, W. R., Friedland, G. W., and Filly, R. A.: Management of children with urinary tract infections. The Stanford Experience. Urology **6:** 273, 1975.
9. Kincaid-Smith, P., and Fairley, K. F.: Controlled trial comparing effect of two and six weeks' treatment in recurrent urinary tract infection. Br. Med. J., **2:** 145, 1969.
10. Kincaid-Smith, P., Friedman, A., and Nanra, R. S.: Controlled trials of treatment in urinary tract infection. In P. Kincaid-Smith and K. F. Fairley (Eds.) Renal Infection and Renal Scarring. Melbourne, Mercedes Publishing Co., 1970, p. 165.
11. Bergstrom, T., Lincoln, K., Redin, B., and Winberg, J.: Studies of urinary tract infections in infancy and childhood. X. Short or long-term treatment in girls with first or second-time urinary tract infections uncomplicated by obstructive urological abnormalities. Acta Paediatr. Scand. **57:** 186, 1968.

12. Grüneberg, R. N., Brumfitt, W.: Single-dose treatment of acute urinary tract infection: A controlled trial. Br. Med. J. **3:** 649, 1967.
13. Williams, J. D., Smith, E. K.: Single-dose therapy with streptomycin and sulfametopyrazine for bacteriuria during pregnancy. Br. Med. J. **4:** 651, 1970.
14. Brumfitt, W., Faiers, M. C., and Franklin, I. N. S.: The treatment of urinary infection by means of a single dose of cephaloridine. Postgrad. Med. J. **46:** Suppl: 65, 1970.
15. Ronald, A. R., Boutros, P., and Mourtada, H.: Bacteriuria localization and response to single-dose therapy in women. J. Am. Med. Assoc. **235:** 1854, 1976.
16. Fang, L. S. T., Tolkoff-Rubin, N. E., and Rubin, R. H.: Efficacy of single-dose and conventional amoxicillin therapy in urinary-tract infection localized by the antibody-coated bacteria technic. N. Engl. J. Med. **298:** 413, 1978.
17. Bailey, R. R., Abbott, G. D.: Treatment of urinary tract infection with a single dose of amoxycillin. Nephron **18:** 316, 1977.
18. Bailey, R. R., Abbott, G. D.: Treatment of urinary tract infection with a single dose of trimethoprim-sulfamethoxazole. Can. Med. Assoc. J. **118:** 551, 1978.
19. Ludwig, P., Buckwold, F., Harding, G., Ronald, A., Thompson, L., Slutchuk, M., and Shaw, J.: Single dose therapy of acute cystitis in adult females: prospective randomized comparison of four regimens (Abstract No. 58). Presented at the 18th Interscience Conference on Antimicrobial Agents and Chemotherapy, Boston, American Society for Microbiology, 1979.
20. Mabeck, C. E.: Treatment of uncomplicated urinary tract infection in non-pregnant women. Postgrad. Med. J. **48:** 55, 1972.
21. Nielsen, M. L., Laursen, H., and Christensen, P.: Control of bacteriuria with sulphamethoxazole-trimethoprim in patients with urinary tract obstruction and chronic infection. Scand. J. Urol. Nephrol. **6:** 239, 1972.
22. Denneberg, T., Ekberg, M., Ericson, C., and Hanson, A.: Co-trimoxazole in the long-term treatment of pyelonephritis with normal and impaired renal function. Scan. J. Infec. Dis. **8:** Suppl. 61, 1976.
23. Stamey, T. A., Condy, M., and Mihara, G.: Prophylactic efficacy of nitrofurantoin macrocrystals and trimethoprim-sulfamethoxazole in urinary infections. Biologic effects on the vaginal and rectal flora. N. Engl. J. Med. **296:** 780, 1977.
24. Fairley, K. F., Hubbard, M., and Whitworth, J. A.: Prophylactic long-term cephalexin in recurrent urinary infection. Med. J. Aust. **1:** 318, 1974.
25. Smolin, E. M., and Rapoport, L.: Hexamethylenetetramine. In A. Weissberger (Consult. Ed.), The Chemistry of Heterocyclic Compounds s-Triazines and Derivatives. Chap. 10, New York, Interscience Publishers, 1959, p. 545.
26. Nicolaier, A.: Ueber die therapeutische verwendung des urotropin (hexamethylentetramin). Detsch. Med. Wochenschr. **21:** 541, 1895.
27. Hanzlik, P. J., and Collins, R. J.: Hexamethylenamine: The liberation of formaldehyde and the antiseptic efficiency under different chemical and biological conditions. Arch. Intern. Med. **12:** 578, 1913.
28. Levy, L. H., and Strauss, A.: A clinical and bacteriological study of hexamethylenamin as a urinary antiseptic. Arch. Intern. Med. **14:** 730, 1914.
29. Shohl, A. T., and Deming, C. L.: Hexamethylenamin: Its quantitative factors in therapy. J. Urol. **4:** 419, 1920.
30. De Eds, F.: Fate of hexamethylenamin in the body and its bearing on systemic antisepsis. Arch. Intern. Med. **34:** 511, 1924.
31. Hinman, F.: An experimental study of the antiseptic value in the urine of the internal use of hexamethylenamin. J. Am. Med. Assoc. **61:** 1601, 1913.
32. Scudi, J. V., and Reinhard, J. F.: Absorption, distribution and renal excretion of Mandelamine (methenamine mandelate). J. Lab. Clin. Med. **33:** 1304, 1948.
33. Knight, V., Draper, J. W., Brady, E. A., and Attmore, C. A.: Methenamine mandelate: Antimicrobial activity, absorption, and excretion. Antibiot. Chemother. **2:** 615, 1952.
34. Gandelman, A. L.: Methenamine mandelate: Antimicrobial activity in urine and correlation with formaldehyde levels. J. Urol. **97:** 533, 1967.
35. Duca, C. J., and Scudi, J. V.: Some antibacterial properties of Mandelamine (methenamine mandelate). Proc. Soc. Exp. Biol. Med. **66:** 123, 1947.
36. Waterworth, P. M.: A misapplication of the sensitivity test: Mandelamine discs. J. Med. Lab. Technol. **19:** 163, 1962.
37. Musher, D. M., and Griffith, D. P.: Generation of formaldehyde from methenamine: effect of pH and concentration, and antibacterial effect. Antimicro. Agents Chemother. **6:** 708, 1974.
38. Heathcote, R. S. A.: Hexamine as an urinary antiseptic. I. Its rate of hydrolysis at different hydrogen ion concentrations. II. Its antiseptic power against various bacteria in urine. Br. J. Urol. **7:** 9, 1935.
39. Tanenbaum, M., and Bricker, C. E.: Microdetermination of free formaldehyde. Anal. Chem. **23:** 354, 1951.
40. Jackson, J., and Stamey, T. A.: The Riker method for determining formaldehyde in the presence of methenamine. Invest. Urol. **9:** 124, 1971.
41. Musher, D. M., Griffith, D. P., and Richie, Y.:

The generation of formaldehyde from methenamine. effect of urinary flow and residual volume. Invest. Urol. **13:** 380, 1976.
42. Miller, H., and Phillips, E.: Antibacterial correlates of urine drug levels of hexamethylenetetramine and formaldehyde. Invest. Urol. **8:** 21, 1970.
43. Pearman, J. W., Peterson, G. J., and Nash, J. B.: The antimicrobial activity of urine of paraplegic patients receiving methenamine mandelate. Invest. Urol. **16:** 91, 1978.
44. Holland, N. H., and West, C. D.: Prevention of recurrent urinary tract infections in girls. Am. J. Dis. Child. **105:** 560, 1963.
45. Harding, G. K. M., and Ronald, A. R.: A controlled study of antimicrobial prophylaxis of recurrent urinary infection in women. N. Engl. J. Med. **291:** 597, 1974.
46. Vainrub, B., and Musher, D. M.: Lack of effect of methenamine in suppression of, or prophylaxis against, chronic urinary infection. Antimicrob. Agents Chemother. **12:** 625, 1977.
47. Rosenheim, M. L., and Camb, M. B.: Mandelic acid in the treatment of urinary infections. Lancet **1:** 1032, 1935.
48. Helmholz, H. F.: The ketogenic diet in the treatment of urinary infections of childhood. J. Am. Med. Assoc. **99:** 1305, 1932.
49. Draskoczy, P., and Weiner, N.: Effect of organic acids on oxidative metabolism of *Escherichia coli.* Fed. Proc. **19:** 140, 1960.
50. Kass, E. H.: Bacteriuria and the diagnosis of infections of the urinary tract; with observations on the use of methionine as a urinary antiseptic. Arch. Intern. Med. **100:** 709, 1957.
51. Kass, E. H., and Zangwill, D. P.: Principles in the long-term management of chronic infection of the urinary tract. In E. L. Quinn and E. H. Kass (Eds.), Biology of Pyelonephritis. Boston, Little, Brown & Co., 1960, p. 663.
52. McDonald, D. F., and Murphy, G. P.: Bacteriostatic and acidifying effects of methionine, hydrolyzed casein and ascorbic acid on the urine. N. Engl. J. Med. **261:** 803, 1959.
53. Travis, L. B., Dodge, W. F., Mintz, A. A., and Assemi, M.: Urinary acidification with ascorbic acid. J. Pediatr. **67:** 1176, 1965.
54. Elliot, J. S., Sharp, R. F., and Lewis, L.: Urinary pH. J. Urol. **81:** 339, 1959.
55. Kasanen, A., Kaarsalo, E., Hiltunen, R., and Soini, V.: Comparison of long-term, low-dosage nitrofurantoin, methenamine hippurate, trimethoprim and trimethoprim-sulphamethoxazole on the control of recurrent urinary tract infection. Ann. Clin. Res. **6:** 285, 1974.
56. Harding, G. K. M., Buckwold, F. J., Marrie, T. J., Thompson, L., Light, R. B., and Ronald, A. R.: Prophylaxis of recurrent uninary tract infection in female patients: efficacy of low-dose thrice-weekly therapy with trimethoprim/sulfamethoxazole. J. Am. Med. Assoc. **242:** 1975, 1979.
57. Louria, D. B., and Brayton, R. G.: The efficacy of penicillin regimens. With observations on the frequency of superinfection. J. Am. Med. Assoc. **186:** 987, 1963.
58. Vosti, K. L.: Recurrent urinary tract infections: prevention by prophylactic antibiotics after sexual intercourse. J. Am. Med. Assoc. **231:** 934, 1975.
59. Petersdorf, R. G., and Sherris, J. C.: Methods and significance of in vitro testing of bacterial sensitivity to drugs. Am. J. Med. **39:** 766, 1965.
60. Massell, B. F., Fyler, D. C., and Hazel, M. M.: Prevention of rheumatic fever and rheumatic heart disease: A brief historical review and a preliminary report of three controlled studies. Heart Center Bulletin of the St. Francis Hospital and Sanatorium **14:** 1, 1957.
61. Symon, W. E.: Penicillin blood levels in patients receiving oral penicillin V, oral penicillin G, and intramuscular aqueous procain (A-P) penicillin G, In H. Welch and F. Marti-Ibanez (Eds.), Antibiotics Annual 1955–1956. New York, Medical Encyclopedia, 1956, p. 473.
62. Putnam, L. E., Wright, W. W., de Nunzio, A., and Welch, H.: Penicillin blood concentrations following oral administration of various dosage forms of penicillin V and comparison with penicillin G, In H. Welch and F. Marti-Ibanez (Eds.), Antibiotics Annual 1955–1956. New York, Medical Encyclopedia, 1956, p. 483.
63. Palmer, J. M., Neal, J. F., and Stamey, T. A.: The use of oral sodium benzyl-penicillin in the urinary tract: A study of urinary levels and in vitro activity. In Progress in Antimicrobial and Anticancer Chemotherapy. Proceedings of the 6th International Congress of Chemotherapy. Baltimore, University Park Press, 1970, Vol. 1, p. 902.
64. Welch, H.: Absorption, excretion, and distribution of terramycin. Ann. N. Y. Acad. Sci. **53:** 253, 1950.
65. Sweeney, W. M., Hardy, S. M., Dornbush, A. C., and Ruegsegger, J. M.: Demethylchlortetracycline: A clinical comparison of a new antibiotic compound with chlortetracycline and tetracycline. Antibiot. Chemother. **9:** 13, 1959.
66. Kunin, C. M., Dornbush, A. C., and Finland, M.: Distribution and excretion of four tetracycline analogues in normal young men. J. Clin. Invest. **38:** 1950, 1959.
67. Williams, D. M., Wimpenny, J., and Asscher, A. W.: Renal clearance of sodium sulphadimidine in normal and uraemic subjects. Lancet **2:** 1058, 1968.
68. Goodhope, C. D.: Thiosulfil in urinary tract infection. J. Urol. **72:** 552, 1954.
69. Garrod, L. P.: Chemotherapy of infections of the

urinary tract. R. Coll. Physicians, Edinburgh. Publ. 11, 1959.

70. Bratton, A. C., and Marshall, E. K., Jr.: A New coupling component for sulfanilamide determination. J. Biol. Chem. **128:** 537, 1939.
71. Bauer, A. W., and Sherris, J. C.: The determination of sulfonamide susceptibility of bacteria. Chemotherapia **9:** 1, 1964.
72. Stamey, T. A., and Bragonje, J.: Resistance to nalidixic acid: a misconception due to underdosage. J. Am. Med. Assoc. **236:** 1857, 1976.
73. Neu, H. C.: Cefoxitin: An overview of clinical studies in the United States. Rev. Infect. Dis. **1:** 233, 1979.
74. Linquist, J. A., Siddiqui, J. Y., and Smith, I. M.: Cephalexin in patients with renal disease. N. Engl. J. Med. **283:** 720, 1970.
75. Kunin, C. M., and Finkelberg, Z.: Oral cephalexin and ampicillin: antimicrobial activity, recovery in urine, and persistence in the blood of uremic patients. Ann. Intern. Med. **72:** 349, 1970.
76. McHenry, M. C., Gavan, T. L., Gifford, R. W., Geurkink, N. A., Van Ommen, R. A., Town, M. A., and Wagner, J. G.: Gentamicin dosages for renal insufficiency. Adjustments based on endogenous creatinine clearance and serum creatinine concentration. Ann. Intern. Med. **74:** 192, 1971.
77. Kunin, C. M.: A guide to use of antibiotics in patients with renal disease. A table of recommended doses and factors governing serum levels. Ann. Intern. Med. **67:** 151, 1967.
78. Kalowski, S., Mathew, T. H., Nanra, R. S., and Kincaid-Smith, P.: Deterioration in renal function in association with co-trimoxazole therapy. Lancet **1:** 394, 1973.
79. Tasker, P. R. W., MacGregor, G. A., and de Wardener, H. E., Thomas, R. D., and Jones, N. F.: Use of co-trimoxazole in chronic renal failure. Lancet **1:** 1216, 1975.
80. Krause, W., Matheis, H., and Wulf, K.: Fungaemia and funguria after oral administration of *Candida albicans*. Lancet **1:** 598, 1969.
81. Hamory, B. H., and Wenzel, R. P.: Hospital-associated candiduria: predisposing factors and review of the literature. J. Urol. **120:** 444, 1978.
82. Howard, R. J., Simmons, R. L., and Najarian, J. S.: Fungal infections in renal transplant recipients. Ann. Surg. **188:** 598, 1978.
83. Schönebeck, J.: Studies on *Candida* infection of the urinary tract and on the antimycotic drug 5-fluorocytosine. Scand. J. Urol. Nephro., Suppl. 11, 1972.
84. Hills, N. H., Bultitude, M. I., and Eykyn, S.: Co-trimoxazole in prevention of bacteriuria after prostatectomy. Br. Med. J. **2:** 498, 1976.
85. Plorde, J. J., Kennedy, R. P., Bourne, H. H., Ansell, J. S., and Petersdorf, R. G.: Course and Prognosis of prostatectomy: with a note on the incidence of bacteremia and effectiveness of chemoprophylaxis. N. Engl. J. Med. **272:** 269, 1965.
86. Genster, H. G., and Madsen, P. O.: Urinary tract infections following transurethral prostatectomy: with special reference to the use of antimicrobials. J. Urol. **104:** 163, 1970.
87. McGuire, E. J.: Antibacterial prophylaxis in prostatectomy patients. J. Urol. **111:** 794, 1974.
88. Morris, M. J., Golovsky, D., Guinness, M. D. G., and Maher, P. O.: The value of prophylactic antibiotics in transurethral prostatic resection: a controlled trial, with observations on the origin of postoperative infection. Br. J. Urol. **48:** 479, 1976.
89. Gonzalez, R., Wright, R., and Blackard, C. E.: Prophylactic antibiotics in transurethral prostatectomy. J. Urol. **116:** 203, 1976.
90. Matthew, A. D., Gonzalez, R., Jeffords, D., and Pinto, M. H.: Prevention of bacteriuria after transurethral prostatectomy with nitrofurantoin macrocrystals. J. Urol. **120:** 442, 1978.
91. Islam, A. K. M. S., and Chapman, J.: Closed catheter drainage and urinary infection—a comparison of two methods of catheter drainage. Br. J. Urol. **49:** 215, 1977.
92. Bultitude, M. I., and Eykyn, S.: The relationship between the urethral flora and urinary infection in the catheterised male. Br. J. Urol. **45:** 678, 1973.
93. Maizels, M., and Schaeffer, A. J.: Decreased incidence of bacteriuria associated with periodic instillations of hydrogen peroxide into the urethral catheter drainage bag. J. Urol. **123:** (June) 1980.
94. Warren, J. W., Platt, R., Thomas, R. J., Rosner, B., and Kass, E. H.: Antibiotic irrigation and catheter-associated urinary-tract infections. N. Engl. J. Med. **299:** 570, 1978.
95. Ansell, J.: Some observations on catheter care. J. Chronic Dis. **15:** 675, 1962.
96. Beeson, P. B.: The case against the catheter. Am. J. Med. **24:** 1, 1958.
97. Cox, C. E., and Hinman, F., Jr.: Retention catheterization and the bladder defense mechanism. J. Am. Med. Assoc. **191:** 171, 1965.
98. Desautels, R. E.: Aseptic management of catheter drainage. N. Engl. J. Med. **263:** 189, 1960.
99. Webb, J. K., and Blandy, J. P.: Closed urinary drainage into plastic bags containing antiseptic. Br. J. Urol. **40:** 585, 1968.
100. Desautels, R. E., Walter, C. W., Graves, R. C., and Harrison, J. H.: Technical advances in prevention of urinary tract infection. J. Urol. **87:** 487, 1962.
101. Finkelberg, Z., and Kunin, C. M.: Clinical evaluation of closed urinary drainage systems. J. Am.

Med. Assoc. **207:** 1657, 1969.

102. Govan, D. E., and Perkash, I.: Urethral catheterization: A method to protect the urinary tract against bacterial contamination and infection. Invest. Urol. **5:** 394, 1968.
103. Guinan, P. D., Bayley, B. C., Metzger, W. I., Shoemaker, W. C., and Bush, I. M.: The case against "the case against the catheter": initial report. J. Urol. **101:** 909, 1969.
104. Kass, E. H., and Schniederman, L. J.: Entry of bacteria into urinary tracts of patients with inlying catheters. N. Engl. J. Med. **256:** 556, 1957.
105. Kunin, C. M., and McCormack, R. C.: Prevention of catheter-induced urinary tract infections by sterile closed drainage. N. Engl. J. Med. **274:** 1155, 1966.
106. Lindan, R.: The prevention of ascending catheter-induced infections of the urinary tract. J. Chronic Dis. **22:** 321, 1969.
107. Martin, C. M., and Bookrajian, E. N.: Bacteriuria prevention after indwelling urinary catheterization: Controlled study. Arch. Intern. Med. **110:** 703, 1962.
108. Martin, C. M., Vaquer, F., Meyers, M. S., and El-Dadah, A.: Prevention of Gram-negative rod bacteremia associated with indwelling urinary tract catheterization. In J. C. Sylvester (Ed.), Antimicrobial Agents and Chemotherapy, 1963. Ann Arbor, American Society for Microbiology, 1964, p. 617.
109. Roberts, J. B. M., Linton, K. B., Pollard, B. R., Mitchell, J. P., and Gillespie, W. A.: Long-term catheter drainage in the male. Br. J. Urol. **37:** 63, 1965

Index